Published and forthcoming Oxford Handbooks

OXFORD MEDICAL PUBLICATIONS

Oxford Handbook of
Anaesthesia

Oxford Handbook of
Anaesthesia

FOURTH EDITION

Edited by

Keith G. Allman

Consultant Anaesthetist,
Royal Devon and Exeter NHS Foundation Trust,
UK

and

Iain H. Wilson

Consultant Anaesthetist,
Royal Devon and Exeter NHS Foundation Trust,
UK

Assistant Editor

Aidan M. O'Donnell

Consultant Anaesthetist,
Waikato Hospital, Hamilton, New Zealand

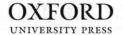

OXFORD
UNIVERSITY PRESS

OXFORD
UNIVERSITY PRESS

Great Clarendon Street, Oxford, OX2 6DP,
United Kingdom

Oxford University Press is a department of the University of Oxford.
It furthers the University's objective of excellence in research, scholarship,
and education by publishing worldwide. Oxford is a registered trade mark of
Oxford University Press in the UK and in certain other countries

© Oxford University Press 2016

The moral rights of the authors have been asserted

First edition 2002
Second edition 2006
Third edition 2011
Fourth edition 2016

Impression: 1

Published in the United States of America by Oxford University Press
198 Madison Avenue, New York, NY 10016, United States of America

British Library Cataloguing in Publication Data

Data available

Library of Congress Control Number: 2015941608

ISBN 978–0–19–871941–0

Printed and bound in China by
C&C Offset Printing Co., Ltd.

This book is dedicated to the memory of Henry Wallace Wilson (1923–2014) and Geoffrey Leslie Allman (1927–2014). Great men, much missed.

Preface

Welcome to the fourth edition of the *Oxford Handbook of Anaesthesia*. We have been delighted with the success of the handbook and hope that this edition will be well received.

The fourth edition contains many changes to take account of the feedback obtained from readers and reviewers. We have involved new authors in different sections of the book, so that the material remains up-to-date and reflects a balanced set of views. In our opinion, each author is an established expert in their field and, more importantly, a good clinical anaesthetist.

The book describes the preparation of the patient for anaesthesia, the implications of concurrent diseases, and the general principles of anaesthetic practice for different subspecialties. A practical approach is suggested where appropriate. There are detailed chapters on obstetric and paediatric anaesthesia, and also emergencies. A comprehensive drug formulary is included. A new section on anaesthesia for weight reduction surgery has been added.

The *Oxford Handbook of Anaesthesia* remains a practical guide to anaesthesia written for those who have mastered basic anaesthetic techniques but need advice for the many common problems encountered in clinical practice.

The *Oxford Handbook of Anaesthesia* has proved popular in many countries throughout the world. A low-cost edition is available in India, Pakistan, and Bangladesh, and translations have been produced in Chinese, Italian, Polish, and Russian. An American edition was produced in 2008.

We are particularly grateful for the expert proofreading skills of Dr Aidan O'Donnell who has provided invaluable support during the preparation of this edition.

Despite all our efforts, it is possible that an occasional error exists; please be careful. We hope that you will enjoy this latest edition of the *Oxford Handbook of Anaesthesia*. Please email us your criticisms and suggestions, so that we can keep improving the book.

Many thanks to our understanding families and authors, and to the landlord and locals of the Bridford Inn during editorial meetings.

Keith and Iain
iain.wilson3@nhs.net
2015

Contents

Contributors

Mark Abou-Samra
Registrar in Anaethesia,
Taunton, UK

Gururaj Arumugakani
Consultant Anaesthetist,
Leeds, UK

Ben Ballisat
Registrar in Anaesthesia,
Bristol, UK

Nicholas Batchelor
Consultant Anaesthetist,
Exeter, UK

Mark Bellamy
Professor of Critical Care and
Anaesthesia, Leeds, UK

Simon Berg
Consultant Anaesthetist,
Oxford, UK

Colin Berry
Consultant Anaesthetist,
Exeter, UK

Hannah Blanshard
Consultant Anaesthetist,
Bristol, UK

Andrew Bodenham
Consultant Anaesthetist,
Leeds, UK

John Bowden
Consultant Maxillofacial Surgeon,
Exeter, UK

Nicholas Bunker
Consultant Anaesthetist,
London, UK

Bruce Campbell
Professor of Vascular Surgery,
Exeter, UK

John Christie
Consultant Gastroenterologist,
Exeter, UK

Tim Cook
Consultant Anaesthetist, Bath, UK

Jules Cranshaw
Consultant Anaesthetist, Bath, UK

Adrian Dashfield
Consultant Anaesthetist, Isle of
Man, UK

Mark Daugherty
Consultant Anaesthetist,
Exeter, UK

John Dean
Consultant Cardiologist,
Exeter, UK

Philippa Dix
Consultant Anaesthetist,
Exeter, UK

James Eldridge
Consultant Anaesthetist,
Portsmouth, UK

Rhys Evans
Consultant Anaesthetist,
Oxford, UK

Pete Ford
Consultant Anaesthetist,
Exeter, UK

Steve Gayer
Consultant Anaesthetist,
Florida, USA

Richard Griffiths
Consultant Anaesthetist,
Peterborough, UK

William Harrop-Griffiths
Consultant Anaesthetist,
London, UK

Lara Herbert
Registrar in Anaesthesia,
Bristol, UK

Graham Hocking
Consultant Anaesthetist, Perth,
Australia

Kath Jenkins
Consultant Anaesthetist,
Bristol, UK

Nick Kennedy
Consultant Anaesthetist,
Taunton, UK

Paul Kerr
Consultant Haematologist,
Exeter, UK

Alex Manara
Consultant Anaesthetist,
Bristol, UK

Alastair Martin
Consultant Anaesthetist,
Exeter, UK

Bruce McCormick
Consultant Anaesthetist,
Exeter, UK

Andrew McIndoe
Consultant Anaesthetist,
Bristol, UK

Alan Merry
Professor of Anaesthesiology,
Auckland, New Zealand

Quentin Milner
Consultant Anaesthetist,
Exeter, UK

Peter Murphy
Consultant Anaesthetist,
Bristol, UK

Paul Myles
Professor of Anaesthesia,
Melbourne, Australia

Jerry Nolan
Consultant Anaesthetist,
Oxford, UK

Aidan O'Donnell
Consultant Anaesthetist, Hamilton,
New Zealand

Fred Roberts
Consultant Anaesthetist,
Exeter, UK

Nicki Ross
Consultant Anaesthetist,
Harrogate, UK

Matt Rucklidge
Consultant Anaesthetist, Perth,
Australia

John Saddler
Consultant Anaesthetist,
Exeter, UK

Samantha Shinde
Consultant Anaesthetist,
Bristol, UK

Adam Shonfeld
Consultant Anaesthetist,
London, UK

Mary Stocker
Consultant Anaesthetist,
Torbay, UK

Mark Stoneham
Consultant Anaesthetist,
Oxford, UK

Andrew Teasdale
Consultant Anaesthetist,
Exeter, UK

Richard Telford
Consultant Anaesthetist,
Exeter, UK

Rhys Thomas
Consultant Anaesthetist,
RAMC, UK

Claire Todd
Registrar in Anaesthesia,
Exeter, UK

Jonathan Warwick
Consultant Anaesthetist,
Oxford, UK

Stu White
Consultant Anaesthetist,
Brighton, UK

Ashleigh Williams
Registrar in Anaesthesia,
Exeter, UK

Joanna Wilson
Registrar in Anaesthesia,
Guildford, UK

Philip Wood
Consultant Anaesthetist,
Leeds, UK

Abbreviations

A&E	accident and emergency
AAA	abdominal aortic aneurysm
AADR	anaesthetic adverse drug reaction
AAGBI	Association of Anaesthetists of Great Britain and Ireland
AAS	atlantoaxial subluxation
ABC	airway, breathing, circulation
ABG	arterial blood gas
AC	alternating current
ACE	angiotensin-converting enzyme
ACF	antecubital fossa
ACoTS	acute coagulopathy of trauma shock
ACT	activated clotting time
ACTH	adrenocorticotrophic hormone
ADH	antidiuretic hormone
ADHD	attention-deficit/hyperactivity disorder
ADP	adenosine diphosphate
AEC	airway exchange catheter
AED	automated external defibrillator
AEP	auditory evoked response
AF	atrial fibrillation
AFE	amniotic fluid embolism
AFOI	awake fibreoptic intubation
AHI	apnoea–hypopnoea index
AICD	automatic implantable cardioverter–defibrillator
AIDS	acquired immunodeficiency syndrome
AIP	acute intermittent porphyria
ALF	acute liver failure
ALI	acute lung injury
ALP	alkaline phosphatase
ALS	advanced life support
ALT	alanine aminotransferase
a.m.	*ante meridiem* (before noon)
ANH	acute normovolaemic haemodilution

AP	anteroposterior
APL	adjustable pressure limiting
APTT	activated partial thromboplastin time
APUD	amine precursor uptake and decarboxylation
AR	aortic regurgitation
ARB	angiotensin receptor blocker
ARDS	acute respiratory distress syndrome
ARF	acute renal failure
art line	arterial line
AS	aortic stenosis
ASA	American Society of Anesthesiologists
ASAP	as soon as possible
ASD	atrial septal defect
ASIS	anterior superior iliac spine
ASRA	American Society of Regional Anesthesia and Pain Medicine
AST	aspartate transaminase
AT	anaerobic threshold
ATD	adult therapeutic dose
ATLS®	Advanced Trauma Life Support®
ATN	acute tubular necrosis
ATR	acute transfusion reaction
AV	atrioventricular
A–V	arteriovenous
AVM	arteriovenous malformation
AVR	aortic valve replacement
AVSD	atrioventricular septal defect
BAHA	bone-anchored hearing aid
BBV	blood-borne virus
BCIS	bone cement implantation syndrome
bd	*bis diem* (twice daily)
BiPAP	bilevel positive airway pressure
BIS	bispectral index
BLS	basic life support
BMHA	British Malignant Hyperthermia Association
BMI	body mass index
BMS	bare-metal stent
BNF	*British National Formulary*

BNFc	*British National Formulary for Children*
BP	blood pressure
bpm	beat per minute
BSE	bovine spongiform encephalopathy
BSS	balanced salt solution
BT	Blalock–Taussig (shunt)
BUN	blood urea nitrogen
BURP	backwards, upwards, and rightwards pressure
Ca^{2+}	calcium ion
CABG	coronary artery bypass grafting
CAD	coronary artery disease
cAMP	cyclic adenosine monophosphate
CBF	coronary blood flow; cerebral blood flow
CC	creatinine clearance
CCD	central core disease
CCF	congestive cardiac failure
CEA	carotid endarterectomy; caudal extradural analgesia
CF	cystic fibrosis
CFTR	cystic fibrosis transmembrane regulator
Ch	Charrière (French) gauge (also FG or Fr)
CHD	congenital heart disease
CI	confidence interval
CICV	cannot intubate, cannot ventilate
CJD	Creutzfeldt–Jakob disease
CK	creatine kinase
Cl^-	chloride ion
CLD	chronic liver disease
cLMA	classic laryngeal mask airway
cm	centimetre
CMACE	Centre for Maternal and Child Enquiries
CMT	combat medical technician
CMV	cytomegalovirus
CNS	central nervous system
CO	carbon monoxide
CO_2	carbon dioxide
COETT	cuffed oral endotracheal tube
COHb	carboxyhaemoglobin

COPD	chronic obstructive pulmonary disease
COPRA	cuffed oropharyngeal airway
CORP	Committee on the Review of Porphyrinogenicity
COX	cyclo-oxygenase
CPAP	continuous positive airway pressure
CPB	cardiopulmonary bypass
CPET	cardiopulmonary exercise testing
CPP	cerebral perfusion pressure
CPR	cardiopulmonary resuscitation
CPSP	chronic post-surgical pain
CRA	continuous regional analgesia
CREST	calcinosis, Raynaud's, oesophageal dysfunction, sclerodactyly, and telangiectasia
CRF	chronic renal failure
CRP	C-reactive protein
CRTZ	chemoreceptor trigger zone
CSE	combined spinal/epidural
CSF	cerebrospinal fluid
CSM	Committee on Safety of Medicines
CT	computed tomography
CVA	cerebrovascular accident
CVC	central venous catheter
CVP	central venous pressure
CVS	cardiovascular system
CXR	chest X-ray
2D	two-dimensional
3D	three-dimensional
d	day
D&C	dilatation and curettage
D&E	dilatation and evacuation
Da	dalton
DAS	Difficult Airway Society
DBD	donor after brain death
DBS	double-burst stimulation
DC	direct current
DCR	dacrocystorhinostomy; damage control resuscitation
DCS	damage control surgery

DES	drug-eluting stent
DHCA	deep hypothermic circulatory arrest
DHPR	dihydropyridine receptor
DHS	dynamic hip screw
DHTR	delayed haemolytic transfusion reaction
DIC	disseminated intravascular coagulation
dL	decilitre
DLCO	diffusing capacity of the lungs for carbon monoxide
DLT	double-lumen (endobronchial) tube
DMARD	disease-modifying antirheumatoid drug
DNAR	Do Not Attempt Resuscitation
DND	delayed neurological deficit
DS	degree of substitution
DVT	deep vein thrombosis
dyn	dyne
EBM	evidence-based medicine
ECF	extracellular fluid
ECG	electrocardiogram
ECMO	extracorporeal membrane oxygenation
ECT	electroconvulsive therapy
ED	external diameter
EEG	electroencephalogram/electroencephalography
EF	ejection fraction
eGFR	estimated glomerular filtration rate
EMA	European Medicines Agency
EMG	electromyogram/electromyography
EMHG	European Malignant Hyperthermia Group
EMI	electromagnetic interference
EMLA®	Eutectic Mixture of Local Anaesthetics®
ENT	ear, nose, and throat
EO	external oblique
EPO	erythropoietin
EPP	exposure-prone procedure
ERAS	enhanced recovery after surgery
ERCP	endoscopic retrograde cholangiopancreatography
ERPC	evacuation of retained products of conception
ESR	erythrocyte sedimentation rate

$ETCO_2$	end-tidal carbon dioxide
ETO_2	end-tidal oxygen
ETT	endotracheal tube
EUA	examination under anaesthesia
EuroSCORE	European System for Cardiac Operative Risk Evaluation
EVD	external ventricular drain
FAST	focused assessment sonogram in trauma
FBC	full blood count
FDA	Food and Drug Administration
FES	fat embolism syndrome
FEV_1	forced expiratory volume in 1 second
FFP	fresh frozen plasma
FG	French gauge (also Fr and Ch)
FGF	fresh gas flow
FHF	fulminant hepatic failure
FiO_2	fractional inspired oxygen content
fLMA	flexible laryngeal mask airway
FPG	fasting plasma glucose
Fr	French gauge (also FG and Ch)
FRC	functional residual capacity
ft	foot (feet)
FTc	corrected flow time
FTSG	full-thickness skin graft
FVC	forced vital capacity
g	gram
G	Gauge (standard wire gauge)
G&S	group and screen
G6PD	glucose-6-phosphate dehydrogenase
GA	general anaesthetic/anaesthesia
GCS	Glasgow Coma Scale
GDC	Guglielmi detachable coil
GEB	gum elastic bougie
GFR	glomerular filtration rate
GI	gastrointestinal
GOLD	Global Initiative for Chronic Obstructive Lung Disease
GP	general practitioner
GT	greater trochanter

GTN	glyceryl trinitrate
GvHD	graft-versus-host disease
H$^+$	hydrogen ion
HAS	human albumin solution
Hb	haemoglobin
HbA1c	glycosylated haemoglobin
HBV	hepatitis B virus
HCO$_3^-$	bicarbonate ion
HCP	hereditary coproporphyria
Hct	haematocrit
HCV	hepatitis C virus
HDL	high-density lipoprotein
HDU	high dependency unit
HELLP	haemolysis, elevated liver enzymes, low platelets
HES	Hospital Episode Statistics; hydroxyethyl starch
HFO	high-frequency oscillation
Hib	*Haemophilus influenzae* type b
HIT	heparin-induced thrombocytopenia
HIV	human immunodeficiency virus
HLA	human leucocyte antigen
HLHS	hypoplastic left heart syndrome
HME	heat and moisture exchanger
HOCM	hypertrophic obstructive cardiomyopathy
HPA	hypothalamic–pituitary–adrenal
hr	hour
HR	heart rate
HRS	Heart Rhythm Society
HRT	hormone replacement therapy
HRUK	Heart Rhythm UK
HTLV	human T cell lymphotropic virus
HVOD	hepatic veno-occlusive disease
Hz	hertz
I:E ratio	inspired:expired ratio
IABP	intra-aortic balloon pump
IBCT	incorrect blood component transfused
IBW	ideal body weight
ICD	implantable cardioverter–defibrillator

ICP	intracranial pressure
ICU	intensive care unit
ID	internal diameter
IDT	intradermal testing
IE	infective endocarditis
IED	improvized explosive device
IHD	ischaemic heart disease
IL	interleukin
ILMA	intubating laryngeal mask airway
IM	intramuscular
IMCAS	independent mental capacity advocacy service
in	inch
INR	international normalized ratio
IO	internal oblique
IOP	intraocular pressure
IP	in-plane
IPPV	intermittent positive pressure ventilation
IT	ischial tuberosity
ITP	idiopathic thrombocytopenic purpura
IU	international unit
IV	intravenous(ly)
IVC	inferior vena cava
IVCT	*in vitro* contracture test
IVI	intravenous infusion
IVRA	intravenous regional anaesthesia
J	joule
JVP	jugular venous pressure
K^+	potassium ion
kcal	kilocalorie
KCl	potassium chloride
kg	kilogram
km	kilometre
kPa	kilopascal
L	litre
LA	lupus anticoagulant; local anaesthetic/anaesthesia
LACA	left atrial circumferential ablation
LAST	local anaesthetic systemic toxicity

LAVH	laparoscopically assisted vaginal hysterectomy
LBW	low birthweight
LCNT	lateral cutaneous nerve of thigh
LDH	lactate dehydrogenase
L-dopa	levodopa
LFT	liver function test
LMA	laryngeal mask airway
LMWH	low-molecular-weight heparin
LP	lumbar puncture
LRTI	lower respiratory tract infection
LSCS	lower-segment Caesarean section
LSD	lysergic acid diethylamide
LV	left ventricle/ventricular
LVEDP	left ventricular end-diastolic pressure
LVEF	left ventricular ejection fraction
LVH	left ventricular hypertrophy
m	metre
M	molar
mA	milliampere
MAC	minimum alveolar concentration
MAGPI	meatal advancement and glanuloplasty
MAO	monoamine oxidase
MAO-A	monoamine oxidase A
MAO-B	monoamine oxidase B
MAOI	monoamine oxidase inhibitor
MAP	mean arterial pressure
MCV	mean corpuscular volume
MDMA	3,4-methylenedioxymethamphetamine
MEAC	minimum effective analgesic concentration
MELD	model for end-stage liver disease
MEN	multiple endocrine neoplasia
MEOWS	Modified Early Obstetric Warning Scoring
MERT	medical emergency response team
MET	metabolic equivalents of task
mg	milligram
Mg^{2+}	magnesium ion
MH	malignant hyperthermia

MHAUS	Malignant Hyperthermia Association of the United States
MHP	massive haemorrhage protocol
MHRA	Medicines and Healthcare Products Regulatory Agency
MHz	megahertz
MI	myocardial infarction
MIBG	*meta*-iodobenzylguanidine
MIC	minimum inhibitory concentration
MILNS	manual in-line neck stabilization
min	minute
mL	millilitre
mm	millimetre
mmHg	millimetre of mercury
mmol	millimole
MMS	masseter muscle spasm
mol	mole
mOsmol	milliosmole
mph	mile per hour
MR	mitral regurgitation
MRI	magnetic resonance imaging
MRSA	meticillin-resistant *Staphylococcus aureus*
ms	millisecond
MSBOS	maximum surgical blood ordering schedule
MSU	midstream urine
mT	millitesla
MTC	major trauma centre; minimum toxic concentration
MUA	manipulation under anaesthesia
MUGA	multigated acquisition scan
MW	molecular weight
6MWT	6-minute walk test
N	newton
Na$^+$	sodium ion
NaCl	sodium chloride
NAP	National Audit Project
NCA	nurse-controlled analgesia
NCEP	National Cholesterol Education Program
NCEPOD	National Confidential Enquiry into Patient Outcome and Death

NDMR	non-depolarizing muscle relaxant
ng	nanogram
NG	nasogastric
NGT	nasogastric tube
NHS	National Health Service
NIBP	non-invasive blood pressure
NICE	National Institute for Health and Care Excellence
NIPPV	non-invasive positive pressure ventilation
NJR	National Joint Registry
nm	nanometre
NMB	neuromuscular blockade
NMDA	N-methyl-D-aspartate
nmol	nanomole
NNT	number needed to treat
NO	nitric oxide
N_2O	nitrous oxide
NSAID	non-steroidal anti-inflammatory drug
NTS	nucleus tractus solitarius
O&D	oesophagoscopy and dilatation
O_2	oxygen
OCP	oral contraceptive pill
OELM	optimal external laryngeal manipulation
OHS	obesity hypoventilation syndrome
OLV	one-lung ventilation
OMV	Oxford miniature vaporizer
OOP	out-of-plane
OPCAB	off-pump coronary artery bypass grafting
OR	odds ratio
ORIF	open reduction and internal fixation
OSA	obstructive sleep apnoea
OSD	ostial segmental disconnection
OSMRS	Obesity Surgery Mortality Risk Score
Pa	pascal
PA	posterior to anterior; pulmonary artery/arterial
PABA	para-aminobenzoic acid
$PaCO_2$	arterial partial pressure of carbon dioxide
PAD	preoperative autologous donation

PAFC	pulmonary artery flotation catheter
PaO_2	arterial partial pressure of oxygen
PAO_2	alveolar partial pressure of oxygen
PAOP	pulmonary artery occlusion pressure
PAP	pulmonary artery pressure
P_{aw}	airway pressure
PAOP	pulmonary artery occlusion pressure
PCA	patient-controlled analgesia
PCC	prothrombin complex concentrate
PCEA	patient-controlled epidural analgesia
PCI	percutaneous coronary intervention
PCR	protein:creatinine ratio; polymerase chain reaction
PCV	packed cell volume
PDA	persistent ductus arteriosus
PDE	phosphodiesterase
PDPH	post-dural puncture headache
PE	phenytoin equivalents; pulmonary embolism
PEA	pulseless electrical activity
PEEP	positive end-expiratory pressure
PEFR	peak expiratory flow rate
PEP	post-exposure prophylaxis
PFT	pulmonary function test
pg	picogram
PICC	peripherally inserted central catheter
PICU	paediatric intensive care unit
p.m.	*post meridiem* (after noon)
pmol	picomole
PNB	peripheral nerve block
PNS	peripheral nerve stimulator
PO	*per os* (oral)
POCD	post-operative cognitive dysfunction
POD	post-operative delirium
PONV	post-operative nausea and vomiting
POSSUM	physiological and operative severity score for enumeration of mortality and morbidity
PPI	proton pump inhibitor
ppo	predicted post-operative

PPV	pulse pressure variation
PR	per rectum
PRBC	packed red blood cell
PRN	*pro re nata* (as required)
PRP	pathogen-reduced plasma
PS	pulmonary stenosis
PSG	polysomnography
PSIS	posterior superior iliac spine
PT	prothrombin time
PTH	parathyroid hormone
PV	polycythaemia vera
PVC	polyvinyl chloride
PVR	pulmonary vascular resistance
qds	*quater die sumendus* (four times daily)
RA	rheumatoid arthritis
RAE	Ring, Adair, and Elwyn (tube)
RALP	robot-assisted laparoscopic prostatectomy
RAST	radioallergosorbent test
RCOG	Royal College of Obstetricians and Gynaecologists
RCT	randomized controlled trial
REM	rapid eye movement
rEPO	recombinant erythropoietin
RFA	radiofrequency ablation
rFVIIa	recombinant factor VIIa
RIMA	reversible inhibitor of monoamine oxidase A
RNA	ribonucleic acid
ROSC	restoration of a spontaneous circulation
RR	risk ratio
RSI	rapid sequence induction
rt-PA	recombinant tissue plasminogen activator
RUQ	right upper quadrant
RV	right ventricle/ventricular
s	second
SAAD	Society for Advancement of Anaesthesia in Dentistry
SAD	supraglottic airway device; substance abuse disorder
SAG-M	saline, adenine, glucose, and mannitol
SAH	subarachnoid haemorrhage

SAM	systolic anterior motion
SaO$_2$	arterial oxygen saturation
SAP	systolic arterial pressure
SC	subcutaneous(ly)
SCD	sickle-cell disease
SCLC	small cell lung cancer
SCM	sternocleidomastoid muscle
ScvO$_2$	central venous oxygen saturation
SGA	small for gestational age
SH	sacral hiatus
SIADH	syndrome of inappropriate antidiuretic hormone (secretion)
SIDS	sudden infant death syndrome
SIRS	systemic inflammatory response syndrome
SLE	systemic lupus erythematosus
SLT	single-lumen tube
SOBA	Society for Obesity and Bariatric Anaesthesia
SpO$_2$	peripheral oxygen saturation
SPT	skin-prick test
SR	sarcoplasmic reticulum
SSG	split skin graft
SSRI	selective serotonin reuptake inhibitor
STEMI	ST-elevation myocardial infarction
STOP	suction termination of pregnancy
SV	spontaneous ventilation
SVC	superior vena cava
SVR	systemic vascular resistance
SVT	supraventricular tachycardia
SVV	stroke volume variation
T	tesla
T$_3$	tri-iodothyronine
T$_4$	levothyroxine
TA	transversus abdominis
TACO	transfusion-associated circulatory overload
TA-GvHD	transfusion-associated graft-versus-host disease
TAP	transversus abdominis plane
TAVI	transcatheter aortic valve implantation
TB	tuberculosis

TBSA	total body surface area
TBW	total body water
TCA	tricyclic antidepressant
TCI	target-controlled infusion
tds	*ter die sumendus* (three times daily)
TEG	thromboelastography
TENS	transcutaneous electrical nerve stimulation
THAM	tris-hydroxymethyl aminomethane
TIA	transient ischaemic attack
TIPSS	transjugular intrahepatic portosystemic shunt
TIVA	total intravenous anaesthesia
TLC	total lung capacity
TLCO	transfer factor of the lungs for carbon monoxide
TLH	total laparoscopic hysterectomy
TMJ	temporomandibular joint
TNF	tumour necrosis factor
TOE	transoesophageal echocardiography
ToF	tetralogy of Fallot
TOF	train-of-four
TOFR	train-of-four ratio
ToGV	transposition of the great vessels
TRALI	transfusion-related acute lung injury
TRAM	transverse rectus abdominis muscle
TSAA	Triservice anaesthetic apparatus
TTP	thrombotic thrombocytopenic purpura
TURP	transurethral resection of the prostate
TUVP	transurethral vaporization of the prostate
U&E	urea and electrolytes
U	unit
UK	United Kingdom
UKOSS	UK Obstetric Surveillance System
UPPP	uvulopalatopharyngoplasty
URTI	upper respiratory tract infection
USS	ultrasound scanning
V/Q	ventilation/perfusion
V	volt
VAE	venous air embolism

VATS	video-assisted thoracoscopic surgery
VC	vital capacity
vCJD	variant Creutzfeldt–Jakob disease
VF	ventricular fibrillation
VIB	vertical infraclavicular block
VIP	vasoactive intestinal peptide
VP	variegate porphyria; venous pressure
VRIII	variable-rate intravenous insulin infusion
vs	versus
VSD	ventricular septal defect
VT	ventricular tachycardia
V_T	tidal volume
VT	ventricular tachycardia
VTE	venous thromboembolism
VTOP	vaginal termination of pregnancy
vWF	von Willebrand factor
WCC	white cell count
WHO	World Health Organization
wk	week
WPW	Wolff–Parkinson–White
X-match	cross-match
yr	year

Chapter 1

General considerations

Good practice

Making anaesthesia safe

- Pay attention to detail.
- Prepare properly, and do not rush.
- Read the notes.
- Correct patient, correct surgery? Use the World Health Organization (WHO) Safe Surgery Checklist actively.
- Assess patient personally—check airway and allergies.
- Check drugs and apparatus.
- Always have a plan B.
- Never leave an anaesthetized patient unattended.
- When ventilating, check the chest is moving.
- Hypotension needs an explanation.
- If in trouble, ask for help.
- Failed intubation—ventilate and oxygenate.
- Difficult ventilation—equipment or patient?
- If in doubt, take it out.
- Never assume.
- Do not panic—remember ABC.
- The anaesthetist, surgeon, and staff are on the same team.
- Know your limits.

Making drug administration safe

Aim to give the right drug, to the right patient, in the right dose, at the right time, by the right route, correctly recorded (the six 'rights').
- Know your pharmacology—if in doubt, check or ask.
- Check the drug history—allergies, drugs given recently, drugs prescribed that still need to be given?
- Tidiness and order matter—mess promotes mistakes.
- Asepsis matters—hand hygiene and alcohol wipes for the ampoules and injection ports.
- Handle one ampoule and one syringe at one time.
- Label the syringe first, then *match* the syringe label with the label on the ampoule while drawing up its contents (matching is more reliable than simply reading).
- Label all syringes—labelling as above assists in checking.
- For the dose—check the order of magnitude: ten times errors tend to harm.
- Double-check with a person or device (e.g. a bar code system), if available—and always when injecting neuraxially.
- Label lines clearly by route—particularly neuraxial lines.
- Keep a physical record, as well as a written one—empty ampoules record what has actually been given for verification at any time.
- Never draw up protamine until you are off bypass: premature protamine ends careers.
- Give prophylactic antibiotics in time (the effective period is up to 60min prior to incision).

Safer anaesthesia and surgery

- Globally, it is estimated that 234 million surgical procedures are performed each year. Of these, 7 million patients suffer harm, and 1 million die. Up to 50% of this harm may be preventable.[1]
- Around 8 million surgical procedures are carried out in England each year, and an estimated 20 000 people die within 30d of surgery.[2]
- Major complications are estimated to occur in 3–17% of inpatient surgical procedures.[3]

Why do complications occur?

- Some adverse outcomes are unavoidable, such as those resulting from complex surgery performed in high-risk patients, but many arise from preventable errors. Common underlying factors include deficiencies in communication, leadership, teamworking, decision-making, and situational awareness. These 'human factors' are increasingly recognized as being important contributing factors to error in the theatre environment.
- During the journey from referral to surgery and discharge, multiple health-care professionals interface with a patient. If one step in care is omitted (such as comprehensive assessment, administration of prophylactic antibiotics, or administration of deep vein thrombosis (DVT) prophylaxis), serious consequences may follow.

How can we improve safety?

- The WHO Second Global Patient Safety Challenge addressed surgical and anaesthesia safety and looked at the evidence base behind surgical complications. The result was a comprehensive clinical review and a 19-point WHO Surgical Safety Checklist intended to focus on key parts of the surgical journey.[4]
- The Checklist was trialled in eight major centres in four high- and four middle- and low-income countries and resulted in a reduction in surgical complications and mortality.[3]
- The Checklist provides a framework to ensure that crucial steps are not omitted in operating room care. It is not intended as a tick box exercise but should change practice in theatre to one of better team communication and a culture of safety.
- WHO indicates that hospitals should modify the Checklist to reflect local practice; eye surgery is different to cardiac surgery. This should be done carefully to avoid making the Checklist more complex or too simple.

A safety culture

- A culture of safety can only be achieved when different individuals in a team are able to support each other. Communication is key. This may be difficult when teams change continually, and it is also well recognized that steep hierarchies between professions may impede effective communication. In poorly functioning teams, members of staff may not feel able to raise concerns, even when patient safety is compromised.

- Many surgeons and anaesthetists have created their own individual safety routines over years of practice, but often there is no consistent team approach. Changing a familiar safety routine is difficult for clinicians, as this challenges a system that they perceive to be working well. However, this diversity of practice between different clinicians and teams represents an inconsistency in the workplace, so that no familiar standard approach to safe care is developed that is applicable to all.
- The WHO Surgical Safety Checklist (Fig. 1.1) offers the opportunity for a consistent approach to theatre checks across national health-care systems.

Briefings and debriefings

- Team briefings before the start and end of an operating list improve communication, teamworking, theatre efficiency, and patient safety. A discussion of the theatre list at the start of the day ensures that each team member knows about the planned operating schedule, the appropriate equipment is available, specific anxieties about individual patients are highlighted, and any last-minute changes are described. A debriefing discussion at the end of the list allows the team to recognize good practice that should become routine, but also to identify factors that need to be improved in future.
- When briefing and debriefing are combined with the WHO Surgical Safety Checklist, a strong safety culture is created to the benefit of patients and clinicians (Table 1.1).

Table 1.1 Suggested components of briefing and debriefing

Briefing	Introduction of team members and roles
	Patients and procedures planned
	Confirmation of order of list
	Specific equipment (anaesthesia and surgery) required
	Any concerns relevant to the day
Debriefing	Thanks to team members for specific actions
	Factors that went well that were useful lessons
	Factors that could be improved for next time

References

1 Weiser TG, Regenbogen SE, Thompson KD, et al. (2008). An estimation of the global volume of surgery: a modelling strategy based on available data. *Lancet*, **372**, 139–44.
2 Department of Health. CMO Annual Report (2009). While you were sleeping. Making surgery safer. In: *On the state of public health: annual report of the Chief Medical Officer 2009*. Chapter 4, pp. 26–33.
3 Haynes AB, Thomas WG, Berry WR, et al. (2009). A surgical safety checklist to reduce morbidity and mortality in a global population. *N Engl J Med*, **360**, 491–9.
4 World Health Organization (2009). *WHO guidelines for safe surgery 2009. Safe surgery saves lives*. http://whqlibdoc.who.int/publications/2009/9789241598552_eng.pdf.

Using the WHO Checklist

The WHO Surgical Safety Checklist (Fig. 1.1) is composed of the Sign In, Time Out, and Sign Out.

Sign In

* The patient identity, planned procedure, and surgical site marking are confirmed against the operating list, the consent form, and the patient. The patient should be actively involved in this process.
* The anaesthesia facilities (machine and drugs) are confirmed as checked, and any added precautions (allergy, airway, anticipated blood loss) identified.
* Suitable monitoring is essential during anaesthesia and should be confirmed as available and functional. In the United Kingdom (UK), the Association of Anaesthetists of Great Britain and Ireland (AAGBI) standards of monitoring should be available; in low-income settings, a pulse oximeter should be the minimum acceptable. Most patients are monitored continuously from the start of anaesthesia, but this may be impractical in some patients such as children or uncooperative adults.

Time Out

* Everyone in theatre should be known by name and role to facilitate teamworking and communication. Introductions should be made where necessary.
* A final confirmation of the patient's identity and planned procedure is undertaken at this point, with reference to imaging where relevant.
* Antibiotics should be administered/confirmed where indicated.
* Any specific concerns relating to the planned procedure should be reviewed by the surgeon, anaesthetist, and nursing staff.
* Many hospitals have added a step to confirm that thromboembolic precautions have been undertaken.

Sign Out

* Swabs and instrument counts are confirmed.
* Specimens are confirmed as correctly labelled (beware of incorrect sticky labels).
* A brief discussion of any specific requirements for post-operative care for the patient should take place at this point.
* The Checklist is a mandatory requirement in several countries. Successful introduction requires a change in theatre culture, and it may be best to trial the Checklist in one theatre first, modify as required by local practice, and then roll out to all other theatres. Leadership from senior clinicians and nurses is important.

Further reading

World Health Organization. *Patient safety*. ℘ http://www.who.int/patientsafety/information_centre/documents/en/index.html.

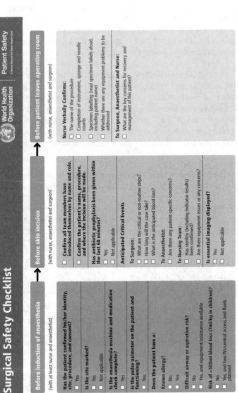

Fig. 1.1 World Health Organization Surgical Safety Checklist.

Preoperative tests

Local protocols for 'routine' preoperative testing should follow National Institute for Health and Care Excellence (NICE) guidance. A test should be done only if the results improve patient information, treatment, and outcomes. Tests should be preceded by a valid consenting process, preferably detailing the chances that a test causes benefit or harm and the positive and negative predictive power for each outcome.[5]

- Start with tests based on surgical grade (Table 1.2) and age (Table 1.3).[6]
- Add tests not yet done, as indicated by disease severity (Table 1.4).
- Local protocols determine whether to undertake a shaded 'NO' (no consensus from NICE). Note there is increasing evidence that routine tests do not benefit patients whose risk of post-operative death or morbidity is low.
- Pregnancy tests to all ♀ who are of menstruating age group.[5]
- Sickle-cell test: African or Afro-Caribbean, Middle Eastern, Asian, East Mediterranean.
- Local protocols should indicate the need for tests not considered by NICE, for instance cardiopulmonary exercise testing (CPET) (see ➲ p. 15).

Table 1.2 Grading surgical procedures

Surgical grades	Examples
Grade 1 (minor)	Excision skin lesion; drainage breast abscess
Grade 2 (intermediate)	Inguinal hernia; varicose vein(s); tonsillectomy; arthroscopy
Grade 3 (major)	Hysterectomy; transurethral resection of the prostate; lumbar discectomy; thyroidectomy
Grade 4 (major +)	Joint replacement; thoracic operations; colonic resection; radical neck dissection

For American Society of Anaesthesiologists (ASA) grading, see ➲ p. 1220.

Table 1.3 Preoperative tests by surgical grade and age

Surgery grade	Age (yr)	CXR	ECG	FBC	INR/ APTT	U&Es/ creat	Random glucose	Urine	Total
One	<16	NO	NO	NO	NO	NO	NO	NO	0
One	16–60	NO	NO	NO	NO	NO	NO	NO	0
One	61–80	NO	NO	NO	NO	NO	NO	NO	0
One	>80	NO	YES	NO	NO	NO	NO	NO	1
Two	<16	NO	NO	NO	NO	NO	NO	NO	0
Two	16–60	NO	NO	NO	NO	NO	NO	NO	0
Two	61–80	NO	NO	YES	NO	NO	NO	NO	1
Two	>80	NO	YES	YES	NO	NO	NO	NO	2
Three	<16	NO	NO	NO	NO	NO	NO	NO	0
Three	16–60	NO	NO	YES	NO	NO	NO	NO	1
Three	61–80	NO	YES	YES	NO	YES	NO	NO	3
Three	>80	NO	YES	YES	NO	YES	NO	NO	3
Four	<16	NO	NO	NO	NO	NO	NO	NO	0
Four	16–60	NO	NO	YES	NO	YES	NO	NO	2
Four	61–80	NO	YES	YES	NO	YES	NO	NO	3
Four	>80	NO	YES	YES	NO	YES	NO	NO	3

Table 1.4 Preoperative tests by disease status

Disease	ASA	CXR	ECG	FBC	INR/ APTT	U&Es/ creat	Blood gases	Lung function	Total
CVS	2	NO	YES	NO	NO	NO	NO	NO	1
CVS	3	NO	YES	NO	NO	YES	NO	NO	2
Lung	2	NO	NO	NO	NO	NO	NO	NO	0
Lung	3	NO	NO	NO	NO	NO	NO	NO	0
Renal	2	NO	NO	NO	NO	YES	NO	NO	1
Renal	3	NO	YES	YES	NO	YES	NO	NO	3

CVS, cardiovascular system.

References

5 National Patient Safety Agency (2010). *Checking pregnancy before surgery.* ℘ http://www.nrls. npsa.nhs.uk/alerts/?entryid45=73838
6 National Institute for Health and Care Excellence (2003). *Preoperative tests. The use of routine pre-operative tests for elective surgery. NICE clinical guideline 3.* ℘ https://www.nice.org.uk/guidance/ cg3/resources/guidance-preoperative-tests-pdf.

Fasting

Background

Pulmonary aspiration of gastric contents, even 30–40mL, is associated with significant morbidity and mortality. Factors predisposing to regurgitation and pulmonary aspiration include inadequate anaesthesia, pregnancy, obesity, difficult airway, emergency surgery, full stomach, and altered gastrointestinal (GI) motility.

Fasting before anaesthesia aims to reduce the volume of gastric contents, and hence the risk should aspiration occur.

Gastric physiology

- Clear fluids (water, fruit juices without pulp, and tea or coffee with <20% of total volume made up of milk) are emptied from the stomach in an exponential manner, with a half-life of 10–20min. This results in complete clearance within 2hr of ingestion.
- Gastric emptying of solids is much slower than for fluids and is more variable. Foods with a high fat or meat content require 8hr or longer to be emptied from the stomach, whereas a light meal, such as toast, is usually cleared in 4hr. Milk is considered a solid, because, when mixed with gastric juice, it thickens and congeals. Cow's milk takes up to 5hr to empty from the stomach. Human breast milk has a lower fat and protein content and is emptied at a faster rate.
- Patients should not have their anaesthesia delayed because of chewing gum, sucking a boiled sweet, or smoking a cigarette immediately before coming to theatre.

Fasting guidelines

Recommendations on preoperative fasting in elective healthy patients were issued by the American Society of Anesthesiologists (ASA) in 1999, followed by similar guidance from the AAGBI (Table 1.5).

Table 1.5 Guidelines for preoperative fasting periods

Ingested material	Minimum fast (hr)
Clear liquids	2
Breast milk	4
Light meal, infant formula, and other milk	6

Delayed gastric emptying

- Delayed gastric emptying due to metabolic causes (e.g. poorly controlled diabetes mellitus, renal failure, sepsis), decreased gastric motility (e.g. head injury), or pyloric obstruction (e.g. pyloric stenosis) will primarily affect emptying of solids, particularly high-cellulose foods such as vegetables. Gastric emptying of clear fluids is affected only in the advanced stages.

- Gastro-oesophageal reflux may be associated with delayed gastric emptying of solids, but emptying of liquids is not affected.
- Raised intra-abdominal pressure (e.g. pregnancy, obesity) predisposes to passive regurgitation.
- Opioids cause marked delays in gastric emptying.
- Trauma delays gastric emptying. The time interval between the last oral intake and the injury is considered as the fasting period, and a rapid sequence induction (RSI) should be used if this interval is short. The time taken to return to normal gastric emptying after trauma has not been established and varies, depending upon the degree of trauma and the level of pain. The best indicators are probably signs of normal gastric motility such as normal bowel sounds and patient hunger.
- Anxiety has not been shown to have any consistent effect on gastric emptying.
- Oral premedication given 1hr before surgery is without adverse effect on gastric volume on induction of anaesthesia. Studies on premedication with oral midazolam 30min preoperatively have not reported any link with gastric regurgitation or aspiration.

Chemical control of gastric acidity and volume

- Antacids can be used to neutralize acid in the stomach, thereby reducing the risk of damage should aspiration occur. Particulate antacids are not recommended. Sodium citrate solution administered shortly before induction is the agent of choice in high-risk cases (e.g. pregnancy).
- H_2 blockers/proton pump inhibitors (PPIs) decrease the secretion of acid in the stomach and should be used for high-risk patients. Ideally, these agents should be administered on the evening before surgery (or early morning for an afternoon list), and a 2nd dose given 2hr preoperatively.
- Gastric motility-enhancing agents, such as metoclopramide, increase gastric emptying in healthy patients, but a clear benefit in trauma patients has not been demonstrated. Metoclopramide is more effective intravenously (IV) than orally (PO).
- Anticholinergic agents do not have a significant effect and are not routinely recommended.
- Pregnant patients should be given ranitidine 150mg on the evening before elective surgery (or at 7 a.m. for an afternoon list), and again 2hr preoperatively (see also ➔ p. 750). During labour, high-risk patients should be given oral ranitidine 150mg 6-hourly. For emergency cases, ranitidine 50mg IV should be given at the earliest opportunity. In addition, 30mL of 0.3M sodium citrate should be given to neutralize any residual gastric acid.
- The ASA does not recommend routine use of these agents in healthy elective patients.

Further reading

Brady M, Kinn S, Ness V, O'Rourke K, Randhawa N, Stuart P (2009). Preoperative fasting for preventing perioperative complications in children. *Cochrane Database Syst Rev*, **4**, CD005285.

Smith I, Kranke P, Murat I, *et al.* (2011). Perioperative fasting in adults and children: guidelines from the European Society of Anaesthesiology. *Eur J Anaesthesiol*, **28**, 556–69.

Prophylaxis of venous thromboembolism

Pulmonary embolism (PE) is responsible for 10% of all hospital deaths. Without prophylaxis, 40–80% of high-risk patients develop detectable DVT, and up to 10% die from PE. Most PEs result from DVTs which start in the venous plexuses of the legs and which then extend proximally. Calf vein DVT is detectable in up to 10% of low-risk patients but seldom extends into proximal veins. DVT and PE are referred to as venous thromboembolism (VTE).

Increased risk of VTE perioperatively is due to:
- Hypercoagulability caused by surgery, cancer, or hormone therapy
- Stasis of blood in the venous plexuses of the legs during surgery and post-operatively
- Interference with venous return (pregnancy, pelvic surgery, pneumoperitoneum)
- Dehydration
- Poor cardiac output.

Any patient confined to bed is at risk of VTE. All patients should be assessed for their risk of VTE on admission to hospital, and prophylaxis should be started without delay. This is particularly important for sick, elderly patients.

Assessing the risk of venous thromboembolism

The risk of VTE is influenced by the type of operation, patient factors, and associated diseases.
- Type and duration of operation:
  - Particularly high-risk procedures include major joint replacements (hip and knee) and surgery to the abdomen and pelvis
  - Operations lasting <30min are considered minor (low-risk), and operations with total surgery and anaesthesia time >90min are high-risk (or >60min for operations on the pelvis or lower limbs).
- Patient factors:
  - Previous history of DVT or PE, thrombophilia (or family history)
  - Pregnancy, puerperium, oestrogen therapy (contraceptive pill, hormone replacement therapy (HRT))
  - Age >60yr (risk increases with age)
  - Obesity and immobility
  - Varicose veins (in abdominal and pelvic surgery; or with phlebitis).
- Associated diseases:
  - Malignancy (especially metastatic or in abdomen/pelvis)
  - Trauma (especially spinal cord injury and lower limb fractures)
  - Heart failure, recent myocardial infarction (MI)
  - Systemic infection
  - Lower limb paralysis (e.g. after stroke)
  - Haematological diseases (polycythaemia, leukaemia, paraproteinaemia)
  - Other diseases, including nephrotic syndrome and inflammatory bowel disease.

Patients can be divided into risk categories in a variety of ways. Stratification into low, medium, or high risk is useful. For example, a slim, fit patient <60yr having minor surgery is low-risk, whereas a fit patient <60yr having major abdominal surgery is moderate-risk, and a patient >60yr having pelvic surgery for cancer is high-risk for VTE.

Patients' risk of bleeding should also be assessed when deciding what methods of VTE prophylaxis to use. Their risks of VTE and of bleeding should be reassessed during their hospital stay.

Methods of prophylaxis

Every hospital should have a policy detailing local practice. General measures which should apply to all patients are:
- Avoidance of prolonged immobility (encourage early mobilization)
- Avoidance of dehydration.

Subcutaneous heparin

Subcutaneous (SC) heparin reduces the incidence of DVT and fatal PE by about two-thirds. Unfractionated (ordinary) heparin has been largely replaced by the newer low-molecular-weight heparins (LMWHs), which may be more effective and cause fewer bleeding complications. They have the added advantage of less frequent administration. Unfractionated heparin may be preferable for patients with renal failure.

Low-molecular-weight heparins

- Normally, start on admission or on the evening before surgery.
- Daily doses are dalteparin 2500–5000U, enoxaparin 2000–4000U, and tinzaparin 3500–4500U.
- The risk of epidural haematoma can be minimized by giving LMWH on the evening before surgery, so that 12hr or more have elapsed before central neuraxial blockade (LMWH plasma half-life is 4hr), or starting prophylaxis post-operatively (see also ➲ p. 1141).

Low-dose unfractionated heparin

- Start 2hr before operation, or on admission if unfit or immobile.
- Dose is 5000U 12-hourly (8-hourly administration may give greater protection and should be used for very high-risk patients).

Fondaparinux sodium

Fondaparinux is a synthetic anticoagulant which is given SC once daily. It has been used increasingly in recent years, especially for patients having major orthopaedic surgery. It should be started after the operation because of the risk of bleeding perioperatively.

Rivaroxaban and dabigatran

These oral anticoagulants are used in hip and knee surgery (see also ➲ p. 215).

Graduated compression stockings (antiembolism stockings)

- These reduce the risk of DVT but are not proven to reduce PE.
- They may give enhanced protection when used in combination with pharmacological prophylaxis.
- Below-the-knee stockings are probably as effective as above-the-knee stockings, but this is controversial.
- Stockings are advisable for all patients having laparoscopic procedures.

Fit with care, and monitor for pressure damage; stockings should be avoided in patients with severe arterial disease of the legs (check the ankle systolic pressure if in doubt), and used with special care in diabetics who may have neuropathy and arterial disease.

Intermittent pneumatic compression devices
- These devices compress the leg (35–40mmHg) for about 10s every minute, promoting venous flow.
- They are as effective as heparin in reducing the incidence of DVT.
- They are used in major surgery, prolonged surgery, and patients with known increased risk for DVT.
- Foot pumps are similar and promote blood flow by compressing the venous plexuses of the feet.

Warfarin, dextran, and aspirin
- Warfarin is used most often in orthopaedic practice where there is good evidence of its efficacy in relation to hip operations. It may be given either as a fixed low dose (2mg/day) or as a monitored dose (target international normalized ratio (INR) 2.0–3.0).
- Dextran (dextran 70/40) is as effective as SC heparin in preventing DVT and PE but is not often used because it requires IV infusion. Fluid overload is a risk, and anaphylaxis can occasionally occur.
- Aspirin and other antiplatelet agents should not be regarded as adequate prophylaxis against VTE. They may increase the risk of bleeding and are sometimes stopped for a few days before surgery (particularly clopidogrel).

Choice of anaesthetic
- Local anaesthesia (LA) eliminates lower limb immobility associated with general anaesthesia (GA).
- Regional anaesthesia (spinal/epidural) appears to be protective in certain kinds of surgery, especially hip/knee replacement.

Oral contraceptive pills and venous thromboembolism
- The risk of spontaneous venous thrombosis is increased in women taking combined oral contraceptive pills (OCPs), particularly 3rd-generation pills containing desogestrel or gestodene.
- OCPs may increase the risk of perioperative thromboembolism by up to 3–4 times, but the evidence is not compelling.
- The risk may decrease, the longer an individual takes a combined OCP.
- Progestogen-only OCPs (and injectable progestogens) do not increase the risk of DVT or PE.

There is no universal consensus on what advice to give. Some guidance recommends considering stopping oestrogen-containing OCPs 4wk before elective surgery. Specialist groups advise that the OCP should not be routinely stopped, because of insufficient evidence and the danger of unwanted pregnancy.

A reasonable policy is as follows:
- There is no need to stop progestogen-only contraceptives for any operation.
- There is no need to stop combined OCPs for minor operations.

For patients on combined OCPs facing major elective surgery, the decision should be made on an individual basis, balancing the risk of thromboembolism (consider other risk factors such as obesity), the possibility of unwanted pregnancy, and the preferences of the patient.

- Patients having intermediate or major surgery when taking the combined OCP should receive SC LMWH and wear antiembolism stockings or receive intermittent pneumatic compression.
- There is no possibility of stopping OCPs for emergency surgery.
- Always record decisions about contraceptives in the case notes, including a record about discussion with the patient.
- If the OCP is stopped, advice must be given about alternative contraceptive measures. In selected cases, consider a change to depot progestogen injections.
- Consider a pregnancy test before operation if there is a possibility of unprotected intercourse having taken place.

Hormone replacement therapy and venous thromboembolism

- HRT increases the incidence of spontaneous VTE, but there are no good data on perioperative risk.
- Stopping HRT may cause recurrence of troublesome menopausal symptoms.
- NICE guidance suggests considering stopping HRT 4wk before major surgery, but it is common practice to continue HRT and to use prophylaxis (pharmacological and stockings).

Further reading

Department of Health (2010). *Venous thromboembolism (VTE) risk assessment.* ℘ http://webarchive.nationalarchives.gov.uk/20130107105354/http:/www.dh.gov.uk/en/Publicationsandstatistics/Publications/PublicationsPolicyAndGuidance/DH_088215.

National Institute for Health and Care Excellence (2010). *Venous thromboembolism: reducing the risk of venous thromboembolism (deep vein thrombosis and pulmonary embolism) in patients admitted to hospital.* ℘ https://www.nice.org.uk/guidance/cg92.

Roderick P, Ferris G, Wilson K, et al. (2005). Towards evidence-based guidelines for the prevention of venous thromboembolism: systematic reviews of mechanical methods, oral anticoagulation, dextran and regional anaesthesia as thromboprophylaxis. *Health Technol Assess*, **9**, iii–iv, ix–x, 1–78.

Cardiopulmonary exercise testing

Survival and the risk of post-operative complications depend upon age, sex, co-morbidity, and severity of surgery. Fitness is measured physically and is the only prognostic variable not routinely recorded in medical notes. Respiratory and cardiac variables at rest, during exercise, and on completion of CPET help define fitness.[7] Where CPET is unavailable, a 6min walk test distance of >563m indicates an anaerobic threshold of >11mL/kg/min.[8]

For CPET, you need:
• An exercise machine (static bicycle or treadmill)
• A computer-controlled ramped increase in workload
• A calibrated pneumotachograph to measure gas flow and composition
• Continuous 12-lead electrocardiogram (ECG) recording and pulse oximetry
• Someone trained to conduct and interpret the test.

Survival correlates with peak values of oxygen (O_2) consumption, power, and heart rate (HR), as well as measurements during CPET, including the anaerobic threshold (AT), ventilatory equivalents for O_2 and carbon dioxide (CO_2), O_2 uptake slope, O_2 pulse, and HR recovery.

Risk stratification and assessment of the cardiorespiratory function using CPET can contribute to:
• Individual estimation of perioperative survival.
• Informed decision-making.
• Perioperative management, including intensive care unit (ICU)/high dependency unit (HDU) requirement.
• Diagnosis and quantification of respiratory and cardiac disease, including occult disease.
• Risk reduction by guiding interventions before, during, and after surgery. Routine CPET is now recommended prior to all abdominal aortic aneurysm (AAA) repairs.[9]

Early work popularized the use of the AT to describe the risk following major surgery (Table 1.6).

Table 1.6 Using anaerobic threshold to predict perioperative mortality

Anaerobic threshold	Mortality rate		
	Test ECG: no ischaemia	Test ECG: ischaemia	Total
>11mL O_2/kg/min	0/107 (0%)	1/25 (4%)	1/132 (0.8%)
<11mL O_2/kg/min	2/36 (5.5%)	8/19 (43%)	10/55 (18%)
All	2/143 (1.4%)	9/44 (20%)	11/187 (6%)

References

7 Hennis PJ, Meale PM, Grocott MP (2011). Cardiopulmonary exercise testing for the evaluation of perioperative risk in non-cardiopulmonary surgery. *Postgrad Med J*, **87**, 550–7.

8 Sinclair RC, Batterham AM, Davies S, Cawthorn L, Danjoux GR (2012). Validity of the 6 min walk test in prediction of the anaerobic threshold before major non-cardiac surgery. *Br J Anaesth*, **108**, 30–5.

9 The Vascular Society (2011). *Elective abdominal aortic aneurysm pre-operative care bundle.* http://www.vascularsociety.org.uk/document/qip-aaa-pre-operative-care-bundle/aaa_pre-operative_care_bundle_updated_july_2011/.

Perioperative medications

Some special considerations have to be made regarding patients' current medications taken for their co-morbidities. These include:

- Anticoagulants and antiplatelet therapies (see ➔ p. 211 and p. 216).
- Diabetic medications (see ➔ p. 151).
- Antipsychotics (see ➔ p. 269).
- Statins should be continued due to their effects on improved endothelial function, enhanced stability of atherosclerotic plaques, and reduced vascular inflammation, causing a reduction in perioperative cardiac events[10].
- Renin–angiotensin system antagonists (angiotensin-converting enzyme (ACE) inhibitors, angiotensin receptor blockers (ARBs)—continuation or cessation depends upon the rationale for their use. If they are being used for left ventricular (LV) dysfunction, they should be continued. If the 1° use is for treatment of hypertension, there is no recommendation either way to stop or continue therapy, and so you should refer to local guidelines.
- There are controversies surrounding the perioperative use of β-blockers following the POISE trial. The latest recommendations suggest that patients already taking β-blockers should remain on them. Patients undergoing high-risk surgery who have evidence of inducible ischaemia, coronary artery disease (CAD), or multiple risk factors for CAD should start low-dose β-blocker treatment at least 1wk preoperatively. For all other patients, the use of β-blockers cannot be recommended. β-blocker therapy should not be started on the day of surgery.[11]

References

10 Schouten O, Boersma E, Hoeks SE, et al. Dutch Echocardiographic Cardiac Risk Evaluation Applying Stress Echocardiography Study Group (2009). Fluvastatin and perioperative events in patients undergoing vascular surgery. N Engl J Med, 361, 980–9.

11 Fleisher LA, Fleischmann KE, Auerbach AD et al. (2014). 2014 ACC/AHA Guideline on Perioperative Cardiovascular Evaluation and Management of Patients Undergoing Noncardiac Surgery. Circulation, 130, e278–e333.

Consent and anaesthetic risk

Kath Jenkins

Consent

- 'It is a legal and ethical principle that valid consent must be obtained before starting treatment, physical investigation, or providing personal care for a patient.'[1] Health professionals who carry out procedures without valid consent are liable to legal action by the patient, and investigation by the General Medical Council or equivalent professional bodies.
- Valid consent implies it is given voluntarily by a competent and informed person not under duress. To have capacity for consent, the patient must be able to comprehend and remember the information provided, weigh up the risks and benefits of the proposed procedure, and consider the consequences of not having the procedure in order to make a balanced decision. Consent may be expressed, either written or verbal, or implied, e.g. holding out one's arm for a blood test.
- Adults are presumed to have capacity to consent, unless there is contrary evidence.[2] Doctors must respect patient autonomy and their right to be involved in decisions that affect them. 'If an adult with capacity makes a voluntary and appropriately informed decision to refuse treatment this decision must be respected. This is the case even when this may result in death of the patient and/or the death of an unborn child, whatever the stage of the pregnancy.'[1]
- Advance decisions: advance refusal of treatment, which may include refusal of life-sustaining treatment, written by a competent individual in case of future incapacity is legally binding in many jurisdictions. Lasting powers of attorney may be appointed by a person with capacity to act on their behalf in health decisions should they lose capacity in the future (England and Wales).[2]
- A new independent mental capacity advocacy service (IMCAS) can provide advice for patients without friends or family in England and Wales.[2]
- Young adults: competent young adults over the age of 16yr can give consent for any treatment, without obtaining separate consent from a parent or guardian.
- Children: those under 16yr who demonstrate the ability to fully appreciate the risks and benefits of the intervention planned can be considered competent to give consent.[3]
- Refusal of treatment: children and young adults who refuse treatment may have their decision overridden by a parent or the court, but the treatment should proceed only if in the child's 'best interests'. When a child lacks capacity for consent, parental consent should be sought. If such a child refuses treatment, judgement needs to be exercised by the parent and the doctor as to the level of restraint that is acceptable, depending on the urgency of the case. Consider postponing the case until adequate premedication can be given.
- In an emergency, verbal consent by telephone is adequate, and essential treatment can be started in the absence of parental authorization, if necessary. Where the child or parent refuses essential treatment, a ward of court order can be obtained, but this should not delay the

emergency management. This enables the doctor to proceed with the treatment lawfully.

- Treatment without consent: in an emergency, consent is not necessary for lifesaving procedures. Unconscious patients may be given essential treatment without consent. It is good practice to consult with the next of kin, but they cannot give or refuse consent for adult patients. Patients who are 'incompetent' may be given treatment, provided it is in their 'best interests'.

- Restricted consent: patients may consent to treatment in general but refuse certain aspects of this treatment, e.g. Jehovah's Witness patients who refuse blood transfusion (see ➲ p. 1050). This must be discussed in full with the patient, so that they are fully aware of the implications of withholding the treatment. The details of the restriction should be carefully documented on the consent form.[4]

- Research and teaching: the same legal principles apply when seeking consent from patients for research or teaching. All clinical research requires ethics committee approval. As research may not have direct benefits for the patients involved, they must receive the fullest possible information about the proposed study, not be pressurized into taking part, and advised they can withdraw at any time without their care being affected. Incompetent patients can be included only in therapeutic research that is considered to be in their best interests or where the therapeutic benefits are genuinely unknown, but there are reasons to believe that there may be advantages from the therapy. Competent children may give consent for clinical research associated with minimal risk. Students should obtain a patient's consent to undertake clinical procedures.

- Documentation: after discussion with the patient in an appropriate environment, the agreed anaesthetic and post-operative plan should be documented in the patient's medical records, including a list of risks explained.[5] Written consent is obtained as part of the overall surgical consent form; separate anaesthetic consent forms are not currently deemed necessary,[6] though they exist in some jurisdictions.

References

1 Department of Health (2009). *Reference guide to consent for examination or treatment*, 2nd edn. ஃ http://webarchive.nationalarchives.gov.uk/20130107105354/http://dh.gov.uk/prod_consum_dh/groups/dh_digitalassets/documents/digitalasset/dh_103653.pdf.

2 *Mental Capacity Act 2005. Chapter 9.* ஃ http://www.legislation.gov.uk/ukpga/2005/9/contents.

3 *Gillick v. West Norfolk and Wisbech Area Health Authority and Department of Health and Social Security; CA 1985* (1986). Appeal Court 112. ஃ http://swarb.co.uk/gillick-v-west-norfolk-and-wisbech-area-health-authority-and-department-of-health-and-social-security-ca-1985/.

4 Association of Anaesthetists of Great Britain and Ireland (2005). *Management of anaesthesia for Jehovah's Witnesses*, 2nd edn. ஃ http://www.aagbi.org/sites/default/files/Jehovah%27s%20Witnesses_0.pdf.

5 General Medical Council (2008). *Consent: patients and doctors making decisions together.* London: General Medical Council. ஃ http://www.gmc-uk.org.

6 Association of Anaesthetists of Great Britain and Ireland (2006). *Consent for anaesthesia*, 2nd edn. ஃ http://www.aagbi.org/publications/guidelines/docs/consent06.pdf.

Anaesthetic risk

Consent is a process. It starts with early provision of written information, including risks, to patients before admission for an elective procedure. Information should also be available in foreign languages, Braille, and large type, and on tape.[7,8]

At the preoperative visit, discussion of risks associated with anaesthesia should be easy to understand and should include all risks that a 'reasonable patient' considers significant. These can range from common, but minor, side effects to rare, but serious, complications.

Communication of risks is important. People vary in how they interpret words and numbers, e.g. a very common side effect of anaesthesia, such as sore throat, may happen on >1 in ten occasions (1:10), whereas death due to anaesthesia is rare (<1:50 000) (Table 2.1). Pictures and diagrams may also be used.

Table 2.1 Communicating risk in simple terms

1 in 10	1 in 100	1 in 1000	1 in 10 000	1 in 100 000
Very common	Common	Uncommon	Rare	Very rare
Someone in a family	Someone in a street	Someone in a village	Someone in a small town	Someone in a large town

The perception of risk is modified by a number of factors:
- Probability of occurrence—true incidence requires a large population sample and may be susceptible to:
  - Regional bias—geographical variation in techniques
  - Exposure bias—catastrophic or dramatic over-publicity
  - Compression/expansion bias—underestimation of large risks, overestimation of small risks.

Both patients' and anaesthetists' perceptions will contribute to the discussion of risks. Anaesthetists should recognize that their bias may frame the presentation of anaesthetic risk and that 'informed consent' may suffer as a consequence.
- Severity—high-severity risks, such as death, paraplegia, and permanent organ failure, even though of very low probability, are perceived as higher overall risks than commoner complications.
- Vulnerability—denial/optimism and a feeling of 'immunity' or 'invincibility' allow us to ignore daily risks.
- Controllability—loss of conscious choice with a feeling of loss of control increases vulnerability. Informed consent with a choice of clinical alternatives is important, as patients who perceive they have had adequate and realistic information with a choice of different anaesthetic options will be less resentful of any subsequent complications.
- Certainty/uncertainty—uncertainty, particularly about the facts, and fear of the uncertain or unknown upset the balance between rational and irrational decisions.

- Familiarity—patients who have had many anaesthetic procedures before will be less worried about any inherent risks, even though these risks may increase with progression of disease. Conversely, patients having their 1st anaesthetic will be more worried.
- Acceptability/dread—anaesthetists fear patient paraplegia more than patient death, stroke, or major MI. Cultural or regional expectations may alter these perceptions, e.g. variations in use of LA techniques.
- Framing or presentation—positive framing is better than negative framing, particularly when relative risks are discussed. For example, '90% survival', rather than '10% mortality', or outcomes are 'twice as good' with one management regimen than with another, although the actual differences may only be between 0.005% and 0.01% mortality. Such 'bias' should not, however, impede discussion of the true incidence or real clinical significance with patients.

The mnemonic BRAN offers a useful approach when assessing the risks of a course of action: benefits, risks, alternatives, and what would happen if nothing were done.

The numerical likelihood of anaesthetic adverse outcomes is presented in Table 2.2.

References

7 Royal College of Anaesthetists and Association of Anaesthetists of Great Britain and Ireland (2008). *Anaesthesia explained*, 3rd edn. ℅ http://www.rcoa.ac.uk/document-store/anaesthesia-explained.

8 Royal College of Anaesthetists (2013). *Risks associated with your anaesthetic—the risk information leaflets*. ℅ http://www.rcoa.ac.uk/document-store/risks-associated-your-anaesthetic-complete-series-2013.

Table 2.2 Risks of anaesthetic adverse outcomes

Risk level (ratio)	Verbal scale	Anaesthetic/medical examples	Example
1:1–9 Single digits	Very common	Pain 1:2 (day surgery)	Heads or tails coin toss 1:2
		Transient ptosis after eye block 1:2 at 24hr (1:5 at 1 month)	
		Sore throat 1:2.5 (ETT)	
		Sore throat 1:5 (LMA)	No pair (poker) 1:2
		Delirium after neck of femur fracture 1:2	
		PONV 1:3	One pair (poker) 1:2.5
		Transient diplopia after eye block 1:4	
		Post-operative cognitive dysfunction (>60yr) 1:4 at 1wk	Rolling a six on a die 1:6
		Shivering 1:4	
		Dizziness 1:5	
		Headache 1:5	
		Backache 1:5 (surgery <1hr), 1:2 (surgery >4hr)	
		Transient arterial occlusion following cannulation 1:5	
		Chest infection after major abdominal surgery 1:5	
		Transient deafness after spinal 1:7	
		30d mortality after emergency laparotomy UK 1:7 (1:4 over 80yr)	
1:10–99 Double digits	Common	Thrombophlebitis 1:10	Getting three balls in UK National Lottery 1:11
		Severe pain (major surgery) 1:10	
		Post-operative cognitive dysfunction (>60yr) 1:10 at 3 months	Two pairs (poker) 1:20

		30d mortality after hip fracture surgery UK 1:14	
		Transient blurred vision after GA 1:20	Rolling a double six on two dice 1:36
		All oral trauma following intubation 1:20	
		CVA or death 1:15 for carotid endarterectomy (symptomatic)	Three of a kind (poker) 1:50
		CVA or death 1:25 for carotid endarterectomy (asymptomatic)	Dying in next 12 months (men 55–64 yr) 1:74
		Disabling CVA or death 1:50 for carotid endarterectomy (all)	
		CVA 1:50 if previous stroke	
		Emergency surgery death 1:40 within 1 month (UK)	
		Difficult intubation 1:50	
		Short-term nerve damage (>48hr) after regional block 1:50–1:100	
		Urinary dysfunction 1:50 (spinal/epidural)	
1:100–999 Hundreds	Moderately common	CVA 1:100 (general surgery)	Dying of any cause in the next year 1:100
		Loss of vision (cardiac surgery) 1:100	
		Awareness during cardiac surgery 1:100	
		Permanent post-operative cognitive dysfunction (>60yr) 1:100	Getting four balls in UK National Lottery 1:206
		Severe headache following epidural 1:100; spinal 1:500 (obstetrics)	
		Permanent complications of arterial cannulation 1:100	
		Arterial puncture at subclavian vein cannulation 1:200	Flush (poker) 1:500
		Awareness during GA for LSCS 1:250	Full house (poker) 1:700
		Perioperative death UK 1:200 (at 1 month)	

(Continued)

Table 2.2 (*Contd.*)

Risk level (ratio)	Verbal scale	Anaesthetic/medical examples	Example
		Minor short-term nerve damage 1:100 (GA)	
		Failure to intubate 1:500	
		Brainstem anaesthesia following ophthalmic block 1:700	
		Post-operative mortality (worldwide) <48hr 1:850	
1:1000–9999 Thousands	Uncommon	Awareness without pain (GA) 1:1000	Exercise stress test death 1:2000
		Post-operative nerve damage >6m 1:2000–1:5000 (regional block)	Four of a kind (poker) 1:4000
		Systemic LA toxicity 1:1000 (regional blocks)	
		Corneal abrasion under GA 1:2800	
		Awareness with pain 1:3000	
		Aspiration pneumonitis 1:3000	Road traffic death in the next year 1:8000
		Cardiac arrest 1:1500 (GA) or 1:3000 (LA)	
		Damage to teeth (GA) requiring treatment 1:4500	
		Retrobulbar haemorrhage following eye block 1:5000	
		Peripheral nerve injury (GA) lasting >3m 1:2000; lasting >1yr 1:5000	
		Failure to intubate/ventilate 1:5000	
		Death related to anaesthesia 1:5000 (ASA 3/4)	

Risk	Category	Anaesthetic risks	Comparison risks
1:10 000–99 999 Tens of thousands	Rare	Anaphylaxis 1:10 000–1:20 000 Spontaneous epidural abscess 1:10 000–1:50 000 Epidural abscess post-epidural insertion (obstetrics) 1:50 000 Globe perforation at eye block 1:10 000 Idiopathic deafness (GA) 1:10 000 Spontaneous sensorineural hearing loss (no anaesthesia) 1:10 000 (GA even rarer) Permanent nerve damage UK (epidural/spinal) 1:23 500–1:50 500 Paraplegia or death UK (epidural/spinal) 1:54 500–1:141 500 Death (related to anaesthesia) 1:50 000–1:100 000 Cranial nerve palsies (spinal) 1:50 000—commonest abducens	Accidental death at home 1:11 000 Getting five balls in UK National Lottery 1:11 098 Straight flush (poker) 1:70 000 Death from hang gliding per flight 1:80 000
1:100 000–999 999 Hundreds of thousands	Very rare	Death (related to anaesthesia) 1:100 000 (ASA 1/2) Meningitis post-epidural insertion (obstetrics) 1:100 000 Paraplegia (spinal/epidural) in obstetrics 1:250 000 Loss of vision (GA) 1:125 000 Epidural haematoma 1:150 000 (epidural), 1:220 000 (spinal) Death due solely to anaesthesia error 1:185 000 Cranial subdural haematoma (after spinal) 1:500 000	Rail accident death 1:500 000 Royal straight flush (poker) 1:650 000
1:1 000 000–9 999 999 Millions	Excessively rare	Spontaneous epidural haematoma (no anaesthesia) 1:1 000 000	Getting six balls in UK National Lottery 1:2 796 763
>1:10 000 000 Tens of millions or billions	Exceptional		Lightning strike 1:10 000 000

Perioperative mortality

- Overall mortality figures (UK) for all non-day-case procedures
  1 month after:
  - Elective surgery 1:177 (~1:200)
  - Emergency surgery 1:34 (~1:40).[9]

Worldwide, post-operative mortality (<48hr) has declined over the last 50yr, from ~1% before the 1970s to 0.12% since the 1990s.

The estimated 1yr post-operative mortality is 5–10%.

Despite the introduction of the Surgical Safety Checklist to focus efforts in reducing surgical morbidity and mortality in both developed and developing countries, post-operative mortality is still 2–3 times higher in developing countries.[10]

- Incidence of death associated with anaesthesia in adult ASA 1 and 2 patients is ~1:100 000, with risk increased 5–10 times for high-risk patients (ASA 3–4) and/or emergency surgery.
- Anaesthetic paediatric mortality is 1:40 000.
- UK death rate associated with anaesthesia for Caesarean sections has decreased from 1:10 000 (1982–84) to 1:100 000 (2000–2002), associated with GA.[11]
- Maternal death rate in the UK attributable to anaesthesia is <1 in 300 000 maternities (2006–2008).[11]
- There are several scoring systems used to predict perioperative risk, including:
  - ASA physical status grading
  - POSSUM—physiological and operative severity score for enumeration of mortality and morbidity. P-POSSUM is used for general surgery (⌘http://www.riskprediction.org.uk/pp-index.php)
  - Operative urgency (UK National Confidential Enquiry into Patient Outcome and Death, NCEPOD).
- National studies of mortality that assess the quality of delivery of care continue to highlight factors that contribute to anaesthetic-related mortality:
  - Inadequate preoperative assessment
  - Inadequate preparation and resuscitation
  - Inappropriate anaesthetic technique
  - Inadequate perioperative monitoring
  - Lack of supervision
  - Poor post-operative care.

References

9 Department of Health (2002). *NHS performance indicators*. ⌘ http://webarchive.national-archives.gov.uk/+/www.dh.gov.uk/en/Publicationsandstatistics/Publications/AnnualReports/Browsable/DH_4992217.

10 Bainbridge D, Martin J, Arango M, et al. (2012). Perioperative and anaesthetic-related mortality in developed and developing countries: a systematic review and meta-analysis. *Lancet*, 380, 1075–81.

11 *Confidential Enquiry into Maternal Deaths in United Kingdom (2000–2002 and 2006–2008)*. ⌘ http://www.hqip.org.uk/cmace-reports/.

Perioperative morbidity

See Table 2.5 for the incidence of various types of anaesthetic morbidity and mortality.

Cardiovascular

(See also **➲** p. 36.)

- Sixty per cent of patients who die within 30d of surgery have evidence of CAD.
- Major non-cardiac surgery is associated with an incidence of cardiac death between 0.5% and 1.5% and of major cardiac complications between 2% and 3.5%.[12]
- In non-cardiac surgery, active cardiac conditions that indicate major clinical risk require intensive management and delay of elective surgery:
  - Unstable coronary syndromes or MI <30d
  - Decompensated heart failure
  - Significant arrhythmias
  - Severe valvular disease.
- Determination of functional capacity: inability to achieve four metabolic equivalents (4 METs—climb flight of stairs, walk at 4mph) is associated with an increased risk of perioperative cardiovascular morbidity (see also **➲** p. 37).
- Clinical risk factors (Table 2.3) include:[13]
  - Ischaemic heart disease (IHD)
  - Compensated or prior heart failure
  - Diabetes mellitus
  - Renal insufficiency
  - Cerebrovascular disease.
- High-risk surgery increases the risk of CVS complications.[13]
- Patients stratified as high- or intermediate-risk require further investigation and consideration of risk reduction prior to planned surgery (Table 2.4).

Table 2.3 Cardiac risk factors and rate of cardiac complications

Number of simple clinical risk factors present	Cardiac risk index	Approximate rate of cardiac complications, including death (%)
0	Class I	~0.5
1	Class II	~1.0
2	Class III	~5.0
3	Class IV	~10.0
4	Class V	~15.00

Table 2.4 Surgical severity and cardiac risk

High-risk surgery (cardiac risk >5%)	Intermediate-risk (cardiac risk 1–5%)	Low-risk surgery (cardiac risk <1%)
Emergency major operations (particularly elderly patients)	Carotid endarterectomy	Endoscopic procedures
	Head and neck surgery	Superficial procedures
Major vascular surgery	Intraperitoneal surgery	
Peripheral vascular surgery	Intrathoracic surgery	Cataract surgery
Prolonged surgery with large fluid shifts	Orthopaedic surgery	Breast surgery
	Prostatic surgery	

The commonest causes for anaesthesia-related cardiac arrest include drug-related events, hypovolaemia, and failure of airway management.[14]

Venous thromboembolism

- In the UK, an estimated 25 000 people die from preventable hospital-acquired VTE every year. The risk of DVT and PE after surgery is substantially increased in the first 12 post-operative weeks and varies considerably by type of surgery. An estimated 1 in 140 middle-aged women undergoing inpatient surgery in the UK will be admitted with VTE during 12wk after surgery (1 in 45 after hip or knee replacement, and 1 in 85 after surgery for cancer), compared with 1 in 815 after day-case surgery and only 1 in 6200 during a 12wk period without surgery.[15]

Respiratory

(See also ➔ p. 85.)

- Post-operative respiratory complications (pneumonia/respiratory failure) remain a major cause of surgical morbidity and mortality—poor post-operative analgesia may often contribute to the aetiology. Predictive factors include abdominal/thoracic surgery, emergency surgery, poor functional status, history of chronic obstructive pulmonary disease (COPD) (forced vital capacity (FVC) <1.5L, forced expiratory volume in 1s (FEV_1)/FVC <50%, $PaCO_2$ >6kPa), increasing age, and raised body mass index (BMI).[16]

Neurological

(See ➔ p. 227.)

Minor

- Incidences of relatively minor morbidity, such as pain and post-operative nausea and vomiting (PONV), have not changed significantly over the last 30yr despite improvements in anaesthetic drugs and techniques.
- Minor sequelae following surgery often have significant impact on patient recovery, leading to decreased function and slower resumption of daily activities following discharge.

Table 2.5 Incidence of anaesthetic morbidity and mortality

Mortality and morbidity	Incidence	Comments
Total perioperative deaths within 30d (UK)	1:200 elective surgery 1:40 emergency surgery	
Total perioperative deaths within 48hr (worldwide)	1:850	
UK 30d perioperative mortality for emergency laparotomies	1:7	1:4 in over 80s
UK 30d perioperative mortality for hip fracture surgery	1:14	
Death		
Related to anaesthesia	1:50 000	1:100 000 (ASA 1–2)
CVS		
Cardiac arrest (GA)	1:1500	
Cardiac arrest (LA)	1:3000	
Respiratory		
Aspiration (GA)	1:3000	× 4 in emergencies, × 3 in obstetrics
Mortality due to aspiration	1:60 000	
Difficult intubation	1:50	
Failure to intubate	1:500	1:250 in obstetrics
Failure to intubate and ventilate	1:5000	
Neurological		
Post-operative cognitive dysfunction (>60yr)	1:4 at 1wk 1:10 at 1 month 1:100 permanent	Irrespective of regional/ general anaesthesia
Post-operative delirium	1:7 general surgery (up to 1:2 elderly neck of femur fracture)	
Cerebrovascular accident	1:50 if previous stroke 1:100 general surgery 1:20 head and neck surgery 1:20 carotid surgery	CVA 1:700 in non-surgical population
Awareness with pain	1:3000	
Awareness without pain	1:1000	
Awareness during cardiac surgery	1:100	
Awareness during GA emergency LSCS	1:250	

(Continued)

Table 2.5 (Contd.)

Mortality and morbidity	Incidence	Comments
Miscellaneous		
Anaphylaxis	1:10 000–1: 20 000	
Pain after major surgery	1:10 severe	
Pain after day surgery	1:3 moderate	
Nausea and vomiting (PONV)	1:2	
Sore throat	1:3	
	1:2.5 tracheal tube	PONV ♀:♂ 3:1
	1:5 laryngeal mask	
	1:10 face mask	
Drowsiness	1:2	
Dizziness	1:5	
Headache	1:5	
Shivering	1:4	
Dental damage	1:100 overall	
	(1:4500 requiring intervention)	
All oral trauma post-intubation	1:20	
Deafness	1:10 000 GA	
	1:7 spinal (transient)	
Loss of vision	1:125 000 GA	
	1:100 cardiac surgery	
	1:100 minor short-term nerve damage	
Peripheral nerve injury (GA)	1:300 ulnar neuropathy	
	1:2000 nerve injury lasting >3m; 1:5000 lasting >1yr	
Regional		
Paraplegia or death after neuraxial block	1:54 500–1:141 500	
Permanent significant nerve injury after neuraxial block	1:23 000–1:50 500	
Temporary nerve damage after obstetric epidural	1:1000	
Permanent nerve damage after obstetric epidural	1:13 000	
Paraplegia after obstetric epidural	1:250 000	
Permanent nerve injury (peripheral block)	1:2000–1:5000	
Transient radicular irritation (spinal)	Up to 1:3 (lidocaine/mepivacaine)	

Table 2.5 (*Contd.*)

Mortality and morbidity	Incidence	Comments
Epidural abscess (obstetrics)	1:50 000	
	1:10 000–1:50 000 (spontaneous abscess)	
Meningitis after epidural (obstetrics)	1:100 000	
Vertebral canal haematoma	1:150 000 epidural	
	1:220 000 spinal	
	1:1 000 000 spontaneous	
Post-dural puncture headache (PDPH)	1:100	
PDPH in day surgery	1:10	
Backache	1:5 if <1hr surgery	
	1:2 if >4hr surgery	
Systemic LA toxicity	1:10 000 epidural	
	1:1500 regional blocks	
Eye blocks		
Retrobulbar haemorrhage	1:250–1:20 000	
Brainstem anaesthesia	1:700	
Globe perforation	1:10 000	
Ptosis (transient)	1:2 at 24hr	
	1:5 at 1 month	

- More than 50% of patients assume that pain is a normal part of the post-operative course/healing process and are prepared to suffer, rather than complain.
- PONV has a multifactorial aetiology, including the type/duration of anaesthesia, drug therapy, type of surgery, and patient characteristics (particularly young, overweight, non-smoking ♀ with a history of motion sickness/previous PONV) (see ➡ p. 1085).

References

12 Poldermans D, Bax JJ, Boersma E, *et al.* (2009). Guidelines for preoperative cardiac risk assessment and perioperative management in non cardiac surgery. *Eur Heart J*, **30**, 2769–812.

13 Fleischer LA, Beckman JA, Brown KA, *et al.* (2007). ACC/AHA 2007 Guidelines on Perioperative Cardiovascular Evaluation and Care for Noncardiac Surgery: Executive Summary: A Report of the American College of Cardiology/American Heart Association Task Force on Practice Guidelines (Writing Committee to Revise the 2002 Guidelines on Perioperative Cardiovascular Evaluation for Noncardiac Surgery): Developed in Collaboration With the American Society of Echocardiography, American Society of Nuclear Cardiology, Heart Rhythm Society, Society of Cardiovascular Anesthesiologists, Society for Cardiovascular Angiography and Interventions, Society for Vascular Medicine and Biology, and Society for Vascular Surgery. *Circulation*, **116**, 1971–96.

14 Lee TH, Marcantonio ER, Mangione CM, *et al.* (1999). Derivation and prospective validation of a simple index for prediction of cardiac risk of major noncardiac surgery. *Circulation*, **100**, 1043–9.

15 Sweetland S, Green J, Liu B, *et al.* (2009). Duration and magnitude of the postoperative risk of venous thromboembolism in middle aged women: prospective cohort study. *BMJ*, **339**, b4583.

16 Arozullah AM, Khuri SF, Henderson WG, Daley J; Participants in the National Veterans Affairs Surgical Quality Improvement Program (2001). Development and validation of a multifactorial risk index for predicting postoperative pneumonia after major noncardiac surgery. *Ann Intern Med*, **135**, 847–57.

Further reading

Adams A (2002). The meaning of risk. In: McConachie I, ed. *Anaesthesia for the high risk patient.* London: Greenwich Medical Media, pp. 239–47.

Jenkins K, Baker AB (2003). Consent and anaesthetic risk. *Anaesthesia*, **58**, 962–84.

Cardiovascular disease

Ischaemic heart disease

Perioperative cardiac morbidity is an important health-care issue. Current Hospital Episode Statistics (HES) data suggest that ~30 000 patients die each year in the UK within 30d of surgery, and ~45% of these deaths (13 500) have a cardiac cause. Many more patients may suffer a cardiac complication. There are 5–10 severe cardiac events for every cardiac death (68–135 000 patients per annum in the UK). IHD is the single main contributory factor. Up to 20% of patients undergoing surgery have preoperative evidence of myocardial ischaemia. The overall rate for perioperative MI is 1% in unselected patients, increasing to 5% for patients undergoing vascular surgery.

Perioperative risk

The key to reducing perioperative CVS morbidity is to identify high-risk patients beforehand (Box 3.1). CVS risk is influenced by patient factors (including functional capacity) and by the nature of the planned surgery (see also ⮕ p. 7).

Box 3.1 Predictors of perioperative risk

Major risk predictors (markers of unstable CAD)	Recent MI (<1 month prior to planned surgery)
	Unstable or severe angina
	Ongoing ischaemia after MI (clinical symptoms or non-invasive testing)
	Decompensated heart failure
	Significant arrhythmias (high-grade AV block, symptomatic arrhythmias, or supraventricular arrhythmias with uncontrolled ventricular rate)
	Severe valvular heart disease (aortic stenosis gradient >40mmHg, valve surface area <1cm^2), mitral stenosis)
	CABG/PCI (BMS <6wk, DES <1yr)
Intermediate risk predictors (markers of stable CAD)	History of IHD
	History of compensated or prior heart failure
	History of cerebrovascular disease
	Abnormal renal function
	Diabetes
Minor risk predictors (increased probability of heart disease)	Advanced (physiological) age
	Abnormal ECG
	Rhythm other than sinus
	Low functional capacity
	Uncontrolled systemic hypertension

AV, atrioventricular; BMS, bare-metal stent; CABG, coronary artery bypass grafting; CAD, coronary artery disease; DES, drug-eluting stent; ECG, electrocardiogram; IHD, ischaemic heart disease; MI, myocardial infarction; PCI, percutaneous coronary intervention.

Patient factors

Functional capacity

Exercise tolerance is a major predictor of perioperative risk. The physiological response to major surgery increases the O_2 demand by up to 40%, requiring a subsequent increase in O_2 delivery. The ability to exercise is an excellent indicator of 'CVS fitness'. It is usually expressed in metabolic equivalents of task (METs) on a scale defined by the Duke Activity Status Index (Box 3.2). One MET is the resting O_2 consumption of a 40-yr-old 70kg ♂ (3.5mL/kg/min). Patients who cannot sustain 4 METs of physical activity frequently have adverse outcomes following high-risk surgery (see also Cardiopulmonary exercise testing, → p. 15).

Box 3.2 Metabolic equivalents of common tasks

1–4 METs	• Eating, dressing, dishwashing, and walking around the house
4–10 METs	• Climbing a flight of stairs, walking on level ground at >6km/hr, running briefly, playing golf
>10 METs	• Strenuous sports: swimming, singles tennis, football

Surgical factors

See Box 3.3.

Box 3.3 Risks of surgery in ischaemic heart disease

High risk: >5% death/non-fatal MI	• Major emergency surgery (especially in elderly) • Aortic/major vascular surgery • Prolonged surgery with large fluid shifts
Intermediate risk: <5% death/non-fatal MI	• Carotid endarterectomy/endovascular aneurysm repair • Head and neck surgery • Intraperitoneal and intrathoracic surgery • Orthopaedic surgery • Prostatic surgery
Low risk: <1% death/non-fatal MI	• Minimally invasive endoscopic surgery • Cataract extraction • Superficial surgery (including breast)

Special investigations

12-lead electrocardiogram

• All patients over 60yr undergoing major surgery and anyone with risk factors for IHD should have a preoperative ECG.

- Arrhythmias and cardiac conduction abnormalities require careful evaluation for underlying cardiopulmonary disease, drug toxicity, and metabolic abnormality.
- Many patients with underlying IHD have a normal resting ECG.

Exercise testing

- Exercise ECG: test of choice in ambulatory patients. Provides an estimate of functional capacity and detects myocardial ischaemia. ST-segment depression is suggestive of myocardial ischaemia. Tachyarrhythmias or significant falls in systolic blood pressure (BP) are also highly suggestive of impaired O_2 delivery to the myocardium. Those patients who are unable to exercise or have pre-existing ECG abnormalities (e.g. left bundle branch block, ventricular hypertrophy/strain, digitalis effect) should have a pharmacological stress test.
- CPET (see also ➲ p. 15): usually performed on a bicycle ergometer using respiratory gas analysis and an ECG. When the anaerobic threshold is reached, excess lactic acid produced by anaerobic metabolism is buffered by the bicarbonate system. This increases CO_2 production, producing an inflection point—the anaerobic threshold. A low anaerobic threshold (<11mL/min/kg), particularly if associated with ECG evidence of ischaemia and high ventilatory equivalents for CO_2, is associated with an increased complication risk in patients presenting for major surgery.

Pharmacological stress testing

- Dipyridamole thallium scintigraphy: uses a coronary vasodilator (dipyridamole) and a radioisotope (thallium) which is taken up by perfused heart muscle. It shows up areas of impaired perfusion as reversible perfusion defects caused by dipyridamole-induced 'steal'. Areas of non-perfused myocardium show up as permanent perfusion defects.
- Dobutamine stress echocardiography: utilizes an increasing dose of dobutamine (to a maximum of 40 micrograms/kg/min), with simultaneous two-dimensional (2D) precordial echocardiography, to look for new or worsening wall motion abnormalities as an indicator of impaired perfusion. The presence of ischaemia, manifested as new wall motion abnormalities at a heart rate of <60% of the age-predicted maximal HR, is associated with an increased risk of perioperative cardiac complications.

Magnetic resonance imaging stress perfusion imaging

- In some hospitals, magnetic resonance imaging (MRI) investigation of myocardial ischaemia will be utilized, although no preoperative studies have yet been reported. Wall motion abnormalities are used as a surrogate for ischaemia.

Patients who have large areas of reversible ischaemia on stress testing should be considered for coronary angiography.

Coronary artery bypass grafting

Occasionally, coronary artery bypass grafting (CABG) may be necessary prior to high-risk non-cardiac surgery. Indications are identical to those for

CABG on prognostic grounds, i.e. significant (>50%) left main stem stenosis, severe (>70%) two- or three-vessel disease (including the proximal left anterior descending), and/or LV systolic dysfunction. Following cardiac surgery, subsequent surgery should be delayed for at least 3 months.

Percutaneous coronary intervention

- Percutaneous coronary intervention (PCI) is very rarely indicated prior to elective surgery. Recent PCI is associated with increased 30d mortality and increased risk of MI.
- PCI causes trauma to the vessel wall, rendering the endoluminal surface thrombogenic until the vessel wall has healed or the stent has re-endothelialized. Dual antiplatelet medication (aspirin/clopidogrel) is necessary to prevent local coronary thrombosis—aspirin for life, clopidogrel for 3wk after balloon angioplasty, 6wk after bare-metal stent (BMS) insertion, or for 12 months when a drug-eluting stent (DES) is used.
- Stopping antiplatelet medication perioperatively is associated with a very high cardiac complication rate and requires careful discussion between the surgeon, who can quantify the risk of perioperative bleeding, and the cardiologist who can assess the likelihood of stent thrombosis.
- DES thrombosis has been reported as late as 1yr after stent insertion when antiplatelet medications have been stopped for surgery. In most patients, the antiplatelet regime should be continued perioperatively, as the risk of stent thrombosis is greater than the risk of bleeding.
- If PCI is considered necessary prior to surgery, careful consideration should be given to the type of PCI performed. For procedures that can be delayed by 12 months, it is reasonable to use a DES. If the procedure can be delayed for 6–8wk, a BMS can be used. If the condition requires surgery to be performed in the next 2–4wk, consideration should be given to performing balloon angioplasty only.
- If a patient taking dual antiplatelet therapy post-PCI needs an operation where bleeding may be problematic (e.g. intracranial surgery, spinal surgery, open aortic surgery), and the operation cannot be deferred for an appropriate time period, consider stopping clopidogrel for 7d preoperatively and bridging the patient with a short-acting platelet IIb/IIIa glycoprotein receptor antagonist (tirofiban, eptifibatide) plus an unfractionated heparin infusion to cover the period prior to surgery. These can be stopped 6hr prior to surgery.
- Where possible, surgery should be deferred for at least 6wk after BMS insertion, or 1yr after DES insertion, irrespective of the antiplatelet regime, as there is a very high risk of cardiac complications (up to 45%).[1]

Choice of perioperative testing

Evaluation of patients with IHD depends on the planned surgery, facilities, and time available. Precise recommendations remain controversial, but careful history, examination, and practical application of preoperative screening tests is important. Little advantage is gained from complex examinations which will not alter management. The positive predictive value of most tests is low. Close liaison with both cardiological and surgical colleagues is required. At times, investigations will indicate the need to consider an alternative less invasive surgical procedure.

Perioperative medical therapy

Approximately 50% of perioperative MIs are caused by an imbalance of O_2 supply and demand. The other 50% are caused by unstable plaque rupture, causing thrombosis and occlusion of a coronary artery. Medical therapy should be continued perioperatively to protect against ischaemic stresses. Drugs should be given IV, where possible, if GI absorption is impaired.

- Chronic β-blockade should be continued. β-blockers have anti-inflammatory properties which stabilize coronary plaques, and this may explain the benefits seen with protracted use.
- Recent evidence suggests that acute perioperative β-blockade may be detrimental. Although acute perioperative β-blockade reduces the risk of non-fatal perioperative MI, it is associated with increased rates of perioperative mortality and stroke.[2]
- There is limited evidence to suggest that very high-risk patients who demonstrate inducible ischaemia on preoperative stress testing may benefit from carefully titrated β-blockade (to a HR of 60–80bpm) started at least 1wk prior to surgery. Low-dose bisoprolol is commonly used.
- A meta-analysis of small randomized trials has suggested that $α_2$-agonists reduce the risk of perioperative cardiac events.[3] Clonidine is the most widely available (up to 300 micrograms daily). Dexmedetomidine has recently been licensed in the UK.
- Nitrates should be continued perioperatively—IV or transdermally, if necessary. There is no evidence that prophylactic administration decreases the risk of perioperative cardiac complications.
- Calcium channel blockers should be continued preoperatively and resumed as soon as possible post-operatively. Verapamil has been shown to confer a small measure of cardiac protection in small randomized controlled clinical trials.
- ACE inhibitors improve survival in patients with LV dysfunction and offer major benefits to patients with vascular disease or diabetes and normal LV function. They do not protect against major perioperative cardiac events. In the perioperative period, they may increase the risk of hypotension (especially with thoracic epidurals or hypovolaemia), requiring more invasive haemodynamic monitoring for major surgery. Some anaesthetists routinely stop administration in the perioperative period—if stopped for several days, restart at a reduced dose.
- Perioperative statin administration has been shown to improve both short-term and long-term cardiac outcome following non-cardiac and coronary bypass surgery.[4,5] Statins enhance plaque stability, making plaque rupture less likely.
- All patients with documented IHD should continue to receive antiplatelet medication to protect against thromboembolic complications.

Anaesthetic considerations

- In addition to standard monitoring, invasive cardiovascular monitoring (arterial line, central venous pressure (CVP) ± cardiac output monitoring) should be used for high-/intermediate-risk patients undergoing major surgery. ECG monitoring should use the 5-lead ECG.
- There is no evidence that any particular technique is superior. Avoid tachycardia and hypotension/hypertension to minimize myocardial ischaemia.
- Good analgesia is important, since uncontrolled pain is a potent cause of tachycardia; regional blocks can be very effective. Central neuraxial blocks ameliorate the hypercoagulable state seen following anaesthesia and surgery.
- Haemoglobin (Hb) levels should be kept >90g/L.
- Myocardial ischaemia may occur during emergence and extubation. Hypertension and tachycardia should be anticipated and avoided. The use of a short-acting β-blocker, e.g. esmolol, should be considered.
- Consider admission to HDU post-operatively for close monitoring.
- Following major surgery, all patients at risk should have supplemental oxygen for 3–4d.[4]

References

1 Spahn DR, Howell SJ, Delebays A, Chassot PG (2006). Coronary stents and perioperative anti-platelet regimen: dilemma of bleeding and stent thrombosis. *Br J Anesth*, **96**, 675–7.
2 POISE Study Group (2008). Effects of extended release metoprolol in patients undergoing non cardiac surgery (POISE Trial): a randomized controlled trial. *Lancet*, **371**, 1839–47.
3 Wijeysundera DN, Naik JS, Beattie WS (2003). Alpha 2 agonists to prevent perioperative cardiovascular complications: a meta-analysis. *Am J Med*, **114**, 742–52.
4 Biccard BM, Sear JW, Foex P (2005). Statin therapy: a potentially useful perioperative intervention in patients with cardiovascular disease. *Anaesthesia*, **60**, 1106–14.
5 Manach Y, Coriat P, Collard CD, Riedel B (2008). Statin therapy within the perioperative period. *Anesthesiology*, **108**, 1141–6.

Further reading

Fleisher LA, Beckman JA, Brown KA, et al. (2009). ACCF/AHA focused update on perioperative beta blockade incorporated into the ACC/AHA 2007 guidelines on perioperative evaluation and care for noncardiac surgery. *J Am Coll Cardiol*, **54**, e13–118.
Hindler K, Shaw AD, Samuels J, Fulton S, Collard CD, Riedel B (2006). Improved perioperative outcomes associated with preoperative statin therapy. *Anesthesiology*, **105**, 1260–72.
Mukherjee D, Eagle KA (2003). Perioperative cardiac assessment for noncardiac surgery: eight steps to the best possible outcome. *Circulation*, **107**, 2771–4.
Poldermans D, Bax JJ, Boersma E, et al. (2009). Guidelines on pre-operative cardiac risk assessment and perioperative cardiac management in non-cardiac surgery. *Eur Heart J*, **30**, 2769–812.

Perioperative acute myocardial infarction

Perioperative MI usually occurs in the 3–4d following surgery. Ten to 20% of patients suffering a perioperative MI will die before hospital discharge. Typical clinical symptoms and signs of acute MI may be masked in the immediate post-operative period by the residual effects of anaesthetic drugs, strong analgesics, and a distracting painful surgical incision. Around half of perioperative MIs are caused by acute plaque rupture, but the severity of the underlying stenosis does not necessarily predict the infarct territory. The remainder are caused by myocardial O_2 supply–demand imbalance. The best markers of myocardial injury are the cardiac troponins T and I which are only found in cardiac muscle and are normally undetectable in the blood. These have very high myocardial tissue specificity and a high sensitivity. When myocardial necrosis occurs, they are detectable in the plasma within 4–12hr. Levels peak at 12–24hr and are detectable for 7–10d. A serum troponin level taken at least 12hr after the onset of chest pain is considered diagnostic of significant myocardial damage if troponin T >0.1 micrograms/L (and highly suspicious of myocardial damage if troponin T = 0.01–0.1 micrograms/L).

- Rapid treatment is essential. Move patients to HDU.
- All patients should receive supplemental O_2.
- Patients should be given sublingual glyceryl trinitrate (GTN) and IV morphine to relieve any chest pain.
- If the patient is not taking an antiplatelet drug, they should receive aspirin (75–300mg), or clopidogrel (75–600mg) if aspirin-intolerant.
- β-blockade should be used to control the HR and to decrease myocardial O_2 demand (metoprolol 1–5mg boluses or esmolol 50–200 micrograms/kg/min loading dose, then 0.05–0.2 micrograms/kg/min). Aim for a rate of 60–80bpm.
- Pulmonary oedema, if present, should be treated with upright posture, IV furosemide (40mg), and IV nitrates. Continuous positive airway pressure (CPAP) should be considered.
- Other therapeutic options are reduced post-operatively. Acute thrombolysis is relatively contraindicated by recent surgery. If available, acute angioplasty of the 'culprit lesion' should be considered—close liaison with a cardiologist is essential.

Heart failure

Heart failure is the commonest cause of admission to hospital in those aged >65yr. Incidence rises with increasing age. It has ~50% 5yr mortality. It is characterized by:
- Fatigue
- Exercise intolerance
- Orthopnoea
- Exertional dyspnoea
- High incidence of ventricular arrhythmias
- Shortened life expectancy.

Perioperatively, heart failure is associated with a substantially increased risk of mortality/morbidity. A patient with uncontrolled heart failure undergoing an emergency laparotomy has a mortality risk of 20–30%.

Medical management
- **Diuretics** reduce peripheral and pulmonary congestion. Aldosterone antagonists (spironolactone, eplerenone) reduce mortality when used in conjunction with ACE inhibitors in patients with severe heart failure (ejection fraction (EF) <25%).
- **Vasodilators** decrease preload and afterload. ACE inhibitors, and to a lesser extent ARBs, improve survival. Hydralazine plus a nitrate may be used in patients who are intolerant of ACE inhibitors and ARBs.
- **β-blockers** (carvedilol, bisoprolol) are indicated to reduce HR and myocardial O_2 demand. Studies show improved survival, but cardiological input is required.
- **Inotropes**: digoxin improves symptoms and may be used to control the ventricular rate of atrial fibrillation (AF) or in patients in sinus rhythm with severe or worsening heart failure.
- **Anticoagulation**: indicated for AF and for those with a history of thromboembolism, LV aneurysm, or with evidence of intracardiac thrombus on echocardiography, to reduce the risk of thromboembolic events.
- Some patients with intractable heart failure may have atrial synchronous biventricular pacing devices inserted in an attempt to make ventricular contraction more synchronous. Known as 'cardiac resynchronization therapy', these devices can improve functional capacity and quality of life.
- Some patients with severely impaired ventricular performance and a history of ventricular tachycardia (VT)/ventricular fibrillation (VF) will have biventricular automatic implantable cardioverter–defibrillators (AICDs) inserted for 2° prevention of arrhythmic death (see p. 81).

Preoperative assessment
- History and examination should identify present or recent episodes of decompensated heart failure (any <6 months adversely affects risk).
- Optimize medical therapy to minimize symptoms of LV dysfunction and maximize functional capacity.
- Continue anti-failure therapy in the preoperative period.

- Consider a period of preoperative 'optimization' in ICU/HDU.
- Treat metabolic abnormalities.
- Treat symptomatic arrhythmias, and attempt to optimize the HR to around 80bpm. Rhythms other than sinus are poorly tolerated (especially AF), as properly timed atrial contractions contribute up to 30% of ventricular filling.

Special investigations

Blood tests (to evaluate aggravating factors)
- FBC, U&Es, liver function tests (LFTs), thyroid function tests, fasting lipids, and glucose.

12-lead electrocardiogram
- Check for arrhythmias. AF may worsen heart failure by reducing the cardiac filling time.

Chest X-ray
- Prominent upper lobe veins (upper lobe diversion), engorged peripheral lymphatics (Kerley B lines), alveolar oedema ('bats' wings').
- Pleural effusions, cardiomegaly.

Transthoracic echocardiography
- Most useful test, particularly when coupled with Doppler flow studies. Will determine whether the primary abnormality is pericardial/myocardial/valvular, systolic/diastolic, segmental/global. Echocardiography also allows the quantitative assessment of the ventricles, atria, pericardium, valves, and vascular structures.
- Alternatives include transoesophageal echocardiography (TOE), radionuclide imaging, and cardiac MRI.
- Modern echocardiography machines generate values for EF (normal range 60–80%) and fractional shortening (normal range 28–44%) which define the degree of LV impairment (Table 3.1).

Table 3.1 Estimating LV impairment from ejection fraction

Ejection fraction 40–50%	Mild LV impairment
Ejection fraction 30–40%	Moderate LV impairment
Ejection fraction <30%	Severe LV impairment

Cardiac catheterization
- This is sometimes performed if significant coronary or valvular heart disease is suspected as a cause of heart failure. Ventricular performance may sometimes be improved if there are areas of ventricular muscle whose contractility may be improved if the blood supply is restored—'hibernating myocardium'.

Perioperative management
- Some patients may be deemed unfit for the proposed surgery. Patients with severe heart failure (EF <30%) are dependent on the preload to maintain ventricular filling. Many also rely on increased sympathetic tone.

Such patients are living 'on a knife edge' and are exquisitely sensitive to small alterations in their physiology.

- Use local or regional techniques for peripheral procedures.
- There is little conclusive evidence of the benefits of GA versus regional anaesthesia for more major surgery.
- Patients should receive all their anti-failure medications on the morning of surgery.
- Digoxin should be given IV post-operatively if the patient is in AF, but, if in sinus rhythm, it can usually be omitted until oral intake resumes. Nitrates can be given transdermally while nil by mouth.
- ACE inhibitors should be resumed as soon as possible post-operatively. If omitted for 3d or more, they should be reintroduced at a low dose to minimize 1st-dose hypotension.
- Whichever anaesthetic technique is chosen, minimize negative inotropy, tachycardia, diastolic hypotension, and systolic hypertension. Careful monitoring of fluid balance is essential. Invasive CVS monitoring, including measurement of cardiac output, should be considered for all major surgery.
- Patients who decompensate in the perioperative period may require treatment with inotropes such as dobutamine and phosphodiesterase inhibitors (milrinone, enoximone).
- Renal perfusion is easily compromised due to markedly impaired glomerular filtration rates (GFRs), and patients are susceptible to renal failure perioperatively. If urine output falls, hypovolaemia should be excluded, and adequate perfusion pressure and cardiac output ensured before diuretics are used. Non-steroidal anti-inflammatory drugs (NSAIDs) are a potent renal insult in these patients, and their use requires care.
- All patients should have supplemental O_2 following surgery.
- Good post-operative analgesia is essential to minimize detrimental effects of catecholamine release in response to pain.
- Have a low threshold for admission to ICU/HDU in the post-operative period.

Further reading

Magner JJ, Royston D (2004). Heart failure. *Br J Anaesth*, **91**, 74–85.

National Institute for Health and Care Excellence (2010). *Chronic heart failure: national clinical guideline for diagnosis and management in primary and secondary care.* ℬ http://guidance.nice.org.uk/CG108/Guidance/pdf/English.

Hypertension

Fifteen per cent of patients are hypertensive (systolic >140mmHg, diastolic >90mmHg). The link between elevated arterial pressure and CVS disease is well established, with the greatest risk associated with the highest arterial pressures.

Traditionally, many patients have had anaesthesia and surgery deferred to allow hypertension to be treated. Evidence that moderately elevated BP is associated with increased perioperative risk is limited, although increased CVS lability under anaesthesia ('alpine anaesthesia') frequently occurs. However, the association of hypertension with end-organ damage (IHD, heart failure, renal failure) contributes significantly to the likelihood of perioperative CVS complications.

Preoperative evaluation

- Is hypertension 1° or 2°? Consider the rare possibility of phaeochromocytoma, hyperaldosteronism, renal parenchymal hypertension, and renovascular hypertension. These will have individual anaesthetic implications.
- Is the hypertension severe? Patients with stage 3 hypertension (systolic >180mmHg, diastolic >110mmHg) should ideally have this treated prior to elective surgery.
- Is there evidence of end-organ involvement? The presence of coronary or cerebrovascular disease, impairment of renal function, signs of LV hypertrophy, and heart failure puts patients in a high-risk category. These conditions may require further investigation and/or treatment, in addition to the control of elevated blood BP.

Perioperative management

Few guidelines exist as to which patients should be cancelled to allow hypertension to be treated or the duration of such treatment prior to surgery. There is little evidence for an association between admission arterial pressures of <180mmHg systolic or <110mmHg diastolic and perioperative CVS complications. A recent meta-analysis of 30 papers involving 12 995 perioperative patients demonstrated an odds ratio (OR) for the association between hypertensive disease and CVS complications of 1.35, which is not clinically significant.[6]

- Do not defer surgery on the basis of a single BP reading on admission to hospital. Obtain several further readings after admission. The general practitioner (GP) may have a record of previous readings.
- Continue preoperative antihypertensive treatment during the perioperative period.
- Stage 1 (systolic 140–159mmHg, diastolic 90–99mmHg) and stage 2 (systolic 160–179mmHg, diastolic 100–109mmHg) hypertension are not independent risk factors for perioperative CVS complications. Surgery should normally proceed in these patients.
- If a patient has stage 3 hypertension (systolic >180mmHg, diastolic >110mmHg), with evidence of damage to the heart or kidneys, defer surgery to allow the BP to be controlled and the aetiology investigated. There is no level 1 evidence as to how long the operation should be

delayed; 4–6wk is usually recommended to allow the autoregulation of cerebral blood flow to return to normal.

- Patients with stage 3 hypertension considered fit for surgery in other respects and with no evidence of end-organ involvement should not be deferred simply on the grounds of elevated BP. Attempt to ensure CVS stability, using invasive monitoring where indicated, and actively control excursions in mean arterial pressure (MAP) >20% from the baseline.
- Patients undergoing major surgery or who are unstable perioperatively should be monitored closely in ICU/HDU.
- Sympatholytic therapies, such as α_2-agonists (clonidine), and thoracic epidural blockade may have a role but also carry risks of hypotension post-operatively.
- Relate perioperative BP readings to the underlying norm—a systolic <100mmHg may represent hypotension in a normally hypertensive patient.[6]

Reference

6 Howell SJ, Sear JW, Foex P (2004). Hypertension, hypertensive heart disease and perioperative cardiac risk. *Br J Anaesth*, **92**, 570–83.

Valvular heart disease

Valvular heart disease is found in 4% of patients over the age of 65yr. Patients with a known valve problem may already be under the care of a cardiologist. Sometimes a murmur may be picked up during preoperative assessment. In each case:

• Assess the significance of the cardiac lesion for the proposed surgery
• Plan anaesthesia according to the haemodynamic picture.

Two-dimensional echocardiography indicates abnormal valvular motion and morphology but does not indicate the severity of stenosis or regurgitation, except in mitral stenosis. Doppler echocardiography identifies an increased velocity of flow across stenotic valves, from which pressure gradients and the severity may be estimated. Doppler flow imaging can also provide estimates of the severity of regurgitant valve disease.

Prosthetic valves

- Most patients will be under the surveillance of a cardiologist.
- Tissue valves do not require anticoagulation. Mechanical valve replacements require lifetime anticoagulation.
- The risk of thromboembolism, if anticoagulation is stopped, depends on the site and type of valve replacement.
- Modern bileaflet aortic valve replacements have a low (<4% per annum) risk of thromboembolism and are best managed by withholding warfarin for 5d preoperatively and administering a prophylactic dose of LMWH.
- Older aortic valve replacements and mechanical mitral valve replacements have a much greater propensity to embolize (>4% per annum). They are best managed by stopping warfarin 5d preoperatively. Bridging therapy with either an IV infusion of unfractionated heparin or therapeutic SC LMWH is recommended when the INR <2. Unfractionated heparin infusions should be stopped 6hr prior to surgery, and therapeutic LMWH stopped the night before surgery.
- IV heparin/therapeutic LMWH can be restarted post-operatively, and warfarin reinstituted when it is safe to do so.

Aortic stenosis

(See also ➋ p. 335.)

- Occasionally congenital (bicuspid valve 2%), mostly due to calcification and rheumatic heart disease. Prevalence increases with age. Anatomical obstruction (Table 3.2) leads to concentric hypertrophy of the LV heart muscle, resulting in decreased diastolic compliance.
- Elevated filling pressures and sinus rhythm are required to fill the non-compliant LV. 'Normal' LV end-diastolic pressure (LVEDP) may reflect hypovolaemia.
- Properly timed atrial contractions contribute as much as 40% to the LV preload in aortic stenosis (AS) patients (normally 20–30%). Arrhythmia may produce a critical reduction in cardiac output.
- High risk of myocardial ischaemia due to increased O_2 demand and wall tension in the hypertrophied LV. Thirty per cent of patients with AS and *normal* coronary arteries have angina. Subendocardial ischaemia may exist, as coronary blood supply does not increase in proportion to the muscular hypertrophy. Tachycardia is detrimental, as it may produce ischaemia. Maintenance of diastolic BP is crucial to maintain coronary perfusion.

Table 3.2 Valve area in aortic stenosis

Normal area	$2.6–3.5cm^2$
Mild	$1.6–2.5cm^2$
Moderate	$1.0–1.5cm^2$
Severe	$<1.0cm^2$

History

- Angina, breathlessness, syncope. The majority of patients with *symptomatic* AS will be dead within 3yr, if not treated. In contrast, age-corrected 10yr survival for patients after successful aortic valve replacement surgery approaches those of the normal population. In the absence of significant co-morbidity, aortic valve replacement is indicated in most, irrespective of age.
- Symptoms do not correlate well with the severity of stenosis; some patients with small valve areas can be asymptomatic.

Examination

- Slow rising pulse with narrow pulse pressure.
- Ejection systolic murmur, maximal at the 2nd intercostal space, right sternal edge, radiating to the neck.

Investigations

- ECG: LV hypertrophy and strain (with 2° ST–T wave abnormalities).
- CXR: normal until the LV begins to fail, post-stenotic dilatation of the aorta, calcified aortic annulus.

- Echocardiogram: enables calculation of the valve gradient (Table 3.3) and assessment of LV performance.
- Cardiac catheterization is also used to estimate the gradient across the valve and to quantify any concurrent CAD.

Table 3.3 LV–aortic gradient

Mild	<20mmHg
Moderate	20–50mmHg
Severe	>50mmHg

Perioperative care

- Symptomatic patients for elective non-cardiac surgery should have aortic valve replacement first, as they are at great risk of sudden death perioperatively.
- Asymptomatic patients for major elective surgery associated with marked fluid shifts (thoracic, abdominal, major orthopaedic) with gradients across the valve >50mmHg should have valve replacement considered prior to surgery.
- Asymptomatic patients for intermediate or minor surgery generally do well if managed carefully.

Haemodynamic goals

- (Low) normal HR.
- Maintain sinus rhythm.
- Adequate volume loading.
- High normal systemic vascular resistance (SVR).

Patients with severe AS have a fixed cardiac output. They cannot compensate for a reduction in the SVR which results in severe hypotension, myocardial ischaemia, and a downward spiral of reduced contractility, causing further falls in BP and coronary perfusion.

The selected technique should maintain afterload and avoid tachycardia, to maintain the balance between myocardial O_2 demand and supply. Titrate drugs carefully. Treat hypotension using direct-acting α-agonists, such as metaraminol and phenylephrine, as these improve systolic and diastolic LV function. Careful fluid balance is essential, guided by invasive monitoring, if required (CVP, oesophageal Doppler, TOE). Direct measurement of arterial BP should be routine, except for very short procedures.

Arrhythmias must be treated promptly, or haemodynamic collapse may ensue. Effective analgesia avoids catecholamine-induced tachycardia and hypertension and the risk of cardiac ischaemia. However, central neuraxial blocks must be used with extreme caution because of the danger of hypotension due to afterload reduction. Limb blocks can be used alone or in conjunction with GA.

Post-operative management

- Have a low threshold for admission to ICU/HDU.
- Meticulous attention must be paid to fluid and pain management.
- Infusions of vasoconstrictors may be required.

Aortic regurgitation

(See also ➋ p. 338.)

- 1° aortic regurgitation (AR) may result from rheumatic heart disease or endocarditis.
- Aortic dissection and connective tissue disorders that dilate the aortic root (tertiary syphilis; Marfan's syndrome, ➋ p. 304; ankylosing spondylitis, ➋ p. 187) result in 2° aortic incompetence.
- Valvular regurgitation usually develops over many years, allowing the heart to adapt to increased volume.
- AR 2° to endocarditis or aortic dissection presents with acute left heart failure and pulmonary oedema. Such patients require emergency valve surgery.

In patients who have chronic AR:
- Afterload and HR determine the degree of regurgitation. Lower aortic pressure decreases LV afterload, augmenting the forward flow
- Vasodilators increase the forward flow by lowering the afterload, decrease the LV size, and enhance the EF
- HRs >90bpm reduce the diastolic 'regurgitation' time and degree of regurgitation
- Aortic diastolic pressure is dependent on the aortic valve and decreases when the valve becomes incompetent.

History
- Dyspnoea, 2° to pulmonary congestion.
- Palpitations.

Examination
- Widened pulse pressure.
- Collapsing ('waterhammer') pulse; Corrigan's sign—visible neck pulsation; de Musset's sign—head nodding; Quincke's sign—visible capillary pulsations in the nail beds.
- Diastolic murmur—2nd intercostal space, right sternal edge.

Investigations
- CXR: cardiomegaly, boot-shaped heart.
- ECG: non-specific LV hypertrophy.
- Echocardiography gives qualitative analysis of the degree of regurgitation.

Perioperative care
Asymptomatic patients usually tolerate non-cardiac surgery well. Patients with poor functional capacity need to be considered for valve replacement surgery.

Haemodynamic goals
- High normal HR—around 90bpm.
- Adequate volume loading.
- Low SVR.
- Maintain contractility.

The selected anaesthetic should maintain afterload in the low normal range to maintain diastolic pressure. Spinal and epidural anaesthesia are well tolerated. Treat perioperative supraventricular tachycardia (SVT)/AF promptly with synchronized direct current (DC) cardioversion (see p. 74 and p. 893), particularly if associated with hypotension. Persistent bradycardia may need to be treated with β-agonist or anticholinergic agents. Intra-arterial pressure monitoring is useful for major surgery. Oesophageal Doppler and other methods of non-invasive cardiac output monitoring are inaccurate.

Mitral stenosis

(See also ➔ p. 340.)

- Rheumatic fever is the commonest cause. A minority have isolated stenosis; the majority have mixed mitral valve disease (stenosis and regurgitation). Mitral valve stenosis underfills the LV and increases both the pressure and volume upstream of the valve (Table 3.4).
- The LV functions normally but is small and poorly filled.
- Initially, the left atrium dilates, keeping the pulmonary artery pressure (PAP) low. As disease progresses, the PAP increases, and medial hypertrophy develops, resulting in chronic reactive pulmonary hypertension. The right heart hypertrophies to pump against a pressure overload, then fails. 2° pulmonary/tricuspid regurgitation develops.
- The pressure gradient across the narrow mitral orifice increases with the square of the cardiac output (note in pregnancy). Rapid HRs, especially with AF, decrease the diastolic filling time and markedly decrease the cardiac output.
- LV filling is optimized by a slow HR.

Table 3.4 Valve area in mitral stenosis

Normal valve surface area	4–6cm²
Symptom-free until	1.6–2.5cm²
Moderate stenosis	1–1.5cm²
Severe stenosis	<1.0cm²

Patients are frequently dyspnoeic due to fluid transudate in the lungs, which reduces lung compliance and increases the work of breathing. Pulmonary oedema may occur if the pulmonary venous pressure exceeds the plasma oncotic pressure. This is especially likely if a large fluid bolus, head-down position, or a uterine contraction raises the pulmonary pressure suddenly.

History

- Dyspnoea, haemoptysis, recurrent bronchitis.
- Fatigue.
- Palpitations.

Examination

- Mitral facies—malar flush on cheeks.
- Peripheral cyanosis.
- Signs of right heart failure (elevated jugular venous pressure (JVP), hepatomegaly, peripheral oedema, ascites).
- Tapping apex beat. Loud 1st heart sound, opening snap (if in sinus rhythm), and low-pitched diastolic murmur heard best at the apex (with the bell of the stethoscope).

Investigations

- ECG: P mitrale (left atrial enlargement) if sinus rhythm. AF usual.
- CXR: valve calcification. Large left atrium (lateral film). Double shadow behind the heart on PA film. Splaying of the carina. Kerley B lines indicating pulmonary congestion.
- Echocardiography: measures the gradient and valve area (Table 3.4).

Perioperative care

Asymptomatic patients usually tolerate non-cardiac surgery well. Patients with poor functional capacity need to be considered for mitral valve replacement.

Haemodynamic goals

- Low normal HR 50–70bpm. Treat tachycardia aggressively with β-blockers.
- Maintain sinus rhythm, if possible. Immediate cardioversion if AF occurs perioperatively.
- Adequate preload.
- High normal SVR.
- Avoid hypercapnia, acidosis, and hypoxia, which may exacerbate pulmonary hypertension.

Anaesthesia—similar to AS, as there is a relatively fixed cardiac output. Maintain an adequate afterload; slow the HR, and avoid hypovolaemia. Measure CVP/pulmonary artery occlusion pressure (PAOP), and maintain an adequate preload. Spinal and epidural anaesthesia may be very hazardous.

Mitral regurgitation

(See also ➋ p. 342.)

- Mitral regurgitation (MR) results from leaflet, chordal, or papillary muscle abnormalities or is 2° to LV dysfunction.
- Leaflet MR is a complication of endocarditis, rheumatic fever, and mitral valve prolapse.
- Chordal MR follows chordae rupture after acute MI or after bacterial endocarditis.
- Papillary muscle MR results from ischaemic posterior papillary muscle dysfunction.
- LV failure leads to varying amounts of MR when the mitral annulus dilates.
- As much as 50% of the LV volume flows into a massively dilated left atrium through the incompetent mitral valve before the aortic valve opens. The LVEF is therefore supranormal.
- Pulmonary vascular congestion develops, followed by pulmonary hypertension.
- The degree of regurgitation is determined by the afterload, size of the regurgitant orifice, and HR. A moderately increased HR (>90bpm) decreases the time for regurgitation in systole and decreases the time for diastolic filling, reducing the LV overload.

History

- Fatigue, weakness.
- Dyspnoea.

Examination

- Displaced and forceful apex (the more severe the regurgitation, the larger the ventricle).
- Soft S_1, apical pansystolic murmur radiating to the axilla, loud S_3.
- AF.

Investigations

- ECG: left atrial enlargement. AF.
- CXR: left atrial and LV enlargement. Mitral annular calcification.
- Echocardiography assesses the degree of regurgitation (TOE particularly useful as mitral valve close to the oesophagus).

Perioperative care

Asymptomatic patients usually tolerate non-cardiac surgery well. Patients with poor functional capacity need to be considered for valve replacement surgery.

Haemodynamic goals

- High normal HR.
- Adequate preload.
- Low SVR.
- Low pulmonary vascular resistance (PVR).

Anaesthesia—aims are similar to AR. Preload can be difficult to estimate; for major non-cardiac surgery, a pulmonary artery catheter may be useful. In advanced disease, pulmonary hypertension is common—avoid factors that increase the PAP (hypoxia, hypercapnia, high inspiratory pressures, acidosis).

Mitral valve prolapse
- Common (incidental finding in 5% of population).
- Usually asymptomatic, but may be associated with atypical chest pain, palpitations, syncope, and emboli.
- Mid-systolic click and late diastolic murmur.
- Echocardiography shows enlarged redundant mitral valve leaflets prolapsing into the left atrium during mid- to late-systole, causing arrhythmias and regurgitation.
- Antiarrhythmics must be continued perioperatively.

Mixed valve lesions
- With mixed regurgitant/stenotic lesions, manage the dominant lesion.

Further reading
Douketis JD, Spyropoulos AC, Spencer FA, et al. (2012). Perioperative management of antithrombotic therapy. Chest, 141, e326S–50S.

The patient with an undiagnosed murmur

Most heart murmurs do not signify cardiac disease. Many are related to physiological increases in blood flow. Assess the functional capacity (Duke Activity Status Index; see ➔ p. 37) and the presence or absence of symptoms. Many asymptomatic children and young adults with a murmur can safely undergo anaesthesia and surgery if they have a good functional capacity and are asymptomatic.

Elderly asymptomatic patients may have an 'aortic' systolic murmur related to sclerotic aortic valve leaflets. Aortic sclerosis is now considered to be an early form of AS (~15% of patients with aortic sclerosis will develop aortic valve stenosis within 7yr) but should not cause clinical problems until progression to stenosis occurs. Factors that differentiate early asymptomatic sclerosis from stenosis include:

- Good exercise tolerance (>4 METs)
- No history of angina/breathlessness/syncope
- Absence of slow rising pulse (normal pulse pressure)
- Absence of LV hypertrophy/LV strain pattern on ECG.

The volume of the murmur does not help.

Take a full history, and examine the ECG/CXR. Patients able to manage 4 METs (able to climb a flight of stairs, walk at 6km/hr on the flat; see ➔ p. 37), with a normal ECG and CXR, will tolerate minor and intermediate surgery but should have an echocardiogram prior to major surgery. Conversely, poor functional capacity in association with an abnormal ECG (such as ventricular hypertrophy or a prior infarction) should be investigated by echocardiography.

Pericardial disease

Acute pericarditis

- Usually a viral condition presenting with chest pain. The diagnosis is supported by widespread ST elevation on ECG.
- Frequently occurs with myocarditis which may increase the likelihood of arrhythmia and sudden death.
- Elective surgery should be postponed for at least 6wk.

Constrictive pericarditis

- This may be post-infective or 2° to an autoimmune disease such as systemic lupus erythematosus (SLE) (see ➋ p. 190). The only effective treatment is pericardectomy which may be dramatically effective.
- Pulsus paradoxus may be evident—a fall in systolic BP with inspiration. The normal maximum fall is 10mmHg.
- Systolic function of the myocardium is well maintained, but diastolic function is severely impaired. When exercise tolerance is reduced, GA carries a significant risk.
- Bradycardia and reduced cardiac filling are poorly tolerated.
- Elevations in intrathoracic pressure, as occur during intermittent positive pressure ventilation (IPPV), can result in profound hypotension.
- If anaesthesia is unavoidable, and regional block is not possible, then a spontaneously breathing technique is preferable to IPPV. Preload should be maintained, and tachycardia avoided.

Cardiomyopathy

Most patients have heart failure and have little reserve for surgery and anaesthesia.

Hypertrophic obstructive cardiomyopathy

- Causes dynamic obstruction of the LV outflow during systole.
- Main feature is asymmetric hypertrophy of the interventricular septum, which obstructs the LV outflow tract when it contracts.
- Ventricular systole is associated with movement of the anterior mitral valve leaflet towards the septum ('systolic anterior motion'—SAM), and the outflow tract is further obstructed. In some patients, this causes MR.
- As with AS, hypertrophic obstructive cardiomyopathy (HOCM) results in a pressure overload of the LV. Diastolic dysfunction is evident on echocardiography.
- Sinus rhythm is crucial to maintain ventricular filling.

The aetiology is unknown but is possibly inherited as an autosomal dominant condition in >50% of cases. Patients present with symptoms similar to AS—angina, dyspnoea, syncope, and palpitations. Sudden death is common. The ECG is abnormal, showing evidence of LV hypertrophy.

Echocardiography is essential to estimate the degree of functional obstruction, asymmetric LV hypertrophy, and SAM of the mitral valve.

Inotropes are contraindicated, as LV obstruction is exacerbated by increased myocardial contractility. Treatment is with β-blockers or verapamil, as they are negatively inotropic. Patients are prone to arrhythmias which are refractory to medical treatment and may require dual-chamber pacing or the insertion of an AICD.

Haemodynamic goals

Maintain a 'large ventricle', since dynamic obstruction is reduced.
- Low normal HR.
- Maintain sinus rhythm.
- Adequate volume loading.
- High normal SVR.
- Low ventricular contractility.

Invasive haemodynamic monitoring is indicated. Measurement of the CVP or use of oesophageal Doppler helps to guide volume resuscitation. Direct-acting α-agonists, such as metaraminol, may be used in an emergency.

Restrictive cardiomyopathy

Rare condition. The commonest cause is myocardial infiltration by amyloid. Characterized by stiff ventricles that impair ventricular filling. Right heart failure often prominent. Echocardiography shows diastolic dysfunction.
- Anaesthesia is hazardous.
- Peripheral vasodilatation, myocardial depression, and reduced venous return may cause catastrophic cardiovascular decompensation and may precipitate cardiac arrest.
- Venous return may be further compromised by positive pressure ventilation. Wherever possible, maintain spontaneous respiration.

- Ketamine may be useful, as it increases myocardial contractility and peripheral resistance.
- Fluids should be given to maintain elevated right heart pressures.

Haemodynamic goals
- Maintain sinus rhythm.
- Adequate volume loading.
- High normal SVR.
- Avoid myocardial depression.

Dilated cardiomyopathy

- Manifests as cardiac failure with an enlarged poorly contractile heart. Stroke volume is initially preserved by dilatation and increased LV end-diastolic volume. Functional mitral and tricuspid incompetence occurs commonly due to dilatation of the valve annulus, exacerbating heart failure.
- The commonest problems are heart failure, arrhythmias, and embolic phenomena.
- Heart failure is treated with diuretics, ACE inhibitors, and vasodilators. Amiodarone is the drug of choice for arrhythmias, as it has the least myocardial depressant effect. Patients are frequently anticoagulated. Synchronized dual-chamber pacing may be used. Some patients may have a biventricular pacing/defibrillator (AICD) in place (see ➔ p. 81).
- Invasive CVS monitoring is required during anaesthesia (arterial and pulmonary arterial catheters and non-invasive methods of cardiac output estimation, e.g. oesophageal Doppler, PiCCO®, LiDCO®).

Haemodynamic goals
- Maintain sinus rhythm.
- Adequate volume loading.
- Normal SVR.
- Avoid myocardial depression; inotropic support is frequently required with dobutamine or phosphodiesterase (PDE) inhibitors.

Further reading

Bovill JG (2003). Anaesthesia for patients with impaired ventricular function. *Sem Cardiothorac Vasc Anesth*, **7**, 49–54.

The patient with a transplanted heart

(See also Anaesthesia after lung transplantation, ➲ p. 116.)

Heart transplantation is increasing in frequency, and patients may present to a non-specialist centre for non-cardiac surgery. Anaesthesia requires attention to:

• Altered physiology
• Effects of immunosuppression
• Medications
• Associated risk factors.

Altered physiology

• The heart is denervated; resting HRs are usually around 85–95bpm. Some patients may have experienced temporary bradyarrhythmias after transplantation. A pacemaker may be *in situ*.
• Normal autonomic system responses are lost (beat-to-beat variation in HR, response to Valsalva manoeuvre/carotid sinus massage).
• Contractility of the heart is close to normal, unless rejection is developing. In the absence of sympathetic innervation, the age-predicted maximal HR is reduced.
• Despite some evidence that reinnervation can occur some years after transplantation, the heart should be viewed as permanently denervated. This results in poor tolerance of acute hypovolaemia.
• If pharmacological manipulation is required, then direct-acting agents should be used; atropine has no effect on the denervated heart; the effect of ephedrine is reduced and unpredictable, and hydralazine and phenylephrine produce no reflex tachy- or bradycardia in response to their 1° action. Adrenaline, noradrenaline, isoprenaline, and β- and α-blockers act as expected.

Immunosuppression

Three classes of drugs are used:

• Immunophilin-binding drugs (ciclosporin, tacrolimus) prevent cytokine-mediated T-cell activation and proliferation
• Nucleic acid synthesis inhibitors (azathioprine) block lymphocyte proliferation
• Steroids block the production of inflammatory cytokines, lyse T-lymphocytes, and alter the function of the remaining lymphocytes.

Anaemia and thrombocytopenia, as well as leucopenia, may result, requiring treatment before surgery. Ciclosporin is associated with renal dysfunction and is the most likely cause of hypertension that affects 40% of heart–lung transplant recipients. It may also prolong the action of non-depolarizing muscle relaxants (NDMRs). Calcium antagonists increase ciclosporin levels variably and are used in some centres to reduce the ciclosporin dose in an attempt to reduce side effects. The effect on blood concentrations must be remembered if calcium antagonists are omitted for any reason perioperatively. Renal dysfunction is also commonly caused by tacrolimus. Steroid supplementation may be required if large doses of prednisolone are being used.

Strict asepsis must be used with all invasive procedures.

Associated risk factors

- Previous, and often repeated, use of central and peripheral vessels can make IV and arterial access difficult.
- Cough may be impaired due to a combination of phrenic and recurrent laryngeal nerve palsies. This increases the risks of sputum retention and post-operative chest infection.
- Heart–lung recipients will have a tracheal anastomosis. It is desirable to avoid unnecessary intubation, but, if it is necessary, use a short tube, and carefully monitor the tracheal cuff pressure. Disrupted lung lymphatic drainage increases the risk of pulmonary oedema.
- The transplanted heart develops CAD.

Choice of technique

There is no evidence to support one anaesthetic technique above another.
- Peripheral surgery under regional block is likely to be well tolerated
- Subarachnoid/epidural block may result in marked falls in BP because of absent cardiac innervation.

Further reading

Toivonen HJ (2000). Anaesthesia for patients with a transplanted organ. *Acta Anaesthesiol Scand*, **44**, 812–33.

Congenital heart disease and non-cardiac surgery

Congenital heart disease (CHD) is common—8:1000 births, with 85% of affected children reaching adult life. Although most of these children will have undergone corrective surgery, many will have residual problems. Studies have reported a high incidence of adverse perioperative events in CHD patients undergoing non-cardiac surgical procedures.

General considerations

Operative procedures for CHD aim to improve the patient's haemodynamic status, although complete cure is not always achieved. Paediatric cardiac surgical procedures can be divided as follows:

- Curative procedures: the patient is completely cured, and life expectancy is normal (e.g. persistent ductus arteriosus (PDA) and atrial septal defect (ASD) closure)
- Corrective procedures: the patient's haemodynamic status is markedly improved, but life expectancy may not be normal (e.g. tetralogy of Fallot repair (ToF); see also ➲ p. 67)
- Palliative procedures: these patients may have abnormal circulations and physiology but avoid the consequences of untreated CHD. Life expectancy is not normal, but many survive to adulthood (e.g. Fontan procedures; see also ➲ p. 67).

Preoperative assessment

Aim to gain an understanding of the anatomy and pathophysiology of the patient's cardiac defect.

- History: define the nature and severity of the lesion. Ask about congestive cardiac failure (CCF)—especially the limitation of daily activities. Consider other associated abnormalities. Check current medication.
- Examination: check for cyanosis, peripheral oedema, hepatosplenomegaly, murmurs, and signs of infection/failure. Check peripheral pulses. Neurological examination for cyanotic patients.
- Investigations: CXR/ECG. Record baseline SpO_2 on air. Laboratory tests depend on the proposed surgery, but most will require FBC, clotting screen, LFTs, and electrolytes. Some patients will need pulmonary function tests (PFTs).
- Consult the patient's cardiologist—a recent echocardiography report and catheter data should be available. Potential risk factors should be considered, along with potential treatment regimes, e.g. inotropes and vasodilators.
- Consider whether the proposed surgery is necessary, with regard to the potential risks, whether admission to ICU/HDU will be required, and whether the patient can or should be moved to a cardiac centre.

Factors indicative of high risk

- Recent worsening of CCF or symptoms of myocardial ischaemia.
- Severe hypoxaemia with SpO_2 <75% on air.
- Polycythaemia (haematocrit, Hct >60%).

- Unexplained dizziness/syncope/fever or recent cerebrovascular accident (CVA).
- Severe AS/pulmonary valve stenosis.
- Uncorrected ToF or Eisenmenger's syndrome.
- Patients with hypoplastic left heart syndrome (HLHS).
- Recent onset of arrhythmias.

Specific problems

- Myocardial dysfunction/arrhythmias: may be due to underlying disease (e.g. hypoplastic LV) or 2° (e.g. due to surgery or medication).
- Air emboli: all CHD patients are at risk from air embolism. Intravascular lines should be free of air.
- Cyanosis has many causes, e.g. shunting of blood from the right to left side of the heart (ToF, Eisenmenger's syndrome) and intracardiac mixing (complete atrioventricular septal defect, AVSD). Cyanosis results in polycythaemia and increased blood volume. Blood viscosity is increased, impairing tissue perfusion. There is often thrombocytopenia and fibrinogen deficiency, leading to a bleeding tendency. An increase in tissue vascularity worsens bleeding problems. Cyanosis can also lead to renal/cerebral thrombosis and renal tubular atrophy.
- Anticoagulant treatment (aspirin or warfarin) is common in CHD patients.
- Antibiotic prophylaxis (see ➲ p. 1211).
- Myocardial ischaemia developing in a patient with CHD is significant and should be investigated.

Specific congenital heart disease lesions

There are over 100 forms of CHD, but eight lesions account for 83% of all congenital cardiac defects. These are ASD, ventricular septal defect (VSD), PDA, pulmonary stenosis (PS), ToF, AS, coarctation of the aorta, and transposition of the great vessels (ToGV). Many of the other cardiac lesions are managed palliatively by producing a Fontan circulation.

Atrial septal defect (secundum type)

- Patients are often asymptomatic.
- Usually results in a left-to-right shunt.
- Can be closed surgically or transcatheter.
- Danger of paradoxical emboli.

Atrial septal defect (primum type)

- Endocardial cushion defect—may involve atrioventricular (AV) valves.
- The more severe form AVSD is associated with Down's syndrome and results in severe pulmonary hypertension (see ⊃ p. 288).
- Surgical repair of these lesions may result in complete heart block.

Ventricular septal defect

- Commonest form of CHD.
- Clinical effects depend on the size and number of VSDs.
- A small single VSD may be asymptomatic with a small left-to-right shunt (pulmonary:systemic flow ratio <1.5:1). In patients who have not had corrective surgery, prevent air emboli and fluid overload.
- Patients with a moderate-sized single VSD often present with mild CCF. They have increased pulmonary blood flow (pulmonary:systemic flow ratio 3:1). If the lesion is not treated, they are at risk of pulmonary hypertension and shunt reversal.
- Patients with a large VSD have equal pressures in their right and left ventricles and present at around 2 months of age with severe CCF. They require early operations. However, if they need anaesthesia for another procedure prior to definitive cardiac surgery, they present severe problems. They should be intubated for all but the most minor procedures, and increases in the left-to-right shunt should be avoided (e.g. avoid hyperventilation and high FiO_2). Care should be taken with fluid administration, and inotropic support is often required.
- Patients with multiple VSDs often require pulmonary artery banding to protect the pulmonary circulation. This band tightens, as the child grows, leading to cyanosis. VSDs often close spontaneously, and then the band may be removed.
- May be closed transcatheter in certain circumstances

Persistent ductus arteriosus

- Patients with PDA may have a moderate left-to-right shunt, and this can result in an elevated PVR, rather like a moderately sized VSD.
- Can be closed surgically or transcatheter.

Tetralogy of Fallot

- PS, VSD, overriding aorta, and right ventricular (RV) hypertrophy.
- Prior to complete repair, ToF may be treated medically with β-blockade or surgically via a Blalock–Taussig (BT) shunt (subclavian to pulmonary artery (PA)).
- In patients without a BT shunt, and prior to definitive surgery, the ratio of SVR:PVR determines both the systemic blood flow and blood O_2 saturation. If they require anaesthesia at this stage, they should be intubated and ventilated in order to maintain a low PVR. Cyanosis should be treated with hyperventilation, IV fluid, and systemic vasopressors such as phenylephrine.
- Total repair of ToF is undertaken in some centres at around 2–6 months of age, although many centres are now performing 1° neonatal repairs.

Eisenmenger's syndrome

- Associated with markedly increased morbidity and mortality.
- Abnormal and irreversible elevation in the PVR, resulting in cyanosis and right-to-left shunting. The degree of shunting depends on the PVR:SVR ratio. Increasing the SVR or decreasing the PVR leads to better arterial SpO_2, as in patients with ToF.
- Avoid reductions in the SVR (epidural/spinal anaesthesia) and rises in the PVR (hypoxia/hypercapnia/acidosis/cold).
- Desaturation episodes can be treated as for ToF (see section above).
- Inotropic support may be required for the shortest of procedures, and an ICU bed should be available.
- Manage patient in a specialist centre, whenever possible.

Fontan procedure

- Palliative procedure, classically for patients with tricuspid atresia, but can be performed for many different cardiac lesions, including HLHS. The Fontan procedure is not a specific operation, but a class of operations that separate the pulmonary and systemic circulations in patients with an anatomical or physiological single ventricle. This separation is accomplished by ensuring that all superior and inferior vena caval blood flows directly into the PA, bypassing the right ventricle and usually the right atrium. Thus, the pulmonary blood flow is dependent solely on the systemic venous pressure. SpO_2 should be normal.
- Leads to elevated systemic venous pressures, liver congestion, protein-losing enteropathy, tendency for fluid overload, ascites, and pleural and pericardial effusions. Hypovolaemia can lead to hypoxia and CVS collapse. Patients are anticoagulated with warfarin.
- In these patients, IPPV results in a fall in cardiac output, and high ventilatory pressures result in poor pulmonary perfusion. Fluid overload is poorly tolerated, as is hypovolaemia.
- CVP monitoring is helpful and is best instituted via the femoral venous route.
- The extracardiac Fontan procedure allows children to survive into the 2nd decade of life, with a 96% survival rate at 14yr post-procedure.

Hypoplastic left heart syndrome

- HLHS accounts for around 2% of congenital cardiac defects and carries a high mortality, with only 65% of patients surviving to 5yr.
- Patients with HLHS undergo a 3-stage repair, which involves an initial neonatal Norwood operation or hybrid procedure, followed later by a Glenn shunt, and finally a Fontan procedure.
- These children are particularly vulnerable and should be managed in a specialist centre, whenever possible.

Adults with congenital heart disease

Anything but the most straightforward situation should be discussed, and the patient referred to a cardiac centre.

Uncorrected disease

- VSD/ASDs may be small and have no symptoms and little haemodynamic effect. With the exception of the potential for paradoxical emboli, small defects present no anaesthetic problems.
- Lesions resulting in large left-to-right shunts will cause progressive pulmonary hypertension and eventual shunt reversal (Eisenmenger's syndrome). Once irreversible pulmonary hypertension has developed, surgical correction is not possible. These patients are high-risk. If surgery is absolutely necessary, it should be performed in a specialist centre.

Corrected disease

- These patients have either had spontaneous resolution or a corrective procedure. They can generally be treated as normal.
- Best assessment of CVS function is generally the exercise tolerance.
- Exclude surgical sequelae/continuing disease.
- Exclude any associated congenital abnormalities.

Palliated disease

- These patients have had operations that improve the functional capacity and life expectancy but do not restore normal anatomy. Operations include Senning and Mustard for ToGV (neonatal switch is now preferred) and Fontan for single-ventricle syndromes (e.g. HLHS and pulmonary atresia).
- An understanding of the underlying physiology is required to avoid disaster when anaesthetizing these patients. At present, management is best provided in specialist cardiac centres.
- In patients with a Fontan circulation, blood leaves a single ventricle, passes through the systemic circulation, and then through the pulmonary circulation, before returning to the heart. The consequences of this are that the CVP is high, providing a pressure gradient across the pulmonary circulation. Any pulmonary hypertension is poorly tolerated and results in reduced ventricular filling. The high venous pressure can result in life-threatening haemorrhage from mucosal procedures such as adenoidectomy (or nasal intubation!).

Further reading

Andropoulos DB, Stayer SA, Russel IA, eds. (2005). *Anesthesia for congenital heart disease*. Malden, MA: Blackwell Futura.

Nichols DG, Cameron DE, Greeley WJ, et al., eds. (1995). *Critical heart disease in infants and children*. St Louis: Mosby.

Thorne S, Clift P (2009). *Adult congenital heart disease*. Oxford: Oxford University Press.

Perioperative arrhythmias

John Dean

See also:

Perioperative arrhythmias

(See also ➔ p. 885.)

Perioperative cardiac arrhythmias are common and may be life-threatening. Whenever possible, they should be controlled preoperatively, as surgery and anaesthesia can cause marked deterioration. Management is easier if the underlying problem has been recognized, investigated, and treated preoperatively. Never give an IV drug for any rhythm disturbance, unless you are in a position to cardiovert immediately.

Practical diagnosis of arrhythmias

Ideally undertaken with a paper printout of the ECG and preferably in a 12-lead format. In theatre, this is often impractical—use the different leads available on the monitor to improve interpretation.

Determine

- What is the ventricular rate?
- Is the QRS complex of normal duration or widened?
- Is the QRS regular or irregular?
- Are P waves present, and are they normally shaped?
- How is atrial activity related to ventricular activity?

Ventricular rate

- Calculate the approximate ventricular rate (divide 300 by the number of large squares between each QRS complex).
- Tachyarrhythmia: rate >100bpm; bradyarrhythmia: rate <60bpm.

QRS complex

- Supraventricular rhythms include nodal rhythms and arise from a focus above the ventricles. Since the ventricles still depolarize via the normal His/Purkinje system, the QRS complexes are of normal width (<0.12s or three small squares) and are termed 'narrow complex rhythms'.
- Arrhythmias arising from the ventricles will be 'broad complex' with a QRS width of >0.12s. In the presence of AV or bundle branch block, a supraventricular rhythm may have broad complexes (2%). This may be present on the 12-lead ECG or develop as a consequence of the arrhythmia—rate-related aberrant conduction.

Regularity

- Irregular rhythm suggests ectopic beats (atrial or ventricular), AF, atrial flutter with variable block, or 2nd-degree heart block with variable block.

P waves

- The presence of P waves indicates atrial depolarization. Absent P waves with an irregular ventricular rhythm suggest AF, whereas a sawtoothed pattern is characteristic of atrial flutter.

Atrial/ventricular activity

- Normally, there will be one P wave per QRS complex. Any change in this ratio indicates a block to conduction between atria and ventricles.

Narrow complex arrhythmias

(See also ➲ p. 893.)

Sinus arrhythmia

Irregular spacing of normal complexes associated with respiration. Constant P–R interval, with beat-to-beat change in the R–R interval. Normal finding, especially in young people.

Sinus tachycardia

Rate >100bpm. Normal P–QRS–T complexes are evident. Causes include:
- Inadequate depth of anaesthesia, pain/surgical stimulation
- Fever/sepsis, hypovolaemia, anaemia, heart failure, thyrotoxicosis
- Drugs, e.g. atropine, ketamine, catecholamines.

Correct the underlying cause where possible. β-blockers may be useful if tachycardia causes myocardial ischaemia but should be used with caution in patients with heart failure or asthma. The sinus nodal blocking agent ivabradine is an alternative.

Sinus bradycardia

Rate <60bpm. May be due to vagal stimulation or normal in athletic patients. Other causes include:
- Drugs, e.g. β-blockers, digoxin, anticholinesterases, halothane, suxamethonium
- MI, sick sinus syndrome
- Raised intracranial pressure (ICP), hypothyroidism, hypothermia.

Unnecessary to correct in a fit person, unless there is haemodynamic compromise (usually when HR <40–45bpm). However, consider:
- Correcting the underlying cause, e.g. stop the surgical stimulus
- Atropine up to 20 micrograms/kg or glycopyrronium 10 micrograms/kg IV
- Patients on β-blockers may be resistant, and an isoprenaline infusion is occasionally required (0.5–10 micrograms/min)—adrenaline is an alternative. Glucagon (50–150 micrograms/kg IV in 5% glucose) can be used—this is an unlicensed indication and dose.

Atrial ectopics

These are common and benign. May occur normally; other causes include:
- Ischaemia/hypoxia
- Light anaesthesia, sepsis, shock
- Anaesthetic drugs.

Correct any underlying cause. Specific treatment unnecessary, unless runs of atrial tachycardia occur.

Arrhythmias due to re-entry

These arrhythmias occur where there is an anatomical branching and rejoining of conduction pathways. If an impulse arrives at a time when the 1st pathway is no longer refractory, it can pass around the circuit repeatedly, activating it. The classical example is Wolff–Parkinson–White (WPW) syndrome where an accessory conduction pathway exists between the atria and ventricles. Other re-entry circuits occur with atrial flutter, AF, SVT, and VT.

Junctional/atrioventricular nodal/supraventricular tachycardia

- ECG usually shows a narrow complex (QRS <0.12s) tachycardia, with a rate of 150–200bpm. A broad complex pattern may occur if anterograde conduction occurs down an accessory pathway or if there is bundle branch block. Rarely causes severe circulatory disturbance in the presence of a structurally normal heart.
- If hypotensive, especially if anaesthetized, the 1st-line treatment is *synchronized* DC cardioversion with 200J.
- Carotid sinus massage may terminate re-entry SVT and may be helpful in differentiating SVT from atrial flutter and fast AF.
- Adenosine blocks AV nodal conduction and is especially useful for terminating re-entry SVT. Give 0.2mg/kg IV rapidly, followed by a saline flush. The effects of adenosine last only 10–15s. It should be avoided in asthma.
- β-blockers, e.g. esmolol by IV infusion at 50–200 micrograms/kg/min, or metoprolol 3–5mg over 10min repeated 6-hourly.
- Verapamil, 5–10mg IV slowly over 2min, is useful in patients with SVT who relapse following adenosine. A further 5mg may be given after 10min, if required. This may cause hypotension—avoid with β-blockers.
- Amiodarone is an alternative when 1st-line drugs have failed.
- Digoxin should be avoided—it facilitates conduction through the AV accessory pathway in WPW syndrome and may worsen tachycardia. AF in the presence of an accessory pathway may allow rapid conduction which can degenerate to VF.

Atrial flutter/atrial tachycardia

The atrial rate is >150bpm; P waves can sometimes be seen superimposed on T waves of the preceding beats. In atrial flutter, there is no flat baseline between P waves, and the typical sawtoothed pattern can be seen. Atrial tachycardia is less common in young adults. Both may occur with any kind of block, e.g. 2:1, 3:1, etc. Same risk of thromboembolism as AF.

- Sensitive to synchronized DC cardioversion—nearly 100% conversion. In the anaesthetized patient with recent onset, this should be the 1st line of treatment.
- Carotid sinus massage and adenosine will slow AV conduction and reveal the underlying rhythm and block where there is any doubt.
- Other drug treatment is as for AF.

Sick sinus syndrome

May coexist with AV nodal disease. Episodes of AV block, atrial tachycardia, atrial flutter, and AF may occur.
- The commonest causes are congenital or old age.
- Can be asymptomatic or present with dizziness or syncope.
- Permanent pacing required if symptomatic.

Atrial fibrillation

Uncoordinated atrial activity, with ventricular rate dependent on AV node transmission—commonly 120–180bpm. Causes of AF include:
- Hypertension, myocardial ischaemia, or heart muscle disease

- Pericarditis/mediastinitis, thoracic surgery
- Mitral valve disease
- Electrolyte disturbance (especially hypokalaemia or hypomagnesaemia)
- Sepsis, thyrotoxicosis, alcohol—especially binge drinking.

Atrial contraction contributes up to 30% of normal ventricular filling. The onset of AF (particularly fast AF) causes a reduction in ventricular filling and cardiac output. Ischaemia often results due to diastolic time reduction and hypotension.

Blood clots may form within the atria and embolize systemically. This risk is highest if there is a return to sinus rhythm after >48hr of AF. In stable AF, the risk of CVA is 4%/yr at 75yr—halved by anticoagulation.

Treatment aims to restore sinus rhythm or control the ventricular rate to <100bpm and prevent embolic complications. In acute AF (<48hr), restoration of sinus rhythm is often possible, whereas, in long-standing AF, control of the ventricular rate is the usual aim. Ideally, the ventricular rate should be controlled by appropriate therapy preoperatively. Occasionally, rapid control of the rate is required perioperatively.

Management of acute atrial fibrillation

Correct precipitating factors, where possible, especially electrolyte disturbances. When AF is 2° to sepsis or thoracic/oesophageal surgery, conversion to sinus rhythm is difficult until the underlying condition is controlled.

Onset <48hr

- Synchronized DC cardioversion at 200J, then 360J (if practical).
- Flecainide 2mg/kg (max 150mg) over 30min IV, or 300mg orally, is the best drug for converting AF to sinus rhythm. It should be avoided in patients with IHD or heart failure. Cardiac monitoring required.

Onset >48hr

Conversion to sinus rhythm is associated with risk of arterial embolization, unless the patient is anticoagulated (at least 3wk)—aim for rate control, unless haemodynamically compromised. Drugs include:

- Digoxin (if K⁺ is normal). IV loading dose of 500 micrograms in 100mL of saline over 20min, repeated at intervals of 4–8hr if necessary, to a total of 1–1.5mg. Lower doses are required for patients already taking digoxin. Digoxin does not convert AF to sinus rhythm or prevent further episodes of paroxysmal AF.
- β-blockers (esmolol, sotalol, metoprolol) may be used to slow the ventricular rate—caution with impaired myocardium, thyrotoxicosis, and avoid with calcium channel blockers. β-blockers can be useful in theatre, until other drugs have taken effect.
- Amiodarone slows the rate and helps sustain sinus rhythm once regained. There are a number of concerns with long-term side effects which include pulmonary fibrosis. Useful in acute AF associated with critical illness and can be combined with digoxin or β-blockers. A loading dose of 300mg (in 5% glucose) IV via a central vein is given over 1hr, and followed by 900mg over 23hr. It may be given peripherally in an emergency, but extravasation is extremely serious. Well tolerated with LV impairment.

- Verapamil 5–10mg IV may be used to slow the ventricular rate in patients unable to tolerate β-blockers. Avoid if there is impaired LV function, evidence of ischaemia, or in combination with β-blockers.

Uncontrolled chronic atrial fibrillation

Ventricular rates >100bpm should be slowed preoperatively to allow adequate time for ventricular filling/myocardial perfusion.

- Digitalization if the patient is not already fully loaded with digoxin. This should usually be done over 1–2d preoperatively. Rapid IV digitalization may be required when the surgery is urgent. Digoxin levels can be measured (therapeutic levels 0.8–2.0 micrograms/L).
- Additional β-blocker (metoprolol, atenolol) or verapamil if good LV function.
- Amiodarone IV if poor LV.

Broad complex arrhythmias

(See also ➲ p. 895.)

Ventricular ectopics

In the absence of structural heart disease, these are usually benign, but, in patients with ventricular disease, they may occasionally herald the onset of runs of VT.

- Correct any contributing causes—ensuring adequate oxygenation, normocapnia, and analgesia.
- If the underlying sinus rate is slow (<50bpm), then 'ectopics' may be ventricular escape beats. Try increasing the rate using IV atropine/ glycopyrronium.

Ventricular tachycardia

The QRS is always wide. P waves may be seen if there is AV dissociation. This is a serious, potentially life-threatening arrhythmia. It may be triggered intraoperatively by:

- Myocardial ischaemia, hypoxia, hypotension
- Fluid overload
- Electrolyte imbalance (low K^+, Mg^{2+}, etc.)
- Injection of adrenaline or other catecholamines.

Management

- Synchronized DC cardioversion (200J) if the patient is haemodynamically unstable. Will restore sinus rhythm in virtually 100% of cases. If the VT is pulseless or very rapid, synchronization is unnecessary. If the patient relapses into VT, lidocaine or amiodarone may be given to sustain sinus rhythm.
- Lidocaine (100mg bolus) restores sinus rhythm in 30–40% of cases and may be followed by a maintenance infusion of 4mg/min for 30min, then 2mg/min for 2hr, then 1mg/min.
- Drugs that may be used if lidocaine fails include:
  - Amiodarone 300mg IV via central venous catheter (CVC) over 1hr, followed by 900mg over 23hr
  - Sotalol 100mg IV over 5min has been shown to be better than lidocaine for acute termination of VT.

Supraventricular tachycardia with aberrant conduction

An SVT may be broad complex due to aberrant conduction between the atria and ventricles. This may appear only at high HRs (rate-related aberrant conduction). SVT caused by an abnormal or accessory pathway (e.g. WPW syndrome) will be of normal width if conduction in the accessory pathway is retrograde (i.e. it is the normal pathway that initiates the QRS complex), but broad complex if conduction is anterograde in the accessory pathway. Adenosine may be used diagnostically to slow AV conduction and may reveal the underlying rhythm in atrial flutter or atrial tachycardia. In the case of SVT, it may also result in conversion to sinus rhythm. In practice, however, all broad complex tachycardias should be treated as VT until proven otherwise.

Acute management of broad complex tachycardia

- If in doubt as to the nature of the rhythm, assume it is VT, rather than SVT (98% will be, especially if there is a history of IHD or cardiomyopathy).
- In the presence of hypotension/CVS compromise—synchronized DC shock with 200J.
- Perform a 12-lead ECG—if possible, both before and after correction, as this will help with retrospective diagnosis.
- If the patient is not acutely compromised, adenosine 0.2mg/kg rapidly IV will be both diagnostic and often curative if it is an SVT.

Ventricular fibrillation

- This results in cardiac arrest. There is chaotic and disorganized contraction of the ventricular muscle, and no QRS complexes can be identified on the ECG.
- Immediate DC cardioversion as per established resuscitation protocol (200J) (see ➲ p. 889).

Action plan in theatre when faced with an arrhythmia

- Assess vital signs—ABC.
- Determine whether the arrhythmia is serious (CVS compromise—BP/cardiac output/HR).

Is there a problem with the anaesthetic?

- Oxygenation?
- Ventilation—check end-tidal CO_2 (ETCO$_2$).
- Anaesthesia too light—alter the inspired volatile agent concentration, and give a bolus of rapid-acting analgesic, e.g. alfentanil.
- Drug interaction/error?

Is there a problem with surgery?

- Vagal stimulation from traction on the eye or peritoneum.
- Loss of cardiac output—air/fat embolism.
- Unexpected blood loss.
- Injection of adrenaline.
- Mediastinal manipulation.

Disturbances of conduction (heart block)

(See also ➔ p. 892.)

First-degree block

Delay in conduction through the AV node to the ventricles. Prolongation of the P–R interval to >0.2s. Normally benign but may progress to 2nd- or 3rd-degree block. 1st-degree heart block is not a problem during anaesthesia.

Second-degree block—Mobitz type I (Wenckebach)

Progressive lengthening of the P–R interval and then failure of conduction of an atrial beat. This is followed by a conducted beat, and the cycle repeats. Common in young athletically trained adults with a high vagal tone. May occur during inferior MI and tends to be self-limiting. Asymptomatic patients do not normally require treatment perioperatively but may require long-term pacing, as Wenckebach block may progress to higher degrees of block.

Second-degree block—Mobitz type II

Intermittent atrial depolarization without a subsequent ventricular beat (2:1 or 3:1 are common forms). This often progresses to complete heart block.

Third-degree block/complete heart block

Complete failure of conduction between the atria and ventricles. Occasionally, a transient phenomenon due to severe vagal stimulation, in which case it often responds to stopping the stimulation, and IV atropine. Very rarely, it may be congenital.

Bundle branch block

If there is a delay in depolarization of the right or left bundle branches, this will cause a delay in depolarization of part of the ventricular muscle, with subsequent QRS widening.

Right bundle branch block

Wide complexes with an 'RSR' in lead V_1 (may appear 'M'-shaped) and a small initial negative downward deflection, followed by a larger upward positive wave, and then a 2nd downward wave in V_6. Often benign.

Left bundle branch block

Septal depolarization is reversed, so there is a change in the initial direction of the QRS complex in every lead. This may indicate heart disease and makes further interpretation of the ECG, other than the rate and rhythm, difficult.

Bifascicular block

Combination of right bundle branch block and block of the left anterior or left posterior fascicle. Right bundle branch block with left anterior hemiblock is commoner and appears as an 'RSR' in V_1, together with left axis deviation. Right bundle branch block with left posterior hemiblock is less common and appears as right bundle branch block with an abnormal degree of right axis deviation. However, other causes for right axis deviation should be considered, and it is a non-specific sign.

Trifascicular block
Sometimes used to indicate the presence of a prolonged P–R interval together with bifascicular block.

Preoperative management

- 1st-degree heart block in the absence of symptoms is common. It needs no specific investigation or treatment.
- 2nd- or 3rd-degree heart block may need pacemaker insertion. If surgery is urgent, this may be achieved quickly by inserting a temporary transvenous wire prior to definitive insertion.
- Bundle branch, bifascicular, or trifascicular block (bifascicular with 1st-degree block) will rarely progress to complete heart block during anaesthesia, and so it is not normal practice to insert a pacing wire, unless there have been episodes of syncope.

Indications for preoperative pacing
- Symptomatic 1st-degree heart block.
- Symptomatic 2nd-degree (Mobitz type I) heart block.
- 2nd-degree (Mobitz type II) heart block.
- 3rd-degree heart block.
- Symptomatic bifascicular block or symptomatic 1st-degree heart block plus bifascicular block (trifascicular block).
- Symptomatic sinus node disease.

Intraoperative heart block

- Atropine is rarely effective but could be tried.
- If hypotension is profound, then an isoprenaline infusion (alternative is adrenaline) can be used to temporize: 1–10 micrograms/min.
  - Dilute 0.2mg in 500mL of 5% glucose, and titrate to effect (2–20mL/min), or
  - Dilute 1mg in 50mL of 5% glucose/glucose–saline, and titrate to effect (1.5–30mL/hr).
- Transcutaneous pacing may be practical in theatre if electrodes can be placed. Oesophageal pacing is also effective. The electrode is passed into the oesophagus, like a nasogastric tube (NGT), and connected to the pulse generator. The position can be adjusted until there is ventricular capture.
- Transvenous pacing is both more reliable and effective, and relatively easy. A PAFC introducer of adequate size to pass the wire is inserted into the internal jugular or subclavian vein (this can be done while other equipment is being collected).
  - Insert balloon-tipped pacing wire to the 20cm mark.
  - Inflate the balloon, and connect the pulse generator at 5V.
  - Advance until ventricular capture. When this happens, deflate the balloon, and insert a further 5cm of catheter.
  - If the 50cm mark is reached, the catheter is coiling up, or not entering the heart, deflate the balloon; withdraw to the 20cm mark, and try again.

Pacemakers and defibrillators

Pacemakers are usually used to treat bradyarrhythmias. However, biventricular systems are used to improve the functional capacity and quality of life in selected patients with severe heart failure.

The Heart Rhythm Society (HRS) and Heart Rhythm UK (HRUK) pacemaker codes are used to describe pacemaker types and function (Box 4.1). The code consists of five letters or positions. The 1st three describe antibradycardia functions and are always stated. The 4th and 5th positions relate to additional functions and are often omitted.

> **Box 4.1 US/UK pacemaker codes**
> - Position 1: chamber-paced (O/V/A/D—none, ventricle, atrium, dual).
> - Position 2: sensing chamber (O/V/A/D).
> - Position 3: response to sensing (O/T/I/D—none, triggered, inhibited, dual).
> - Position 4: programmability or rate modulation (O/P/M/R—none, simple programmable, multiprogrammable, rate modulation).
> - Position 5: antitachycardia functions (O/P/S/D—none, pacing, shock, dual).

Implications for anaesthesia and surgery

- Patients with pacemakers should attend follow-up clinics. The most recent visit should confirm an adequate battery life and normal function of the pacemaker system. A preoperative ECG will provide confirmation of the expected function, e.g. AV synchronicity, polarity of pacing, and baseline rate.
- The main source of concern is electromagnetic interference (EMI). Possible responses include inappropriate triggering or inhibition of a paced output, asynchronous pacing, reprogramming (usually into a backup mode), and damage to device circuitry. Pacing wires may also act as aerials and cause heating where they contact the endocardium. Diathermy is the commonest source of EMI found in the operating theatre.
- Bipolar diathermy is safe. If conventional diathermy is necessary, position the plate so that most of the current passes away from the pacemaker. In an emergency, most pacemakers can be changed to asynchronous ventricular pacing (V00) by placing a magnet over the box. There is a theoretical risk of inducing VF, as the magnet-induced asynchronous pacing may result in stimulation during a vulnerable period and induce an arrhythmia—'competitive pacing'. In modern pacemakers, the switch to asynchronous pacing is coupled with the next cardiac cycle to avoid this.
- For patients with severe heart failure, where loss of AV synchrony may precipitate haemodynamic compromise, there should be a telemetric programmer and cardiac technician close at hand.

Implantable cardioverter–defibrillators

ICDs should be deactivated prior to surgery where diathermy might be used (the ICD will detect the signal as VF and deliver a shock). The patient should be monitored throughout surgery, and then the device reactivated afterwards.

Further reading

Poldermans D, Bax JJ, Boersma E, *et al.* (2010). Guidelines for pre-operative cardiac risk management and perioperative cardiac management in non-cardiac surgery. *Eur J Anaesthesiol*, **27**, 92–137.

Salukhe TV, Dob D, Sutton R (2004). Pacemakers and defibrillators: anaesthetic implications. *Br J Anaesth*, **93**, 95–104.

Respiratory disease

Lara Herbert and Bruce McCormick

Effects of surgery and anaesthesia on respiratory function

Effects of surgery

- Upper abdominal operations are associated with pulmonary complications in 20–40% of the general surgical population.
- Incidence with lower abdominal surgery is 2–5%.
- Upper abdominal or thoracic surgery is associated with profound reductions in lung volume; vital capacity (VC) is reduced by 50–60%, and functional residual capacity (FRC) reduced by about 30%.
- Diaphragmatic dysfunction plays an important role in these changes, but pain and splinting are also factors.
- Reductions in lung volumes are not seen with surgery on the extremities.

Effects of anaesthesia

- On induction of anaesthesia, FRC decreases by 15–20% (~450mL); the diaphragm relaxes and moves cranially, and the rib cage moves inward.
- FRC may be reduced by 50% of the awake supine value in morbidly obese patients. Positive end-expiratory pressure (PEEP) may reduce these effects. FRC is relatively maintained during ketamine anaesthesia.
- Under anaesthesia, the closing capacity (the lung volume at which airway closure begins) encroaches upon the FRC, and airway closure occurs, contributing to the risk of atelectasis, pneumonia, and ventilation/perfusion (V/Q) mismatching. This happens more readily in smokers, the elderly, and those with underlying lung disease.
- Chest computed tomography (CT) shows atelectasis in the dependent zones of the lungs in >80% of anaesthetized subjects. Microatelectasis results in areas of the lungs that are perfused but not ventilated, leading to impaired gas exchange and consequent post-operative hypoxaemia.
- Intubation halves the dead space by circumventing the upper airway.
- The ventilatory response to hypercapnia is blunted, and the acute responses to hypoxia and acidaemia almost abolished by anaesthetic vapours at concentrations as low as 0.1 minimum alveolar concentration (MAC).
- Inhibition of cough and impairment of mucociliary clearance of respiratory secretions contribute to the risk of post-operative infection.
- Most of these adverse changes are more marked in patients with lung disease but usually improve within a few hours post-operatively. After major surgery, they may last several days.

Predicting post-operative pulmonary complications

- Post-operative pulmonary complications include atelectasis, infection, prolonged mechanical ventilation, respiratory failure, exacerbation of underlying chronic lung disease, and bronchospasm.[1]
- Post-operative pulmonary complications are as prevalent as cardiac complications and contribute similarly to morbidity and mortality.
- Preoperative identification of patients with pre-existing respiratory dysfunction reduces post-operative complications.
- Even for patients with severe pulmonary disease, surgery that does not involve the abdominal or chest cavities is inherently of low risk for serious perioperative pulmonary complications.
- Large and rigorous studies to identify risk factors for pulmonary complications are lacking (in contrast to those identifying cardiac risk).

Factors shown to predict perioperative pulmonary complications

Patient factors

- Increasing age (>50yr).
- Chronic obstructive lung disease.
- Smoking within 8wk of surgery.
- Obstructive sleep apnoea (OSA).[2]
- Pulmonary hypertension.[3]
- ASA grade 2 or greater.
- CCF.
- Functional dependence.
- Serum albumin <30g/dL.

Procedure-related factors

- Prolonged surgery.
- Residual neuromuscular blockade (NMB).[4]
- Upper abdominal and thoracic surgery.
- Neurosurgery, head and neck surgery.
- Vascular surgery, especially aortic aneurysm repair.
- Emergency surgery.

References

1 Smetana GW, Lawrence VA, Cornell JE; American College of Physicians. Preoperative pulmonary risk stratification for noncardiothoracic surgery: systematic review for the American College of Physicians (2006). Ann Intern Med, 144, 581–95.
2 Memtsoudis S, Liu SS, Ma Y, et al. (2011). Perioperative pulmonary outcomes in patients with sleep apnea after noncardiac surgery. Anesth Analg, 112, 113–21.
3 Price LC, Montani D, Jaïs X, et al. (2010). Noncardiothoracic nonobstetric surgery in mild-to-moderate pulmonary hypertension. Eur Respir J, 35, 1294–302.
4 Murphy GS, Szokol JW, Marymont JH, et al. (2008). Residual neuromuscular blockade and critical respiratory events in the postanesthesia care unit. Anesth Analg, 107, 130–7.

Assessment of respiratory function

- A complete history and physical examination are the most important elements of preoperative risk assessment.[5,6]

History

- Significant risk factors for post-operative pulmonary complications should be identified (see ➔ p. 85).
- Details of hospital admissions with respiratory disease should be noted, particularly if the patient was admitted to intensive care.
- If the patient has chronic lung disease, compare the current respiratory function with previous disease trends.
- Explore symptoms such as cough and sputum production. Send a sputum specimen for culture and sensitivity.
- Note past and present cigarette consumption.
- Review current treatment, reversibility of symptoms with bronchodilators, and steroid intake.
- There is no evidence that screening for sleep apnoea affects surgical complication rates, but it is advisable to question obese patients about symptoms suggestive of OSA prior to major surgery (see ➔ p. 112).[7]
- Any history suggesting unrecognized chronic lung disease or heart failure, such as exercise intolerance, unexplained dyspnoea, or cough, requires further consideration.
- Dyspnoea can be described using Roizen's classification. Undiagnosed dyspnoea of grade II or worse may require further investigation (Box 5.1).

Box 5.1 Roizen's classification of dyspnoea

Grade 0:   No dyspnoea while walking on the level at normal pace

Grade I: 'I am able to walk as far as I like, provided I take my time'

Grade II: Specific street block limitation—'I have to stop for a while after one or two blocks'

Grade III: Dyspnoea on mild exertion—'I have to stop and rest, going from the kitchen to the bathroom'

Grade IV: Dyspnoea at rest

Examination

- Abnormal findings on clinical examination are predictive of pulmonary complications after abdominal surgery.[5]
- Physical examination should be directed toward evidence for obstructive lung disease. Signs, such as decreased breath sounds, wheeze, or prolonged expiratory phase, are important.
- Measurement of O_2 saturation by oximetry helps to stratify risk and is useful before high-risk surgery.[8]
- A formal assessment of exercise tolerance, such as stair climbing or the 6-minute walk test (6MWT), correlates well with PFTs and provides a reliable test of pulmonary function. However, it also reflects the CVS status, cooperation, and determination and is an impractical assessment for those with limited mobility.

Investigations

(See ➡ p. 88.)

- All candidates for lung resection should have preoperative PFTs performed.
- For all other procedures, laboratory tests serve as adjuncts to the clinical evaluation and should be obtained only in selected patients.

References

5 Lawrence VA, Dhanda R, Hilsenbeck SG, Page CP (1996). Risk of pulmonary complications after elective abdominal surgery. *Chest*, **110**, 744–50.

6 Brooks-Brunn JA (1997). Predictors of postoperative pulmonary complications following abdominal surgery. *Chest*, **111**, 564–71.

7 Chung F, Yegneswaran B, Liao P, et al. (2008). STOP questionnaire: a tool to screen patients for obstructive sleep apnea. *Anesthesiology*, **108**, 812–21.

8 Canet J, Gallart L, Gomar C, et al. (2010). Prediction of postoperative pulmonary complications in a population-based surgical cohort. *Anesthesiology*, **113**, 1338–50.

Respiratory investigations

Peak expiratory flow rate (PEFR or peak flow)
- A useful test for COPD or asthma.
- Measured on the ward, using a peak flow meter (best of three attempts); technique is important. For normal values, see ➔ p. 1223.
- The patient's daily record gives a good indication of current fitness.
- Coughing is ineffective if the peak flow is <200L/min.

Spirometry
- Useful to quantify the severity of ventilatory dysfunction and to differentiate between restrictive and obstructive defects.
- Measured in the respiratory function laboratory or at the bedside using a bellows device.
- Normally, FVC, FEV_1, and the ratio FEV_1/FVC (as a percentage) are reported. The results of these tests are given with normal values calculated for that individual. A normal FEV_1/FVC ratio is 70% (see ➔ p. 1223).
- In those with an obstructive picture (low FEV_1/FVC ratio), reversibility with a bronchodilator should be tested. Spirometry after a course of steroids (prednisolone 20–40mg daily for 7d) should be repeated.
- Previously used to assess risk in patients with significant respiratory disease scheduled for major surgery. However, recent evidence suggests that spirometry does not predict pulmonary complications, even in patients with severe COPD.
- Spirometry should not be used as the 1° factor to deny surgery. Despite poor preoperative spirometry, series of patients successfully undergoing thoracic and major non-thoracic surgery are being increasingly reported. An FEV_1 <1000mL indicates that post-operative coughing and secretion clearance will be poor and increases the likelihood of needing respiratory support following major surgery.
- Spirometry should not be ordered routinely prior to abdominal or other high-risk surgery.
- Specific subgroups of patients who may benefit from spirometry are:
  - Those with dyspnoea or exercise intolerance that remains unexplained after clinical evaluation. In this case, the differential diagnosis may include cardiac disease. Spirometry results may change preoperative management
  - In patients with COPD or asthma if the clinical evaluation cannot determine if the patient is at their best baseline and that airflow obstruction is optimally reduced. Spirometry may identify patients who will benefit from more aggressive preoperative management
  - Patients in whom functional ability cannot be assessed because of lower extremity disability.
- Spirometry also forms part of the assessment of patients for lung parenchymal resection (see ➔ p. 356).

Flow–volume loops

- Measured in the respiratory function department.
- Peak flows at different lung volumes are recorded. Although more complex to interpret, loops provide more accurate information regarding ventilatory function. They provide useful data about the severity of obstructive and restrictive respiratory disease.
- Used in the assessment of airway obstruction from both extrinsic (e.g. thyroid) and intrinsic causes (e.g. bronchospasm).

Transfer factor, TLCO (diffusing capacity, DLCO)

- Measures the diffusion of carbon monoxide (CO) into the lung, using a single breath of gas containing 0.3% CO and 10% helium held for 20s.
- With restrictive disease, DLCO helps to differentiate between intrinsic lung disease (DLCO usually reduced) and other causes of restriction (DLCO usually normal). With obstructive disease, the DLCO helps to differentiate between emphysema and other causes of chronic airway obstruction.
- Normal value is 17–25mL/min/mmHg; however, most use the percentage value compared to the predicted.

Arterial blood gas analysis

- Measure baseline blood gases in air for any patient breathless on minimal exertion. Compare with previous results if the patient has had previous arterial blood gas (ABG) measurements.
- Detects CO_2 retention. A resting $PaCO_2$ >6.0kPa (45mmHg) is predictive of pulmonary complications and suggests ventilatory failure.
- Demonstrates the usual level of oxygenation, which indicates the severity of disease and is useful to set realistic parameters post-operatively.

Chest X-ray

- There is insufficient evidence to determine which patients will benefit from a preoperative CXR.
- It is reasonable to obtain a CXR in patients with known cardiopulmonary disease and in those over the age of 50, undergoing high-risk surgical procedures, including upper abdominal, aortic, oesophageal, and thoracic surgery.
- An abnormality predicts the risk of pulmonary complications.
- Reveals lung pathology, cardiac size and outline, and provides a baseline should post-operative problems develop.

CT thorax

- Chest CT is required in a few patients with lung cysts/bullae to accurately assess the size and extent of their disease.
- Impingement of mass lesions on the major airways and the likely extent of lung resection can be assessed.
- May demonstrate anterior or posterior pneumothorax and interstitial disease, such as lung fibrosis, not seen on CXR.
- Spiral CT chest investigations can detect PE and dissecting aortic lesions.

Ventilation/perfusion scan

- Reports the likelihood of PE. Difficult to interpret in the presence of other pathology.
- Useful in the assessment of patients for lung parenchymal resection to predict the effect of resection on overall pulmonary performance (resecting a non-ventilated/perfused lung will reduce shunt and should improve oxygenation).

Cardiopulmonary exercise testing

(See also ➜ p. 15.)

- Has been studied most extensively in preparation for lung resection.
- CPET, with a calculation of the maximum O_2 uptake and anaerobic threshold, may have a role in the evaluation of patients undergoing non-cardiopulmonary surgery with unexplained dyspnoea.
- Both measurements have been shown to predict survival and overall post-operative complications.[9]
- Studies have not measured post-operative pulmonary complications as a separate outcome.

Reference

9 Smith TB, Stonell C, Purkayastha S, Paraskevas P (2009). Cardiopulmonary exercise testing as a risk assessment method in non cardio-pulmonary surgery: a systematic review. *Anaesthesia*, **64**, 883–93.

Pulmonary risk indices

- Cardiac risk indices have been used widely since 1977. Until recently, no similar indices have been developed for risk stratification of pulmonary complications.
- Two important proposed pulmonary risk indices include the Arozullah and Canet indices. They provide a simplified approach to preoperative pulmonary risk estimation and are useful tools to stratify risk and to identify those patients most likely to benefit from risk reduction strategies.

Arozullah risk index

- Used to predict post-operative respiratory failure.[10]
- Points are assigned to factors that predict post-operative respiratory failure, such as type of surgery, emergency surgery, COPD, albumin <30g/dL, blood urea nitrogen (BUN) >30mg/dL, dependent functional status, and advanced age (60–69yr and >70yr).
- Procedure-related risk factors dominate the index, with type of surgery and emergency surgery being the most important predictors.

Canet risk index

- Risk index to predict post-operative pulmonary complications.[11]
- Seven risk factors are used to stratify risk into low, intermediate, and high risk for post-operative pulmonary complications.
- Risk factors include advanced age, low preoperative O_2 saturation, respiratory infection within the past month, preoperative anaemia, upper abdominal or thoracic surgery, surgery lasting >2hr, and emergency surgery.

References

10 Arozullah AM, Daley J, Henderson WG, Khuri SF (2000). Multifactorial risk index for predicting postoperative respiratory failure in men after major noncardiac surgery. The National Veterans Administration Surgical Quality Improvement Program. *Ann Surg*, **232**, 242–53.
11 Canet J, Gallart L, Gomar C, *et al*. (2010). Prediction of postoperative pulmonary complications in a population-based surgical cohort. *Anesthesiology*, **113**, 1338–50.

Strategies to reduce post-operative pulmonary complications

Preoperative

- Smoking cessation as early as possible; stopping smoking for 8wk or longer is more likely to be beneficial.[12]
- Regular ipratropium or tiotropium for all patients with clinically significant COPD.
- Inhaled β-agonists, as required, for patients with COPD or asthma who have wheeze or dyspnoea.
- Preoperative glucocorticoids for patients with COPD or asthma who are not optimized and whose airway obstruction has not been maximally reduced.
- Delay elective surgery if respiratory tract infection is present.
- Antibiotics only for patients with lower respiratory tract infection (LRTI).
- Preoperative inspiratory muscle training and chest physiotherapy. This involves breathing exercises, aerobic exercise, incentive spirometry (deep breathing facilitated by a simple mechanical device), education on active breathing, and forced expiration techniques.[13,14]

Intra-operative

- Choose an alternative procedure lasting <4hr when possible.
- Surgery other than upper abdominal or thoracic when possible. For example, percutaneous cholecystostomy could be substituted for open cholecystectomy in a critically ill, high-risk patient with acute cholecystitis.
- Regional anaesthesia—if an option in very high-risk patients.
- Epidural or spinal anaesthesia may confer lower risk than GA, though this remains an area of debate.
- Avoid long-acting muscle relaxants in very high-risk patients. Residual NMB is associated with post-operative hypoventilation which may increase post-operative complications.
- Choosing laparoscopic, rather than open, surgery may be beneficial.
- Lung protective ventilation. A lung protective strategy of low tidal volume (V_T) ventilation (6–8mL/kg of ideal body weight (IBW), PEEP at 6–8cmH$_2$O, and recruitment manoeuvres every 30min) is associated with a reduction in adverse pulmonary events (see ➲ p. 94).[15]

Post-operative

- If possible, aim for upright posture post-operatively. Respiratory performance, FRC, and clearance of secretions are improved when sitting or standing, compared with the supine position.
- Early mobilization reduces the incidence of thromboembolic disease.
- Ensure regular clinical review, and monitor the respiratory rate and O_2 saturation. Respiratory deterioration may present in a non-specific way (confusion, tachycardia, fever, malaise). Regular review allows urgent investigation and aggressive therapy. Seek assessment and advice of the intensive care/outreach team early if the patient does not respond to initial treatment.

- Early post-operative chest physiotherapy, including incentive spirometry and breathing exercises, aids clearance of secretions and reduces atelectasis.
- Administer supplemental O_2 for up to 72hr post-operatively, particularly if the patient is receiving opioids. Anaesthetic agents exert a dose-dependent depression on the sensitivity of central chemoreceptors, reducing the stimulatory effect of CO_2. This effect can occur for up to 72hr post-operatively and is commonest at night. Preoperative measurement of PaO_2, SaO_2, and $PaCO_2$ is essential to establish a realistic target for each patient.
- Patients who chronically retain CO_2 (advanced COPD) may be dependent on hypoxaemia as their main ventilatory drive due to downregulation of central chemoreceptors. The concentration of delivered O_2 should be controlled (e.g. by Venturi mask) and titrated, in order to optimize oxygenation and prevent hypoventilation. Adequate monitoring should be available, ideally using serial ABG measurement (pulse oximetry shows only SpO_2).
- Humidification of O_2 aids physiotherapy and sputum clearance.
- Accurate management and documentation of fluid balance is essential. Adequate intravascular filling is required to maintain perfusion of organs such as the kidney and gut. However, patients with lung disease are at increased risk of pulmonary oedema. (A dilated right ventricle may mechanically compromise the function of the left ventricle.) Fluid overload is poorly tolerated in these patients, and a high index of suspicion should be maintained.
- Good analgesia is essential for the maintenance of efficient respiratory function, compliance with physiotherapy, early mobilization, and minimizing cardiac stress. Regular PO or IV paracetamol and, where not contraindicated, NSAIDs should be prescribed. NSAIDs should be used with caution in the elderly, as renal function may be compromised and they may induce fluid retention.
- Patients with lung dysfunction may benefit from local or regional anaesthesia. The surgeon may be able to place a catheter for regional anaesthesia at the time of operation (e.g. paravertebral catheter for thoracotomy). The benefits of opioid-based analgesia (patient control, mobility, and avoidance of bladder catheterization) should be weighed against the benefits of regional analgesia (avoidance of high-dose systemic opioids, preservation of respiratory function) and discussed with the patient preoperatively.
- Involve the pain management team early in the post-operative period, requesting at least daily reviews.

References

12 Celli BR (1993). Perioperative respiratory care of the patient undergoing upper abdominal surgery. *Clin Chest Med*, **14**, 253–61.
13 Valkenet K, van de Port IG, Dronkers JJ, et al. (2011). The effects of preoperative exercise therapy on postoperative outcome: a systematic review. *Clin Rehabil*, **25**, 99–111.
14 Hulzebos EH, Smit Y, Helders PP, van Meeteren NL (2012). Preoperative physical therapy for elective cardiac surgery patients. *Cochrane Database Syst Rev*, **11**, CD010118.
15 Futier E, Constantin JM, Paugam-Burtz C, et al. (IMPROVE Study Group) (2013). A trial of intraoperative low-tidal-volume ventilation in abdominal surgery. *N Engl J Med*, **369**, 428–37.

Lung protective ventilation

- In 2000, the ARDSNet study showed that the use of low V_T (6–8mL/kg IBW) during mechanical ventilation significantly reduced mortality in acute respiratory distress syndrome (ARDS).[16]
- The IMPROVE study randomized 400 patients undergoing elective abdominal surgery into two groups.[17] One group received low V_T ventilation: 6–8mL/kg IBW, PEEP 6–8cmH$_2$O, and recruitment manoeuvres every 30min. The other group received standard mechanical ventilation (10–15mL/kg with PEEP and recruitment manoeuvres provided, according to the anaesthetist's discretion). In both groups, the anaesthetists tried to keep plateau pressures under 30cmH$_2$O. The rate of post-operative pulmonary complications was significantly lower in the group receiving low V_T ventilation.

References

16 The Acute Respiratory Distress Syndrome Network (2000). Ventilation with lower tidal volumes as compared with traditional tidal volumes for acute lung injury and the acute respiratory distress syndrome. The Acute Respiratory Distress Syndrome Network. *N Engl J Med*, **342**, 1301–8.
17 Futier E, Constantin J-M, Paugam-Burtz C, *et al.*; for the IMPROVE Study Group (2013). A trial of intraoperative low-tidal-volume ventilation in abdominal surgery. *N Engl J Med*, **369**, 428–37.

Post-operative admission to HDU/ICU

- Ideally, admission to ICU or HDU should be planned preoperatively.
- Patients may require admission for ventilatory support (CPAP, bilevel positive airway pressure (BiPAP), invasive ventilation) or increased levels of monitoring and nursing care that are not available on the surgical ward.

The precipitating reasons for admission to the ICU or HDU may be predictable or unpredictable (Table 5.1).

Table 5.1 Reasons for post-operative ICU or HDU admission

Predictable	Unpredictable
Borderline or established failure of gas exchange preoperatively	Unexpected perioperative complications (e.g. fluid overload, haemorrhage)
Intercurrent respiratory infection (with urgent surgery)	Inadequate or ineffective regional analgesia with deterioration in respiratory function
Chest disease productive of large amounts of secretions (e.g. bronchiectasis)	Unexpectedly prolonged procedure
Major abdominal or thoracic surgery	Acidosis
Major surgery not amenable to regional analgesia and necessitating systemic opioids	Hypothermia
Long duration of surgery	Depressed conscious level/slow recovery from anaesthetic/poor cough

Respiratory tract infection and elective surgery

(For paediatric implications, see ➔ p. 795.)

- Patients who have respiratory tract infections producing fever and cough with or without chest signs on auscultation should not undergo elective surgery under GA due to the increased risk of post-operative pulmonary complications.
- Adult patients with simple coryza are not at significantly increased risk of developing post-operative pulmonary problems, unless they have pre-existing respiratory disease or are having major abdominal or thoracic surgery.[18]
- Laryngospasm may be more likely in patients with a recent history of upper respiratory tract symptoms who are asymptomatic at the time of surgery.
- Compared with asymptomatic children, children with symptoms of acute or recent upper respiratory tract infection (URTI) are more likely to suffer from transient post-operative hypoxaemia (SpO_2 <93%). This is most marked when intubation is necessary.[19]

References

18 Fennelly ME, Hall GM (1990). Anaesthesia and upper airway respiratory tract infections—a non-existent hazard? *Br J Anaesth*, **64**, 535–6.

19 Levy L, Pandit UA, Randel GI, Lewis IH, Tait AR (1992). Upper respiratory tract infections and general anaesthesia in children. *Anaesthesia*, **47**, 678–82.

Smoking

- Cigarette smoke contains nicotine, a highly addictive substance, and at least 4700 other chemical compounds, of which 43 are known to be carcinogenic. Long-term smoking is associated with serious underlying problems such as COPD, lung neoplasm, IHD, and vascular disorders.[20]
- Respiratory tract mucus is produced in greater quantities, but mucociliary clearance is less efficient. Smokers are more susceptible to respiratory events during anaesthesia and to post-operative atelectasis/pneumonia. Abdominal or thoracic surgery and obesity increase these risks.
- Carboxyhaemoglobin (COHb) levels may reach 5–15% in heavy smokers, causing reduced O_2 carriage by the blood. COHb has a similar absorption spectrum to oxyhaemoglobin and will cause falsely high O_2 saturation readings.
- Increased airway irritability increases coughing, laryngospasm, and desaturation during induction and airway manipulation (e.g. laryngeal mask insertion). Avoid by using a less irritant volatile (e.g. sevoflurane) and deepening anaesthesia slowly.
- Maintaining spontaneous breathing via an endotracheal tube (ETT) or laryngeal mask airway (LMA) may be awkward due to airway irritation—consider LA to the vocal cords, opioids, relaxants, and IPPV.

Risk reduction

- Abstinence from smoking for 8wk is required to decrease morbidity from respiratory complications to a rate similar to that of non-smokers.
- Smokers unwilling to stop preoperatively will still benefit by refraining from smoking for 12hr before surgery. During this time, the effects of nicotine (activation of the sympathoadrenergic system with raised coronary vascular resistance) and COHb will decrease.

Reference

20 Warner DO (2007). Tobacco dependence in surgical patients. *Curr Opin Anesthesiol*, **20**, 279–83.

Asthma

Asthma[21–23] is a disorder of variable severity, which causes symptoms resulting from airway obstruction, inflammation, and hyper-responsiveness. Symptoms of asthma are most frequently a combination of shortness of breath, wheeze, cough, and sputum production.

Bronchial wall inflammation is a fundamental component and results in mucus hypersecretion, epithelial damage, and an increased tendency for airways to constrict.

Asthma can be differentiated from COPD by the presence of childhood symptoms, diurnal variation, specific trigger factors (especially allergic), absence of smoking history, and response to previous treatments.

General considerations
- Most well-controlled asthmatics tolerate anaesthesia and surgery well.
- The incidence of perioperative bronchospasm and laryngospasm in asthmatic patients undergoing routine surgery is <2%, especially if routine medication is continued.
- The frequency of complications is increased in patients >50yr and in those with active disease.
- Poorly controlled asthmatics are at risk of perioperative problems (bronchospasm, sputum retention, atelectasis, infection, respiratory failure).
- Do not anaesthetize a patient for elective surgery whose asthma is not optimally controlled.

Preoperative assessment
- Patients and doctors frequently underestimate the severity of asthma, especially if it is long-standing.
- Key indicators of severe disease include a history of frequent exacerbations, hospital visits, and most importantly prior tracheal intubation and mechanical ventilation to manage a severe attack.
- Document any allergies/drug sensitivities, especially the effect of aspirin/NSAIDs. The prevalence of aspirin-induced asthma (measured by oral provocation) is 21% in adult asthmatics, and 5% in paediatric asthmatics. Much lower rates are quoted if verbal history is used to assess prevalence (3% and 2%, respectively).
- Ask about trigger factors and recent respiratory tract infections.
- The type, dose, frequency, and degree of benefit of therapy provide important clues about the severity and control of the disease.
- Examination is often unremarkable but should focus on detecting signs of acute bronchospasm, active lung infection (which should defer surgery), chronic lung disease, and right heart failure.
- Treatment options prior to surgery are based on the level of the severity of the disease.
- Advise patients to stop smoking at least 2 months prior to surgery.
- Patients with mild asthma (peak flow >80% of predicted and minimal symptoms) rarely require extra treatment prior to surgery. Consider adding a short-acting β_2-agonist just prior to surgery.

- Moderately controlled patients should add inhaled corticosteroids to their β₂-agonists 1wk prior to surgery.
- Poorly controlled asthmatics (>20% variability in PEFR) may need to add oral corticosteroids to their regimen such as oral prednisolone 20–40mg daily for 1wk. Consider preoperative review by a chest physician.
- Emphasize the benefits of good compliance with treatment prior to surgery (Table 5.2).
- Viral infections are potent triggers of asthma, so postpone elective surgery if symptoms suggest URTI.
- There is an association with nasal polyps in atopic patients.

Table 5.2 Perioperative recommendations for asthma medications

Class of drug	Examples	Perioperative recommendation	Notes
β₂-agonists	Salbutamol, terbutaline, salmeterol	Convert to nebulized preparation	High doses may lower K^+. Cause tachycardia and tremor
Anticholinergic drugs	Ipratropium	Convert to nebulized form	
Inhaled steroids	Beclometasone, budesonide, fluticasone	Continue inhaled formulation	If >1500 micrograms/d of beclometasone, adrenal suppression may be present
Oral steroids	Prednisolone	Continue as IV hydrocortisone until taking orally	If >10mg/d, adrenal suppression is likely (see ➋ p. 165)
Leukotriene receptor antagonist (anti-inflammatory effect)	Montelukast, zafirlukast	Restart when taking oral medications	
Mast cell stabilizer	Disodium cromoglicate	Continue by inhaler	
Phosphodiesterase inhibitor	Aminophylline	Continue where possible	In severe asthma, consider converting to an infusion perioperatively

Investigations

- Serial home measurements of peak flow are more informative than a single reading. Measure the response to bronchodilators, and look for 'early morning dip' in peak flow (this suggests control is not optimal).
- Spirometry helps to detect the chronic residual effects of acute asthma and helps to stratify the severity of the disease. Results of peak flow and

spirometry are compared with predicted values based on age, sex, and
height (see p. 1223).

- Blood gases are only necessary in assessing patients with severe
  asthma (poorly controlled, frequent hospital admissions, previous ICU
  admission), particularly prior to major surgery.
- ECG may show right atrial or ventricular hypertrophy, acute strain, right
  axis deviation, and right bundle branch block.
- CXRs reveal flattened diaphragms if the lungs are hyperinflated and are
  useful to evaluate for pulmonary congestion, oedema, or infiltrates.

Conduct of anaesthesia

- The overriding goal is to avoid bronchospasm.
- For major surgery, start chest physiotherapy preoperatively.
- Consider premedicating the patient with an anticholinergic agent, such
  as glycopyrronium or atropine, to dry out secretions and suppress
  upper airway vagal responses.
- Add nebulized salbutamol 2.5mg to the premedication.
- Consider the need for an arterial line intra-operatively in high-risk cases
  to facilitate ABG measurement.
- No definitive evidence shows that one method is superior to another.
- When asthma is poorly controlled, regional techniques are ideal for
  peripheral surgery. Spinal anaesthesia or plexus/nerve blocks are
  generally safe, provided the patient is able to lie flat comfortably.
- Where GA is necessary, use short-acting anaesthetic agents.
  Short-acting opioid analgesics (e.g. alfentanil, remifentanil) are
  appropriate for procedures with minimal post-operative pain or when a
  reliable regional block is present (Table 5.3).
- Intubation may provoke bronchospasm. Consider potent opioid cover
  (alfentanil). LA to the cords may help. Only instrument the airway when
  the patient is in a deep plane of anaesthesia. The use of an LMA may
  be preferable to tracheal intubation in asthmatic patients; however, the
  benefits of these must be weighed up against the risks of an unsecured
  airway.
- Ventilatory strategies, such as limiting peak inspiratory pressures and
  V_T and lengthening the I:E ratio, assist in avoiding air trapping and
  auto-PEEP.
- Avoid histamine-releasing drugs or use with care (morphine,
  d-tubocurarine, atracurium, mivacurium).
- Inspired gases should be humidified to avoid airway irritation.
- Stimulating manoeuvres, such as airway suctioning, should be avoided or
  only performed while the patient is deeply anaesthetized.
- Reversal of neuromuscular-blocking agents using acetylcholinesterase
  inhibitors should be used with caution in asthmatics due to their
  muscarinic side effects such as bronchospasm.
- Prophylactic use of antiemetic agents or antacids should be considered
  to avoid aspiration, which can trigger severe bronchospasm.

Table 5.3 Drugs considered safe for asthmatics

Induction	Propofol, etomidate, ketamine, midazolam
Opioids	Pethidine, fentanyl, alfentanil, remifentanil
Muscle relaxants	Suxamethonium, vecuronium, rocuronium, pancuronium, cisatracurium
Volatile agents	Halothane, isoflurane, enflurane, sevoflurane

Severe bronchospasm during anaesthesia
(See ➲ p. 909.)

Post-operative care

- Patients with severe asthma (previous ICU admissions, brittle disease) undergoing major abdominal or thoracic surgery should be admitted to HDU/ICU for post-operative observation.
- If acute bronchospasm persists at the end of the operation, or if it has been severe, or if the patient has a difficult airway, trauma, or full stomach, consideration should be given to a period of post-operative mechanical ventilation to avoid having to reverse the NMB and to allow time for airway recovery.
- Ensure all usual medications are prescribed after surgery.
- Following major abdominal or thoracic surgery, good pain control is important, and epidural analgesia is frequently the best choice, provided widespread intercostal blockade is avoided.
- For patient-controlled analgesia (PCA), consider fentanyl if morphine has previously exacerbated bronchospasm.
- Prescribe O_2 for the duration of epidural or PCA.
- Prescribe regular nebulizer therapy, with additional nebulized bronchodilators as needed.
- Review the dose and route of administration of steroid daily.
- Regular NSAIDs can be used if tolerated in the past. Avoid in brittle and poorly controlled asthmatics.
- If there is increasing dyspnoea and wheeze following surgery, consider other possible contributing factors (LV failure and PEs are potent triggers of bronchospasm). Also consider fluid overload and pneumothorax (check for recent central line).

References

21 British Thoracic Society, Scottish Intercollegiate Guidelines Network (2008). *British guideline on the management of asthma. A national clinical guideline, revised 2012.* ℰ https://www.brit-thoracic.org.uk/document-library/clinical-information/asthma/btssign-guideline-on-the-management-of-asthma/.

22 Woods BD, Sladen RN (2009). Perioperative considerations for the patient with asthma and bronchospasm. *Br J Anaesth*, **103** (suppl 1), i57–65.

23 Applegate R, Lauer R, Lenart J, Gatling J, Vadi M (2013). The perioperative management of asthma. *J Allergy Ther*, **S11**, 007.

Chronic obstructive pulmonary disease

- COPD[24-27] is a common, preventable, and treatable disease. It is characterized by airflow obstruction that is usually progressive and associated with an enhanced chronic inflammatory response in the airways and the lung to noxious particles or gases.
- The more familiar terms 'chronic bronchitis' and 'emphysema' are now included within the COPD diagnosis.
- Chronic bronchitis is defined as a chronic, productive cough for 3 months in each of two successive years in a patient in whom other causes of cough (e.g. bronchiectasis) have been excluded. Small airway inflammation causes obstruction and air trapping, which results in V/Q mismatching and poor respiratory muscle mechanics.
- Emphysema is a histological diagnosis of abnormal and permanent enlargement of the airspaces distal to the terminal bronchioles without obvious fibrosis. Loss of alveolar structural integrity leads to decreased gas transfer as well as V/Q mismatching.
- Often it is not possible to distinguish between the two subtypes, and the relative contribution of each varies from patient to patient.
- There is no single diagnostic test for COPD. Diagnosis relies on a combination of history, examination, and confirmation of airflow obstruction using spirometry.
- Both NICE and Global Initiative for Chronic Obstructive Lung Disease (GOLD) provide guidelines for the diagnosis and assessment of COPD.
- The most important risk factor for COPD is cigarette smoking. Other factors associated with COPD include occupational exposure to dusts and atmospheric pollution, poor socio-economic status, repeated viral infections, α-1 antitrypsin deficiency, and regional variation. Genetic factors may also be implicated.
- A diagnosis of COPD should be considered in patients over the age of 35, who have a risk factor (generally smoking) and who present with exertional breathlessness, chronic cough, regular sputum production, frequent winter 'bronchitis', or wheeze. The presence of airflow obstruction should be confirmed by performing post-bronchodilator spirometry. Airflow obstruction defined by an FEV_1/FVC ratio of <0.7 is used to diagnose COPD.
- There is no single test to assess the severity of COPD. Instead, it is assessed using a range of factors, including measurement of the degree of airflow obstruction, the level of disability, the frequency of exacerbations, FEV_1, TLCO, the degree of breathlessness, exercise tolerance, and BMI.

General considerations

- Patients with a diagnosis of COPD have an increased risk of perioperative pulmonary complications.
- Frequent exacerbations of COPD can occur, causing a rapid and sustained worsening of the patient's symptoms beyond normal day-to-day variations.
- COPD is not an absolute contraindication to any surgery.

- The further the procedure from the diaphragm, the lower the complication rate.
- COPD is associated with a number of co-morbidities such as lung cancer and pulmonary hypertension.

Preoperative assessment

- Preoperative assessment should include a careful history, physical examination, and assessment of functional capacity.
- Close attention should be paid to a history of smoking, dyspnoea, cough, and sputum production.
- Establish the exercise tolerance—ask specifically about hills and stairs. Simple exercise tests, such as stair climbing and the 6MWT, are safe and simple to perform, and correlate well with more formal exercise testing.
- Enquire as to the frequency of exacerbations, timings of the most recent course of antibiotics or steroids, hospital admissions, and previous requirements for invasive and non-invasive ventilation.
- Assess the nutritional status. Poor nutritional status with a serum albumin <35g/L is a strong predictor of post-operative pulmonary complications.
- Decreased breath sounds, prolonged expiration, and wheeze are predictive of post-operative pulmonary complications.
- Surgery should, if possible, be postponed and appropriate treatment started if symptoms and signs of an active respiratory infection are found.

Investigations

- Preoperative spirometry is useful if clinical evaluation cannot determine whether the patient is at their best baseline and that airflow obstruction is optimally reduced. It also aids the assessment of severity of COPD. Identification of severe airflow obstruction may be particularly important in patients who are candidates for upper abdominal or thoracic surgical procedures.
- Check ABGs in patients with moderate to severe COPD. Useful to determine post-operative respiratory parameters.
- ECG may reveal right heart disease (RV hypertrophy or strain) or concomitant IHD. Consider echocardiography.
- CXR is not mandatory. It should be considered if there is clinical evidence of current infection or recent deterioration in symptoms, as it is useful in excluding an LRTI or malignancy.

Preoperative optimization

- Every effort should be made to assist patients in stopping smoking. Smoking cessation at least 8wk preoperatively is optimal.
- All patients with symptomatic COPD should receive daily inhaled ipratropium or tiotropium.
- Inhaled β-agonists should be used, as needed, for symptoms and wheezing in the perioperative period.
- Continue patients' usual inhaled medication in the perioperative period.
- Patients with COPD, persistent wheeze, and functional limitations, despite bronchodilators, should be treated with perioperative glucocorticoids. Ideally, these patients should be reviewed by a respiratory physician preoperatively.

- If patients have severe COPD, post-operative respiratory failure is likely after abdominal or thoracic surgery. Plan for elective HDU/ICU admission.
- Consider preoperative chest physiotherapy in patients with copious sputum production. This may reduce the incidence of intra-operative bronchial plugging or pneumonitis.
- Pulmonary rehabilitation, in the form of patient education, exercise training, and behavioural interventions, is not currently routine in the preoperative management of these patients but may become commonplace in the near future.
- Consider the need for preoperative nutritional supplementation.

Conduct of anaesthesia

- GA, and in particular tracheal intubation and IPPV, is associated with adverse outcomes in patients with COPD. Such patients are prone to bronchospasm, laryngospasm, CVS instability, barotrauma, hypoxaemia, and increased rates of post-operative pulmonary complications.
- Consider avoiding GA by using a regional anaesthetic technique, where possible. This may be limited by some patients' inability to lie flat.
- Consider using an arterial line for both beat-to-beat BP analysis and repeated blood gas analysis.
- Where GA cannot be avoided, preoxygenation should be used in any patient who is hypoxic on air prior to induction.
- Avoid intubation where possible. Some patients, however, are unsuitable for a spontaneously breathing technique (particularly those who are obese, breathless, and require long operations). Patients with heavy sputum production may benefit from endotracheal toilet.
- If using IPPV, consider using PEEP and allowing more time for exhalation by decreasing the respiratory rate or the I:E ratio (typically 1:3–1:5). These approaches may help to reduce air trapping and the development of intrinsic PEEP, both of which can cause an increase in intrathoracic pressure, which can lead to CVS instability. Harmful effects of air trapping include pulmonary barotrauma, hypercapnia, and acidosis.
- Ensure the neuromuscular agent is fully reversed, the patient is warm and well oxygenated, and has a $PaCO_2$ close to the patient's normal preoperative values prior to extubation.
- Extubate in the sitting position.
- Bronchodilator treatment may be helpful peri-extubation.
- Extubation of the high-risk patient directly onto non-invasive ventilation may reduce the work of breathing and air trapping.

Post-operative care

- Those patients with severe disease or significant co-morbidities should be managed in a high-dependency setting capable of regular ABG measurements and the provision of non-invasive ventilation.
- Hypoventilation as a result of residual anaesthesia or opioids should be avoided, as this may lead to hypercapnia and hypoxia.
- Encourage early mobilization.
- Use of saline nebulization, suctioning, and physiotherapy are useful to prevent atelectasis and to encourage sputum production.

- Continue with nebulized salbutamol (2.5mg qds) and ipratropium (500 micrograms qds) until fully mobile. Change back to inhalers at least 24hr before discharge.
- Effective analgesia is a significant determinant of post-operative pulmonary function. Epidural anaesthesia is an attractive option, as it reduces the risk of respiratory failure because of excessive sedation from opioids. It should therefore be considered, if appropriate.

References

24 National Institute for Health and Care Excellence (2010). *Chronic obstructive pulmonary disease: management of chronic obstructive pulmonary disease in adults in primary and secondary care (partial update)*. NICE *clinical guideline* **101**. ℳ https://www.nice.org.uk/guidance/cg101/resources/guidance-chronic-obstructive-pulmonary-disease-pdf guidance.nice.org.uk/cg101.

25 Global Initiative for Chronic Obstructive Lung Disease (GOLD) (2015). *Global strategy for the diagnosis, management, and prevention of chronic obstructive pulmonary disease*. ℳ http://www.goldcopd.org/uploads/users/files/GOLD_Report_2015_Feb18.pdf.

26 Lumb A, Biercamp C (2013). Chronic obstructive pulmonary disease and anaesthesia. *Contin Educ Anaesth Crit Care Pain*, doi:10.1093/bjaceaccp/mkt023.

27 American Thoracic Society (2005). *COPD guidelines for health professionals*. ℳ http://www.thoracic.org/go/copd.

Bronchiectasis

Bronchiectasis has similar features to COPD, including inflamed and easily collapsible airways, obstruction to airflow, and frequent hospitalizations. The diagnosis is usually established clinically on the basis of a chronic daily cough with thick, mucopurulent sputum production, and radiographically by the presence of bronchial wall thickening and dilatation of the bronchi and bronchioles on chest CT scans.

It is an acquired disorder that is characterized by permanent abnormal dilatation and destruction of the bronchial and bronchiolar walls. This pathology is caused by an infectious insult, impairment of drainage, airway obstruction, and/or a defect in host defence.

There are multiple aetiologies that can lead to the pathophysiological processes that cause bronchiectasis. These include airway obstruction (e.g. foreign body aspiration), defective host defences, cystic fibrosis (CF), rheumatic diseases, dyskinetic cilia, smoking, pulmonary infections, and allergic bronchopulmonary aspergillosis.

General considerations

- Patients with bronchiectasis need to be as fit as possible before undergoing any major surgery, which will inhibit coughing and impair respiratory function.
- Once established, bacterial infections can be difficult or impossible to eradicate. *Pseudomonas aeruginosa* is a common pathogen that may be present for many years and be associated with intermittent exacerbations of respiratory symptoms.
- The mainstay of treatment for bronchiectasis is regular physiotherapy, frequent courses of appropriate antibiotics, and treatment of any asthmatic symptoms.

Preoperative assessment

- Before elective surgery, the patient should be as fit as possible. This may mean a planned admission for IV antibiotics and physiotherapy prior to surgery.
- Consultation with the patient's chest physician is essential.
- Send a sputum sample for culture before surgery. A course of IV antibiotics and physiotherapy for 3–10d immediately prior to surgery may be necessary. Prior to major surgery, consider starting IV antibiotics on admission. Use current or most recent sputum cultures, with advice from the microbiologist/local protocols, to guide appropriate prescribing. If in doubt, assume that the patient has *P. aeruginosa*.
- Maximize bronchodilation by converting to nebulized bronchodilators.
- Increase the dose of prednisolone by 5–10mg/d if on long-term oral steroids.
- Postpone elective surgery if the patient has more respiratory symptoms than usual.

Investigations

- In patients with severe disease, check spirometry and blood gases.
- Send a sputum sample for culture.

Conduct of anaesthesia

- Choose regional above GA where possible.
- Although it is desirable to avoid intubation, this will be necessary for all but the shortest operations to facilitate intra-operative removal of secretions.
- Use short-acting anaesthetic and analgesic agents where post-operative pain is minimal or regional analgesia can be used.
- Extubate and recover in the sitting position.
- Ensure that the patient receives physiotherapy immediately post-operatively.

Post-operative care

- Ensure that regular physiotherapy is available—three times daily (tds), and at night if severely affected.
- Monitor SpO_2, giving supplemental O_2 to achieve adequate oxygenation (guided by preoperative value).
- Continue appropriate IV antibiotics for at least 3d post-operatively or until discharged.
- Maintain adequate nutrition, especially if any malabsorption.
- Refer to the respiratory physician early if there is any deterioration in respiratory symptoms.

Cystic fibrosis

CF[28–30] is a multisystem, autosomal recessive disease and is the commonest lethal genetic disease in Caucasians. The disease is caused by mutations in a single gene—the CF transmembrane regulator (*CFTR*) gene on chromosome 7.

The CFTR is a chloride (Cl^-) channel found at the apical border of epithelial cells, which line most exocrine glands in the body. All mutations causing CF lead to abnormal Cl^- conductance through the CFTR channel. This results in loss of Cl^- transport and a disturbance of the sodium (Na^+)/Cl^- balance needed to maintain a normal thin mucus layer. In CF, the mucus is viscid and is less well cleared by the cilia.

The clinical manifestations of CF include progressive lung disease (frequent LRTI, chronic hypoxaemia, and cor pulmonale), nasal problems (chronic sinusitis and nasal polyps), hepatobiliary system disease due to obstruction of bile ductules (focal biliary cirrhosis, portal hypertension, multinodular biliary cirrhosis), meconium ileus, recurrent abdominal pain, pancreatic exocrine insufficiency and CF-related diabetes, infertility, and osteoporosis.

General considerations

- Patients with severe disease are best managed in a major centre with multidisciplinary input.
- Neonates may present for surgical treatment of meconium ileus.
- Nasal polypectomy, enteral feeding, or vascular access device placement are commonly performed as elective surgical procedures for CF patients.
- Almost all patients with CF have symptoms of bronchiectasis (see p. 106).
- The perioperative complication rate in CF is ~10% (mostly pulmonary), but half of this is for minor ear, nose, and throat (ENT) procedures.
- Day-case surgery is uncommon in CF patients; however, it is possible in patients with stable disease and a good baseline functional status.

Preoperative assessment

- Gain a history of therapy, medications, and exacerbations.
- Exclude or treat active chest infection.
- Ascertain the patient's functional ability.
- Note details of the non-respiratory components.
- Always inform the patient's physician of an admission to a surgical ward.

Investigations

- FBC, U&Es, coagulation study, LFTs, and blood glucose should be performed.
- Respiratory assessment tests include CXR, baseline ABG analysis, and spirometry.
- Spirometry generally shows an obstructive pattern, with a decrease in FEV_1 and the FEV_1/FVC ratio.
- In advanced disease, an ECG and echocardiogram are useful to diagnose cor pulmonale.

- A 6MWT forms part of the pre-lung transplant work-up in many centres. The results of this may be available when patients present for non-transplant surgery.
- CPET may prove to be a useful indicator of physiological reserve.

Conduct of anaesthesia

- Consider placing an arterial line to facilitate frequent ABG analysis.
- Consider using cardiac output monitoring in patients with cor pulmonale who present for major surgery.
- For short or non-abdominal or non-thoracic procedures, an LMA with a spontaneously breathing patient may minimize the adverse effects of GA on respiratory mechanics.
- An ETT, however, allows bronchial toilet and improved control of gas exchange.
- Avoid nasal intubation, where possible, due to the high incidence of nasal polyposis.
- Keep airway pressures as low as possible when using positive pressure ventilation. Monitor for pneumothorax.
- Use humidified gases.
- Short-acting drugs should be used, wherever possible, to facilitate rapid emergence.
- Patients are often cachectic, so careful positioning and padding is important.
- Consider a regional anaesthetic technique, where appropriate, to avoid airway manipulation and to optimize post-operative analgesia.

Post-operative care

- Aim to minimize the risk of development of a post-operative respiratory tract infection.
- Aim to extubate early.
- Ensure NMB is fully reversed.
- For patients who use home non-invasive ventilation, ensure that the patient's own equipment is available immediately post-operatively.
- Chest physiotherapy should be resumed as early as possible.
- It is appropriate for patients with advanced disease to be monitored in a high dependency setting.
- For patients with FEV_1 <1L, PaO_2 <9.3kPa, or $PaCO_2$ >6.6kPa, consider a period of post-operative ventilation.
- Eighty per cent of CF patients have pancreatic malabsorption. Maintaining adequate nutrition after surgery is essential, as is the advice of an experienced dietitian.

References

28 Della Rocca G (2002). Anaesthesia in patients with cystic fibrosis. *Curr Opin Anesthesiol*, **15**, 95–101.
29 Huffmyer JL, Littlewood KE, Nemergut EC (2009). Perioperative management of the adult with cystic fibrosis. *Anesth Analg*, **109**, 1949–61.
30 Fitzgerald M, Ryan D (2011). Cystic fibrosis and anaesthesia. *Contin Educ Anaesth Crit Care Pain*, doi:10.1093/bjaceaccp/mkr038.

Restrictive pulmonary disease

- Restrictive lung disease is characterized by a reduced lung volume, due to disease of either the lung parenchyma or the pleura, chest wall, or neuromuscular apparatus. There is a reduction in total lung capacity (TLC), VC, and resting V_T.
- The many disorders that cause a reduction of lung volume may be classified into intrinsic and extrinsic pulmonary disease.

Diffuse parenchymal lung disease

- A diverse group of disorders (often referred to as interstitial lung disease) that are classified together because of similar clinical, radiographic, physiological, or pathological manifestations.
- Results in decreased lung compliance and impaired gas exchange.
- An initial inflammatory reaction in the alveoli impairs gas exchange. This is followed by collagen deposition and fibrosis, resulting in lungs that are smaller in volume and less compliant to inflation.
- Diffuse parenchymal lung diseases are divided into those that are associated with known causes and those that are idiopathic.
- The commonest identifiable causes include exposure to occupational and environmental agents, especially to inorganic or organic dusts, drug-induced pulmonary toxicity (e.g. amiodarone, chemotherapy agents, and paraquat poisoning), and radiation-induced lung injury. Diffuse parenchymal lung disease can also complicate the course of most connective tissue disorders (e.g. dermatomyositis, rheumatoid arthritis (RA), SLE, and scleroderma).
- Idiopathic causes include sarcoidosis, cryptogenic organizing pneumonia, and the idiopathic interstitial pneumonias.
- A variety of infections can cause interstitial opacities on CXR, including fungal pneumonias, atypical bacterial and viral pneumonias. These infections often occur in immunocompromised hosts.
- Treatment is usually with oral steroids, but other immunosuppressive therapy may be used, and young patients may be considered for lung transplantation if severely affected.

Extrinsic conditions of the chest wall

- The components of the chest wall include the bony structures (ribs, spine), respiratory muscles, and nerves connecting the central nervous system (CNS) with the respiratory muscles.
- Disease that alters the structure of the chest wall will affect the mechanics of ventilation and may result in respiratory compromise or failure.
- Examples of conditions that affect the chest wall include ankylosing spondylitis, congenital deformities (such as pectus excavatum, flail chest, kyphoscoliosis), thoracoplasty, abdominal processes (such as morbid obesity and ascites), and chest wall tumours.

General considerations

- The work of respiration is optimized by rapid shallow breaths and is easier in the sitting position.

- Many patients are stable and only slowly deteriorate over some years. These patients may tolerate surgery relatively well.

Preoperative assessment

- Should focus on determining the degree of respiratory impairment and the underlying disease process to establish the extent of involvement of other organs.
- A history of exertional dyspnoea (or at rest) should be evaluated further with ABGs and PFTs.
- Discuss seriously affected patients with a respiratory physician.

Investigations

- ABGs—often remain normal until late. Reduced PaO_2 reflects significant disease, and CO_2 retention is a late sign, implying impending ventilatory failure.
- Obtain PFTs, including spirometry, lung volumes (all are reduced), and gas transfer, if these have not been done within the previous 6–8wk. A VC of <15mL/kg is indicative of severe dysfunction.
- CXR changes will be according to the underlying condition.

Conduct of anaesthesia

- As for other pathologies, consider regional techniques, and minimize positive pressure ventilation and airway instrumentation as far as possible. Spinal disease may preclude subarachnoid or epidural blocks.
- Where IPPV is necessary, minimize peak airway pressure using pressure-controlled ventilation with high rate and low V_T.
- Check the need for additional steroid cover at induction for those patients on regular steroid therapy (see ➜ p. 165).
- Maintain a high index of suspicion for pneumothorax.

Post-operative care

- Consider post-operative ICU/HDU admission following major surgery. May be suitable for elective training in CPAP/non-invasive positive pressure ventilation (NIPPV) techniques preoperatively.
- Extubate in a sitting position.
- Give supplemental O_2, and maintain SpO_2 >92%.
- Good physiotherapy and analgesia are vital to achieve sputum clearance. With severe disease, minor respiratory complications may precipitate respiratory failure.
- Mobilize early.
- Treat respiratory infection vigorously.
- Ensure steroid cover continues in appropriate formulation.

Sleep apnoea syndrome

(See also ➔ p. 630.)

Sleep apnoea[31–33] is defined as cessation of airflow at the mouth and nose for at least 10s. Sufferers develop intermittent respiratory arrest and hypoxaemia during rapid eye movement (REM) sleep. Respiration resumes due to hypoxic stimulation.

- The majority of sufferers are overweight, middle-aged men, who present with complaints of snoring with periods of apnoea, disturbed sleep, excessive daytime drowsiness, and headache.
- Two types of sleep apnoea are recognized:
  - OSA (85%). This results from obstruction of the upper airway
  - Central apnoea (5%). This is due to intermittent loss of respiratory drive.
- Five per cent of patients have both types.
- The condition can often be diagnosed using history and examination alone, but, for standardization and a qualitative diagnosis, more formal investigations are required. A sleep study with polysomnography (PSG) will establish the extent and severity of OSA. PSG examinations include recordings of ECG, electroencephalography (EEG), eye movements, and electromyography. Snoring volume, oronasal airflow, and peripheral pulse oximetry are usually also recorded.
- The two most widely available treatment options for OSA include weight loss and CPAP.

General considerations

- There is an increased perioperative risk in OSA patients. This is likely due to increased upper airway collapse and OSA-related co-morbidities.
- OSA is an independent risk factor for serious neurocognitive, endocrine, and CVS morbidity and mortality in all age groups. For example, OSA patients are at increased risk of cerebrovascular accidents, depression, psychosocial problems, impaired glucose tolerance, dyslipidaemia, hypertension, and arrhythmias.
- Biventricular dysfunction, pulmonary hypertension, and CCF significantly increase the risk of haemodynamic instability in the perioperative period.
- In children, OSA is most commonly associated with adenotonsillar hypertrophy, but the severity of OSA is not always proportional to the size of the tonsils and adenoids.
- Patients with sleep apnoea syndrome are at risk of perioperative airway obstruction and respiratory failure, while under the effects of sedative drugs.

Preoperative assessment

- OSA is undiagnosed in ~80% of patients. Preoperative evaluation should include a review of previous medical records, a history from the patient and/or family, and a physical examination.
- Check for airway difficulty with previous anaesthetics, hypertension, or other CVS problems. Ask about snoring, apnoeic episodes, disturbed sleep, morning headaches, and daytime somnolence.

- Several screening tools have been developed and validated to identify potential surgical patients with OSA: the Berlin questionnaire, the ASA checklist, and the STOP-Bang questionnaire.
- While these questionnaires have been validated as screening tools for OSA in the surgical population, formal preoperative testing with PSG in patients with clinical risk factors for OSA is still useful to diagnose and determine the severity of OSA.
- Ideally, patients with OSA should be risk-stratified to assess whether PSG (an expensive resource, which is often scarce and often has long waiting times) is required to assess severity, whether they are suitable for day-case surgery, and whether they require high dependency care post-operatively.
- Factors to take into consideration when assessing the level of risk in these patients include patient and surgical factors and the perioperative sedation risk.
- Patient factors include the severity of OSA, presence of craniofacial abnormalities, compliance with CPAP, and obesity.
- Surgical factors include the site and duration of surgery, whether it can be performed laparoscopically, and whether it can be done using a regional anaesthetic technique.
- High perioperative sedation risk includes patients who are likely to require high doses of opioids in the perioperative period.
- Among preoperative patients in whom it is determined that diagnostic evaluation for OSA is warranted, clinicians need to decide whether to defer surgery until after a formal sleep evaluation or to manage the patient presumptively.
- Early liaison with the surgical team, respiratory physicians, and intensive care is important in high-risk patients.
- A period of preoperative CPAP may be beneficial, particularly in high-risk patients.
- OSA should be considered in all children presenting for adenotonsillectomy.
- Ensure that management of associated conditions, such as obstructive airway disease, hypertension, and cardiac failure, is optimal.
- Ask patients to bring their own CPAP machine and mask for post-operative use. Ensure that ward staff are familiar with the set-up and running of equipment.

Investigations
- In known OSA, perform FBC (polycythaemia), pulse oximetry, and ECG (right heart strain).
- If ECG shows RV strain (3% of children presenting for adenotonsillectomy), echocardiography is indicated to exclude RV hypertrophy.
- Obtain baseline ABGs.
- Consider referral for PSG in high-risk patients.

Conduct of anaesthesia
- If the patient is on inhalers, change to nebulized bronchodilators.
- Avoid night sedation or sedative premedication, as patients with OSA are susceptible to the central respiratory effects of benzodiazepines,

opioids, and neuroleptics. Also, by enhancing the relaxation of the pharyngeal muscles during sleep, these drugs compound the symptoms of OSA.

- Anticipate that mask ventilation and intubation may be difficult, and prepare for this.
- Regional anaesthesia/analgesia and post-operative analgesia will avoid or minimize the use of GA agents and sedative opioid analgesics. Reduce doses of all sedative/anaesthesia drugs. Use short-acting anaesthetic/ analgesic agents where post-operative pain is minimal.
- GA, preceded by preoxygenation, with tracheal intubation and mechanical ventilation is preferred to sedation or a GA with spontaneous ventilation (SV).
- Give NSAIDs and paracetamol.

Post-operative care

- Ensure NMB is fully reversed, and extubate fully awake in the sitting position.
- Nurse sitting up whenever possible.
- High-risk patients may require admission to HDU/ICU. A few hours of post-operative ventilation may be required after major surgery.
- Administer supplementary O_2, and ensure continuous pulse oximetry monitoring on the ward.
- Unless contraindicated by the surgical procedure, CPAP should be administered continuously to patients who were using it preoperatively. Compliance may be improved if patients bring their own equipment into hospital.
- Aim to maintain the O_2 saturation that the patient had preoperatively, titrating O_2 to the minimum required. A few patients may develop CO_2 retention with O_2 therapy. Serial blood gas analysis may be necessary in drowsy patients at risk of CO_2 retention.

References

31 Martinez G, Faber P (2011). Obstructive sleep apnoea. *Contin Educ Anaesth Crit Care Pain*, **11**, 5–8.

32 Weinberg L, Tay S, Lai CF, Barnes M (2013). Perioperative risk stratification for a patient with severe obstructive sleep apnoea undergoing laparoscopic banding surgery. *BMJ Case Rep*, pii, bcr2012008336.

33 Gross JB, Bachenberg KL, Benumof JL, *et al*.; American Society of Anesthesiologists Task Force on Perioperative Management (2006). Practice guidelines for the perioperative management of patients with obstructive sleep apnea: a report by the American Society of Anesthesiologists Task Force on Perioperative Management of patients with obstructive sleep apnea. *Anesthesiology*, **104**, 1081–93.

Sarcoidosis

A multisystem disease of unknown aetiology, characterized by the formation of non-caseating granulomata, which occur in any body tissue and heal with fibrosis. It occurs at all ages, with the highest prevalence at 20–40yr. It is commoner in black individuals in the US.

General considerations

- Pulmonary changes occur in 50% of cases. Pleural, peribronchial, and alveolar granulomata are replaced by fibrosis. Hilar lymphadenopathy may cause bronchial obstruction and distal atelectasis. Infiltration of the bronchial mucosa may cause stenosis. Mucosal infiltration of the nose, nasopharynx, tonsils, palate, or larynx may occur.
- Cardiac effects (in 20%). Right ventricular failure 2° to lung disease. Myocardial and valvular granulomata are rare. Conduction abnormalities, VT, and sudden death have been reported.
- Other effects include skin involvement, uveitis/iritis, and hypercalcaemia.

Preoperative assessment

- Pulmonary and cardiac features are most important.
- May have extensive pathology, but only minor symptoms.
- Note steroid treatment or other immunosuppressive drugs.

Investigations

- Preoperative respiratory function tests may reveal a restrictive defect. TLCO (DLCO) may be reduced. ABGs will determine the level of hypoxaemia.
- ECG may show RV hypertrophy or arrhythmias.
- Check serum calcium (Ca^{2+}) for hypercalcaemia (treat with systemic steroids).

Conduct of anaesthesia

- Consider avoidance of GA and the use of local/regional anaesthesia, where possible, if respiratory function is impaired clinically.
- Consider regional analgesia for abdominal surgery if significant respiratory disease.
- Give appropriate steroid cover, if needed.

Post-operative care

- Nurse the patient sitting upright.
- Good post-operative analgesia.
- Chest physiotherapy/breathing exercises.

Anaesthesia after lung transplantation

(See also ⊃ The patient with a transplanted heart, p. 62.)

Lung transplantation[34,35] was first performed in 1963; outcomes have improved since the introduction of ciclosporin A in 1981. Surgery may be indicated for:
- Complications related to transplant
- Complications of immunosuppressive treatment
- The underlying condition (emphysema, α-1 antitrypsin deficiency, pulmonary fibrosis, 1° pulmonary hypertension, CF)
- Unrelated reasons.

General considerations
- The loss of afferent and efferent innervation distal to the bronchial anastomosis results in loss of the cough reflex (i.e. to stimuli distal to the anastomosis) and neurally mediated changes in the bronchomotor tone.
- Airway reactivity does not appear to be increased.
- Mucociliary clearance is impaired in the pulmonary allograft, which, together with immunosuppression and impaired cough, places the patient at increased risk for perioperative pneumonia.
- Hypoxic vasoconstriction is unimpaired, so, during an episode of acute rejection, pulmonary blood flow may be directed away from the transplanted lung.
- Lymphatic drainage is severed but then re-established 2–4wk post-transplantation. Transplanted lungs are at particular risk of pulmonary oedema, especially in the early post-operative period.
- Allograft function may be compromised at any time by episodes of acute rejection, which are often difficult to distinguish clinically from pulmonary infection.
- In double-lung transplant, the heart may be denervated and has a higher resting HR (90–100bpm). It may be more susceptible to arrhythmias.

Preoperative assessment
- Assess the status of the transplanted lung(s). Have there been any episodes of rejection and increased immunosuppression?
- Look for evidence of rejection or infection. All but the most urgent procedures should be delayed if there is a reversible complication present.
- In patients with single-lung transplants, careful attention should be paid to establish the extent of disease and the degree of compromise in the native lung, because these factors may have implications for the provision of mechanical ventilation. For example, differential lung ventilation requiring a double-lumen tube may be required.
- Symptoms, such as dry cough and dyspnoea, 8–12 months post-operatively may indicate obliterative bronchiolitis, the predominant feature of chronic transplant rejection. This is characterized by progressive narrowing of the small airways.
- Evaluate the extent of any residual systemic disease and the effects of immunosuppressive drugs on other organ function.

- Assess for airway narrowing or compromise. Previous tracheostomy may have caused a degree of subglottic stenosis.
- Coordinate with transplant or respiratory services. Make a plan for whether they will need to review the patient perioperatively.

Conduct of anaesthesia

- The interaction of immunosuppressive drugs (ciclosporin, steroids, azathioprine) with anaesthetic drugs is more theoretical than clinical.
- Stress doses of steroids will be required in most cases.
- Attention to aseptic techniques is important, as immunosuppression occurs with most chemotherapeutic drugs.
- There is no evidence to suggest that placing CVCs on the side opposite the transplanted lung is safer.
- Monitor neuromuscular function, and avoid high doses of opioid in order to achieve early extubation.
- Intubation should be performed to leave the tube just through the cords, and the cuff carefully inflated and checked intraoperatively, to minimize the risk of damage to the tracheal/bronchial anastomosis. If a double-lumen tube is required, it should be placed under direct vision using a fibrescope.
- The basic goal in ventilation is ensuring adequate oxygenation and ventilation while minimizing peak airway pressures and O_2 administration.
- A mask or LMA is not contraindicated, although there is a risk of silent aspiration in patients with no carinal cough reflex.
- Strict attention to fluid balance is required.
- Aim for early return of pulmonary function and extubation.

Post-operative care

- Post-operative admission to ICU is only indicated when anaesthesia is complicated by inadequate recovery of respiratory function, the surgical condition, or the presence of rejection or infection.
- Chest physiotherapy, postural drainage, and incentive spirometry in the post-operative period may be beneficial.

References

34 Haddow GR (1997). Anaesthesia for patients after lung transplantation. *Can J Anaesth*, **44**, 182–97.
35 Elsharkawy H, Lewis B, Farag E (2008). Anesthetic challenges in patients after lung transplantation. *The Internet Journal of Anesthesiology*, **20**, Number 1.

Renal disease

Quentin Milner

See also:

Creatinine clearance

Preoperative renal dysfunction is an independent risk factor for post-operative morbidity and mortality. Creatinine is a product of skeletal muscle metabolism and undergoes little renal tubular secretion, so creatinine clearance reflects the GFR (normal GFR = 125mL/min). Plasma creatinine shows a rectangular hyperbolic relationship with creatinine clearance. This means:

- GFR must be reduced by 50% before serum creatinine starts to rise
- Small changes in serum creatinine in the low (normal) range imply a large change in GFR, making the test very sensitive
- GFR falls by 1% per annum after 30yr of age
- Low muscle mass (e.g. small elderly lady) means little creatinine to clear, so normal plasma creatinine may not mean a normal renal function
- Creatinine clearance (CC) can be more accurately estimated from the serum creatinine by using the Cockcroft–Gault formula (Fig. 6.1).

$$\text{Creatinine clearance (mL/min)} = \frac{(140 - \text{age}) \times \text{weight (kg)}}{0.814 \times \text{serum creatinine (micromoles/L)}} \quad (\times\, 0.85 \text{ for women)}.$$

Fig. 6.1 The Cockcroft–Gault formula.

Chronic renal failure

Chronic renal failure (CRF) (Box 6.1) is a multisystem disease. Patients often have complex medical histories, take a multitude of drugs, and may have severe systemic complications. Dialysis is usually required when the GFR is <15mL/min.

> **Box 6.1 Main causes of CRF**
>
> | | |
> |---|---|
> | Diabetes mellitus | 30% |
> | Hypertension | 24% |
> | Glomerulonephritis | 17% |
> | Chronic pyelonephritis | 5% |
> | Polycystic renal disease | 4% |
> | Unknown cause | 20% |

Classification of chronic renal failure

- Stage 1, normal GFR—other evidence of renal damage.
- Stage 2, GFR 60–90mL/min—other evidence of renal damage.
- Stage 3, GFR 30–60mL/min—moderate CRF.
- Stage 4, GFR 15–30mL/min—severe CRF.
- Stage 5, GFR <15mL/min—end-stage renal failure. Dialysis-dependent.

Preoperative

- These patients are high-risk, particularly diabetics with CRF.
- Determine the underlying cause, previous surgery, including transplantation, and drug therapy.
- Check for hypertension, diabetes, and anaemia. IHD is very common and often silent, especially in diabetics. Incidence of calcific valvular heart disease and LV failure is increased. Autonomic neuropathy is common. Pericardial effusions are rare if dialysis is effective.
- Check the type of dialysis: peritoneal or haemodialysis—line or fistula.
- Determine the residual urine output per day.
- Examine for fluid overload (dependent oedema, basal crepitations, dialysis record, weight) or hypovolaemia (postural hypotension, low JVP, thirst, skin turgor, urine output).
- Allow 4–6hr to elapse after haemodialysis before surgery. This allows fluid compartment equilibration and metabolism of residual heparin. Indications for urgent dialysis include hyperkalaemia, fluid overload, acute acidosis, and symptomatic uraemia. If volume overload occurs post-operatively, the patient will need extra dialysis.
- If major surgery, plan post-operative care with renal/ICU team.

Investigations

- FBC: usually well-compensated normochromic normocytic anaemia due to decreased erythropoiesis and red cell survival and GI losses. Aim for Hb 8–10g/dL; transfusion can worsen hypertension and precipitate heart failure.
- Electrolytes: a recent serum K^+ is essential—if >6.0mmol/L, dialysis will be required. Drugs causing raised K^+ include suxamethonium, NSAIDs, β-blockers, ACE inhibitors, spironolactone, tacrolimus, and ciclosporin. Na^+ may be low due to water retention. Hypocalcaemia and hyperphosphataemia are common, but rarely symptomatic. A mild metabolic acidosis is frequent, and the ability to compensate further acidosis is poor.
- Coagulation: INR, APTT, and platelet count usually normal; uraemia affects platelet function and causes a prolonged bleeding time. Dialysis improves coagulation once heparin has worn off. Thrombocytopathy is not corrected by platelet transfusion but may be improved by cryoprecipitate or desmopressin (0.3 micrograms/kg in 30mL of saline over 30min). Tendency to thrombosis in fistula in stage 5 CRF on haemodialysis.

Perioperative care

- Venous access and fistulae: many patients have an upper limb arteriovenous (A–V) fistula. Avoid cannulation and non-invasive BP (NIBP) in this arm. Wrap the fistula arm in padding for protection. Wherever possible, cannulate the dorsum of the hand to avoid damage to the veins in the forearm and antecubital fossa needed for future fistulae. Use dialysis catheters for IV access only as a last resort, and remember that the dead space may contain high-dose heparin (at least 1000IU/mL). Aspirate and discard.
- Fluid and electrolyte balance must be carefully managed. Many patients have some residual renal function and urine output. Normovolaemia is ideal. Replace fluid losses promptly. Avoid hypotension.
- If large fluid shifts are likely, CVP or oesophageal Doppler monitoring is useful. These patients may have had multiple CVP lines—use ultrasound. Avoid the femoral vein in patients suitable for transplants, and the subclavian vein in those needing dialysis, as the incidence of stenosis is high.
- Avoid fluids containing K^+; generally use 0.9% sodium chloride (NaCl) or Gelofusine®. Significant blood loss should be replaced.
- Suxamethonium elevates serum K^+ by 0.5mmol/L. Hyperkalaemia is also worsened by acidosis, so avoid hypoventilation and hypercapnia.
- Delayed gastric emptying (autonomic neuropathy) and increased gastric acidity make gastric reflux more likely. Most patients are on H_2 antagonists/proton pump inhibitors (PPIs) (cimetidine may cause confusion and should be avoided). In practice, rapid sequence induction (RSI) is reserved for patients who have not fasted or who have symptomatic reflux and a normal serum K^+.

- Immunity: sepsis is a leading cause of death in CRF. Inhibition of humoral and cell-mediated immunity occurs. Careful attention to asepsis is required for all invasive procedures.
- Hepatitis B and C are common.

Post-operative

- Liaise carefully with the renal unit about the timing/need for dialysis post-operatively. Use epidurals with caution.
- Prescribe analgesics carefully (see ➲ p. 124).
- Pay attention to fluid balance. In oliguria, hourly fluid maintenance should replace fluid losses plus 30mL/hr for insensible losses. Avoid nephrotoxic drugs and periods of hypotension.

Anaesthetic drugs in chronic renal failure

Most drugs are excreted by the kidneys, either unchanged or as metabolites. Loading doses of drugs are often unchanged, but maintenance doses should be reduced or the dosing interval prolonged. Hypoalbuminaemia and acidosis increase the free drug availability of highly protein-bound drugs (e.g. induction agents). Most anaesthetic drugs and techniques reduce renal blood flow, GFR, and urine output (Table 6.1).

Table 6.1 Anaesthetic drugs and chronic renal failure

	Drugs safe in CRF	Drugs safe in limited or reduced doses	Drugs contraindicated in CRF
Premedication	Lormetazepam, midazolam, temazepam		
Induction	Propofol	Ketamine, etomidate, thiopental	
Maintenance	Isoflurane, desflurane, halothane, propofol	Sevoflurane	Enflurane
Muscle relaxants	Suxamethonium, atracurium, cisatracurium	Vecuronium, rocuronium	Pancuronium
Opioids	Alfentanil, remifentanil	Fentanyl, morphine, oxycodone	Pethidine, codeine, tramadol
Local anaesthetics	Bupivacaine, lidocaine (reduce dose by 25%)		
Analgesics	Paracetamol		NSAIDs

- Analgesics: most opioids are excreted by the kidney and so have a prolonged duration of action in CRF. The long-acting morphine metabolite morphine-6-glucuronide has far greater potency than morphine itself. Avoid pethidine, as norpethidine can cause convulsions. Fentanyl has inactive metabolites but accumulates with prolonged use. Alfentanil and remifentanil may be used in normal doses. Half-lives of codeine and dihydrocodeine are prolonged five times—avoid. Oxycodone has active metabolites—reduce the dose, and increase the interval. Tramadol and its active metabolites are renally excreted. The manufacturer does not recommend its use in end-stage renal failure.
- PCA morphine or fentanyl (10 micrograms bolus, 5min lockout time) can be used, but with caution. In theory, the reduction in excretion increases the plasma concentration, causing negative feedback and thus reducing subsequent demand.
- Paracetamol is safe in normal doses. Avoid NSAIDs, even in anuric patients.

- Induction agents: reduce the doses of benzodiazepines, thiopental, and etomidate by ~30% because of changes in protein-binding, volume of distribution, and cardiac function. However, the dose of propofol required for a bispectral index (BIS) of 50 is increased. Wake-up following infusion is faster.
- The elimination of volatile anaesthetic agents is not dependent on the renal function. Isoflurane, halothane, and desflurane are all safe. Sevoflurane is safe for induction but will produce inorganic fluoride ions with prolonged use (avoid >4 MAC hours total). Enflurane is worse.
- Muscle relaxants: suxamethonium is discussed on ➲ p. 1024; plasma cholinesterase activity is unchanged in CRF. Atracurium and cisatracurium are logical choices. Vecuronium and rocuronium can be used as single doses, with prolonged duration of action. Mivacurium clearance is decreased. Always use a peripheral nerve stimulator. Sugammadex is excreted in the urine unchanged, but its action does not depend on renal excretion. It appears to be safe to use in CRF but is not recommended for GFR <30mL/min.[1] It is unpredictably removed by dialysis.
- The excretion of neostigmine and glycopyrronium is prolonged in CRF.
- The duration of action of LAs is reduced. Reduce maximum doses by 25% because of decreased protein binding and a lower CNS seizure threshold. Epidurals and spinals work well, but consider the increased risks of hypovolaemia post-dialysis, haemorrhage, and spinal haematoma formation.
- Anaesthesia for A–V fistula formation: ask the surgeon where the fistula is to be formed. Local infiltration works well for a brachiobasilic fistula. Axillary/supraclavicular brachial plexus block is recommended for a brachiocephalic fistula, and evidence shows a better fistula outcome. Patient may need extra LA in the axilla. Avoid hypotension to prevent fistula thrombosis. The fistula may be used for dialysis after 3–4wk. Synthetic grafts can be used immediately but do not last as long.
- Peritoneal dialysis uses the large surface area of the peritoneum to exchange fluid and metabolites via temporary (hard) or permanent Tenckhoff (soft) catheters in the lower abdomen. This type of dialysis is inefficient but can run continuously. Catheter placement or removal usually requires a mini-laparotomy. Dialysis fluid should be drained before anaesthesia to prevent respiratory function compromise. Patients can usually omit 24–48hr of dialysis, but a period of haemodialysis may be needed if undergoing bowel surgery.
- Most antibiotics are excreted by the kidney. It is common to use a normal loading dose, with reduced and/or delayed maintenance doses. If in doubt, check in the *British National Formulary* (*BNF*) or with a microbiologist.

Reference

1 Staals LM, Snoeck MM, Driessen JJ, Flockton EA, Heeringa M, Hunter JM (2008). Multicentre, parallel-group, comparative trial evaluating the efficacy and safety of sugammadex in patients with end-stage renal failure or normal renal function. *Br J Anaesth*, **101**, 492–7.

Renal transplantation

- Renal transplantation is the treatment of choice for stage 5 renal failure, with greatly increased survival and quality of life. There are insufficient organs available, and patients should be pre-optimized.
- All the rules for anaesthesia in patients with CRF apply (induction agents, analgesics, muscle relaxants, volatile anaesthetics) (see ➋ p. 124).
- Early onset of urine output is directly correlated with graft survival. The evidence for dopamine (3 micrograms/kg/min), mannitol 0.5g/kg, and furosemide 250mg (rate of 4mg/min) is sparse but these may be requested perioperatively by the transplant team.
- Major operation which may last 2–4hr.
- Blood loss not usually great.
- Steroid dose prior to reperfusion.
- Protect A–V fistulae—may be needed post-operatively.
- CVP monitoring and access for dopamine are used (see ➋ p. 122). Maintain CVP at 10–12mmHg. This may require 60–100mL/kg of fluid. Cardiac output montoring is recommended.
- LA blocks (transversus abdominis plane, TAP) and wound catheters are useful. Normal doses of paracetamol (no NSAIDs) and PCA morphine/fentanyl. Post-operative pain is often inversely related to graft function.
- Post-operative care is managed in close conjunction with nephrologists/surgeons. Aim for urine output of 0.5mL/kg/hr. Fluid replacement is 30mL plus losses plus urine output/hr. Avoid hypotension.
- Make sure thromboprophylaxis is prescribed.

Anaesthesia in a patient with a renal transplant

- The serum creatinine may be normal, but renal function and creatinine clearance are not. The transplanted kidney never works perfectly and has only half the number of nephrons.
- Immunosuppression decreases the function further (ciclosporin).
- Patients are immunosuppressed, and strict asepsis must be applied. Immunosuppression must be continued—discuss with the nephrologist.
- CVS depression may compromise kidney function; avoid hypovolaemia and hypotension.
- Avoid nephrotoxic drugs. Do not use NSAIDs, but paracetamol is safe in normal doses.
- The new kidney is placed superficially in the abdomen and can be damaged by patient positioning (i.e. prone position) or supports.

Living donor transplant nephrectomy

- Best results for kidney transplantation. Donor mortality 0.02%.
- Often laparoscopic in the lateral position.
- Post-operative pain may be problematic: PCA ± LA wound catheter or TAP/paravertebral block.
- Post-operative renal function improves with time to ~75% of normal.
- Avoid NSAIDs. Maintain fluid volume and urine output.
- Ensure thromboprophylaxis.

Acute renal failure

Acute renal failure (ARF) developing in the perioperative period has a high mortality (Table 6.2). It is diagnosed by oliguria and a rising serum creatinine. Occasionally, ARF may occur with normal volumes of urine, but with poor creatinine clearance (high-output ARF).

Table 6.2 Risk factors for perioperative ARF

Pre-existing problem	Renal compromise, diabetes, advanced age
Perioperative	Sepsis, hypotension/hypovolaemia, dehydration
Drugs	Nephrotoxins: antibiotics, NSAIDs, ACE inhibitors, lithium, chemotherapy agents, radiological contrast media
Trauma	Rhabdomyolysis (myoglobinaemia from crush injuries)
Surgery	Biliary surgery in the presence of obstructive jaundice (hepatorenal syndrome) (see ➲ p. 134)
	Renal and abdominal vascular surgery
Intra-abdominal hypertension	Any cause of abdominal distension
Urinary obstruction	

Assessment of renal function

- Measure hourly urine output (remember catheters can block). Urinary electrolytes may help differentiate hypoperfusion (Na^+ <20mmol/L, urine osmolality >500mOsmol/kg) from acute tubular necrosis (Na^+ >20mmol/L, urine osmolality <500mOsmol/kg). These results are meaningless if diuretics have been given.
- Serum creatinine is the main initial measurement. Serum urea is much less specific, since it is increased in dehydration, GI bleeding, sepsis, and excessive diuretic use.
- Check electrolytes before surgery (especially serum K^+).
- Contrast-induced nephropathy. Minimize doses of radiological contrast. Prevent by prescribing IV sodium bicarbonate 1.26% 3mL/kg/hr for 1hr preoperatively, and then 1mL/kg/hr until 6hr post-operatively. Acetylcysteine PO/IV may also be added.

Perioperative considerations

- Aim to prevent further deterioration of renal function, and maintain an adequate urine output (>0.5mL/kg/hr).
- Preoperative rehydration is essential, and any fluid deficit should be corrected before surgery. Invasive monitoring may be needed.
- Remember that an adequate BP is needed for renal perfusion. Aim for an MAP >70mmHg (>85mmHg in hypertensives). Inotropes may be required.

- The outcome from polyuric ARF is better than oliguric ARF. There is no place for diuretics (furosemide) until adequate filling and arterial BP have been achieved.
- Furosemide is given initially as an IV bolus of 20–40mg. In patients with established renal failure, furosemide 250mg may be infused over 1hr.
- There is no evidence to support the use of low-dose ('renal') dopamine; it may even be harmful.
- Mannitol (0.5g/kg IV) may improve urine flow.
- Check serum K^+ regularly.
- Seek advice from the renal unit/ICU about post-operative care and dialysis.

Post-operative care
- Avoid NSAIDs in all patients at risk of renal failure.
- Avoid dehydration.
- Closely monitor hourly urine output. If oliguria occurs (<0.5mL/kg/hr), try a fluid challenge of 250–500mL of 0.9% NaCl/Gelofusine®.
- Intra-abdominal hypertension (pressure >20mmHg) is common following major abdominal surgery and causes anuria by direct compression of the renal pelvis and reduced renal perfusion.

Emergency management of hyperkalaemia
See ➜ p. 122.

Further reading
Craig RC, Hunter JM (2008). Recent developments in the perioperative management of adult patients with chronic kidney disease. *Br J Anaesth*, **101**, 296–310.

Martinez BS, Gasanova I, Adesanya AO (2013). Anesthesia for kidney transplantation—a review. *J Anesth Clin Res*, **4**, 270.

Merten GJ, Burgess WP, Gray LV, et al. (2004) Prevention of contrast-induced nephropathy with sodium bicarbonate. *JAMA*, **291**, 2328–34.

Milner QJW (2003). Pathophysiology of chronic renal failure. *BJA CEPD Reviews*, **3**, 130–3.

O'Brien B (2012). Anaesthesia for living donor transplant nephrectomy. *Contin Educ Anaesth Crit Care Pain*, **12**, 317–21.

Toivonen HJ (2000). Anaesthesia for patients with a transplanted organ. *Acta Anaesthesiol Scand*, **44**, 812–33.

Hepatic disease

Ashleigh Williams and John Christie

Acute hepatic disease

Acute liver failure (ALF) is the development of hepatocellular dysfunction associated with coagulopathy and encephalopathy in patients without prior known liver disease (Table 7.1). It is associated with a high mortality (rates of 10–100% have been described) and often rapidly progresses to multi-organ failure.

Previously well patients with ALF rarely present for anaesthesia and surgery.

Table 7.1 Subtypes of acute liver failure

Subtype	Onset	Transplant-free survival (%)
Hyperacute	Within 7d	30
Acute	8–28d	33
Subacute	28d to 6 months	14

Causes of acute liver failure

- The commonest cause in the UK is paracetamol excess (up to 70% cases).
- Viral hepatitis: types A–G, cytomegalovirus (CMV), herpes simplex/ Epstein–Barr virus, and serology-negative hepatitis (non-A to E)
- Autoimmune hepatitis.
- Less commonly—toxins, including carbon tetrachloride, *Amanita phalloides* mushrooms.
- Others: acute fatty infiltration of pregnancy, HELLP (haemolysis, elevated liver enzymes, low platelets) syndrome, Wilson's disease, Reye's syndrome.

Acute liver disease is characterized by encephalopathy, cerebral oedema, and severe coagulopathy with active fibrinolysis. Metabolic derangement leads to hypoglycaemia, hypokalaemia, hyponatraemia, and metabolic acidosis. There is a high cardiac output state with reduced SVR and risk of raised ICP, ARDS, and renal failure.

Management

- Active acute hepatitis is a contraindication to elective surgery. Due to high perioperative mortality, patients should have all surgery postponed (unless true emergency) until at least 30d after LFTs have returned to normal.
- Hepatitis B and C are highly contagious via parenteral inoculation to theatre personnel, and universal precautions must be strictly followed.
- Patients with abnormal LFTs and coagulopathy should be closely monitored—intensive care management is often required.
- Electrolyte disturbance and hypoglycaemia should be corrected.
- Patients with encephalopathy, deteriorating INR, hypoglycaemia, or acidosis should be discussed with a specialist liver unit (for King's College criteria for liver transplant, see Table 7.2).

- Patients with grades 3/4 encephalopathy need intubation to protect their airway.
- Hypovolaemia and hypotension should be treated with IV fluids and inotropes/vasopressors (noradrenaline as 1st choice) (see fluids section, ◐ p. 1053).
- Bicarbonate-buffered haemofiltration and ICP monitoring are often required.
- Aetiology-specific treatment should be instigated: acetylcysteine infusion in paracetamol overdose, delivery of fetus if pregnancy-related.
- Orthotopic liver transplantation may be a definitive treatment in some cases.
- Reversal of coagulopathy should not be routinely carried out, as prothrombin time (PT) provides a surrogate marker of hepatic function. Reversal is indicated for invasive procedures or active bleeding.

Table 7.2 King's College criteria for transplant referral in acute liver disease

Paracetamol
pH <7.3
Or ALL of the following:
Grades 3–4 encephalopathy
Creatinine >300
PT >100 or INR >6.5
Non-paracetamol
PT >100
Or any three of the following:
Age <10 or >40
PT >50
Bilirubin >300

Data from O'Grady J, Alexander G, Hayllar K, Williams R (1989). Early indicators of prognosis in fulminant hepatic failure. *Gastroenterology* **97**(2), 439–45.

Chronic hepatic disease

Chronic hepatitis is any hepatitis lasting >6 months. Inflammation can lead to hepatic fibrosis, and, in some patients, there is progression to cirrhosis, characterized by nodular regeneration and disruption of the architecture of the liver, which can lead to portal hypertension. Liver function can still be maintained in cirrhosis (compensated cirrhosis), but ongoing damage or an acute precipitant, such as infection, can lead to a deterioration in liver function (decompensated cirrhosis). Treatment of the underlying cause of the liver disease can result in improvement in liver function and reversal of liver fibrosis. Where the underlying disease is not amenable to treatment and cirrhosis remains decompensated, then liver transplantation is considered.

Chronic liver disease (CLD) is far more prevalent than acute liver disease.

- Cirrhosis is most commonly caused by alcohol, hepatitis B virus (HBV), hepatitis C virus (HCV), and fatty liver disease.
- It is less commonly attributed to inherited causes (haemochromatosis, Wilson's disease, and α-1 antitrypsin deficiency), immune-mediated (primary biliary cirrhosis, primary sclerosing cholangitis, and autoimmune hepatitis), vascular disease (Budd–Chiari, veno-occlusive disease), and drugs (isoniazid, methyldopa).
- There is a risk of developing chronic HBV if infected at birth (95%). It is widespread in the Far East/Africa and infects 300 million people worldwide due to vertical transmission. However, worldwide vaccination of babies is leading to falling numbers of infections.
- Chronic HBV develops in 3% of those infected as an adult. High-risk groups include homosexuals, IV drug users, haemophiliacs, haemodialysis patients, and those in institutional care.
- Chronic HCV develops in 75% of those infected. The main risk factor is IV drug use. Blood products were previously responsible for many cases of hepatitis C, but now all donors are screened.
- Non-alcoholic liver disease has become a major cause of cirrhosis in the West due to rising levels of obesity, particularly in patients with type 2 diabetes and hypertension.
- Chronic alcohol ingestion places patients at high risk of alcohol withdrawal syndromes and delirium tremens. This may present either pre- or post-operatively. For management, see substance abuse section, → p. 264.
- Assessment of risk for surgery and anaesthesia in CLD may be estimated by Child's classification (Table 7.3), or perhaps more accurately by the model for end-stage liver disease (MELD) score. Surgical risk in CLD depends on the extent of hepatic impairment, in addition to the urgency and type of surgery. Common causes of mortality in the perioperative period include sepsis, renal failure, bleeding, and worsening liver failure with encephalopathy.

Table 7.3 Surgical risk assessment: Child's classification, as modified by Pugh

Mortality	Minimal (<5%)	Modest (5–50%)	Marked (>50%)
Bilirubin (micromol/L)	<25	25–40	>40
Albumin (g/L)	>35	30–35	<30
PT (s, prolonged)	1–4 (INR <1.7)	4–6 (INR 1.7–2.3)	>6 (INR >2.3)
Ascites	None	Moderate	Marked
Encephalopathy (see ➋ p. 134)	None	Grades 1 and 2	Grades 3 and 4
Nutrition	Excellent	Good	Poor

INR, international normalized ratio; PT, prothrombin time.

MELD is a statistical model initially developed to predict survival in cirrhotic patients undergoing liver transplant but may be more accurate in predicting outcome in the non-transplant setting than Child–Pugh.

$$MELD = 3.78 \left[\log_e \text{serum bilirubin (mg/dL)}\right] + 11.2 \left[\log_e \text{INR}\right] + 9.57 \left[\log_e \text{serum creatinine (mg/dL)}\right] + 6.43$$

Online calculators are available at ⅏ http://www.esot.org/resources/tools.

Patients with a MELD score <10 are considered low-risk for elective surgery, 10–15 intermediate-risk, and >15 signifies an unacceptable mortality likelihood and non-essential surgery should be postponed.

Further reading

Hanje AJ, Patel T (2007). Preoperative evaluation of patients with liver disease. *Nat Clin Pract Gastroenterol Hepatol*, **4**, 266.

Complications and physiological changes of liver disease

CLD presents to the anaesthetist and surgeon more frequently than acute liver disease. However, the complications and physiological considerations for both are largely the same.

- **Bleeding**: the liver plays a pivotal role in coagulation; it synthesizes all clotting factors, except factor VIII. Coagulopathy features prominently in liver disease and is associated with an increased morbidity and mortality in the surgical setting.
- Coagulopathy is attributed to several mechanisms:
  - Decreased synthesis of clotting factors
  - Quantitative (thrombocytopenia) and qualitative platelet abnormalities
  - Decreased clearance of activated clotting factors
  - Hyperfibrinolysis.

Preoperative clotting studies and FBC must be carefully checked. Jaundice may lead to vitamin K deficiency, resulting in a prolonged PT. There are no reliable assays of vitamin K, and so a therapeutic trial of IV vitamin K determines if there is vitamin K deficiency. PT will improve if the cause of the coagulopathy is vitamin K deficiency, but not if it is impaired liver synthetic function.

Reversal of coagulopathy may be achieved with fresh frozen plasma (FFP), cryoprecipitate, and platelet transfusion. Adequate provision must be made for cross-matched blood and clotting products.

Liver disease is also associated with thrombotic complications. PT only reflects one part of the clotting cascade; thus, the coagulation studies must be carefully interpreted. The increasing availability of thromboelastography (TEG) may be useful in assessing coagulation defects in the perioperative setting.

- **Encephalopathy**: in severe liver failure, toxic products build up (particularly ammonia, due to deranged amino acid metabolism), leading to a progressive encephalopathy (Box 7.1). This may be precipitated by sedatives, GI bleeding, infection, surgical operations, trauma, hypokalaemia, and constipation. Intubation is required if a decreased level of consciousness compromises the airway or if cerebral oedema develops.

Box 7.1 Grades of hepatic encephalopathy

Grade 0	Alert and orientated
Grade I	Drowsy and orientated
Grade II	Drowsy and disorientated
Grade III	Rousable stupor, restlessness
Grade IV	Coma—unresponsive to deep pain

- **Hypoglycaemia**: patients with liver disease have impaired hepatic glycogen storage and are prone to hypoglycaemia. Check blood glucose levels regularly. Give 10% glucose infusions if <2mmol/L, and monitor plasma K^+.
- **Ascites**: fibrotic changes in the liver lead to portal hypertension, and, in combination with salt/water retention 2° to hyperaldosteronism, splanchnic vasodilation, and a low serum albumin, fluid accumulates in the peritoneal cavity. Spironolactone is used in the management of ascites but may exacerbate electrolyte disturbances and renal dysfunction (see fluids section, ➲ p. 143).
- **Infection**: immune function is depressed, and infections of the respiratory and urinary tract are common. In the presence of ascites, spontaneous bacterial peritonitis may cause significant sepsis. Intraoperative antibiotic prophylaxis should be given where indicated.
- **CVS**: portosystemic, pulmonary, and cutaneous shunting (spider angiomata) contributes to a hyperdynamic, high cardiac output state, often increased by up to 50%. There is, in addition, a low SVR and arterial pressure, increased HR, and volume expansion 2° to an activated renin–angiotensin system. Alcohol excess is associated with cardiomyopathy, and concurrent smoking is a risk factor for CAD.
- **Renal**: impairment is most commonly due to dehydration, sepsis, or nephrotoxic drugs. Renal failure in the context of liver failure confers a high mortality; the precipitating cause should be investigated and treated. Up to 50% of patients presenting with ALF will also have ARF.
  - **Hepatorenal syndrome** is a diagnosis of exclusion and occurs exclusively in patients with cirrhotic liver disease as a consequence of altered renovascular tone. It is subdivided into type 1 which is rapidly progressive, and type 2 which is slower in onset and associated with diuretic-resistant ascites. Both are associated with poor prognosis, and liver transplantation may be the only definitive treatment. Diagnostic criteria are:
    — Urinary Na <10mmol/L
    — Urine: plasma osmolality and creatinine ratios >1
    — Normal CVP and no diuresis on central volume expansion
    — Underlying CLD and ascites.

Prevention requires adequate hydration (see fluids section, ➲ p. 143) and optimization of renal blood flow. The use of cardiac output monitoring and goal-directed fluid management may be useful.

Tense ascites may impair renal blood flow and give a falsely high CVP. Intra-operative hypotension should be avoided, and a urine output of 1mL/kg/hr maintained. Avoidance of nephrotoxic drugs is important.

- **Respiratory**: hypoxia is common and multifactorial. Ascites causes splinting of the diaphragm, basal atelectasis, and collapse.
  - **Hepatopulmonary syndrome** occurs when intrapulmonary vascular dilations contribute to hypoxia in liver disease, possibly 2° to increased production or decreased clearance of vasodilators such as N_2O. Intra-pulmonary shunting further contributes to V/Q mismatch, increased A–a gradient, and low PaO_2. The only definitive treatment is liver transplantation.

- **Pulmonary hypertension** is a serious complication present in 0.25–4% of all patients with cirrhosis. It is thought to occur due to local pulmonary production of vasoconstrictors that occurs while systemically vasodilation predominates.
- **Low plasma proteins**: impaired hepatic synthetic function leads to low albumin and plasma proteins. This contributes to oedema/ascites and has implications for drug protein-binding.
- **Anaemia**: is contributed to by chronic blood loss, hypersplenism, haemolysis, chronic illness, and malnutrition.
- **Portal hypertension and oesophageal varices**: portal hypertension occurs in cirrhosis and conditions where there is disruption of hepatic blood flow. Portal hypertension leads to engorgement of the anastomoses between portal and systemic circulations, leading to varices at the gastro-oesophageal junction, haemorrhoids, and dilated abdominal wall veins (caput medusae).
- Patients with varices are at risk of acute bleeding which is associated with a high mortality rate (see Anaesthetic management of acute oesophageal variceal haemorrhage, ⊃ p. 144).

Further reading

Amitrano L, Guardascione A, Brancaccio V, Balzano A (2002). Coagulation disorders in liver disease. *Semin Liver Dis*, **22**, 83–96.

Machicao VI, Balakrishnan M, Fallon MB (2014). Pulmonary complications in chronic liver disease. *Hepatology*, **59**, 1627–37.

Trotter JF (2009). Practical management of acute liver failure on ITU. *Curr Opin Crit Care*, **15**, 163–7.

Drug metabolism and liver disease

- The vast majority of drugs, including anaesthetic drugs, are metabolized by the liver (Table 7.4).
- Most drugs are initially metabolized by the cytochrome P450 system. In phase I, they are either oxidized or reduced, and, in phase II, they are conjugated with a glucuronide, glycine, or sulphate to enhance water solubility and excretion in bile or urine.
- In early alcoholic liver disease, the cytochrome P450 system is often induced, leading to rapid metabolism of drugs, whereas this is reversed in end-stage disease.
- The liver has a large functional reserve, so these functions are usually preserved until end-stage disease.
- Pharmacodynamics and the sensitivity of target organs for sedatives and anaesthetics may be altered, with coma easily induced in end-stage liver disease.
- Advanced liver disease may prolong the half-life and potentiate the clinical effects of alfentanil, morphine, vecuronium, rocuronium, mivacurium, and benzodiazepines.
- Liver disease reduces the synthesis of plasma cholinesterase. This may lead to prolongation of the action of suxamethonium.

Table 7.4 Causes of altered drug pharmacokinetics in liver failure

Liver problem	Pharmacological effect
Decreased portal blood flow in hepatic fibrosis	Decreased first-pass metabolism
Hypoalbuminaemia	Increased free drug in plasma
Ascites and sodium/water retention	Increased volume of distribution
Biotransformation enzymes	Activity may increase or decrease
Reduced liver cell mass	Reduced activity
Obstructive jaundice	Decreased biliary excretion of drugs

Anaesthetic management of the patient with liver failure

Patients with liver disease have a high perioperative risk, which is proportional to the degree of hepatic dysfunction. All patients should have a thorough preoperative assessment, including signs, symptoms, and risk factors for liver disease.

- **Symptoms**: anorexia, malaise, weight loss, easy bruising, itching, right upper quadrant (RUQ) pain.
- **Signs**: jaundice, palmar erythema, spider naevi, caput medusae, gynaecomastia, ascites, hepatosplenomegaly, testicular atrophy.
- **Risk factors**: alcohol excess, IV drug abuse, obesity, autoimmune conditions, haemodialysis, haemophilia, homosexuality, family history, and previous blood transfusion.

Preoperative laboratory investigations

- FBC and clotting studies. PT is a good marker of liver function.
- Electrolytes and creatinine. The urea is often falsely low due to decreased hepatic production. Hyponatraemia and hypokalaemia are common, and diuretic use may further exacerbate electrolyte disturbances.
- Glucose—hepatic stores of glycogen and glucose utilization are often affected.
- LFTs (see ➲ p. 139).
- Urinalysis.
- Hepatitis screening (although universal precautions should always be observed).

Assessment of liver function

- Serum LFTs (Table 7.5) are rarely specific, but PT, albumin, and bilirubin are sensitive markers of overall liver function. Serial measurements are useful and indicate trends. Avoid giving FFP, unless treating active bleeding, as the PT is an excellent guide to overall liver function.
- Liver transaminases (aspartate transaminase (AST), alanine aminotransferase (ALT)) are sensitive to even mild liver damage and have no role in mortality prediction. Levels may decrease in severe disease.
- Alkaline phosphatase is raised with biliary obstruction.
- Imaging techniques: ultrasound is the main initial investigation of obstructive jaundice. Other useful investigations include endoscopic retrograde cholangiopancreatography (ERCP), CT, and MRI cholangiograms.
- LFTs must always be interpreted alongside a careful history and examination. The liver has a large functional reserve and can often withstand considerable damage before LFTs become deranged.

Table 7.5 Liver function tests

Test	Normal range	Raised
Bilirubin	2–17 micromoles/L	Haemolysis
		Gilbert's syndrome
		Acute and chronic liver failure
		Biliary obstruction
Aspartate transaminase (AST)	0–35IU/L	Non-specific (found in liver, heart, muscle, etc.)
		Hepatocellular injury
Alanine aminotransferase (ALT)	0–45IU/L	Specific
		Hepatocellular injury
		Degree of elevation can point to aetiology:
		>1000: acute viral hepatitis, drugs, autoimmune hepatitis, and ischaemia
		100–200: acute viral hepatitis, alcohol and non-alcoholic fatty liver disease
Alkaline phosphatase (ALP)	30–120IU/L	Physiological (pregnancy, adolescents, familial)
		Bile duct obstruction (stones, drugs, cancer)
		Primary biliary cirrhosis
		Metastatic liver disease
		Bone disease
γ-glutamyl transpeptidase (γ-GT)	0–30IU/L	Non-specific (found in heart, pancreas, kidneys)
		Useful to confirm hepatic source for ↑ ALP (always raised if liver source of ↑ ALP)
		Alcoholic liver disease
Albumin	40–60g/L	Non-specific (affected by nutritional status, catabolism, and urinary and GI losses)
		Prognostic in chronic liver disease
Prothrombin time and international normalized ratio (INR)	10.9–12.5s (INR 1.0–1.2)	Non-specific (vitamin K deficiency, warfarin therapy, DIC)
		However, best prognostic marker in acute liver failure

Preoperative investigations

Cardiac
- ECG is essential—electrolyte abnormalities may precipitate arrhythmias, and alcohol excess may result in AF and cardiomyopathy. Prolonged QTc is relatively common, and hyperbilirubinaemia may precipitate bradyarrhythmias.
- Echocardiography—cardiomyopathy may develop in association with causes of CLD, particularly alcohol excess. Pericardial effusions and diastolic dysfunction also develop in cirrhosis. Smoking is associated with alcohol excess and is an independent risk factor for CAD.

Respiratory
- CXR to assess for pleural effusion.
- ABG—hypoxia is common in liver disease (see physiology section, 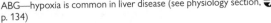 p. 134)

Nutrition
- CLD is associated with a poor nutritional state and predisposes to increased incidence of post-operative complications. Preoperative nutrition may help to reduce this in major elective surgical procedures.

Other
- The presence of varices in patients with known liver disease must be established, as this is a contraindication for the use of oesophageal Doppler probes and oesophageal temperature probes.

Reversal of coagulopathy
- Prior to invasive surgical procedures, coagulopathy should be reversed, depending on the urgency and extent of the derangement (see Chapter 10).

Perioperative considerations
- **Premedication:** PPIs or H_2 antagonists should be used preoperatively. RSI will further reduce the risks of gastric aspiration. Sedative medication may precipitate or worsen encephalopathy.
- **Monitoring:** standard monitoring should be used, with consideration given to invasive arterial and CVP monitoring, depending on the severity of the underlying liver disease and the extent of planned surgery. Perioperative haemodynamic instability can worsen hepatic function; mean BP should be maintained within 10–20% of preoperative levels—particularly in the hypertensive patient. Hepatic blood flow and O_2 delivery should be maintained; cardiac output monitoring may be useful. The presence of varices contraindicates the use of oesophageal Doppler.
- **Drug effects:** even in severe liver disease, the problem is usually one of exaggerated effects of drugs on the CNS, rather than poor liver metabolism (Table 7.6). Hepatic blood flow is altered by anaesthetic drugs (including α- and β-agonists/antagonists), positive pressure ventilation, PEEP, and surgical technique. In most cases, anaesthesia reduces hepatic blood flow, particularly if halothane is used. Isoflurane, sevoflurane, and desflurane are the preferred volatile agents, as

enflurane and particularly halothane have marked effects in decreasing hepatic blood flow and inhibiting drug metabolism. Desflurane best preserves hepatic blood flow, is least metabolized, and has a quicker emergence time.

- **Regional techniques**: can be used as long as coagulation is not deranged, and it should be remembered that all LAs are metabolized by the liver.
- **Other considerations**: intramuscular (IM) and SC injections risk haematoma formation if coagulopathic or thrombocytopenic. Care with positioning; the skin may be fragile—weight loss and muscle wasting may leave patients prone to neuropraxia and pressure damage.

Table 7.6 Anaesthetic drugs in liver failure

	Drugs safe in liver failure	Drugs to be used with caution (may need reduced dosage)	Drugs contraindicated in liver failure
Premedication	Lorazepam	Midazolam, diazepam	
Induction	Propofol, thiopental, etomidate		
Maintenance	Desflurane, sevoflurane, isoflurane, nitrous oxide	Enflurane	Halothane (possibly)[1]
Muscle relaxants	Atracurium, cisatracurium	Rocuronium, vecuronium, suxamethonium	
Opioids	Remifentanil	Fentanyl, alfentanil, morphine, pethidine	
Analgesics	Paracetamol	NSAIDs, lidocaine, bupivacaine	

[1] Halothane has been rarely reported to cause hepatitis (see ➲ p. 142).

Post-operative considerations

- Patients with advanced liver disease will need post-operative intensive care or high dependency care.
- Post-operative decompensation of CLD carries a high mortality.
- Constipating analgesics, such as opioids, should be prescribed with concurrent lactulose to prevent encephalopathy.
- Post-operative ileus may also precipitate encephalopathy in cirrhotic patients.
- Complications include delayed wound healing, sepsis, renal impairment, and bleeding.
- Fluid balance should be carefully monitored post-operatively, aiming for a urine output of 1mL/kg/hr.
- Coagulopathy increases the risk of post-operative bleeding and haematoma formation.

Post-operative liver dysfunction or jaundice

Although post-operative jaundice (Table 7.7) is relatively common, significant liver dysfunction is relatively rare in previously healthy patients. Dysfunction has a varied aetiology and often resolves without treatment. It should be remembered that hepatitis due to volatile agents is extremely rare and is largely a diagnosis of exclusion.

- Common causes include hepatic O_2 deprivation from intra- and post-operative hypoxia and hypotension.
- Benign post-operative intrahepatic cholestasis mimics biliary obstruction and usually occurs after major surgery associated with hypotension, hypoxaemia, and multiple transfusions.
- The surgical procedure should also be considered, and significant haematoma resolution is a common cause.

Table 7.7 Causes of post-operative liver dysfunction or jaundice

Bilirubin overload (haemolysis)	Blood transfusion
	Haematoma resorption
	Haemolytic anaemia (sickle-cell, prosthetic heart valve, glucose-6-phosphate dehydrogenase deficiency)
Hepatocellular injury	Exacerbation of pre-existing liver disease
	Hepatic ischaemia: hypovolaemia, hypotension, cardiac failure
	Septicaemia
	Drug-induced (antibiotics, halothane)
	Hypoxia
	Viral hepatitis
Cholestasis	Intrahepatic (benign, infection, drug-induced, e.g. cephalosporins, carbamazepine, erythromycin)
	Extrahepatic (pancreatitis, gallstones, bile duct injury)
Congenital	Gilbert's syndrome

Halothane hepatitis

The use of halothane has largely been superseded by other volatile agents so is becoming a historical phenomenon. Halothane has been linked to post-operative liver dysfunction. Two syndromes are recognized:

- The first is associated with a transient rise in LFTs and low morbidity, often after initial exposure
- The second is thought to occur after repeated exposure and has an 'immune' mechanism with the development of fulminant hepatic failure (FHF) and high mortality. It is rare, with an incidence of 1:35 000 anaesthetics

- Antibodies specific to FHF patients exposed to halothane are found in 70% of such patients. It is postulated that a halothane oxidative metabolite binds to liver cytochromes to form a hapten and induce a hypersensitivity reaction. All patients exposed to halothane have altered liver proteins, but it is unknown why only a few develop liver failure.

Other inhalational anaesthetic agents

- The chance of an 'immune' reaction to a volatile agent occurring is thought to relate to the amount it is metabolized. Halothane is 20% metabolized.
- Enflurane is 2% metabolized and should therefore cause ten times fewer reactions. Products of enflurane metabolism have been shown to alter liver proteins, and there have been rare case reports linking enflurane with liver damage. There is a theoretical basis for cross-reactivity with previous halothane exposure.
- Isoflurane is 0.2% metabolized. There is therefore a theoretical risk of reaction, and indeed there have been a few case reports. These, however, have been contested, and isoflurane is considered safe for use in patients at risk of hepatic failure, as are sevoflurane and desflurane.

Intravenous fluids in liver disease

- It is important to maintain adequate peri- and post-operative hydration, as there is high risk of acute kidney injury.
- Five or 10% glucose is unsuitable as a resuscitation or maintenance fluid, as it provides little intravascular volume replacement and may exacerbate hyponatraemia and cerebral oedema. It is useful in the correction of hypoglycaemia.
- Normal saline 0.9% or Hartmann's solution are both good choices of crystalloid, although Hartmann's may present an external lactate load, and the high sodium load in normal saline 0.9% may worsen ascites.
- Human albumin solution (HAS) 4.5% is a useful colloid, especially if synthetic liver function is impaired and serum albumin is low.
- If oliguria persists despite adequate fluid resuscitation, IV terlipressin 0.5–2mg IV qds, in conjunction with daily HAS, may improve renal function.
- Perioperative removal of ascites will result in post-operative re-accumulation. This should be accounted for in the fluid balance.

Anaesthetic management of acute oesophageal variceal haemorrhage

Acute variceal haemorrhage is a medical emergency, commonly presenting with haematemesis or melaena on a background of cirrhotic liver disease. Patients are often significantly haemodynamically compromised and coagulopathic.

Thirty per cent of patients with varices bleed, with an associated mortality of 40%.

Treatment

- Initial management is to correct hypovolaemia, stop the bleeding, and reverse the coagulopathy.
- Two large-bore IV lines and a CVP line should be inserted. Invasive arterial monitoring should be considered.
- Drugs that may cause or exacerbate the bleeding, e.g. aspirin, should be stopped.
- Early endoscopy is warranted to confirm the diagnosis and control the bleeding. Band ligation appears more effective than sclerosant injection for variceal haemorrhage. Ulcers may be injected with adrenaline. However, 70% of patients will rebleed, most within 6wk. Intubation with RSI is almost always required, as there is a high risk of aspiration.
- Vasoactive drugs (terlipressin 2mg 6-hourly, or less commonly vasopressin 0.2–0.4U/min for 24–48hr) constrict vessels in the mesenteric beds but may cause coronary constriction and angina. GTN patches or infusion may help. Terlipressin causes less angina than vasopressin.
- Somatostatin (a hypothalamic hormone) 250 micrograms/hr and octreotide (an analogue) 50 micrograms/hr for 2–5d (as well as terlipressin/vasopressin), in combination with endoscopic therapy, may be more effective than either alone and should be started, while waiting for an experienced endoscopist.
- Balloon tamponade with an oesophageal and gastric balloon can provide temporary haemostasis but should be used only where endoscopic and drug treatments have failed. There is a high risk of fatal complications (aspiration, oesophageal tear/rupture, and airway obstruction), and therefore this should be used only in HDU/ICU.
- In the case of acute bleed and failed banding, transjugular intrahepatic portosystemic shunt (TIPSS) procedure should be the treatment of choice. This achieves shunting without the need for surgical intervention.
- Prophylactic β-blockade (propranolol 40–160mg twice daily (bd)) can decrease portal pressure in the chronic situation and may decrease the rebleed rate from 70% to 50%, but may mask the early signs of hypovolaemia and exacerbate hypotension during rebleeding.
- Banding can also be performed on an elective basis, in which case IV sedation may be used.

Anaesthesia for transjugular intrahepatic portosystemic shunt procedure

TIPSS is indicated in refractory variceal bleeding and ascites resistant to diuretic therapy. There is increasing evidence that early TIPSS in variceal bleeding improves outcome.

- A stent is positioned radiologically between the hepatic and portal veins, allowing blood to bypass the dilated oesophageal and gastric veins.
- Patients should be adequately resuscitated, and variceal bleeding controlled with balloon tamponade.
- Complications of the procedure include pneumothorax (if the internal jugular route is used), cardiac arrhythmias, and massive bleeding 2° to hepatic artery puncture or hepatic capsular tear. TIPSS may precipitate acute cardiac failure, as the shunt leads to an increased venous return and preload. This risk is exaggerated in the context of cardiomyopathy. A pre-procedural echocardiography should be considered.
  Post-procedural worsening of jaundice or encephalopathy may be seen.
- The anaesthetic technique involves having a cardiovascularly stable patient with good IV access, invasive arterial line monitoring, and inotropes and blood products easily available.
- TIPSS is contraindicated if there is any clinical or EEG evidence of encephalopathy.

Further reading

American Association for the Study of Liver Diseases (AASLD). ℛ http://www.aasld.org.

British Society of Gastroenterology (BSG). ℛ http://www.bsg.org.uk.

European Association for the Study of the Liver (EASL). ℛ http://www.easl.eu.

Garcia-Pagan AC, Di Pascoli M, Caca K, et al. (2013). Use of early-TIPS for high-risk variceal bleeding: results of a post-RCT surveillance study. *J Hepatol*, **58**, 45–50.

Kam PCA, Williams S, Yoong FFY (2004). Vasopressin and terlipressin: pharmacology and clinical relevance. *Anaesthesia*, **59**, 993–1001.

Lai WK, Murphy N (2004). Management of acute liver failure. *Contin Educ Anaesth Crit Care Pain*, **4**, 40–2.

Lentschener C, Ozier Y (2003). What anaesthetists need to know about viral hepatitis. *Acta Anaesthesiol Scand*, **47**, 794–803.

Ng CK, Chan MH, Tai MH, Lam CW (2007). Hepatorenal syndrome. *Clin Biochem Rev*, **28**, 11–17.

Vaja R, McNichol L, Sisley I (2010). Anaesthesia for patients with liver disease. *Contin Educ Anaesth Crit Care Pain*, **10**, 15–19.

Endocrine and metabolic disease

Hannah Blanshard

Diabetes mellitus

Insulin is necessary, even when fasting, to maintain glucose homeostasis and balance stress hormones (e.g. adrenaline). It has two classes of action:
- Excitatory—stimulating glucose uptake and lipid synthesis
- Inhibitory (physiologically more important)—inhibits lipolysis, proteolysis, glycogenolysis, gluconeogenesis, and ketogenesis.

Lack of insulin is associated with hyperglycaemia, osmotic diuresis, dehydration, hyperosmolarity, hyperviscosity predisposing to thrombosis, and increased rates of wound infection. Sustained hyperglycaemia is associated with increased mortality, hospital stay, and complication rates.

Diabetes mellitus is present in 5% of the population.
- Type 1 diabetes (20%): immune-mediated and leads to absolute insulin deficiency. Patients cannot tolerate prolonged periods without exogenous insulin. Glycogenolysis and gluconeogenesis occur, resulting in hyperglycaemia and ketosis. Treatment is with insulin.
- Type 2 diabetes (80%): a disease of adult onset, associated with insulin resistance. Patients produce some endogenous insulin, and their metabolic state often improves with fasting. The treatment may be diet control, oral hypoglycaemics, and/or insulin.

General considerations

Many diabetic patients are well informed about their condition and have undergone previous surgery. Discuss management with them. Hospital diabetic teams can be useful for advice. The overall aims of perioperative diabetic management are to maintain physiological glucose levels (above hypoglycaemic levels, but below those at which deleterious effects of hyperglycaemia become evident) and prevent hypokalaemia, hypomagnesaemia, and hypophosphataemia.

Preoperative assessment

- CVS: the diabetic is prone to hypertension, IHD (may be 'silent'), cerebrovascular disease, MI, and cardiomyopathy. Autonomic neuropathy can lead to tachy- or bradycardia and postural hypotension.
- Renal: 40% of diabetics develop microalbuminuria, which is associated with hypertension, IHD, and retinopathy. This may be reduced by treatment with ACE inhibitors.
- Respiratory: diabetics are prone to perioperative chest infections, especially if they are obese and smokers.
- Airway: thickening of soft tissues (glycosylation) occurs, especially in ligaments around joints, leading to limited joint mobility syndrome. Intubation may be difficult if the neck is affected or there is insufficient mouth opening.
- GI: 50% of patients have delayed gastric emptying and are prone to reflux.
- Diabetics are prone to infections.

Investigations

- Ensure that diabetic control is optimized prior to surgery.
- Measure glycosylated Hb (HbA$_{1c}$), a measure of recent glycaemic control (normal 20–48mmol/mol, 4–6.5%). If HbA$_{1c}$ is >69mmol/mol (8.5%), refer to the team who manages their diabetes for optimization. Surgery may then proceed with caution. A value >85mmol/mol (10%) suggests inadequate control. Refer to the diabetic team, and only proceed if surgery is urgent.
- Patients with hypoglycaemic unawareness should be referred to the diabetes specialist team, irrespective of HbA$_{1c}$.

Preoperative management

- Make an individualized diabetes management plan, agreed with the patient, for the pre-admission and perioperative period.
- Ensure that co-morbidities are recognized and optimized prior to admission.
- Place the patient first on the operating list, if possible.
- Individuals with type 1 diabetes should NEVER go without insulin, as they are at risk of diabetic ketoacidosis.
- The Enhanced Recovery Partnership Programme recommends high-carbohydrate drinks prior to surgery. This may compromise blood sugar control and is not recommended for people with insulin-treated diabetes.
- Avoid overnight preoperative admission to hospital wherever possible.
- Patients with a planned short starvation period (no more than one missed meal in total) should be managed by modification of their usual diabetes regime, avoiding a variable-rate IV insulin infusion (VRIII) wherever possible.
- Patients expected to miss >1 meal should have a VRIII.
- For suggested perioperative management of insulin, see Table 8.1. For suggested perioperative management of non-insulin diabetic medication, see Table 8.2.

Perioperative management

- Monitor blood glucose on admission, and hourly during the day of surgery. Aim for blood glucose level of 6–10mmol/L; 4–12mmol/L is acceptable.
- If blood glucose is >12mmol/L either pre- or post-surgery, check capillary blood ketones or urinary ketones. If capillary blood ketones are >3mmol/L or urinary ketones > +++, cancel surgery.
- Consider an RSI if gastric stasis is suspected.
- Regional techniques may be useful for extremity surgery and to reduce the risk of undetected hypoglycaemia. Document any existing nerve damage.
- Autonomic dysfunction may exacerbate the hypotensive effect of spinals and epidurals.

Table 8.1 Perioperative management of insulin therapy

	Day of surgery	
	Patient for a.m. surgery	Patient for p.m. surgery
Once daily (evening)	No dose change	
Once daily (morning)	No dose change	
Twice daily	Halve the usual morning dose	
	Leave the evening meal dose unchanged	
Twice daily—separate injections of short-acting and intermediate-acting	Calculate the total dose of both morning insulins, and give half as intermediate-acting only in the morning	
	Leave the evening meal dose unchanged	
3–5 injections daily	**Basal bolus regimens:** Omit the morning and lunchtime short-acting insulins. Keep the basal unchanged, unless patient grazes all day when consider reducing by a third	Take usual morning insulin dose(s) Omit lunchtime dose
	Premixed a.m. insulin Halve morning dose, and omit lunchtime dose	

Reproduced from Dhatariya, K. et al., NHS Diabetes perioperative management guideline, Appendix 2, *Diabetic Medicine* © Crown Copyright 2012.

Perioperative adjustment of *insulin* (short starvation period—no more than ONE missed meal)

Insulin should be taken as usual on the day before surgery.

Check blood glucose on admission.

Perioperative adjustment of *non-insulin medication* (short starvation period—no more than ONE missed meal)

For well-controlled patients (HbA$_{1c}$ <69mmol/mol) undergoing surgery with a short starvation period (one missed meal) and preoperative hyperglycaemia (blood glucose >12mmol/L):
- Type 1 diabetes: give SC rapid-acting insulin analogue. Assume that 1U will drop blood glucose by 3mmol/L, but take advice from the patient wherever possible. Recheck blood glucose hourly. If surgery cannot be delayed, commence VRIII.
- Type 2 diabetes: give 0.1U/kg of SC rapid-acting insulin analogue, and recheck blood glucose 1hr later to ensure it is falling. If surgery cannot be delayed or the response is inadequate, commence VRIII.

Table 8.2 Perioperative management of oral diabetic medication

	Day of surgery	
	Patient for a.m. surgery	Patient for p.m. surgery
Acarbose	Omit morning dose if NBM	Give morning dose if eating
Meglitinide (repaglinide or nateglinide)	Omit morning dose if NBM	Give morning dose if eating
Metformin (if procedure not requiring use of contrast media*)	Take as normal	Take as normal
Sulfonylurea	Once daily a.m. omit	Once daily a.m. omit
(e.g. glibenclamide, gliclazide, glipizide, etc.)	Twice daily, omit a.m.	Twice daily, omit a.m. and p.m.
Pioglitazone	Take as normal	Take as normal
DDP-4 inhibitor (e.g. sitagliptin, vildagliptin, saxagliptin)	Omit on day of surgery	Omit on day of surgery
GLP-1 analogue (e.g. exenatide, liraglutide)	Omit on day of surgery	Omit on day of surgery

* If contrast medium is to be used and estimated GFR <50mL.min/1.73², metformin should be omitted on the day of surgery and for the following 48hr.

a.m., morning; DDP-4, dipeptidyl peptidase-4; GLP-1, glucagon-like peptide-1; NBM, nil by mouth; p.m., afternoon.

Reproduced from Dhatariya, K. *et al.*, NHS Diabetes perioperative management guideline, Appendix 3, *Diabetic Medicine* © Crown Copyright 2012.

Patients undergoing surgery with a long starvation period (i.e. two or more missed meals)

* Commence VRIII on admission.
* If patient is already on a long-acting insulin analogue, these should be continued, even if planning to use a VRIII through the perioperative period.
* Glucose/insulin infusions should be administered through the same cannula to prevent accidental administration of insulin without glucose. Both infusions should be regulated by volumetric pumps, with an anti-reflux valve on the IV glucose line.
* Hartmann's solution should be used in preference to 0.9% saline in those patients not requiring a VRIII.

Hypoglycaemia

- Blood glucose <4mmol/L is the main danger to diabetics perioperatively. Fasting, recent alcohol consumption, liver failure, and septicaemia commonly exacerbate this.
- Characteristic signs are tachycardia, light-headedness, sweating, and pallor. This may progress to confusion, restlessness, incomprehensible speech, double vision, convulsions, and coma. If untreated, permanent brain damage will occur, made worse by hypotension and hypoxia.
- Anaesthetized patients may not show any of these signs. Monitor blood sugar regularly, and suspect hypoglycaemia with unexplained changes in the patient's condition.
- If hypoglycaemia occurs, give 75mL of 20% glucose over 15min or 150mL of 10% glucose, and repeat the blood glucose after 15min. Alternatively, give 1mg of glucagon (IM or IV); 10–20g (2–4 teaspoons) of sugar by mouth or an NGT is an alternative.

Variable-rate intravenous insulin infusion

- The recommended 1st-choice solution for VRIII is 0.45% NaCl with 5% glucose, and either 0.15% potassium chloride (KCl) or 0.3% KCl; however, this is not always available.
- 4% glucose and 0.18% NaCl, 10% glucose, or 5% glucose are acceptable. Whenever giving hypotonic parenteral fluids, beware of hyponatraemia. Preferably give 10% glucose at 60mL/hr, rather than 5% glucose at 120mL/hr (prevents water overload, particularly in the elderly).
- If K^+ <4.5mmol/L, add 10mmol KCl to each 500mL bag of glucose.
- Start VRIII using a syringe pump. Adjust according to the sliding scale in Table 8.3. Test blood glucose hourly initially. Patients on >100U of insulin/day will need higher doses of insulin by infusion.

Transferring from a variable-rate intravenous insulin infusion to subcutaneous insulin or oral treatment

Restarting oral hypoglycaemic medication

- Recommence oral hypoglycaemic agents once the patient is ready to eat and drink.
- Be prepared to withhold or reduce sulphonylureas if the food intake is likely to be reduced.
- Metformin should only be recommenced if the estimated GFR (eGFR) >50mL/min/1.73^2.

Restarting subcutaneous insulin for patients already established on insulin

- Conversion to SC insulin should be delayed until the patient is able to eat and drink without nausea and vomiting.
- It should take place when the next meal-related SC insulin dose is due, e.g. with breakfast or lunch.

Table 8.3 VRIII sliding scale

Blood glucose (mmol/L)	Initial rate of insulin infusion (U/hr)	Insulin infusion rate if blood glucose not maintained <10mmol/L (U/hr)
<4.0	0.5 (0.0 if a long-acting background insulin has been continued), and treat as for hypoglycaemia	0.5 (0.0 if a long-acting background insulin has been continued), and treat as for hypoglycaemia
4.1–7.0	1.0	2.0
7.1–9.0	2.0	3.0
9.1–11.0	3.0	4.0
11.1–14.0	4.0	5.0
14.1–17.0	5.0	6.0
17.1–20.0	6.0	8.0
>20	Check infusion running, and seek diabetes team or medical advice)	Check infusion running, and seek diabetes team or medical advice

- Restart the normal pre-surgical regime. Be aware that insulin requirement may change due to post-operative stress, infection, or altered food intake.
- Consult the diabetes team if blood sugar is outside the acceptable range (4–12mmol/L) or if a change in diabetic management is needed.
- Ensure overlap between the VRIII and the 1st injection of the fast-acting insulin. The fast-acting insulin should be injected SC with the meal, and the VRIII discontinued 30–60min later.

For patients on basal bolus insulin
- If the patient was previously on a long-acting insulin analogue, such as Lantus® or Levemir®, this should have been continued, and so the patient only needs to restart their normal short-acting insulin at the next meal.

For patients on a twice-daily fixed-mix regimen
- The insulin should be only reintroduced before breakfast or before the evening meal.

For patients on continuous subcutaneous insulin
- Commence the SC insulin infusion at their normal basal rate as long as not at bedtime.
- VRIII should be continued until the next meal bolus has been given.

Intensive care unit admissions

- Manage patients admitted to ICU post-operatively to ensure blood glucose between 5 and 10mmol/L. Previous evidence from Van den Berghe et al.[1] for tighter glucose control (4.4–6.1mmol/L), leading to improved mortality and morbidity, has not been borne out by recent evidence from the Glucontrol study[2] and the VISEP study.[3] These showed no difference in outcomes, but significantly more hypoglycaemia and the need for more nursing input to achieve this level of glycaemic control safely.

Glucose–potassium–insulin regime (GKI or Alberti)

This is an alternative, simpler regime which does not require infusion pumps, but may provide less accurate control of blood sugar. The original regime, as described by Alberti,[4] consists of:
- 500mL of 10% glucose
- Add 10–15U of soluble insulin, plus 10mmol of KCl per 500mL bag
- Infuse at 100mL/hr
- Provides insulin 2–3U/hr, K$^+$ 2mmol/hr, and glucose 10g/hr.

Glucose 10% is not always available, so the following regime with 5% glucose can be used—infuse 5% glucose (500mL bags) at the calculated rate for the patient's fluid maintenance requirements. Insulin and K$^+$ should be added to each bag, as per Table 8.4. The bag may be changed according to 2-hourly blood glucose measurements.

Table 8.4 GKI infusions based on 5% glucose solution

Blood glucose (mmol/L)	Soluble insulin (U) to be added to each 500mL bag of 5% glucose	Blood K$^+$ (mmol/L)	KCl (mmol) to be added to each 500mL bag of 5% glucose
<4	5	<3	20
4–6	10	3–5	10
6.1–10	15	>5	None
10.1–20	20		
>20	Review	If potassium level not available, add 10mmol KCl to each bag	

References

1 Van den Berghe G, Wouters P, Weekers F, et al. (2001). Intensive insulin therapy in critically ill patients. *N Engl J Med*, **345**, 1359–67.

2 Preiser JC, Devos P, Ruiz-Santana S, et al. (2009). A prospective randomized multi-centre controlled trial on tight glucose control by intensive insulin therapy in adult intensive care units: the Glucontrol study. *Intensive Care Med*, **35**, 1738–48.

3 Brunkhorst FM, Engel C, Bloos F, et al. (2008). Intensive insulin therapy and pentastarch resuscitation in severe sepsis. *N Engl J Med*, **358**, 125–39.

4 Alberti KGMM (1991). Diabetes and surgery. *Anesthesiology*, **74**, 209–11.

Further reading

Dhatariya K, Levy N, Kilvert A, et al. (2011). NHS Diabetes guideline for the peri-operative management of the adult patient with diabetes. *Diabet Med*, **29**, 420–33.

Lobo DN, et al. (2012). The peri-operative management of the adult patient with diabetes. http://www.asgbi.org.uk.

Rehman HU, Mohammed K (2003). Peri-operative management of diabetic patients. *Curr Surg*, **60**, 607–11.

Simpson AK, Levy N, Hall GM (2008). Perioperative IV fluids in diabetic patients—don't forget the salt. *Anaesthesia*, **63**, 1043–5.

Sonksen P, Sonksen J (2000). Insulin: understanding its action in health and disease. *Br J Anaesth*, **85**, 69–79.

Acromegaly

A rare clinical syndrome caused by overproduction of growth hormone from the anterior pituitary. Patients may present for pituitary surgery (see ❷ p. 399) or require surgery unrelated to their pituitary pathology.

Preoperative assessment

- CVS: cardiac assessment for hypertension (30%), IHD, cardiomyopathy, heart failure, conduction defects, and valvular disease.
- Airway: difficult airway management/intubation may occur—check for large jaw, head, tongue, lips, and general hypertrophy of the larynx and trachea. Also vocal cord thickening or strictures and chondrocalcinosis of the larynx. Consider direct/indirect laryngoscopy preoperatively if vocal cord or laryngeal pathology is suspected. Snoring and daytime somnolence may indicate sleep apnoea. Look for enlargement of the thyroid (25%) which may compress the trachea.
- Drugs: somatostatin analogues (octreotide, lanreotide) may cause vomiting and diarrhoea. Bromocriptine, a long-acting dopamine agonist, is often used to lower growth hormone levels. It can cause severe postural hypotension.
- Neurological: symptoms and signs of raised ICP.

Investigations

- ECG as routine. Echocardiogram if patient symptomatic or has murmurs.
- CXR if cardiorespiratory problems.
- Blood glucose—25% of cases are diabetic.

Conduct of anaesthesia

- Large face masks and long-bladed laryngoscopes may make airway management and intubation easier. Awake fibreoptic intubation (AFOI) is the technique of choice for patients with anticipated difficult intubation but is seldom required (see ❷ p. 969). Elective tracheostomy should be considered in those with severe respiratory obstruction.
- Positioning may be difficult. A long table may be required.
- Nerve compression syndromes are common, so take care to protect vulnerable areas (ulnar nerve at the elbow, median nerve at the wrist, and common peroneal nerve below the knee).
- Experience shows more problems with extubation than intubation.
- If evidence of sleep apnoea, extubate the patient awake and sitting up.

Post-operative care

If major surgery, consider ventilating the patient with sleep apnoea for a few hours in ICU, until they are stable to wean from the ventilator.

Further reading

Nemergut EC, Dumont AS, Barry UJ, Lawes ER (2005). Perioperative management of patients undergoing transsphenoidal pituitary surgery. *Anesth Analg*, **101**, 1170–81.

Seidman PA, Kofke WA, Policare R, Young M (2000). Anaesthetic complications of acromegaly. *Br J Anaesth*, **84**, 179–82.

Thyroid disease

May present for thyroidectomy (see ➔ p. 574) or non-thyroid surgery.

General considerations for non-thyroid surgery

Hypothyroidism

- Commonly due to autoimmune thyroid destruction.
- CVS complications include decreased blood volume, cardiac output, and HR, with a predisposition to hypotension and IHD. Pericardial effusions also occur.
- Also associated with anaemia, hypoglycaemia, hyponatraemia, and impaired hepatic drug metabolism.
- If clinical evidence of hypothyroidism, delay elective surgery to obtain a euthyroid state. Liaise with the endocrinologist. Suggest levothyroxine (T_4) (starting dose 50 micrograms, increasing to 100–200 micrograms PO over several weeks). The elderly are susceptible to angina and heart failure, with increasing cardiac work caused by thyroxine, so start with 25 micrograms, and increase by 25 micrograms at 3- to 4-weekly intervals.
- If surgery is urgent, then liothyronine (T_3) (10–50 micrograms slow IV with ECG monitoring, or 5–20 micrograms in patients with known or suspected cardiac disease, followed by 10–25 micrograms 8-hourly) can be used, but this is more controversial.
- Be cautious in interpreting low serum thyroid hormones in sick or surgical patients, as it is important to distinguish between hypothyroidism and the 'euthyroid sick syndrome'. There is no clear evidence to give thyroid hormone replacement in the latter.

Hyperthyroidism (thyrotoxicosis)

- Typically presents with weight loss, hypertension, sweating, and cardiac arrhythmias (especially AF). Treatment is with carbimazole (30–45mg PO daily for 6–8wk). This inhibits iodination of tyrosyl residues in thyroglobulin. Occasionally, in severe cases with a large thyroid, Lugol's iodine is substituted 10d preoperatively to reduce gland vascularity.
- β-blockade (propranolol 30–60mg tds) is also started if there are signs of tremor or palpitations. The non-cardioselective β-blockers, such as propranolol, are more effective than the selective ones. $β_1$-adrenergic blockade treats the symptoms of tachycardia, but $β_2$-adrenergic blockade prevents the peripheral conversion of T_4 to T_3.

Preoperative assessment

- Thyroid function: check the patient is euthyroid (HR <80bpm, no hand tremor)—delay surgery, if possible, until achieved. Patients with subclinical hypothyroidism usually have no anaesthetic problems, and elective surgery can proceed without special preparation.[5]
- Airway: look for tracheal deviation—a large goitre can cause respiratory obstruction. This is a particular problem when the gland extends retrosternally. Ask the patient about positional dyspnoea and dysphagia. Look for evidence of tracheal compression with shortness of breath, dysphagia, and stridor (occurs with 50% compression). Infiltrating

carcinoma may make any neck movement difficult and is an independent predictor of difficult intubation.
- Superior vena cava (SVC) obstruction can occur. Look for distended neck veins that do not change with respiration.
- Check for other autoimmune disorders.

Investigations
- FBC, U&Es, serum calcium, thyroid function tests.
- CXR/thoracic inlet views essential to assess tracheal compression.
- If tracheal compression present, perform CT or MRI scan to reveal the site and length of narrowing and also the presence of any calcification.
- Refer to the ENT surgeon for indirect laryngoscopy to document any preoperative vocal cord dysfunction.

Conduct of anaesthesia

Hypothyroid patients
- Give all drugs slowly. Susceptible to profound hypotension, which may be relatively resistant to the effects of catecholamine therapy.
- Low metabolic rate predisposes to hypothermia, so actively warm.
- Controlled ventilation is recommended—tendency to hypoventilate.
- Drug metabolism can be slow. Monitor twitch response, and reduce the dose of relaxants and opioids.

Hyperthyroid patients
- Continue β-blockade perioperatively to reduce the possibility of a thyroid storm.

Special considerations

Thyroid storm
- A life-threatening exacerbation of the hyperthyroid state, with evidence of decompensation in one or more organ systems—mortality 20–30%.
- Usually presents 6–24hr post-surgery with fever (>40°C), sweating, sinus tachycardia (>140bpm), coma, nausea, vomiting, diarrhoea.
- Rehydrate with IV saline and glucose.
- Treat hyperthermia with tepid sponging and paracetamol. Do not give NSAIDs or aspirin, as these displace thyroid hormone from serum binding sites.
- Give propranolol (1mg increments, up to 10mg), with CVS monitoring, to decrease the pulse rate to <90bpm. Alternatively, give esmolol (loading dose 250–500 micrograms/kg, followed by 50–100 micrograms/kg/min).
- Give hydrocortisone (200mg IV qds) to treat adrenal insufficiency and to decrease T_4 release and conversion to T_3 at very high levels.
- Give propylthiouracil (1g loading dose via NGT, followed by 200–300mg qds). This inhibits thyroid hormone release and also decreases the peripheral conversion of T_4 to T_3.
- After blockade by propylthiouracil, give sodium iodide (500mg tds IV), potassium iodide (five drops qds via NGT), or Lugol's iodine (5–10 drops qds via NGT).[5]

Hypothyroid coma

- A rare form of decompensated hypothyroidism—mortality 15–20%.
- Characterized by coma, hypoventilation, bradycardia, hypotension, and a severe dilutional hyponatraemia.
- Precipitated by infection, trauma, cold, and CNS depressants.
- Rehydrate with IV glucose and saline.
- Stabilize cardiac and respiratory systems, as necessary. May require ventilation.
- Sudden warming may lead to extreme peripheral vasodilatation, so use cautious passive external warming.
- Give levothyroxine 200–400 micrograms IV bolus, followed by 100 micrograms the next day. Use smaller doses in patients with CVS disease.
- Patients should first receive stress-dose steroids (e.g. hydrocortisone 100mg qds IV), in case they have concomitant 1° or 2° adrenal insufficiency, a common result of hypothyroidism.
- Consider a combination of IV T_3 and T_4, particularly if urgent surgery required.[6] The conversion of T_4 to T_3 is suppressed in hypothyroid coma, and T_3 is more active than T_4. For doses of IV T_3, see ➲ p. 157.
- Transfer to ICU.

References

5 Bennett-Guerrero E, Kramer DC, Schwinn DA (1997). Effect of chronic and acute thyroid hormone reduction on perioperative outcome. *Anesth Analg*, **85**, 30–6.
6 Mathes DM (1998). Treatment of myxedema coma for emergency surgery. *Anesth Analg*, **86**, 445–51.

Further reading

Bahn RS, Burch HB, Cooper DS, *et al.* (2011). Hyperthyroidism and other causes of thyrotoxicosis: management guidelines of the American Thyroid Association and American Association of Clinical Endocrinologists. *Thyroid*, **21**, 593–646.
Farling PA (2000). Thyroid disease. *Br J Anaesth*, **85**, 15–28.
Langley RW, Burch HB (2003). Perioperative management of the thyrotoxic patient. *Endocrinol Metab Clin North Am*, **32**, 519–34.
Manzullo EF, Ross DS (2014). *Non-thyroid surgery in the patient with thyroid disease*. ℘ http://www.uptodate.com/contents/nonthyroid-surgery-in-the-patient-with-thyroid-disease.
Stathalos N, Wartoskky L (2003). Perioperative management of patients with hypothyroidism. *Endocrinol Metab Clin North Am*, **32**, 503–18.

Parathyroid disorders

General considerations

The parathyroid glands secrete parathyroid hormone (PTH), which acts on the bones and kidneys to increase serum calcium and decrease serum phosphate. It stimulates osteoclasts to release calcium and phosphate into the extracellular fluid (ECF) and simultaneously increases phosphate excretion and calcium reabsorption in the kidney. Patients may present for parathyroidectomy (see ➲ p. 578) and non-parathyroid-related surgery.

Hyperparathyroidism

- 1° hyperthyroidism: usually an adenoma causing a high PTH, high calcium, and low phosphate. Associated with familial multiple endocrine neoplasia (MEN) type 1. Tumours rarely palpable and are located at surgery. Methylthioninium chloride (methylene blue) up to 1mg/kg is often given preoperatively to localize the parathyroid gland.
- Presentation—50% of cases are asymptomatic, and presentation is often subtle. May present with anorexia, dyspepsia, nausea, vomiting and constipation, hypertension, shortened QT interval, polydipsia, polyuria, renal calculi, depression, poor memory, and drowsiness.

Hypercalcaemic crisis

- Occurs most commonly in the elderly with undiagnosed hyperparathyroidism and with malignant disease. Dehydration results in anorexia and nausea/vomiting which exacerbates the cycle. Also characterized by weakness, lethargy, mental changes, and coma.
- Serum calcium >4.5mmol/L is life-threatening and can be rapidly, but transiently, lowered with phosphate (500mL of 0.1M neutral solution over 6–8hr).
- Rehydrate (4–6L of fluid often required).
- Pamidronate (60mg in 500mL of saline over 4hr) is the 1st-line treatment. Bisphosphonates are potent inhibitors of osteoclastic bone resorption. Effect is rapid and long-lasting.
- Calcitonin (3–4U/kg IV, then 4U/kg SC bd). Causes a rapid, but temporary, decrease in skeletal release of calcium and phosphate.
- 2nd-line treatment, once volume repletion has been achieved, is with forced saline diuresis with furosemide (40mg IV every 4hr). Loop diuretics decrease the proximal tubular resorption of calcium. Consider central pressure monitoring in the elderly at risk of LV failure.
- Hydrocortisone (200–400mg IV daily) in patients with malignancy.
- Dialysis is reserved for patients with renal failure.

Secondary hyperparathyroidism

- Results from compensatory parathyroid hypertrophy due to chronic low calcium. Complicates CRF.
- Parathyroid hyperplasia causes a high PTH, normal or low calcium level, and a high phosphate level.
- Usually presents as excessive bone resorption (seen earliest in the radial aspect of the middle phalanx of the 2nd digit) or soft tissue calcification of the vascular and soft tissues, including kidneys, heart, lungs, and skin.

- Treat medically with dietary phosphate restriction, calcium, and vitamin D supplements. Medical therapy fails in 5–10% of patients on long-term dialysis, and surgery becomes necessary.
- Risks of surgery are bleeding, recurrent hyperparathyroidism, hypoparathyroidism, and injury to the recurrent laryngeal nerves. Patients should undergo dialysis within 1d of surgery and then 48hr post-operatively or as required.
- Watch for post-operative hypocalcaemia and hypomagnesaemia.

Tertiary hyperparathyroidism

- Parathyroid hyperplasia progresses to autonomous secretion, behaving like an adenoma. Excessive secretion of PTH continues, despite correction of renal failure. Only a few cases require operation.

Perioperative plan

- Restore intravascular volume with 0.9% NaCl. If the patient has normal CVS and renal systems, a normal ECG, and a total serum calcium <3mmol/L, then proceed with the operation. If the serum calcium is >3mmol/L, the ECG is abnormal, or the patient has CVS or renal impairment, the operation should be postponed until after treatment.
- Careful monitoring of NMB should be undertaken if NDMRs are used.

Hypoparathyroidism

- Usually caused by parathyroidectomy, but post-radiotherapy and idiopathic cases also occur. Patients with a history of extensive neck dissection in the past should have serum calcium measured before further surgery.
- Results in hypocalcaemia—ionized calcium <0.9mmol/L, total calcium (corrected for albumin) <2.2mmol/L. Trough level usually occurs at 20hr following parathyroidectomy and typically normalizes by days 2–3.
- The presenting features are due to low calcium levels and manifest as carpopedal spasm, tetany, dysrhythmia, hypotension, and prolonged P–R interval on ECG.
- Treat with calcium (calcium gluconate 10mL 10% IV over 10min, followed by 40mL in 1L of saline over 8hr).
- Low serum magnesium is also common and can be treated with magnesium sulfate (1–5mmol IV slowly).

To adjust calcium concentration for albumin level:

Add 0.1mmol/L to calcium for each 5g/L that albumin is below 40g/L.

Further reading

Mihai R, Farndon JR (2000). Parathyroid disease and calcium metabolism. *Br J Anaesth*, **85**, 29–43.
Sasidharan P, Johnston IG (2009). *Parathyroid physiology and anaesthesia. Anaesthesia tutorial of the week.* ♪ http://www.anaesthesiauk.com.

Adrenocortical insufficiency

Primary (Addison's disease)

- Destruction of adrenal cortex by autoimmune disease (75%), infection (TB), septicaemia, acquired immune deficiency syndrome (AIDS), haemorrhage, metastases, surgery. Associated with glucocorticoid and mineralocorticoid deficiency.

Secondary

- Insufficient adrenocorticotrophic hormone (ACTH) to stimulate the adrenal cortex due to pituitary suppression by exogenous steroids or generalized hypopituitarism usually from pituitary or hypothalamic tumours. Associated with glucocorticoid deficiency only.

Acute adrenal crisis

- Due to stress in patients with chronic adrenal insufficiency without adequate steroid replacement, acute adrenal haemorrhage, or pituitary apoplexy (apoplexy is defined as a sudden neurologic impairment, usually due to a vascular process, i.e. infarction or haemorrhage).

Clinical features of chronic adrenal insufficiency

- Weakness, fatigue (100%), skin hyperpigmentation (90%—1° only), postural hypotension (90%—pronounced in 1°), nausea, vomiting, diarrhoea, weight loss (60%), myalgia, joint pain, salt craving (1° only), pale skin (2° only).

Investigations

- Low serum glucose, low Na^+ (90%), raised K^+ (70%), raised urea and creatinine (1° only), raised Ca^{2+} (1° only) (Table 8.5).

Table 8.5 Biochemical diagnosis of adrenal insufficiency

Test	Normal range	Definite adrenal insufficiency	
		1°	2°
Early morning cortisol	165–680nmol/L	Cortisol <165nmol/L and ACTH >22.0pmol/L	Cortisol <100nmol/L
Early morning ACTH	1.1–11.0pmol/L		Not diagnostic
Standard short Synacthen® test[1]	Peak cortisol >500nmol/L	Peak cortisol <500nmol/L	Peak cortisol <500nmol/L
Insulin tolerance test[2]	Peak cortisol >500nmol/L		Peak cortisol <500nmol/L

[1] Serum cortisol at 0 and 30min after 250 micrograms of Synacthen® IV.

[2] Serum glucose and cortisol 0, 15, 30, 45, 60, and 90min after insulin (0.1–0.15U/kg IV). Test only valid if symptomatic hypoglycaemia (serum glucose <2.2mmol/L) is achieved. Gold standard test—close supervision mandatory.

Treatment
- Hydrocortisone (20mg in the morning and 10mg at night PO).
- Fludrocortisone (0.1mg PO) to replace aldosterone (1° deficiency only)

Perioperative management of patients with long-standing Addison's disease (according to ⌘ http://www.Addisons.org.uk)
- Give all medication on the morning of surgery.
- For any nil-by-mouth regime, give IV saline to prevent dehydration, and maintain mineralocorticoid stability, e.g. 100mL every 8hr if >50kg.
- IM hydrocortisone is preferable to IV administration, as it gives more sustained stable cover. It may alternatively be given by an infusion pump, e.g. hydrocortisone 25mg bolus, then 5mg/hr in glucose 5%.
- Give hydrocortisone 100mg IM just before anaesthesia, and continue every 6hr until the patient is eating and drinking normally. Then double the oral dose for 48hr if major surgery, and 24hr if minor surgery. Then return to normal dose.
- If any post-operative complications arise, e.g. fever, delay the return to normal dose.
- Four-hourly blood glucose and daily electrolytes.
- Joint care with an endocrinologist is advisable.
- With respect to mineralocorticoid potency, 20mg hydrocortisone is equivalent to 0.05mg fludrocortisone, so, with hydrocortisone doses of 50mg or more, mineralocorticoid replacement in 1° adrenal insufficiency can be reduced.

Adrenal crisis (Addisonian crisis)
Classically presents as hypotension, hyponatraemia, hyperkalaemia, and hypoglycaemia with abdominal pain. Characteristically resembles hypovolaemic shock but can also mimic septic shock with fever, peripheral vasodilatation, and a high cardiac output. In patients with type 1 diabetes, deterioration of glycaemic control with recurrent hypoglycaemia can be the presenting sign of adrenal insufficiency.
- 100% O_2 and ventilatory support if necessary. Refer to ICU/HDU.
- IV fluids. Colloid to restore blood volume, saline to replace Na^+ deficit initially at 1000mL/hr, and glucose for hypoglycaemia.
- Hydrocortisone 200mg stat, followed by 100mg qds. If hydrocortisone is given IV, please administer over a minimum of 10min to prevent vascular damage. Baseline cortisol and ACTH prior to administration of hydrocortisone. Dexamethasone (4mg IV) can be used if the diagnosis has not been confirmed, since this does not interfere with the measurement of cortisol and ACTH stimulation testing.
- Inotropes/vasopressors, as required. May be resistant in the absence of cortisol replacement.
- Ascertain and treat the precipitating cause.

Relative adrenal insufficiency in the critically ill

- Relative hypoadrenalism in ICU patients occurs in ~30–50% of septic patients. Consider in patients who are increasingly vasopressor-dependent or require prolonged mechanical ventilation. Treat if suspected—200mg hydrocortisone IV.
- Abnormal response to a short Synacthen® test is a poor prognostic indicator.

Further reading

Annane D, Bellissant E, Bollaert PE, Briegel J, Keh D, Kupfer Y (2004). Corticosteroids for severe sepsis and septic shock: a systematic review and meta-analysis. *BMJ*, **329**, 480–4.

Arlt W, Allolio B (2003). Adrenal insufficiency. *Lancet*, **361**, 1881–93.

Wass J, Howlett T, Arlt W, Pearce S (2014). *Glucocorticoid medication requirements for surgery and dentistry*. ℜ http://www.addisons.org.uk/comms/publications/surgicalguidelines-colour.pdf.

The patient on steroids

Steroids are used as replacement therapy in adrenocortical insufficiency or to suppress inflammatory and immunological responses. Patients on steroids requiring surgery may develop complications from their underlying disease or from a potentially impaired stress response due to hypothalamic–pituitary–adrenal (HPA) suppression. Classically, these patients were given additional large doses of steroids perioperatively; however, recent research suggests that smaller physiological replacement doses are more than adequate (Table 8.6).

Table 8.6 Perioperative steroid replacement therapy

<10mg prednisolone/day	Assume normal HPA axis	No additional steroid cover required
>10mg prednisolone/day	Minor surgery, e.g. hernia	Routine preoperative steroid or hydrocortisone 25mg IV at induction
	Intermediate surgery, e.g. hysterectomy	Routine preoperative steroid plus hydrocortisone 25mg IV at induction, and then 6-hourly for 24hr
	Major surgery, e.g. cardiac	Routine preoperative steroid plus hydrocortisone 25mg IV at induction, then 6-hourly for 48–72hr
High-dose immunosuppression	Should continue usual immunosuppressive dose until able to revert to normal oral intake, e.g. 60mg prednisolone/24hr = 240mg hydrocortisone/24hr	
Patient formerly taking regular steroids	<3 months since stopped steroids—treat as if on steroids >3 months since stopped steroids—no perioperative steroids necessary	

Hypothalamic–pituitary–adrenal suppression

- Endogenous cortisol (hydrocortisone) production is of the order of 25–30mg/24hr (following a circadian pattern). During stress induced by major surgery, it rises to 75–100mg/d and can remain elevated for a variable period of time (up to 72hr following cardiac surgery).
- Prednisolone is a synthetic glucocorticoid with the general properties of the corticosteroids. Prednisolone exceeds hydrocortisone in glucocorticoid and anti-inflammatory activity, being ~3–4 times more potent on a weight basis than the parent hormone, but is considerably less active than hydrocortisone in mineralocorticoid activity. Therefore, it is often given for chronic conditions to limit water retention and is found only as an oral preparation. In contrast, the relatively high mineralocorticoid activity of hydrocortisone and the resulting fluid retention make it unsuitable for disease suppression on a long-term basis; however, hydrocortisone can be given as an oral or IV preparation, which is why it is often used perioperatively, instead of prednisolone.

- Low-dose steroid treatment (<10mg prednisolone per day) usually carries little danger of HPA suppression. Treatment with >10mg prednisolone (or equivalent) risks HPA suppression. This may occur after treatment via the oral, topical, parenteral, nebulized, and inhaled routes. These patients must be assumed to be suffering from an inability to mount a normal endogenous steroid response to stress and be supplemented accordingly.
- HPA suppression can be measured using various methods. In practice, the short Synacthen® test (corticotropin test) is reliable, cheap, and safe. Patients are given Synacthen® (synthetic corticotropin) (250 micrograms IV), and serum cortisol is measured at 0, 30, and 60min. Normal peak cortisol levels range from 420 to 700nmol/L and indicate the ability of the patient to mount a stress response. If the result is equivocal, an insulin tolerance test can be performed under the supervision of an endocrinologist.

For beclometasone and adrenal suppression, see ➜ p. 99.

Prednisolone 5mg is equivalent to:
- Hydrocortisone 20mg
- Methylprednisolone 4mg
- Betamethasone 750 micrograms
- Dexamethasone 750 micrograms
- Cortisone acetate 25mg
- Deflazacort 6mg
- Triamcinolone 4mg.

Fludrocortisone is available only in the oral preparation. It may be withheld on the day of surgery and while the patient is receiving stress doses of hydrocortisone (20mg hydrocortisone has equivalent mineralocorticoid potency of 0.05mg fludrocortisone).

Further reading

Nicholson G, Burrin JM, Hall GM (1998). Peri-operative steroid replacement. *Anaesthesia*, **53**, 1091–104.

Cushing's syndrome

A syndrome due to excess plasma cortisol caused by iatrogenic steroid administration (commonest), pituitary adenoma (Cushing's disease—80% of remainder), ectopic ACTH (15% of remainder—e.g. oat cell carcinoma of lung), adrenal adenoma (4% of remainder), adrenal carcinoma (rare).

Clinical features

- Moon face, truncal obesity, proximal myopathy, and osteoporosis.
- Easy bruising and fragile skin, impaired glucose tolerance, diabetes.
- Hypertension, LV hypertrophy, sleep apnoea.
- High Na^+, bicarbonate (HCO_3^-), and glucose; low K^+ and Ca^{2+}.
- GI reflux.

Diagnosis

- High plasma cortisol and loss of diurnal variation (normal range ~165–680nmol/L; trough level at ~ midnight, peak level at ~6.00 a.m.).
- Increased urinary 17-(OH)-steroids.
- Loss of suppression with dexamethasone 2mg.
- ACTH level:
  - Normal/high—pituitary
  - Low—adrenal, ectopic cortisol administration
  - Very high—ectopic ACTH.

Preoperative assessment

- Many patients have ECG abnormalities (high-voltage QRS and inverted T waves) which may make IHD difficult to exclude, but they will revert to normal after curative surgery. These ECG changes seem to be related to the Cushing's disease itself.
- Eighty-five per cent of patients are hypertensive and are often poorly controlled.
- Sleep apnoea and gastro-oesophageal reflux are common.
- Sixty per cent of patients have diabetes or impaired glucose tolerance, and a sliding scale should be started before major surgery if glucose is >10mmol/L.
- Patients are often obese with difficult veins!
- Patients are at risk of peptic ulcer disease, so give prophylactic antacid medication.

Conduct of anaesthesia

- Position the patient carefully intraoperatively due to increased risk of pressure sores and fractures secondary to fragile skin and osteoporosis.

Further reading

Sheeran P, O'Leary E (1997). Adrenocortical disorders. *Int Anesthesiol Clin*, **35**, 85–98.
Smith M, Hirsch NP (2000). Pituitary disease and anaesthesia. *Br J Anaesth*, **85**, 3–14.

Conn's syndrome

Excess of aldosterone produced from either an adenoma (60%), benign hyperplasia of the adrenal gland (35–40%), or adrenal carcinoma (rare).

General considerations

Aldosterone promotes active reabsorption of Na^+ and excretion of K^+ through the renal tubules. Water is retained with Na^+, resulting in an increase in extracellular fluid (ECF) volume. To a lesser extent, there is also tubular secretion of hydrogen (H^+) ions and Mg^{2+}, resulting in a metabolic alkalosis.

Clinical features

• Refractory hypertension, hypervolaemia, metabolic alkalosis.
• Spontaneous hypokalaemia (K^+ <3.5mmol/L); moderately severe hypokalaemia (K^+ <3.0mmol/L) during diuretic therapy despite oral K^+.
• Muscle weakness or paralysis, especially in ethnic Chinese (2° to hypokalaemia).
• Nephrogenic diabetes insipidus 2° to renal tubular damage (polyuria).
• Impaired glucose tolerance in ~50% of patients.

Preoperative assessment for adrenalectomy

• Spironolactone (competitively inhibits aldosterone production) is usually given to reverse the metabolic and electrolyte effects. It also allows the patient to restore normovolaemia. Doses of up to 400mg/d may be required.
• The patient should have normal serum K^+ and HCO_3^-, but this may be difficult to achieve.
• Hypertension is usually mild and well controlled on spironolactone, but features of end-organ damage, e.g. LV hypertrophy, should be excluded.
• Calcium channel blockers, such as nifedipine, are effective antihypertensive agents with aldosterone-secreting adenomas. This is a specific action.

Investigations

• Aldosterone (pg/mL) to renin (ng/mL/hr) ratio >400.
• 2° hyperaldosteronism has a raised serum aldosterone with a normal ratio.
• Important to distinguish between adenoma and hyperplasia, as adenoma is usually treated surgically and hyperplasia medically.
• Adrenal vein sampling, radiolabelling tests, CT, and MRI are all used.

Conduct of anaesthesia for adrenalectomy

Unilateral adrenalectomy can be done laparoscopically or via laparotomy, and an appropriate method of analgesia should be discussed. Handling of the adrenal gland during surgery can cause CVS instability but is not as severe as with a phaeochromocytoma (see p. 580).

• A short-acting α-blocker should be available (phentolamine 1mg boluses IV).
• Check blood glucose perioperatively.

- Chronic hypokalaemia has an antagonistic action upon insulin secretion/release and may result in abnormal glucose tolerance with the stress of surgery.

Post-operative care

- Give hydrocortisone IV post-operatively until the patient can tolerate oral hydrocortisone and fludrocortisone.
- Hypertension may persist after removal of the adenoma, due presumably to permanent changes in vascular resistance.

Management of patients with Conn's syndrome for non-adrenal surgery

Such patients usually have bilateral hyperplasia of the zona glomerulosa. Hypertension is usually more severe and may require additional therapy (ACE inhibitors are useful). Try to restore K^+ to normal value preoperatively. Perform CVS assessment as for any hypertensive patient.

Further reading

Winship SM, Winstanley JH, Hunter JM (1999). Anaesthesia for Conn's syndrome. *Anaesthesia*, **54**, 564–74.

Apudomas

Tumours of amine precursor uptake and decarboxylation (APUD) cells which are present in the anterior pituitary gland, thyroid, adrenal medulla, GI tract, pancreatic islet, carotid bodies, and lungs. Apudomas include phaeochromocytoma, carcinoid tumour, gastrinoma, VIPomas, and insulinoma and may occur as part of the MEN syndrome.

Phaeochromocytoma

See ⊃ p. 580.

Carcinoid tumours

- Carcinoid tumours are derived from argentaffin cells and produce peptides and amines. Most occur in the GI tract (75%), bronchus, pancreas, and gonads. Tumours are mainly benign, and, of those that are malignant, only about a quarter release vasoactive substances into the systemic circulation, leading to the carcinoid syndrome.
- Mediators are metabolized in the liver; therefore, only tumours with hepatic metastases or a 1° tumour with non-portal venous drainage lead to the carcinoid syndrome.
- Vasoactive substances include serotonin, bradykinin, histamine, substance P, prostaglandins, and vasoactive intestinal peptide (VIP).
- Patients with an *asymptomatic* carcinoid tumour have simple carcinoid disease and do not present particular anaesthetic difficulties. Patients with *carcinoid syndrome* can be extremely difficult to manage perioperatively.

Carcinoid syndrome

Affects about 10% of patients with carcinoid tumours.
Patients may have symptoms related to:
- The 1° tumour, causing intestinal obstruction or pulmonary symptoms, e.g. haemoptysis and respiratory compromise
- Vasoactive peptides, resulting in intermittent flushing (90%), especially of the head, neck, and torso, or diarrhoea (78%), which may lead to dehydration and electrolyte disturbances. Other symptoms include bronchospasm (20%), hypotension, hypertension, tachycardia, hyperglycaemia, and right heart failure 2° to endocardial fibrosis affecting the pulmonary and tricuspid valves (mediators are metabolized in the lung before reaching the left heart).

Preoperative assessment

- Treat symptomatically—antidiarrhoeals, bronchodilators, correction of dehydration/electrolyte imbalance, treatment of heart failure.
- Prevent the release of mediators—octreotide (100 micrograms SC tds) for 2wk prior to surgery, and octreotide (100 micrograms IV, slowly diluted to 10 micrograms/mL) at induction.
- Avoid factors that may trigger carcinoid crises—catecholamines, anxiety, and drugs that release histamine, e.g. morphine.

Investigations
- Check FBC, electrolytes (may show the effects of chronic diarrhoea), LFTs, and clotting if metastases present.
- Ensure rapid cross-matchable blood is available.
- ECG (may show RV hypertrophy).
- Echocardiography to exclude right-sided cardiac disease.
- CXR and lung function tests, if indicated.

Conduct of anaesthesia
This is best managed by centres familiar with the difficulties. Major complications anticipated in the perioperative period include severe hypotension, severe hypertension, fluid and electrolyte shift, and bronchospasm.
- Premedication: anxiolytic (benzodiazepine) and octreotide (100 micrograms (50–500 micrograms) SC 1hr preoperatively), if not already treated; otherwise continue with preoperative regime.
- Monitoring should include invasive BP pre-induction (both induction and surgical manipulation of the tumour can cause large swings), CVP, regular blood glucose, and blood gases. Cardiac output monitoring will guide fluid therapy and help in managing hormone-induced preload and afterload variations, particularly if cardiac complications present.
- Consider an epidural. Benefits include a reduced risk of a carcinoid crisis with decreased stress response 2° to good analgesia; however, low doses of LA should be used (avoiding hypotension, as this may elicit bradykinergic crisis).
- Induction: prevent pressor response to intubation. Suxamethonium has been used safely for RSI, although fasciculations may theoretically stimulate hormone release by increasing the intra-abdominal pressure.
- Maintenance: both total IV anaesthesia (TIVA) and inhalation techniques have been used successfully.
- Octreotide (10–20 micrograms boluses IV) to treat severe hypotension.
- Avoid all histamine-releasing drugs (atracurium, morphine) and catecholamines (release serotonin and kallikrein, which activate bradykinins).
- Labetalol, esmolol, or ketanserin (5-HT$_2$ receptor blocker) can be used for hypertension.

Post-operative
- ICU or HDU is required.
- Patients may waken very slowly (thought to be due to serotonin).
- Avoid morphine, and use either PCA with fentanyl or pethidine, or an epidural.
- Hypotensive episodes may occur, as surgery may have reduced, rather than eliminated, the tumour, thus requiring further IV boluses of octreotide (10–20 micrograms).
- Wean octreotide over 7–10d following tumour resection.

Gastrinoma

Excess production of gastrin by benign adenoma, malignancy, or hyperplasia of the D cells of the pancreatic islets. Gastrin stimulates acid production from gastric parietal cells. Leads to Zollinger–Ellison syndrome, severe peptic ulceration, and diarrhoea. May also have GI bleeds, perforation, electrolyte disturbance, and volume depletion. Treatment includes PPIs (e.g. omeprazole), H_2 receptor antagonists, and octreotide. May present for surgery related to gastrinoma, e.g. perforation, or pancreatic resection of the tumour, or a totally unrelated pathology.

• FBC to look for anaemia from bleeding gastric ulceration.
• Check clotting screen and LFTs, since alterations in fat absorption may influence clotting factors, and hepatic function may be affected by liver metastases.
• Antacid prophylaxis preoperatively and RSI.
• Invasive pressure monitoring for major surgery.
• Continue omeprazole post-operatively, as the gastric mucosa may have become hypertrophied, producing excess acid.

VIPoma

Rare tumour secreting VIP which leads to Verner–Morrison syndrome. Characterized by profuse watery diarrhoea, intestinal ileus, abdominal distension, confusion, drowsiness, hypokalaemia, achlorhydria, hypomagnesaemia, hyperglycaemia, metabolic alkalosis, and tetany.

• VIP inhibits gastrin release; therefore, give H_2 receptor-blocking drugs preoperatively to prevent rebound gastric acid hypersecretion.
• Replace fluids and electrolytes.
• Treat medically with somatostatin analogues (octreotide). If this fails, try steroids (such as methylprednisolone) and indometacin (a prostaglandin inhibitor).
• Sixty per cent become malignant with liver metastases, so all warrant resection.
• Use invasive pressure monitoring for major surgery.
• Frequent measurement of ABGs to check the acid–base status and electrolytes.

Insulinoma

Rare tumour of β cells of the pancreas which secrete insulin—diagnosis made by the Whipple's triad—symptoms of hypoglycaemia, low plasma glucose, and relief of symptoms when glucose is given.

• Diagnosis also made by a fasting blood glucose <2.2mmol/L, increased insulin, increased C-peptide, and absence of sulphonylurea in the plasma.
• Medical treatment is used to reduce symptoms. Diazoxide (a non-diuretic benzothiazide which inhibits the release of insulin and stimulates glycogenolysis) has been used where surgery has failed but has unpredictable efficacy. Octreotide is also used. It binds with the somatostatin receptors on insulinomas and decreases insulin secretion in 40–60% of patients.
• Tumours are usually non-malignant, but, if malignant, hepatic resection may be required.
• Start 10% glucose and K^+ infusion preoperatively, and monitor blood glucose closely perioperatively, particularly at the time of tumour manipulation.

Glucagonoma

Tumour of the α cells of the pancreas. Glucagon stimulates hepatic glycogenolysis and gluconeogenesis, resulting in increased blood glucose and diabetes mellitus. Ketoacidosis is rare, since insulin is also increased. Characterized by a rash (necrotizing migratory erythema which presents in the groin/perineum and migrates to the distal extremities).

- Associated with weight loss, glossitis, stomatitis, anaemia, and diarrhoea.
- Patients usually have liver metastases at presentation.
- Treatment consists of surgical debulking and somatostatin analogues.
- Increased incidence of venous thrombosis, so give prophylactic antithrombotic therapy.

Further reading

Holdcraft A (2000). Hormones and the gut. *Br J Anaesth*, **85**, 58–68.

Mancuso K, Kaye AD, Boudreaux JP, *et al.* (2011). Carcinoid syndrome and perioperative anesthetic considerations. *J Clin Anesth*, **23**, 329–41.

Powell B, Al Mukhtar A, Mills GH (2011). Carcinoid: the disease and its implications for anaesthesia. *Contin Educ Anaesth Crit Care Pain*, **11**, 9–13.

Hypokalaemia

Defined as plasma K^+ <3.5mmol/L.

• Mild	3.0–3.5mmol/L
• Moderate	2.5–3.0mmol/L
• Severe	<2.5mmol/L

Causes
- Decreased intake.
- Increased K^+ loss—vomiting or nasogastric suctioning, diarrhoea, pyloric stenosis, diuretics, renal tubular acidosis, hyperaldosteronism, Mg^{2+} depletion, leukaemia.
- Intercompartmental shift—insulin, alkalosis (0.1 increase in pH decreases K^+ by 0.6mmol/L), β_2-agonists, and steroids.

Clinical manifestations
- ECG changes—T wave flattening and inversion, prominent U wave, ST-segment depression, prolonged P–R interval.
- Dysrhythmias, decreased cardiac contractility.
- Skeletal muscle weakness, tetany, ileus, polyuria, impaired renal concentrating ability, decreased insulin secretion, growth hormone secretion, aldosterone secretion, negative nitrogen balance.
- Encephalopathy in patients with liver disease.

Management
- Check U&Es, creatinine, Ca^{2+}, phosphate, Mg^{2+}, HCO_3^-, and glucose if other electrolyte disturbances suspected. Hypokalaemia resistant to treatment may be due to concurrent hypomagnesaemia.
- Exclude Cushing's and Conn's syndromes.
- Oral replacement is safest, up to 200mmol/d, e.g. KCl (Sando-K®) two tablets qds = 96mmol K^+.
- IV replacement—essential for patients with cardiac manifestations, skeletal muscle weakness, or where oral replacement not appropriate.
- Aim to increase K^+ to 4.0mmol/L if treating cardiac manifestations.
- Maximum concentration for peripheral administration is 40mmol/L (greater concentrations than this can lead to venous necrosis); 40mmol KCl can be given in 100mL of 0.9% NaCl over 1hr, but only via an infusion device, with ECG monitoring, in HDU/ICU/theatre environment, and via a central vein. Plasma K^+ should be measured at least hourly during rapid replacement. K^+ depletion sufficient to cause 0.3mmol/L drop in serum K^+ requires a loss of ~100mmol of K^+ from total body store.

Anaesthetic considerations

The principal problem is the risk of arrhythmia. The rate of onset is important—chronic, mild hypokalaemia is less significant than that of rapid onset.

Patients must be viewed individually, and the decision to proceed should be based on the chronicity and level of hypokalaemia, the type of surgery, and any other associated pathologies. The ratio of intracellular to extracellular K^+ is of more importance than isolated plasma levels.

- Classically, K^+ <3.0mmol has led to postponement of elective procedures (some controversy exists about this in the fit, non-digitalized patient who may well tolerate chronically lower K^+ levels, e.g. 2.5mmol/L, without adverse events).
- For emergency surgery, if possible, replace K^+ in the 24hr prior to surgery. Aim for levels of 3.5–4.0mmol/L. If this is not possible, use an IV replacement regime, as documented earlier, intra-/perioperatively.
- If HCO_3^- is raised, then the loss is probably long-standing with low intracellular K^+, and will take days to replace.
- May increase sensitivity to NMB; therefore, need to monitor.
- Increased risk of digoxin toxicity at low K^+ levels. Aim for K^+ of 4.0mmol/L in a digitalized patient.

Further reading

Freshwater-Turner D (2006). *Sodium, potassium and the anaesthetist.* ℘ http://www.frca.co.uk/article.aspx?articleid=100676.

Gennari FJ (2002). Disorders of potassium homeostasis. Hypokalaemia and hyperkalaemia. *Crit Care Clin*, 18, 273–88.

Hyperkalaemia

Defined as plasma K^+ >5.5mmol/L.

• Mild	5.5–6.0mmol/L
• Moderate	6.1–7.0mmol/L
• Severe	>7.0mmol/L

Causes

- Increased intake—IV administration, rapid blood transfusion.
- Decreased urinary excretion—renal failure (acute or chronic), adrenocortical insufficiency, drugs (K^+-sparing diuretics, ACE inhibitors, ciclosporin, etc.).
- Intercompartmental shift of K^+—acidosis (H^+ is taken into the cell, in exchange for K^+), rhabdomyolysis, trauma, malignant hyperthermia (MH), suxamethonium (especially with burns or denervation injuries), familial periodic paralysis.
- Pseudohyperkalaemia—due to *in vitro* haemolysis

Clinical manifestations

- ECG changes, progressing through peaked T waves, widened QRS, prolonged P–R interval, loss of P wave, loss of R wave amplitude, ST depression, VF, asystole. ECG changes potentiated by low Ca^{2+}, low Na^+, and acidosis.
- Muscle weakness at K^+ >8.0mmol/L.
- Nausea, vomiting, diarrhoea.

Management

Treatment should be initiated if K^+ >6.5mmol/L or ECG changes present. Unlike hypokalaemia, the incidence of serious cardiac compromise is high, and therefore intervention is important. Treat the cause, if possible. Ensure IV access and cardiac monitor.

- Insulin (10U in 50mL of 50% glucose IV over 30–60min). This has the fastest onset of action and is very effective in reducing serum K^+ by shifting the K^+ into the cells. Beware rebound occurs within 2hr.
- β_2-agonist—salbutamol (5–10mg nebulized—beware tachycardia). Should see a response at 30min and has a longer duration of action than insulin.
- Ca^{2+} (5–10mL of 10% calcium gluconate or 3–5mL of 10% calcium chloride). Ca^{2+} stabilizes the myocardium by increasing the threshold potential. Rapid onset, short-lived.
- If acidotic, give HCO_3^- (50mmol IV).
- Ion exchange resin—calcium resonium (15g PO or 30g per rectum (PR) 8-hourly). This binds K^+ in the gut.
- If initial management fails, consider dialysis or haemofiltration.

Anaesthetic considerations

Do not consider elective surgery. If life-threatening surgery, treat hyperkalaemia first.

Avoid Hartmann's solution and suxamethonium, if possible. If there is a compelling case for rapid intubation conditions without long-term paralysis, suxamethonium has been used safely with a preoperative K+ of >5.5mmol/L.[7] However, rocuronium, followed by its reversal agent sugammadex, is an excellent alternative and widely available now. Monitor NMB, since effects may be accentuated.

- Avoid hypothermia and acidosis.
- Control ventilation to prevent respiratory acidosis.
- Monitor K+ regularly.

Reference

7 Schow AJ, Lubarsky DA, Olson RP, Gan TJ (2002). Can succinylcholine be used safely in hyperkalaemic patients? *Anesth Analg*, **95**, 119–22.

Further reading

Elliot MJ, Ronksley PE, Clase CM, Ahmed SB, Hemmelgarn BR (2010). Management of patients with acure hyperkalaemia. *CMAJ*, **182**, 1631–5.
Nyirenda MJ, Tang JI, Padfield PL, Seckl JR (2009). Hyperkalaemia. *BMJ*, **339**, 1019–24.

Hyponatraemia

Defined as serum Na^+ <135mmol/L.

- Mild   125–134mmol/L
- Moderate   120–124mmol/L
- Severe   <120mmol/L

ECF volume is directly proportional to total body Na^+ content. Renal Na^+ excretion ultimately controls the ECF volume and total body Na^+ content. To identify the causes of abnormalities of Na^+ homeostasis, it is important to assess plasma and urinary Na^+ levels, along with the patient's state of hydration (hypo-/eu-/hypervolaemic).

Causes

Hypovolaemic hyponatraemia

Urinary Na^+ <30mmol/L suggests an extrarenal cause, i.e. diarrhoea, vomiting, burns, pancreatitis, trauma.

Urinary Na^+ >30mmol/L suggests a 1° renal problem, i.e. diuretic excess, osmotic diuresis, mineralocorticoid deficiency, salt-wasting nephropathy, proximal renal tubular acidosis.

Euvolaemic hyponatraemia

Hypotonic fluid replacement post-surgery, hypothyroidism, glucocorticoid deficiency, syndrome of inappropriate antidiuretic hormone secretion (SIADH), psychogenic polydipsia.

Hypervolaemic hyponatraemia

ARF or CRF, CCF, cirrhosis, nephrotic syndrome, transurethral resection of the prostate (TURP) syndrome.

Presentation

- Important to differentiate between acute and chronic hyponatraemia. Speed of onset is much more important for the manifestation of symptoms than the absolute Na^+ level. Rare to get clinical signs if Na^+ >125mmol/L.
- Na^+ 125–130mmol/L causes mostly GI symptoms, i.e. nausea/vomiting.
- Na^+ <125mmol/L—neuropsychiatric symptoms, nausea/vomiting, muscular weakness, headache, lethargy, psychosis, raised intracranial pressure, seizures, coma, and respiratory depression. Mortality high, if untreated.

Treatment of symptomatic hyponatraemia

- Acute symptomatic hyponatraemia (develops in <48hr), e.g. TURP syndrome, hysteroscopy-induced hyponatraemia, SIADH. Aim to raise serum Na^+ by 2mmol/L/hr until symptoms resolve. Complete correction is unnecessary, although not unsafe. Infuse hypertonic saline (3% NaCl) at a rate of 1.2–2.4mL/kg/hr through a large vein. Measure Na^+ levels hourly. In cases of fluid excess, give furosemide (20mg IV) to promote diuresis. If there are severe neurological symptoms (seizures, coma) 3% NaCl may be infused at 4–6mL/kg/hr. Electrolytes should be carefully monitored (see also ➲ p. 593).

- Chronic symptomatic hyponatraemia (present for >48hr or duration unknown). Aim to correct serum Na$^+$ by 5–10mmol/d. Rapid correction (serum Na$^+$ rise of >0.5mmol/L/hr) can lead to central pontine myelinolysis, subdural haemorrhage, and cardiac failure. If hypovolaemia is present, correct with 0.9% NaCl. This removes the antidiuretic hormone (ADH) response that accentuates the Na$^+$/water imbalance. If hypervolaemic, treat with fluid restriction and furosemide. Monitor electrolytes and urine output every 12hr. For SIADH—fluid-restrict, and give demeclocycline (300–600mg daily).
- Consult with an endocrinologist.
- Watch for resolution of symptoms.
- Treat the cause.

Asymptomatic hyponatraemia (often chronic)
- Fluid-restrict to 1L/d.
- Treat the cause.

Anaesthetic implications
- No elective surgery if Na$^+$ <120mmol/L or symptomatic hyponatraemia.
- Emergency surgery: consider risk to benefits. Consult an endocrinologist.

Hypernatraemia

Defined as serum Na^+ >145mmol/L.

- Mild   145–150mmol/L
- Moderate   151–160mmol/L
- Severe   >160mmol/L

Caused by excessive salt intake or, more frequently, inadequate water intake. Important to assess the volume status.

Causes

Hypovolaemic
- *Renal*—loop/osmotic diuretics, intrinsic renal disease, post-obstruction
- *Extrarenal*—diarrhoea/vomiting, burns, excessive sweating, fistulae.

Euvolaemic
- Diabetes insipidus, insensible losses.

Hypervolaemic
- Na^+ ingestion/administration of hypertonic saline, Conn's syndrome, Cushing's syndrome.

Presentation

CNS symptoms likely if serum Na^+ >155mmol/L due to hyperosmolar state and cellular dehydration, e.g. thirst, confusion, seizures, and coma. Features depend on the cause, e.g. water deficiency will present with hypotension, tachycardia, and decreased skin turgor.

Management

Correct over at least 48hr to prevent occurrence of cerebral oedema and convulsions. Treat the underlying cause. Give oral fluids (water), if possible.
- Hypovolaemic (Na^+ deficiency): 0.9% NaCl until hypovolaemia corrected, then consider 0.45% saline.
- Euvolaemia (water depletion): estimate the total body water (TBW) deficit; treat with 5% glucose.
- Hypervolaemic (Na^+ excess): diuretics, e.g. furosemide (20mg IV) and 5% glucose; dialysis if required.
- Diabetes insipidus—replace urinary losses, and give desmopressin (1–4 micrograms daily SC/IM/IV).

Anaesthetic implications

- No elective surgery if Na^+ >155mmol/L or hypovolaemic.
- Urgent surgery—use CVP monitoring if the volume status is uncertain or may change rapidly intraoperatively, and be aware of dangers of rapid normalization of electrolytes.

Further reading

Bagshaw SM, Townsend DR, McDermid RC (2009). Disorders of sodium and water balance in hospitalized patients. *Can J Anaesth*, **56**, 151–67.
Kaye AD, Kucera IJ (2005). Sodium physiology (in Chapter 46, Intravascular fluid and electrolyte physiology). In: Miller RD, ed. *Anesthesia*, 6th edn. Philadelphia: Churchill Livingstone, pp. 1764–8.

Bone, joint, and connective tissue disorders

Colin Berry

Rheumatoid arthritis

RA is a chronic, systemic inflammatory disorder, mainly involving joints, but with extra-articular effects. Overall prevalence in the UK is 1.5 per 100 000 in ♂, and 3.6 per 100 000 in ♀, with a peak incidence in the 7th decade. It also affects children as Still's disease. Patients are often frail, in chronic pain, and taking medications with adverse effects. Airway problems are common. There is a higher than average mortality due to both the disease itself and the presence of concurrent disorders (Table 9.1).

Preoperative assessment

Articular

- **Temporomandibular**: assess for limited mouth opening.
- **Cricoarytenoid**: fixation of the cricoarytenoid joints may lead to voice changes, hoarseness, or even rarely to stridor from glottic stenosis. The larynx can also be obstructed by amyloid or rheumatoid nodules. Minimal oedema may lead to airway obstruction post-operatively.
- **Atlantoaxial subluxation (AAS)** occurs in ~25% of severe rheumatoid patients, but, of these, only a quarter will have neurological signs or symptoms. Enquire about tingling hands or feet and neck pain, and assess the range of neck movement. Excessive movement during anaesthesia may lead to cervical cord compression.
  - Anterior AAS: comprises 80% of all AAS. C1 forward on C2 from destruction of the transverse ligament. Significant if there is a gap of >3mm between the odontoid and the arch of the atlas in lateral flexion radiographs. Worsened by neck flexion.
  - Posterior AAS: this is rare. C1 backward on C2, resulting from destruction of the odontoid peg. Can be seen on lateral extension radiographs. Worsened by neck extension (e.g. from direct laryngoscopy).
  - Vertical AAS: arises from destruction of lateral masses of C1. The odontoid moves upward through the foramen magnum to compress the cervicomedullary junction.
  - Lateral AAS: uncommon. Arises from the involvement of the C1/ C2 facet joints. More than 2mm difference in the lateral alignment is significant. Causes spinal nerve compression and vertebral artery compression. Requires a frontal open mouth odontoid view to assess.
- **Subaxial subluxation** (i.e. below C2):
  - More than 2mm loss of alignment is significant.
  - Look for this particularly if the patient has undergone previous fusion at a higher level.
- **Other joints**: assess joint deformities with a view to positioning and possible anaesthetic technique (if planning an axillary block, can the patient abduct their arm?). Manual dexterity may be important if planning to use standard PCA apparatus after surgery. Special adaptations are available, e.g. trigger by blowing.

Non-articular

- CVS: association with CAD. Systemic vasculitis may lead to arterial occlusion in various organs and Raynaud's. Myocardial disease due to fibrosis, amyloid or nodular involvement. Pericarditis and pericardial effusions uncommon. Aortic incompetence and endocarditis rare.
- Respiratory: fibrosing alveolitis (restrictive defect), frequently asymptomatic. Acute pneumonitis rare. Pleural effusions and/or nodules in pleura may show on X-ray. Association with obliterative bronchiolitis. Costochondral disease gives reduced chest wall compliance.
- Anaemia: NSAID-associated blood loss. Normocytic, normochromic anaemia of chronic disease. Drug-associated bone marrow depression. Felty's syndrome is a combination of splenomegaly and neutropenia and may be associated with anaemia and thrombocytopenia.
- Nervous system: peripheral and compression neuropathies occur. Cord compression may be atlantoaxial or subaxial. Neurological changes may be chronic or acute (trauma).
- Infections: common both from the disease itself and drug effects.
- Renal and hepatic: CRF from drugs is common, as is decreased albumin, increased fibrinogen and α-1 acid glycoprotein (acute phase protein).
- Thin skin and difficult venous access.

Investigations

- All patients should have FBC, U&Es, ECG, and CXR. Consider LFT, ABGs, and coagulation studies.
- Cervical spine radiographs: the role of preoperative cervical spine flexion/extension views is controversial, and interpretation is difficult. The automatic reordering of radiographs in all patients is unnecessary. Flexion/extension views are mandatory in all patients with neurological symptoms or signs, and in those with persistent neck pain. Stabilization surgery may be necessary before other elective surgery is undertaken. Preoperative cervical spine radiographs may help determine management, but only in association with a full clinical review. Specialist radiological advice should be sought. Unless it is certain that the cervical spine is stable, all rheumatoid patients should be treated as if they might have an unstable spine. This may involve AFOI or manual in-line stabilization when undertaking direct laryngoscopy/LMA insertion/ moving the patient. MRI and CT may be useful in assessing cord compression.
- PFTs should be carried out for patients with unexplained dyspnoea or radiological abnormalities.
- An ENT opinion should be sought, and nasendoscopy performed if there is hoarseness or symptoms/signs of respiratory obstruction.
- Echocardiography is needed if there is valvular or pericardial involvement and in symptomatic cardiac disease.

Drugs in the perioperative period

- Steroid supplementation, if indicated (see ➔ p. 165).
- NSAIDs: continue, as this enables early mobilization. Stop if post-operative bleeding is a potential problem, hypotension, or deterioration in renal function.
- Disease-modifying antirheumatoid drugs (DMARDs): these drugs include gold, penicillamine, and immunosuppressant drugs such as methotrexate, azathioprine, cyclophosphamide, anakinra, ciclosporin, leflunomide, and sulfasalazine. Usually continue, as mobilization is important, and there is little evidence that omission reduces post-operative complications (wound infections). If leucopenic, consult with the rheumatologist.
- Tumour necrosis factor (TNF)-α blockers (biologics): infliximab, certolizumab, etanercept, adalimumab—belong to the class of drugs blocking the effects of TNF-α, an inflammatory mediator. Other 2nd-line drugs directly target specific monoclonal antibodies and interleukin (IL)-6 (e.g. rituximab). There are suggestions of potential for increased rate of operative infection, but no consensus on whether to discontinue perioperatively.
- DVT prophylaxis (see ➔ p. 11): early mobilization.
- GI agents: continue H_2 antagonists and PPIs prior to, and after, surgery, especially for patients on NSAIDs.

Operative considerations

- Take care of the neck, and maintain in a neutral position at all times, especially on transfer and turning. Use manual in-line stabilization during airway manipulation while the patient is unconscious (unless it is certain that the spine is stable). If intubation is necessary, consider fibreoptic intubation if difficulties are anticipated (see ➔ p. 969), particularly if there is posterior AAS (rare) and/or predicted difficulty. If direct laryngoscopy is undertaken, consider using manual in-line stabilization and a gum elastic bougie (GEB).
- Ensure careful positioning and padding/protection of vulnerable areas on the operating table. Note comfortable position before induction, then try to maintain this during surgery.
- Regional techniques may be difficult. Patient discomfort from prolonged immobilization may favour GA, perhaps in combination with regional techniques.
- Normothermia is especially important, as hypothermia may increase the risk of wound infections.
- Strict asepsis with invasive procedures, as increased risk of infection.

Post-operative

- Adequate pain control allows early mobilization. PCA may be impractical due to impaired hand function.
- Continue NSAIDs unless contraindicated.
- Physiotherapy and mobilization are important.
- Continue DVT prophylaxis until the patient is fully mobile.
- Maintain fluid intake, and monitor renal function.
- Restart DMARDs to avoid exacerbation of joint immobility.

Ankylosing spondylitis

Inflammatory arthritis of the sacroiliac joints and spine, leading to anky-losis and 'bamboo spine'. Associated with HLA-B27 in >90% of cases. Commoner in ♂, with peak age onset in the 3rd decade. Important anaes-thetic implications are both articular and non-articular (Table 9.1).

Articular

- Progressive kyphosis and fixation of the spine may hinder intubation. Conventional intubation and tracheostomy may be impossible. AAS and myelopathy can occur rarely. There may be limited mouth opening from temporomandibular involvement. Use of intubating LMA (ILMA) described, but fibreoptic intubation usually preferred.
- At risk of occult cervical fracture with minimal trauma—ensure the head is supported and not left self-supporting.
- Cricoarytenoid arthritis may make cords susceptible to trauma.
- Axial skeletal involvement may make neuraxial block difficult or impossible. Spinal anaesthesia using a paramedian approach appears to be the most practical technique for neuraxial block. Possible increased risk of epidural haematoma with epidural block.
- Limited chest expansion may lead to post-operative pulmonary complications. Effective external cardiac massage may be impossible.
- Deformity leads to difficulty with positioning, particularly if a prone position is required.

Non-articular

- Fibrosing alveolitis may occur, exacerbating post-operative hypoxia.
- AR (1%). Mitral valve involvement and conduction defects are rare.
- Amyloid may cause renal involvement.
- Cauda equina syndrome may occur in long-standing cases.
- Associated use of NSAIDs and DMARDs (see ➡ p. 186).

Table 9.1 Connective tissue disorders and anaesthesia

	Rheumatoid arthritis	Ankylosing spondylitis	Systemic lupus erythematosus	Systemic sclerosis
Prevalence (%)	1	0.15	0.03	0.001
Airway and intubation	C-spine instability/ankylosis, cricoarytenoid arthritis, temporomandibular joint arthritis	Cervical kyphosis, temporomandibular joint arthritis, occult fractures		Limited mouth opening
Respiratory	Fibrosing alveolitis, pleural effusions, nodules on CXR	Fixed chest wall, apical fibrosis	Chest infections, pulmonary emboli, pleuritis	Fibrosing alveolitis
Cardiovascular	Ischaemic heart disease (association)	Aortic regurgitation (1%)	Raynaud's, hypertension, coronary ischaemia, pericarditis, endocarditis (Libman Sacks)	Raynaud's >90%, hypertension, pulmonary hypertension, myocardial fibrosis, arrhythmias, pericardial effusions
Neurological	Peripheral neuropathy, radiculopathy, myelopathy	Cauda equina syndrome (rare)	Peripheral neuropathy Psychosis, convulsions	
Renal	Mild renal impairment common		Glomerulonephritis	Chronic impairment Hypertensive renal crisis

Gastrointestinal	Drug-related gastritis	Drug-related gastritis	Abdominal pain / Nausea / Mesenteric vasculitis	Reflux invariable
Haematology	Anaemia—drug-related and disease-related / Felty's syndrome (splenomegaly and leucopenia)	Anaemia—drug-related and disease-related	Antiphospholipid syndrome, anaemia, thrombocytopenia	
Neuraxial block	Often difficult, infection risk	Difficult—consider lateral approach, increased risk of epidural haematoma	Check coagulation, infection risk	

Systemic lupus erythematosus

This is a chronic multisystem disease, commonest in young ♀, especially in pregnancy. It is characterized by the presence of numerous antibodies, including antinuclear antibody, and immune-mediated tissue damage. Although joints may be affected, there is no deformity or bony erosion and no specific airway implications. The main anaesthetic implications are CVS disease, renal disease, coagulation status, and increased risk of infection (Table 9.1).

Preoperative assessment

- Skin and joint involvement is common, as are oral and pharyngeal ulcerations.
- CVS: pericarditis in 15% of cases. Myocarditis and endocarditis are less common. Raynaud's phenomenon 30%. CAD from atherosclerosis and other mechanisms common.
- Respiratory system: infections and PEs common. Pleuritis and pleural effusion. Pulmonary fibrosis less common.
- Neurological: cranial and peripheral nerve lesions may occur, 2° to arteritis and ischaemia. Transverse myelitis, leading to weakness or paraplegia, occurs rarely. Depression, psychosis, and fits.
- Renal: glomerulonephritis is a serious complication and may lead to nephrotic syndrome and renal failure.
- Haematological: clotting disorders or hypercoagulable states can occur. Check FBC and clotting status. Immune thrombocytopenia or circulating anticoagulants (e.g. antibodies to factor VIII) may be present. Up to a third of patients with SLE may demonstrate features of antiphospholipid syndrome (see → p. 226). This is a hypercoagulable state which paradoxically may be associated with the presence of lupus anticoagulant and a prolonged APTT. Since a prolonged APTT may indicate either a clotting disorder or a hypercoagulable state, further haematological advice should be sought.
- Higher risk of stroke with antiphospholipid antibodies.
- Steroids and other immunosuppressant drugs are used.

Anaesthesia

- There may be absolute or relative contraindications to neuraxial blocks in patients taking anticoagulants or in patients with coagulopathy (see → p. 1141). The presence of a peripheral nerve lesion may be a relative contraindication to neuraxial/regional nerve blockade.
- Maintenance of normothermia may reduce the risk of infection, as well as lessening the impact of Raynaud's phenomenon, if present.
- Laryngeal erythema and oedema are common—try to minimize trauma to the airway.
- Consider hourly urine output and invasive monitoring.
- Steroid supplementation (see → p. 165).
- Strict asepsis with invasive procedures, as increased risk of infection.

Systemic sclerosis (scleroderma)

The limited cutaneous form, comprising calcinosis, Raynaud's, oesophageal dysfunction, sclerodactyly, and telangiectasia (CREST), is commoner (60% of cases) than the more aggressive diffuse cutaneous form, which has more widespread effects and a high mortality (see → p. 188) (Table 9.1).

The following may be relevant to anaesthesia:

- CVS: Raynaud's, pericarditis, or myocardial fibrosis. Conduction defects. Pulmonary hypertension common.
- Pulmonary: fibrosing alveolitis in both forms (40% in diffuse form).
- Renal: may develop renal crisis associated with malignant hypertension.
- GI: oesophageal reflux invariable.
- Airway: may have mouth narrowing and tightened skin around the neck, leading to difficult intubation.
- No consensus on GA versus regional.

Scoliosis

Progressive lateral curvature of the spine with added rotation. Scoliosis may lead to an increasing restrictive ventilatory defect which, in turn, leads to hypoxia, hypercapnia, and pulmonary hypertension. Corrective surgery may be carried out in the teens to arrest these changes. Scoliosis may be idiopathic (~75%) or 2° to other conditions with anaesthetic implications:
- Muscular dystrophies
- Poliomyelitis
- Cerebral palsy
- Friedreich's ataxia (see ➋ p. 292).

Conduct of anaesthesia
- Formal PFTs are mandatory in severe cases.
- Check for pulmonary hypertension and right heart failure.
- Some muscular dystrophies may be associated with cardiac abnormalities. Consider echocardiography (see ➋ p. 251).
- Intraoperative spinal cord monitoring may be indicated.
- Regional techniques (e.g. paravertebral blocks), where possible, ± GA.
- Plan for high dependency or intensive care in complex cases.

Achondroplasia

The commonest form of dwarfism is caused by premature ossification of bones, combined with normal periosteal bone formation, giving a characteristic appearance of short limbs and a relatively normal cranium. The following should be noted:

- The larynx may be small, and intubation is occasionally difficult. Have a range of tube sizes and a difficult intubation trolley available. Laryngoscopy may be compromised by pectus carinatum.
- Foramen magnum stenosis is common. Avoid hyperextension during intubation.
- Central and peripheral venous access is often difficult.
- Use an appropriately sized BP cuff.
- OSA is common (see ➔ p. 630).
- Restrictive ventilatory defects may occur and can lead to pulmonary hypertension.
- Regional techniques may be difficult.
- The back may be normal. The epidural space is often narrowed with spinal canal stenosis. The volume of LA needed for an epidural is reduced.
- It is difficult to predict the volume needed for a single-injection spinal. Use of an incremental spinal catheter technique is suggested, but single-dose spinal anaesthesia is reported. Websites giving medical advice for achondroplastics suggest that spinal anaesthesia should not be used.
- The patient is of normal intelligence.

Further reading

Carrillo S, Gantz E, Baluch A, Kaye R, Kaye A (2012). Anesthetic considerations for the patient with systemic lupus erythematosus. *Middle East J Anaesthesiol*, **21**, 483–92.

Mitra S, Nilanjan D, Gomber K (2007). Emergency caesarian section in a patient with achondroplasia: an anaesthetic dilemma. *J Anesth Clin Pharmacol*, **23**, 315–18.

Samanta R, Shoukrey K, Griffiths R (2011). Rheumatoid arthritis and anaesthesia. *Anaesthesia*, **66**, 1146–59.

Woodward LJ, Kam PCA (2009). Ankylosing spondylitis: recent developments and anaesthetic implications. *Anaesthesia*, **64**, 540–8.

Haematology: drugs, tests, and disorders

Paul Kerr and Pete Ford

Anaemia

Anaemia results when Hb is below normal for age and sex. Conventionally, this is <130g/dL in an adult ♂ and <120g/dL in an adult ♀. Common causes of anaemia in the surgical patient are:
- Blood loss: acute or chronic (usually resulting in iron deficiency)
- Bone marrow failure: infiltration by tumour or suppression by drugs
- Megaloblastic anaemias: folate or vitamin B12 deficiency
- Complex anaemias: effects on production and breakdown, e.g. renal failure, RA, and hypothyroidism
- Haemolytic anaemias: either inherited (thalassaemia, sickle-cell disease (SCD), spherocytosis), acquired (autoimmune, drugs, infections), or physical (mechanical heart valves, disseminated intravascular coagulation (DIC), prolonged marching ('march haemoglobinuria')).

Clinical
- Associated with fatigue, dyspnoea, palpitations, headaches, and angina. Severity often reflects the speed of onset more than the degree of anaemia, as there is less time for adaptation.
- Symptoms of the commonest causes should be elicited, including relevant family history; always enquire about NSAIDs and alcohol.
- Respiratory and CVS history may be worsened by the anaemia or make its impact greater.

Investigations
- Measure Hb prior to surgery in appropriate patients (see ➋ p. 8), including all those at risk of anaemia undergoing major surgery and anyone with other significant medical problems, especially heart or lung disease.
- Much can be deduced from the Hb and mean corpuscular volume (MCV) alone, but, in many instances, a blood film gives additional useful information.
- Confirmatory tests, such as ferritin, B12/folate levels, reticulocyte count, direct Coombs test, erythrocyte sedimentation rate (ESR), liver/renal function, and bone marrow, should be requested, as appropriate.

Preoperative preparation
- Ideally, patients scheduled for elective surgery should have FBC checked in the weeks approaching the operation, so that abnormalities can then be investigated and corrected in time.
- When delay to surgery is possible, it is more appropriate and safer to treat the underlying cause and raise the Hb slowly with simple, effective measures, e.g. oral iron, B12 injections. Transfusing a patient with pernicious anaemia may precipitate heart failure.
- Patient compliance with oral iron is poor; IV preparations are now available that can be given IV over a few minutes and will render a patient immediately iron-replete; the Hb will take an average of 10d to respond to IV iron.
- Preparations include iron sucrose, iron polymaltose and iron carboxymaltose. Some have been associated with serve adverse

reactions such as anaphylaxis. The doses and infusion rates vary: check your local protocol or discuss with haematologist.

Perioperative blood transfusion

(See also ➲ p. 1040.)

Recent randomized controlled trials (RCTs) have confirmed that transfusion is not required for mild anaemia, even in the presence of CVS disease. In some of these trials, the use of a lower 'transfusion trigger' has been associated with a lower mortality. The following are accepted levels for transfusion:

- Red cell transfusion is indicated if the Hb level is <70g/L.
- Checking a HemoCue® reading gives comparable results to a Coulter® counter and can help to avoid a transfusion if >80g/L.
- Each case must be assessed with a view to coexistent disease, expected intraoperative blood loss, and whether acute or chronic.
- For patients with IHD:
  - Mild (angina rarely): accept Hb 70–80g/L
  - Moderate (angina regularly, but stable): accept Hb 80–90g/L
  - Severe (recent MI, unstable angina): accept Hb 100g/dL or higher.

Sickle-cell disease

SCD is caused by inheriting sickling haemoglobinopathies, either in the homozygous state (HbSS—sickle-cell anaemia), heterozygous (HbSA—sickle-cell trait), or in combination with another Hb β chain abnormality such as Hb C (HbSC disease), Hb D (HbSD disease), or β-thalassaemia (HbS/β-thal). It is estimated that there are now over 10 000 patients with SCD in Britain. SCD is endemic in parts of Africa, the Mediterranean, the Middle East, and India. The highest incidence is from equatorial Africa; all patients from areas with a high prevalence should have a sickle test preoperatively. The pathology of SCD is primarily a result of vaso-occlusion by sickled red cells, leading to haemolysis and tissue infarction. This can be precipitated by hypoxia, hypothermia, pyrexia, acidosis, dehydration, or infection. Other variant haemoglobins Hb C and Hb D-Punjab, in association with HbS, enhance the sickling process, whereas HbF (fetal Hb) impedes it.

- Susceptibility to sickling is proportional to the concentration of HbS. In the heterozygous state (sickle-cell trait), sickling is extremely uncommon—HbS concentration is <50%.
- These patients have a positive sickle solubility test, but normal blood film and Hb level. This can be confirmed by Hb electrophoresis, but, in an emergency, a normal blood film should suffice.
- These patients do not need special treatment, other than avoidance of extreme hypoxia, dehydration, infection, acidosis, and hypothermia.

Clinical features

- The manifestations of SCD do not become apparent before 3–4 months of age, when the main switch from fetal to adult Hb occurs.
- There is great variability, not only between patients, but also within individual patients at different periods of life. Many remain well most of the time.
- Vaso-occlusive crises are the commonest cause of morbidity and mortality. The presentation may be dramatic with an acute abdomen, 'acute chest syndrome' (acute pneumonia-like), stroke, priapism, and painful dactylitis. By the time patients reach adulthood, most will have small, fibrotic spleens and are functionally asplenic, with the associated risk of overwhelming septicaemia. A less acute complication is proliferative retinopathy due to retinal vessel occlusion and neovascularization (commoner in HbSC disease).
- Aplastic crises are characterized by temporary shutdown of the marrow, manifested by a precipitous fall in Hb and an absence of reticulocytes. Infection with parvovirus B19 and/or folate deficiency are the two precipitating factors.
- Sequestration crises occur mainly in children. Sudden massive pooling of red cells in the spleen can cause hypotension and severe exacerbation of anaemia, with fatal consequences, unless transfusion is given in time.
- Haemolytic crises manifest by a fall in Hb and rise in reticulocytes/ bilirubin, and usually accompany vaso-occlusive crises. Chronic haemolysis leads to gallstones in virtually all patients with SCD, though many remain asymptomatic.

Laboratory features

- Hb is usually 6–9g/dL (often lower than suggested by the clinical picture). Reticulocytes are almost always increased, and the film shows sickled cells and target cells. Howell–Jolly bodies are present if the spleen is atrophic. Leucocytosis and thrombocytosis are common reactive features. In the sickle-cell trait, the Hb and film are normal.
- Screening tests for sickling which rely on deoxygenation of HbS are positive in both HbSS and HbAS.
- Hb electrophoresis distinguishes SS, AS, and other haemoglobinopathies. Measurement of the HbS level is important in certain clinical situations where a level of <30% is aimed for. It is not necessary to wait for the results of electrophoresis before embarking on emergency surgery; clinical history, Hb level, a positive sickle test, and the blood picture usually allow distinction between SCD and the sickle-cell trait.

Management

- As no effective routine treatment exists for SCD, care is directed towards prophylaxis, support, and treatment of complications. Folic acid supplements, pneumococcal/*Haemophilus influenzae* type b (Hib) vaccinations, and penicillin prophylaxis (to protect from the susceptibility to infection caused by decreased splenic function) are recommended from an early age, preferably within a comprehensive care programme.
- For crises—rest, rehydration with oral/IV fluids, antibiotics if infection is suspected; maintain PaO_2; keep warm; prompt and effective analgesia (traditionally diamorphine/morphine is used over pethidine; regional anaesthesia very effective).
- Blood transfusions may be lifesaving, but the indications are limited. Exchange transfusions have a role in some vaso-occlusive crises (acute chest syndrome, stroke). Always discuss with a haematologist. For patients with high perioperative risk, transfusing to achieve an HbS level of <30% may decrease complications but is controversial.

Preoperative preparation

- Always seek expert advice from a haematologist well before surgery. A sample for group and antibody screening should be sent well in advance, as previously transfused sickle-cell patients often have red cell antibodies.

Perioperative and post-operative care

- Special attention must be given to hypoxia, dehydration, infection, acidosis, hypothermia, and pain. These considerations should be continued well into the post-operative period.
- Dehydration: allow oral fluids as late as possible, and pre- and post-operative IV fluids.
- Hypoxia: pulse oximetry and prophylactic O_2.
- Prophylactic antibiotic cover should always be considered because of increased susceptibility to infection.
- Positive pressure ventilation may be required to achieve normocapnia and avoid acidosis.

- Hypothermia should be avoided by warming the operating room, using a fluid warmer and active warming such as a Bair Hugger®. Core temperature should be monitored.
- Regional anaesthesia is not contraindicated, and tourniquets can be used if limbs are meticulously exsanguinated prior to inflation.

Haemoglobin SC disease

- Results from compound heterozygosity for HbS and HbC.
- Affects 0.1% of African Americans.
- Causes SCD—phenotype may be milder than homozygous HbSS.
- Patients develop anaemia, splenomegaly, jaundice, aseptic necrosis of the femoral head, hepatic disease, retinal disease, and bone marrow and splenic infarcts.
- Myocardial necrosis has been described after GA.
- Management principles are as for SCD.
- Patients with SC disease are more prone to retinal disease, and often maintain splenic function into adult life.

Porphyria

The porphyrias are a group of diseases in which there is an enzyme defect in the synthesis of the haem moiety, leading to an accumulation of precursors that are oxidized into porphyrins. There are hepatic and erythropoietic varieties. Only the three acute hepatic forms, inherited in an autosomal dominant manner (although with variable expression), affect the administration of anaesthesia:

- Acute intermittent porphyria (AIP). Common in Sweden—have increased urinary porphobilinogen and d-aminolevulinic acid
- Variegate porphyria (VP). Common in Afrikaners, a Southern African ethnic group descended from predominantly Dutch settlers—have increased copro- and protoporphyrin in the stool. Dermal photosensitivity
- Hereditary coproporphyria (HCP). Very rare—have increased urinary porphyrins. Dermal photosensitivity.

Porphyric crises

- Attacks occur most frequently in women in the 3rd to 4th decades.
- Acute porphyric crises may be precipitated by drugs, stress, infection, alcohol, menstruation, pregnancy, starvation, and dehydration.
- Symptoms include acute abdominal pain, vomiting, motor and sensory peripheral neuropathy, autonomic dysfunction, cranial nerve palsies, mental disturbances, coma, convulsions, and pyrexia.

General principles

- Patients may never have had an attack; therefore, a positive family history must be taken seriously.
- Individuals may have normal biochemical tests between attacks.
- Patients may present with unrelated pathology, e.g. appendicitis.
- Symptoms may mimic surgical pathologies, e.g. acute abdominal pain, acute neurology.
- Any patient giving a strong family history of porphyria must be treated as potentially at risk. Latent carriers may exhibit no signs, be potentially negative to biochemical screening, but still be at risk from acute attacks.

Anaesthetic management

- Many commonly used drugs are thought to have the potential to trigger porphyric crises. However, it is difficult to be definitive, as crises can also be triggered by infection or stress, which often occur simultaneously. Drugs that are considered to be definitely unsafe to use, probably safe, and controversial are documented in Table 10.1.
- Up-to-date information is available from the *BNF*, the Committee on the Review of Porphyrinogenicity (CORP),[1] the Welsh Medicines Information Centre,[2] and online resources: ✍ http://www. porphyria-europe.com and ✍ http://www.cardiff-porphyria.org/.

Suggested anaesthetic techniques

- Premedication—important to minimize stress: use temazepam/ midazolam.

Table 10.1 Anaesthetic drugs and porphyria

	Definitely unsafe	Probably safe	Controversial
Induction agents	Barbiturates, etomidate	Propofol	Ketamine
Inhalational agents	Enflurane	N_2O, ether, cyclopropane	Halothane, isoflurane, sevoflurane
Neuromuscular-blocking agents	Alcuronium	Suxamethonium, tubocurarine, gallamine, vecuronium	Pancuronium, atracurium, rocuronium, mivacurium
Neuromuscular reversal agents		Atropine, glycopyrronium, neostigmine	
Analgesics	Pentazocine	Alfentanil, aspirin, buprenorphine, codeine, fentanyl, paracetamol, pethidine, morphine, naloxone	Diclofenac, ketorolac, sufentanil
Local anaesthetics	Mepivacaine, ropivacaine	Bupivacaine, prilocaine, procainamide, procaine	Cocaine, lidocaine
Sedatives	Chlordiazepoxide, nitrazepam	Lorazepam, midazolam, temazepam, chlorpromazine, chloral hydrate	Diazepam
Antiemetics and H_2 antagonists	Cimetidine, metoclopramide	Droperidol, phenothiazines	Ondansetron, ranitidine
Cardiovascular drugs	Hydralazine, nifedipine, phenoxybenzamine	Adrenaline, α-agonists, β-agonists, β-blockers, magnesium, phentolamine, procainamide	Diltiazem, disopyramide, sodium nitroprusside, verapamil
Others	Aminophylline, oral contraceptive pill, phenytoin, sulfonamides		Steroids

- Minimize preoperative fasting. Use glucose/saline IV (avoid dextrose alone due to the frequency of hyponatraemia).
- Regional anaesthesia—bupivacaine is considered safe for epidural anaesthesia, but, in the context of any peripheral neuropathy, detailed preoperative examination and documentation are essential. In acute porphyric crises, regional anaesthesia should be avoided, as neuropathy may be rapid in onset and progressive.
- GA—propofol is the induction agent of choice. Maintenance with N_2O and/or propofol infusion. There are numerous case reports of the safe use of halothane and isoflurane.
- NMB—suxamethonium and vecuronium are considered safe (atracurium controversial). Fentanyl, morphine, and pethidine all considered safe.
- Monitoring—invasive BP during acute crisis, as hypovolaemia is common, and autonomic neuropathy may cause labile BP. Perform CVP monitoring, if clinically indicated.

Problems during anaesthesia
- Hypertension and tachycardia—treat with β-blockers such as metoprolol.
- Convulsions—treat with diazepam, propofol, or magnesium sulfate (avoid barbiturates and phenytoin).

Post-operative management
- ICU/HDU if a crisis is suspected.
- Remember that the onset of a porphyric crisis may be delayed for up to 5d.

Treatment of acute porphyric crises
- Withdraw drugs that may have precipitated the crisis.
- Give haem arginate 3mg/kg IV once daily for 4d (leads to negative feedback to ALA synthetase—the initial enzyme responsible for haem production). Treat infection, dehydration, and electrolyte imbalance, and give glucose (20g/hr).
- Treat symptoms with 'safe' drugs.
- Monitor the patient appropriately.

References
1 CORP Secretariat, Lennox Eales Porphyria Laboratories, MRC/UCT Liver Research Centre, University of Cape Town Medical School, Observatory 7925, South Africa. Fax: 010-27-21448-6815.
2 Welsh Medicines Information Centre, University Hospital of Wales, Cardiff CF14 4XW, UK. Tel. +44-029-20742979.

Rare blood disorders

Hereditary spherocytosis

- An autosomal dominant condition, in which erythrocytes have a smaller surface to volume ratio and are abnormally permeable to Na^+.
- The inflexible red cells are phagocytosed in the spleen, resulting in a microspherocytic anaemia with marked reticulocytosis. The blood film is usually diagnostic.
- Splenomegaly is common. Splenectomy leads to a 50–70% increase in red cell survival.
- Splenectomy should not be performed in children <6yr of age and should ideally be preceeded by pneumococcal, meningococcal, and Hib vaccines and lifelong oral penicillin, to help avoid infection.
- There are no particular anaesthetic considerations.

Glucose-6-phosphate dehydrogenase deficiency

- X-linked trait with variable penetrance in African Americans and people from the Mediterranean.
- The disease may afford some protection against malaria and is prevalent in endemic areas.
- The glucose-6-phosphate dehydrogenase (G6PD) enzyme is responsible for the production of NADPH, which is involved in the cell's defence against oxidative stresses such as infections (usually viral, but also septicaemia, malaria, and pneumonia) or oxidative drugs (aspirin, quinolones, chloramphenicol, isoniazid, probenecid, primaquine, quinine, sulfonamides, naphthalene, and vitamin K).
- Additionally, drugs producing methaemoglobinaemia, such as nitroprusside and prilocaine, are contraindicated, as patients are unable to reduce methaemoglobin, thereby diminishing the O_2-carrying capacity.
- Classically, ingestion of broad (fava) beans results in haemolysis (favism).
- Usually the haemolysis of red cells occurs 2–5d after exposure, causing anaemia, haemoglobinaemia, abdominal pain, haemoglobinuria, and jaundice.
- Diagnosis is made by demonstration of Heinz bodies and red cell G6PD assay (G6PD levels may be falsely raised/normal in acute haemolysis).
- Treatment includes discontinuation of the offending agent, and transfusion may be required.

Thalassaemias

Thalassaemias are due to absent or deficient synthesis of α- or β-globin chains of Hb. The severity of these disorders is related to the degree of impaired globin synthesis.

- The hallmark of β-thalassaemia is anaemia, presenting in the 1st year of life.
- α-thalassaemia is more commonly associated with hydrops fetalis.
- Diagnosis is confirmed by Hb electrophoresis and/or globin chain analysis.

- The disease is prevalent in people of Mediterranean (mainly β), African (β and non-deletional α), and Asian (deletional α) extraction.
- Regardless of the underlying chain involved, thalassaemia is classified as major, intermediate, or minor.
- Those with thalassaemia major are transfusion-dependent.
- Iron from transfused blood builds up in the reticuloendothelial system, until it is saturated, when iron is deposited in parenchymal tissues, principally the liver, pancreas, endocrine, and heart.
- Preoperative preparation should include assessment of the degree of major organ impairment (heart, liver, pancreas, endocrine) 2° to iron overload.
- High-output CCF with intravascular volume overload is common in severe anaemia and should be treated preoperatively by transfusion.
- Previous transfusion exposure may cause antibody production, and therefore cross-matching may be delayed.
- The exceedingly hyperplastic bone marrow of the major thalassaemias may cause overgrowth and deformity of the facial bones, leading to airway problems and making intubation difficult. Modern management of thalassaemia should, however, avoid skeletal malformation.

Coagulation disorders

For regional anaesthesia and coagulation abnormalities, see ⮕ p. 1141.

The classical separation of coagulation into extrinsic and intrinsic pathways is overly complicated and is now not thought to occur *in vivo*. Instead there is a common pathway of initiation (Fig. 10.1). Tissue factor from damaged vascular beds combines with factor VIIa and activates factors IX and X, which leads to the generation of small amounts of thrombin (IIa), followed by amplification. This then activates further factors (V and VIII), leading to the massive production of thrombin and generation of fibrin from fibrinogen.

- Congenital disorders of clotting may not present until challenged by trauma or surgery in adult life.
- Acquired disorders are due to lack of synthesis of coagulation factors, increased loss due to consumption (e.g. DIC, massive blood loss, and the production of substances that interfere with their function.
- A family history may be elicited (haemophilia A and B—sex-linked recessive; von Willebrand's disease—autosomal dominant with variable penetrance) but cannot be relied upon (absent in 30% of haemophiliacs).
- Response to previous haemostatic challenges (tonsillectomy, dental extractions) may indicate the severity of the coagulopathy, e.g. in severe haemophilia A (factor VIII <2%), bleeding occurs spontaneously; in mild haemophilia A (factor VIII 5–30%), bleeding occurs only after trauma.

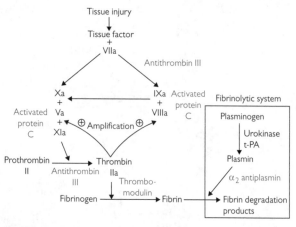

Fig. 10.1 Coagulation cascade (colour indicates inhibitor).
t-PA, tissue plasminogen activator.

- Concurrent and past medical problems, such as liver disease, malabsorption (vitamin K deficiency), infection, malignancy (DIC), autoimmune disease (SLE, RA), as well as medications (anticoagulants, aspirin, and NSAIDs), may be relevant.
- Abnormalities due to liver disease and vitamin K deficiency—give daily vitamin K (phytomenadione) 10mg IV slowly. FFP (15mL/kg) may be needed, in addition, if the presenting symptom is bleeding. Coagulation tests may be misleading in the presence of liver disease, over-emphasizing the bleeding risk; consider using TEG to evaluate the true underlying coagulopathy.[3]

For blood test results in common coagulation disorders, see Table 10.2.

Reference

3 Stravitz RT, Lisman T, Luketic VA, et al. (2012). Minimal effects of acute liver injury/acute liver failure on hemostasis as assessed by thromboelastography. *J Hepatol*, **56**, 129–36.

Table 10.2 Blood results in common coagulation disorders

Disorder	Platelet count	INR	APTT	TT	Fibrinogen	Other
Haemophilia A	Normal	Normal	↑	Normal	Normal	↓ VIII
Haemophilia B	Normal	Normal	↑	Normal	Normal	↓ IX
von Willebrand's disease	Normal (usually)	Normal	↑	Normal	Normal	↓ VIII, vWF, ↑ bleeding time
Liver disease	Normal or ↓	↑	↑	Normal	Normal or ↓	↓ V
Vitamin K deficiency	Normal	↑	↑	Normal	Normal	↓ II, VII, IX, X
DIC	Normal or ↓	↑	↑	↑	Normal or ↓	↑ FDPs, D-dimers ↓ II, V, VIII
Massive transfusion	↓	↑	Normal or ↑	Normal or ↑	Normal or ↓	Normal FDPs
Heparin (unfractionated)	Normal (rarely ↓)	Normal or ↑	↑	↑	Normal	↑ anti-Xa
Heparin (LMWH)	Normal (rarely ↓)	Normal	Normal	Normal	Normal	↑ anti-Xa
Warfarin	Normal	↑	↑	Normal	Normal	↓ II, VII, IX, X
Lupus anticoagulant	Normal	Normal or ↑	↑	Normal	Normal	DRVVT +ve, cardiolipin antibody

DRVVT, dilute Russell's viper venom test; FDPs, fibrin degradation products; vWF, von Willebrand factor.

Haemophilia and related clotting disorders

Inherited disorders of blood coagulation include haemophilia A (X-linked defect in factor VIII activity), von Willebrand's disease (autosomal defect in von Willebrand factor (vWF)), and haemophilia B (X-linked defect in factor IX).

- Haematological advice should always be sought.
- Previously untreated mild haemophilia requires strenuous efforts at avoiding blood products. Desmopressin infusion of 0.3 micrograms/kg in 50–100mL of 0.9% NaCl over 30min, with the use of tranexamic acid, can be used for mild disease or where there is low risk of bleeding.
- In elective cases, factor levels should be obtained prior to surgery. Depending on the type of surgery, the factor level should be 50–100% of normal and maintained for 2–7d post-procedure. If factors are necessary, the treatment of choice is now recombinant factor, in accordance with established guidelines. Always involve a haemophilia specialist.
- Cryoprecipitate (contains factor VIII) and FFP (contains factor IX) should be used to correct these clotting factors only in an emergency, when concentrate is unavailable, due to their chance of transmitting infection.
- NSAIDs, other anticoagulants, antiplatelet drugs, and IM injections should be avoided.
- von Willebrand's disease is divided into four subtypes: types 1, 2, and 3, and platelet type. Type 2 has four subtypes 2A, 2B, 2M, and 2N. Desmopressin is given to types 1 and 2A prior to surgical procedures and works by stimulating the release of vWF from endothelial cells. A rise in vWF is seen 30–60min after the infusion and maintained for about 6hr. Desmopressin should not be given to type 2B because of thrombocytopenia and thrombotic complications. Desmopressin is not effective in types 2M and 2N. The treatment of choice for patients who are non-responders to desmopressin is virus-inactivated factor VIII concentrate of intermediate purity. A haematologist should be involved in the planning of surgery in all such patients.

Thrombocytopenia

Defined as a platelet count $<150 \times 10^9$/L.

Spontaneous bleeding is uncommon, until the count falls below $10–20 \times 10^9$/L. The causes of thrombocytopenia are many, including:

- Failure of platelet production, either selectively (hereditary, drugs, alcohol, viral infection) or as part of general marrow failure (aplasia, cytotoxics, radiotherapy, infiltration, fibrosis, myelodysplasia, megaloblastic anaemia)
- Increased platelet consumption, with an immune basis (idiopathic thrombocytopenic purpura (ITP), drugs, viral infections, SLE, lymphoproliferative disorders) or without an immune basis (DIC, thrombotic thrombocytopenic purpura (TTP), cardiopulmonary bypass (CPB))
- Dilution, following massive transfusion of stored blood
- Splenic pooling (hypersplenism)
- Unexpected thrombocytopenia should always be confirmed with a 2nd sample and a blood film.

Preoperative preparation

- Unexplained thrombocytopenia should be investigated before elective surgery, as the appropriate precautions will be determined by the underlying cause.
- Minor procedures, such as bone marrow biopsy, may be performed without platelet support, provided adequate pressure is applied to the wound.
- For procedures, such as insertion of central lines, transbronchial biopsy, liver biopsy, lumbar puncture, or laparotomy, the platelet count should be raised to at least 50×10^9/L.
- For epidural/spinal anaesthesia, a platelet count of 80×10^9/L is adequate.
- Operations in critical sites, such as the brain or eyes, the platelet count should be raised to 100×10^9/L (see also p. 1141 and p. 758).
- In ITP, platelet transfusions should be reserved for major haemorrhage, since platelet survival is extremely short-lived. Preparation for surgery entails the use of steroids or high-dose immunoglobulins initially.

Post-operative management

- If microvascular bleeding continues, despite a platelet count of $>50 \times 10^9$/L, suspect DIC. If confirmed by coagulation tests, give FFP and cryoprecipitate, as appropriate.
- IM injections and analgesics containing aspirin or NSAIDs should be avoided.
- Desmopressin 0.3 micrograms/kg in 50–100mL of saline over 30min may improve platelet function in renal failure.

Anticoagulants

For anticoagulants and central neuraxial block/regional anaesthesia, see ➔ p. 758 (obstetrics) and p. 1141.

The main indications for anticoagulation are to prevent stroke in AF and patients with mechanical heart valves, and for the treatment and prevention of venous thrombosis and PEs (Table 10.3, Fig. 10.2).

Table 10.3 Suggested patient risk stratification for perioperative arterial and venous thromboembolism

Risk	Indication for therapy		
	Mechanical heart valve	Atrial fibrillation	VTE
High	Any mitral valve prosthesis	CHADS* score of 5 or 6	Recent (within 3 months) VTE
	Any caged ball or tilting disc aortic valve prosthesis	Recent (within 3 months) stroke or transient ischaemic attack	Severe thrombophilia (e.g. deficiency of protein C, protein S, antithrombin, antiphospholipid antibodies, multiple abnormalities)
	Recent (within 6 months) stroke or transient ischaemic attack	Rheumatic valvular heart	
Moderate	Bileaflet aortic valve prosthesis and one of the following: AF, prior stroke or transient ischaemic attack, hypertension, diabetes, congestive heart failure, age >75yr	CHADS score of 3 or 4	VTE within the past 3–12 months
			Non-severe thrombophilic conditions (e.g. heterozygous factor V Leiden mutation, heterozygous factor II mutation)
			Recurrent VTE
			Active cancer (treated within 6 months or palliative)
Low	Bileaflet aortic valve prosthesis without AF and no other risk factors for stroke	CHADS score of 0–2 (and no prior stroke or transient ischaemic attack)	VTE >12 months previous and no other risk factors

* For CHADS score, see ➔ p. 214.

AF, atrial fibrillation; VTE, venous thromboembolism.

Reproduced from Douketis JD et al. (2012). The perioperative management of antithrombotic therapy: American College of Chest Physicians evidence-based clinical practice guidelines, 9th edn. Chest, 141(2)(Suppl):e326S–e350S with permission from American College of Chest Physicians.

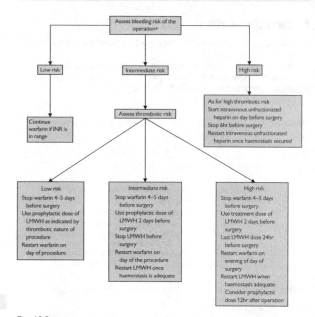

Fig. 10.2 Perioperative management of anticoagulation based on risk assessment.
Reproduced with permission from Figure 1, p.1440, Thachil J et al. (2008). Mangement of surgical patients receiving anticoagulation and antiplatelet drugs. *British Journal of Surgery*, **95**, 1437–48.

Warfarin

- Oral anticoagulant that results in the liver synthesizing non-functional coagulation factors II, VII, IX, and X, as well as proteins C and S, by interfering with vitamin K metabolism. Prolongs the PT, and monitoring is achieved by comparing this with a control, i.e. the INR.
- Recommended targets:
  - INR 2–2.5 for prophylaxis of DVT
  - INR 2.5 for treatment of DVT/PE, prophylaxis in AF, cardioversion
  - INR 3.5 for recurrent DVT/PE (despite warfarin in the therapeutic range) or mechanical heart valves.
- Reversal of a high INR can be achieved in several ways, depending on the circumstances. In the absence of bleeding, with an INR <5, reducing or omitting a dose is usually sufficient; if INR is 5–9, give vitamin K 1–2mg orally in addition. If there is minor bleeding or a grossly raised INR >9, give a small PO or IV dose of vitamin K (2–5mg). Life-threatening bleeding requires slow IV vitamin K (10mg) and prothrombin complex concentrate (PCC); PCC is a pooled blood product and prothrombotic, and can be associated with DIC (see ➋ p. 220).

- Warfarin pharmacokinetics and dynamics can be affected by a multitude of other drugs (see *BNF* for a fuller discussion). The important anaesthetic interactions include:
  - Potentiation (by inhibition of metabolism): alcohol, amiodarone, cimetidine, ciprofloxacin, co-trimoxazole, erythromycin, indometacin, metronidazole, omeprazole, paracetamol
  - Inhibition (by induction of metabolism): barbiturates, carbamazepine
  - In addition, drugs that affect platelet function can increase the risk of warfarin-associated bleeding, e.g. aspirin and NSAIDs.

Warfarin and surgery/anaesthesia

The perioperative management of patients taking anticoagulants poses significant challenges for surgeons and anaesthetists. The lack of evidence, along with the wide variety of clinical scenarios, requires individual decision-making. Anaesthetists should assess the risk of perioperative thrombotic events and the risk of perioperative bleeding and balance these risks for each individual case. Recent recommendations have been published by the American College of Chest Physicians (9th edition, 2012)[4] and are summarized in Table 10.3.

The risk of thromboembolism can be calculated by the CHADS score (Box 10.1) and considered in terms of the proposed surgery. Fig. 10.2 guides further management. Important considerations include:

- Some minor surgery may be performed without stopping warfarin.
- Limited evidence suggests that patients having surgery without discontinuation of oral anticoagulation have a perioperative major bleeding risk of 10% (one-third needing transfusion).
- The risk of thromboembolism from a mechanical heart valve in the mitral or aortic region without oral anticoagulation has an estimated annual incidence of 17% or ~0.4% for an 8d perioperative period.
- The perioperative risk of arterial thromboembolism in patients who have AF and no anticoagulation is ~1%.
- The risk stratification for patients with prior VTE is different to the arterial thromboembolism of mechanical heart valves and AF. Embolic stroke is fatal or associated with significant neurological deficit in 70% of cases. Recurrent VTE is fatal in 4–9%, with less morbidity. In addition, low-dose anticoagulation has been shown to be effective in 'bridging therapy' for recurrent VTE, but not for arterial embolism.
- Warfarin should be stopped at least 5d prior to elective surgery to allow the INR to decrease below 1.5—the level usually considered to be safe for surgery (may need to be <1.2 for high-risk surgery).
- Once the INR is <2, alternative pre- and post-operative prophylaxis should be considered.
- In patients at high risk of bleeding, a continuous IV infusion of unfractionated heparin should be started at 1000U/hr and adjusted to keep the APTT between 1.5 and 2.5. This should be stopped 6hr prior to surgery and restarted 12hr afterwards. This should be continued until INR >2.0.
- Warfarin therapy should be restarted within 12–24hr and may take up to 48hr to become therapeutic.

- For cases with a low or intermediate risk of bleeding, IV heparin can usually be replaced by the use of SC LMWH (prophylactic or treatment dose). Again this should be continued until warfarin is restarted and the INR >2.0.
- In patients who are receiving bridging anticoagulation with therapeutic-dose LMWH, there is no established role for routine perioperative monitoring of antifactor Xa levels, as in certain non-operative settings.
- Alternative methods of embolism prophylaxis should be considered such as compression stockings, and compression pumps should be considered in all cases (see ➐ p. 11).
- If the risk of VTE is very high (e.g. very recent thromboembolism) and effective anticoagulation cannot be undertaken, the insertion of a caval filter should be considered.
- In emergency surgery, there is too little time to withdraw warfarin, and specialist haematological advice should be sought. PCCs (such as Octaplex® or Beriplex®) have replaced FFP as first-line treatment. The dose varies, depending on the initial INR. Vitamin K 5–10mg IV slowly should also be given. FFP (10–15mL/kg) is a cheaper and viable alternative, but is not as effective.
- CHADS: CCF, Hypertension, Age 75yr or older, Diabetes mellitus, and a history of Stroke or transient ischaemic attack (TIA). The stroke rate per 100 patient-years without antithrombotic therapy increases by a factor of 1.5 for each one-point increase in CHADS score.

Box 10.1 CHADS score[4]

Assign one point each for:
- Presence of congestive heart failure
- Hypertension
- Age 75yr or older
- Diabetes mellitus
  Assign two points for history of stroke or TIA.

Heparin

- A parenterally active anticoagulant that acts by potentiating antithrombin; can be used for both prophylaxis and the treatment of thromboembolism.
- Unfractionated heparin is given by IV bolus or infusion. It is monitored by prolongation of the APTT (maintain at 1.5–2.5 times the normal laboratory value).
- A validated regime is to give a bolus of 80U/kg, followed by an infusion of 18U/kg/hr, and check the first APTT after 6hr.
- It has a narrow therapeutic window with complex pharmacokinetics and great inter-patient variation in dose requirements.
- Half-life is 1–2hr, so stopping it is usually enough to reverse excessive anticoagulation or bleeding. If bleeding is severe, protamine can be used.

- Protamine sulfate counteracts heparin. If given within 15min of heparin, 1mg of protamine IV neutralizes 100U of heparin. After this, less protamine is required, as heparin is rapidly excreted. It should be given slowly to avoid hypotension
- Complications of heparin include heparin-induced thrombocytopenia (HIT), which can cause serious venous and arterial thrombosis. Patients on heparin for 5d or more should have their platelet counts checked. This is less of a problem with LMWH.
- LMWH has largely replaced unfractionated heparin for both prophylaxis and the treatment of thromboembolism and unstable CAD. Administered once daily by SC injection, it needs no monitoring (although antifactor Xa levels can be measured in renal failure). Many patients with DVT are now managed as outpatients.
- LMWH is renally excreted so should be used with caution in renal failure.
- The reversal of LMWH is more difficult. The neutralizing effect of protamine on the inhibition of factor Xa is 95% for unfractionated heparin, but only 55% for LMWH. 1mg of enoxaparin = 100U: 1mg of protamine. Halve the dose if >8hr since administration.

Hirudins (lepirudin)

- Lepirudin, a recombinant hirudin, can be used for anticoagulation in patients who have type II (immune) HIT.
- Dose is monitored according to APTT, and reduced in renal failure.

Epoprostenol

- Prostaglandin, which inhibits platelet aggregation and is used in renal haemodialysis or haemofiltration and 1° pulmonary hypertension.
- Given by continuous IV infusion, as half-life is ~3min.

Newer anticoagulants

Direct thrombin inhibitors may take over from warfarin, without the need for routine anticoagulant monitoring. Many of these powerful new drugs do not have specific reversal agents.

Dabigatran and rivaroxaban

- Dabigatran (direct thrombin inhibitor) and rivaroxaban (anti-Xa inhibitor) are now licensed for extended VTE prophylaxis after hip and knee replacement surgery, and to reduce the risk of stroke and systemic embolism in patients with non-valvular AF.

Fondaparinux

- Fondaparinux sodium is a synthetic pentasaccharide that inhibits activated factor X.
- Licensed for the prophylaxis of VTE in immobilized medical patients; as VTE prophylaxis after hip and knee replacement surgery or abdominal surgery; treatment of DVT and PE; treatment of unstable angina or MI.
- The initial dose should not be given until 6hr after surgical closure.

Reference

4 Douketis JD, Spyropoulos AC, Spencer FA, et al. (2012). Perioperative management of antithrombotic therapy: Antithrombotic Therapy and Prevention of Thrombosis, 9th edn: American College of Chest Physicians Evidence-Based Clinical Practice Guidelines. Chest, **141**(2 Suppl), e326S–50S.

Antiplatelet drugs

These decrease platelet aggregation and may inhibit thrombus formation in the arterial circulation where anticoagulants have little effect.

Aspirin

- Binds irreversibly to platelets and prevents the production of thromboxane by inactivating cyclo-oxygenase (COX), the enzyme that catalyses the 1st committed step in prostaglandin synthesis. New platelets have to be formed to reverse its effects.
- Should be given immediately in acute MI.
- Low-dose aspirin is a mainstay for 2° prevention of thrombotic vascular events in vascular and cardiac disease.
- May also be used in angina, post-coronary bypass surgery, intermittent claudication, AF, and 1° prevention of IHD.
- If aspirin is to be stopped, it takes 7–9d for platelet function to return to normal.
- There are few published trials looking at perioperative bleeding due to aspirin.
- In CABG, aspirin increases perioperative bleeding but increases graft patency.
- In transurethral prostatectomy, aspirin considerably increases perioperative bleeding.
- Minor surgery to skin or cataract surgery does not require aspirin to be stopped.
- On balance, aspirin should be stopped for at least 7d prior to surgery when the risks of perioperative bleeding are high (major surgery) or where the risks of even minor bleeding are significant (retinal and intracranial surgery). This risk of bleeding must be balanced against the possibility of precipitating a thromboembolic event, particularly in patients with unstable angina.

Dipyridamole

- Used with low-dose aspirin for post-coronary artery surgery and valve replacement.
- Also used for 2° prevention of stroke and TIAs.
- Dipyridamole needs to be stopped at least 7d prior to surgery but probably has less effect than aspirin.

Clopidogrel

- Binds irreversibly with the adenosine diphosphate (ADP) receptor on platelets.
- Used with aspirin in acute coronary syndrome and for the prevention of ischaemic events in symptomatic patients. Also commonly used after coronary stents to maintain patency.
- Can be used in peripheral arterial disease or post-ischaemic stroke.
- Needs to be stopped 7d prior to surgery to avoid antiplatelet effect.
- If rapid reversal is necessary for bleeding or emergency surgery, platelet transfusions have been used with some success. However, as it is a prodrug and undergoes biotransfomation, these may be ineffective

if given just after a dose—therefore, try to delay surgery for 24hr. If impossible, case reports have suggested that aprotinin may be useful.

Glycoprotein IIb/IIIa inhibitors

- Prevent platelet aggregation by blocking the binding of fibrinogen to receptors on platelets via the GP IIb/IIIa receptor.
- Abciximab is licensed as an adjunct to aspirin and heparin in percutaneous transluminal coronary intervention.
- Eptifibatide and tirofiban are used to prevent early MI in unstable angina and non-ST-segment elevation MI.
- These drugs are potent inhibitors of platelet function. Abciximab binds strongly to platelets and has a half-life of several days. Platelet transfusions will be needed to control profound bleeding.
- Eptifibatide and tirofiban are renally eliminated. Therefore, if renal function is normal, full reversal will occur within 4–8hr from discontinuation of therapy. For more rapid reversal, platelet transfusions are less helpful, as free drug is circulating (but the addition of FFP may be beneficial).
- For elective surgery, as the half-life of abciximab is several days, it should be discontinued a week prior to surgery. Eptifibatide and tirofiban need only 8hr if the renal function is normal.

Perioperative management of antiplatelet drugs

An increasing number of patients are receiving antiplatelet drugs for the 1° and 2° prevention of MI or stroke or for the prevention of coronary stent thrombosis after placement of a BMS or DES.

- Evidence shows that dual antiplatelet therapy with aspirin and clopidogrel is needed for 1yr after DES insertion to preserve patency. Then aspirin alone (or clopidogrel in those intolerant) is continued for life.
- Evidence is also increasing that the risks of stopping antiplatelet therapy during the perioperative period are far higher than the risks of bleeding.
- The American Heart Association and European Society of Cardiology have recommended that all elective surgery is postponed until after the 12-month period of dual therapy.
- If surgery cannot be postponed, then ideally it would proceed with the continuation of dual (or at the very least single) therapy.
- Early discontinuation of antiplatelet therapy is the most significant determinant of stent thrombosis which can have a mortality of up to 50%.
- Any acute bleeding can be reversed with platelet transfusion.
- All cases must be discussed on a case-by-case basis between the cardiologist, surgeon, and anaesthetist.
- The risk of stent thrombosis associated with stopping antiplatelet agents is also influenced by factors such as the nature of the lesion and timing of the procedure. It is likely to be highest when multiple recently implanted stents are present, particularly involving arterial bifurcations, and in patients with renal impairment, diabetes, and dehydration.

Fibrinolytics

- Act as thrombolytics by activating plasminogen to plasmin; this degrades fibrin and therefore dissolves thrombi.
- Alteplase (recombinant tissue plasminogen activator, rt-PA) and streptokinase by continuous infusion.
- Reteplase and tenecteplase by bolus injection (making them ideal for early community injection).
- Used for acute MI where benefits outweigh risks.
- Benefit greatest with early injection, ECG changes with ST elevation or new bundle branch block, and anterior infarction.
- Alteplase, reteplase, and streptokinase need to be given within 12hr of symptom onset, ideally within 1hr; use after 12hr requires specialist advice. Tenecteplase should be given as early as possible and usually within 6hr of symptom onset.
- Should be used in combination with antithrombin (LMWH) and antiplatelet (aspirin) therapy to reduce early reinfarction.
- Alteplase, streptokinase, and urokinase can be used for other thromboembolic disorders such as DVT and PE. Alteplase is also used for acute ischaemic stroke. Treatment must be started promptly.
- Contraindications include any risk of bleeding, especially trauma (including prolonged cardiopulmonary resuscitation, CPR), recent surgery, GI tract and intracerebral pathology.
- Streptokinase can cause allergic reactions and should be used only once due to the production of antibodies.
- Serious bleeding calls for the discontinuation of therapy and may require coagulation factors. Cryoprecipitate (high levels of factor VIII and fibrinogen) and FFP (factors V and VIII), as well as platelets, may all be required. Antifibrinolytics, such as aminocaproic acid, tranexamic acid, and aprotinin, may also be useful.
- Bleeding times are prolonged for up to 24hr after these drugs. In emergency, surgery reversal will be required.
- Urokinase is also licensed to restore the patency of occluded IV catheters and cannulae blocked with fibrin clots. Inject directly into the catheter or cannula 5000–25 000U dissolved in a suitable volume of NaCl 0.9% to fill the catheter or cannula lumen; leave for 20–60min, then aspirate the lysate; repeat, if necessary.

Antifibrinolytics/haemostatic drug therapy

Tranexamic acid (and aminocaproic acid)

- Both these drugs are synthetic derivatives of the amino acid lysine and reversibly bind to plasminogen, thereby blocking its binding to fibrin.
- Tranexamic acid is ten times more potent than aminocaproic acid.
- Following CRASH 2,[5] tranexamic acid was found to decrease the risk of death in people who have significant bleeding due to trauma.
- Recently, there has been increased interest in the use of tranexamic acid during joint arthroplasty where it has been shown to decrease blood loss and reduce transfusion requirements.
- Other uses include post-operative bleeding in prostatectomy and dental extractions (particularly in haemophiliacs), cardiac and craniofacial surgery, and menstrual bleeding.
- Also useful in the reversal of thrombolytics.
- Contraindicated in DIC and ureteric bleeding (risk of clot uropathy).
- Usual dose of tranexamic acid is 1g tds PO.

Aprotinin

- The drug was temporarily withdrawn worldwide following the Blood Conservation Using Antifibrinolytics in a Randomized Trial (BART) trial,[6] after studies suggested that its use increased the risk of complications or death in cardiac surgery. In February 2012, the European Medicines Agency (EMA) reverted its previous standpoint regarding aprotinin and recommended that the suspension be lifted.
- The drug is still available—Nordic became the manufacturer.
- It is contraindicated for repeated use within a year due to anaphylaxis.
- It can cause renal failure and is contraindicated in renal insufficiency.
- The drug is useful during the anhepatic phase of liver transplantation where its use is guided by TEG.

Desmopressin

- An analogue of arginine vasopressin which induces the release of vWF from the vascular endothelium to increase both vWF and factor VIII.
- Can be used (0.3 micrograms/kg given in 50–100mL of saline over 30min) for haemophilia A and von Willebrand's disease to double or quadruple the levels of vWF or factor VIII.
- Platelet function may also be improved in patients with renal failure and aspirin-induced platelet dysfunction.

Factor VIIa

- Recombinant factor VIIa (rFVIIa) acts at the 'tissue factor–factor VIIa' complex at the site of endothelial damage.
- This effect appears localized to the area where the vessel is damaged, leading to few systemic side effects.
- Numerous case reports have shown rFVIIa to have potent haemostatic effects, even when other treatments have failed and whatever the cause of bleeding. Its use to stop bleeding during operations is

off-licence, however. These potential benefits have to be weighed up against its thrombogenic risk; a Cochrane review (updated February 2011) concluded the data supporting the off-licence use of rFVII were weak, and the use of rFVIIa outside its current licensed use—haemophilia and inhibitory allo-antibodies and for prophylaxis and treatment of patients with congenital factor VII deficiency—should be restricted to clinical trials.

- Dosing and mode of delivery (IV bolus or continuous infusion) have still not been established (20–40 micrograms/kg has been used).

Prothrombin complex concentrates (PCCs)

- Dried prothrombin complex is prepared from human plasma and contains factor IX, together with variable amounts of factors II, VII, and X.
- Indications are treatment and prophylaxis of congenital or acquired deficiency of factors II, VII, IX, and X (such as during warfarin treatment).
- Contraindications are angina, recent MI, and history of HIT.
- Side effects include thrombosis and hypersensitivity/anaphylaxis.

References

5 Roberts I, Shakur H, Coats T, et al. (2013). The CRASH-2 trial: a randomised controlled trial and economic evaluation of the effects of tranexamic acid on death, vascular occlusive events and transfusion requirement in bleeding trauma patients. *Health Technol Assess*, **17**, 1–79.

6 Henry D, Carless P, Fergusson D, Laupacis A (2009). The safety of aprotinin and lysine-derived antifibrinolytic drugs in cardiac surgery: a meta-analysis. *CMAJ*, **180**, 183–93.

Haematological management of the bleeding patient

(See also ➜ p. 1049.)
- Establish whether the cause of bleeding is surgical or a coagulopathy.
- A coagulopathy is more likely if bleeding is simultaneous from several sites or is slow in onset.
- A single site or sudden massive bleeding suggests a surgical source.
- Coagulation tests may help but often take some time to be obtained.
- Remember blood products also take time to arrive.
- Treatment should be aimed primarily at the removal or control of the underlying cause, while support is given to maintain tissue perfusion and oxygenation.
- Abnormal coagulation parameters in the presence of bleeding or the need for an invasive procedure are indications for haemostatic support. Further useful information can often be gained from a TEG where available (see ➜ p. 222). Transfusion of platelets and FFP (15mL/ kg initially or 4U in an average adult) should help restore platelets, coagulation factors, and the natural anticoagulants antithrombin III and protein C. Cryoprecipitate (two pools or 10U initially) may also be necessary if the fibrinogen level cannot be raised above 1g/L by FFP alone.
- Indications for heparin, concentrates of antithrombin, and protein C are not established. Antifibrinolytics, such as tranexamic acid, are generally contraindicated in DIC; conversely, tranexamic acid is beneficial for bleeding 2° to trauma and should routinely be considered in the heavily bleeding patient.
- Massive transfusion of stored blood perioperatively may cause significant coagulation disorders due to the lack of factors V, VIII, and XI. DIC and thrombocytopenia may also be present. Therapy consists of replacement FFP, cryoprecipitate, and platelets, as guided by coagulation tests and TEG. A haematologist should be consulted.
- Several case reports (see ➜ p. 219) have shown good results from giving factor VIIa in cases of uncontrollable haemorrhage.

Disseminated intravascular coagulation

- Acute DIC is probably the commonest cause of a significant coagulation abnormality in the surgical setting, especially in the peri- and post-operative phase.
- It is associated with infections (especially Gram-negative bacteraemia), placental abruption, amniotic fluid embolism (AFE), major trauma, burns, hypoxia, hypovolaemia, and severe liver disease.
- Haemorrhage, thrombosis, or both may occur.
- Chronic DIC is associated with aneurysms, haemangiomas, and carcinomatosis.
- Laboratory abnormalities are variable, depending on the severity of the DIC, and reflect both the consumption of platelets and coagulation factors, as well as hyperplasminaemia and fibrinolysis.
- Discuss treatment options with a haematologist.

Coagulation tests

Standard coagulation tests

- Activated clotting time (ACT), APTT, INR, fibrinogen, platelets.
- In the bleeding coagulopathic patient, pH, temperature, and ionized Ca^{2+} can also be measured for correction.

Viscoelastic tests: thromboelastography/thromboelastometry

- TEG/thromboelastometry measure the viscoelastic properties of blood. The traditional technique involves blood being placed in a rotating cup, into which a pin is inserted. As a clot forms, rotational forces from the cup are transmitted to the pin and recorded by an electrical transducer. Fig. 10.3 gives an explanation of the trace.
- In 1996, thromboelastograph and TEG became registered trademarks of Haemoscope Corporation, and these terms are now used to describe the assay performed on their machine. Tem Innovations GmbH makes another machine, using slightly different technology, and uses the terms thromboelastometry and ROTEM.
- The TEG uses whole blood and kaolin to activate the test. Once the sample is taken from the patient, it must be tested within about 5min.
- The ROTEM uses a citrated sample and a number of different activating reagents (INTEM, EXTEM, HEPTEM, FIBTEM, and APTEM). Once the sample is taken from the patient and placed in a citrated bottle, it must be tested within 4hr.

Advantages compared with routine coagulation tests

- Routine coagulation tests PT and APTT poorly represent the cell-based model of haemostasis. The PT and APTT are based on the time taken for the initiation of clot formation to occur. Viscoelastic tests, such as TEG, are a better representation of the cell-based model. TEG gives information on the time taken for clot formation to begin, but also

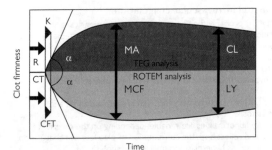

Fig. 10.3 A TEG and ROTEM trace.

on the speed of clot formation, the strength of clot formation, and whether excessive clot lysis is occurring.
- Routine coagulation tests are performed in the laboratory and therefore may take up to 45min to be completed and reported. TEG machines are usually placed in a clinical location, allowing the evolving trace to be viewed and consequentially results obtained rapidly.

Limitations of thromboelastography

Standard TEG is unable to measure the effects of antiplatelet drugs. The thrombin produced during the test is such a potent platelet activator that it overwhelms the effects of other weaker platelet activators (arachidonic acid and ADP), on which the antiplatelet drugs aspirin and clopidogrel work.

Nomenclature and normal values

Parameters differ between the two machines by name and by their normal values (due to the different reagents used) (Fig. 10.3 and Box 10.2).

Box 10.2 Nomenclature and normal values for the TEG and the ROTEM

	TEG	ROTEM
Clotting time (time to 2mm amplitude)	R (reaction time) (kaolin-activated) 4–8min	CT (clotting time) (citrated, INTEM) 137–246s, (citrated, EXTEM) 42–74s
Clot kinetics (2–20mm amplitude)	K (kinetics) (kaolin-activated) 1–4min	CFT (clot formation time) (citrated, INTEM) 40–100s, (citrated, EXTEM) 46–148s
Clot strengthening (α angle)	(kaolin-activated) 47–74°	(citrated, INTEM) 71–82°, (citrated, EXTEM) 63–81°
Maximum strength	MA (maximum amplitude) (kaolin-activated) 55–73mm	MCF (maximum clot firmness) (citrated, INTEM) 52–72mm, (citrated, EXTEM) 49–71mm
Lysis (at fixed time)	CL30, CL60	LI30, ML(maximum lysis)

Interpretation of results

- Similar to learning how to interpret an ECG. A stepwise approach is used initially.
- **Prolongation of the CT/CFT or R/K times.** Could there be a heparin effect? If YES, do CT/CFT or R/K times correct with heparinase (hepTEM assay using the ROTEM)? If YES, consider protamine. If NO, results are due to clotting deficiencies—consider FFP.
- **Reduced MA or MCF.** Perform a FIBTEM (ROTEM) or a functional fibrinogen test (TEG) (both reagents contain strong platelet inhibitors). Is MA or MCF reduced using these tests? If YES, the result is due to

fibrinogen deficiency—consider using cryoprecipitate. If NO, the result is due to platelet deficiency—consider giving a platelet transfusion.
- **Increased CL30/CL60 (TEG) or LI30/LI60 (ROTEM).** If YES, the result is due to excessive fibrinolysis—consider an antifibrinolytic. An APTEM (ROTEM) test will inhibit fibrinolysis, bringing LI30 and LI60 back to normal limits, confirming the result.
- Eventually, the traces can be interpreted by pattern recognition (Fig. 10.4).

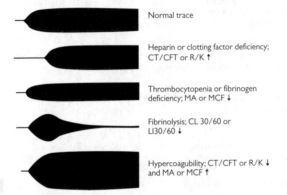

Normal trace

Heparin or clotting factor deficiency; CT/CFT or R/K ↑

Thrombocytopenia or fibrinogen deficiency; MA or MCF ↓

Fibrinolysis; CL 30/60 or LI30/60 ↓

Hypercoagulability; CT/CFT or R/K ↓ and MA or MCF ↑

Fig. 10.4 Characteristic TEG traces.

Hypercoagulability syndromes

Polycythaemia

A pattern of red blood cell changes that usually results in Hb >17.5g/dL in ♂ and >15.5g/dL in ♀. This is accompanied by a corresponding increase in the red cell count to 6.0 and 5.5 × 10^{12}/L and an Hct of 55% and 47%, respectively.

Causes

- 1°: polycythaemia vera (PV).
- 2°: due to compensatory erythropoietin (EPO) increase (high altitude, cardiorespiratory diseases—especially cyanotic, heavy smoking, methaemoglobinaemia) or inappropriate EPO increase (renal diseases—hydronephrosis, cysts, carcinoma; massive uterine fibromyomata; hepatocellular carcinoma; cerebellar haemangioblastoma).
- Relative: 'stress' or 'spurious' polycythaemia. Dehydration or vomiting.
- Plasma loss: burns, enteropathy.

Polycythaemia vera

- Presenting features include headaches, dyspnoea, chest pain, vertigo, pruritus, epigastric pain, hypertension, gout, and thrombotic episodes (particularly retinal).
- Splenomegaly.
- Thrombocythaemia in 50% of cases.
- Differential diagnosis is with other causes of polycythaemia. These can be excluded by history, examination, and blood tests, including bone marrow aspiration, ABGs, and EPO levels.
- Genetic testing can reveal the JAK 2 mutation in 90–95% of patients with PV, and 50% of patients with myelofibrosis.
- Therapy is aimed at maintaining a normal blood count by venesection and myelosuppression with drugs.
- Thrombosis is a potential cause of death, and 10% of cases develop myelofibrosis and rarely acute leukaemia.

Essential thrombocythaemia

- Megakaryocyte proliferation and overproduction of platelets are the dominant features, with a sustained platelet count >450 × 10^9/L.
- Closely related to PV, with recurrent haemorrhage and thrombosis as the principal clinical features.
- Abnormal large platelets or megakaryocyte fragments may be seen on a blood film.
- Differential diagnosis is from other causes of a raised platelet count, e.g. haemorrhage, chronic infection, malignancy, PV, myelosclerosis, and chronic granulocytic leukaemia.
- Platelet function tests are consistently abnormal.
- Hydroxycarbamide is the mainstay of therapy, but some treatments are more toxic.

Antiphospholipid syndrome

This is a rare, but increasingly recognized, syndrome resulting in arterial or venous thrombosis or recurrent miscarriage, with a positive laboratory test for antiphospholipid antibody and/or lupus anticoagulant (LA). It may present with another autoimmune disease such as SLE (2°) or as a 1° disease. The main feature of the disease is thrombosis, with a spectrum from subacute migraine and visual disturbances to accelerated cardiac failure and major stroke. Arterial thrombosis helps distinguish this from other hypercoagulable states. Paradoxically, the LA leads to a prolongation of coagulation tests, such as the APTT, but detailed testing is needed before the diagnosis can be confirmed. Patients may present for surgery because of complications (miscarriage, thrombosis) or for incidental procedures. Initially, patients are started on aspirin, but, after a confirmed episode of thrombosis, they usually remain on lifelong warfarin. High risk of thrombosis in these patients means that, if warfarin needs to be stopped for surgery, IV heparin should be commenced both pre- and post-operatively.

Anaesthesia and surgery in the hypercoagulable patient

- There are no published guidelines, but it seems prudent that elective patients who are polycythaemic should be venesected to a normal blood count to decrease the risk of perioperative thrombosis.
- Antithrombotic stockings and intermittent compression devices should be used with SC heparin.
- Haematological advice may be required.

Further reading

Association of Anaesthetists of Great Britain and Ireland (2005). *Blood transfusion and the anaesthetist: blood component therapy.* ℘ http://www.aagbi.org/sites/default/files/bloodtransfusion06.pdf.

Bombeli T, Spahn DR (2004). Updates in perioperative coagulation: physiology and management of thromboembolism and haemorrhage. *Br J Anaesth*, **93**, 275–87.

British Committee for Standards in Haematology, Blood Transfusion Task Force (2003). Guidelines for the use of platelet transfusions. *Br J Haematol*, **122**, 10–23.

Douketis JD, Spyropoulos AC, Spencer FA, et al. (2012). Perioperative management of antithrombotic therapy: Antithrombotic Therapy and Prevention of Thrombosis, 9th edn: American College of Chest Physicians Evidence-Based Clinical Practice Guidelines. *Chest*, **141**(2 Suppl), e326S–50S.

Firth PG, Head CA (2004). Sickle cell disease and anesthesia. *Anesthesiology*, **101**, 766–85.

Henry D, Carless P, Fergusson D, Laupacis A (2009). The safety of aprotinin and lysine-derived antifibrinolytic drugs in cardiac surgery: a meta-analysis. *CMAJ*, **180**, 183–93.

James MFM, Hift RJ (2000). Porphyrias. *Br J Anaesth*, **85**, 143–53.

Kraai EP, Lopes RD, Alexander JH, Garcia D (2009). Perioperative management of anticoagulation: guidelines translated for the clinician. *J Thromb Thrombolysis*, **28**, 16–22.

Mackman N (2009). The role of tissue factor and factor VIIa in hemostasis. *Anesth Analg*, **108**, 1447–52.

Mahdy AM, Webster NR (2004). Perioperative systemic haemostatic agents. *Br J Anaesth*, **93**, 842–58.

Murphy MF, Wallington TB, Kelsey P, et al. (2001). Guidelines for the clinical use of red cell transfusions. *Br J Haematol*, **113**, 24–31.

O'Shaughnessy DF, Atterbury C, Bolton Maggs P, et al. (2004). Guidelines for the use of fresh frozen plasma, cryoprecipitate and cryosupernatant. *Br J Haematol*, **126**, 11–28.

Spahn DR, Cassutt M (2000). Eliminating blood transfusions. *Anesthesiology*, **93**, 242–55.

Tanaka KA, Key NS, Levy JH (2009). Blood coagulation: hemostasis and thrombin regulation. *Anesth Analg*, **108**, 1433–46.

Thachil J, Gatt A, Martlew V (2008). Management of surgical patients receiving anticoagulation and antiplatelet drugs. *Br J Surg*, **95**, 1437–48.

Neurological and muscular disorders

Andrew Teasdale

Jane Halsall

Epilepsy

Epilepsy is a disorder characterized by chaotic brain dysfunction, leading to symptoms ranging from behavioural disorder through to life-threatening convulsions. Most epileptic patients will be on seizure-modifying drug therapy.

General considerations

- Maintain GI function to avoid metabolic disturbance and interference with drug therapy.
- Make provision for therapy if oral antiepileptic medication cannot be given.

Preoperative assessment

- Nature, timing, and frequency of seizures should be recorded.
- Full drug history, including timing of antiepileptic therapy, should be noted.
- The effect of the condition on lifestyle and the eligibility to hold a driver's licence should be noted.

Investigations

- Electrolyte and glucose measurement. Disturbance will alter seizure potential.

Conduct of anaesthesia

- Avoid prolonged fasting.
- Sedative premedication, if necessary, may be achieved with benzodiazepines. Long-acting drugs, such as diazepam (10mg PO) or lorazepam (2–4mg PO), are useful.
- Maintain antiepileptic therapy up to the time of surgery.
- All currently used anaesthetic agents are anticonvulsant in conventional doses. Thiopental is powerfully anticonvulsant and may be a preferred induction agent in the poorly controlled epileptic.
- Muscle relaxation is best achieved by drugs without a steroid nucleus (e.g. atracurium, cisatracurium), since enzyme induction by all commonly used anticonvulsant drugs (especially phenytoin, carbamazepine, and the barbiturates) will lead to rapid metabolism of vecuronium and rocuronium.
- Avoid hyperventilation and consequent hypocarbia, since this will lower the seizure threshold.
- Regional anaesthesia may assist in the preservation of, or early return to, oral intake. Be aware of maximum LA doses.
- Use antiemetic agents unlikely to produce dystonias (e.g. cyclizine 50mg IV/IM, domperidone 30–60mg PR, ondansetron 4mg IV).
- Record any epileptiform activity in the perioperative period carefully. The misdiagnosis as epilepsy, of postoperative shivering/dystonic movements on induction, may have profound implications.
- Day-case anaesthesia is suitable for those with well-controlled epilepsy (seizure free for 1yr or nocturnal seizures only). Patients should be warned of the potential for perioperative convulsions.

Drug issues

The following drugs (Table 11.1) should be used with caution in epileptics.

Table 11.1 Drugs to be used with caution in epilepsy

Drug	Notes
Methohexital	Reported to produce seizures in children. Increased EEG evidence of spike activity during administration. No longer marketed in the UK
Ketamine	Avoided because of cerebral excitatory effects, although it has been used, without incident, in many epileptics
Etomidate	Associated with a high incidence of myoclonus (not centrally mediated). May be confused with epileptic activity
Antiemetics: phenothiazines (e.g. prochlorperazine), central dopamine antagonists (e.g. metoclopramide), butyrophenones (e.g. droperidol)	High incidence of dystonic reactions may lead to confusion with epileptic activity
Inhalational agents: enflurane	Associated with abnormal EEG activity after administration—especially in presence of hyperventilation. No longer available in the UK
Neuromuscular blockers: steroid-based (e.g. vecuronium, rocuronium)	Pharmacodynamic resistance due to enzyme activation

Propofol

- Propofol is reported to be associated with abnormal movements during both induction and emergence from anaesthesia. This is unlikely to represent true seizure activity (EEG studies fail to demonstrate epileptiform activity during these episodes).
- Epileptic patients may be prone to seizures during the rapid emergence from propofol anaesthesia.
- Profound suppression of abnormal EEG activity is usually noted during propofol infusion.
- Propofol has also been reported to be effective in status epilepticus in ICU.

Caution is advised in the administration of propofol to epileptics (particularly those holding driving licences), unless there is an overwhelming clinical need for its administration. Co-induction with benzodiazepine (e.g. midazolam 2–3mg IV) may reduce its potential to produce abnormal movements and reduce the potential for post-operative seizure.

Driving and epilepsy

At present, UK law mandates the withdrawal of a driving licence from an epileptic until at least 6 months from the last seizure. The implications of a single convulsion in the post-operative period on a previously well-controlled epileptic cannot be overstated. Up-to-date advice on fitness to drive is available from the DVLA (Driver and Vehicle Licensing Agency, % http://www. dvla.gov.uk).

What if oral or nasogastric therapy is not possible?

The following drugs (Table 11.2) are available in parenteral or rectal formulations. In general, IM administration of antiepileptic medication should be avoided because of unpredictable absorption post-operatively and the irritant nature of the formulations.

Drug levels should be measured during parenteral therapy or after changing the route of administration.

Table 11.2 Common anticonvulsant drugs and doses

Drug	Notes
Carbamazepine	125mg PR, equivalent to 100mg PO. Maximum 1g daily in four divided doses
Phenobarbital	200mg IM repeated 6-hourly. Child 15mg/kg. IV administration associated with sedation. Slow infusion of dilute preparation recommended
Phenytoin	Loading dose 15mg/kg IV at rate of no greater than 50mg/min. Maintenance dose (same IV as PO) bd. Infusion usually under ECG and BP control
Fosphenytoin	A prodrug of phenytoin. Less irritation and CVS instability on injection. Absorbed very slowly after IM injection, although non-irritant. Dose—same dose (in phenytoin equivalents*) and frequency as oral phenytoin
Sodium valproate	IV dose same as oral dose, bd. Dose to be injected over 3–5min
Clonazepam	IV infusion in high dependency area only—facilities for airway control available. Child (any age) 500 micrograms. Adult 1mg

* See ➍ p. 1157.

Cerebrovascular disease

Stroke is the 3rd leading cause of death in the industrialized world (after heart disease and cancer). Cerebrovascular disease[1] is manifested by either global cerebral dysfunction (multi-infarct dementia) or a focal ischaemic disorder ranging from TIA to major stroke.

Transient ischaemic attacks

- These are defined as focal neurological deficits that occur suddenly and last for several minutes to hours, but never >24hr. Residual neurological deficit does not occur.
- They are thought to be related to embolism of platelet and fibrin aggregates released from areas of an atherosclerotic plaque. The risk of stroke in untreated patients is said to be ~5% per annum, with a mortality of ~30% per episode.
- Patients with a history of TIA should be investigated and assessed by a specialist vascular service, if practical. Doppler flow studies, with or without angiography, are indicated in all cases of recurrent TIAs or those that have occurred despite aspirin therapy.
- Delay of all, but urgent or emergency, surgery is warranted until Doppler studies are performed. At present, only those with a history of TIA with good recovery and a surgically accessible lesion of either >80% stenosis or 'ragged' plaque are routinely referred for carotid surgery. Crescendo TIA is considered by some as an indication for urgent carotid surgery.

General considerations

Cerebrovascular disease is associated with hypertension, diabetes, obesity, and smoking. The incidence rises with age. Medical management is based on the treatment of the underlying disorder, cessation of smoking, and antiplatelet/anticoagulant therapy.

Signs of concurrent cardiac and renal dysfunction should be sought.

When to operate

- Operation within 6wk of a cerebral event is associated with an up to 20-fold increase in the risk of post-operative stroke.
- Hemiplegia of <6–9 months' duration is associated with exaggerated hyperkalaemic response to suxamethonium.

It therefore seems prudent to delay all, but lifesaving, surgery for at least 6wk following a cerebral event, and preferably to wait 3–6 months before considering elective surgery.

Preoperative assessment

- Measure BP (both arms), and test blood glucose. The therapeutic aims are for normotension and normoglycaemia.
- Take a full drug history—continue antihypertensive drugs until the operation.
- Warfarin should be discontinued and substituted with heparin (unfractionated or LMWH, as per local protocol), if necessary.

- Aspirin is discontinued only if the consequences of haemorrhage are significant (e.g. tonsillectomy, neurosurgery).
- Document the nature of any ischaemic events and any residual neurological deficit. These may range from transient blindness (amaurosis fugax) to dense hemiplegia. This will help in differentiating new lesions arising in the perioperative period that may require urgent therapy.
- Ask about precipitating events. Vertebrobasilar insufficiency is most likely to be precipitated by postural changes and neck positioning.

Conduct of anaesthesia

- Ensure that antihypertensive medication (with the possible exception of ACE inhibitors for major surgery or when thoracic epidurals are planned) is continued to the time of operation. ACE inhibitors may predispose to profound, resistant hypotension under anaesthesia (see ⮕ p. 40).
- Thromboprophylaxis is advisable, unless contraindicated (e.g. low-dose LMWH).
- Ensure that pressor and depressor agents are available prior to induction. Use agents with which you are familiar. Maintain BP as close as practical to preoperative levels to maintain cerebral blood flow. Useful pressors are ephedrine/metaraminol; useful depressors are opioids/labetalol/esmolol/GTN.
- BP may 'swing' excessively during surgery due to the interactions of anaesthesia, antihypertensives, and the surgical stimulation on a relatively rigid vascular system. IV fluid replacement should be proactive, rather than reactive, with large-bore IV access. Non-invasive cardiac output monitoring may be useful if large fluid shifts are expected.
- Ensure that neck positioning is neutral and avoids movements associated with syncope.
- Induction of anaesthesia may result in dangerous hypotension, followed by extreme hypertension on intubation. Careful IV induction is indicated. Cover for intubation may be provided by opioids (e.g. alfentanil 500–1000 micrograms or fentanyl 150–250 micrograms).
- Avoid hyperventilation. Hypocarbia is associated with reduced cerebral blood flow, and therefore cerebral ischaemia. The combination of hypotension and hypocarbia must be avoided.
- Examine the patient early in the post-operative period to determine any change in the neurological status. New neurological signs will require urgent referral to a neurologist/vascular surgeon and urgent treatment, if possible.

Reference

1 Selim M (2007). Perioperative stroke. *N Engl J Med*, **356**, 706–13.

Parkinson's disease

General considerations

- Parkinsonism is a syndrome characterized by tremor, bradykinesia, rigidity, and postural instability. The aetiology of Parkinson's disease is unknown, but parkinsonism may be precipitated by drugs (especially neuroleptic agents) or be post-traumatic/post-encephalitic.
- Parkinsonism is due to an imbalance of the mutually antagonistic dopaminergic and cholinergic systems of the basal ganglia. Pigmented cells in the substantia nigra are lost, leading to reduced dopaminergic activity. There is no reduction in cholinergic activity.
- Drug therapy of parkinsonism is aimed at restoring this balance by either increasing dopamine or dopamine-like activity or reducing cholinergic activity within the brain.
- Drug therapy in parkinsonism is limited by severe side effects (nausea and confusion), especially in the elderly. Up to 20% of patients will remain unresponsive to drug therapy.

Drug therapies

Dopaminergic drugs

- Levodopa (L-dopa) is an inactive precursor of dopamine, which is converted by decarboxylases to dopamine within the brain. It is more useful in patients with bradykinesia and rigidity than those with tremor and is usually administered with decarboxylase inhibitors (e.g. benserazide, carbidopa) that do not cross into the brain, reducing peripheral conversion into dopamine.
- Monoamine oxidase B (MAO-B) inhibitors (e.g. selegiline) act by reducing the central breakdown of dopamine. Selegiline has fewer drug interactions than the non-specific MAO inhibitors but may cause a hypertensive response to pethidine and dangerous CNS excitability with selective serotonin reuptake inhibitors (SSRIs) and tricyclic antidepressants (see ➜ p. 267).
- Ergot derivatives, such as bromocriptine, cabergoline, lisuride, and pergolide, act by direct stimulation of dopamine receptors. They are usually reserved for adjuvant therapy in those already on L-dopa or those intolerant of the side effects of L-dopa.
- Entacapone is an adjuvant agent capable of reducing the dose of L-dopa and increasing the duration of its effect. It is usually reserved for those experiencing 'end-of-dose' deterioration after long-term dopaminergic therapy.
- Other adjuvant dopaminergic agents are ropinirole, rotigotine pramipexole, amantadine, apomorphine, and tolcapone.
- Apomorphine is the only agent available in a parenteral formulation. Rotigotine is sometimes used as monotherapy as a transdermal patch.

Anticholinergic (antimuscarinic) drugs

- The most commonly used agents in this group are benzatropine, procyclidine, trihexyphenidyl, and orphenadrine.

- These agents are indicated as 1st-line therapy only when symptoms are mild and tremor predominates. Rigidity and sialorrhoea may be improved by these agents, but bradykinesia will not be affected.
- This class of drug is useful for drug-induced parkinsonism, but not in tardive dyskinesia.
- Parenteral formulations exist for procyclidine and benzatropine, making these useful for acute drug-induced dystonias.

Surgical therapies

Surgery for treatment of Parkinson-induced disability is increasing in popularity. It is normally performed in the awake patient using stereotactic guided probes.

- Thalamotomy is used in those with tremor as the predominant disability, especially if the tremor is unilateral. Anterior thalamotomy is sometimes used for rigidity.
- Pallidotomy is primarily for those with rigidity and bradykinesia, although the tremor (if present) may also be reduced.
- Deep brain stimulation using implantable devices is becoming more commonplace. There is little literature at present relating to incidental anaesthesia in patients with these devices, but it would seem prudent to contact the manufacturer or team responsible for insertion of the device before using diathermy. If diathermy is necessary, bipolar should be used, as far as practical from the device or lead. Device function should be checked after surgery.

Preoperative assessment

Ideally, patients with severe disease should be under the care of a physician with a special interest in Parkinson's disease, who should be involved in the perioperative care.

The following assessment is of particular interest:

- A history of dysphagia or excessive salivation (sialorrhoea) is evidence of increased risk of aspiration and possible failure to maintain an airway in the perioperative period. Gastro-oesophageal reflux is common in this group of patients.
- Postural hypotension may be evidence of both dysautonomia and drug-induced hypovolaemia and should warn of possible hypotension on induction or position changes during surgery.
- Drug-induced arrhythmias, especially ventricular premature beats, are common, although they are usually not clinically significant.
- Respiratory function may be compromised by bradykinesia and muscle rigidity, as well as by sputum retention. Chest radiograph, lung function tests, and blood gases may be indicated.
- Difficulty in voiding may necessitate urinary catheterization. Post-operative urinary retention may be a potent cause of post-operative confusion.
- The severity of the underlying disease should be determined, and other likely problems anticipated, e.g. akinesia, muscle rigidity, tremor, confusion, depression, hallucinations, and speech impairment.

Drug interactions

Most patients with severe disease are on several maintenance drugs, many of which have potentially serious interactions (Table 11.3).

Table 11.3 Drugs interactions in parkinsonism

Class of drug	Interaction	Notes
Pethidine	Hypertension and muscle rigidity with selegiline	May resemble malignant hyperthermia
Synthetic opioids, e.g. fentanyl, alfentanil	Muscle rigidity	More apparent in high doses
Inhalational agents	Potentiate L-dopa-induced arrhythmias	
Antiemetics, e.g. metoclopramide, droperidol, prochlorperazine	May produce extrapyramidal side effects or worsen parkinsonian symptoms	Metoclopramide may increase plasma concentration of L-dopa—use domperidone/ondansetron
Antipsychotics, e.g. phenothiazines, butyrophenones, piperazine derivatives	May produce extrapyramidal side effects or worsen Parkinson's symptoms	Better to use atypical antipsychotics such as sulpiride, clozapine, risperidone
Antidepressants: tricyclics (e.g. amitriptyline), serotonin reuptake inhibitors (e.g. fluoxetine)	Potentiate L-dopa-induced arrhythmias (tricyclics only). Hypertensive crises and cerebral excitation with selegiline (tricyclics and SSRIs)	
Antihypertensives (all classes)	Marked antihypertensive effect in treated and untreated parkinsonism. Related to postural hypotension and relative hypovolaemia	Most marked with clonidine and reserpine

Conduct of anaesthesia

- Treatment for parkinsonism should be continued up to the start of anaesthesia. Distressing symptoms may develop as little as 3hr after a missed dose. Acute withdrawal of drugs may precipitate neuroleptic malignant syndrome (see p. 269).
- Premedication is usually unnecessary, unless distressing sialorrhoea is present. Consider glycopyrronium (200–400 micrograms IM) as an antisialogogue.
- The presence of preoperative sialorrhoea or dysphagia is a sign of GI dysfunction. Airway control with intubation by RSI may be indicated.
- Maintain normothermia to avoid shivering.
- There is no evidence that any anaesthetic technique is superior to any other.
- Analgesia: IV morphine is useful if regional or local analgesia is not possible (PCA may prove difficult for the patient). Oral analgesia may be difficult to administer with coexisting dysphagia (a nasogastric tube may be necessary).

Post-operative care

- In principle, the more disabled the patient preoperatively, the greater the need for post-operative high dependency and respiratory care.
- Post-operative physiotherapy should be arranged if rigidity is disabling.
- NGT insertion may be needed if GI dysfunction is present to allow early return of oral medication.
- Prolonged GI dysfunction post-operatively may lead to severe disability, since no parenteral dopaminergic therapy is currently available.

Special considerations

Antiemetic therapy may prove problematic. The following are useful:
- Domperidone (10–20mg 4–6-hourly PO or 30–60mg 4- to 6-hourly PR). The drug of 1st choice for PONV in Parkinson's patients. It does not cross the blood–brain barrier to a significant degree and is thus not associated with significant extrapyramidal effects
- Serotonin antagonists, e.g. ondansetron 4mg IV and granisetron 1mg IV slowly, may be useful rescue agents in PONV if domperidone alone is ineffective
- Antihistamine derivatives (e.g. cyclizine 50mg IV/IM).

Further reading

Nicholson G, Pereira A, Hall G (2002). Parkinson's disease and anaesthesia. *Br J Anaesth*, **89**, 904–16.
Stotz M, Thümmler D, Schürch M, Renggli JC, Urwyler A, Pargger H (2004). Fulminant neuroleptic malignant syndrome after perioperative withdrawal of antiParkinsonian medication. *Br J Anaesth*, **93**, 868–71.

Anaesthesia in spinal cord lesions

There are ~40 000 patients in the UK with spinal cord injuries. Most are young adults. Fertility in affected ♀ approaches that of the non-injured population, and obstetric services are regularly required.

Pathophysiology of spinal cord injury

Spinal injury can be divided into three distinct phases:

- The initial phase: very short (minutes) period of intense neuronal discharge caused by direct cord stimulation. This leads to extreme hypertension and arrhythmias, with risk of LV failure, MI, and pulmonary oedema. Steroid usage in acute spinal cord injury remains controversial. If used, steroids must be given within 8hr of injury, in high dosage (e.g. 30mg/kg of methylprednisolone)
- Spinal shock follows rapidly and is characterized by hypotension and bradycardia due to loss of sympathetic tone. It is commonest after high cord lesions (above T7). There is associated loss of muscle tone and reflexes below the level of the lesion. Vagal parasympathetic tone continues unopposed, causing profound bradycardia or asystole—especially on tracheal suction/intubation. This phase may last from 3d to 8wk. Paralytic ileus is common
- Reflex phase: as neuronal 'rewiring' occurs, efferent sympathetic discharge returns, along with muscle tone and reflexes.

Autonomic dysreflexia

This is characterized by massive, disordered autonomic response to stimulation below the level of the lesion. It is rare in lesions lower than T7. Incidence increases with higher lesions. It may occur within 3wk of the original injury. The dysreflexia and its effects are thought to arise because of a loss of descending inhibitory control on regenerating presynaptic fibres.

Hypertension is the commonest feature but is not universal. Other features include headache, flushing, pallor (may be manifest above the level of the lesion), nausea, anxiety, sweating, bradycardia, and penile erection. Less commonly, pupillary changes or Horner's syndrome occur. Dysreflexia may be complicated by seizures, pulmonary oedema, coma, and death and should be treated as a medical emergency. The stimulus required to precipitate the condition varies but is most commonly:

- Urological: bladder distension, UTI, catheter insertion
- Obstetric: labour, cervical dilation, etc.
- Bowel obstruction/faecal impaction
- Acute abdomen
- Fractures
- Rarely, minor trauma to the skin, cutaneous infection (bedsores).

Management of dysreflexia

- Discover the cause, if possible, and treat.
- If no apparent cause, examine carefully for unrevealed trauma or infection; catheterize, and check for faecal impaction.

- If simple measures fail, consider:
  - Phentolamine 2–10mg IV, repeated if necessary
  - Transdermal GTN
  - Clonidine (150–300 micrograms) if there is hypertension and spasticity
  - β-blockers are indicated only if there is associated tachycardia—esmolol 10mg IV, repeated.

Systemic complications of spinal cord lesions

- Reduced blood volume—may be as little as 60mL/kg, a 20% reduction.
- Abnormal response to the Valsalva manoeuvre with continued drop in BP (no plateau) and no overshoot with release.
- Profound postural hypotension, with gradual improvement after the initial injury (never to normal). Changes in cerebral autoregulation reduce its effect on the cerebral blood flow and consciousness in the non-anaesthetized patient.
- Lesions above C3—apnoea.
- Lesions at C3/4/5—possible diaphragmatic sparing, some respiratory capacity. Initial lesions may progress in height with shock and oedema, with recovery as the oedema improves, leading to a marked improvement in respiratory capacity.
- Below C5—phrenic sparing, intercostal paralysis. Recruitment of accessory muscles is necessary to improve respiratory capacity (this may take up to 6 months).
- Paralysis of abdominal muscles severely affects the ability to force expiration, reducing the ability to cough.
- The FVC is better in the horizontal or slight head-down position due to increased diaphragmatic excursion.
- Bronchial hypersecretion may occur.
- Poor thermoregulation due to isolation of central regulatory centres from information pathways, inability to use muscle to generate heat, and altered peripheral blood flow.
- Muscle spasms and spasticity occur due to intact reflexes below the level of the lesion. They can be caused by minor stimuli. Baclofen and diazepam may be used, the former increasingly via epidural infusion.
- Reduced bone density, leading to increased risk of fractures. There is heterotopic calcification around the joints in up to 20% of patients.
- Poor peripheral perfusion—pressure sores and difficult venous access.
- Anaemia, usually mild.
- Tendency to thrombosis and PE. Some centres warfarinize tetraplegics 5d after initial presentation.
- There is delayed gastric emptying in tetraplegics (up to five times longer).

Suxamethonium in chronic spinal cord lesions

- After upper motor neuron denervation, the motor endplate effectively extends to cover the entire muscle cell membrane. With the administration of suxamethonium, depolarization occurs over this extended endplate, leading to massive K^+ efflux and potential cardiac arrest.

- Recommendations vary as to the period of potential risk. Practically, avoid suxamethonium from 72hr following the initial injury. There are no reports of clinically significant hyperkalaemia with suxamethonium after 9 months.

Conduct of anaesthesia

Spinal shock phase

Surgery is usually confined to the management of life-threatening emergencies and coexisting injury. Anaesthesia should reflect this.

- Severe bradycardia or even asystole may complicate intubation—give atropine (300 micrograms IV) or glycopyrronium (200 micrograms IV) prior to intubation.
- Extreme care should be taken if cervical spine injury is suspected.
- Preload with fluid (500–1000mL of crystalloid) to reduce hypotension.
- Central line insertion may be necessary to manage fluid balance and guide appropriate inotrope therapy.

Reflex phase

Previous anaesthetic history is vital—many procedures in these patients are multiple and repeated. Pay close attention to the following:

- Is there a sensory level, and is it complete? (Risk of autonomic dysreflexia is greater in complete lesions.)
- If complete, is the proposed surgery below the sensory level? (Is anaesthesia necessary?)
- Has there been spinal instrumentation? (Potential problems with spinal/ epidural anaesthesia.)
- Is the cervical spine stable/fused/instrumented? (Potential intubation difficulty.)
- Is postural hypotension present? (Likely to be worsened by anaesthesia.)
- Is there a history of autonomic dysreflexia (paroxysmal sweating and/or headache), and, if so, what precipitated it?
- In cervical lesions, what degree of respiratory support is necessary?
- Are there contractures or pressure sores?

Investigations

- FBC—anaemia.
- U&Es—renal impairment.
- LFTs—possible impairment with chronic sepsis.
- PFTs (FVC)—mandatory with all cervical lesions due to potential respiratory failure.

Is anaesthesia necessary?

In principle, if the planned procedure would require anaesthesia in a normal patient, it will be required for a cord-injured patient.

- Minor peripheral surgery below a complete sensory level is likely to be safe without anaesthesia.
- Even with minor peripheral surgery, minimal stimulation may provoke muscular spasm that may require anaesthesia to resolve. LA infiltration may prevent its occurrence.
- Care should be taken with high lesions (T5 and above) or patients with a history of autonomic dysreflexia undergoing urological procedures.

- If the decision is made to proceed without anaesthesia, IV access is mandatory, and ECG, NIBP, and pulse oximeter should be applied.
- An anaesthetist should be present on 'standby' for such procedures.

General anaesthesia

- Monitoring should be applied prior to induction, and BP measured before and after every position change. Invasive monitoring should be performed with the same considerations as normal.
- Despite the theoretical risk of gastro-oesophageal reflux, there appears to be no increased risk of aspiration. If intubation is necessary for the desired procedure, anticholinergic pre-treatment is recommended.
- Those with cervical cord lesions are likely to require assistance with ventilation under GA. If IPPV is performed in tetraplegics, BP may drop precipitously. Fluid preloading and vasopressors (e.g. ephedrine) may be required.
- With the exception of paralysis to facilitate intubation, NMB is unlikely to be necessary, unless troublesome muscular spasm is present.
- Care should be taken to preserve the body temperature (wrapping or forced-air warming blankets). Position with respect to pressure areas.
- Fluid management may be difficult, as blood volume is usually low, and, with high cord lesions, reflex compensation for blood loss is absent. Fluid preloading, coupled with aggressive replacement of blood losses with warmed fluid, is recommended.

Central neuraxil anaesthesia

Advantages

- Prevents autonomic dysreflexia.
- Unlikely to cause CVS instability, since the sympathetic tone is already low prior to blockade.
- No reported adverse effect of spinal injection of LAs or opioids on neurological outcome.
- Avoids risks of GA.
- Spinal anaesthesia is commoner than epidural anaesthesia, as it is technically easier and more reliable in preventing autonomic dysreflexia. Use standard doses of LA agents (bupivacaine 'heavy' or plain). Intrathecal opioids appear to confer no advantage.

Disadvantages

- May be technically difficult to perform. Spinal anaesthesia is usually possible, but epidural techniques are likely to fail in the presence of spinal instrumentation or previous spinal surgery.
- There is difficulty in determining the success or level of blockade in complete lesions. Incomplete lesions are tested as usual.

Post-operative care

- Tetraplegics are best nursed supine or only slightly head-up due to improved ventilatory function in this position.
- Temperature should be monitored, and hypothermia actively treated.
- Analgesia should be provided by conventional means.
- Dysreflexia may occur and require drug treatment after removal of precipitating causes (such as pain and urinary retention).

Obstetric anaesthesia

Effect of pregnancy on spinal cord injury

- Exaggerated postural hypotension and worsened response to caval occlusion.
- Reduced respiratory reserve, with increased risk of respiratory failure and pneumonia. Increased O_2 demand.
- Increased anaemia due to haemodilution.
- Labour is a potent cause of autonomic dysreflexia in those with lesions above T5 (dysreflexia may be the 1st sign of labour in such patients).

Effect of spinal injury on pregnancy

- Increased risk of infection (urinary infection and pressure sores).
- Increased risk of premature labour (increasing risk with higher level injury).
- Increased risk of thromboembolic complications.
- Labour pains will not be felt in complete lesions above T5. Lesion between T5 and T10—some awareness of some contractions.

Management of labour

- All cord-injured patients should be reviewed early in pregnancy, and a plan formulated for the likely need for analgesia. The relative risks and difficulties of epidural catheter insertion should be predicted and discussed with the patient. A plan for anaesthesia, in the event of a Caesarean section, should also be formulated and recorded in the patient notes.
- Epidural analgesia is usually possible in those with high cord lesions without vertebral instrumentation at the level of catheter insertion.
- Spinal anaesthesia is usually possible for an elective Caesarean section and may be achievable with both single-shot and microcatheter techniques, irrespective of the presence of spinal instrumentation.
- GA may proceed with the precautions outlined on ➲ p. 240.

Epidural analgesia in labour

- The most effective preventive measure for autonomic dysreflexia is adequate epidural analgesia. Those with high lesions may have an epidural commenced prior to induction of labour.
- Hypotension is not usually a problem after adequate fluid preloading (at least 1L of crystalloid or colloid). However, hypotension from any cause should be treated aggressively in those with high lesions due to the lack of compensatory mechanisms and a tendency to progressive hypotension. Aortocaval compression should be avoided by careful positioning for the same reasons.
- Autonomic dysreflexia has been reported up to 48hr after delivery. If a successful block is achieved, it would appear prudent to leave the epidural *in situ* for this time.
- Failure to establish an adequate epidural blockade may necessitate drug treatment of autonomic dysreflexia (see ➲ p. 237).

Further reading

Hambly PR, Martin B (1998). Anaesthesia for chronic spinal cord lesions. *Anaesthesia*, **53**, 273–89.
Raw DA, Beattie JK, Hunter JM (2003). Anaesthesia for spinal surgery in adults. *Br J Anaesth*, **91**, 886–904.

Myasthenia gravis

Myasthenia gravis is characterized by muscle weakness and fatigability. It is caused by autoimmune disruption of post-synaptic acetylcholine receptors at the neuromuscular junction, with up to 80% of functional receptors lost. The disease may occur at any age but is commonest in the elderly where it may be underdiagnosed. It may be associated with thymus hyperplasia, with ~15% of affected patients having thymomas.

- Symptoms range from mild ptosis to life-threatening bulbar palsy and respiratory insufficiency.
- Management is usually with oral anticholinesterase medication, with or without steroid therapy.
- Severe disease may require immunosuppressant therapy, plasmapheresis, or immunoglobulin infusion.

General considerations

- All patients with myasthenia are sensitive to the effects of NDMRs (Table 11.4).
- Plasmapheresis depletes plasma esterase levels, prolonging the effect of suxamethonium, mivacurium, ester-linked LAs, and remifentanil.
- Suxamethonium may have an altered effect—patients may be resistant to depolarization due to reduced receptor activity, requiring an increased dose. This, in conjunction with treatment-induced plasma esterase deficiency, leads to an increased risk of non-depolarizing (phase II) block.

Table 11.4 Specific drugs of interest in myasthenia gravis

Drug	Interaction	Notes
Non-depolarizing neuromuscular-blocking agents	Marked sensitivity	Avoid use if possible. Start with 10% normal dosage. Always monitor neuromuscular function. Use short- and intermediate-acting agents only
Suxamethonium	Resistance to depolarization and delayed onset of action	No reported clinical ill effects using 1.5mg/kg. Delayed recovery in patients with induced esterase deficiency (plasmapheresis, anticholinesterase treatment). Follow with non-depolarizing agents only when full recovery of neuromuscular function noted
Inhalational anaesthetics	All inhalational agents reduce neuromuscular transmission by up to 50%	Avoiding need for neuromuscular-blocking agents
IV anaesthetics	No discernible clinical effect on neuromuscular transmission	TIVA with propofol may be useful if neuromuscular function is precarious

Table 11.4 (Contd.)

Drug	Interaction	Notes
LAs	Prolonged action and increased toxicity in ester-linked agents with anticholinesterase therapy and plasmapheresis. Exacerbation of myasthenia reported	Use minimum dosage required for adequate block. Monitor respiratory function as with general anaesthesia
Drugs dependent on esterases for elimination	Prolonged effect and increased toxicity if patient on plasmapheresis or (theoretically) anticholinesterase therapy	Suxamethonium, remifentanil, mivacurium, ester-linked LAs, esmolol, etc.
Antibiotics	Neuromuscular-blocking effects may become clinically important	Avoid aminoglycosides (e.g. gentamicin). Similar effects reported with erythromycin and ciprofloxacin
Miscellaneous	All the following agents have a reported effect on neuromuscular transmission: procainamide, β-blockers (especially propranolol), phenytoin, magnesium	
Pyridostigmine	Adult: 30–120mg at suitable intervals (usually 4- to 6-hourly). Do not exceed total daily dose of 720mg. Child: <6yr initial dose 30mg; 6–12yr initial dose 60mg. Total daily dose 30–360mg Neonate: 5–10mg every 4hr, 30–60min before feeds	Useful duration of action. No parenteral preparation available. Less potent and slower onset than neostigmine
Neostigmine (SC/IM)	Adult: 1–2.5mg at suitable intervals (usually 2- to 4-hourly). Total daily dose 5–20mg Child: 200–500 micrograms 4-hourly Neonate: 50–250 micrograms 4-hourly	IV usage increases side effects and has reduced duration of action. If IV usage is necessary, anticholinergic agents (atropine/glycopyrronium) should be administered
Neostigmine (oral)	Adult: 15–30mg PO at suitable intervals (up to 2-hourly). Total daily dose 75–300mg Child: <6yr initial dose 7.5mg PO; 6–12yr initial dose 15mg PO. Total daily dose 15–90mg Neonate: 1–5mg PO 4-hourly, 30min before feeds	More marked GI effects than pyridostigmine. Useful if parenteral therapy indicated but more likely to require antimuscarinic (atropine or glycopyrronium) cover if used by this route

(Continued)

Table 11.4 (*Contd.*)

Drug	Interaction	Notes
Edrophonium	Adult: 2mg by IV injection, followed after 30s by 8mg if no adverse reaction Child: 20 micrograms/kg IV, followed by 80 micrograms/kg after 30s if no adverse reaction	Use limited to diagnosis of myasthenia and differentiation of myasthenic and cholinergic crises
Distigmine	Adult: 5mg daily 30min before breakfast. Maximum 20mg daily	Very long-acting with risk of cholinergic crisis due to dosage accumulation. Not recommended in small children or neonates

Preoperative assessment

- Assess the degree of weakness and the duration of symptoms. Those with isolated ocular symptoms of long standing are unlikely to have progressive disease. Those with poorly controlled symptoms should have their condition optimized.
- Any degree of bulbar palsy is predictive of the need for both intra- and post-operative airway protection.
- Those who have significant respiratory impairment are more likely to require post-operative ventilation.
- Take a full drug history, and determine the effect of a missed dose of anticholinesterase. Those with severe disease may be very sensitive to dose omission.

Conduct of anaesthesia

- Maintain anticholinesterase therapy up to the time of induction. Although theoretical inhibition of neuromuscular blockade is possible, this has never been reported.
- Premedication should be minimal.
- Avoid the use of neuromuscular-blocking drugs, if possible. Intubation/ventilation is often achievable using non-paralysing techniques.
- Non-depolarizing drugs should be used sparingly. Monitor the response with a nerve stimulator. Initial doses of ~10–20% of normal are usually adequate.
- Consider a topical LA to the airway.
- Avoid ester-linked LAs (prilocaine), since anticholinesterase treatment may interfere with metabolism.
- Bupivacaine and ropivacaine appear safe for use in epidural analgesia.
- Short- and intermediate-duration non-depolarizing drugs, such as atracurium, mivacurium, vecuronium, and rocuronium, are preferable to longer-acting drugs.
- Reversal of neuromuscular-blocking drugs should be achievable with standard doses of neostigmine if preoperative symptom control has been good (see ➔ p. 1024). Avoidance of reversal with neostigmine is

preferred, since further doses of anticholinesterase may introduce the risk of overdose (cholinergic crisis). Drugs with spontaneous reversal (e.g. atracurium) or those with novel reversal (e.g. rocuronium/ sugammadex) are optimal.

• Consider the insertion of an NGT if difficulty with bulbar function is anticipated and early return of oral therapy required.
• Extubation is possible if the neuromuscular function is assessed as adequate using nerve stimulation. Beware of preoperative bulbar function abnormality. The best predictor of safe extubation is >5s head lift.
• Regional anaesthesia may reduce the need for post-operative opioids and the risks of respiratory depression.
• Facilities for post-operative ventilation should be available.

Principles of perioperative cholinesterase management

• An easy conversion for oral pyridostigmine to parenteral (IV, IM, or SC) neostigmine is to equate every 30mg of oral pyridostigmine to 1mg of parenteral neostigmine.
• Reversal of NMB is possible with neostigmine, if indicated by a nerve stimulator—in general, no twitches on train of four means no reversal possible.
• Initial dosage of neostigmine should be used under nerve stimulator control, starting with a 2.5–5mg bolus, and increasing if necessary with a 1mg bolus every 2–3min to a maximum equivalent dose to the oral pyridostigmine dose (1:30). For example, if the pyridostigmine dose is 120mg 3- to 4-hourly, then the maximum neostigmine dose should be 4mg (to be repeated after 2–4hr if necessary).
• Consider the use of sugammadex (see ➲ p. 1029).

Rapid sequence induction

• Suxamethonium may be used if indicated—doses of 1.5mg/kg are usually effective.
• If doubt exists as to the ease of intubation, consider awake techniques.
• If suxamethonium is used, do not use any other NMB until muscle function has returned and no fade is present.

Post-operative care

• Rapid return of drug therapy is mandatory. Use an NGT if necessary.
• In the event of GI failure, parenteral therapy is indicated.

Preoperative predictors of need for post-operative ventilation

• Major body cavity surgery.
• Duration of disease >6yr.
• A history of coexisting chronic respiratory disease.
• Dose requirements of pyridostigmine >750mg/d.
• A preoperative VC of <2.9L.
• Blood loss >1000mL.

- The best monitors of post-operative respiratory capacity are:
  - Repeated peak flow measurements
  - VC should be at least twice the tidal volume to allow for cough.

Blood gases and pulse oximetry may be normal up to the point of respiratory failure.

Special considerations

Thymectomy

- Consensus now favours thymectomy in all adults with generalized myasthenia gravis. Remission rates are high, and improvement of symptoms is almost universally attainable (96% gain benefit, regardless of preoperative characteristics).
- Best results are achieved in those with normal or hyperplastic thymus.
- The approach most commonly used is trans-sternal. Transcervical approaches provide less satisfactory access for surgery.
- Thoracoscopic thymectomy is gaining acceptance, although its reputed benefit of reduced complications and need for post-operative ventilation is yet to be proven.
- Anaesthetic management follows the same general principles outlined on ➋ p. 244, although all patients need post-operative care in HDU or require ventilation for a short period in the early post-operative period.
- Fewer than 8% of patients requiring sternotomy for thymectomy need ventilation for >3hr post-operatively.
- Almost all patients will require a degree of muscle relaxation if preoperative preparation has been optimal. Post-operative analgesia can be achieved satisfactorily with epidural or PCA.

Eaton–Lambert syndrome

Eaton–Lambert syndrome (myasthenic syndrome) is a proximal muscle weakness associated with cancer (most often small cell carcinoma of the lung).

- The condition is thought to be due to a reduction in the release of acetylcholine (prejunctional failure).
- It is not reversed by anticholinesterase therapy, and muscle weakness is improved by exercise.
- Associated dysautonomia may manifest as dry mouth, impaired accommodation, urinary hesitance, and constipation.
- Unlike myasthenia gravis, patients with myasthenic syndrome are sensitive to both depolarizing and non-depolarizing neuromuscular-blocking drugs.
- Reduced doses should be used if the disease is suspected. Maintain a high index of suspicion in those undergoing procedures related to the diagnosis and management of carcinoma of the lung.

Further reading

Blichfeldt-Lauridsen L, Hansen BD (2012). Anaesthesia and myasthenia gravis. *Acta Anaesthesiol Scand*, **56**, 17–22.
Mirakhur RK (2009). Sugammadex in clinical practice. *Anaesthesia*, **64**, 45–54.
Wainwright AP, Brodrick PM (1987). Suxamethonium in myasthenia gravis. *Anaesthesia*, **42**, 950–7.

Multiple sclerosis

An acquired disease of the CNS characterized by demyelinated plaques within the brain and spinal cord. The onset of symptoms usually occurs in early adulthood, with 20–30% of cases following a benign course and 5% a rapid deterioration. It is commonest in geographical clusters within Europe, North America, and New Zealand.

General considerations

This is an incurable disease, but steroids and interferon have been associated with improved symptom-free intervals. Most patients suffer from associated depression. Baclofen and dantrolene are useful for painful muscle spasm.

- Symptoms range from isolated visual disturbance and nystagmus to limb weakness and paralysis.
- Respiratory failure due to both respiratory muscle failure and bulbar palsy may be a feature in end-stage disease.
- Symptoms are characterized by symptomatic episodes of variable severity, with periods of remission, for several years.
- Permanent weakness and symptoms develop in some patients, leading to increasingly severe disability.
- Demyelinated nerve fibres are sensitive to heat. A temperature rise of 0.5°C may cause a marked deterioration in symptoms.

Preoperative assessment and investigation

- Preoperative evaluation must include a history of the type of symptoms suffered and a detailed neurological examination. This will allow comparison with the post-operative state to elucidate any new lesions.
- Respiratory function may be affected. Bulbar palsy causes an increased risk of aspiration and reduced airway reflexes in the post-operative period.

Conduct of anaesthesia

- GA does not affect the course of multiple sclerosis.
- Regional anaesthesia does not affect neurological symptoms, but it may be medicolegally prudent to document the discussion of relative risks before embarking on a nerve or plexus blockade.
- Centroneuraxial blockade has been associated with recurrence of symptoms. However, this is reduced by the use of minimal concentrations of LA/opioid in combination.
- Epidural analgesia for labour is not contraindicated—keep LA concentration to a minimum. There is widespread use of spinal anaesthesia for Caesarean section in patients with multiple sclerosis in the UK.
- Suxamethonium is associated with a large efflux of K^+ in debilitated patients and should be avoided.
- Response to non-depolarizing drugs is normal, although caution and reduced dosages are indicated in those with severe disability.
- Careful CVS monitoring is essential, since autonomic instability leads to marked hypotensive responses to drugs and sensitivity to hypovolaemia.

- Temperature is important and should be monitored in all patients. Pyrexia must be avoided and should be treated aggressively with antipyretics (paracetamol 1g PR/PO), tepid sponging, and forced-air blowers. Hypothermia may delay recovery from anaesthesia.

Further reading

Drake E, Drake M, Bird J, Russell R (2006). Obstetric regional blocks for women with multiple sclerosis: a survey of UK experience. *Int J Obstet Anesth*, **15**, 115–23.

Guillain–Barré syndrome

Guillain–Barré syndrome is an immune-mediated progressive demyelinating disorder, characterized by acute or subacute proximal skeletal muscle paralysis. The syndrome is often preceded by limb paraesthesiae/back pain and, in more than half of affected patients, by a viral illness. No single viral agent has been implicated.

More than 85% of patients achieve a full recovery, although this may take several months. The use of steroids in the management of this condition remains controversial.

- One-third of patients will require ventilatory support.
- The more rapid the onset of symptoms, the more likely the progression to respiratory failure. Impending respiratory failure may be evidenced by difficulty in swallowing and phonation due to pharyngeal muscle weakness.
- Inability to cough is a marker of severe respiratory impairment and usually indicates the need for intubation and ventilation.
- Autonomic dysfunction is common.

Conduct of anaesthesia

- Respiratory support is likely to be necessary, both during surgery and in the post-operative period.
- Autonomic dysfunction leads to potential severe hypotension during induction of anaesthesia, initiation of positive pressure ventilation, and postural changes under anaesthesia or recovery.
- Hydration should be maintained with wide-bore IV access and pressor agents (ephedrine 3–6mg bolus IV) prepared prior to induction.
- Tachycardia due to surgical stimulus may be extreme, and atropine may elicit a paradoxical bradycardia.
- Suxamethonium should be avoided due to potential catastrophic K^+ efflux. The risk of hyperkalaemia may persist for several months after clinical recovery.
- NDMRs may not be needed and should be used cautiously.
- Epidural analgesia is useful and may avoid the need for systemic opioid analgesia. Epidural opioids have been used to manage distressing paraesthesiae in these patients.

Motor neuron disease (amyotrophic lateral sclerosis)

Amyotrophic lateral sclerosis is one of a family of motor neuron diseases, which are degenerative disorders of upper and lower motor neurons in the spinal cord. It manifests initially with weakness, atrophy, and fasciculation of peripheral muscles (usually those of the hand) and progress to axial and bulbar weakness.

- Progression is relentless, with death from respiratory failure usually occurring within 3yr of diagnosis.
- Patients remain mentally competent up to the point of terminal respiratory failure, leading to ethical and moral difficulty in the provision of long-term ventilation.

Conduct of anaesthesia

- Bulbar palsy increases the risk of sputum retention and aspiration. Intubation may be necessary. Many patients with advanced disease will have a long-term tracheostomy for airway protection and episodes of mechanical ventilation.
- Respiratory support is likely to be necessary, both during surgery and in the post-operative period.
- Autonomic dysfunction leads to potentially severe hypotension during induction of anaesthesia, initiation of positive pressure ventilation, and postural changes under anaesthesia or recovery.
- Hydration should be maintained with wide-bore IV access if necessary, and pressor agents (ephedrine/metaraminol) prepared prior to induction.
- Suxamethonium should be avoided due to potential catastrophic K^+ efflux.
- Non-depolarizing agents should be used in reduced dosage if necessary, and their action monitored with a nerve stimulator.

Dystrophia myotonica

Dystrophia myotonica (myotonic dystrophy, myotonia atrophica) is the commonest of the dystonias (1:20 000), the others being myotonia congenita and paramyotonia. It is an autosomal dominant disease, presenting in the 2nd or 3rd decade of life.

General considerations

- Persistent contraction of the skeletal muscle follows stimulation. It is characterized by prefrontal balding and cataracts.
- The main clinical features are related to muscular atrophy, especially of facial, sternomastoid, and peripheral muscles.
- Progressive deterioration/atrophy of the skeletal, cardiac, and smooth muscle over time leads to a deterioration in cardiorespiratory function and (possibly severe) cardiomyopathy.
- Further respiratory deterioration occurs due to degeneration of the CNS, leading to central respiratory drive depression.
- Progressive bulbar palsy causes difficulty in swallowing/clearing secretions and an increased risk of aspiration.
- Degeneration of the cardiac conduction system causes dysrhythmia and AV block.
- Mitral valve prolapse occurs in ~20% of patients.
- There is mental deterioration after the 2nd decade.
- Endocrine dysfunction may lead to diabetes mellitus, hypothyroidism, adrenal insufficiency, and gonadal atrophy.
- Death usually occurs in the 5th or 6th decade.
- Pregnancy may aggravate the disease, and Caesarean section is commoner due to uterine muscle dysfunction.
- Therapy is supportive, using antimyotonic medications such as procainamide, phenytoin, quinine, and mexiletine.

Preoperative assessment

- Assess the respiratory reserve, including signs of bulbar palsy (difficulty with cough or swallowing).
- Seek signs of cardiac failure and dysrhythmia.
- Gastric emptying may be delayed. Premedication with an antacid (ranitidine 150–300mg PO) or a prokinetic (metoclopramide 10mg PO) may be indicated.

Investigations

- CXR, spirometry, and ABGs if indicated by respiratory symptoms.
- ECG to exclude conduction defects, and echocardiography for myocardial dysfunction.
- U&Es and glucose to exclude endocrine dysfunction.

Conduct of anaesthesia

- Suxamethonium produces prolonged muscle contraction (and K^+ release) and should be avoided. Contraction may make intubation, ventilation, and surgery difficult.

- Non-depolarizing drugs are safe to use but do not always cause muscle relaxation. Use of a nerve stimulator may provoke muscle contraction, leading to misdiagnosis of tetany.
- Reversal with neostigmine may also provoke contraction. Non-depolarizing agents with short action and spontaneous reversal (atracurium, mivacurium) are preferred.
- Reversal of rocuronium and vecuronium is possible without the use of neostigmine, using sugammadex.
- Intubation and maintenance of anaesthesia can often be achieved without the use of any muscle relaxant.
- Invasive arterial monitoring is indicated for significant CVS impairment.
- Even small doses of induction agents can produce profound cardiorespiratory depression.
- Bulbar palsy increases the need for intubation under GA.
- Regional anaesthesia does not prevent muscle contraction. Troublesome spasm may be helped by infiltration of an LA directly into the affected muscle. Quinine (600mg IV) and phenytoin (3–5mg/kg IV slowly) have been effective in some cases.
- High concentrations of inhaled anaesthetics should be avoided because of their effect on myocardial contraction and conduction.
- Patient warmth must be maintained. Post-operative shivering may provoke myotonia.

Post-operative care
- High dependency care is indicated after anything but minor peripheral surgery. Discharge to low dependency areas should be considered only if the patient is able to cough adequately and maintain oxygenation on air or simple supplemental O_2.
- Analgesia is best provided, if possible, by regional or local block to avoid the systemic depressant effects of opioids.

Myotonia congenita
This develops in infancy and early childhood, and is characterized by pharyngeal muscle spasm leading to difficulty in swallowing. It improves with age, and patients have a normal life expectancy.

Paramyotonia
This is extremely rare. It is characterized by cold-induced contraction, only relieved by warming the affected muscle. Anaesthetic management is the same as for myotonic dystrophy. Patient warmth is paramount.

Further reading
Imison AR (2001). Anaesthesia and myotonia—an Australian experience. *Anaesth Intensive Care*, 29, 34–7.

Muscular dystrophy

The muscular dystrophies comprise a range of congenital muscular disorders characterized by progressive weakness of affected muscle groups. They can be classified, according to inheritance:

• X-linked: Duchenne, Becker
• Autosomal recessive: limb-girdle, childhood, congenital
• Autosomal dominant: facioscapulohumeral, oculopharyngeal.

Duchenne muscular dystrophy

This is the commonest and most severe form.

General considerations

• Sex-linked recessive trait, clinically apparent in ♂.
• Onset of symptoms of muscle weakness at 2–5yr.
• The patient is usually confined to a wheelchair by 12yr.
• Death usually by 25yr due to progressive cardiac failure or pneumonia.
• Cardiac: myocardial degeneration, leading to heart failure and possible mitral valve prolapse. Evidence of heart failure is often apparent by 6yr (reduced R wave amplitude and wall motion abnormalities). Isolated degeneration of the left ventricle may lead to right outflow obstruction and right heart failure.
• Respiratory: progressive respiratory muscle weakness, leading to a restrictive ventilation pattern, inadequate cough, and eventual respiratory infection and failure.
• Possible vascular smooth muscle dysfunction, leading to increased bleeding during surgery.
• Associated progressive and severe kyphoscoliosis.
• Disease progression may be tracked by serum creatinine kinase (CK) levels. These are elevated early in the disease but reduce to below normal as muscles atrophy.

Other muscular dystrophies (Becker, facioscapulohumeral, and limb-girdle dystrophy) are less severe than Duchenne dystrophy, with onset at a later age and slower progression of the disease. Isolated ocular dystrophy is associated with a normal lifespan.

Preoperative assessment and investigations

• Patients are usually under the care of specialist paediatricians.
• CXR, spirometry, and blood gases may be indicated by respiratory symptoms.
• Echocardiography is mandatory if the patient is wheelchair-bound—myocardial and valve function can be assessed.
• Reduced gut muscle tone leads to delayed gastric emptying and increased risk of aspiration.

Conduct of anaesthesia

• Antacid premedication (H_2 receptor blocker or PPI) with a prokinetic, such as metoclopramide, may be useful to reduce the risk of aspiration.
• An antisialogogue, such as glycopyrronium, may be needed if secretions are a problem.

- Careful IV induction of anaesthesia with balanced opioid/ induction agent.
- Potent inhalational anaesthetics should be used cautiously in these patients because of the risk of myocardial depression.
- Current opinion would suggest that non-triggering anaesthesia (e.g. TIVA with propofol) may be indicated because of the risk of anaesthetic-induced rhabdomyolysis.
- Suxamethonium should be avoided because of K^+ efflux and potential cardiac arrest.
- Non-depolarizing neuromuscular blockers are safe, although reduced doses are required. Nerve stimulator monitoring should be used.
- Respiratory depressant effects of all anaesthetic drugs are enhanced, and post-operative respiratory function should be monitored carefully. Those with pre-existing sputum retention and inadequate cough are at high risk of post-operative respiratory failure and may need prolonged ventilatory support.
- Regional analgesia is useful to avoid opioid use and potential respiratory depression after painful surgery. Caudal epidural may be technically easier to perform than lumbar epidural in those with kyphoscoliosis.

Further reading

Almenrader N (2006). Spinal surgery in children with non-idiopathic scoliosis: is there a need for routine post operative ventilation? *Br J Anaesth*, **97**, 851–7.

Hayes J, Veyckemans F, Bissonnette B (2008). Duchenne muscular dystrophy: an old anesthesia problem revisited. *Paediatr Anaesth*, **18**, 100–6.

Malignant hyperthermia

Aetiology

- MH is a pharmacogenetic disease of the skeletal muscle induced by exposure to all potent volatile anaesthetic agents and the depolarizing muscle relaxant suxamethonium.
- It is inherited as an autosomal dominant condition and caused by the loss of normal Ca^{2+} homeostasis at some point along the excitation–contraction coupling process on exposure to triggering agents. Any defect along this complex process could result in the clinical features of MH and may explain why differing chemical agents trigger MH and the heterogeneity seen in DNA studies.
- The most likely site is the triadic junction between the T tubules, involving the voltage sensor of the dihydropyridine receptor (DHPR), and the ryanodine receptor, a Ca^{2+} efflux channel on the sarcoplasmic reticulum (SR).
- About 70% of MH families are linked to the *RYR1* gene located on chromosome 19q. Over 200 mutations have been identified in *RYR1*, but only 29 have evidence of causality. Other loci have been identified (e.g. chromosomes 1, 3, and 7), but only for small numbers of families.

Epidemiology

- Incidence is about 1:10 000–15 000, but difficult to estimate. All races are affected.
- Mortality rates have fallen dramatically from 70–80% to 2–3% due to increased awareness, improved monitoring standards, and the availability of dantrolene.
- Commonly seen in young adults, ♂ > ♀, but this may be a lifestyle, rather than a true sex, difference.
- Used to be more frequent in minor operations, e.g. dental/ENT, due to anaesthetic technique, i.e. when suxamethonium and vapour were commonly used.
- Previous uneventful anaesthesia with triggering agents does not preclude MH; 75% of MH probands (index cases) have had previous anaesthesia prior to their MH crisis.
- Annual UK incidence of confirmed MH cases is falling (currently approximately 10–15/yr) due to changes in anaesthetic techniques, e.g. decreased use of suxamethonium, increased use of TIVA and LA. However, there is an increased referral rate due to an increased index of suspicion.

Clinical presentation

- The clinical diagnosis can be difficult, as the presentation of MH varies considerably, and no one sign is unique to MH. It can be a florid dramatic life-threatening event or have an insidious onset. Rarely, it can develop 2–3d post-operatively with massive myoglobinuria and/or renal failure due to severe rhabdomyolysis.

Clinical signs

- Signs of increased metabolism: tachycardia, dysrhythmias, increased CO_2 production, metabolic acidosis, pyrexia, DIC. Often called a 'metabolic storm'. Pyrexia develops as a consequence of metabolic stimulation, so it occurs after other signs. A pyrexia developing after recovery from normal anaesthesia is not indicative of MH.
- Muscle signs: masseter spasm after suxamethonium, generalized muscle rigidity, hyperkalaemia, high CK, myoglobinuria, renal failure.
- The two most important early signs are unexplained, unexpected, increasing HR and $ETCO_2$.

Masseter muscle spasm

- Masseter muscle spasm (MMS) after suxamethonium defined as impeding intubation and persisting for ~2min; 30% of patients presenting with MMS alone, even when anaesthesia has proceeded uneventfully, prove to be MH-susceptible.
- If possible, abandon surgery; if not, convert to 'MH-safe' technique (volatile-free); allow ~15min to ensure that the patient is stabilized. Monitor $ETCO_2$ and temperature, and consider an arterial line.
- Additional MH signs increase the likelihood of MH significantly: 50–60% if metabolic signs present, 70–80% if muscle signs present.
- Investigations that are particularly useful are the initial and 24hr CK and examination of the 1st voided specimen for myoglobinuria, indicating evidence of muscle damage.
- Prolonged severe muscle stiffness greatly in excess of the 'normal suxamethonium pains' may occur.
- MMS may be the 1st indication of a previously unsuspected muscle disease, particularly the myotonic conditions. Perform resting CK and electromyography (EMG). Consider neurological opinion.

Treatment of a crisis

(See ➲ p. 918.)
- '*Guidelines for the treatment of an MH crisis*' is available from the AAGBI for display in theatres.

After treating a suspected malignant hyperthermia crisis

- If MH was suspected clinically, refer the patient to an MH unit with all the relevant clinical details/anaesthetic chart/laboratory results. The timing of various events is important.
- In the meantime, warn the patient and family of the potential implications of MH.
- MH is not a diagnosis to be made lightly without adequate follow-up.
- Unless MH can be clearly excluded on clinical grounds, the patient/ family will be offered screening to confirm or refute the clinical diagnosis.
- The proband is always screened, even if the clinical reaction is undoubted. If the proband cannot be screened (e.g. died or too young), the most appropriate relative is screened (e.g. parents of a young child).

Diagnosis of malignant hyperthermia susceptibility

- Muscle biopsy using the *in vitro* contracture test (IVCT) remains the gold standard of MH diagnosis. This is an open invasive procedure, usually performed under an ultrasound-guided femoral nerve block, to remove 8–10 muscle specimens, ~3–4cm long, from the vastus medialis muscle. As living samples are used, the patient has to travel to the MH centre.
- The IVCT follows a European Malignant Hyperthermia Group (EMHG) protocol, exposing muscle tissue to halothane and separately to caffeine under preset conditions in a dedicated laboratory.
- The diagnosis is considered positive if the muscle contracts in response to halothane and/or caffeine.
- There is a potential for 'false positive' MH diagnoses in order to ensure the accuracy of the MH-negative diagnosis. The combined EMHG data indicate a specificity of 93.6% and sensitivity of 99%.
- If the proband is confirmed as MH-susceptible by IVCT, they are screened for the 29 *RYR1* mutations currently used for diagnostic purposes by the EMHG for DNA testing of MH.
- If a mutation is identified in the proband, family members can be offered an initial DNA blood test for the familial mutation; if a mutation carrier, they are classified as MH-susceptible without a muscle biopsy; if mutation-negative, a confirmatory biopsy is required for reasons of safety, because MH is complex with a small incidence (~5–10%) of discordant results within families.
- If a mutation is not identified in the proband, family members are offered IVCT only.
- Family screening is organized on the basis of the autosomal dominant pattern of inheritance, so relatives with a 50% risk are screened first, i.e. parents, siblings, and children; the latter are not screened until aged 10–12yr.
- The purpose of family screening is to identify the small number of individuals in a family who are susceptible to MH, rather than labelling the whole family. Screening will involve only a small proportion of the family.
- Once identified as MH-susceptible, the MH unit can provide written information about MH, warning cards/discs, and information about the British Malignant Hyperthermia Association (BMHA), a patient support charity.
- MH centres should coordinate family screening to ensure the appropriate method of testing is offered.

Anaesthesia for known or suspected malignant hyperthermia-susceptible patients

- MH patients should not be denied necessary surgery solely because of MH.
- Preoperative questioning about personal and family anaesthetic history is essential to identify potential MH patients.
- It is not absolutely essential to screen suspected cases prior to surgery, provided careful individual assessment has been made of the risks involved.

- An MH-'safe' technique, i.e. avoiding suxamethonium and all anaesthetic volatile agents, may not pose any additional risk in many circumstances but will do so in certain situations, e.g. when the preferred technique would have necessitated the use of these agents (Table 11.5).
- All LA agents are safe.
- Dantrolene is not required prophylactically, because of its side effects, but should be readily available.
- Standard monitoring is adequate, i.e. ECG, NIBP, SaO$_2$, ETCO$_2$. A baseline core temperature should be established before the procedure and monitored ~4hr post-operatively.
- If no volatile-free machine is available, remove all vaporizers and circuitry from the machine and ventilator, including soda lime, and purge with O$_2$ for 20–30min. Use new circuits/soda lime/LMAs/ETT, etc.
- The MH unit can be contacted for further advice, if required.

Table 11.5 Anaesthesia for the MH-susceptible patient

MH 'triggering' agents	Avoid suxamethonium and all anaesthetic vapours/volatiles
MH-'safe' agents	All induction agents, including ketamine, all analgesics, all non-depolarizing agents, all LAs
	Atropine/glycopyrronium/neostigmine
	Ephedrine and other vasopressors
	Metoclopramide/droperidol
	N$_2$O, benzodiazepines
Monitoring	ECG, NIBP, ETCO$_2$, core temperature
	Check temp 2hr preoperatively to establish baseline and 4–6hr post-operatively
Anaesthetic equipment	If no vapour-free machine is available, remove the vaporizers, and flush both the anaesthetic machine and the ventilator with oxygen for 20–30min. Use fresh clean tubing/masks/ETTs/soda lime, etc. If possible, select a ventilator with little inner tubing, e.g. Nuffield Penlon
Dantrolene	This is not required prophylactically, as no reaction should occur. It is unpleasant for the patient and markedly prolongs the action of NDMRs. However, it should be readily available

Anaesthesia for a patient with a known or suspected family history of malignant hyperthermia

- Establish the family history and the relationship of your patient to the named proband or other tested family members. The MH centre will then be able to advise about the risk to your patient and the need for further investigation.
- If anaesthesia is urgent and more details unavailable, proceed as for an MH-susceptible patient.

Suspicious previous anaesthetic history

- Unexplained/unexpected cardiac arrest/death during anaesthesia carries a 50% risk of MH.
- History of post-operative myoglobinuria (red/black urine).
- Renal failure in otherwise healthy patient.
- Post-operative pyrexia. Establish the timing of the pyrexia in relation to surgery. If the intraoperative/immediate recovery period was uneventful, with the pyrexia developing later on the ward, MH is not implicated. If the timing is unclear, the likelihood of MH is low but cannot be excluded.
- Take a thorough history of the event. If possible, obtain old records, and seek further advice from the MH centre. If surgery is urgent, proceed as if MH-susceptible, and resolve the problem later.

Obstetric patients

- Baby of susceptible parent:
  - Has 50% chance of being affected if one parent is MH-susceptible, so should be treated as potentially MH-susceptible.
- Mother MH-susceptible:
  - Plans for any emergency situation should be prepared with an obstetric anaesthetist prior to the estimated date of delivery
  - It is essential to anticipate airway problems and consider other options, e.g. awake intubation
  - Regional techniques preferred
  - For GA, use an MH-safe technique, substituting suxamethonium with a rapid-onset NDMR, e.g. rocuronium, and maintaining anaesthesia with a propofol infusion
  - Ephedrine, oxytocin, and ergometrine can be used.
- Father MH-susceptible (fetus at risk):
  - Avoid MH-triggering agents which cross the placenta, i.e. inhalational agents, until after delivery of the baby
  - Suxamethonium, being highly charged, can be used, as it does not cross the placenta to any great extent.

Associated conditions

- Central core disease (CCD) is a non-progressive inherited condition, causing peripheral muscle weakness and occasionally musculoskeletal and cardiac problems. It is the only condition known to be associated with MH, but this is not invariable. CCD patients should be treated as potentially MH-susceptible but offered screening because of the discordant association. Other muscle diseases are not thought to be related to MH but clearly cause anaesthetic problems in their own right.
- Heatstroke and King–Denborough syndrome remain controversial (see ⮀ p. 300).
- Neuroleptic malignant syndrome and sudden infant death syndrome are not associated with MH (see ⮀ p. 269).

Malignant hyperthermia centres and the British Malignant Hyperthermia Association

- There is only one MH centre in the UK: Dr P. J. Halsall, MH Investigation Unit, Clinical Sciences Building, St James's University Hospital, Leeds LS9 7TF. Tel: 0113 2065274; Fax: 0113 2064140; hotline: 07947 609601 (usually available for medical emergencies only).
- BMHA is a charitable patient support group which provides the 'hotline', warning cards/discs, translations for travel abroad, and newsletters, as well as fundraising for research. Secretary: Mrs A. Winks, 11 Gorse Close, Newthorpe, Nottingham NG16 2BZ. Tel: 01773 717901.
- There are 16 MH centres in Europe. Contact the EMHG Secretary Dr P. J. Halsall for further details, or see the EMHG website at ℘ http://www.emhg.org.
- For the US and Canada, contact Malignant Hyperthermia Association of the United States (MHAUS), 39 East State St, PO Box 1069, Sherburne, NY 13460, USA. Tel: in North America, 1-800-MH-Hyper; outside North America, 1-315-464-7079; ℘ http://www.mhaus.org. Hotline: 1-800-98-MHAUS.
- For Australia, contact Dr Neil Street, Anaesthetic Dept, The New Children's Hospital, Westmead, NSW, PO Box 3515, Parramatta 2124. Tel: (02) 9845 0000; Fax: (02) 9845 3489.
- For New Zealand, contact Dr Neil Pollock, Anaesthetic Dept, Palmerston North Hospital, 50 Ruahine St, Palmerston North 4442. Tel: (06) 3569169; Fax: (06) 3508566.

Further reading

Association of Anaesthetists of Great Britain and Ireland. *Guidelines for the treatment of a malignant hyperthermia crisis*. London: Association of Anaesthetists of Great Britain and Ireland. ℘ http://www.aagbi.org.

Davis PJ, Brandon BW (2009). The association of malignant hyperthermia and unusual disease: when you're hot you're hot or maybe not. *Anesth Analg*, **109**, 1001–3.

Ellis FR, Halsall PJ, Christian AS (1990). Clinical presentation of suspected malignant hyperthermia during anaesthesia in 402 probands. *Anaesthesia*, **45**, 838–41.

Halsall PJ, Hopkins PM (2003). Inherited disease and anaesthesia. In: Healy TEJ, Knight PR, eds. *A practice of anaesthesia*, 7th edn. London: Arnold, pp. 363–76.

MacLennan DH, Phillips MS (1992). Malignant hyperthermia. *Science*, **256**, 789–94.

Urwyler A, Deufel T, McCarthy T, West S; European Malignant Hyperthermia Group (2001). Guidelines for the molecular genetic testing of susceptibility to malignant hyperthermia. *Br J Anaesth*, **86**, 283–7.

Psychiatric disorders and drugs

Aidan O'Donnell

See also:

Psychiatric disorders

Some form of psychiatric illness is present in about 10% of the UK population at any time. The commonest psychiatric disorder is depression, and most psychiatric patients are well controlled most of the time. Many patients are on long-term drug therapy which should be continued perioperatively where possible.

Major psychiatric illness affects about 1% of the population and carries a significant risk of self-harm or suicide. Alcohol and drug misuse is also common among the psychiatric population. The stress of hospitalization for surgery may exacerbate coexisting psychiatric problems.

The anaesthetic implications of psychiatric illness include:
- Capacity of the patient to give consent may be impaired (e.g. dementia, mania, psychosis)
- Where the psychiatric illness itself also causes physical illness (e.g. anorexia nervosa)
- Where the psychiatric medication may interact with anaesthetic drugs and techniques (e.g. antidepressants).

Consent
- Most patients can give consent normally (see ➲ p. 20). In England and Wales, the Mental Capacity Act (2005) and, in Scotland, the Adults with Incapacity Act (2000) clarify capacity and consent issues. Patients who are detained under the Mental Health Act (1983) may only be compelled to accept psychiatric treatment under the terms of the Act.

Anxiety
- Anxiety in the anaesthetic room is extremely common and usually best managed with explanation, reassurance, oral premedication, or IV sedation (e.g. midazolam 1–2mg) titrated to effect. Anxiety disorder may be acute or chronic (symptoms are similar) or occur as part of other disorders (e.g. depression). Extreme agitation may make cannulation difficult. Patients may hyperventilate and have high levels of circulating catecholamines.

Dementia
- Dementia refers to an irreversible global deterioration in higher mental functioning. Fifty per cent of cases are due to Alzheimer's disease.
- Prevalence: 1% aged 65–74, rising to 10% aged >75, and 25% aged >85yr. Slightly commoner in women.
- Mean life expectancy is approximately 7yr from diagnosis.
- Patients may be unable to give informed consent; an incapacity form should be completed by the consultant responsible.
- Patients are usually confused and may be agitated (occasionally violent) or profoundly withdrawn.
- Patients with mild to moderate dementia are commonly treated with antidementia drugs. Donepezil, rivastigmine, and galantamine are all anticholinesterases, which may prolong the action of suxamethonium and partially antagonize the effects of non-depolarizing neuromuscular-blocking drugs.

- Regional anaesthesia may still be desirable if significant co-morbidity; ketamine (e.g. 5–20mg IV) may facilitate this and preserves airway reflexes and BP (titrate to effect). (Midazolam may cause disinhibition, which may paradoxically worsen agitation.)
- Patients with dementia may be at increased risk of post-operative cognitive dysfunction (POCD).

Anorexia nervosa

Anorexia nervosa is a chronic, severe, multisystem disorder which carries the highest morbidity and mortality rate of any psychiatric disorder. Up to 20% of patients may die prematurely.[1–4]

- Anorexia (abnormal body image with deliberate weight loss through food restriction) is present in 0.3% of young women and is commoner in teenagers. Bulimia nervosa (uncontrolled binge eating and purging) is commoner (~1%). In both disorders, patients are about 90% ♀.
- Typically, anorexics are 25% below their ideal weight (bulimics may be normal or even overweight). One diagnostic criterion is BMI <17.5.
- Many patients have psychiatric co-morbidity such as depression, anxiety, and obsessive–compulsive disorder.
- Misuse of laxatives, emetics, diuretics, and other substances to increase weight loss is common. Patients are evasive about their behaviour. A well-documented history (e.g. from the GP) is valuable.
- Clinical features are those of malnutrition and starvation: cachexia, hair loss, amenorrhoea, and osteoporosis. Immunocompetence is usually preserved until >50% of the normal body weight is lost. Endocrine derangements cause amenorrhoea and impaired thyroid function and glycaemic control, and may mimic panhypopituitarism.
- CVS: significant bradycardia and hypotension are common (e.g. systolic BP <100mmHg). ECG changes may be present in up to 80% of patients (AV block; ST depression; T wave inversion and prolonged QT (associated with significant risk of sudden death)). Arrhythmias are common. Myocardial impairment may occur. Patients are at risk of cardiac failure if overfilled intraoperatively.
- Respiratory system: prolonged starvation causes loss of lung elasticity. Airway pressures may be high.
- Renal: GFR is reduced. Two-thirds of patients have proteinuria. Excessive losses of Na^+, K^+, Cl^-, and H^+ from the stomach result in hypochloraemic metabolic alkalosis and hypokalaemia. Severe hypokalaemia is uncommon but should be corrected with caution preoperatively. Hypocalcaemia may accompany hypokalaemia.
- GI: anorexics/bulimics may have paradoxically delayed gastric emptying. Fasting is not a reliable way of ensuring an empty stomach.
- Anaesthetic management: patients need more laboratory tests than their age alone would suggest. Check FBC, U&Es, LFTs, glucose, Ca^{2+}, Mg^{2+}, phosphate, and ECG. Rehydrate the patient preoperatively, and correct any abnormal electrolyte levels, but refeeding is dangerous and should not be attempted. RSI is recommended. Hypokalaemia and hypocalcaemia may potentiate NMB. Patients are prone to hypothermia. Patients should be positioned carefully because of their risks of pressure necrosis and nerve palsies.

- Hypoalbuminaemia may cause elevated levels of unbound drugs in the plasma, and drug metabolism and elimination may be slowed. Avoid hyperventilation (this exacerbates hypokalaemia). Avoid large infusions, which may precipitate pulmonary oedema.
- Reversal of NMB with neostigmine may provoke rhythm instability. Always use a nerve stimulator, and consider sugammadex or allowing the block to wear off spontaneously.

Alcohol

Alcohol use is common and causes problems as a result of both acute intoxication and the health effects of chronic consumption.[5] Ask all adults about alcohol consumption, although their answers may be unreliable.

- Acute alcohol intoxication causes problems with consent. Non-emergency surgery should be avoided. If surgery is unavoidable, ensure adequate rehydration, with careful attention to electrolyte and glucose disturbances. Consider IV B-vitamins (e.g. Pabrinex® slow IV bd for 3–5d).
- Acute intoxication may cause vomiting, hypoglycaemia, and delayed gastric emptying. RSI is advised.
- Chronic alcohol excess induces tolerance to GA and is associated with a 2- to 5-fold increase in post-operative complications.
- Alcoholic cardiomyopathy is characterized by a dilated, hypokinetic LV and decreased EF. Patients may present with CCF and oedema, exacerbated by low serum albumin. Consider echocardiography.
- Alcoholic liver disease: the earliest form is reversible fatty liver, progressing to alcoholic hepatitis (abdominal pain, weight loss, jaundice, fever) and later cirrhosis (jaundice, ascites, portal hypertension, hepatic failure). Correct clotting abnormalities preoperatively. Transfuse appropriately, if required. Patients with liver failure require intensive care if surgery is planned (see also ❷ p. 138).
- Ketoacidosis may present after binge drinking, in association with vomiting and fasting. Blood alcohol levels may already have normalized.
- Anticipate alcohol withdrawal symptoms. Most patients can tolerate 24hr abstinence perioperatively. Do not complicate management by attempting alcohol withdrawal perioperatively. Prescribe regular benzodiazepines, e.g. chlordiazepoxide.
- Seizures most commonly seen 6–48hr after cessation of drinking, typically tonic–clonic. Several fits over a period of a few days are common. Low K^+ and Mg^{2+} predispose. Seizures may be preceded by disorientation and agitation (*delirium tremens*). Treat with benzodiazepines, e.g. diazepam 10mg IV, repeated as required.

References

1 Seller CA, Ravalia A (2003). Anaesthetic implications of anorexia nervosa. *Anaesthesia*, **58**, 437–43.
2 Denner AM, Townley SA (2009). Anorexia nervosa: perioperative implications. *Contin Educ Anaesth Crit Care Pain*, **9**, 61–4.
3 Morris J, Twaddle S (2007). Anorexia nervosa. *BMJ*, **334**, 894–8.
4 Hirose K, Hirose M, Tanaka K, et al. (2014). Perioperative management of severe anorexia nervosa. *Br J Anaesth*, **112**, 246–54.
5 Chapman R, Plaat F (2009). Alcohol and anaesthesia. *Contin Educ Anaesth Crit Care Pain*, **9**, 10–13.

Antidepressant drugs

The aetiology of depression is complex and multifactorial. The monoamine theory of depression postulates that depression is caused by functional deficiency of serotonin and noradrenaline in the CNS. Manipulation of CNS monoamines remains the most successful pharmacological approach to depression. Several families of drugs have this effect.

Tricyclic antidepressants

Formerly the mainstay of treatment of depressive illness, tricyclic antidepressants (TCAs) have largely been superseded by SSRIs (fewer side effects and safer in overdose). They may be used in the treatment of other problems, e.g. chronic pain. They need to be given for 2–4wk to become effective.

- TCAs block reuptake of monoamines (e.g. serotonin, noradrenaline) from the synaptic cleft by competing for a transport protein.
- Most have atropine-like side effects: dry mouth, blurred vision, urinary retention, and constipation. Other common side effects are sedation and postural hypotension.
- They are strongly bound to plasma proteins, and their effects may be enhanced by competing drugs (e.g. aspirin, warfarin, digoxin).
- In overdose, TCAs are extremely toxic, producing agitation, delirium, respiratory depression, and coma. Cardiac arrhythmias with prolongation of the QT interval are frequent. There is no specific antidote, and treatment is supportive, although intensive care may be required. Alkalinization of plasma reduces the amount of free drug.
- It is not necessary (and may be harmful) to withdraw TCAs perioperatively.
- Increased sensitivity to catecholamines may result in hypertension and arrhythmias, following the administration of sympathomimetic drugs (adrenaline, noradrenaline). Indirect sympathomimetics (e.g. ephedrine, metaraminol) should be avoided.
- Ventricular arrhythmias may occur with high concentrations of volatile agents, especially halothane.
- TCAs may delay gastric emptying.
- Anticholinergic drugs (e.g. atropine) which cross the blood–brain barrier may precipitate post-operative confusion.
- Tramadol increases risk of CNS toxicity.

St John's wort (Hypericum perforatum)

- Extract of the plant contains several alkaloids which are similar in structure to TCA drugs.[6]
- Useful and safe as monotherapy in mild depressive illness.
- May induce certain cytochrome P450 enzymes, thereby enhancing the metabolism of many drugs, including warfarin, digoxin, theophylline, ciclosporin, tacrolimus, HIV protease inhibitors, and oral contraceptive drugs.
- May interact with other drugs, e.g. SSRIs, to cause serotonin syndrome (see p. 266). Consider withdrawing 5d preoperatively.

Selective serotonin reuptake inhibitors

SSRIs are the most commonly prescribed antidepressants worldwide and are increasingly being prescribed for other conditions (e.g. panic disorder, obsessive–compulsive disorder). They are highly specific inhibitors of pre-synaptic reuptake of serotonin from the synaptic cleft and are much less toxic in overdose than TCAs. Common examples include fluoxetine, venla-faxine, and mirtazapine.

- Common side effects affect the GI tract (nausea, vomiting, diarrhoea, upper GI bleeding) and the CNS (insomnia, agitation, tremor, headache, sexual dysfunction). CVS side effects are rare (occasional reports of bradycardia).
- In patients with pre-existing IHD, SSRIs may precipitate coronary vasoconstriction.
- SIADH has been described with the use of SSRIs, especially in the elderly, and may present with hyponatraemia (see ➔ p. 178).
- High doses of SSRIs may impair platelet aggregation and cause prolonged bleeding times.
- SSRIs inhibit cytochrome P450 enzymes, which may prolong or enhance the activity of other drugs, notably warfarin, theophylline, phenytoin, carbamazepine, tolbutamide, benzodiazepines (diazepam, midazolam), type 1c antiarrhythmics (e.g. flecainide), TCAs, and some NSAIDs.
- Serotonin syndrome[7,8] is a toxic crisis resulting from increased synaptic levels of serotonin in the brainstem and spinal cord due to overdose of SSRIs or a combination of other drugs affecting serotonin (especially TCAs, monoamine oxidase inhibitors (MAOIs), pethidine, and tramadol). It presents as an alteration in behaviour (agitation, confusion), motor activity (rigidity, myoclonus, hyperreflexia), and autonomic instability (pyrexia, tachycardia, diarrhoea, unstable BP). It may progress to seizures, oculogyric crises, DIC, rhabdomyolysis, myoglobinuria, ARF, arrhythmia, coma, and death. It may mimic the neuroleptic malignant syndrome (see ➔ p. 269). The patient is likely to require intensive care. Treatment is mainly supportive, and the episode usually lasts <24hr.

Anaesthesia for patients on selective serotonin reuptake inhibitors

- Abrupt withdrawal of SSRIs can precipitate a withdrawal syndrome.
- Check U&Es to exclude hyponatraemia, especially in the elderly.
- A coagulation screen should be assessed and corrected, if necessary.
- Benzodiazepines should be used cautiously, as their effects may be prolonged. Pethidine, tramadol, pentazocine, and dextromethorphan should be avoided.

References

6 Mills E, Montori VM, Wu P, et al. (2004). Interaction of St John's wort with conventional drugs: systematic review of clinical trials. *BMJ*, **329**, 27–30.
7 Chinniah S, French JLH, Levy D (2008). Serotonin and anaesthesia. *Contin Educ Anaesth Crit Care Pain*, **8**, 43–5.
8 Jones D, Story DA (2005). Serotonin syndrome and the anaesthetist. *Anaesth Intensive Care*, **33**, 181–7.

Monoamine oxidase inhibitors

MAOIs are 3rd-line antidepressants, used in refractory cases.[9,10] The enzyme monoamine oxidase (MAO) is present on mitochondrial membranes where it deaminates (thereby inactivating) monoamine neurotransmitters in the cytoplasm. It has two isoenzymes A and B.

- MAO-A preferentially metabolizes serotonin, noradrenaline, and adrenaline, and predominates in the CNS. MAO-B preferentially metabolizes non-polar aromatic amines such as phenylethylamine and methylhistamine. It predominates in the liver, lungs, and non-neural cells; 75% of all MAO activity is due to MAO-B.
- Tyramine (a monoamine found in cheese and other foods) and dopamine are substrates for both A and B.
- **Indirect sympathomimetics**, which are metabolized by MAO, may have greatly exaggerated effects. They may displace noradrenaline from neurotransmitter vesicles in such high amounts that a fatal hypertensive crisis may be precipitated.
- Older drugs (**tranylcypromine, phenelzine, isocarboxazid**) bind covalently to the MAO enzyme and are non-selective for A and B. Regeneration of new enzyme takes 2–3wk.
- Newer drugs are reversible and selective for MAO-A, known as reversible inhibitors of monoamine oxidase A (RIMAs). **Moclobemide** is the only RIMA available in the UK.
- **Linezolid** (antibacterial used against methicillin-resistant *Staphylococcus aureus*, MRSA) is a non-selective, but reversible, MAOI—treat patients as if on a classical MAOI.
- **Selegiline** is an MAO-B inhibitor used in Parkinson's disease.
- Methylthioninium chloride (methylene blue) has MAOI properties.

Preoperative withdrawal

- If the patient is taking tranylcypromine, phenelzine, or isocarboxazid, ideally it must be stopped at least 2wk prior to surgery to be of benefit. This may provoke drastic relapses in symptoms and should not be done without consultation with a senior psychiatrist. If stopped for <2wk, patients should be considered as still on MAOI.
- If the patient is taking moclobemide, it can be omitted safely for 24hr preoperatively, and restarted afterward.
- It is not necessary to stop selegiline if taken in doses of <10mg/d. At this dose, there is no reaction with sympathomimetics. Pethidine, however, should still be avoided.

Anaesthesia for a patient on monoamine oxidase inhibitor

- GA can be provided with caution to patients who are taking an MAOI (Table 12.1).
- The most dangerous interactions are with indirect sympathomimetics and some opioids (especially pethidine, which is absolutely contraindicated with any MAOI).
- **Indirect sympathomimetics** (ephedrine, metaraminol, amphetamine, cocaine, tyramine), which release stored noradrenaline from vesicles,

may precipitate potentially fatal hypertensive crises, and are absolutely contraindicated with any MAOI.
- **Direct sympathomimetics** (e.g. noradrenaline, adrenaline, phenylephrine, methoxamine, dopamine, dobutamine, isoprenaline) may have an exaggerated effect and should be used with caution.
- Treat hypotension initially with IV fluid, then cautious doses of phenylephrine (e.g. 10–20 micrograms).
- Opioid drugs which have serotoninergic properties (including **pethidine** and dextromethorphan) may precipitate serotonin syndrome (see ➲ p. 269).
- MAOIs can inhibit hepatic microsomal enzymes, prolonging the action of all opioids and enhancing their effect. This can be treated with naloxone.
- Phenelzine decreases plasma cholinesterase levels and prolongs the action of suxamethonium. This is specific to phenelzine and is not typical of MAOIs.
- Pancuronium releases stored noradrenaline and should be avoided.
- Safe drugs: induction agents propofol, thiopental, and etomidate; non-depolarizing neuromuscular-blocking drugs (except pancuronium); volatile agents and N_2O; NSAIDs; benzodiazepines.
- LA drugs (except cocaine) are safe (caution if contain adrenaline). Axial and regional blocks are ideal; however, hypotension should be treated cautiously. Felypressin is a satisfactory alternative to adrenaline if a vasoconstrictor is required.
- Anticholinergic drugs (atropine, glycopyrronium) are safe.
- Morphine is the opioid of choice and should be titrated cautiously to effect. However, there is no direct evidence of problems with fentanyl, alfentanil, remifentanil, or sufentanil.

Table 12.1 Drug interactions with MAOIs

Drugs to be avoided	Reason	Suitable alternative
Pethidine, tramadol, dextromethorphan	Risk of serotonin syndrome	Morphine, fentanyl
Ephedrine, metaraminol, cocaine	Hypertensive crises	Phenylephrine, noradrenaline
Pancuronium	Releases stored noradrenaline	Vecuronium, atracurium
Suxamethonium	Phenelzine only (decreased cholinesterase activity)	Mivacurium, rocuronium

References

9 Luck JF, Wildsmith JAW, Christmas DMB (2003). Monoamine oxidase inhibitors and anaesthesia. *Royal College of Anaesthetists Bulletin*, **21**, 1029–34.
10 Peck T, Wong A, Norman E (2010). Anaesthetic implications of psychoactive drugs. *Contin Educ Anaesth Crit Care Pain*, **10**, 177–81.

Antipsychotic drugs and lithium

Antipsychotic drugs

- Antipsychotic drugs (formerly known as major tranquillizers or neuroleptics) include haloperidol, chlorpromazine, olanzapine, quetiapine, and risperidone, and are used in the treatment of schizophrenia and similar disorders. Their main action is antagonism at CNS dopamine (D_2) receptors.
- Most antagonize other receptors, including histamine (H_1), serotonin ($5-HT_2$), acetylcholine (muscarinic), and α-adrenergic receptors.
- Main side effects include sedation, extrapyramidal motor disturbances, and the development of tardive dyskinesia with chronic use. Other side effects include gynaecomastia, weight gain, postural hypotension, antimuscarinic effects, obstructive jaundice (uncommon), and agranulocytosis (rare, but severe). Most are powerful antiemetics.
- Many drugs prolong the QT interval, especially when combined with other drugs which may do the same (e.g. antidepressants).
- Clozapine is associated with a risk of agranulocytosis.
- Neuroleptic malignant syndrome[11] is a rare idiosyncratic reaction to antipsychotic drugs which resembles MH (see ➡ p. 918). Typical patients are young ♂. Features include hyperthermia, tachycardia, extrapyramidal dysfunction (rigidity, dystonia), and autonomic dysfunction (sweating, labile BP, salivation, urinary incontinence). CK and white cell count (WCC) are raised. Patients should be treated in ICU. Mortality is ~20%.
- Abrupt withdrawal of antipsychotic medication is dangerous.
- Antipsychotic drugs potentiate sedative and hypotensive effects of anaesthetic agents (including opioids).

Lithium

- Lithium is an inorganic ion used as a mood stabilizer in the treatment of bipolar affective disorder. It has a low therapeutic ratio, with an optimal plasma concentration of 0.4–1.0mmol/L.
- Lithium mimics Na^+ in excitable tissues, being able to permeate voltage-gated ion channels, and accumulates inside cells, causing slight loss of intracellular K^+ and partial depolarization.
- Chronic use causes weight gain, renal impairment, and hypothyroidism.
- Lithium toxicity occurs at >1.5mmol/L and is exacerbated by hyponatraemia, diuretic therapy, and renal disease. Features include lethargy/restlessness, nausea/vomiting, thirst, tremor, polyuria, renal failure, ataxia, convulsions, coma, and death. Haemodialysis is effective.
- Lithium potentiates both depolarizing and non-depolarizing NMB; nerve stimulator monitoring should be used.
- Lithium may cause T wave flattening or inversion, but clinically important CVS effects are rare.
- NSAIDs should be used with caution (risk of exacerbating renal impairment and causing toxicity).

Reference

11 Adnet P, Lestavel P, Krivosic-Horber R (2000). Neuroleptic malignant syndrome. Br J Anaesth, 85, 129–35.

Sedation of agitated patients on the ward

Anaesthetists may be asked to help with sedation of agitated patients on general wards and are more likely to be familiar with the effects of sedation than junior medical or surgical staff.

- Patients are likely to be in an acute confusional state—exacerbated by pain, unfamiliar/threatening surroundings, and strangers. They may be disoriented, agitated, disinhibited, or violent, and may experience visual or auditory hallucinations.
- When presentation is acute in a previously lucid patient, the cause is usually organic. Establishing and treating the cause may remove the need for sedation.
- Exclude hypoglycaemia, hypoxia, pain, alcohol withdrawal, and a full bladder.
- Differential diagnosis includes infection (chest, urine, lines), drugs (cocaine, LSD, sedatives, analgesics), and metabolic derangement (e.g. hyponatraemia, hypoglycaemia). Less frequently: head injury, stroke, acute psychiatric disorder (e.g. mania), acute porphyria.

Approach to the patient

- Ensure the safety of yourself and other staff. A calm and reassuring approach will help the patient and any onlookers.
- If physical restraint is necessary, ensure plenty of help is available (hospital security, porters, and even police), and discuss with a psychiatrist.
- Establish venous access, if possible, and bandage the cannula.
- Aim to render the patient calm and cooperative, rather than unconscious.
- Do not leave a sedated patient unattended.

Drug therapy

- Haloperidol 5mg IV initially (reduce dose in the elderly, e.g. 1mg). Repeat after 5min if no effect. Titrate to effect. Maximum dose: 18mg/24hr, according to *BNF*, but higher doses are occasionally warranted.
- Midazolam 1–2mg IV may also be useful (titrate to effect). May cause paradoxical disinhibition, especially in the elderly.
- Alcohol withdrawal: give diazepam 5–10mg IV (or chlordiazepoxide 50mg PO), and repeat as required. Ketamine is useful in emergencies if the patient is extremely violent or dangerous. Give 0.5–1mg/kg IV (or 5–10mg/kg IM).
- Do not use propofol (too short-acting), opioids (respiratory depression), or drugs you may be unfamiliar with.
- In accident and emergency (A&E), or where the history is unknown, further investigation (e.g. CT scan) may be appropriate. In this circumstance, RSI of anaesthesia with full monitoring may be required.

Anaesthesia for drug-misusing patients

General considerations

- In the UK, around 10% of adults have used an illegal drug in the past year. Misuse of street drugs occurs in all socio-economic groups. Drug misuse causes the following specific problems:[12,13]
  - Acute intoxication may impede informed consent. In addition, the effects of the drug may counteract (stimulants) or enhance (sedatives) the effects of anaesthetic drugs. Consider drug misuse in all patients with a reduced conscious level or requiring emergency surgery and anaesthesia.
  - Chronic drug misuse is associated with poor nutrition, medical and psychiatric co-morbidity, and the presence of viral infections.
  - IV drug users often have no accessible veins. IV drug misuse is associated with IV infective complications. HIV and viral hepatitis are the commonest. Bacterial endocarditis is rare, but serious, and associated with pulmonary abscesses, embolic phenomena from vegetations, and vasculitis.
  - Drugs in common use fall into four groups (Table 12.2). Combinations of drugs are common, often with alcohol.

Table 12.2 Street drugs in common use

Drug	Clinical signs
Cannabis	Tachycardia, abnormal affect (e.g. euphoria, anxiety, panic, or psychosis), poor memory, fatigue
Stimulants: cocaine, amphetamines, ecstasy	Tachycardia, labile BP, excitement, delirium, hallucinations, hyperreflexia, tremors, convulsions, mydriasis, sweating, hyperthermia, exhaustion, coma
Hallucinogens: LSD, phencyclidine, ketamine	Sympathomimetic, weakly analgesic, altered judgement, hallucinations, toxic psychosis, dissociative anaesthesia
Opioids: morphine, heroin, oxycodone	Euphoria, respiratory depression, hypotension, bradycardia, constipation, pinpoint pupils, coma

Anaesthesia

- Keep a high index of suspicion—especially in trauma.
- Difficult venous access—IV drug users may be able to direct you to a patent vein. May need central venous cannulation or cut-down, or consider use of ultrasound scanning (USS) for vein location. Consider inhalational induction.
- Take full precautions against infection risk.
- Plan post-operative analgesia with the patient preoperatively.
- Do not attempt drug withdrawal perioperatively.

Opioids

- Patients who misuse opioids should expect the same quality of analgesia as other patients. Recovering opioid users may be taking methadone.
- If opioids are the only method of providing analgesia, they should be administered in the same way as for normal patients, with doses titrated to effect (large doses may be required—see ⊃ p. 1080 for a suitable dosing regime). Combinations of regional nerve blocks and NSAIDs may avoid the need for opioids.
- Opioid-addicted surgical patients should be supported by specialist addiction services during the perioperative period (usually contactable via the local psychiatric services).
- A small group of 'ex-addicts' may have fears about being prescribed opioids precipitating relapse. This should not become an obstacle to treating post-operative pain, but opioids should not be given without first obtaining consent.

Cocaine and crack cocaine

- Cocaine is usually 'sniffed' in powder form. Free-base ('crack') cocaine is heat-stable and can be smoked.
- Cocaine toxicity is mediated by central and peripheral adrenergic stimulation. Presenting symptoms include tachycardia, hypertension, aortic dissection, arrhythmias, accelerated CAD, coronary spasm, infarction, and sudden death. Intracerebral vasospasm can lead to stroke, rigidity, hyperreflexia, and hyperthermia. Inhalation of cocaine can cause alveolar haemorrhage and pulmonary oedema.
- Psychiatric symptoms range from elation and enhanced physical strength to full toxic paranoid psychosis.
- Patients who need surgery following ingestion of cocaine may need intensive care while they are stabilized. Most of the life-threatening side effects of cocaine are due to vasospasm and can be reversed, using combinations of vasodilators, antiarrhythmic agents, and α/β-blockers titrated against effect, using full invasive monitoring.
- Combination LA/vasoconstrictors (or any vasopressor) should be avoided. Tachycardia or hypertensive crisis may result. If vasopressors are required in theatre, use very small doses, and titrate against response.
- Intra-arterial injections of cocaine have led to critical limb and organ ischaemia. Successful treatment has included regional plexus blockade, IV heparin, stellate ganglion block, intra-arterial vasodilators, urokinase, and early fasciotomy.

Ecstasy (3,4-methylenedioxymethamphetamine, MDMA)

- Ecstasy is a stimulant drug related to amphetamine. It is usually taken in tablet form. ~30 people die from taking ecstasy annually in the UK.
- Hyperthermia (>39°C), DIC, and dehydration are common features.
- Excessive ADH release (or water ingestion) may also cause hyponatraemia, leading to coma.
- Carefully monitor fluid and electrolyte replacement.

References

12 Jenkins BJ (2002). Drug abusers and anaesthesia. *BJA CEPD Reviews*, **2**, 15–19.
13 Roberts TN, Thompson JP (2013). Illegal substances in anaesthetic and intensive care practices. *Contin Educ Anaesth Crit Care Pain*, **13**, 42–6.

Anaesthesia for electroconvulsive therapy

Procedure	Electrically induced seizure
Time	5–10min
Pain	±
Position	Supine
Blood loss	Nil
Practical technique	Short IV GA, face mask only, bite block

General considerations

Electroconvulsive therapy (ECT) is safe and effective in the treatment of mental disorders, most commonly severe depression unresponsive to drugs, catatonia, or where there is a high risk of suicide or self-neglect. ECT is commonly carried out in an isolated site; ensure skilled assistance, adequate monitoring, and resuscitation facilities. Anaesthetic equipment may be old or unfamiliar.

Physiological effects of electroconvulsive therapy

- During the seizure, there is parasympathetic hyperactivity—bradycardia and hypotension, lasting about 15s, followed by a more prolonged (5min) sympathetic stimulation: tachycardia, hypertension, dysrhythmias, increased myocardial O_2 requirement.
- CNS: increased ICP, cerebral blood flow, and cerebral O_2 requirement.
- Other: hypersalivation, increased intragastric pressure, increased intraocular pressure (IOP), occasionally incontinence.

Preoperative

- A careful preoperative assessment (including investigations) should be undertaken, as for any GA.
- Consent is normally arranged by the psychiatrist responsible.
- ECT is usually given twice weekly for several weeks, reducing in frequency as the patient improves. Read the notes for documentation of previous problems.
- Absolute contraindications: recent MI or cerebrovascular accident (CVA), phaeochromocytoma, intracranial mass lesion, intracranial or aortic aneurysm.
- Relative contraindications: uncontrolled angina, CCF, severe osteoporosis, major bone fracture, glaucoma, retinal detachment. ECT in pregnancy is acceptable.
- Avoid sedative premedication, which is anticonvulsant.
- Glycopyrronium (0.1–0.3mg IV) may be used to reduce secretions and to counteract bradycardia. Consider antacids if history of reflux.

Perioperative

- Efficacy of ECT is dependent on seizure duration and quality, as measured by EEG-derived variables. However, there is no further benefit beyond about 60s.
- Good technique provides short GA, muscle relaxation to lessen the risk of trauma, attenuation of physiological effects, and rapid recovery.
- Thorough preoxygenation is recommended.
- All GAs shorten the seizure in a dose-related fashion; use light doses.
- Propofol, thiopental, etomidate, and ketamine (less suitable) may all be used for induction. Propofol attenuates the sympathetic response but shortens the seizure more than the others. Etomidate shortens the seizure less, but the sympathetic response may be more pronounced. Inhalational sevoflurane is effective but takes longer.
- The combination of a small dose of propofol with remifentanil (1 microgram/kg) is effective.
- Suxamethonium (0.5–1mg/kg) is given to 'modify' the seizure (reduce muscle power to prevent injury). Mivacurium (0.2mg/kg) may be used instead but will probably require reversal. The combination of rocuronium and sugammadex is also effective.
- Insert a bite-block to prevent damage to the mouth and teeth.
- Maintain the airway with a face mask and/or oral airway. Hand-ventilate the patient with O_2 until breathing resumes afterward.
- The psychiatrist may titrate the magnitude of the stimulus to the length of seizure; be prepared to maintain the anaesthetic with further boluses of induction agent if a 2nd stimulus is required.
- Sympathetic response may also be attenuated with alfentanil (10 micrograms/kg) or esmolol (e.g. 0.25mg/kg). Labetalol, sodium nitroprusside, and hydralazine have also been used.
- Seizure augmentation: both caffeine and theophylline lower the seizure threshold and prolong the seizure. Moderate hyperventilation with bag and mask before the seizure is also effective.
- If the seizure lasts longer than 60s, it should be terminated, e.g. with propofol titrated to response.

Post-operative

- Post-ictal agitation, confusion, or aggression may occur in some patients. They should be nursed in a calm environment and may occasionally require sedation (e.g. midazolam 1mg IV).
- Headache and muscle pains are commonly reported and usually respond to simple analgesics.
- Drowsiness and cognitive impairment are very common but typically resolve within a few hours.
- No evidence of memory loss is demonstrable at 6 months. However, patients sometimes complain of memory loss for specific life events.
- Other complications include nausea, exacerbation of IHD, fractures/dislocations, dental/oral injury, and laryngospasm.
- ECT does not increase the risk of other types of seizure.
- Overall mortality is about 1 per 80 000 treatments.

Further reading

Ding Z, White PF (2002). Anesthesia for electroconvulsive therapy. *Anesth Analg*, **94**, 1351–64.

Flood S, Bodenham A (2010). Lithium: mimicry, mania, and muscle relaxants. *Contin Educ Anaesth Crit Care Pain*, **10**, 77–80.

Hooten WM, Rasmussen KG Jr (2008). Effects of general anesthetic agents in adults receiving electroconvulsive therapy: a systematic review. *J ECT*, **24**, 208–23.

Jackson P, Gleeson D (2010). Alcoholic liver disease. *Contin Educ Anaesth Crit Care Pain*, **10**, 66–71.

Tess AV, Smetana GW (2009). Medical evaluation of patients undergoing electroconvulsive therapy: current concepts. *N Engl J Med*, **360**, 1437.

Uppal V, Dourish J, Macfarlane A (2010). Anaesthesia for electroconvulsive therapy. *Contin Educ Anaesth Crit Care Pain*, **10**, 192–6.

Walker SC, Bowley CJ, Walker HAC (2013). Anaesthesia for ECT. In: Waite J, Easton A, eds. *The ECT handbook*, 3rd edn. London: Royal College of Psychiatrists, pp. 14–27.

Uncommon conditions

Graham Hocking

A

Aarskog–Scott syndrome

Cervical spine hypermobility/odontoid anomaly, mild/moderate short stature, cleft lip/palate, skin and skeletal anomalies/laxity, interstitial pulmonary disease, pectus excavatum. △ Difficult intubation.[1]

Achalasia of the cardia

Motor disorder of the distal two-thirds of the oesophagus, failure of relaxation of the lower oesophageal sphincter → dilatation, dysphagia, regurgitation, and risk of malignant change. △ ↑ Gastric reflux.[2]

Achondroplasia

Dwarfism, normal-sized trunk, short limbs, disproportionately large head, flat face, possible small larynx, bulging skull vault, and kyphoscoliosis. Spinal stenoses in the canal/foramen magnum can occur. ↑ risk of OSA. △ Difficult intubation. Care on neck flexion (cord compression). Central neural blocks may have unpredictable spread (use smaller amounts).[3,4] (See also ⊃ p. 1135.)

Acromegaly

See also ⊃ p. 156.

Enlarged jaw/tongue/larynx, nerve entrapment syndromes, respiratory obstruction, including sleep apnoea, diabetes mellitus, hypertension, cardiac failure, thyroid and renal impairment, possible narrow cricoid ring, associated organ dysfunction, perioperative glucose intolerance. △ Difficult intubation and airway maintenance.[5,6]

Alagille's syndrome (syndromic bile duct paucity)

Paucity of interlobular bile ducts, chronic cholestasis, coagulopathy. Pre-treat with vitamin K. Splenomegaly may cause thrombocytopenia, cardiac/musculoskeletal/ocular/facial abnormalities, pathological fractures, neuropathies (vitamin deficiencies), retinopathy, CVS assessment (stenosis/hypoplasia common), sagittal spinal cleft, and cerebellar ataxia. Document pre-existing peripheral neuropathy. △ ↑ Gastric reflux (abdominal distension).[7]

Albers–Schönberg disease (marble bones)

See Osteopetrosis.

Albright's osteodystrophy (pseudohypoparathyroidism type 1a)

Resistance of target tissues to PTH, short stature, round face, short neck, short 4th and 5th metacarpals, hypocalcaemia (may → neuromuscular irritability, convulsions), hyperphosphataemia, and inappropriately high PTH.

Albright's syndrome (McCune–Albright syndrome)

Defective regulation of cyclic adenosine monophosphate (cAMP), multiple unilateral bone lesions, skin pigmentation, ♀ sexual precocity, bony deformity (including skull), fractures, spinal cord compression, acromegaly, thyrotoxicosis. Cushing's syndrome may coexist. Identify endocrine abnormalities. ⚠ May need larger-than-expected ETT. Cardiac arrhythmias and bony deformity may complicate regional blocks.[8]

Alport syndrome

Hereditary nephropathy, predominantly ♂, characterized by nephritis → renal failure, hypertension, sensorineural deafness, myopia, thrombocytopenia with giant forms of platelets. ► Check renal function and clotting.[9]

Alstrom syndrome

Obesity from infancy, nystagmus, sensitivity to light, progressive visual impairment with blindness by 7yr, sensorineural hearing loss, diabetes mellitus and renal failure in early adult life, cardiac disease, problems associated with obesity/organ dysfunction.[10]

Alveolar hypoventilation

Central hypoventilation due to midbrain lesion/severance of spinal tracts from the midbrain (Ondine's curse), periods of prolonged apnoea, hypoxia, hypercapnia, abnormal respiratory drive, take care with oxygen supplements if relying on hypoxic drive, cor pulmonale, polycythaemia, autonomic dysfunction. ⚠ Re-establishing spontaneous ventilation may be difficult; consider regional techniques, post-operative respiratory failure.[11,12]

Amyloidosis

Abnormal deposition of hyaline material in tissues, macroglossia. Beware laryngeal amyloid. Unexpected cardiac or renal failure can occur. Associated with other pathologies; assess to detect systems affected and risk of post-operative organ failure.[13]

Amyotonia congenita

See *Spinal muscular atrophy*.

Amyotrophic lateral sclerosis

Progressive degeneration of lower motor neurons, motor nuclei of the brainstem, descending pathway of the upper motor neurons, atrophy and weakness involving most skeletal muscles, including tongue, pharynx, larynx, and chest wall muscles, fasciculation, sensation normal, impaired ventilation. ⚠ Altered response to muscle relaxants, aspiration risk (laryngeal incompetence), sensitive to respiratory depressants (see also ➔ p. 250).[14,15]

Analbuminaemia

Deficiency of albumin. Sensitivity to all protein-bound drugs—titrate drugs carefully.[16]

Andersen's disease

See *Glycogenoses, type IV*.

Andersen's syndrome

Triad of K⁺-sensitive periodic paralysis/ventricular arrhythmias/dysmorphic features, long QT, spontaneous attacks of paralysis with acute K⁺ changes; baseline level may be hypokalaemia/normokalaemia/hyperkalaemia.[17]

Anhidrotic/hypohidrotic ectodermal dysplasia (Christ–Siemens–Touraine syndrome)

Hypodontia, hypotrichosis, hypohidrosis, heat intolerance, recurrent chest infections (poor mucus formation). △ Difficult intubation.[18]

Ankylosing spondylitis

Asymmetric oligoarthropathy, total vertebral involvement, cardiomegaly, aortic regurgitation, cardiac conduction abnormalities, pulmonary fibrosis, bamboo spine. △ Difficult airway/neuraxial blockade.[19,20] (See also ➔ p. 187.)

Antley–Bixler syndrome

Autosomal recessive, multiple bone/cartilaginous abnormalities, mid-face hypoplasia, significant craniosynostosis, choanal stenosis/atresia, femoral bowing, radiohumeral synostosis, multiple joint contractures, CVS/renal/GI malformations. △ Potential difficult airway. Extremity deformities may complicate vascular access and positioning.[21]

Apert's syndrome

Craniosynostosis, high forehead, maxillary hypoplasia, relative mandibular prognathism, cervical synostosis, visceral malformations, congenital heart anomalies. Assess for other organ involvement and ↑ ICP. △ Airway difficulties, perioperative respiratory problems (especially wheezing).[22]

Arnold–Chiari malformation

Group of congenital hindbrain anomalies causing downward displacement of the pons and medulla, with variable neurological sequelae. ▶ Preoperative assessment of CNS function and response to neck movement and ICP, careful neuroanaesthetic (usual potential problems).[23]

Arthrogryposis (congenital contractures)

Skin and SC tissue abnormalities, contracture deformities, micrognathia, cervical spine and jaw stiffness, CHD (10%); hypermetabolic response is probably not MH. △ Difficult airway and venous access, sensitive to thiopental.[24,25]

Asplenia syndrome

Complex congenital heart defects, asplenia, visceral anomalies secondary to abnormal lateralization, cardiac failure, hiatus hernia/reflux, recurrent pneumonias. Part of the heterotaxy group of syndromes.[26]

Ataxia telangiectasia

Progressive cerebellar ataxia, conjunctival telangiectasia, progressive neurological degeneration, recurrent chest and sinus infections, bronchiectasis, malignancies (leukaemias), sensitivity to X-rays/radiotherapy (cellular damage), premature ageing.[27]

Axenfeld–Rieger syndrome

Ocular and dental defects, maxillary hypoplasia, heart defects, short stature, mental deficiency. △ Airway problems.[28]

References

1 Teebi AS, et al. (1993). Am J Med Genet, **46**, 501–9.
2 Spechler SJ (2013). ✆ http://www.uptodate.com/contents/achalasia-beyond-the-basics.
3 Krishnan BS, et al. (2003). Paediatr Anaesth, **13**, 547–9.
4 Wardall GJ, Frame WT (1990). Br J Anaesth, **64**, 367–70.
5 Seidman PA, et al. (2000). Br J Anaesth, **84**, 179–82.
6 Khan ZH, Rasouli MR (2009). Eur J Anaesthesiol, **26**, 354–5.
7 Yildiz TS, et al. (2007). Paediatr Anaesth, **17**, 91–2.
8 Langer RA, et al. (1995). Anesth Analg, **80**, 1236–9.
9 Kashtan CE (1999). Medicine, **78**, 338–60.
10 Lynch GM, et al. (2007). Anaesth Intensive Care, **35**, 305–6.
11 Wiesel S, Fox GS (1990). Can J Anaesth, **37**, 122–6.
12 Strauser LM, et al. (1999). J Clin Anesth, **11**, 431–7.
13 Fleming I (2012). Contin Educ Anaesth Crit Care Pain, **14**, 72–7.
14 Rowland LP, Schneider NA (2001). N Engl J Med, **344**, 1688–700.
15 Prabhakar A (2013). J Anesthesia, **27**, 909–18.
16 Koot BG (2004). Eur J Pediatr, **163**, 664–70.
17 Young DA (2005). Paediatr Anaesth, **54**, 1019–20.
18 Singh AK, Saini A (2010). ✆ http://bja.oxfordjournals.org/forum/topic/brjana_el%3B5895.
19 Woodward LJ, Kam PC (2009). Anaesthesia, **64**, 540–8.
20 Lu PP, et al. (2001). Can J Anaesth, **48**, 1015–19.
21 Gencay I (2013). J Craniofac Surg, **24**, 21–3.
22 Hutson LR, et al. (2007). J Clin Anesth, **19**, 551–4.
23 Choi CK, Tyagaraj K (2013). Case Reports in Anesthesiology, Article ID 512915.
24 Chowdhuri RJ (2011). Anaesthesiol Clin Pharmacol, **27**, 244–6.
25 Nguyen NH, et al. (2000). J Clin Anesth, **12**, 227–30.
26 Uchida K, et al. (1992). Masui, **41**, 1793–7.
27 Lockman JL, et al. (2012). Paediatr Anaesth, **22**, 256–62.
28 Asai T, et al. (1998). Paediatr Anaesth, **8**, 444.

B

Bardet–Biedl syndrome
See also *Laurence–Moon syndrome*.

Obesity, retinitis pigmentosa, polydactyly, mental retardation, hypogonadism, renal failure.[29]

Bartter syndrome
Growth retardation, hypertrophy and hyperplasia of the juxtaglomerular apparatus, ADH antagonism by prostaglandins, hyperaldosteronism, hypokalaemic alkalosis, normal BP, ↓ response to vasopressors, platelet abnormalities. ▶ Maintain CVS stability, control serum K⁺, meticulous fluid balance, caution with renally excreted drugs; neuraxial anaesthesia may be hazardous (stature, clotting, pressor response).[30]

Beckwith–Wiedemann syndrome (infantile gigantism)
Macroglossia, microcephaly, omphalocele, perinatal/post-natal gigantism, possible CHD (ASD/VSD/PDA/hypoplastic LV), neonatal hypoglycaemia (hyperinsulinism). ⚠ Abnormal airway anatomy; extubate awake.[31,32]

Behçet's syndrome
Chronic multisystem vasculitis of unknown aetiology, triad of recurring iritis/mouth ulceration/genital ulceration, possible altered fibrinolysis; vasculitis may involve other organ systems. ▶ Fully assess other organ functions. ⚠ Prior oral ulceration/scarring may complicate airway management; minimize needle punctures (diffuse inflammatory skin reaction); autonomic hyperreflexia may occur with spinal cord involvement.[33]

Bernard–Soulier syndrome (giant platelet syndrome)
Congenital lack of membrane glycoprotein GP1b, ↓ number of huge platelets, ↑ bleeding time, severe bleeding tendency, possibly improves with age; platelet infusions may be needed.[34]

Blackfan–Diamond syndrome (congenital red cell aplasia)
Congenital hypoplastic anaemia, growth retardation, CCF, hepatosplenomegaly (↓ FRC), hypersplenism, thrombocytopenia.[35]

Bland–White–Garland syndrome
Anomalous origin of the left coronary artery from the pulmonary trunk, chronic myocardial ischaemia/subendocardial fibrosis/LV dilation/valvular insufficiency (papillary muscle damage), CCF. ⚠ Often difficult to wean ventilation; beware perioperative myocardial failure.[36]

Bloom's syndrome
Rare autosomal recessive disorder, chromosome breakage/recombination, short stature, photosensitive, facial telangiectasic erythema, predisposition to malignant diseases. Limit X-rays (may damage cells). ⚠ Potential difficulties with mask fit and laryngoscopy.[37]

Brugada syndrome

Abnormal human cardiac Na^+ channel, right bundle branch block/ST elevation in leads V1–V3, sudden death from VF (up to 1 in 1000 young South East Asian ♂), may have underlying cardiac structural abnormality, tachyarrhythmias not responsive to medical therapy. ► May have ICD if pre-existing syncope (requires usual care during surgery); treat intraoperative tachyarrhythmias by cardioversion; avoid neostigmine (worsens ST elevation—risk of VT/VF); safety of techniques needing high doses of local anaesthetics not yet tested; spinal anaesthesia appears safe.[38]

Buerger's disease (thromboangiitis obliterans)

Peripheral vascular disease with ulceration, Raynaud's phenomenon, hyperhidrosis, bronchitis, emphysema; NIBP may over-read.

Bullous cystic lung disease

Non-communicating lung cysts may be more compliant than normal lung. ► Risk of pneumothorax with IPPV; avoid nitrous oxide (N_2O); high-frequency jet ventilation used successfully.[39]

Burkitt's lymphoma

Undifferentiated lymphoblastic lymphoma most commonly affecting the jaw (also abdominal organs/breasts/testes). ⚠ Difficult intubation.[40]

References

29 Mahajan R, et al. (2007). Minerva Anesthesiol, 73, 191–4.
30 Bhaskar BS (2010). Indian J Anaesth, 54, 327–30.
31 Kimura Y, et al. (2008). J Anesth, 22, 93–5.
32 Gurkowski MA, Rasch DK (1989). Anesthesiology, 70, 711–12.
33 Gupta A, et al. (2013). Anesth Essays Res, 7, 279–81.
34 Kostopanagiotou G, et al. (2004). J Clin Anesth, 16, 458–60.
35 Daniela Maria Arturi Foundation. ℜ http://diamondblackfananemia.org/about/facts/.
36 Kleinschmidt S, et al. (1996). Paediatr Anaesth, 6, 65–8.
37 Aono J, et al. (1992). Masui, 41, 255–7.
38 Carey S, Hocking G (2011). Anaesth Intensive Care, 39, 571–7.
39 Normandale JP, et al. (1985). Anaesthesia, 40, 1182–5.
40 Palmer CD, et al. (1998). Paediatr Anaesth, 8, 506–9.

C

Cantrell's pentalogy
Defect of supraumbilical abdominal wall, agenesis of lower part of sternum/anterior portion of diaphragm, absence of diaphragmatic part of pericardium, cardiac malformation (VSD/ASD), hypoplastic lungs. ▶ Check for R → L shunting; avoid pressure to lower thorax/abdomen.[41]

Carpenter's syndrome
Cranial synostosis, small mandible, CHD (PDA/VSD), obesity, umbilical hernia, mental retardation, cerebrospinal malformations (narrowed foramen magnum, hypoplastic posterior fossa, kinked spinal cord). △ Difficult intubation.[42]

Central core disease
See *Congenital myopathy*.

Cerebrocostomandibular syndrome
Micrognathia, cleft palate, tracheal anomalies, rib defects/microthorax, mental deficiency, early death from respiratory complications. △ Difficult intubation.[43]

Chagas' disease (American trypanosomiasis)
Many patients are asymptomatic. Malaise, anorexia, fever, hepatomegaly, mega-colon/mega-oesophagus, unilateral oedema, cardiac failure, chronic myocarditis, associated organ dysfunction. △ ↑ Gastric reflux.[44]

Charcot–Marie–Tooth disease (peroneal muscular atrophy)
Chronic peripheral neuromuscular denervation/atrophy, spinal/lower limb deformities, ↑ K⁺, may affect respiratory muscles (restrictive pattern); evidence suggests low MH risk. ▶ Avoid suxamethonium.[45]

CHARGE association
Coloboma/Heart anomaly/choanal Atresia/Retardation/Genital/Ear anomalies. △ Difficult intubation (micrognathia).[46]

Chediak–Higashi syndrome
Albinism, photophobia, nystagmus, weakness, tremor, thrombocytopenia, susceptible to infection.[47]

Cherubism
Tumorous mandibular and maxillary lesions, intraoral masses, may develop acute respiratory distress, profuse bleeding; tracheostomy may be needed. △ Difficult intubation.[48]

Chronic granulomatous disease
Rare genetically transmitted disorder, recurrent life-threatening infections with catalase-positive microorganisms, excessive inflammatory reactions, granuloma formation, multiple organ system involvement, including pulmonary granulomata, long-term prophylactic antibiotics. △ Regurgitation/aspiration risk (GI granulomata).[49]

Cockayne's syndrome

Rare autosomal recessive condition, failure of DNA repair, dysmorphic dwarfism, mental retardation in infancy/childhood, hypertension, hepatic deficiencies, osteoporosis, deafness, blindness, other effects of premature ageing (see *Progeria*). ⚠ Airway management problems, ↑ risk of gastric aspiration, weight-appropriate equipment.[50]

Congenital adrenal hyperplasia (adrenogenital syndrome)

Congenital disorders—defects in cortisol biosynthesis, ↑ ACTH, disordered androgens, may mimic pyloric stenosis in neonate, electrolyte abnormalities. ► Adequate perioperative fluid/steroid therapy.[51]

Congenital analgesia

Hereditary disorder → self-mutilation, defective thermoregulation, vasomotor control, sensitivity to anaesthetic drugs. ► Careful positioning.[52]

Congenital myopathy (central core disease)

Non-progressive extremity weakness (lower > upper), difficulty rising from sitting, ↑ lumbar lordosis, ptosis, most test positive for MH *in vitro*. ⚠ Avoid trigger factors; ventilatory weakness, sensitive to muscle relaxants.[53,54]

Conradi–Hunermann syndrome (chondrodysplasia punctata)

Epiphyseal calcifications, short stature, hypertelorism, saddle nose, short neck, tracheal stenosis, scoliosis, renal and congenital heart disease. ⚠ Ventilatory failure due to airway and thoracic deformities, renal impairment, skin protection (use patient's creams/padding), attention to thermoregulation (lose heat quickly).[55]

Cornelia de Lange syndrome

Duplication/partial trisomy chromosome 3, psychomotor retardation, skeletal craniofacial deformities, VSD, GI anomalies; assess cardiorespiratory function, susceptible to infections. ⚠ Possible difficult airway, ↑ gastric reflux.[56,57]

Costello syndrome

Mental and growth retardation, short neck, macroglossia, hypertrophied tonsillar/supraglottic tissues, laryngeal papillomata, choanal atresia, cardiac arrhythmias, hypertrophic cardiomyopathy, talipes, scoliosis. ⚠ Potential airway difficulties, ↑ gastric reflux, arrhythmias.[58]

CREST syndrome

Also see ➋ p. 191.

Form of scleroderma, widespread necrotizing angiitis with granulomata, Calcinosis/Raynaud's phenomenon/oEsophageal dysfunction/Sclerodactyly/Telangiectasia, multiple organ involvement, nerve compression syndromes, arrhythmias, contractures, pulmonary fibrosis. ⚠ Airway difficulties, ↑ gastric reflux.

Cretinism

Congenital hypothyroidism, neurological and intellectual damage, muscle weakness, cardiomyopathy, respiratory complications, steroid cover, glucose and electrolyte abnormalities. ► Steroid cover. ⚠ Intubation problems (macroglossia), sensitive to anaesthetic drugs.

Creutzfeldt–Jakob disease (CJD)

One of the transmissible spongiform encephalopathies. Progressive fatal encephalopathy, responsible for recent changes in surgery/anaesthesia relating to re-use/sterilization of equipment. Four types: *sporadic CJD* (85–90% cases, older patients, rapidly progressive over few months); *familial CJD* (5–10%, due to gene mutation); *iatrogenic CJD* (<5%, transmission from surgical instruments/implants/growth hormone); *variant CJD* (young patients, slowly progressive 1–2yr); caused by prions (small proteinaceous infectious particles resistant to inactivation—contain abnormal isoform of a cellular protein), highest concentration in CNS/eye/lymphoid tissue, progressive neurological signs—psychiatric symptoms/altered sensation/visual loss/ataxia/weakness/involuntary movements/cognitive impairment/aphasia. ► Involve staff from communicable diseases; follow protocols for handling fluids/waste; remove unnecessary equipment/staff from theatre; universal precautions; consider antisialogogue to reduce secretions; portable suction to stay with patient throughout entire theatre visit/recovery; consider recovering in theatre—send directly back to ward; quarantine all used equipment (ventilator, etc.); use disposable equipment where possible; bipolar diathermy plume may contain inhalable prions (monopolar better); warn laboratory staff.[59]

Cri-du-chat syndrome

Inherited disease resulting in mental retardation, abnormal cry (due to abnormal larynx), laryngomalacia, microcephaly, micrognathia, macroglossia, spasticity, CHD (30%), hypotonia (possible airway obstruction by soft tissues). ⚠ Potential airway problems, long curved epiglottis, narrow diamond-shaped glottis, temperature instability.[60]

Crouzon's disease

Craniosynostosis, hydrocephalus, ↑ ICP, maxillary hypoplasia, mandibular prognathism, prominent nose, coarctation. Assess other organ involvement/ICP. ⚠ Airway difficulty, post-operative respiratory obstruction; correction procedures can bleed profusely.[61,62]

Cutis laxa (elastic degeneration)

Defective elastin cross-linking probably 2° to copper deficiency, extreme laxity of facial/trunk skin, no retraction after stretching, fragile skin/blood vessels, respiratory infections/emphysema common. ► Pendulous pharyngeal/laryngeal mucosa may obstruct the airway, careful positioning.[63]

Cystic hygroma

Benign multilocular lymphatic tumour of the neck/oral cavity/tongue causing local pressure symptoms, including airway compromise. ⚠ Oral intubation often impossible (enlarged tongue); partially obstructed airway in awake patient may totally obstruct on induction; tracheostomy complicated by submandibular involvement.[64]

References

41 Laloyaux P, et al. (1998). *Paediatr Anaesth*, **8**, 163–6.
42 Bhardwaj M, et al. (2013). *Int J Obstet Anaesth*, **22**, 251–4.
43 Georgiou AP, Gatward J (2008). *Br J Anaesth*, **100**, 567.
44 Fernandez Gil M, et al. (2009). *Rev Esp Anesthesiol Reanim*, **56**, 262–5.
45 Pasha TM, et al. (2013). *Br J Anaesth*, **110**, 1061–3.
46 Rashmi J, et al. (2008). *J Anaesth Clin Pharmacol*, **24**, 215–16.
47 Ulsoy H, et al. (1995). *Middle East J Anesthesiol*, **13**, 101–5.
48 Maydew RP, Berry FA (1985). *Anesthesiology*, **62**, 810–12.
49 Wall RT, et al. (1990). *J Clin Anesth*, **2**, 306–11.
50 Raghavendran F, et al. (2008). *Paediatr Anaesth*, **18**, 360–1.
51 Mudaraddi R, Areti Y. (2012). *Internet J Anesthesiol*, **30**, 3.
52 Nagasako EM, et al. (2003). *Pain*, **101**, 213–19.
53 Johi RR, et al. (2003). *Br J Anaesth*, **91**, 744–7.
54 Farbu E, et al. (2003). *Acta Anaesthesiol Scand*, **47**, 630–4.
55 Pandit JJ, Evans FE (1996). *Anaesthesia*, **51**, 992–3.
56 Corsini LM, et al. (1998). *Paediatr Anaesth*, **8**, 159–61.
57 Hirai T, et al. (2006). *Masui*, **55**, 454–6.
58 Shukry M, et al. (2008). *Paediatr Anaesth*, **18**, 567–8.
59 Porter MC, Leemans M (2013). *Contin Educ Anaesth Crit Care Pain*, **13**, 119–24.
60 Brislin RP, et al. (1995). *Paediatr Anaesth*, **5**, 139–41.
61 Padmanabhan V, et al. (2011). *Contemp Clin Dent*, **2**, 211–14.
62 Martin TJ, et al. (2008). *Int J Obstet Anesth*, **17**, 177–81.
63 Pandey R, et al. (2008). *Paediat Anaesth*, **18**, 907–9.
64 Esmaeili MRH, et al. (2009). *J Res Med Sci*, **14**, 191–5.

D

Dandy–Walker syndrome

Congenital obstruction to foramina of Luschka/Magendie, progressive head enlargement, hydrocephalus, craniofacial abnormalities, cardiac/renal/skeletal malformations, altered medullary respiratory control, usually requires CSF shunt. △ Control ICP; risk of respiratory failure/recurrent apnoea post-operatively. Consider ICU.[65]

Delleman syndrome (oculocerebrocutaneous syndrome)

Somatic mutation of autosomal dominant gene only compatible with life in mosaic form, multiple brain/skin/eye/bony abnormalities, hydrocephalus, vertebral anomalies, seizures can occur under general anaesthesia (seen as unexplained autonomic changes), aspiration pneumonitis. △ Difficult intubation, post-operative apnoea monitoring.[66,67]

Dermatomyositis (polymyositis)

Inflammatory myopathy, skeletal muscle weakness → dysphagia/recurrent pneumonia/aspiration, myocarditis, cardiomyopathy (arrhythmias/cardiac failure), steroid supplementation, anaemia. △ Restricted mouth opening, enhanced/delayed effect of muscle relaxant.[68]

di George syndrome (velocardiofacial/CATCH 22 syndrome)

Caused by 22q11.2 deletion. Cardiac abnormalities/Abnormal facies/Thymic hypoplasia/Cleft palate/Hypocalcaemia/chromosome 22 affected, immune deficiency, recurrent chest infections, hypotonia. △ Upper airway problems/stridor, obstructive apnoea, hyperventilation-induced seizures ($\downarrow$ Ca^{2+}), gastro-oesophageal reflux.[69]

Down's syndrome

Commonest congenital abnormality (1.6 per 1000 deliveries), higher morbidity and mortality, characteristic dysmorphic features, impaired global development, congenital cardiac defects (40%—predominantly endocardial cushion defects/VSD), Eisenmenger's syndrome (especially if there is associated OSA), recurrent respiratory tract infection (relative immune deficiency and a degree of upper airway obstruction from tonsillar/adenoidal hypertrophy), atlantoaxial instability (30%, but frequently asymptomatic—routine X-ray not indicated), epilepsy (10%), obesity and potentially difficult venous access, hypothyroidism (40%), careful airway assessment (relatively large tongue, crowding of mid-facial structures, high arched narrow palate, micrognathia, short broad neck), careful cardiorespiratory assessment (including investigation), as indicated—beware asymptomatic disease, optimize where possible, reduced threshold for post-operative HDU/ICU, often uncooperative (sedative premed often helpful—caution if airway obstructed), drying agents useful if hypersalivation (caution—may have exaggerated sensitivity to mydriatic/cardiac effects of atropine), $\uparrow$ incidence of gastro-oesophageal reflux, avoid excessive neck movement, prone to hypoventilation—consider IPPV, post-operative pain management may be problematic (consider regional blocks/local anaesthesia, PCA possible in selected patients), parents/carers often indispensable in managing post-operative agitation, hypotonia (up to 75%) may compromise airway, prone to atelectasis/respiratory tract infections—consider humidified oxygen/physiotherapy.[70]

Dubowitz syndrome

Retarded growth, microcephaly, craniofacial deformations, dysmorphic extremities, psychomotor development varies—normal/retarded, thin hair, cryptorchidism, hyperactivity, thorough assessment required since the condition may involve the cutaneous, dental, digestive, musculoskeletal, ocular, urogenital, CVS, neurological, haematological, and immune systems. ⚠ Difficult intubation.[71]

Dwarfism

Manifestation of over 100 syndromes, disproportionate short stature ('midgets' are proportionate), large tongue, atlantoaxial instability, spinal stenosis and/or compression, thoracic dystrophy (ventilatory problem/frequent pneumonia), scoliosis/kyphoscoliosis, congenital cardiac disease, evaluate and protect the cervical spine, document pre-existing neurological deficit if central blockade considered. ⚠ Difficult airway.[72]

Dyggve–Melchior–Clausen syndrome

Autosomal recessive, mental retardation, small stature (short vertebral column), thoracic kyphosis, protruding sternum, reduced articular mobility, microcephaly. ⚠ Difficult intubation.[73]

Dysautonomia (Riley–Day syndrome)

One of the hereditary sensory and autonomic neuropathies. Emotional lability, autonomic instability may → dysautonomic crisis (sweating, vomiting, unstable HR/BP), poor thermoregulation, gastric reflux/drooling, sensitivity to respiratory depressants with reduced hypoxic drive (need IPPV), reduced somatic pain sensitivity but visceral/muscle sensation intact, volatile agents can cause hypotension and bradycardia.[74]

References

65 Ewart MC, Oh TE (1990). *Anaesthesia*, **45**, 646–8.
66 Sadhasivam S, Subramaniam R (1998). *Anesth Analg*, **87**, 553–5.
67 Jamieson BD, Kuczkowski KM (2005). *Ann Fr Anesth Reanim*, **24**, 830.
68 Sharma S, et al. (2007). *Indian J Anaesth*, **51**, 43–6.
69 Yotsui-Tsuchimochi H, et al. (2006). *Paediatr Anaesth*, **16**, 454–7.
70 Association of Anaesthetists of Great Britain and Ireland (2009). ℬ http://www.aagbi.org/node/889.
71 Lee MK, et al. (2010). *Korean J Anesthesiol*, **58**, 495–9.
72 Morrow MJ, Black IH (1998). *Br J Anaesth*, **81**, 619–21.
73 Eguchi M, et al. (2001). *Masui*, **50**, 1116–67.
74 Mustafa HI, et al. (2012). *Anesthesiology*, **116**, 205–15.

E–F

Eaton–Lambert syndrome

See *Myasthenic syndrome* (also see ➲ p. 306).

Ebstein's anomaly (tricuspid valve disease)

CHD, downward displacement of deformed tricuspid valve, atrialization of right ventricle, may be no obvious clinical signs, association with Wolff–Parkinson–White syndrome, risk of SVT with induction/light anaesthesia or fluid and electrolyte imbalance.[75]

Edward's syndrome (trisomy 18)

Craniofacial anomalies, CHD, mental/physical delays, pain assessment difficult, only less severe cases survive.[76]

Ehlers–Danlos syndrome

Group of conditions with defective collagen cross-linking, variable features depending upon the tissue distribution of different collagens, extensible fragile skin, joint laxity/hypermobility, recurrent dislocations, prolonged/spontaneous bleeding, rupture of cerebral/other vessels, bowel perforation, ocular abnormalities, kyphoscoliosis, spontaneous pneumothorax. ► Careful positioning/padding, beware undiagnosed pneumothorax, intubation may cause severe tracheal bruising.[77]

Eisenmenger's syndrome (pulmonary hypertension, VSD, right ventricular failure)

See also ➲ p. 67.

Cyanotic CHD, usually uncorrectable, pulmonary hypertension/VSD/right ventricular failure, medical therapy may prolong life (thirties), high mortality in pregnant patients due to ↓ SVR and ↑ shunt (termination has been advocated), prevent increases in right-to-left shunt (caused by e.g. ↓ PVR/↑ SVR from volatiles/histamine release, etc.). ► Avoid dehydration, consider pancuronium (sympathetic stimulation beneficial), air from infusions/syringes can cross VSD, risk of asystole under general anaesthesia, slow equilibration of inhaled gases.[78]

Ellis–Van Creveld disease (chondroectodermal dysplasia)

Dwarfism, pulmonary/cardiac abnormalities (ASD/VSD/single atrium), polydactyly, hepatic/renal involvement, airway anomalies, respiratory failure.[79]

Epidermolysis bullosa

Extreme bullae formation of skin and mucosa, dystrophic nails, flexion contractures/deformities, carious teeth, small mouth caused by scarred lip contractures are characteristic, avoid skin/mucous membrane trauma, shearing force worse than direct pressure. ► Care with positioning, electrodes (consider using defib pads as an interface), tape, padding below BP cuff, longest acceptable inflation interval, lubricate everything well, keep upper airway manipulations to a minimum, consider post-operative ICU.[80,81]

Erythema multiforme

Acute self-limiting condition of skin and mucous membranes—consider drug-related cause, concentric rings of erythematous papules/bullae (epidermal necrosis), severe cases can be fatal (Stevens–Johnson syndrome). ▶ Beware post-intubation laryngeal oedema.

Fabry syndrome

α-galactosidase deficiency, deposition of glycosphingolipid in most organs, IHD/LV hypertrophy/abnormal conduction, hypertension, renal failure, autonomic instability (may ↑ with neuraxial block), abnormal thermoregulation, hyperhidrosis, pain 2° to nerve infiltration. ▶ Document any neurological deficit prior to regional techniques, monitor/control core temperature.[82]

Factor V Leiden mutation

Resistance to anticoagulant effect of protein C, high risk of PE ▶ Careful control of anticoagulation.[83]

Familial dysautonomia

See *Dysautonomia*.

Familial periodic paralysis

See also *Hypokalaemic familial periodic paralysis*.
   Muscular weakness related to K^+ changes (absolute K^+ value is not important).

Fanconi's anaemia

Congenital aplastic anaemia, growth retardation, hyperpigmentation, defective DNA regeneration. Limit exposure to X-rays (sensitive).[84]

Fanconi syndrome (renal tubular acidosis)

Generalized defect in proximal tubular function, glycosuria, polyuria, polydipsia, phosphate/K^+/HCO_3^- wasting, aminoaciduria, muscle weakness, acidosis, dwarfing, osteomalacia, usually 2° to other disease. ▶ Correct/maintain careful fluid/electrolyte balance.[85]

Farber's disease (lipogranulomatosis)

Ceramidase deficiency, hoarse cry, painful swollen joints, periarticular nodules, pulmonary infiltrates, mental handicap, thickened heart valves, cardiomyopathy, renal/hepatic failure, usually die by 2yr (airway problems), laryngeal granulomata may complicate intubation. ⚠ Difficult intubation, post-extubation laryngeal oedema/bleeding, anatomical neck deformity may complicate urgent tracheostomy.[86]

Felty's syndrome

Hypersplenism in RA, pancytopenia, haemolysis due to red cell sequestration, ↑ plasma volume. (See also ➜ p. 184.)

Fibrodysplasia ossificans progressiva

Progressive bony infiltration of tendons/muscles/fascia/aponeuroses, leading to joint ankylosis throughout the body. ▶ Permanent ankylosis of the jaw may follow minimal soft tissue trauma, AAS possible, restrictive pulmonary disease, cardiac conduction abnormalities. ⚠ Intubation difficulties.[87]

Fibromatosis (including juvenile and hyaline forms)

Large cutaneous nodules (especially head/neck/lips), joint contractures, gingival hypertrophy, osteolytic lesions. ⚠ Potential airway problems.[88]

Fraser syndrome (cryptophthalmos—'hidden eye')

Cryptophthalmos, laryngeal atresia/hypoplasia, fixed posterior arytenoids, cleft lip/palate, genitourinary abnormalities, possible CHD/neurological abnormalities. ⚠ Potential airway problems.[89]

Freeman–Sheldon (craniocarpotarsal dysplasia or 'whistling face') syndrome

Progressive congenital myopathy, multiple deformities of face/hands/feet, microstomia with pursed lips, micrognathia, anterior larynx, neck rigidity, post-operative respiratory complications. ⚠ Difficult intubation, difficult venous access, possible MH risk.[90]

Friedreich's ataxia

Autosomal recessive progressive ataxia, myopathy, cardiomyopathy with failure/arrhythmias (may have ICD), diabetes, peripheral neuropathy. ► Kyphoscoliosis → respiratory failure, ?suxamethonium sensitivity—not supported by the evidence.[91]

References

75 Khatib SK, et al. (2012). *Anaesth Pain Intensive Care*, **16**, 60–3.
76 Courreges P, et al. (2003). *Paediatr Anaesth*, **13**, 267–9.
77 Lane D (2006). *Anaesth Intensive Care*, **34**, 501–5.
78 Jones HG, Stoneham MD (2006). *Anaesthesia*, **61**, 1214–18.
79 Abeles AI, Tobias JD (2008). *J Clin Anaesth*, **20**, 618–21.
80 Saraf SV, et al. (2013). *J Anaesthesiol Clin Pharmacol*, **29**, 390–3.
81 Edler AA, et al. (2008). *Paediatr Anaesth*, **18**, 1107–9.
82 Wooley J, Pichel AC (2008). *Anaesthesia*, **63**, 101–2.
83 Donahue BS (2004). *Anesth Analg*, **98**, 1623–34.
84 Dogan Z, et al. (2014). *Braz J Anesthesiol*, in press.
85 Pandey R, et al. (2010). *J Clin Anesth*, **22**, 635–7.
86 Asada A, et al. (1994). *Anesthesiology*, **80**, 206–9.
87 Gorji R, et al. (2011). *J Clin Anesth*, **23**, 558–61.
88 Norman B, et al. (1996). *Br J Anaesth*, **76**, 163–6.
89 Mohan VK, et al. (2013). *Saudi J Anaesth*, **7**, 102–3.
90 Ma LL, et al. (2012). *Chin Med J*, **125**, 390–1.
91 Schmitt HJ, et al. (2004). *Br J Anaesth*, **92**, 592–6.

G

Gaisbock's syndrome

Relative polycythaemia due to ↓ plasma volume in middle-aged obese, smoking, hypertensive ♂, arterial thrombotic risk, myocardial/cerebral ischaemia. Consider venesection to normal haematocrit.

Gardner's syndrome (familial polyposis coli)

Multiple colonic polyps (risk of malignant change), soft tissue tumours, osseous neoplasms. ► Possible laryngeal polyps.

Gaucher's disease

Autosomal recessive disorder of lipid catabolism, end-organ dysfunction from glycosphingolipid accumulation, three variants differ in onset/CNS involvement, seizures, hypersplenism, thrombocytopenia, anaemia, gastro-oesophageal reflux, chronic aspiration. ► Possible upper airway obstruction (bulbar involvement/infiltration of upper airway). Check and correct haematological parameters, if required.[92,93]

Gilbert's disease

Asymptomatic familial unconjugated non-haemolytic hyperbilirubinaemia. Perioperative jaundice may be precipitated by stress/surgery/starvation.[94]

Glanzmann's disease (thrombasthenia)

Lack of membrane protein GPIIb and GPIIIa, normal number/sized platelets, no clot retraction, defective aggregation, moderately severe bleeding diathesis, platelet transfusions sometimes ineffective due to antiplatelet antibodies.[95]

Glomus jugulare tumours

Highly vascular benign tumour of glomus body, invades locally, may affect cranial nerves (progressive deafness/tinnitus), may need to sacrifice local structures (carotid, etc.). ⚠ Sudden severe haemorrhage during excision (?hypotensive technique). Consider cerebral protection measures.[96,97]

Glucagonoma

Rare tumour of pancreatic islet α-cells, usually ↑ blood glucagon/glucose levels (↓ glucose also reported), potential significant metabolic/myocardial dysfunction, control blood glucose—large amounts of glucagon can be released during tumour handling. ► Careful evaluation of nutrition/fluid/electrolytes, thromboembolic prophylaxis.[98]

Glucose-6-phosphate-dehydrogenase deficiency (favism)

Predominantly ♂ (X-linked hereditary defect), attacks of haemolytic anaemia precipitated by infections/some drugs (including aspirin, methylthioninium chloride (methylene blue), phenytoin, vitamin K, chloramphenicol), chronic anaemia (increased 2,3-diphosphoglycerate) of 5–10g/dL.[99]

Glycogenoses (glycogen storage diseases)

Type I (von Gierke's disease)

Mental retardation, hepatosplenomegaly, renal enlargement, hypoglycaemic convulsions, stomatitis, bleeding diathesis, leucopenia, tendency to hypoglycaemia during fasting, lactic acidosis, cautious attention to metabolic/homeostatic derangements, abdominal distension may affect ventilation.[100]

Type II (Pompe's disease)

Wide spectrum of severity: neonatal acyanotic cardiac death to normal life. Cardiomegaly/cardiomyopathy, progressive cardiac failure, outflow obstruction, generalized hypotonia, neurological deficits, macroglossia, normal glucose tolerance, post-operative respiratory insufficiency, potential exaggerated hyperkalaemic response to suxamethonium. Consider local anaesthetic alternatives.[101]

Type III (Forbes' disease)

Perioperative hypoglycaemia.

Type IV (Andersen's disease)

Hepatosplenomegaly, cirrhosis, hepatic dysfunction, severe growth retardation, death before 3yr, muscular hypotonia, muscle relaxants generally unnecessary, ↓ doses of IV drugs, prone to perioperative hypoglycaemia/heat loss.

Type V (McArdle's disease)

Muscle weakness, exercise-induced myoglobinuria, renal failure, perioperative hypoglycaemia, no firm clinical association with MH.[102]

Goldenhar syndrome (oculoauriculovertebral syndrome, hemifacial microsomia)

Eye/ear abnormalities, micrognathia, maxillary hypoplasia, cleft/high arched palate, cervical synostosis, congenital heart anomalies (Fallot/VSD), craniovertebral anomalies, atropine-resistant bradycardia. ⚠ Difficult intubation.[103]

Goltz–Gorlin syndrome (focal dermal hypoplasia)

Dental/facial asymmetry, stiff neck, hypertension, airway papillomatosis. ⚠ Difficult airway.[104]

Goodpasture's syndrome

Severe repeated intrapulmonary haemorrhages with fibrosis, restrictive lung defect, hypertension, anaemia, renal failure.

Gorham syndrome ('disappearing bone disease')

Massive osteolysis—replacement of bone by fibrovascular tissue (commonest in 2nd/3rd decades), pathological fractures, lymphangiomatosis, respiratory and neurological deficits, relapsing pleural effusions, chylothorax/pericardium. ▶ Assess respiratory function, check cervical spine (often involved), avoid suxamethonium (may cause/worsen pathological fractures), careful positioning, consider post-operative ICU respiratory support, poor prognosis.[105]

References

92 Kita T, et al. (1998). Masui, **47**, 69–73.

93 Ioscovich A, et al. (2005). Can J Anesth, **52**, 845–7.

94 Nag DS, et al. (2011). J Anaesthesiol Clin Pharm, **27**, 253–5.

95 Monte S, Lyons G (2002). Br J Anaesth, **88**, 734–8.

96 Braude BM, et al. (1986). Anaesthesia, **41**, 861–5.

97 Mather SP, Webster NR (1986). Anaesthesia, **41**, 856–60.

98 Gin VC, Zacharias M (2009). Anaesth Intensive Care, **37**, 329–30.

99 Cappellini MD, Fiorelli G (2008). Lancet, **371**, 64–74.

100 Huang IR, et al. (2006). Acta Anaesthesiol Taiwan, **44**, 51–3.

101 Kishnani PS, et al. (2006). Gen Med, **8**, 267–88.

102 Bollig G (2013). Paediatr Anaesth, **23**, 817–23.

103 Sukhupragarn W, Rosenblatt WH (2008). J Clin Anesth, **20**, 214–17.

104 Gosavi SG, et al. (2012). Indian J Anaesth, **56**, 394–6.

105 Sahoo RK, et al. (2013). Indian J Anaesth, **56**, 391–3.

H–I

Haemochromatosis ('bronze diabetes')

Iron deposits in liver/pancreas/joints/skin/heart, cirrhosis, diabetes, arthritis, late cardiac failure, may be having weekly venesections.[106]

Haemolytic–uraemic syndrome

Triad of renal failure/haemolytic anaemia/thrombocytopenia, multisystem disorder may also involve CVS/respiratory/CNS/hepatic systems.[107]

Haemorrhagic telangiectasia (Osler–Weber–Rendu syndrome)

Familial telangiectasia of mucous membranes (nose/oropharynx/viscera/skin), GI bleeding, repeated haemorrhages, bleeding difficult to control, may have pulmonary AV fistulae. ► Avoid trauma, invasive procedures complicated (poor tissues).[108]

Hallermann–Streiff syndrome

Oculomandibulodyscephaly, dwarfism. ⚠ Direct laryngoscopy may be hazardous/difficult (brittle teeth, temporomandibular joint dislocation).[109]

Hallervorden–Spatz disease

Rare progressive disorder of basal ganglia, myotonia/dystonic posturing, scoliosis, dementia, trismus, volatile agents relieve the posturing (returns after discontinuation). ⚠ Difficult intubation.[110]

Hand–Schuller–Christian disease (histiocytic granulomata)

Diabetes insipidus, hepatic failure, respiratory failure, pancytopenia, electrolyte problems. ⚠ Difficult intubation (small larynx).

Hartnup disease

Defective tubular/jejunal reabsorption of most neutral amino acids, leading to tryptophan malabsorption/nicotinamide deficiency, pellagra, psychiatric disorders, cerebellar ataxia.

Hay–Wells syndrome

Maxillary hypoplasia/micrognathia/palatal hypoplasia. ⚠ Difficult intubation.

Hecht–Beals syndrome (trismus pseudocamptodactyly/Dutch–Kentucky syndrome)

Arachnodactyly, kyphoscoliosis, multiple joint contractures, crumpled ears, ventilatory defect, mitral valve prolapse, aortic root dilatation. ⚠ Difficult intubation (restricted mouth opening).[111,112]

Henoch–Schönlein purpura

Multisystem IgA-mediated vasculitis, rash, arthralgia, abdominal pain, normal platelet count (?abnormal aggregation), haemorrhagic risk, nephritis (30%) may → renal failure.[113]

Holt–Oram syndrome (hand–heart syndrome)

Rare disorder combining congenital cardiac anomalies (ASD/VSD/occasionally others) and upper limbs (hypoplastic thumbs/clavicles), dysrhythmias frequent, even with normal anatomy, risk of sudden death, hypoplastic vasculature. ▶ Potentially difficult venous access (especially central), restrictive lung disease, renal dysfunction, often previous cardiac surgery.[114]

Homocystinuria

Homocysteine excreted in urine, mental handicap, Marfan-like syndrome, venous/arterial thrombotic episodes, PEs (requiring heparinization), renal failure, hypoglycaemia.[115]

Hunter syndrome (mucopolysaccharidosis II)

See *Mucopolysaccharidoses*.

Huntington's chorea/juvenile Huntington's disease

Similar conditions, progressive degenerative involuntary choreoathetoid movements and dementia, dysphagia/regurgitation → ⚠ pulmonary aspiration, poor respiratory function, possible associated autonomic neuropathy, depression/apathy → cachexia and malnutrition.[116]

Hurler syndrome (gargoylism, mucopolysaccharidosis I)

Most severe mucopolysaccharidosis, death at early age. See *Mucopolysaccharidoses*.[117]

Hutchinson–Gilford syndrome (premature ageing syndrome)

See *Progeria*.

Hyperviscosity syndrome (Waldenström's macroglobulinaemia, multiple myeloma)

Thrombotic risk, preoperative plasmapheresis may be needed.

Hypokalaemic familial periodic paralysis

Attacks of severe muscle weakness/flaccid muscle paralysis with ↓ serum K^+, perioperative attack may compromise spontaneous ventilation, avoid drugs known to cause K^+ shifts (e.g. β-agonists), arrhythmias, sensitive to muscle relaxants.[118,119]

Hypoplastic left heart syndrome

Hypoplasia of LV/mitral valve/ascending aorta, aortic valve atresia. Previously 100% mortality, survival depends upon PDA, balance of PVR and SVR (both circulations in parallel supplied by single ventricle), control of pulmonary blood flow. ▶ VF may occur with surgical manipulation.[120]

Ichthyosis

Hyperkeratotic plates of flaky/fissured skin. ▶ Difficulty placing and securing catheters/cannulae/electrodes (consider bandaging), perioperative temperature control.[121]

Idiopathic thrombocytopenic purpura

See also ➔ p. 210.

Thrombocytopenia <50 × 10⁹/L, petechiae, consider platelet infusions, beware rebound thrombosis after splenectomy. ▶ Minimize airway trauma (consider LMA), avoid regional blocks, avoid heparin/aspirin.[122]

Isaac's syndrome (continuous muscle fibre activity syndrome, neuromyotonia, quantal squander)

Autoimmune condition, continuous involuntary muscle fibre activity, fasciculation, delayed relaxation, ataxia, incoordination, anticonvulsants effective, regional blocks acceptable. ⚠ Exaggerated response to muscle relaxants, ↑ risk of aspiration (bulbar involvement).[123]

Ivemark syndrome

See *Asplenia syndrome*.

References

106 Shander A, et al (2012). *J Clin Anesth*, **24**, 419–25.
107 Tobias JD (2007). *Paediatr Anaesth*, **17**, 584–7.
108 Peiffer KM (2009). *AANA J*, **77**, 115–18.
109 Krishna MH, et al. (2012). *Paediat Anaesth*, **22**, 497–8.
110 Hurtado P, et al. (2009). *Rev Esp Anestesiol Reanim*, **56**, 180–4.
111 Kumar A, et al. (2012). *Indian J Anaesth*, **56**, 591–2.
112 Vaghadia H, Blackstock D (1988). *Can J Anaesth*, **35**, 80–5.
113 Sedeek KA, Liu J (2009). *Paediatr Anaesth*, **19**, 811–12.
114 Babu GN, et al. (2010). *J Anesthesiol Clin Pharmacol*, **26**, 541–3.
115 Yamada T, et al. (2005). *J Clin Anesth*, **17**, 565–7.
116 Kivela JE, et al. (2010). *Anesth Analg*, **110**, 515–23.
117 Spinello CM, et al. (2013). *ISRN Anesthesiology*, Article ID 791983.
118 Chitra S, Korula G (2009). *Indian J Anaesth*, **53**, 226–9.
119 Abbas H, et al. (2012). *Natl J Maxillofac Surg*, **3**, 220–1.
120 Walker A, et al. (2009). *Paediatr Anaesth*, **19**, 119–25.
121 Hegde HV, et al. (2012). *Paediatr Anaesth*, **22**, 492–4.
122 Trimmings AJ, Walmsley AJ (2009). *Anaesthesia*, **64**, 226–7.
123 Sim YK, et al. (2013). *Korean J Anaesth*, **64**, 164–7.

J

Jervell–Lange–Nielsen syndrome

Congenital prolonged QT interval/enlarged T wave, deafness. ⚠ Prone to ventricular arrhythmias/cardiac arrest, consider pacemaker insertion/β-blockade (for CVS stability), select drugs/technique known to minimize catecholamine levels.[124]

Jeune's syndrome (asphyxiating thoracic dystrophy)

Pulmonary hypoplasia, severe thoracic defect preventing normal intercostal function, renal dysfunction, myocardial dysfunction in older patients. ► Minimize ventilator pressures.[125]

Joubert syndrome

Abnormal respiratory control (brainstem/cerebellar hypoplasia), hypotonia, ataxia, mental retardation, sensitive to respiratory depressant effects of anaesthetic agents (including N_2O). ► Spontaneously breathing general anaesthetic may be problematic, special care with opioids (↑ apnoea time), close post-operative observation.[126,127]

References

124 Ryan H (1988). *Can J Anaesth*, **35**, 422–4.
125 Saletti D, et al. (2012). *Rev Bras Anesthesiol*, **62**, 424–31.
126 Bhaskar P, et al. (2013). *J Clin Anaesth*, **25**, 488–90.
127 Galante D, et al. (2009). *Acta Anaesthesiol Scand*, **53**, 693–4.

K

Kartagener's syndrome

Abnormal cilia → sinusitis, bronchiectasis, and situs inversus in 50% of cases, dextrocardia (usually structurally normal in situs inversus), immunoincompetence, chronic/recurrent chest infections. Fully assess CVS/respiratory system function, preoperative physiotherapy. ▶ Reverse ECG lead position/defibrillator paddles, etc., right lateral displacement (obstetrics), humidify gases, local/regional block preferred.[128]

Kawasaki disease (mucocutaneous lymph node syndrome)

Acute childhood (<5yr) febrile illness → coronary arteritis, aneurysms/thrombotic occlusions/arrhythmias/sudden death, accelerated atherosclerosis → IHD. Degree of CVS dysfunction determines technique. ⚠ Invasive lines have ↑ complication risk.[129]

Kearns–Sayre syndrome

Mitochondrial myopathy, cardiac conduction abnormalities common (range from bundle branch block to third-degree AV block), sudden death, generalized CNS degeneration, progressive external ophthalmoplegia, progressive skeletal muscle weakness → respiratory failure (care with opioids). ▶ Possible sensitivity to induction agents/muscle relaxants, consider inhalation induction with deep anaesthesia intubation, may need rapid cardiac pacing.[130]

Kelly–Paterson syndrome

See *Plummer–Vinson syndrome*.

Kenny–Caffey syndrome

Proportional dwarfism, macrocephaly, eye anomalies, dysmorphic facies, mandibular hypoplasia, episodic hypocalcaemic tetany, may be associated with Mounier–Kuhn syndrome, hypocalcaemia, anaemia, thoracic/skeletal abnormalities. ⚠ Difficult airway.[131]

King–Denborough syndrome

Slowly progressive myopathy, short stature, kyphoscoliosis, pectus carinatum, cryptorchidism, characteristic facial appearance. ⚠ ?MH risk.[132]

Klinefelter's syndrome

Chromosomal abnormality 47XXY, poor sexual development, tall stature, reduced intelligence, vertebral collapse from osteoporosis, may have ↓ muscle bulk/power. ▶ Care during positioning.[133]

Klippel–Feil syndrome

Three main types differ in severity. Congenital fusion of cervical and/or thoracic vertebrae, short neck, limited range of motion, possible cervical cord compression, syncope on sudden rotation of head, kyphoscoliosis, cardiac/respiratory/renal anomalies. ⚠ Difficult intubation, keep neck in neutral axis (basilar insufficiency).[134]

Klippel–Trenaunay syndrome (angio-osteohypertrophy)

Generalized haemangiomas, soft tissue hypertrophy, bone overgrowth, and/or AV malformations → high-output cardiac failure, consumptive coagulopathy. ⚠ Possible airway problems, possible epidural/subdural vascular malformations (consider neurovascular imaging before neuraxial block).[135,136]

Kniest syndrome

Dwarfism, tracheomalacia, micrognathia, cleft palate, stiff atlanto-occipital instability. ⚠ Difficult intubation.[137]

Kugelberg–Welander syndrome (spinal muscular atrophy type III)

See *Spinal muscular atrophy*.

References

128 Dylan Bould M, Gothard JW (2006). *Paediatr Anaesth*, **16**, 977–80.
129 To L, et al. (2013). *Ochsner J*, **13**, 208–13.
130 Baldwin MK, Nembhard VN (2009). *Paediatr Anaesth*, **19**, 639–40.
131 Janke EL, et al. (1996). *Paediatr Anaesth*, **6**, 235–8.
132 Habib AS, et al. (2003). *Can J Anaesth*, **50**, 589–92.
133 Lanfranco F, et al. (2004). *Lancet*, **364**, 273–83.
134 Khawaja OM, et al. (2009). *Anesth Analg*, **108**, 1220–5.
135 Barbara DW, Wilson JL (2011). *Anesth Analg*, **113**, 98–102.
136 Sivaprakasam MJ, Dolak JA (2006). *Can J Anaesth*, **53**, 487–91.
137 Min HW, et al. (2012). *J Genet Med*, **9**, 93–7.

L

Larsen's syndrome

Multiple congenital dislocations, unstable cervical spine, subglottic stenosis, prominent forehead, flattened face, chronic respiratory disease from kyphoscoliosis. ⚠ Difficult intubation.[138]

Laurence–Moon syndrome

See also *Bardet–Biedl syndrome*.

Mental retardation, spastic paraplegia, retinitis pigmentosa, hypogonadism, obesity. ▶ Possible difficult venous access, difficult intubation.[139]

Leber's hereditary optic neuropathy

Mitochondrial DNA mutation → optic nerve atrophy. ▶ Possible idiopathic hypoventilation, sensitivity to sedatives/opioids reported.[140]

Leigh syndrome

Necrotizing encephalomyelopathy, abnormal mitochondrial function, abnormal central respiratory control, cardiomyopathy, hypotonia, seizures, ↑ reflux/aspiration. ⚠ Post-operative respiratory failure, muscle relaxants may have prolonged effect, risk of lactic acidosis.[141,142]

LEOPARD syndrome

Rare inherited progressive disorder related to Noonan's syndrome. Lentigines/ECG abnormality/Ocular hypertelorism, obstructive cardiomyopathy/Pulmonary valve stenosis/Abnormal ♂ genitalia/Retarded growth/Deafness. ▶ CVS assessment will determine technique, cardiomyopathy may be occult.[143]

Leprechaunism (Donohue syndrome)

'Gnome' facies, dwarfism, cutis laxa, acanthosis nigricans, adipose tissue atrophy, extreme wasting, dysphagia requiring parenteral feeding, mentally defective (see *Cutis laxa* ➲ p. 286, *Dwarfism* ➲ p. 289), abnormal insulin receptor → hyperinsulinism. ▶ Maintain blood sugar during fasting.[144]

Lesch–Nyhan syndrome (hyperuricaemia)

Disorder of purine metabolism, hyperuricaemia, spasticity, choreoathetosis, dystonia, self-injurious behaviour, aggression, mental retardation, seizures, possible atlantoaxial instability, sudden unexplained death, abnormalities in respiration, apnoea, chronic pulmonary aspiration, abnormal adrenergic pressor response—severe bradycardia. ▶ Caution with exogenous catecholamines, ↑ incidence of vomiting/regurgitation, propofol beneficial due to ↑ uric acid excretion, difficulty positioning.[145]

Letterer–Siwe disease (histiocytosis X)

Histiocytic granulomata in viscera/bones, similar clinical course to acute leukaemia, pancytopenia, anaemia, purpura, haemorrhage, pulmonary infiltration, hepatic involvement, tooth loss.[146]

Lipodystrophy (total lipoatrophy)

Generalized loss of body fat, fatty fibrotic liver, hepatic failure, portal hypertension, splenomegaly, hypersplenism, anaemia, thrombocytopenia, nephropathy, renal failure, diabetes mellitus. ▶ Care with temperature.[147]

Long QT syndrome

Mutations in cardiac ion channels, prolonged ventricular repolarization, genetic/drug-induced, 60% of patients are symptomatic (syncope, seizure-like episodes, cardiac arrest). ▶ Should have preoperative cardiology assessment, high risk of perioperative malignant ventricular arrhythmias (may be refractory), preoperative β-blockade, normalize all electrolytes, prevent sympathetic activation (pain, sedative premed, laryngoscopy, extubation, normocapnia, etc.), invasive monitoring advisable, maintain temperature (hypothermia prolongs QT), adequate analgesia essential, torsade de pointes may be self-limiting/require cardioversion/Mg^{2+}/pacing, consider post-operative ICU.[148]

Lowe syndrome (oculocerebrorenal syndrome)

Metabolic acidosis due to renal tubular dysfunction, renal failure, convulsions, mental retardation, abnormal skull shape, bone fragility, hypotonia, hypocalcaemia, glaucoma/cataracts.[149]

References

138 Malik P, Choudhry DK (2002). *Paediatr Anaesth*, **12**, 632–6.
139 Dhulkhed VK, *et al.* (2013). *Anesth Essays Res*, **7**, 276–8.
140 Adler M, *et al.* (2002). *J Neurol Neurosurg Psychiatry*, **73**, 347–8.
141 Terkawi AS, *et al.* (2012). *Saudi J Anaesth*, **6**, 181–5.
142 Footitt EJ, *et al.* (2008). *Br J Anaesth*, **100**, 436–41.
143 Yeoh TY, *et al.* (2014). *J Cardiothorac Vasc Anaesth*, **14**, in press.
144 Garcia-Candel A, *et al.* (2007). *Rev Esp Anestesiol Reanim*, **54**, 256–7.
145 Salhotra R, *et al.* (2012). *J Anaesthesiol Clin Pharmacol*, **28**, 239–41.
146 Broscheit J, *et al.* (2004). *Eur J Anaesthesiol*, **21**, 919–21.
147 Bennett T, Alford M (2012). *Paediatr Anaesth*, **22**, 299–300.
148 Hunter JD, *et al.* (2008). *Contin Educ Anaesth Crit Care Pain*, **8**, 67–70.
149 Pandey R, *et al.* (2010). *J Clin Anaesth*, **22**, 635–7.

M

Maffucci syndrome

Progressive condition. Enchondromatosis and multiple soft tissue haeman-giomata (including airway/cervical spine), ↑ risk of malignancy, intracranial lesions, anaemia, coagulopathy, pathological fractures, GI bleeding. ▶ ↑ risk of epidural haematoma (spinal lesions), assess for ↑ ICP, may be sensitive to vasodilating drugs.[150]

Mandibulofacial dysostosis (Treacher–Collins syndrome)

Mandibulofacial dysostosis, deafness, hypoplasia of facial bones (mandible/maxilla/cheek), characteristic facies, CVS malformations. ▶ Post-operative laryngeal/pharyngeal oedema may develop, ~50% have grade 4 laryngeal view—worsens with increasing age, sleep apnoea, respiratory distress, sudden death all reported.[151]

Maple syrup urine disease

Branched-chain ketoacid decarboxylase deficiency, failure to thrive, fits, cerebral degeneration, neonatal acidosis.[152]

Marchiafava–Micheli syndrome

Autoimmune haemolytic anaemia, VTE, paroxysmal nocturnal dyspnoea.

Marfan's syndrome

Autosomal dominant disorder of connective tissue metabolism, tall with long/thin fingers, dilation of ascending aorta, dissecting aneurysms, aortic/mitral regurgitation, coronary thrombosis, cataracts/retinal detachment/lens dislocation, emphysema, spontaneous pneumothorax, pectus excavatum, beware possible tracheomalacia, OSA, easy joint dislocation, cervical spine bony/ligamentous abnormality (routine X-ray not indicated), high arched palate, crowded teeth, kyphoscoliosis. ▶ Control BP, perioperative β-blockade if not already treated, minimize sympathetic response, consider invasive monitoring, central blocks are acceptable (see also ➔ p. 52).[153]

Maroteaux–Lamy syndrome (mucopolysaccharidosis VI)

See *Mucopolysaccharidoses*.

Marshall–Smith syndrome

Accelerated bone maturation, dysmorphic facial features, airway abnormalities, including possible atlantoaxial instability, laryngomalacia/tracheomalacia, patients often die in early infancy from respiratory complications. ▶ Face mask ventilation may be impossible, maintain spontaneous breathing if possible, consider elective use of nasopharyngeal airway during induction/emergence.[154,155]

Meckel's syndrome (Meckel–Gruber syndrome)

Microcephaly, micrognathia, cleft epiglottis/palate, congenital CVS disease, polycystic kidneys, renal failure, encephalocele. ⚠ Difficult intubation.[156]

Meig's syndrome

Large ovarian cyst in peritoneal space (space/pressure effects) and pleural effusion, may → respiratory distress, poor nutrition. ▶ Intravascular volume correction.[157]

Menkes' disease

Suppression of copper-dependent enzymes resulting from copper deficiency, kinky hair, bone/connective tissue lesions, hypothermia, seizures, mental retardation. ⚠ ↑ gastro-oesophageal reflux, airway complications (poor pharyngeal motor tone).[158,159]

MERRF syndrome

Myoclonic epilepsy with ragged red fibres. Mitochondrial encephalomyopathy, mixed seizures, myoclonus, progressive ataxia, spasticity, mild myopathy, growth retardation, deafness, dementia.[160]

Mikulicz's syndrome

Salivary/lacrimal gland enlargement, anticholinergics probably best avoided. ▶ Glandular tissue may complicate airway management.

Miller–Fisher syndrome (variant of Guillain–Barré syndrome)

See ➋ p. 249.

Miller's syndrome

Rare congenital disorder, facies similar to Treacher–Collins syndrome, CHD (ASD/VSD/PDA), limb abnormalities. ▶ Consider early tracheostomy for airway maintenance (especially if repeated procedures planned), difficult venous access, ↑ gastric reflux.

Moebius syndrome

Multiple cranial nerve palsies, orofacial malformations, limb anomalies, ↑ incidence of other anomalies (congenital cardiac/spinal/alveolar hypoventilation/peripheral neuropathies), ↑ risk of aspiration (↑ drooling/gastric reflux). ⚠ Difficult intubation, ↑ risk of post-operative respiratory failure.[161]

Morquio syndrome (mucopolysaccharidosis IV)

Short stature, short neck, hypoplastic odontoid/atlantoaxial instability (compression of long tracts/paraplegia can occur), potential narrowed tracheal lumen (infiltration), sleep apnoea, loss of muscle tone, hypermobility/loose skin, aortic incompetence, prominent sternum, end-organ dysfunction, respiratory and cardiac failure in early adult life. ⚠ Difficult airway.[162] See also *Mucopolysaccharidoses.*[163]

Mounier–Kuhn syndrome

Diffuse tracheobronchomegaly, communicating paratracheal cysts. ▶ Intubate trachea/pack pharynx if ventilation needed.[164]

Moyamoya disease (in the German literature 'Nishimoto–Takeuchi–Kudo–Suzuki's disease')

Severe internal carotid artery stenosis, fine network of vessels around basal ganglia, CNS deterioration can follow general anaesthesia. ▶ Optimize cerebral perfusion (BP/CO_2, etc.), consider regional anaesthesia options.[165]

Mucopolysaccharidoses (Hunter, Hurler, Morquio, Maroteaux–Lamy, Scheie syndromes)

Abnormal mucopolysaccharide metabolism (lack of lysosomal enzyme), anatomical abnormalities/organ dysfunction from progressive deposition in tissues, upper airway obstruction (infiltration of lips/tongue/epiglottis/tonsils/adenoids) and lower airway, obstructive/restrictive ventilatory defects (abnormal laryngeal/tracheal cartilage, copious airway secretions, vertebrae/thoracic deformities), recurrent infection, protruberant abdomen, ↑ muscle tone, CVS abnormalities (coronary infiltration/valvular disease/myocardial insufficiency). ⚠ Difficult intubation (craniofacial abnormalities—short neck/stiffened temporomandibular joints/large tongue/anterior larynx), difficulty increases with age, generally die from pneumonia/cardiac complications. (See also Further reading and *Morquio syndrome*.)[166]

Multiple myeloma

Neoplastic proliferation of plasma cells characterized by immunoglobulin disorders, renal failure, haemorrhagic tendency, hyperviscosity syndrome, anaemia, ↑ susceptibility to infections, hypercalcaemia, pathological fractures → care positioning.[167]

Myasthenic syndrome (Eaton–Lambert syndrome)

See also ➔ p. 246.

Paraneoplastic condition, defective acetylcholine release at neuromuscular junctions, proximal muscle weakness, including ocular/bulbar muscles, post-tetanic facilitation, respiratory complications, autonomic dysfunction. ▶ Impaired oesophageal motility, sensitive to muscle relaxants.[168,169]

Myositis ossificans

See *Fibrodysplasia ossificans progressiva*.

Myotonia congenita (Thomsen's disease)

See also ➔ p. 251.

Defective skeletal muscle Cl^- channel → failure of muscle relaxation, can be precipitated by cold, surgery, diathermy, anticholinesterases. Widespread dystrophy and/or hypertrophy, palatopharyngeal dysfunction, ↑ aspiration risk, cardiomyopathy. ⚠ Suxamethonium may cause myotonia with difficult intubation/ventilation, normal response to non-depolarizing muscle relaxants, no absolute association with MH.[170]

References

150 Chan SK, *et al.* (1998). *Anaesth Intensive Care*, **26**, 586–9.

151 Hosking J, *et al.* (2012). *Paediatr Anaesth*, **22**, 752–8.

152 Fuentes-Garcia D, Falcon-Arana L (2009). *Br J Anaesth*, **102**, 144–5.

153 Singh SI, *et al.* (2008). *Can J Anaesth*, **55**, 526–31.

154 Antila H, *et al.* (1998). *Paediatr Anaesth*, **8**, 429–32.

155 Dernedde G, *et al.* (1998). *Can J Anaesth*, **45**, 660–3.

156 Miyazu M, *et al.* (2005). *J Anesth*, **19**, 309–10.

157 Hahm TS, *et al.* (2010). *Korean J Anesthesiol*, **58**, 202–6.

158 Passariello M, *et al.* (2008). *Paediatr Anaesth*, **18**, 1225–6.

159 Langley A, Dameron CT (2013). *Anesthesiology Res Pract*, 2013, 750901.

160 Footitt EJ, *et al.* (2008). *Br J Anaesth*, **100**, 436–41.

161 Gondipalli P, Tobias JD (2006). *J Clin Anesth*, **18**, 55–9.

162 Theroux MC, *et al.* (2012). *Paediatr Anaesth*, **22**, 901–7.

163 Dias PJ, Gopal S (2009). *Anaesthesia*, **64**, 444–6.

164 Min JJ, *et al.* (2011). *Korean J Anesthesiol*, **61**, 83–7.

165 Parray T, *et al.* (2011). *J Neurosurg Anesthesiol*, **23**, 100–9.

166 Walker R, *et al.* (2013). *J Inherit Metab Dis*, **36**, 211–19.

167 Wake M, *et al.* (1995). *Masui*, **44**, 1282–4.

168 Itoh H, *et al.* (2001). *Anaesthesia*, **56**, 562–7.

169 Lee CJ, *et al.* (2010). *Korean J Anesthesiol*, **59**, 45–8.

170 Marsh S, *et al.* (2012). *Contin Educ Anaesth Crit Care Pain*, **11**, 115–18.

N

Nager syndrome

Oromandibular hypogenesis (like Treacher–Collins syndrome), vertebral malformations (cervical spine involvement), congenital cardiac defects. △ Mandibular/mid-face manifestations may complicate perioperative/post-operative airway management.[171]

Nance–Insley syndrome (otospondylomegaepiphyseal dysplasia 'OSMED')

Disrupted cartilaginous growth leading to mid-face hypoplasia/micrognathia/cleft palate, disproportionate short stature/short limbs, progressive sensorineural deafness, joint contractures, vertebral abnormalities. △ Difficult airway.[172]

Nemaline myopathy

Congenital myopathy, non-progressive hypotonic symmetrical muscle weakness (including skeletal/diaphragm, sparing cardiac/smooth), rarely cardiomyopathy, skeletal deformities, facial dysmorphism, chronic aspiration, poor respiratory function (restrictive). △ Abnormal drug responses (including relaxants), MH not described.[173,174]

Nesidioblastosis (congenital hyperinsulinism)

Autonomous insulin secretion unaffected by blood glucose, neonatal/infantile apnoea, hypoglycaemia, hypotonia, seizures, usually require total pancreatectomy. ▶ Monitor blood glucose.[175]

Neurofibromatosis

Café-au-lait spots, cutaneous neurofibromas, occult phaeochromocytoma (5% of patients) in neurofibromatosis type 1, intracranial/neuraxial tumours commoner in neurofibromatosis type 2. Multisystem involvement requires thorough preoperative assessment. △ Airway neurofibromas may → difficult airway, CNS imaging before neuraxial techniques, avoid proconvulsants.[176,177]

Niemann–Pick disease

Sphingomyelin accumulation in organs (liver/spleen/bone marrow), progressive central/peripheral nervous system degeneration, respiratory failure, mental retardation, anaemia, hepatosplenomegaly, thrombocytopenia. △ Difficult intubation/ventilation, seizures.[178]

Noonan's syndrome

Short stature, cardiac defects (pulmonary stenosis/hypertrophic cardiomyopathy/VSD), mental retardation, micrognathia, short webbed neck, pectus excavatum, vertebral anomalies, lymphoedema, platelet/coagulation defects, renal failure. △ Difficult intubation.[179]

References

171 Groeper K, et al. (2002). *Paediatr Anaesth*, **12**, 365–8.
172 Denton R (1996). *Anaesthesia*, **51**, 100–1.
173 Asai T, et al. (1992). *Anaesthesia*, **47**, 405–8.
174 Klingler W, et al. (2009). *Anesth Analg*, **109**, 1167–73.
175 Hardy OT, Litman RS (2007). *Paediatr Anaesth*, **17**, 616–21.
176 Bagam KR, et al. (2010). *J Anaesthesiol Clin Pharmacol*, **26**, 553–4.
177 Oliveira VM, et al. (2010). *European J Anaesth*, **47**, 134.
178 Miao N, et al. (2012). *J Child Neurol*, **27**, 1541–6.
179 Bajwa SJS, et al. (2011). *Saudi J Anaesth*, **5**, 345–7.

O

Ondine's curse/Ondine–Hirschsprung disease
See *Alveolar hypoventilation*.

Opitz–Frias syndrome (hypospadias dysphagia syndrome)
Recurrent pulmonary aspiration of intestinal contents, achalasia of the oesophagus, subglottic stenosis, hypertelorism, micrognathia, high arched palate.[180]

Osler–Weber–Rendu syndrome
See *Haemorrhagic telangiectasia*.

Osteogenesis imperfecta (brittle bone disease)
Inherited connective tissue disorder. Four types ranging in severity, bone fragility, frequent fractures, and/or deformities, blue sclera (not all types), excessive bleeding. ▶ Teeth easily damaged, tendency to hyperthermia—probably not MH.[181]

Osteopetrosis (Albers–Schönberg disease)
Group of disorders. Increased bone density, changes in modelling with overgrowth, range of severity, brittle bones, nerve compression syndromes, mental retardation, hearing loss, leucoerythroblastic anaemia (bone marrow involvement), thrombocytopenia, hepatosplenomegaly (↓ FRC), ↓ myocardial contractility (hypocalcaemia). △ Head/mandibular involvement may affect intubation, cervicomedullary stenosis (cord trauma during intubation). Take care moving and positioning—risk of fractures.[182]

References
180 Bolsin SN, Gillbe C (1985). *Anaesthesia*, **40**, 1189–93.
181 Oakley I, Reece LP (2010). *AANA J*, **78**, 47–53.
182 Burgoyne LL, *et al.* (2010). *Paediatr Anaesth*, **20**, 1046–51.

P

Paramyotonia congenita (Eulenburg's disease)

Variant of hyperkalaemic periodic paralysis, cold-induced myotonia, flaccid paralysis, worsened by exercise. Assess sensitivity to cold/frequency of myotonic episodes. ▶ Warm theatre/fluids/patient, probably normal response to non-depolarizing muscle relaxants, avoid suxamethonium ($\uparrow$ K⁺), central neural blocks safe, no clear MH tendency (see also ➔ p. 176).[183,184]

Patau's syndrome (trisomy 13)

Multiple craniofacial/cardiac/neurological/renal anomalies, 'rockerbottom feet', thoracic kyphoscoliosis, possible neural tube defects, ineffective cough, full cardiac assessment (severe malformations in 80% of cases), impaired renal function, polycythaemia, platelet dysfunction. △ Difficult airway, post-operative respiratory problems, apnoeic episodes.[185]

Pemphigus vulgaris

Autoimmune disease, impaired cell adhesion within epidermis, bullous eruptions of skin/mucous membrane, possible ulceration/bullae/oedema of glottis after intubation. ▶ Lubricate everything well, take care with fluid/electrolyte balance (include losses from bullae), perioperative steroids to reduce exacerbation, regional/general anaesthetic acceptable, avoid friction (airway manipulation/monitors/positioning lines, etc.).[186]

Pendred's syndrome

Genetic defect in thyroid hormone synthesis. Hypothyroidism, goitre, deafness. Treat as hypothyroidism.[187]

Pfeiffer syndrome (acrocephalosyndactyly type V)

Growth/developmental retardation, sagittal craniosynostosis, hypertelorism, low-set ears, micrognathia with mandibular ankylosis, congenital heart defects, genital anomalies, solid cartilaginous trachea lacking rings may be present.[188]

Pharyngeal pouch (Zenker's diverticulum)

Epithelial-lined diverticulum above the upper oesophageal sphincter, often asymptomatic, dysphagia. Empty pouch manually (by patient) prior to induction or carefully with large-bore NGT, consider intubation in head-up position or under local anaesthetic, avoid coughing. ▶ Tracheal soiling not prevented by cricoid pressure.[189]

Phenylketonuria

Defective phenylalanine-4-hydroxylase, mental retardation, cerebral damage, epilepsy, sensitive to opioids/barbiturates. Consider inhalation induction, may have B12 deficiency. ▶ Avoid N_2O and proconvulsants.[190]

Pickwickian syndrome

Morbid obesity, episodic somnolence, hypoventilation, hypoxaemia, polycythaemia, pulmonary hypertension, cardiac failure, prone to wound infection, DVT/PE risk. ► Difficult IV access/positioning, sensitive to respiratory depressants, regional anaesthesia ideal for peripheral surgery, alert ICU following major surgery, CPAP beneficial.[191]

Pierre–Robin syndrome

Cleft palate, micrognathia, mandibular hypoplasia, receding mandible fails to hold tongue forward—falls against posterior pharyngeal wall, CHD. ⚠ Difficult airway.[192]

Plott's syndrome

Laryngeal abductor paralysis, retardation, 6th nerve palsy, stridor at rest, cyanosis during crying/exertion. ► ↑ risk of post-operative stridor/coughing.[193]

Plummer–Vinson syndrome
(Paterson–Brown–Kelly syndrome)

Upper oesophageal web, dysphagia, regurgitation risk, iron deficiency anaemia, glossitis, angular stomatitis, ↑ risk of post-cricoid carcinoma. ⚠ Regurgitation risk.[194]

Pneumatosis cystoides intestinalis

Multiple intramural gas-filled cysts in gut, disturbed bowel function, systemic sclerosis association. ► Avoid N_2O.[195]

Pompe's disease

See *Glycogenoses, type II.*

Post-poliomyelitis syndrome

New neuromuscular symptoms occurring >15yr after clinical stability attained in patients with prior history of symptomatic poliomyelitis, limb atrophy, slow progression with periods of stabilization, bulbar dysfunction, cold intolerance. ⚠ Respiratory muscle involvement, sleep apnoea, sensitive to sedatives and muscle relaxants, prolonged emergence, increased post-operative pain due to 'wind-up', autonomic dysfunction.[196]

Potter's syndrome (bilateral renal agenesis)

Incompatible with life. Pulmonary hypoplasia, characteristic facial features. ⚠ Ventilation may be impossible despite intubation.

Prader–Willi syndrome

Mental retardation, severe obesity, polyphagia, dental caries, muscle hypotonia, short stature, hypogonadism, CVS anomalies, arrhythmias, altered thermoregulation, convulsions. ► Difficult venous access, blood glucose should be maintained IV during fasting, perioperative respiratory problems may occur.[197]

Progeria

Premature ageing of skin, bones, and CVS → arthritis/IHD/hypertension/cardiomyopathy at young chronological age. Plan technique around 'physiological age'. ⚠ Micrognathia, small mouth, abnormal dentition may → difficult ventilation/intubation.[198]

Progressive external ophthalmoplegia (PEO)

Progressive mitochondrial myopathy, ptosis, diabetes mellitus, hypothyroidism, hyperparathyroidism, short stature. ▶ Sensitive to all induction agents, possible MH risk.[199]

Proteus syndrome

Congenital progressive hamartomatous disorder, partial gigantism, hemihypertrophy (often whole side of the body), macrocephaly, scoliosis, cervical spine abnormalities, cystic lung changes, (probably explains 'the Elephant Man'). △ Difficult airway, avoid N_2O (see also *Bullous cystic lung disease*; *Klippel–Trenaunay syndrome*).[200]

Prune belly syndrome (Eagle–Barrett syndrome)

Almost exclusively ♂. Absent abdominal muscles, genitourinary malformations/bilateral undescended testes, pulmonary hypoplasia, weak cough, CHD, skeletal anomalies, imperforate anus, careful fluid balance, renal failure may coexist. △ Difficult airway (micrognathia), beware post-operative respiratory distress.[201]

Pseudoxanthoma elasticum (Grönblad–Strandberg disease)

Hereditary disorder of elastic tissue. Four types—variable features, fragile connective tissue, vascular complications (slow progressive occlusive arterial disease), retinal changes with early blindness/myopia, blue sclera, high arched palate, lungs not affected, valvular disease/hypertension/IHD/arrhythmias. ▶ Fragile tissue—haemorrhage with minor trauma (including airway), care in fixing IV lines.[202]

Pulmonary cysts

Can ↑ in size and rupture during anaesthesia (especially with N_2O).

References

183 Kaneda T, et al. (2007). J Anesth, 21, 500–3.
184 Rosenbaum HK, Miller JD (2002). Anesthesiol Clin N Am, 20, 623–64.
185 Pollard RC, et al. (1996). Paediatr Anaesth, 6, 151–3.
186 Bansal A, et al. (2000). Saudi J Anaesth, 6, 165–8.
187 Kandasamy N, et al. (2011). Eur J Endocrinol, 165, 167–70.
188 Moore MH, et al. (1995). Cleft Palate Craniofac J, 32, 62–70.
189 Cope R, Spargo P (1990). Anesth Analg, 71, 312.
190 Dal D, Celiker V (2004). Paediatr Anaesth, 14, 701–2.
191 Chau EHL, et al. (2013). Sleep Med Clin, 8, 135–47.
192 Semjen F, et al. (2008). Anaesthesia, 63, 147–50.
193 McDonald D (1998). Paediatr Anaesth, 8, 155–7.
194 Novacek G (2006). Orphanet J Rare Dis, 1, 36.
195 Sutton DN, Poskitt KR (1984). Anaesthesia, 39, 776–80.
196 Lambert DA, et al. (2005). Anesthesiology, 103, 638–44.
197 Lirk P, et al. (2004). Eur J Anaesthesiol, 21, 831–3.
198 Nguyen NH, Mayhew JF (2001). Paediatr Anaesth, 11, 370–1.
199 Guasch E, et al. (2003). Anaesthesia, 58, 607–8.
200 Cekmen N, et al. (2004). Paediatr Anaesth, 14, 689–92.
201 Baris S, et al. (2001). Paediatr Anaesth, 11, 501–4.
202 Douglas MJ, et al. (2003). Int J Obstet Anesth, 12, 45–7.

R

Refsum's disease

Defective metabolism of phytanic acid, sensorimotor polyneuropathy, ataxia, retinal damage, deafness. ► Document any neurology before performing regional blocks.

Rett syndrome

Devastating disabling ♀ neurological disease, 2nd commonest cause of mental retardation in ♀ after Down's. Long QT, sudden death, abnormal respiratory control when awake (hyperventilation/apnoea), respiratory pattern normal under general anaesthesia, full respiratory assessment ideal but may be technically difficult, ↑ pain threshold (abnormal processing), scoliosis, may be sensitive to sedative drugs/resistant to muscle relaxants, prolonged weaning. Consider depth of anaesthesia monitoring.[203]

Rigid spine syndrome

Very limited spinal flexion, generalized proximal limb weakness, limb contractures, progressive scoliosis, restrictive ventilatory defect, cardiomyopathy, conduction defects, pulmonary hypertension, right ventricular failure. ⚠ Difficult intubation, flexible ETT provides better fit in hyperextended trachea, avoid suxamethonium (↑ K⁺), low MH risk, care with muscle relaxants, careful positioning/padding, consider post-operative HDU/ICU.[204]

Riley–Day syndrome

See *Dysautonomia*.

Romano–Ward syndrome

Congenital delay of cardiac depolarization, prolonged QT interval, risk of sudden death during induction of anaesthesia. ► Consider preoperative pacing.[205]

Rubinstein–Taybi syndrome

Microcephaly, craniofacial abnormalities, mental retardation, broad thumbs/toes, recurrent respiratory infections/chronic lung disease, CHD (33% of cases), arrhythmias. ⚠ Difficult airway.[206]

Russell–Silver syndrome

Short stature, facial/limb asymmetry, mandibular hypoplasia, micrognathia, macroglossia, sweating, fasting hypoglycaemia, intelligence usually normal, CHD. ⚠ Difficult airway (including mask fit), monitor neuromuscular block (normal doses may overdose), care with temperature control (minimal body fat) and blood glucose.[207]

References

203 Nho JS, et al. (2011). *Korean J Anesthesiol*, **61**, 428–30.
204 Kanniah S (2006). *Can J Anaesth*, **53**, 739–40.
205 Staikou C, et al. (2012). *Br J Anaesth*, **108**, 730–44.
206 Park CH, et al. (2012). *Korean J Anesthesiol*, **63**, 571–2.
207 Scarlett MD, Tha MW (2006). *West Indian Med J*, **55**, 127–9.

S

Saethre–Chotzen syndrome
Craniosynostosis, micrognathia, renal failure. △ Difficult intubation.[208]

Scheie syndrome (mucopolysaccharidosis V)
See *Mucopolysaccharidoses*.

Scimitar syndrome
Anomalous venous drainage of right lung into inferior vena cava (IVC), right lung hypoplasia. Scimitar-shaped radiographic shadow of the anomalous vein gives syndrome its name.

Seckel syndrome
'Bird-headed dwarfism', microcephaly, mental retardation, micrognathia, beak-like nose, laryngeal stenosis. ▶ Potential difficult airway.[209]

Sheehan's syndrome (post-partum pituitary necrosis)
Pituitary infarction following post-partum haemorrhage, variable degree of pituitary insufficiency. Assess endocrine derangement.

Shy–Drager syndrome (central nervous and autonomic degeneration)
Progressive neurovegetative disorder with 1° autonomic failure, severe orthostatic hypotension/syncope, anhidrosis, disordered thermoregulation, impotence/urinary incontinence, respiratory obstruction/sleep apnoea. △ ↑ aspiration risk (gut motility disorder plus laryngeal weakness), IPPV may cause CVS instability (reduced venous return—ensure normovolaemia), regional blocks used successfully, consider fludrocortisone to sustain plasma volume, vasopressin may be drug of choice for severe unresponsive hypotension.[210,211]

Sipple syndrome (multiple endocrine neoplasia type IIa)
See also ➔ p. 580 and p. 574.

Phaeochromocytoma, medullary carcinoma of thyroid with or without parathyroid hyperplasia. Assess degree of endocrine dysfunction, treat as for phaeochromocytoma.[212]

Sjögren's syndrome (keratoconjunctivitis sicca)
Dry eyes without RA, may also have other autoimmune disease, dysphagia/abnormal oesophageal motility, renal defects, pulmonary hypertension, peripheral neuropathy, vasculitis, assess for other systemic conditions. ▶ Worsened by anticholinergic drugs, improved by humidification, increased risk of mucous plugs.[213]

Smith–Lemli–Opitz syndrome

Abnormal cholesterol biosynthesis, severe growth failure, congenital anomalies affecting most organ systems, early death, developmental delay, self-injurious/ritualistic behaviour, typical dysmorphic facial features (micrognathia/cleft palate/small and abnormally hard tongue), thymic hypoplasia, intrinsic lung disease, ↑ gastric reflux and aspiration, possibly susceptible to infection. ⚠ Difficult intubation.[214]

Spinal muscular atrophy

See also ➲ p. 250.

Peripheral motor neurons affected, upper motor neurons spared, ↓ rate of progression through types I–IV, muscular wasting (see also *Amyotrophic lateral sclerosis*), proximal/respiratory muscle weakness (IPPV advisable), kyphoscoliosis, restrictive chest defects, bulbar dysfunction. Regional blocks may be technically difficult, beware altered distribution of local anaesthetics. ⚠ Difficult intubation (spinal deformity/aspiration risk), avoid suxamethonium (chronic denervation/K^+), abnormal reaction to muscle relaxants (if essential, monitor blockade and ensure full reversal), post-operative respiratory support may be indicated, ↑ risk of pulmonary aspiration.[215]

Strümpell's disease (hereditary spastic paraplegia)

Progressive spastic paresis predominantly of the lower extremities, poor respiratory function/reserve. ▶ Avoid suxamethonium, possible sensitivity to non-depolarizing muscle relaxants, regional anaesthesia probably acceptable.[216]

Sturge–Weber syndrome

Unilateral angiomatous lesions of the leptomeninges/upper face, contralateral hemiparesis, seizures, mental retardation, evaluate for associated abnormalities. ▶ Careful intubation/extubation (angiomas of mouth/upper airway), prevent ↑ ICP/intraocular pressure.[217]

References

208 Easely D, Mayhew JF (2008). *Paediatr Anaesth*, **18**, 81.
209 Arora S, et al. (2012). *J Anaesthesiol Clin Pharm*, **28**, 398–9.
210 Malinovsky JM, et al. (2003). *Can J Anaesth*, **50**, 962–3.
211 Ricardo V, et al. (2002). *Anesth Analg*, **95**, 50–2.
212 Grant F (2005). *Curr Opin Anesthesiol*, **18**, 345–52.
213 Fox R (2014). ℘ http://www.uptodate.com/contents/sjogrens-syndrome-beyond-the-basics.
214 Matveevskii A, et al. (2006). *Paediatr Anaesth*, **16**, 322–4.
215 Islander G (2013). *Paediatr Anaesth*, **23**, 804–16.
216 McIver T, et al. (2007). *Int J Obstet Anesth*, **16**, 190–1.
217 Gandhi M, et al. (2009). *Indian J Anaesth*, **53**, 64–7.

T

Takayasu's disease (pulseless disease, occlusive thromboaortopathy, or aortic arch syndrome)

Chronic autoimmune inflammatory disease. Elastic tissue replaced by fibrous tissue, leading to blood vessel narrowing/occlusion/aneurysms (preferentially large arteries—aorta and branches), often self-limiting, hypertension (usually renovascular), IHD, cerebrovascular disease, NIBP measurements may be inaccurate, many have post-operative CVS complications from poorly controlled hypertension. ► Maintain organ perfusion (BP, CO_2, etc.), consider regional blocks (care—CVS effect of spinal).[218]

Tangier disease (familial α-lipoprotein deficiency)

Deficient high-density lipoprotein (HDL) apoprotein, accumulation of cholesterol in reticuloendothelial tissue, enlarged orange tonsils, hepatosplenomegaly, corneal opacities, polyneuropathy, IHD, anaemia, thrombocytopenia. ► Sensitivity to muscle relaxants.[219]

TAR syndrome (thrombocytopenia, absent radius)

May also have ToF. (See also ➲ p. 67)

Tay–Sachs disease ('familial amaurotic idiocy')

Accumulation of GM2 gangliosides in CNS/peripheral nerves, progressive cerebral degeneration/seizures/dementia/blindness, usually die <2yr, characteristic macular cherry spot appearance, progressive neurology leads to respiratory complications.

Thrombotic thrombocytopenic purpura

Rare severe disease pentad of haemolytic anaemia/consumptive thrombocytopenia/CNS dysfunction/renal impairment/fever. May need therapeutic splenectomy. Triad of haemolytic anaemia/consumptive thrombocytopenia/CNS dysfunction, renal disease, bleeding risk, often need splenectomy (rebound thrombocytosis). ► Padding/positioning important. Preferably postpone elective surgery until remission. ► Check coagulation (usually normal)/renal/liver function, consider prophylactic antiplatelet drugs/corticosteroids, platelet transfusion contraindicated (may worsen disease), use packed cells/FFP, strict asepsis (often immunocompromised), avoid IM route/nasal intubation, control BP (renal/cerebral perfusion), take care with positioning (see also ➲ p. 210).[220]

Tourette syndrome

Profane vocalizations, repetitious speech, muscle jerking. Sedating premedication beneficial, continue normal medication. ► Do not confuse tic-like behaviour with seizure activity on induction/emergence, pimozide may cause prolonged QT, beware interaction of psychotropic drugs and sympathomimetics.[221]

Toxic epidermal necrolysis ('scalded skin syndrome')

Split at level of stratum granulosum, epidermal erythema/blistering/necrosis, made worse by lateral shearing forces, can be drug-related. ▶ Prevent friction (monitors/lines/airway manipulation/positioning, etc.), consider fluid losses from blisters/exposed areas of dermis, manage like severe second-degree burn.[222]

Treacher–Collins syndrome

See *Mandibulofacial dysostosis*.

Trisomy 13

See *Patau's syndrome*.

Trisomy 18

See *Edward's syndrome*.

Trisomy 21

See *Down's syndrome*.

Tuberous sclerosis (Bourneville's disease)

Neurocutaneous syndrome, facial angiofibromas, seizures, mental retardation, CVS/CNS/renal hamartomas, may affect airway/lungs/CVS—spontaneous rupture/bleeding, spontaneous pneumothoraces. ▶ Careful positioning/padding, avoid proconvulsants, consider full preoperative CVS assessment (cardiac rhabdomyoma in 30–50% of patients).[223]

Turner's syndrome

XO karyotype, micrognathia, short webbed neck, often ↑ gastric reflux, diabetes, hypothyroidism, coarctation/dissecting aortic aneurysms/pulmonary stenosis, renal anomaly (50% of patients). ⚠ Possible difficult intubation.[224]

References

218 Kiran S, et al. (2012). *Egyptian J Anaesth*, **28**, 287–9.
219 Mentis SW (1996). *Anesth Analg*, **83**, 427–9.
220 Benington SR, et al. (2009). *Anaesthesia*, **64**, 1018–21.
221 Sener EB, et al. (2006). *Int J Obstet Anesth*, **15**, 163–5.
222 Lee JH, et al. (2010). *Korean J Anesthesiol*, **59**, S167–S171.
223 Causse-Mariscal A, et al. (2007). *Int J Obstet Anesth*, **16**, 277–80.
224 Mashour GA, et al. (2005). *J Clin Anesth*, **17**, 128–30.

U–Z

Urbach–Wiethe disease (lipoid proteinosis)
Type of histiocytosis (see *Hand–Schuller–Christian disease*), hyaline deposits in larynx and pharynx—hoarseness/aphonia. ⚠ Cautious intubation, laryngeal opening may be small.[225] (See also *Letterer-Siwe disease*.)

von Recklinghausen's disease
See *Neurofibromatosis*.

von Willebrand's disease (pseudohaemophilia)
See ➲ p. 206.

WAGR syndrome
Wilms' tumour/Aniridia/Genitourinary abnormalities/Retardation, may also have cardiomyopathy or cardiac defects—consider preoperative echocardiography.[226]

Weaver syndrome
Unusual craniofacial appearance, micrognathia, may have large stature in adulthood. ⚠ Airway problems (may ↓ with age as mandible grows).[227]

Weber–Christian disease
Global fat necrosis (including retroperitoneal/pericardial/peritoneal/meningeal), associated organ dysfunction (e.g. adrenals, constrictive pericarditis). ► Avoid trauma to superficial fat during movement/positioning during surgery (cold, heat, pressure).

Wegener's granulomatosis
Necrotizing granulomata in inflamed vessels of multiple organ systems (CNS/CVS/renal/respiratory systems), pneumonia, bronchial destruction, valvular dysfunction, abnormal cardiac conduction, arteritis (cerebral aneurysms, arterial line difficulty), IHD, renal failure, peripheral neuropathy. ⚠ Consider possible laryngeal stenosis.[228]

Welander's muscular atrophy
Peripheral muscular atrophy. ► Sensitive to thiopental/muscle relaxants/opioids, good prognosis.

Werdnig–Hoffman disease (spinal muscular atrophy type I acute, and type II chronic)
See *Spinal muscular atrophy*.

Wermer's syndrome (multiple endocrine neoplasia type I)
Parathyroid/pituitary/adrenal/thyroid adenomas, pancreas islet cell tumours. Assess endocrine dysfunction.

Werner syndrome (premature ageing syndrome)
See *Progeria*.

Wiedemann–Rautenstrauch syndrome

See *Progeria*.

Williams' syndrome

Characteristic elfin facies, CHD (aortic/pulmonary stenosis), hypercalcae-mia, feeding problems, severe gag reflex, dental abnormalities, stellate blue eyes, retardation but social personality, hyperacusis. ⚠ Potential difficult mask ventilation/intubation.[229]

Wilson's disease

Inborn error of copper metabolism. Basal ganglia degeneration, neurological symptoms, trismus, weakness, hepatic and renal failure. ▶ Respiratory com-plications, difficulty reversing muscle relaxants.[230]

Wiskott–Aldrich syndrome

Faulty presentation of antigen to macrophages. Thrombocytopenia, coagu-lopathy, anaemia, immunodeficiency, recurrent infections.

Wolf–Hirschhorn syndrome

Rare chromosomal abnormality. Variable psychomotor retardation, seiz-ures, VSD/ASD, characteristic facies, midline fusion abnormalities, 34% die by age 2 (cardiac failure/bronchopneumonia). Assess for system dysfunc-tion, MH risk unproven.[231]

Wolfram syndrome (DIDMOAD syndrome)

Diabetes Insipidus, Diabetes Mellitus, Optic Atrophy, Deafness. ▶ Fluid/electrolyte control important.[232]

Wolman's syndrome

Familial xanthomatosis, adrenal calcification, hepatosplenomegaly, hyper-splenism, anaemia, thrombocytopenia. Platelet transfusion may only be successful after splenectomy.

Zellweger syndrome (cerebrohepatorenal syndrome)

Reduced/absent peroxisomes in brain/liver/kidney, flat/round face, micro-gnathia, cleft palate, polycystic kidneys, impaired adrenal function, apnoeas, congenital heart defects, hypotonia, areflexia, seizures, hepatomegaly/bil-iary dysgenesis. ⚠ Difficult intubation, care with muscle relaxants.[233]

References

225 Kelly JE, et al. (1989). Br J Anaesth, **63**, 609–11.
226 Yanagidate F, et al. (2001). Anesthesia, **56**, 1203–16.
227 Crawford MW, Rohan D (2005). Paediatr Anaesth, **15**, 893–6.
228 Rookard P, et al. (2009). Middle East J Anesthesiol, **20**, 21–9.
229 Asegaonkar B, et al. (2013). Open J Anesthesiol, **3**, 57–60.
230 Langley A, Dameron CT (2013). Anesthesiology Res Pract, **2013**, 750901.
231 Choi JH, et al. (2011). Korean J Anesthesiol, **60**, 119–23.
232 Rohayem J, et al. (2011). Diabetes Care, **34**, 1503–10.
233 Platis CM, et al. (2006). Paediatr Anaesth, **16**, 361–2.

Further reading

Baum VC, O'Flaherty JE (2007). *Anesthesia for genetic, metabolic and dysmorphic syndromes of childhood*, 2nd edn. Philadelphia: Lippincott Williams & Wilkins.

Benumof JL (1998). *Anesthesia and uncommon diseases*, 4th edn. Philadelphia: WB Saunders.

Butler MG, Hayes BG, Hathaway MM, Begleiter ML (2000). Specific genetic diseases at risk for sedation/anesthesia complications. *Anesth Analg*, **91**, 837–55 [good review].

Hines RL, Marschall K (2008). *Stoelting's anesthesia and co-existing disease*, 5th edn. Philadelphia: WB Saunders.

Russell SH, Hirsch NP (1994). Anaesthesia and myotonia. *Br J Anaesth*, **72**, 210–16.

For online information about rare conditions, try:

Diseases Database. ℘ http://www.diseasesdatabase.com.

MedlinePlus. ℘ http://www.nlm.nih.gov/medlineplus/healthtopics.html. [Extensive information from the National Institutes of Health and other trusted sources on over 650 diseases and conditions.]

National Organization for Rare Disorders. ℘ http://www.rarediseases.org/.

Online Mendelian Inheritance in Man, OMIM (TM). McKusick-Nathans Institute for Genetic Medicine, Johns Hopkins University (Baltimore, MD) and National Center for Biotechnology Information, National Library of Medicine (Bethesda, MD) (2000). ℘http://www.ncbi.nlm.nih.gov/omim/. [Click on 'Search the OMIM Database', and enter the name of the condition in the search field.]

Cardiac surgery

Rhys Evans

See also:

Determinants of myocardial oxygen supply and demand

Coronary blood flow (CBF) to the LV occurs only during diastole. Increased HR decreases the diastolic interval, with little change in the length of systole.

Myocardial O_2 **supply** depends upon:
- O_2 content of arterial blood (Hb and SaO_2)
- Myocardial (coronary) blood flow; this is further determined by:
  - Diastolic BP (dependent upon systolic pressure, arterial compliance, aortic valve competence, and HR)
  - Diastolic interval (length of diastole, again dependent upon HR)
  - Blood viscosity (decreased on CPB)
  - Coronary vascular resistance (variable coronary vascular tone and fixed atheromatous lesions)
  - LVEDP (higher pressures decrease flow).

Myocardial O_2 **demand** depends upon:
- Myocardial wall tension (systolic BP)
- Number of contractions per minute (i.e. HR):
  - 'Physiological' HRs and systemic arterial pressures provide optimal coronary flow
  - Bradycardia provides long diastolic intervals, and hence more time for CBF, together with few contractions demanding O_2, but falling diastolic pressure during prolonged diastole decreases the coronary perfusion pressure, and hence CBF becomes limited in late diastole
  - Tachycardia increases the mean diastolic pressure, and hence coronary perfusion pressure, but allows relatively little time for the flow to occur; increased numbers of contractions also increase myocardial O_2 consumption
- High BP provides higher diastolic pressures for improved coronary perfusion, and hence O_2 supply, but the generation of increased systolic pressures increases O_2 consumption
- Low BPs are generated by low myocardial wall tension, and hence low systolic pressures and O_2 demand, but the associated low diastolic pressure limits CBF, and hence O_2 supply.

Risk scoring

The EuroSCORE (European System for Cardiac Operative Risk Evaluation) is a simple method for calculating predicted operative mortality for patients undergoing cardiac surgery (Table 14.1). For each risk factor, a weight or number is assigned—these weights are then added to give an *approximate percentage of predicted perioperative mortality*. In very high-risk patients, this simple additive model may underestimate the risk; the original 'additive' EuroSCORE was replaced by the more comprehensive 'logistic' version of EuroSCORE, and, since 2011, the further refined 'EuroSCORE II' may be used to give a more accurate prediction (see ℗ http://www.euroscore.org/calculators. htm). This assessment includes a score for diabetics requiring insulin.

Table 14.1 EuroSCORE method of predicting mortality following cardiac surgery

Factors	Definitions	Score
Patient-related factors		
Age	Per 5yr or part thereof over 60yr	1
Sex	♀	1
Chronic pulmonary disease	Long-term use of bronchodilators or steroids for lung disease	1
Extracardiac arteriopathy	Any one or more of the following: claudication, carotid occlusion, >50% stenosis, previous or planned intervention on the abdominal aorta, limb arteries, or carotids	2
Neurological dysfunction	Severely affecting ambulation or day-to-day functioning	2
Previous cardiac surgery	Requiring opening of the pericardium	3
Serum creatinine	>200 micromoles/L preoperatively	2
Active endocarditis	Patient still under antibiotic treatment for endocarditis at the time of surgery	3
Critical preoperative state	Any one or more of the following: VT, fibrillation, aborted sudden death, preoperative cardiac massage, preoperative ventilation before arrival in the anaesthetic room, preoperative inotropic support, intra-aortic balloon counterpulsation, preoperative ARF (anuria or oliguria <10mL/hr)	3
Cardiac-related factors		
Unstable angina	Rest angina requiring IV nitrates until arrival in the anaesthetic room	2
LV dysfunction	Moderate or LVEF 30–50%	1
	Poor or LVEF <30%	3

(Continued)

Table 14.1 (*Contd.*)

Factors	Definitions	Score
Recent MI	<90d	2
Pulmonary hypertension	Systolic PAP >60mmHg	2
Operation-related factors		
Emergency	Carried out on referral before the beginning of the next working day	2
Other than isolated CABG	Major cardiac procedure other than, or in addition to, CABG	2
Surgery on thoracic aorta	For disorder of ascending arch or descending aorta	3
Post-infarct septal rupture		4

Cardiopulmonary bypass

- CPB replaces the function of heart and lungs, while the heart is arrested, allowing for a bloodless and stable surgical field.
- Membrane oxygenators are most commonly used. These contain minute hollow fibres, giving a large surface area for gas exchange ($2–2.5m^2$). Gas exchange occurs down concentration gradients; increasing the gas flow to the oxygenator removes more CO_2, and increasing FiO_2 increases oxygenation.
- Prior to CPB, full anticoagulation of the patient with heparin is required, with an ACT recorded at >400s.
- The bypass circuit is primed with crystalloid (e.g. Hartmann's solution), heparin, and occasionally mannitol and HCO_3^-. The bypass machine normally delivers non-pulsatile flow of $2.4L/min/m^2$ (to correspond to a typical cardiac index).
- MAP is normally maintained between 50 and 70mmHg by altering SVR.
- Volume, as crystalloid/colloid/blood, can be added to the pump reservoir or removed by ultrafiltration, to maintain an Hct of 20–30%.
- CPB causes haemolysis, platelet damage, and consumption of coagulation factors. This is usually minimal for the first 2hr.
- Other problems include poor venous drainage, aortic dissection, and gas embolization.
- Risk of a CVA ranges from 1% to 5% and is associated with increasing age, hypertension, aortic atheroma, previous CVA, diabetes, and the type of surgery (aortic arch replacement > valve replacement > coronary artery surgery).
- Hypoperfusion and emboli are the main aetiological factors. Strategies to reduce cerebral injury (thiopental, steroids, mannitol, use of arterial filters in the bypass circuit) lack an evidence base. Maintaining optimum perfusion pressures, normoglycaemia, scrupulous surgical de-airing of the heart, and careful temperature control may decrease the incidence of neurological sequelae.

Instituting cardiopulmonary bypass

- Baseline ABG, ACT, and TEG should be measured.
- Prior to instituting bypass, the patient should be anticoagulated with heparin 300IU/kg (use central, rather than peripheral, line for administration to minimize risk of delivery failure). ACT must be confirmed at >400s prior to aortic cannulation.
- Before cannulation, systolic BP should be decreased (to 80–100mmHg) to reduce the risk of aortic dissection.
- Blood cardioplegia is commonly administered by the perfusionist through the pump; some centres use crystalloid cardioplegia administered by the anaesthetist. If cold crystalloid cardioplegia is to be used, prepare and pressurize cardioplegia to 300mmHg, ensuring a bubble-free circuit.
- Once bypass is established, the ventilator is turned off, and an IV anaesthetic (e.g. propofol 6mg/kg/hr) started. A benzodiazepine (e.g. midazolam) or a volatile agent administered by a vaporizer mounted

on the bypass machine are suitable alternatives. Adjunct opioid (e.g. morphine bolus) may also be administered during CPB.
- The perfusionist maintains a perfusion pressure of 50–70mmHg by the use of vasoconstrictors (e.g. metaraminol) and vasodilators (e.g. GTN, phentolamine).
- Blood gases and ACT are checked every 30min. Beware heparin resistance in patients who have been on heparin infusion (e.g. for acute coronary syndrome) preoperatively.
- Tranexamic acid may be administered (2g at the commencement of CPB, 1g after CPB, or as an infusion). High-dose tranexamic acid administration is used in some centres (30mg/kg at induction; 20mg/kg on commencing CPB; an infusion of 16mg/kg/hr throughout the procedure). This regime should be used with caution in patients predisposed to epilepsy.
- The patient's temperature is actively lowered, or allowed to drift, to 28–34°C, depending on the type of surgery and surgical preference.

Coming off bypass
- This is a team effort between the surgeon, anaesthetist, and perfusionist. The aim is to wean the patient from the bypass machine, allowing the heart and lungs to re-establish normal physiological function.
- Before coming off bypass:
  - The nasopharyngeal temperature should have returned to 37°C
  - K^+ should be 4.5–5mmol/L
  - Hct should be >20%
  - Acid/base should be in the normal range.
- The HR should be 70–100bpm and sinus rhythm (if possible). Epicardial pacing may be required. Defibrillate, and use atropine/isoprenaline/adrenaline as necessary.
- Ventilate with 100% O_2, and ensure the lung bases are expanded.
- The venous line is progressively clamped, and the heart gradually allowed to fill/eject. It is usual practice to come off bypass with the heart relatively 'underfilled'. This avoids overdistension of the ventricles, which may not yet function normally (impaired Frank–Starling relation).
- The perfusionist will transfuse 100mL of perfusate boluses, as required. Be vigilant—watch the heart performance and filling carefully. If the ventricle is performing poorly, commence inotropic support (e.g. adrenaline).
- Do not draw up protamine (1mg/100IU heparin—usually 3mg/kg) until off CPB. When the surgeon requests protamine, clearly inform the perfusionist to turn off the suction, and administer slowly IV (ideally peripherally, though maintaining wide-bore venous access protamine-free for fluid administration). Protamine may cause systemic hypotension and pulmonary hypertension. Rapid volume administration may be required.

Following bypass
- Ensure adequate anaesthesia and analgesia with a volatile agent (e.g. isoflurane) and an opioid.

- Systolic BP should be controlled at 80–140mmHg by careful filling and adjustments of vasodilator/inotrope infusions, as necessary.
- Maintain serum K^+ levels at 4–5mmol/L. Hypokalaemia should be treated with aliquots of 20mmol KCl (in 100mL over 30min).
- Check ABG, ACT, and TEG.
- The perfusionist may have blood left over in the circuit reservoir—this will be bagged and handed to the anaesthetist to be transfused. Remember this blood is heparinized and of low Hct. Occasionally, the perfusionist will infuse this 'pump' blood through a cell saver first.

Cardioplegia

- Based on the Ringer's solution containing K^+ (20mmol/L), Mg^{2+} (16mmol/L), and procaine.
- When rapidly infused (1L), this renders the heart asystolic.
- Cold (4°C) cardioplegia affords myocardial protection against ischaemia. Further doses (500mL) are repeated every 20min or when electrical activity returns.
- Can be blood or crystalloid-based. The advantages of blood cardioplegia are largely theoretical and based on the assumption that Hb will carry O_2 and thus help reduce myocardial damage. Reperfusion (warm blood) cardioplegia is sometimes used towards the end of bypass to wash out products of metabolism.
- Cardioplegia is usually administered anterograde (via the coronary arteries), but retrograde cardioplegia may be delivered via the coronary sinus (in which case, monitor the infusion pressure—the CVP transducer may be used for this—and take care not to let the infusion pressure rise).

Temperature management

- During bypass, the patient's nasopharyngeal temperature may be allowed to 'drift' down to 34°C, or the patient can be actively cooled to a lower temperature (28–34°C).
- Generally, a cooler temperature allows better cerebral protection but requires longer periods on CPB for rewarming.
- Different centres vary in approach, but marked hypothermia is usually reserved for more complex cases.

Intermittent cross-clamping and fibrillation

- Coronary arterial grafts can be undertaken, using either cardioplegia (asystole) or intermittent cross-clamping with fibrillation.
- In intermittent cross-clamping, the aorta is clamped, and a fibrillator pad placed underneath the heart to induce VF. The graft bottom-end anastomosis can then be sutured. After each graft, the cross-clamp is removed, and the heart cardioverted into sinus rhythm; the graft top-end anastomosis is then completed.
- Advantages are that no cardioplegia is used (hence a lower incidence of complete heart block), and, after each graft is attached, the ECG can be inspected for ischaemia.
- As the heart is not protected by cardioplegia, the surgical time needs to be kept to a minimum (<10min) to avoid myocardial damage.

Volatile agents and cardiopulmonary bypass

- All volatile agents cause vasodilatation, cardiac depression, and bradycardia in a dose-dependent manner.
- Isoflurane has been shown in the animal model to cause coronary 'steal' phenomenon, but this has not been convincingly demonstrated in man.
- Desflurane has a very similar cardiodynamic profile to isoflurane but may cause slightly greater stimulation of sympathetic outflow.
- Effects of volatile agents on ischaemia–reperfusion injury are probably not clinically significant.
- There is probably little to choose between different anaesthetic agents in terms of morbidity and mortality.

Coronary artery bypass grafting

Procedure	Bypassing a coronary artery stenosis with an arterial or venous graft
Time	4hr
Pain	+++/++++
Position	Supine ± crucifix
Blood loss	Moderate (X-match 2U)
Practical techniques	ETT, IPPV, arterial/CVP, urinary catheter, temperature monitoring, usually on CPB. Large-bore IV access. Consider pulmonary artery flotation catheter and TOE

Preoperative

- Commonly associated medical problems include hypertension, COPD/smoking, diabetes, cerebrovascular disease, and renal dysfunction. Often have had previous PCI/stents.
- History of angina, recent MI, or CVA.
- Investigations: recent FBC, U&Es, clotting screen, CXR, ECG. PFTs and ABGs may be appropriate.
- Careful assessment of LV function:
  - Orthopnoea and paroxysmal dyspnoea are important symptoms of LV failure
  - Exercise ECG
  - Coronary angiography within past 12 months
  - Echocardiography assessment (transthoracic or transoesophageal)
  - A useful assessment of LV function is exercise tolerance.
- EuroSCORE scoring system (see p. 325).
- Premedication with IM opioid and anticholinergic (e.g. morphine/hyoscine 10mg/0.4mg for an adult ♂, which is very amnesic, soporific, and analgesic; alternatively an oral anxiolytic, but this lacks analgesia for awake line placement). Prescribe O_2 supplementation from the time of premedication.
- Continue cardiac medication preoperatively (most centres stop aspirin/antiplatelet drugs/ACE inhibitors).

Echocardiography

EF 40–50%	Mild LV impairment
EF 30–40%	Moderate LV impairment
EF <30%	Severe LV impairment

Perioperative

- Insert peripheral venous and arterial lines pre-induction, preoxygenate, and induce with fentanyl 10–15 micrograms/kg and a cardiostable induction agent. Paralyse with an NDMR; intubate, and maintain anaesthesia with a volatile agent in an O_2 and air mixture. Insert internal jugular lines and a urinary catheter.
- Five-lead ECG with ST segment monitoring is advised (lead II for rhythm and V_5 for ischaemia).
- Use a nasopharyngeal temperature probe.
- Indications for a pulmonary artery flotation catheter (PAFC) include:
  - LVEF <30%
  - Mitral valve dysfunction, as filling and PAP monitoring are important post-operatively
  - Patients with raised preoperative creatinine
  - A preoperative alternative is to insert a left atrial line or use TOE to assess filling and ventricular function.
- Avoid hyper- or hypotension and tachy- or bradycardia. Aim for CVS stability with volume, GTN infusion, and careful boluses of a vasoconstrictor (e.g. metaraminol 0.5–1mg).
- Prophylactic antibiotics timed to coincide with skin incision:
  - Flucloxacillin 2g IV (ceftriaxone 2g IV if penicillin allergy; teicoplanin 800mg IV if MRSA risk)
  - Gentamicin 1.5mg/kg
- Stop ventilation, and anticipate BP surge during sternotomy; cover with fentanyl/volatile supplements and/or GTN, and restart ventilation once the sternum is opened.
- Give heparin 300IU/kg, and ensure ACT >400s pre-bypass.
- Maintain systolic BP in range 80–100mmHg for aortic cannulation.
- Continue as for CPB (see ➲ p. 327).
- Once the chest is closed and the patient is stable, transfer intubated to the recovery unit.
- Patients require optimal filling post-operatively, particularly in the presence of bleeding, diuresis, and vasodilatation caused by warming. If cardioplegia has been used, temporary pacing wires will be inserted, and temporary pacing may be needed.

Post-operative

- Check FBC, TEG/clotting, and ABG, and ensure blood loss is <100mL/hr.
- Once warm, awake, weaned, and not bleeding (i.e. a stable patient), extubate. Administer morphine (0.02mg/kg/hr) with GTN to keep systolic BP <140mmHg—to protect the graft anastomoses and reduce bleeding.

Special considerations

- For severe left main stem disease, adequate myocardial perfusion must be preserved by maintaining the diastolic pressure and diastolic interval (i.e. HR) at preoperative values.
- Unstable angina with poor ventricle: consider insertion of PAFC and an intra-aortic balloon pump (IABP) in the anaesthetic room (see ➲ p. 334).

- Thoracic epidurals are used in some centres, claiming improved haemodynamic stability and excellent post-operative pain relief, but this is controversial due to the perceived risk of epidural haematoma and paraplegia following anticoagulation for CPB.
- Arterial grafts (internal mammary/radial artery) are prone to spasm; therefore, maintain GTN infusion post-operatively. Avoid noradrenaline, if possible.

Off-pump coronary artery bypass grafting

Management is as for CABG, but without bypass and using a 'stabilizer' to keep the heart as still as possible.

- The patient is usually heparinized in case of urgent need for instituting CPB.
- Anaesthetic regime is as for pre-bypass (fentanyl and volatile agent).
- Keep the patient well filled with crystalloid.
- Keep the patient warm (blood/fluid warmer, warming mattress/blanket, heat and moisture exchanger (HME), etc.).
- May need vasoconstrictor when the surgeon manipulates the heart to maintain adequate BP.
- Consider TOE or oesophageal Doppler probe.
- The patient may still require full- or half-dose heparin (surgical preference).
- If patient unstable, may need to go on bypass (1–10% of cases).
- For right/posterior descending coronary artery grafts, the patient is placed in the Trendelenburg position to increase venous return.
- Post-operatively: as for CABGs on bypass.

Emergency coronary artery bypass graft (failed percutaneous coronary intervention)

Preoperative

- The patient will be collapsed in peri-arrest, with the need for urgent surgery to correct ischaemia.
- Should have good arterial access from the 'cath lab' (femoral lines).
- The patient will probably need inotropes, if not already started. Ideally, attain some degree of stability, or cardiac arrest may follow induction.
- An IABP can help poor coronary perfusion by increasing diastolic pressure, plus improve LV function by offloading the heart.
- Consider placement of central venous access under LA before induction (administration of cardioactive drugs in case of cardiac arrest during induction).
- Patient may have had streptokinase, clopidogrel, abciximab, or other antiplatelet drug and may require platelets and antifibrinolytics post-bypass.

Perioperative

- May need a PAFC, but do not waste time if speed is important. It can be inserted later during the case.
- Cautious induction with a reduced dose of fentanyl (250–500 micrograms) and etomidate (4–6mg). CVS stability is essential.
- Adrenaline should be prepared to be given as a bolus, 10 or 100 micrograms/mL, as appropriate.
- Do not forget to give heparin (300IU/kg) before aortic cannulation.
- Institute CPB as soon as possible.

Post-operative

- Inotropes should be maintained post-CPB; restart IABP if placed preoperatively, and consider insertion of IABP if not.
- There is no urgency to extubate the patient. A period of stability is required.
- There is a high risk of renal failure.
- Consider additional antibiotics if the operation was non-sterile.

Intra-aortic counterpulsation balloon pump

- Inserted percutaneously; triggered by arterial pressure or (preferably) ECG.
- Inflation (with helium) during diastole 'augments' diastolic pressure and improves CBF and O_2 delivery, without increasing O_2 demand.
- Deflation during systole reduces the afterload and offloads the LV, improving LV ejection.
- Requires heparinization; check the distal femoral pulses.
- Position must be checked by CXR (tip just distal to the left subclavian artery) or echocardiography.
- Indications include: myocardial ischaemia, cardiac failure/cardiogenic shock, weaning from CPB, MR, and VSD.
- Contraindications include: AR, AAA, and aortic dissection.

Aortic valve replacement: stenosis

(See also ➔ p. 50.)

Procedure	Replacement of aortic valve
Time	4hr
Pain	+++/++++
Position	Supine
Blood loss	Moderate (X-match 2U)
Practical techniques	As for CABG + TOE

The anatomical problems and consequences of particular valve lesions should be understood to appreciate the physiological requirements necessary for the forward flow of blood before and after valve replacement. The LV is pressure-overloaded with myocardial hypertrophy and high wall tension.

Mechanical valves tend to be used in younger patients, as they are longer-lasting; however, anticoagulation (warfarin) is needed to prevent clot formation around the valve. In elderly patients, biological tissue (homograft) valves can be used, as long-term anticoagulation is not needed. These valves probably only last for ~15yr.

Preoperative

- A sudden change in heart rhythm (e.g. AF) can precipitate LV failure.
- Perform echocardiography and angiography to assess LV function and CBF.
- AS causes LV hypertrophy, with no increase in LV volume and a stiff non-compliant ventricle with poor diastolic function (relaxation). This increases O_2 demand and requires higher filling pressures. If long-standing, the LV fails; LVEDP increases (causing MR and a high PAP), and there is ultimately RV failure.

- An LV–aorta gradient exceeding 40mmHg or an aortic orifice of <0.8cm represents significant obstruction to LV outflow.
- Surgery is indicated if gradient >70mmHg with good LV (>50mmHg with poor LV).
- If a known gradient is decreasing, this is a sign of LV failure.

Perioperative

- HR: 'aortic stenosis—always slow'. Tachycardia is not well tolerated, as it shortens diastole, hence time for CBF, and increases O_2 demand. The atrial contraction of sinus rhythm improves the filling of a stiff LV.
- Preload: should be maintained/increased to aid filling of a stiff LV; beware vasodilators reducing the preload and cardiac output.

- SVR: the afterload must be meticulously maintained with α_1-agonists (e.g. metaraminol, noradrenaline). A reduction in diastolic pressure may critically reduce CBF to a hypertrophic LV; again, use extreme caution with vasodilators.
- Contraction: the stiff and thickened LV may require adrenaline.
- TOE routinely performed at the end of CPB, once the heart is closed and beating, permits assessment of valve haemodynamics.

Post-bypass

- Pacing may be required (damage to the AV node).
- Preload: volume remains essential for adequate filling and perfusion of a stiff LV; consider sequential AV pacing to stimulate atrial contraction and augment ventricular filling. TOE post-bypass is helpful to assess cardiac function and filling.
- SVR: an infusion of noradrenaline may be required once well filled.
- Contraction: inotropic support (e.g. adrenaline) may be required to improve LV performance.

Special considerations

- Consider a PAFC, as filling is crucial, particularly in the post-operative period. Pre-bypass, the high PAP in long-standing AS may underestimate LV filling.
- Good myocardial protection for a hypertrophied ventricle by meticulous cardioplegic technique during CPB is the key to a good outcome.

Transcatheter aortic valve implantation

- Common procedure to avoid operative aortic valve replacement (AVR) in frail and elderly patients.
- May be performed transapically (mini-thoracotomy) or transfemorally (percutaneous).
- Set up as for CPB: arterial line, CVP, large-bore IV access, urinary catheter, external defibrillator pads.
- Typically target-controlled infusion (TCI) (e.g. remifentanil, propofol, relaxant; intubate and ventilate with O_2/air/volatile agent).
- Consider noradrenaline infusion to maintain systemic BP.
- Procedure involves rapid atrial pacing to permit valvotomy and placement of the prosthetic valve—maintain BP (>100mmHg) before this starts, and have adrenaline (1:10 000) drawn up, as the heart may be stunned immediately following this; stop ventilating when the valve is being positioned to stabilize the field.
- Infiltrate the wounds with LA, IV paracetamol for post-operative pain relief; consider paravertebral block for mini-thoracotomy.
- For transfemoral procedures, some centres use LA if the valve type used does not require TOE.
- For the transapical approach, more analgesia is required; blood should be available in the angiography suite for the LV apical ventriculotomy, and consider cell salvage. Have hypotensive agents (e.g. esmolol, GTN) available post-valve insertion, as hypertension can be marked.
- Early extubation is feasible following transcatheter aortic valve implantation (TAVI).

Aortic valve replacement: regurgitation

(See also ➔ p. 52.)

Procedure	Replacement of aortic valve
Time	4hr
Pain	+++/++++
Position	Supine
Blood loss	Moderate (X-match 2U)
Practical techniques	As for CABG + TOE

Preoperative

- AR may be associated with aortic root dilatation or dissection. There may be a history of endocarditis, although these patients are not usually operated on when acutely septic.
- In AR, the LV is volume-overloaded, with LV dilatation. There is increased sympathetic drive, causing tachycardia, increased contractility, peripheral vasoconstriction, and fluid retention to increase the preload.
- Surgery is indicated once symptomatic; angina is a late symptom indicating end-stage disease.

Perioperative

- 'Full, fast, and forward for a regurgitant lesion.'
- HR: the cardiac output is rate-dependent; increasing the rate reduces regurgitation during diastole and encourages forward flow. Avoid bradycardia, and aim for a rate of 90bpm. Collapsing the diastolic pressure due to AR also decreases coronary perfusion, so again keep the HR up to maintain the mean diastolic pressure, and hence CBF.
- Preload: the LV is stiff with an increased volume; therefore, maintain adequate filling. Sinus rhythm is of benefit, but patients are often in AF. Consider AV sequential pacing.
- SVR: anaesthesia causes a reduction in SVR, reducing the regurgitant fraction and encouraging forward flow. Vasodilators have similar effects but may also reduce the venous return/preload. Pre-bypass, beware of excessive systemic vasodilatation decreasing the diastolic pressure and hence coronary perfusion.
- Contraction: if LV function is poor, inotropic support/inodilators may be required.

Severity of AR is assessed by echocardiography with colour-flow Doppler; the dimensions of the jet into the LV cavity on apical five-chamber view indicate severity. A jet width >60% at cusp level indicates severe AR (the 5th chamber is the aortic root).

Post-bypass
- Before coming off CPB, the heart/valve is assessed by TOE.
- Preload: because of LV dilatation, adequate filling is essential and must be maintained.
- SVR: a reduction will encourage forward flow, particularly if the LV is impaired.
- Contraction: inotropic support may be required. An inodilator (e.g. milrinone, enoximone) will both reduce the SVR and improve LV function.

Special considerations
- An IABP (see → p. 334) is contraindicated in AR but may be useful post-bypass when the aortic valve is competent to offload the LV and optimize the cardiac output, and to augment the diastolic pressure and hence CBF.
- Careful control of BP is needed pre-bypass in patients with aortic root dilatation or dissection. Aim to keep systolic BP <120mmHg with vasodilators/volatile agents.

With mixed regurgitant/stenotic lesions, manage the dominant lesion.

Mitral valve replacement: stenosis

(See also ➔ p. 54.)

Procedure	Replacement of aortic valve
Time	4hr
Pain	+++/++++
Position	Supine
Blood loss	Moderate (X-match 2U)
Practical techniques	As for CABG + PAFC and TOE

Prosthetic mitral valves are often mechanical—most patients are anticoagulated anyway because of chronic AF.

Preoperative
- Frail, flushed, often in AF and on warfarin, with a fixed cardiac output and possible pulmonary hypertension.
- Almost always due to rheumatic heart disease, normally asymptomatic for >20yr.
- Surgery required if dyspnoea on mild exertion/at rest.
- Continue antiarrhythmic therapy, and convert those on warfarin to heparin preoperatively.
- Echocardiography and angiography to assess PAP, ventricular function, and coronary arteries.
- Opioid/anticholinergic premedication with O_2 supplementation.

Normal valve surface area	4–6cm^2
Symptom-free until	1.6–2.5cm^2
Moderate stenosis	1–1.5cm^2
Severe stenosis	<1.0cm^2

Perioperative
- HR: the mitral flow is relatively fixed; keep <100bpm and sinus rhythm, if possible, to maximize the time for diastole and CBF.
- Preload: does not normally need to be augmented pre-bypass.
- SVR: because of fixed cardiac output, the SVR is often raised—avoid reducing it, as the diastolic pressure will fall and, with it, CBF. Venodilatation will also reduce the cardiac return and cardiac output, for which the heart cannot compensate.

- PVR: pulmonary hypertension 2° to raised PVR and PAPs may be at least partially reversible. Avoid pulmonary vasoconstriction, and consider techniques to improve pulmonary vasodilatation:
  - Maintain filling pressures
  - Avoid hypoxia/hypercapnia, even at the expense of raised mean intrathoracic pressures
  - Check ABGs regularly—avoid acidosis
  - Pulmonary vasodilators if PAP > two-thirds systemic pressure—nitric oxide (NO) is the 1st-line choice, alternatively inhaled epoprostenol (prostacyclin), and consider PDE inhibitors (milrinone, sildenafil).
- Contraction: severe mitral stenosis leads to pulmonary hypertension and, with it, RV failure. The LV is normally unaffected until end-stage disease. Inotropic support (e.g. adrenaline) may be required if the RV is very dilated and failing.
- HR: disruption of conducting pathways from surgery can cause heart block and arrhythmias, requiring pacing and/or chronotropic agents (e.g. atropine, isoprenaline).

Post-bypass

- TOE, following valve insertion, will check valve and heart function.
- Preload: keep well filled, as obstruction to flow has been removed (pulmonary artery occlusion pressure, PAOP 13–16mmHg).
- SVR: a reduction will now encourage forward flow.
- PVR: maintain pulmonary vasodilatation to optimize pulmonary blood flow and left-sided filling.
- Contraction: inotropic support (e.g. adrenaline) may be required if the RV is failing, in order to optimize the cardiac output.

Special considerations

- Use a PAFC to assess PAP, PVR, filling, and requirement for inotropes.
- PAPs take several days/weeks to decrease; avoid hypoxia, hypercapnia, and acidosis. NO/pulmonary vasodilators may help. Use vasoconstrictors only with caution.
- Catastrophic AV disruption (rupture) in the early post-operative period is rare and usually fatal.

Mitral valve replacement: regurgitation

(See also ➽ p. 54.)

Procedure	Replacement or repair of mitral valve
Time	4hr
Pain	+++/++++
Position	Supine
Blood loss	Moderate (X-match 2U)
Practical techniques	As for CABG + PAFC and TOE

Preoperative

- May result from papillary muscle rupture due to MI; therefore, IHD may coexist. If acute, may cause pulmonary oedema.
- Seventy-five per cent of cases have AF. Continue antiarrhythmic therapy, and change warfarin to heparin. The LV is volume-overloaded; MR increases PAP and may cause RV failure.

Perioperative

- 'Full, fast, and forward for a regurgitant lesion.'
- HR: avoid bradycardia; maintain HR >70/min (increases forward flow but also increases regurgitation).
- Preload: keep the patient well filled, again to encourage forward flow.
- SVR: an increase in SVR increases the regurgitant fraction. Vasoconstrictors should be avoided if there is a drop in BP—fluids should be given to supplement the circulating blood volume. Avoid bradycardia.
- PVR: avoid pulmonary vasoconstriction, and attempt to decrease PVR (see Mitral valve replacement: stenosis, ➽ p. 340). PAP monitoring is useful.
- Contraction: inotropes are rarely needed pre-bypass; however, with acute MR, an IABP decreases the afterload and improves the cardiac output.

Severity of MR relates to the regurgitant fraction and PVR.
- Echocardiography with colour-flow Doppler:
    - If regurgitant jet fills area of left atrium >8cm^2 = severe MR
    - If regurgitant jet fills area of left atrium <4cm^2 = mild MR.
- Raised PAP = chronic significant MR (pulmonary hypertension).

Post-bypass

- LV function is often overestimated preoperatively in MR, as the pulmonary circulation provides a low-pressure release system for a poor ventricle. On replacing the valve, the LV has to work harder, which may precipitate failure and the need for inotropes/inodilators.
- Preload: adequate filling is still essential.

- SVR: afterload reduction will benefit the forward flow and cardiac output.
- PVR: the pulmonary vasculature is often highly reactive and prone to vasoconstrictive spells. Avoid factors causing pulmonary vasoconstriction (hypoxia, hypercapnia, acidosis), and consider pulmonary vasodilators. Although IPPV raises the mean intrathoracic pressure, and hence PVR, this is more than offset by the pulmonary vasodilatation resulting from optimized ABGs (see also ➔ p. 340). Inadequate circulatory filling will collapse pulmonary blood vessels, increasing PVR.
- Contraction: inotropic support may be required for a failing LV.

Special considerations

- A PAFC is indicated in MR, as PAP monitoring and correct ventricular filling are essential.
- An IABP may also be of use in the short term for a failing LV (see ➔ p. 334).
- Pacing may be required if the conduction system has been surgically damaged.
- Mitral valve repair is increasingly attempted in these patients. Anaesthetic management is similar to mitral valve replacement; TOE following repair and before coming off CPB is mandatory.

Thoracic aortic surgery

Procedure	Replacement of ascending aorta/aortic arch with a tubular graft
Time	3–6hr
Pain	+++/++++
Position	Supine
Blood loss	Moderate/severe (X-match 6U)
Practical techniques	As for CABG ± deep hypothermic circulatory arrest

General considerations
- Thoracic aortic aneurysms and dissection are usually due to atherosclerosis. They can be divided into two groups: those with hypertension and those with hereditary conditions such as Marfan's syndrome.
- More than 66% have coexisting IHD, and dilatation of the aortic root with AR is common.
- They are classified as type A, involving the ascending aorta to the brachiocephalic artery, and type B, the arch/descending aorta.
- Type A and those involving the arch are treated surgically; the remainder of type B (descending lesions) are treated medically.
- Arch involvement, although rare, is treated surgically under deep hypothermic circulatory arrest.
- They may present as elective or emergency procedures.

Preoperative
- For emergency dissections, control of BP and bleeding, and fluid resuscitation are the main priorities. Wide-bore venous access is essential; consider inserting a PA catheter sheath (for rapid transfusion through the side-arm and later placement of PAFC), though beware distressing a conscious patient and causing hypertension. An arterial line should be inserted under LA pre-induction; be aware of unequal pulses.
- Cross-match 6U of red cells urgently; warn the laboratory regarding the need for clotting factors, platelets, and more blood later.
- Vasodilators (e.g. GTN, labetalol) may be required to keep the systolic pressure <120mmHg.

- Managing hospital transfer of patient for emergency thoracic aortic surgery.
- Adequate analgesia.
- O_2.
- Wide-bore IV access.
- Monitoring: invasive BP plus NIBP monitoring on contralateral arm, SpO_2, ECG.
- BP control/antihypertensive therapy (e.g. labetalol infusion)

Perioperative

- It is essential to avoid hypertension during induction, as this can rupture the thoracic aorta.
- Once stable, patients should be treated as those with AR (see ➔ p. 342)—avoid bradycardia and reduced afterload, and keep well filled.
- Inotropes/vasoconstrictors should be avoided, as any dissection can extend or rupture.
- Be aware that a dissection and surgical clamps may interfere with invasive arterial monitoring.
- Tranexamic acid (see Cardiopulmonary bypass, ➔ p. 327) should be administered to decrease thrombolysis. Clotting should be monitored with TEG.
- Femoral artery cannulation is usually required, as the ascending aorta is to be resected; administer heparin (300IU/kg), and ensure adequate anticoagulation (ACT >400s) before femoral cannulation.
- If the aortic root is involved, the aortic valve may need to be replaced, and the coronary arteries reimplanted.
- Perform regular ABGs, and monitor acid–base for indices of organ perfusion.
- Inotropic support (e.g. adrenaline) may be required before coming off bypass.

Post-bypass

- Bleeding and control of the arterial pressure are major problems.
- Following administration of protamine, check coagulation; if indicated, administer clotting factors (FFP, platelets, cryoprecipitate).
- Meticulous control of systolic pressure at <120mmHg.
- Aortic dissection may involve renal and mesenteric vessels—monitor indices of kidney/gut perfusion.

Special considerations

Circulatory arrest

- Protection of the CNS by deep hypothermia during prolonged periods of circulatory arrest is necessary if the arch of the aorta is to be operated on (during this procedure, it is not possible to perfuse the cerebral vessels reliably on bypass).
- Hypothermia depresses the metabolic rate and O_2 consumption in the brain and also seems to protect the cerebral integrity during reperfusion. The maximum safe duration of **deep hypothermic circulatory arrest (DHCA)** is thought to be ~45min at 18°C. In neonates, this can be extended to 60min.
- Most centres do not rely solely on hypothermia to protect the brain; the head can be packed in ice, and consider adding thiopental (7mg/kg) or steroid, e.g. methylprednisolone (15mg/kg), and mannitol (0.5g/kg) to the pump prime, in an effort to decrease the cerebral metabolic demand further and protect against ischaemic damage.
- The shorter the period of DHCA, the better. The incidence of post-operative neurological problems is directly proportional to the time of DHCA.

- To aid rapid cooling, and to ensure that the brain is cooled, a vasodilator (e.g. GTN) is given. This prevents localized vasoconstriction due to hypothermia.
- Once the circulation has been arrested, all infusions and pumps are stopped.
- It is essential to measure both the core (rectal) and skin temperature and to make sure the core temperature reaches <20°C; measurement of the nasopharyngeal or tympanic temperature may be regarded as the cerebral temperature.
- On rewarming, remove head ice packs; switch on warming blankets, but do not set to >10°C above the patient temperature in order to avoid burns. Start propofol infusion (3–6mg/kg/hr, as tolerated); check coagulation, and, if necessary, order FFP (4U) and platelets (one pooled donor pack), as these patients frequently encounter bleeding problems. A vasodilator (e.g. GTN), if tolerated, may be used to maintain vasodilatation and help rewarming.
- Mannitol (0.5g/kg) may also be given to encourage diuresis.
- When the core temperature reaches 35°C, start an inotrope (e.g. adrenaline) to improve the cardiac function.
- A steep head-down tilt is used to allow air out of the aortic graft. Keeping the patient warm is difficult, as it takes a considerable time to warm thoroughly. Skin temperature must be >33°C, with a core temperature of ≥37°C, before attempting to come off bypass. Do not rush, as rebound cooling occurs in recovery, which will exacerbate poor myocardial function and any coagulopathy.

Pulmonary thromboembolectomy

Procedure	Removal of clot/tumour from PA
Time	2–3hr
Pain	++/+++
Position	Supine
Blood loss	Moderate (X-match 4U)
Practical techniques	As for CABG

Preoperative

- The patient is often collapsed—resuscitation may be in progress.
- Presentation with tachycardia, tachypnoea, hypoxia, cyanosis with distended neck veins, haemoptysis, and signs of RV failure.
- A healthy heart requires 50–80% of the pulmonary trunk to be obstructed before RV failure.
- The patient may have recently received thrombolytic therapy.
- Urgent CPB to re-establish oxygenation is the priority, so rapid decision-making is essential.

Perioperative

- Once the decision is taken to operate, speed is the key—allow no delays. Do not forget to give heparin (300IU/kg).
- Intubate, and ventilate with 100% O_2, maintaining perfusion with inotropes, as necessary, and institute CPB as soon as possible.
- There may be substantial airway haemorrhage from pulmonary infarction. Ventilation may be difficult, and the ETT may require frequent suctioning. A double-lumen ETT may be helpful to control pulmonary bleeding and aid ventilation.
- The surgeons should consider placing an IVC filter post-embolectomy.

Post-bypass

- Inotropic support is likely to be needed; keep well filled, and reduce SVR with vasodilators, if tolerated.
- Pulmonary vascular reactivity is often increased post-embolectomy. NO, inhaled epoprostenol, or a PDE inhibitor (e.g. milrinone, sildenafil) may help reduce a raised PAP. Adrenaline may be required to support RV function. Delay heparinization (following CPB) for 24hr to reduce surgical bleeding.

Special considerations

- Very high right-sided pressures may open the foramen ovale and cause right-to-left shunting. This will worsen hypoxia and may allow paradoxical emboli, causing a CVA.
- With significant PEs, the capnograph will detect very little or no expired CO_2. Following embolectomy, if successful, this should show dramatic improvement, as the pulmonary circulation is re-established.

Pulmonary embolism

Diagnosis
- Chest pain, dyspnoea, tachypnoea, haemoptysis, cyanosis, tachycardia, dysrhythmia, raised JVP, hypotension, oliguria, collapse, arrest.
- ABGs: hypoxia, hypo-/hypercapnia, metabolic acidosis.
- CXR: oligaemic lung fields, prominent PA.
- ECG: $S_1Q_3T_3$, RV strain, normal in 50% of cases.
- Te/Xe V/Q lung scan, pulmonary angiography, spiral CTPA.

Assessment of severity
- Minor (<30% pulmonary obstruction, no RV dysfunction):
  - Non-specific symptoms, pleuritic chest pain, dyspnoea, tiredness
  - Specific treatment: anticoagulation (heparin, then warfarin).
- Moderate (30–50% pulmonary obstruction, some RV dysfunction, but normotensive):
  - Haemoptysis, tachypnoea → respiratory alkalosis, raised JVP, tachycardia
  - Specific treatment: thrombolysis.
- Massive (>50% pulmonary obstruction, severe RV failure, and haemodynamic impairment/collapse):
  - Severe chest pain, dyspnoea, hypotension, hypoxia, syncope, shock, arrest
  - Specific treatment: embolectomy.

General treatment
- O_2, IV access, fluid resuscitation, analgesia, inotropic support, ventilatory support, as required. Specific treatment (see Assessment of severity above), according to severity.

CTPA, computed tomography pulmonary angiography.

Redo cardiac surgery

Preoperative

- There is often poor LV function.
- Venous/arterial access as for CABG, but often more difficult.
- Cross-match 6U of blood.

Perioperative

- Place external defibrillator pads on the patient, as VF is a risk at sternotomy and during the dissection of adhesions. This can be a problem with extensive use of diathermy, as it obscures the ECG, and, with VF, all you may notice is a flat arterial trace (be vigilant).
- Femoral cannulation may be required for CPB; give heparin (300IU/kg) before femoral artery cannulation.
- There is a risk of torrential bleeding, as the RV may be stuck by adhesions to the underside of the sternum. Ensure adequate wide-bore venous access (e.g. PAFC sheath), and have blood checked and available in theatre. In the event of uncontrolled RV haemorrhage on sternotomy, it may be necessary to go on to femoral CPB urgently.
- Damage to a previous coronary graft during dissection of adhesions is also possible, leading to myocardial ischaemia. Monitor the ECG.
- Coagulopathy is common. Monitor TEG, and consider giving tranexamic acid (see Cardiopulmonary bypass, ➲ p. 327).

Post-operative

- There is increased risk of post-operative bleeding. After administering protamine, check coagulation, and administer appropriate clotting factors, if indicated.
- There may be problems related to poor LV function.

Cardioversion

Procedure	DC shock to convert an arrhythmia back to sinus rhythm
Time	5–10min
Pain	–
Position	Supine
Blood loss	Nil
Practical techniques	Monitor ECG/SpO$_2$/NIBP; IV access; propofol ± LMA; ETT if full stomach

Preoperative

- AF is the commonest arrhythmia—acute or chronic.
- Often a remote site, with patients who are cardiovascularly unstable.
- If possible, transfer to an anaesthetic room in theatre with help nearby.
- Treat as for any surgical procedure, and have a physician ready to cardiovert the patient. K$^+$ should be in the normal range, as the myocardium may become unstable.
- If in AF >24hr and not anticoagulated, the left atrium should be checked for clot with TOE before cardioversion. This can be done under propofol sedation. If a clot is present, anticoagulation for 4wk is required, and then check again. If clear, continue with propofol, and secure the airway, as appropriate.

Perioperative

- Attach monitoring; depending on the model of the defibrillator, if necessary, connect ECG leads through the defibrillator, and synchronize to the R wave.
- Any 'day-case' GA suitable, including sevoflurane by inhalation.
- Preoxygenate; induce slowly with, e.g., a minimal dose of propofol. Maintain the airway using a face mask. RSI/ETT if risk of aspiration.
- Consider etomidate if haemodynamically unstable.
- Opioids/muscle relaxants are not usually necessary.
- Obese patients and those who are likely to have an awkward airway can be defibrillated in the lateral position.
- Safety during defibrillation—follow the advanced life support (ALS) protocol. Remove O$_2$ during shock.
- AF—start at 150J biphasic defibrillator, 200J standard defibrillator. Atrial flutter—start with 50J, and increase by increments of 50J (depending on the model of the defibrillator, some advise full shock to start).

Post-operative

- Turn the patient into the recovery position, with supplemental O$_2$, and recover with full monitoring as for any anaesthetic.

Special considerations

- Digoxin increases the risk of arrhythmia—omit on the day.
- Amiodarone improves the success of cardioversion to sinus rhythm.

Anaesthesia for implantable defibrillators

Procedure	Implanting pacemaker/defibrillator
Time	1–3hr
Pain	+
Position	Supine
Blood loss	Nil
Practical techniques	LA + sedation; GA: ETT/IPPV or LMA/SV ± invasive arterial monitoring

General considerations

- Implantable defibrillators are placed in patients who are at risk of sudden death due to malignant cardiac arrhythmias. Patients range from young and otherwise fit adults with normal cardiac contractility to extremely compromised cardiac patients.
- The procedure may be straightforward, when two venous wires (sensing and shocking) are positioned transvenously, or complex when pacemakers are replaced or the coronary sinus is catheterized to gain access to the LV myocardium.
- In many units, cardiologists provide their own sedation service.
- During the procedure, VF is induced on a number of occasions to test the device. The patient needs to be sedated during this phase.
- Invasive monitoring (arterial line) is advisable for any patients with impaired contractility.
- The cardiologist usually gains access via the left cephalic vein and uses fluoroscopy to guide the position of the leads.
- Careful asepsis is important to avoid infection of the prosthesis.
- Prophylactic IV antibiotics are indicated.
- Monitor the total dose of LA used by the cardiologist.

Preoperative

- Careful assessment is required to assess the functional cardiac reserve. Use LA and sedation for anyone who is compromised. Check the coagulation status, as patients in paroxysmal dysrhythmia may be warfarinized.
- Ensure resuscitation drugs and equipment are available, as well as an external defibrillator.
- Draw up vasopressors and vagolytic drugs ready for use (e.g. ephedrine/metaraminol/glycopyrronium). Have dedicated, skilled assistance.
- Give a good explanation to the patient of what will happen.

Perioperative

- If sedation is planned, give small doses of a short-acting sedative (e.g. midazolam) and an opioid (e.g. fentanyl) until comfortable, cooperative,

but sleepy. Administer O_2. Deepen the sedation immediately before defibrillator testing—propofol TCI is ideal at minimal doses.
- If the defibrillator is to be placed under the muscle, it is often difficult to get fully effective regional anaesthesia, and a short period of deeper sedation/anaesthesia may be required.
- If GA is planned, ensure recovery is organized preoperatively. Use light anaesthesia with careful induction, as many of these patients have limited cardiac reserve. An X-ray table may not tip, and induction may be safer on a tilting trolley.
- ECG is recorded by the cardiologist.
- Antibiotics will be required, according to local protocols.

Special considerations
- During VF testing, if the device does not work, do not allow the heart to be stopped for long. Repeated shocks may be required.
- After VF and defibrillation, the BP may remain low for a short period. Vasopressors may be required.
- If the patient has an existing pacemaker to be changed, and the cardiologist is using diathermy, loss of pacemaker function can occur.
- Cardiac catheter laboratories are difficult places to work in—space may be at a premium. Do not allow yourself to be distracted by the range of other activities taking place.
- A large plastic sheet (similar to an awake carotid set-up) allows the anaesthetist access to the patient's airway without compromising sterility. Infection is a serious complication.
- Broadly similar anaesthetic considerations apply to transcatheter ablation procedures for chronic AF. These may be pulmonary vein ostial segmental disconnection (OSD) or left atrial circumferential ablation (LACA). These procedures (typically >3hr) are performed in the cardiac angiography suite; light GA, with ETT/IPPV, TCI (e.g. propofol, remifentanil), and full monitoring are appropriate. Ensure patients are kept warm.

Further reading

Andropoulos DB, Stayer SA, Russell IA, Mossad EB, eds. (2010). *Anesthesia for congenital heart disease.* Hoboken: Wiley Blackwell.

Berton C, Cholley B (2002). Equipment review: new techniques for cardiac output measurement—oesophageal Doppler, Fick principle using carbon dioxide, and pulse contour analysis. *Crit Care,* **6**, 216–21.

Braithwaite S, Kluin J, Buhre WF, de Waal EE (2010). Anaesthesia in the cardiac catheterization laboratory. *Curr Opin Anaesthesiol,* **23**, 507–12.

Chamorro C, Borrallo JM, Romera MA, Silva JA, Balandin B (2010). Anesthesia and analgesia protocol during therapeutic hypothermia after cardiac arrest: a systematic review. *Anesth Analg,* **110**, 1328–35.

Falk SA (2011). Anesthetic considerations for the patient undergoing therapy for advanced heart failure. *Curr Opin Anaesthesiol,* **24**, 314–19.

Feussner M, Mukherjee C, Garbade J, Ender J (2012). Anaesthesia for patients undergoing ventricular-assist device implantation. *Best Pract Res Clin Anaesthesiol,* **26**, 167–77.

Frogel J, Galusca D (2010). Anesthetic considerations for patients with advanced valvular heart disease undergoing non-cardiac surgery. *Anesthesiol Clin,* **28**, 67–85.

Haas S, Richter HP, Kubitz JC (2009). Anesthesia during cardiologic procedures. *Curr Opin Anaesthesiol,* **22**, 519–23.

Habicher M, Perrino A, Spies CD, von Heymann C, Wittkowski U, Sander M (2011). Contemporary fluid management in cardiac anesthesia. *J Cardiothorac Vasc Anesth*, **25**, 1141–53.

Hemmerling TM, Romano G, Terrasini N, Noiseux N (2013). Anesthesia for off-pump coronary artery bypass surgery. *Ann Card Anaesth*, **16**, 28–39.

Hensley FA, Gravlee GP, Martin DE, eds. (2012). *A practical approach to cardiac anesthesia*, 5th edn. Philadelphia: Lippincott, Williams & Wilkins.

Huffmyer J, Raphael J (2011). The current status of off-pump coronary bypass surgery. *Curr Opin Anaesthesiol*, **24**, 64–9.

Kaplan JA, Reich DL, Savino JS, eds. (2011). *Kaplan's cardiac anesthesia: the echo era*, 6th edn. St Louis: Saunders-Elsevier.

Kertai MD, Whitlock EL, Avidan MS (2012). Brain monitoring with electroencephalography and the electroencephalogram-derived bispectral index. *Anesth Analg*, **114**, 533–46.

Klein A, Vuylsteke A, Nashef SAM, eds. (2008). *Core topics in cardiothoracic critical care*. Cambridge: Cambridge University Press.

Schonberger RB, Haddadin AS (2010). The anaesthesia patient with acute coronary syndrome. *Anesthesiol Clin*, **28**, 55–66.

Stone KR, McPherson CA (2004). Assessment and management of patients with pacemakers and implantable cardioverter defibrillators. *Crit Care Med*, **32**, S155–65.

Timperley J, Leeson P, Mitchell ARJ, Betts T, eds. (2007). *Pacemakers and ICDs (Oxford Specialist Handbooks in Cardiology)*. Oxford: Oxford University Press.

Wasnick JD, Hillel Z, Kramer D, Littwin S, Nicoara A, eds. (2011). *Cardiac anesthesia and transesophageal echocardiography*. New York: McGraw-Hill Medical.

Thoracic surgery

Claire Todd and Bruce McCormick

General principles

Successful thoracic anaesthesia requires the ability to control ventilation of the patient's two lungs independently, skilful management of the shared lung and airway, and a clear understanding of planned surgery. Good communication between the surgeon and anaesthetist is essential.

Patients undergoing thoracic surgery are commonly older and less fit than other patients (30% >70yr, 50% > ASA 3). Long-term smoking, bronchial carcinoma, pleural effusion, cardiac disease, oesophageal obstruction, and cachexia are all common and can significantly reduce the cardiorespiratory physiological reserve.

General considerations

- Discuss the planned procedure and any potential problems with the surgeon. The surgical procedure may change during the case because of intraoperative findings.
- Optimize lung function before elective surgery—try to stop patients smoking; arrange preoperative physiotherapy and incentive spirometry. Optimize bronchodilator therapy, and consider a course of oral steroids.
- The lateral decubitus position with the operating table 'broken' to separate the ribs is used for the majority of procedures.
- Post-operative mechanical ventilation stresses pulmonary suture lines and increases air leaks and the risk of chest infection, so avoid, if possible.
- Minimize post-operative respiratory dysfunction by providing good analgesia and physiotherapy.
- Prescribe post-operative O_2 therapy routinely to compensate for increased V/Q mismatch. Warmed humidified 40% O_2 via a face mask is recommended after pulmonary surgery. Nasal cannulae delivering O_2 at 3L/min are better tolerated and satisfactory for most other patients.

Preoperative assessment

- Patients require a standard assessment, with particular emphasis on the cardiorespiratory reserve.
- Examine the most recent CXR and CT scans. Check for airway obstruction and tracheal or carinal distortion/compression, which can cause difficulties with double-lumen tube placement. Examine for other lung pathology, such as bullae and effusions, which will impact on the patient's response to ventilation and lung isolation.
- Discuss scans with the surgeon—tumours impinging on the chest wall, crossing fissures, or in proximity to major vessels have implications for the surgery performed.
- Patients with significant cardiac disease form a high-risk group.

Lung resection

Based on history, examination, and simple PFTs, patients may be classified as:[1,2]

- Clinically fit with good exercise tolerance and normal spirometry—accept for surgery

- Major medical problems, minimal exercise capacity, and grossly impaired PFTs—high risk for surgery; consider alternative treatment
- Reduced exercise capacity (short of breath on climbing two flights of stairs) and abnormal spirometry, with or without moderate coexisting disease—require careful evaluation of risks/benefits of surgery.

PFTs (see ➍ p. 88 and p. 1223) are often used to determine suitability for lung resection surgery by estimating the post-operative lung function. Always consider the results in the context of the patient's general health and proposed resection.

- Spirometry reflects the 'bellows' function of the respiratory system, while tests of diffusion capacity (e.g. DLCO) assess the ability to transfer O_2 to the circulation. It is important to realize that patients with diffuse alveolar lung disease can have severely impaired gas transfer with relatively normal spirometry (see also ➍ p. 89).
- Generally accepted minimum preoperative values of FEV_1 for the following procedures are: pneumonectomy >55%, lobectomy >40%, wedge resection >35% of the patient's predicted value.
- Predicted post-operative (ppo) value of PFTs is preoperative value × (5 − number of lobes resected)/5. The goal is for ppoFEV_1 and ppoDLCO >40% of the predicted normal (FEV_1 0.8–1.0L for the average ♂).
- If preoperative DLCO <40% predicted normal, ppoFEV_1 <800mL, or ppoFVC <15mL/kg, it is likely that post-operative ventilation will be needed (poor cough with an FVC <1L).
- Ventilation scans may be used to account for non-functional lung (e.g. atelectasis beyond an obstructing tumour).
- CPET is used in the preoperative assessment of thoracic patients. It is particularly useful for 'borderline cases'.
- A multidisciplinary approach is essential and should involve the anaesthetist, surgeon, respiratory physician, and radiologist.

Important scenarios encountered by thoracic anaesthetists

- **Subglottic obstruction** of the trachea/carina from extrinsic compression (retrosternal thyroid, lymph node masses, etc.) or invasion of the lumen, usually by a bronchial or oesophageal carcinoma.
- **Dynamic hyperinflation** of the lungs following positive pressure ventilation in patients with severe emphysema, bullae, lung cysts, or in the presence of an airway obstruction acting as a 'flap valve' resulting in gas trapping. Progressive lung distension creates the mechanical equivalent of a tension pneumothorax. The increase in intrathoracic pressure compromises the venous return and RV function, dramatically reducing the cardiac output. 'Pulseless electrical activity (PEA) arrest' may follow. Emergency treatment is to disconnect the patient from the ventilator, open the tracheal tube (TT) to the atmosphere, relieve any airway obstruction, and support RV function. Remember, 'if in doubt, let it (the trapped gas) out!'[3]
- **Significant mediastinal shifts** can occur due to large pleural effusions, tension pneumothorax, and lateral positioning, leading to a severe

reduction in the cardiac output. Prompt recognition and correction of the underlying cause is vital.

- **Sudden falls in cardiac output** presenting as acute severe hypotension can be **caused by surgical manipulation** within the chest, obstructing the venous return or cardiac filling. The effects can be reduced by volume-loading the patient, but the surgeon or assistant should be advised and requested to 'stop squashing the heart!'

Miscellaneous thoracic procedures

Table 15.1 presents the important information for these procedures that are not covered in the individual topics within this chapter.

References

1 Lim E, Baldwin D, Beckles M, *et al.*; British Thoracic Society; Society for Cardiothoracic Surgery in Great Britain and Ireland (2010). Guidelines on the radical management of patients with lung cancer. *Thorax*, **65** (Suppl 3), iii1–27.
2 Gould G, Pearce A (2006). Assessment of suitability for lung resection. *Contin Educ Anaesth Crit Care Pain*, 97–100.
3 Conacher I (1998). Dynamic hyperinflation—the anaesthetist applying a tourniquet to the right heart. *Br J Anaesth*, **81**, 116–17.

Table 15.1 Miscellaneous thoracic procedures

Operation	Description	Time	Pain	Position/approach	Blood loss/ X-match	Notes
Fibreoptic bronchoscopy	Visual inspection of tracheobronchial tree ± biopsy and bronchial brushings/lavage	5–10min	+	Supine	None	GA rarely used. Single-lumen tube (SLT) (8–9mm) with bronchoscopy diaphragm on angle piece. IPPV with relaxant appropriate to duration. Expect high airway pressures while scope in ETT. Suction can empty breathing system
Lung biopsy	Diagnostic sampling of lung tissue for localized or diffuse abnormality	30–60min	+++/++++	Lateral/VATS or mini-thoracotomy	Minor/ G&S: X-match if anaemic	DLT and OLV facilitate VATS procedures. Patients with diffuse disease can have very poor lung function—risk of ventilator dependence and significant mortality
Oesophagoscopy and dilatation (O&D)	Visual inspection of oesophagus via rigid or fibreoptic scope ± dilatation of stricture with flexible bougies or balloon	5–20min	−/+	Supine	None	Regurgitation risk, so RSI advised. SLT on left side of mouth—watch for airway obstruction and ETT displacement during procedure. Flexible oesophagoscopy often done under IV sedation

(Continued)

Table 15.1 (Contd.)

Operation	Description	Time	Pain	Position/approach	Blood loss/X-match	Notes
Oesophageal stent insertion	Endoscopic placement of tubular stent through oesophageal stricture	10–30min	+/++	Supine	None	Often emaciated, may be anaemic. Preoperative IV fluids to correct dehydration. RSI, SLT, and awake extubation in lateral position. Small risk of oesophageal rupture
Fundoplication/hiatus hernia repair	'Anti-reflux' procedure—fundus of stomach wrapped round lower oesophagus, may require a gastroplasty to lengthen oesophagus	2–3 hr	++++/+++++	Supine/laparotomy. Lateral/left thoracotomy. Now often done laparoscopically	Moderate/G&S; if Hb <12, X-match 2U	Fundoplication patients often obese—check respiratory function. RSI or AFOI mandatory. NGT required. DLT helpful for thoracic approach. Epidural or paravertebral catheter and PCA recommended
Pectus excavatum/carinatum repair	Correction of 'funnel chest'/'pigeon chest' deformity of sternum	3–5hr	+++/++++	Supine—arms to sides/midline sternal incision	Moderate to severe/X-match 2U	Primarily cosmetic unless deformity severe. Usually young fit adults. GA, IPPV via SLT, and mid-thoracic epidural recommended. Risk of pneumothoraces. Minimally invasive technique for pectus excavatum repair is becoming increasingly popular—epidural still recommended, although some centres use PCA

| Thymectomy | Excision of residual thymic tissue and/or thymoma from superior and anterior mediastinum | 2–3hr | ++/+++ | Supine—arms to sides/median sternotomy | Moderate/ X-match 2U | Usually for myasthenia gravis. Check for airway compression, other autoimmune diseases, thyroid function, and steroid, immunosuppressive, and anticholinesterase therapy (see ⊕ p. 242). GA, IPPV via SLT, IV anaesthesia, minimal or no relaxant, and monitoring of neuromuscular transmission. May need post-operative ventilatory support |

Analgesia

- Thoracotomy incisions are extremely painful. Inadequate pain relief increases the neurohumoral stress response and impairs mobilization and respiration, leading to an increase in respiratory complications.
- Chronic pain syndrome after thoracic surgery occurs in 25–60% of patients.[4] The multiple pathogenic mechanisms proposed include pre-, intra-, and post-operative factors.
- Effective analgesia is crucial, and a technique combining paracetamol, NSAIDs, a regional block, intraoperative opioids, and regular or post-operative PCA is recommended.
- Perioperative intercostal nerve blocks or percutaneous paravertebral blocks are useful for thoracoscopic procedures, with oral or opioid PCA post-operatively.
- Unless specifically contraindicated, patients undergoing thoracotomy or thoracoabdominal incisions should receive continuous thoracic epidural or paravertebral regional analgesia. These techniques have equivalent analgesic efficacy, and similar effects on the stress response and respiratory function. Paravertebral blockade is associated with fewer adverse events (hypotension, urinary retention, and PONV).[5]
- With either technique, it is imperative to match the level of block to that of the incision—usually T5/6 or T6/7.
- Perioperative epidural blockade should be established cautiously (3–4mL of 0.25% bupivacaine), as an extensive thoracic sympathetic block can cause a major reduction in the cardiac output and severe hypotension.
- Percutaneous paravertebral injection of 0.5% bupivacaine (0.3mL/kg) may be performed. A continuous post-operative infusion of bupivacaine (0.5% for 24hr, then 0.25% for 3–4d) at 0.1mL/kg/hr via a surgically placed paravertebral catheter provides excellent post-thoracotomy analgesia.

References

4 Wildgaard K, Ravn J, Kehlet H (2009). Chronic post-thoracotomy pain: a critical review of pathogenic mechanisms and strategies for prevention. *Eur J Cardiothorac Surg*, **36**, 170–80.
5 Gulbahar G, Kocer B, Muratli SN, *et al.* (2010). A comparison of epidural and paravertebral catheterization techniques in post-thoracotomy pain management. *Eur J Cardiothorac Surg*, **37**, 467–72.

Isolation of the lungs

- Achieving independent ventilation of the lungs is not always straightforward.
- One-lung ventilation (OLV)[6] is associated with a number of complications and should be used only when the benefits outweigh the risks.

Advantages of one-lung ventilation

- Protects the dependent lung from blood and secretions.
- Allows independent control of ventilation to each lung.
- Improves surgical access and reduces lung trauma.

Disadvantages of one-lung ventilation

- Inevitably creates a shunt and usually causes hypoxia.
- Acute lung injury (ALI) occurs in 2–5% of cases.
- Increases technical and physiological challenge.

Indications for isolation and separation of the two lungs

- To avoid contamination of a lung in cases of infection, massive pulmonary haemorrhage, or bronchopulmonary lavage.
- To control the distribution of ventilation in massive air leaks or severe unilateral lung disease (e.g. giant bullae and lung cysts).
- Improving access for surgery is a *relative* indication for OLV. If isolation of the lung proves difficult, the need to pursue OLV should be discussed with the surgeon, since satisfactory access can often be achieved by careful lung retraction.

Techniques

- **Double-lumen endobronchial tubes** (DLTs) are the commonest and most versatile approach.
- **Bronchial blockers** (Univent tube or Arndt endobronchial blocker). Useful in experienced hands, especially in patients who are difficult to intubate or have a distorted tracheobronchial anatomy/tracheostomy.
- DLT and bronchial blockers have been shown to be clinically equivalent in the provision of OLV.[7]
- Single-lumen endobronchial tubes are rarely used.

Double-lumen endobronchial tubes

- Traditional, reusable, red rubber DLTs are still used in some specialist centres, but disposable plastic (polyvinyl chloride—PVC) tubes are in wider general use.
- Described as 'right' or 'left', according to the main bronchus they are designed to intubate.
- Right-sided tubes have a hole or slit in the wall of the endobronchial section to facilitate ventilation of the right upper lobe.
- Sizes of plastic DLTs are given in Charriere (Ch) gauge (equivalent to French gauge), which is the external circumference of the tube in mm. Thus, a 39Ch tube has an external diameter of about 13mm. Note that the diameter of the bronchial segment of the tubes varies between manufacturers (for the same tube gauge).

- The lumens of DLTs are small, compared with standard single-lumen tubes used in adults. The internal diameters of the lumens of the 39 and 35Ch 'Broncho-Cath' DLTs are only 6.0 and 4.5mm, respectively.
- Bronchoscopic placement and checking require a narrow scope (<4mm in diameter), ideally with an integral battery light source for ease of manipulation.
- A major contraindication to the use of a DLT is a very distorted tracheobronchial anatomy or an intraluminal lesion—placement is likely to be difficult and possibly dangerous.

Types of double-lumen endobronchial tube

- Carlens (left-sided): has a carinal 'hook' to aid correct placement.
- White's (right-sided): has a carinal hook and slit in the tube wall for the right upper lobe.
- Robertshaw (right- and left-sided): D-shaped lumens; traditionally a red rubber, reusable tube, now available as a single-use version in small, medium, and large sizes.
- Single-use PVC (right- and left-sided): high-volume, low-pressure cuffs; bronchial cuff and pilot tube coloured blue; radiopaque marker stripe running to the tip of the bronchial lumen; available in sizes 28–41Ch, e.g. 'Broncho-Cath' (Mallinckrodt) and 'Sheribronch' (Sheridan).

Selection of double-lumen endobronchial tube

- Use the largest DLT that will pass easily through the glottis. A 41Ch- or 39Ch-gauge PVC tube (large or medium Robertshaw) for ♂, a 37Ch-gauge PVC tube (medium Robertshaw) for ♀. Small individuals may need a 35Ch-gauge or small Robertshaw tube.
- It is common practice to choose a left-sided tube, unless the surgery involves a proximal left lobar resection or left pneumonectomy, or an abnormal bronchial anatomy is likely to obstruct intubation of the left main bronchus. A left-sided tube is less likely to block a lobar bronchus and gives a greater tolerance to shifts in tube position, which inevitably occur when the patient is moved.
- Where indicated, use a right-sided tube. Placement is generally straightforward if bronchoscopically guided.

Placement of double-lumen endobronchial tube

- Assess the risks/benefits of using a DLT. Examine the X-rays, CT scans, and any previous bronchoscopy reports for tracheobronchial anatomy and lung pathology—is there distortion or narrowing which will interfere with bronchial intubation?
- Check the Y connector, and ensure that 15mm connectors are inserted into the proximal ends of the DLT ('Broncho-Caths' come with these connectors separately wrapped).
- Most plastic DLTs are supplied with a malleable stylet which can be used to adjust the curve of the tube to facilitate intubation.
- Commence intubation with the concavity of the endobronchial section of the DLT facing anteriorly—once the tip is past the glottis, partially withdraw the stylet, and rotate the tube 90° to bring the oropharyngeal

curve into the sagittal plane. Turn the patient's head to the side opposite to the bronchus to be intubated (i.e. to the right for a left-sided DLT), and gently slide the tube down the trachea until resistance is felt to further advancement.

- At this stage, treat DLT as an ordinary ETT—inflate only the tracheal cuff to achieve a seal, and confirm ventilation of both lungs.
- It is easy to push plastic DLTs in too far. The patient's height is the main determinant of correct insertion depth—the usual insertion depth to the corner of the mouth in a patient 170cm (5ft 7in) tall is 29cm (the depth changes by 1cm for every 10cm (4in) change in the patient's height).[8]
- The diameter of a DLT makes intubation more difficult than with a standard tube, even with a good view of the larynx. Alternative strategies in difficult intubation include intubation over an airway exchange catheter (AEC), intubation with a standard tube followed by change to a DLT over an AEC, or use of a bronchial blocker (see ➔ p. 366).[9] Where available, a fibreoptic laryngoscope (e.g. the C-MAC®) can aid placement.

Clinical confirmation of double-lumen endobronchial tube position

- Check the tube position, and establish isolation of lungs. Beware of pathology affecting clinical signs—compare with preoperative clinical examination findings and radiology. It is easy to get confused, so check the tube position by achieving the lung isolation required for the surgery.
- Check that you can achieve ventilation on the non-operative lung first. Clamp off the gas flow to the operative lung at the Y connector, and allow the lung to deflate by opening the sealing cap on this lumen.
- *Look* for chest movement—is there appropriate unilateral expansion on the non-operative side?
- *Listen*—auscultate both lungs, and listen over the end of the open tube. A leak indicates air passing around the deflated bronchial cuff. Listen while inflating the bronchial cuff, 1mL at a time (use a 5mL syringe), until the leak stops. If a reasonable seal cannot be obtained with <4mL of air, the tube is either incorrectly placed or too small for the patient. Check specifically that all lobes are ventilated, especially the right upper if using a right-sided DLT.
- *Feel*—assess compliance by 'bagging' the right, left, and both lungs. Very poor compliance (high inflation pressures) which is not explained by the patient's pathology suggests malposition—peak pressure on OLV should be <35cmH$_2$O.
- Close the sealing cap, and remove the Y connector clamp. Some anaesthetists then confirm it is possible to isolate and achieve OLV of the opposite (operative) lung via the tracheal lumen.
- Remember that the operative lung will only partially collapse until the pleural cavity is opened.
- ETTs often move when the patient is placed in the lateral position. Recheck isolation and OLV once the patient is in position and before surgery starts.

Fibreoptic bronchoscope
- Ideally, the position of every DLT should be checked bronchoscopically. At the very least, a suitable bronchoscope must be immediately available to assess DLT placement if there are clinical problems with the tube or with OLV.
- This is invaluable where bronchial intubation is difficult and can be used to 'railroad' the tube into the correct main bronchus. Insert the bronchoscope via the bronchial lumen; partially withdraw the DLT, so its tip lies in the trachea, and locate the carina. Left–right recognition is aided by looking for the longitudinal trachealis muscle that runs along the posterior wall of the trachea. Advance the scope into the appropriate main bronchus, then slide the tube into position.
- Several bronchoscopic studies have shown that up to 80% of DLTs are malpositioned to some extent, even when clinical signs are satisfactory. The upper surface of the bronchial cuff (blue) should lie just below the carina when visualized via the tracheal lumen.
- Always confirm positioning of the right-sided tube by bronchoscopy. The lateral 'slit' in the wall of the distal bronchial lumen should be aligned with the right upper lobe bronchus.

Bronchial blocker technique
- A balloon-tipped catheter ('blocker') is manipulated through a single-lumen TT into the appropriate main (or lobar) bronchus with the aid of a narrow fibreoptic bronchoscope.
- Good lubrication of both the bronchoscope and blocker is essential.
- The position of the blocker should be rechecked after the patient has been positioned for surgery.
- Placement is usually straightforward in the supine position but can be awkward in the lateral position.
- The lung or lobe is isolated from ventilation by inflating the balloon within the bronchus. The isolated lung slowly collapses, as the trapped gas is absorbed or escapes via the blocker's narrow central lumen.
- Collapse can be accelerated by ventilating with 100% O_2 for a few minutes and then inflating the blocker at end-expiration when lung volume is at its minimum.
- Reinflation of the collapsed lung requires deflation of the blocker, and consequently loss of isolation of the lungs. (A correctly positioned DLT will maintain separation of the airways to each lung until extubation.)
- During pneumonectomy or sleeve resection (bronchial reanastomosis), the blocker has to be withdrawn to allow surgical access to the bronchus.

There are two modern forms of bronchial blocker:
- Univent tube: a single-lumen tube with an internal channel in its wall, containing an adjustable blocker bearing a high-volume, low-pressure cuff
- Arndt wire-guided endobronchial blocker (Cook™): a stiff catheter with a cylindrical cuff and an adjustable 'wire' loop at its tip which guides the blocker along the outside of a fibreoptic bronchoscope into the required bronchus. Supplied with a special adapter which

allows it to be deployed through a conventional single-lumen or cuffed tracheostomy tube.

Indications for using a bronchial blocker

- On the rare occasions when isolation of a lobar bronchus is required (localized bronchiectasis or haemorrhage, lung abscess, bronchopleural fistula, previous lung resection, and poor tolerance of OLV).
- In patients who are difficult to intubate or have a permanent tracheostomy.
- To avoid the reintubation required to change to or from a DLT in patients receiving pre- or post-operative IPPV.

References

6 Dr Gallagher's Neighborhood. *Lung isolation.* http://www.youtube.com/watch?v=9oV_0AbTW6s#t=229.
7 Brodsky JB, Benumof JL, Ehrenwerth J, Ozaki GT (1991). Depth of placement of left double-lumen endobronchial tubes. *Anesth Analg*, 73, 570–2.
8 Brodsky (2009). Lung separation and the difficult airway. *Br J Anaesth*, 103(Suppl 1), i66–75.
9 Campos JH (2003). Which device should be considered the best for lung isolation: double-lumen endotracheal tube versus bronchial blockers. *Curr Opin Anaesthesiol*, 20, 27–31.

Management of one-lung ventilation

The physiology is complex, and some aspects remain controversial.[10] OLV inevitably creates a shunt through the unventilated lung, and the crucial factor in managing OLV is to minimize the effects of this shunt.

Initiating one-lung ventilation

- Start with typical ventilator settings during two-lung ventilation (FiO_2 0.33, V_T 6–8mL/kg, and peak airway pressure (P_{AW}) ≤25cmH$_2$O).
- Increase FiO_2 to 0.5 before initiating OLV. Note the P_{AW} generated by this V_T.
- Clamp the Y connection to the operative (non-dependent) lung, and open the sealing cap on that lumen of the DLT to allow the gas to escape.
- Observe the airway pressure closely. It will increase by 30–40% (about 7–10cmH$_2$O) if OLV is achieved. If the operative lung was non-functioning prior to anaesthesia (collapse 2° to bronchial obstruction or massive effusion), the pressure may not change.
- If P_{AW} is excessive (>35cmH$_2$O) or rises abruptly with each inspiration, exclude mechanical causes (e.g. kinked connector, clamp incorrectly placed) and DLT malposition or obstruction (e.g. ventilating the lobe, rather than the lung, sputum plugs, opening of the tracheal lumen against the wall of the trachea).
- Adjust V_T and ventilation profile to limit P_{AW} to ≤35cmH$_2$O, and ideally to ≤30cmH$_2$O. Incidence of ALI is reduced by employing a 'protective ventilation strategy'—lower P_{AW}, PEEP.
- Some monitoring systems allow you to compare the spirometry loop before and during OLV.
- Observe SpO_2 and $ETCO_2$ closely. If necessary, increase the ventilatory rate to maintain an acceptable minute volume and CO_2 clearance.
- Check with the surgeon that the lung is collapsing (may take a few minutes in patients with obstructive airways disease) and that the mediastinum has not 'sunk' into the dependent hemithorax.

Failure to achieve one-lung ventilation

- If inflation pressure does not increase when OLV is attempted, be suspicious that OLV has not been achieved. The DLT is likely not to be in far enough and should be advanced under fibrescopic guidance.
- If the surgeon says the lung has not collapsed, but the DLT position appears satisfactory, suction down the operative lumen to clear secretions, and hasten lung collapse (particularly in emphysematous lungs).

Hypoxia on one-lung ventilation

- Hypoxia is a frequent complication of OLV,[11] and is commoner when the right lung is collapsed.
- It usually occurs after a few minutes of OLV (as O_2 in the non-ventilated lung is absorbed).
- SpO_2 dips but then often rises again a few minutes later, as the non-ventilated lung collapses more completely and blood flow through it decreases.

- Increase FiO_2, and try to ensure an adequate cardiac output.
- Confirm correct positioning of the DLT—are all lobes ventilated? Check with the fibreoptic bronchoscope, if unsure.
- If partial collapse of the ventilated (dependent) lung is suspected ('sinking' mediastinum), try 5–10cmH$_2$O PEEP on that lung—this may help, but the effect is unpredictable, and PEEP may be limited by P_{AW}. Peak P_{AW} may be limited by changing from volume-controlled to pressure-controlled ventilation.
- If still hypoxic, warn the surgeon; partially reinflate the non-dependent lung, and then apply 5–10cmH$_2$O CPAP via a simple reservoir bag/ adjustable pressure limiting (APL) valve arrangement (CPAP System, Mallinckrodt™) supplied with 100% O_2 from an auxiliary O_2 flowmeter or cylinder at 5L/min. This will reliably improve saturations—simply insufflating O_2 into the collapsed non-dependent lung will not.
- If hypoxia persists, use intermittent inflation of the non-dependent lung with O_2 breaths from the CPAP circuit—this needs to be coordinated with surgical activity.
- If these manoeuvres are not successful, return to two-lung ventilation.
- The surgeon may clamp the appropriate PA, thus eliminating the shunt and improving oxygenation.
- Persisting with OLV in the face of continuing hypoxia (SpO$_2$ <90%) is dangerous and can rarely be justified.

Returning to two-lung ventilation

- Gently suction the non-ventilated lung to clear any blood or pus—use the long suction catheters supplied with the DLT.
- Close the sealing cap on the lumen to the non-ventilated lung and remove the clamp on the Y connector.
- Switch to manual ventilation, and reinflate the collapsed lung under direct vision. Long, sustained ventilation breaths are effective, and inflation pressures up to 35–40cmH$_2$O are often required to fully re-expand all areas of the lung.
- The surgeon will commonly observe for air leaks at this point and may ask for a specific airway pressure to be generated.
- Return the patient to mechanical ventilation, and, unless significant volumes of the lung have been resected, return to the original two-lung ventilator settings and FiO_2.
- Adjust the respiratory rate to maintain normocapnia.
- Always be prepared to return to OLV immediately, should problems occur, e.g. large air leak from the operated lung.
- Many anaesthetists advocate deflating the bronchial cuff as soon as possible to prevent bronchial wall necrosis.

References

10 Wilson WC, Benumof JL (2005). Physiology of one lung ventilation. In: Miller RD, ed. *Miller's anesthesia*, 6th edn. Philadelphia: Elsevier Churchill Livingstone, pp. 1890–4.
11 Karzai W, Schwarzkopf K (2009). Hypoxemia during one lung ventilation: prediction, prevention and treatment. *Anesthesiology*, **110**, 1402–11.

Rigid bronchoscopy and stent insertion

Procedure	Endoscopic inspection of tracheobronchial tree— ± biopsy, stents, removal of foreign body
Time	5–20min
Pain	+
Position	Supine with head and neck extended
Blood loss	Usually minimal
Practical techniques	TIVA with propofol boluses/TCI, alfentanil/remifentanil, intermittent suxamethonium
	IPPV through bronchoscope with O_2 via Venturi needle and Sanders injector

Preoperative

- Check for airway obstruction—stridor, tracheal tumour on CT scan, or history of foreign body inhalation.
- Suitable as a day-case procedure in appropriate patients.
- Warn about post-operative coughing, haemoptysis, and suxamethonium myalgia.
- Often combined with mediastinoscopy to assess suitability for lung resection.
- The airway will be unprotected, so patients at risk of regurgitation should be pre-treated to reduce the volume and acidity of gastric secretions (omeprazole 40mg PO the night before, and 40mg 2–6hr before the procedure). Ranitidine is an alternative.

Perioperative

- Give full preoxygenation.
- Confirm the surgeon is in theatre before inducing the patient.
- Boluses of midazolam (2–3mg) and alfentanil (500–1000 micrograms) facilitate induction and may reduce risk of awareness.
- Normally induce in the anaesthetic room; transfer to theatre with a face mask, and give suxamethonium just prior to bronchoscopy.
- An alternative to muscle relaxation is a remifentanil infusion.
- If there is potential airway obstruction (foreign body or tracheal compression), inhalation induction in theatre with sevoflurane in O_2 is recommended until the airway is secure.
- Coordinate ventilation with surgical activity.
- Observe or palpate the abdomen to detect recovery of muscle tone if a muscle relaxant has been used.
- Suction the upper airway, and confirm adequate muscle power before removing the scope.

Post-operative

- Turn the patient, biopsied side down, to avoid bleeding into the normal lung.
- Sit fully upright as soon as awake.
- A blood clot can cause severe lower airway obstruction, requiring immediate intubation, suction, and repeat bronchoscopy.

Special considerations

- The procedure is very stimulating and can generate a marked hypertensive response.
- Extreme CVS responses need to be obtunded, and profound relaxation provided, but with prompt return of laryngeal reflexes and spontaneous respiration.
- Vocal cords can be sprayed with LA (4% topical lidocaine), but this will not prevent carinal reflexes and may impair post-operative coughing.
- Rarely, a biopsy can precipitate a life-threatening airway bleed.
- Stent insertion can be technically difficult and may involve periodic loss of airway control.
- A short-acting NDMR can be employed, but it is difficult to achieve the profound paralysis required using mivacurium. Some patients will also undergo superior mediastinoscopy, and so longer-acting agents can be used.
- Bradycardias caused by repeat doses of suxamethonium are rarely seen during rigid bronchoscopy in adults. Atropine should be drawn up, but routine administration is not recommended since this will exacerbate any tachycardia.
- Use of rocuronium followed by reversal with sugammadex, is an alternative.

Superior/cervical mediastinoscopy

Procedure	Inspection and biopsy of tumours and lymph nodes in superior and anterior mediastinum via small suprasternal or anterior intercostal incision
Time	20–30min
Pain	+
Position	Supine or slightly head-up, arms by sides, and head ring with bolster under shoulders
Blood loss	Usually minimal, but potential for massive haemorrhage, G&S
Practical techniques	IPPV via single-lumen tube

Preoperative
- Suitable as day-case procedure in appropriate patients.
- Check for SVC obstruction and tracheal deviation or compression due to large mediastinal masses.
- Often preceded by rigid bronchoscopy ('Bronch & Med').

Perioperative
- Tape the eyes, and check the tracheal tube connectors, as the head will be obscured by drapes.
- Give boluses of IV fentanyl during surgery.
- Insert 16-gauge (G) cannula in the lower leg vein after induction (see **⬆** Special considerations, p. 372).
- Watch for surgical compression of the trachea—monitor V_T and airway pressures.
- Monitor BP in the left arm, and put the pulse oximeter on the right hand (see **⬆** Special considerations, p. 372).

Post-operative
- Paracetamol and NSAID.

Special considerations
- There is the potential for massive haemorrhage from the great vessels—the risk is increased in patients with SVC obstruction (hence cannula in the leg)—may require immediate median sternotomy.
- The brachiocephalic artery can be compressed by the mediastinoscope, restricting blood flow to the right arm and carotid artery, creating a risk of cerebral ischaemia. Place the pulse oximeter on the right hand to monitor perfusion.
- Mediastinotomy can cause a pneumothorax.

Lung surgery: wedge resection, lobectomy, and pneumonectomy

Procedure	Excision of pulmonary tissue either selectively (wedge resection or lobectomy) or a whole lung (pneumonectomy)
Time	2–4hr
Pain	+++++
Position	Lateral decubitus with table 'broken', elbows flexed to bring forearms parallel to face, with upper arm in gutter support
Blood loss	200–800mL—occasionally significantly more; G&S for lobectomy/pneumonectomy
Practical techniques	IPPV via DLT using OLV during resection phase. Epidural or paravertebral regional anaesthesia with catheter for post-operative analgesia, arterial line

Preoperative

- Cancer is the commonest indication for lung resection—others include benign tumours, bronchiectasis, and TB.
- Assess the cardiorespiratory reserve, and estimate the post-resection lung function (see ➲ p. 356).
- Assess the airway with respect to placement of the DLT.
- Plan the post-operative analgesia regime.

Perioperative

- Select the appropriate DLT, and check lung isolation carefully after intubation.
- Use a left-sided tube, unless the surgery involves a proximal left lobectomy or pneumonectomy, or an abnormal bronchial anatomy is likely to obstruct intubation of the left main bronchus.
- IV infusion in the non-dependent arm—14G to 16G cannula.
- Radial arterial lines function better in the dependent arm, as that wrist is usually extended.
- CVP monitoring is unreliable in the lateral position with an open chest. Central lines are not recommended for routine use but may be indicated for access purposes or post-operative monitoring. Similarly, oesophageal Doppler monitoring is unhelpful, since the lateral position and an open chest prevent a steady signal for analysis.
- OLV facilitates surgery and prevents soiling of the dependent lung.
- Continuous display of the airway pressure/volume loop is a valuable adjunct to monitoring and managing OLV.
- Surgical manipulation often causes cardiac and venous compression, which reduces the cardiac output/BP and may cause arrhythmias.

- Suction the airway to the collapsed lung prior to reinflation.
- The bronchial suture line is 'leak-tested' under saline by manual inflation to 40cmH$_2$O.
- Titrate IV fluids to losses and duration of surgery. Avoid excessive fluid replacement, especially in pneumonectomy.
- Preoperative epidural or paravertebral block with a surgically inserted catheter. Epidural can be used preoperatively, but cautious incremental boluses are recommended (3mL of 0.25% bupivacaine ± opioid).

Post-operative

- Aim to extubate the patient awake and sitting at the end of the procedure.
- Prescribe continuous supplementary O$_2$—humidified is preferable, but nasal cannulae are more likely to stay on the patient in the ward.
- Ensure good analgesia is achieved.
- A CXR is usually required in the recovery room.

Special considerations

- Occasionally, patients with bronchial carcinoma may have 'non-metastatic' manifestations (Eaton–Lambert myasthenic syndrome or ectopic hormone production). See p. 167, p. 170, and p. 242.
- Perioperative mortality from pneumonectomy is 5%. ALI occurs in 2–5% of resections and is three times commoner after pneumonectomy when the mortality is 25–50%.[12] Additional risk factors include the inflammatory response to surgery, chronic alcohol abuse, genetic predisposition, intraoperative plateau pressures >15cmH$_2$O, and >4000mL of IV fluid in first 24hr.[13] Incidence may be reduced by the intraoperative use of lung-protective strategies (as established in ARDS—management) and goal-directed fluid therapy.
- Arrhythmias, especially AF, are quite common after pneumonectomy, and many advocate prophylactic digitalization (digoxin 500 micrograms IV over 30min given during surgery, followed by 250 micrograms/d orally for 4–5d).

References

12 Licker M, de Perrot M, Spiliopoulos A, *et al.* (2003). Risk factors for acute lung injury after thoracic surgery for lung cancer. *Anesth Analg*, **97**, 1558–65.
13 Slinger PD (2006). Postpneumonectomy pulmonary edema: good news, bad news. *Anesthesiology*, **105**, 2–5.

Thoracoscopy and video-assisted thoracoscopic surgery procedures

Procedure	Inspection of thoracic cavity via scope passed through intercostal incision. Used for drainage of effusions, lung and pleural biopsy, pleurectomy/pleurodesis, pericardial biopsy/window
Time	30–120min
Pain	++/+++
Position	Lateral decubitus with table 'broken', elbows flexed to bring forearms parallel to face, with upper arm in gutter support
Blood loss	Minimal to 200mL, G&S
Practical techniques	IPPV and OLV via left-sided DLT. Percutaneous paravertebral block/catheter or intercostal blocks, ± art line

Preoperative

- Assess as for a thoracotomy, but this procedure is less invasive, with less post-operative deterioration of lung function.
- Discuss regional analgesia and, where appropriate, PCA.

Perioperative

- Consider invasive arterial pressure monitoring for high-risk or compromised patients.
- IV infusion in the upper arm; an arterial line in the radial artery of the dependent arm.
- Boluses of fentanyl (50–100 micrograms) for intraoperative analgesia.
- Commence OLV (using left-sided DLT) before the insertion of a trocar.
- Good collapse of the lung is required for surgical access.
- Intercostal or paravertebral blocks. A paravertebral catheter can be inserted under thoracoscopic guidance for more extensive procedures.

Post-operative

- Extubate; sit up, and start supplementary O_2 in theatre before transfer to recovery.
- CXR in recovery is required to confirm full lung re-expansion.
- Patients need balanced analgesia, as for lung resection. PCA morphine may be required for 24–48hr for more painful procedures such as pleurectomy, pleurodesis, and wedge resections.
- Encourage early mobilization.

Special considerations

- There is always the possibility of conversion to an open thoracotomy.
- Epidural is not usually necessary, but worth considering if bilateral.

Lung volume reduction surgery and bullectomy

Procedure	Non-anatomical resection of regions of hyperinflated and poorly functioning pulmonary tissue
Time	2–5hr
Pain	+++/+++++
Position	Median sternotomy (bilateral surgery)—supine with arms to sides. Thoracotomy—lateral decubitus (as for lung resection)
Blood loss	200–800mL, G&S
Practical techniques	Thoracic epidural pre-induction. GA with TIVA, relaxant, DLT—extreme care with IPPV and OLV

Lung volume reduction surgery is a surgical treatment for selected patients with severe respiratory failure 2° to emphysema. The aim is to reduce the total lung volume to more physiological levels by resecting most diseased areas, thereby improving the respiratory function. Most of these patients belong to a group in which GA would normally be avoided at any cost. The procedure is also considered for those with bullous disease and recurrent pneumothoraces.

Preoperative
- Patients require intensive assessment, careful selection, and optimization prior to surgery.
- Cardiac assessment for lung volume reduction surgery often includes coronary angiography and right heart catheterization to evaluate IHD, ventricular function, and PAPs.
- Patients are often on corticosteroids—perioperative supplementation is required.
- A clear understanding of the pathophysiology and adequate thoracic experience is essential to safe anaesthetic management.[14]

Perioperative
- Surgery may be performed via sternotomy, thoracotomy, or by video-assisted thoracoscopic surgery (VATS).
- There is a serious risk of rupturing emphysematous bullae with IPPV, causing leaks and tension pneumothorax.
- N_2O is contraindicated, and, since an increased alveolar–arterial gradient may exist for volatile agents, TIVA with remifentanil and propofol is recommended.[15]
- Continuous spirometry, and invasive arterial and CVP monitoring are essential.
- Clinical assessment of DLT placement is difficult—verify the position bronchoscopically.

- Limit the risk of 'gas trapping' and dynamic pulmonary hyperinflation (see ➔ 357) by deliberate hypoventilation and permissive hypercapnia ($PaCO_2$ up to 8.5kPa). Recommend V_T 6–7mL/kg, 10–12bpm, I:E ratio 1:4, and P_{AW} <30cmH$_2$O.
- Disconnect from the ventilator intermittently to allow the lungs to 'empty'.
- Bronchospasm and sputum retention with mucus plugging can be a problem.
- Use colloids for fluid replacement to minimize the risk of pulmonary oedema.

Post-operative

- HDU or ICU care will be required—extubate as soon as possible.
- Anticipate and accept raised $PaCO_2$ (7–9kPa), and adjust FiO_2 to maintain SaO_2 in the range of 90–92%.
- Watch closely for air leaks—use a maximum of 10cmH$_2$O suction on intercostal drains.
- Requires excellent pain relief, skilled physiotherapy, and a pulmonary rehabilitation programme.

Special considerations

- Commonest complication is prolonged air leak: >7 days in 50% of patients.
- Mortality from recent series is 5–10%.
- The National Emphysema Treatment Trial demonstrated that lung volume reduction surgery benefits patients with predominantly upper lobe disease and a low baseline exercise capacity.[14]
- Patients with an isolated congenital bulla or 'lung cyst' require the same careful intraoperative anaesthetic management but are usually much fitter and do not normally require invasive cardiological assessment.

References

14 Hillier J, Gillbe C (2003). Anaesthesia for lung volume reduction surgery. *Anaesthesia*, **58**, 1210–19.

15 Purugganan RV (2008). Intravenous anesthesia for thoracic procedures. *Curr Opin Anesthesiol*, **21**, 1–7.

Drainage of empyema and decortication

Procedure	Surgical removal of pus (empyema) and organized thick fibrinous pleural membrane (decortication)
Time	Drainage 20–40min; decortication 2–3hr
Pain	+++/+++++
Position	Lateral decubitus for thoracotomy
Blood loss	Simple drainage: minimal Decortication: 500–2000mL, X-match 2U
Practical techniques	GA with IV induction, relaxant, intubation, IPPV DLT advised for decortication (risk of air leaks); single-lumen tube adequate for drainage procedures; art line/CVP

Preoperative
- Intrapleural infection usually 2° to pneumonia, intercostal drains, and chest surgery.
- Patients are often debilitated by infection and may be frankly septic.
- Respiratory function often already compromised by pneumonia or prior lung resection.
- Check for bronchopleural fistula created by erosion into the lung.

Perioperative
- Empyema usually drained by rib resection and insertion of a large-bore intercostal drain.
- Thoracoscopy may be used to break down a loculated effusion or empyema and free pleural adhesions.
- Decortication requires 'thoracotomy' anaesthetic with epidural analgesia, since paravertebral catheter usually not possible due to loss of pleura.
- Decortication frequently causes significant haemorrhage.
- Arterial line/CVP monitoring are advisable for all but the fittest of patients.

Post-operative
- Balanced analgesia with regular paracetamol, NSAID, regional block (intercostal blocks useful for drainage procedures), and opioids.
- High dependency care is recommended for debilitated patients undergoing decortication.

Special considerations
- The surgical principle is to remove infected tissue, including pleural 'peel', fully re-expand the lung, and obliterate the infected pleural space.
- Air leaks are common following decortication of the visceral pleura, and lobectomy is occasionally required if a massive air leak or severe parenchymal lung damage occurs.
- Decortication is a major procedure which requires careful evaluation of risks and benefits in elderly, frail, and sick patients.

Repair of bronchopleural fistula

Procedure	Closure of communication between pleural cavity and trachea or bronchi
Time	2–3hr (for thoracotomy approach)
Pain	++++/+++++
Position	Keep sitting upright, with affected side tilted down until good lung isolated, then lateral decubitus for thoracotomy
Blood loss	300–800mL, G&S, X-match 2U if anaemic
Practical techniques	IV induction and fibreoptic-guided endobronchial intubation with DLT. Awake fibreoptic-guided intubation with DLT. Intubation with DLT under deep inhalation anaesthesia with SV

Preoperative

- Features are productive cough, haemoptysis, fever, dyspnoea, SC emphysema, and falling fluid level in the post-pneumonectomy space on the CXR.
- The severity of symptoms is proportional to the size of the fistula—big fistulae with large air leaks cause severe dyspnoea and may necessitate urgent respiratory support.
- Patients are often debilitated, with the respiratory function compromised by infection and prior lung resection.
- Check previous anaesthetic charts for ease of intubation and the type of DLT used.
- Check the anatomy of the lower airway carefully on CXR—it is often distorted by previous surgery.
- Patients require supplementary O_2, a functioning chest drain, IV antibiotics, and fluids.

Perioperative

- Key principles are to protect the 'good' lung from contamination and to control the distribution of ventilation. Failure to adequately isolate the lungs after induction will put the patient at grave risk.
- Small or moderate fistulae are usually assessed by bronchoscopy and may be amenable to sealing with tissue glue.
- Commence invasive arterial pressure monitoring before induction.
- Traditionally, awake intubation under LA has been recommended as the safest option, but ultimately the technique should be selected to give the best balance of risks and benefits for each patient. Many thoracic anaesthetists use a modified RSI and advance the DLT under direct vision with a fibreoptic bronchoscope to ensure correct placement in the bronchus contralateral to the fistula, before ventilation is

commenced. The potential exists to enlarge the fistula by inappropriate placement of the DLT.
- IPPV increases gas leakage, causing loss of V_T and the risk of tension pneumothorax.
- TIVA is recommended—delivery of volatile agents may be unreliable with large gas leaks. Ketamine may be useful in high-risk patients.

Post-operative
- Plan HDU/ICU care for all but the most straightforward cases.
- Minimize airway pressures during ventilation, and extubate as soon as possible.
- Use standard post-thoracotomy analgesic regimen, but watch the renal function with NSAIDs.

Special considerations
- Most fistulae are post-operative complications of pneumonectomy or lobectomy, but some are 2° to pneumonia, lung abscesses, and empyema.
- Anaesthesia for repair of a bronchopleural fistula is challenging and not recommended for an 'occasional' thoracic anaesthetist!

Tips for controlling a massive air leak
(i.e. unable to ventilate effectively)
If a DLT cannot be positioned satisfactorily, these are worth attempting:
- Intubate with an uncut, cuffed, 6mm-diameter single-lumen tube—pass the fibreoptic bronchoscope through the tube into the intact main bronchus, and 'railroad' the tube into the bronchus to isolate and ventilate the good lung
- Ask the surgeon to pass a rigid bronchoscope into the intact main bronchus, and slide a long flexible bougie or Cook™ AEC (which allows jet ventilation) into the bronchus—remove the bronchoscope, and railroad the single-lumen tube
- If all else fails, an Arndt endobronchial blocker or a large Fogarty embolectomy catheter passed into the fistula via a rigid bronchoscope may control the leak temporarily.

Pleurectomy/pleurodesis

Procedure	Stripping of parietal pleura from inside of chest wall (pleurectomy). Production of adhesions between parietal and visceral pleura either chemically (talc, tetracycline) or by physical abrasion (pleurodesis)
Time	Pleurectomy 1–2hr; pleurodesis 20–40min
Pain	+++/++++
Position	Lateral decubitus for open thoracotomy or VATS. May be supine for pleurodesis
Blood loss	Minimal if thoracoscopic; up to 500mL for thoracotomy, G&S
Practical techniques	IPPV, DLT, and OLV advised for open/VATS procedures. A single-lumen tube is usually adequate for talc pleurodesis

Preoperative

- Patients fall into two groups: the relatively young and fit with recurrent pneumothoraces (check for asthma) and older patients compromised by COPD or recurrent pleural effusions (check respiratory reserve).
- Check a recent CXR for pneumothorax and/or effusion.
- A preoperative intercostal drain is advised if pneumothorax present.
- Check the planned surgical approach.
- Discuss post-operative analgesia and the regional technique.

Perioperative

- Keep airway pressures as low as possible in patients with a history of pneumothorax.
- Be alert for pneumothoraces, as they can tension rapidly on IPPV, even with a drain *in situ*, and can be on the 'healthy' side.
- Avoid N_2O.
- Collapse the lung during instillation of the irritant to facilitate pleural coating. If using a single-lumen tube, preoxygenate, and then briefly disconnect the lungs from the ventilator.
- Aim for full expansion of the lung at the end of the procedure to appose the parietal and visceral pleurae.

Post-operative

- Extubate, and sit the patient upright before transfer to the recovery room.
- A CXR is needed to check full lung expansion. Suction on intercostal drains is often prescribed to assist expansion. Pleural inflammation usually causes severe pain, particularly when abrasion of the pleura is performed.

- Use regular paracetamol, but avoid NSAIDs which may make pleurodesis less effective.
- Thoracic epidural is recommended for a pleurectomy, especially bilateral procedures, and is sited and used as for a thoracotomy. A combination of morphine PCA with intercostal blocks is an alternative. Paravertebral blocks are usually unsuitable due to damage to the pleura.

Special considerations

- Pleurectomy is usually performed for recurrent pneumothorax, combined with stapling of the lung tissue responsible for recurrent air leaks (usually apical 'blebs' or small bullae).
- Pleurodesis is often used to manage malignant pleural effusions (mesothelioma, metastatic carcinoma)—there may be large volumes of fluid causing significant respiratory compromise.
- Patients with massive pleural effusions (more than two-thirds of the hemithorax on CXR or >2000mL) should have these 'tapped' and partially drained at least 12hr before surgery, because rapid intraoperative reinflation of the collapsed lung can precipitate unilateral post-operative 're-expansion' pulmonary oedema.
- Patients with extensive effusions are also at risk of circulatory collapse when turned 'effusion side up' for surgery. The mechanism is probably a combination of mediastinal shift and high intrathoracic pressure on IPPV reducing the venous return and cardiac output. If this occurs, return the patient to the supine position, and drain the effusion before proceeding.

Oesophagectomy

Procedure	Total or partial excision of oesophagus with mobilization of stomach (occasionally colon) into chest
Time	3–6hr
Pain	+++++
Position	Supine with arms by sides and/or lateral decubitus for thoracotomy
Blood loss	500–1500mL; X-match 2U
Practical techniques	IPPV, DLT useful if thoracotomy, art/CVP lines, urinary catheter, thoracic epidural, or paravertebral catheter for thoracoabdominal incision

Preoperative

- Establish the indication for surgery—usually oesophageal cancer, but occasionally for non-malignant disease (benign stricture, achalasia).
- The anaesthetic plan requires an understanding of the surgical approach:
  - **Transhiatal**: laparotomy and cervical anastomosis
  - **Ivor–Lewis**: laparotomy and right thoracotomy
  - **Thoracoabdominal**: left thoracotomy crossing the costal margin and diaphragm
  - **McKeown 3 stage**: laparotomy, right thoracotomy, and cervical anastomosis
  - **Minimally invasive**: thoracoscopic oesophageal mobilization, laparoscopic gastric mobilization, and cervical anastomosis.
- Preoperative malnutrition or cachexia is common and associated with higher risk of post-operative morbidity and mortality. Requires careful cardiorespiratory assessment.
- Plan for the duration of surgery and the need to reposition the patient during the procedure.
- Preoperative adjuvant chemotherapy may leave residual immunosuppression but can dramatically improve dysphagia.
- Reflux is a risk. Give preoperative ranitidine or omeprazole if the patient can swallow.
- Book HDU or ICU, according to the patient's fitness and local protocols.

Perioperative

- Consider all patients with oesophageal disease to be at risk of regurgitation, so RSI with cricoid pressure advised.
- If thoracotomy is planned, use a DLT and OLV to facilitate surgical access and reduce trauma to the lung.
- Plan regional anaesthesia, according to the surgical approach. Paravertebral LA infusion with morphine PCA for the thoracoabdominal approach. For laparotomy/thoracotomy, a mid-thoracic epidural (using

3mL boluses of 0.25% bupivacaine perioperatively and post-operative infusion).
- An NGT will be required initially. It is removed for resection and reinserted under surgical guidance following anastomosis.
- Do not put an internal jugular line on the side required for cervical anastomosis.
- Monitor the core temperature, and be obsessional about keeping the patient warm (efficient fluid warmer and forced-air warming blanket).
- Stay ahead with fluid replacement—for open procedures, aim for 10mL/kg/hr of crystalloid plus colloid or red cells to replace blood loss.
- Check Hb (HemoCue® ideal) and blood gases intraoperatively—watch for metabolic acidosis suggesting inadequate tissue perfusion.
- Arrhythmias and reduced cardiac output causing hypotension may occur during intrathoracic oesophageal mobilization.
- Change the DLT to a single-lumen tube to improve surgical access prior to cervical anastomosis (if performed).

Post-operative
- Patients require intensive and experienced post-operative nursing care in a specialist ward, HDU, or ICU.
- If cold (<35.5°C) or haemodynamically unstable, ventilate until the condition improves.
- Aim for a minimum urine output of 1mL/kg/hr.
- Use a jejunostomy or nasoduodenal tube for early enteral feeding.

Special considerations
- Oesophagectomy has one of the highest perioperative mortality rates of all elective procedures (up to 5%, even in specialist centres).
- Sixty-six per cent of deaths are from systemic sepsis 2° to respiratory complications or anastomotic breakdown.
- Over 30% of patients suffer from a major complication.
- In some centres, minimally invasive (endoscopic) oesophagectomy is replacing the traditional open approaches. Beware 'tension capnothorax' if the pleura is breached during laparoscopic hiatal dissection.
- Occasional practice in anaesthesia (or surgery) for oesophagectomy is not recommended.

Chest injury

The emergency diagnosis and initial treatment of major thoracic trauma are described on ➲ p. 856. This section deals with the anaesthetic management for the definitive repair of ruptures of the diaphragm, oesophagus, and tracheobronchial tree.

General considerations

- Serious chest injuries are frequently associated with major head, abdominal, and skeletal injuries, and appropriate attention and priority must be given to their management (cervical spine immobilization, laparotomy to arrest bleeding, splintage of limb fractures).
- Fewer than 30% of patients with thoracic trauma require a thoracotomy, but persistent bleeding from intercostal drains exceeding 200mL/hr is an indication for urgent surgery.
- Most deaths from thoracic trauma are due to exsanguination. Good IV access with two large-bore cannulae will allow rapid infusion.
- Emergency thoracotomy in the resuscitation room is seldom indicated and rarely associated with a favourable outcome.
- Standard principles of emergency anaesthesia should be applied.
- Maintain a high index of suspicion for tension pneumothorax during IPPV, as an intercostal drain does not guarantee protection.
- Massive air leaks usually indicate significant tracheobronchial injury (see ➲ p. 386).
- Patients with major thoracic trauma are at high risk of multiple organ failure and require post-operative management in an ICU.

Repair of ruptured diaphragm

- Clinical features and diagnosis are described on ➲ p. 857.
- May present as a chronic condition or as intestinal obstruction of a herniated bowel, so check preoperative fluid and electrolyte status.
- The defect should be closed promptly, but this seldom needs to be done as an emergency.
- The surgical approach is via a standard lateral thoracotomy or a thoracoabdominal incision.
- Intraoperative management is as for a fundoplication (see ➲ p. 359).
- Avoid N_2O, as it distends the bowel and may make reduction of the hernia more difficult.
- DLT and OLV facilitate surgical access for repair.
- An NGT should be used to decompress the stomach.

Repair of ruptured oesophagus

- Clinical features and diagnosis are described on ➲ p. 858—surgical emphysema and pleural effusions are frequently present.
- Other causes of oesophageal rupture include excessive abdominal straining and uncoordinated vomiting (Boerhaave's syndrome). Oesophageal perforation can be caused by foreign bodies but is often iatrogenic (during endoscopic procedures).

- Mediastinitis is followed rapidly by sepsis and a systemic inflammatory response syndrome (SIRS), with associated problems of circulatory shock, renal failure, and ARDS.
- The principles of surgical management are initially drainage and prevention of further contamination.
- Careful endoscopic assessment will determine the extent of oesophageal disruption.
- Small tears in unfit, frail patients may be managed conservatively with chest drainage and nasogastric suction, but normally urgent surgery is required.
- Patients should be stabilized preoperatively in ICU with chest drainage, IV fluid replacement, analgesia, invasive monitoring, and inotropic support.
- Intraoperative management is as for oesophagectomy (see ⟴ p. 383).
- Upper and lower oesophageal injuries require right and left thoracotomy, respectively.
- 1° closure may be possible if the oesophagus is healthy; if not, oesophagectomy will be required.
- Arrhythmias are common, particularly AF, due to mediastinitis.
- Change the DLT for a single-lumen tube before transfer to intensive care for post-operative ventilation.
- Even patients who are stable at the end of the repair procedure remain at high risk of major complications for several days.
- Early post-operative feeding—feeding jejunostomy or parenterally.
- There is a significant incidence of dehiscence, resulting in an oesophagopleurocutaneous fistula with high mortality.

Repair of tracheobronchial injury

- Most patients with significant tracheal/bronchial disruption do not reach hospital alive.
- Clinical features of laryngeal and tracheobronchial injuries are described on ⟴ p. 858.
- The priority is 100% O_2 and relief of tension pneumothorax, which may require two large-bore intercostal drains with independent underwater seals.
- If ventilation and oxygenation are acceptable, call for thoracic surgical assistance, and try to assess and identify the site of airway injury by fibreoptic bronchoscopy before intubation.
- Airway management and anaesthetic principles apply as for a large bronchopleural fistula (see ⟴ p. 379).
- Adequate positive pressure ventilation may be impossible with a single-lumen tube.
- A torn bronchus can be isolated by fibreoptic-guided intubation of the contralateral intact main bronchus with an appropriate DLT.
- An uncut single-lumen tube can be guided past an upper tracheal tear with a bronchoscope, so its cuff lies distal to the injury.
- Once the airway is secure and ventilation is stabilized, proceed to an urgent thoracotomy for repair.

- Carinal disruption may require CPB to maintain oxygenation during repair.
- Inappropriate management can lead to later stenosis and long-term airway problems.

Further reading

Ghosh S, Latimer RD (1999). *Thoracic anaesthesia principles and practice.* London: Butterworth-Heinemann.

Wilson WC, Benumof JL (2005). Anesthesia for thoracic surgery. In: Miller RD, ed. *Miller's anesthesia*, 6th edn. Philadelphia: Elsevier Churchill Livingstone, pp. 1847–930.

Neurosurgery

Alex Manara and Samantha Shinde

General principles

Intracranial pressure

Normal ICP is 5–12mmHg. Changes in ICP reflect changes in the volume of intracranial contents held within the confines of the skull (brain substance 1200–1600mL, blood 100–150mL, CSF 100–150mL, ECF <75mL). Compensatory mechanisms initially reduce the effect of an intracranial space-occupying lesion on ICP by displacing the CSF into the spinal subarachnoid space, increasing the absorption of CSF and reducing intracranial blood volume. Eventually, these mechanisms are overwhelmed, and further small increases in intracranial volume result in a steep rise in ICP (Fig. 16.1). If a lesion develops slowly, it may reach a relatively large volume before causing a significant rise in ICP. A lesion that appears relatively small on a CT scan may have developed quickly, allowing little time for compensation.

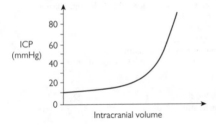

Fig. 16.1 Intracranial pressure and volume.

Causes of raised intracranial pressure
- Increased brain substance: tumour, abscess, haematoma.
- Increased CSF volume: hydrocephalus, benign intracranial hypertension, blocked shunt.
- Increased blood volume:
  - Increased cerebral blood flow (CBF): hypoxia, hypercapnia, volatile anaesthetic agent
  - Increased cerebral venous volume: increased thoracic pressure, venous obstruction in the neck, head-down tilt, coughing.
- Increased ECF: cerebral oedema.

Cerebral perfusion pressure
Cerebral perfusion pressure (CPP) is the effective pressure that results in blood flow to the brain.

$$CPP = MAP - (ICP + VP)$$

Venous pressure (VP) at the jugular bulb is usually zero or less, and therefore CPP is related to ICP and MAP alone. The CPP therefore varies with the patient's MAP, but CBF is maintained constant by autoregulation.

Cerebral blood flow

Autoregulation maintains CBF between a MAP of 50 and 140mmHg. Outside these limits, CBF varies passively with perfusion pressure. In patients with chronic hypertension, the lower and upper limits of autoregulation are higher than normal, so that a MAP that may be adequate in a normal patient may lead to cerebral ischaemia in the hypertensive patient. Autoregulation is also impaired or abolished acutely in the presence of brain tissue acidosis, i.e. with hypoxia, hypercapnia, acute intracranial disease, and following head injury.

CBF varies with:

- Metabolism: CBF is primarily determined by the metabolic demands of the brain. It increases during epileptic seizures and with pain/anxiety. It is reduced in coma, hypothermia, and with anaesthetic agents
- CO_2 tension: hypocapnia results in cerebral vasoconstriction and a reduction in CBF. The greatest effect is at normal $PaCO_2$ where a change of 1kPa (7.5mmHg) results in a 30% change in blood flow. MAP modifies the response of CBF to hyperventilation. High perfusion pressures increase the responsiveness to hyperventilation, whereas hypotension of 50mmHg abolishes the effect of $PaCO_2$ on CBF
- O_2 tension: PaO_2 is not an important determinant of CBF, a value of <7kPa (53mmHg) being required before cerebral vasodilatation occurs
- Temperature: hypothermia reduces cerebral metabolism by ~5% per °C, thereby reducing CBF
- Viscosity: there is no effect on CBF when the Hct is between 30% and 50%. CBF will increase with reduced viscosity outside this range
- Anaesthetic agents: see ➲ p. 392.

Measuring intracranial pressure

- Ventricular: a catheter inserted into a lateral ventricle via a burr hole is the gold standard for measuring ICP. This also allows drainage of CSF as a treatment option. Risks include haemorrhage at insertion and ventriculitis with prolonged use. Insertion may be difficult in patients with cerebral oedema and small ventricles.
- Intraparenchymal: micro-miniature silicone strain gauge monitors can be inserted into the brain parenchyma to monitor ICP. They are accurate and relatively easy to insert, even by non-neurosurgical staff. They are currently the commonest technique used to measure ICP.

Anaesthesia in the presence of raised intracranial pressure

Symptoms and signs to identify patients with a raised ICP preoperatively:
- Early: headache, vomiting, seizures, focal neurology, papilloedema
- Late: increasing BP and bradycardia. Agitation, drowsiness, coma, Cheyne–Stokes breathing, apnoea. Ipsilateral, then bilateral, pupillary dilatation; decorticate, then decerebrate posturing
- Investigations: evaluate CT/MRI scans for the presence of generalized oedema, midline shift, acute hydrocephalus, and site/size of any lesion.

Management aims

Do not increase ICP further.
- Avoid increasing CBF by avoiding hypercapnia, hypoxia, hypertension, and hyperthermia. Use IPPV to control $PaCO_2$, and ensure good oxygenation, adequate analgesia, and anaesthetic depth.

- Avoid increasing VP. Avoid coughing and straining, the head-down position, and obstructing neck veins with ETT ties.
- Prevent further cerebral oedema. While patients are generally fluid-restricted, it is important to maintain intravascular volume and CPP. Do not use hypotonic solutions—fluid flux across the blood–brain barrier is determined mainly by plasma osmolality, not oncotic pressure. Maintenance of a high normal plasma osmolality is essential.
- Maintain CPP: hypotension will decrease CPP in the presence of a raised ICP. Control BP using fluids and vasopressors, as necessary. Aim for a CPP >60mmHg.
- Avoid anaesthetic agents that increase ICP (see below).

Specific measures to decrease intracranial pressure
- Reduce cerebral oedema using osmotic or loop diuretics, or both. Give mannitol 0.25–1g/kg over 15min or 5% saline (100mL) and furosemide 0.25–1mg/kg. Insert a urinary catheter in patients receiving diuretics.
- Modest hyperventilation to $PaCO_2$ of 4.0–4.5kPa (30–34mmHg) has a transient effect in reducing ICP for 24hr. Excessive hyperventilation results in cerebral ischaemia and a loss of autoregulation. Note: $ETCO_2$ is lower than $PaCO_2$.
- Corticosteroids reduce oedema surrounding tumours and abscesses but have no role in head injury. They take several hours to work. Dexamethasone 4mg 6-hourly is often given electively preoperatively.
- CSF may be drained via a ventricular or lumbar drain.
- Position the patient with a head-up tilt of 30° to reduce CVP. Ensure that MAP is not significantly reduced, as the overall result could be a reduction in CPP.

Anaesthetic agents and intracranial pressure
- Volatile agents uncouple metabolism and flow, reducing cerebral metabolism, while increasing CBF and ICP. They abolish autoregulation in sufficient doses. Halothane causes the greatest increase in ICP, and isoflurane the least. ICP is unaffected by concentrations of <1 MAC of isoflurane, sevoflurane, and desflurane. Enflurane may cause seizures and has no place in neuroanaesthesia. N_2O is a weak cerebral vasodilator increasing CBF, and therefore ICP. It has also been shown to increase cerebral metabolic rate.
- IV anaesthetic agents all decrease cerebral metabolism, CBF, and ICP, with the exception of ketamine. Ketamine has some neuroprotective properties but is considered contraindicated in neurosurgery. CO_2 reactivity and autoregulation of the cerebral circulation are well maintained during propofol/thiopental anaesthesia.
- Other drugs:
  - Suxamethonium causes a rise in ICP through muscle fasciculation, increasing VP. This effect is of little clinical relevance. Suxamethonium should still be used when rapid intubation is required in the presence of a potentially full stomach (e.g. head injury)
  - Opioid analgesics have little effect on CBF and ICP if hypercapnia is avoided. CO_2 reactivity is maintained.

Craniotomy

Procedure	Excision or debulking of tumour, brain biopsy, drainage of cerebral abscess
Time	1–12hr
Pain	+/+++
Position	Supine, head-up tilt, or lateral decubitus
Blood loss	0–2000mL, G&S, or X-match 2U
Practical techniques	ETT, IPPV, art line, CVP

Preoperative

- Assess the patient for symptoms and signs of raised ICP. Document any neurological deficits. Assess the gag reflex.
- Intracranial tumours may be metastatic; 1° sites include the lung, breast, thyroid, and bowel.
- Check CT/MRI scans—the duration and complexity of the procedure are determined by the size, site, and vascularity of lesions being excised.
- Patients receiving diuretics or who have been vomiting may have disordered electrolytes. Patients receiving dexamethasone may be hyperglycaemic.
- Restrict IV fluids to 30mL/kg/d if cerebral oedema present. Avoid glucose-containing solutions. They may cause hyperglycaemia, which is associated with a worse outcome after brain injury. They also reduce osmolality, resulting in increased cerebral oedema.
- Ensure graduated compression stockings are fitted to prevent DVT.
- Prophylactic or therapeutic phenytoin may be required (a loading dose of 15mg/kg, followed by a single daily dose of 3–4mg/kg).

Perioperative

- Patients undergoing burr hole biopsy require standard monitoring. Those scheduled for craniotomy also need an arterial line/CVP, neuromuscular monitoring, and core temperature. Insert a urinary catheter for long procedures and in patients who receive diuretics.
- Induce with thiopental 3–5mg/kg or propofol 2–3mg/kg combined with remifentanil (0.2–0.5 micrograms/kg/min). Give IV induction agents slowly to avoid reducing BP and CPP. A non-depolarizing relaxant is used to facilitate intubation. Remifentanil usually attenuates the hypertensive response to intubation—if not, use additional agents such as lidocaine 1.5mg/kg or a β-blocker (labetalol 5mg increments). Use an armoured ETT to prevent kinking, and secure in place with tapes, as ties may cause venous obstruction. Protect the eyes.
- Avoid N₂O. Maintain anaesthesia using either a volatile agent (sevoflurane/isoflurane <1 MAC) or TCI propofol (3–6 micrograms/mL). Remifentanil infusion is continued at a lower rate (0.15–0.25 micrograms/

kg/min), titrated to response. Top-up doses of muscle relaxants are rarely required when remifentanil is used. In the absence of remifentanil, use fentanyl 5 micrograms/kg at induction, followed by top-up doses, as required, or an alfentanil infusion (25–50 micrograms/kg/hr).

- Patients may be placed in the supine or lateral position. Avoid extreme neck flexion or rotation, which may impair cerebral venous return, and maintain a head-up tilt. If the head is turned for surgery, support the shoulder to reduce the effect on neck veins.
- Application of the Mayfield 3-point fixator to secure the head can cause a marked hypertensive response. Pin sites can be infiltrated with LA, and, if necessary, give a further dose of remifentanil (0.5–1 microgram/kg) or propofol (0.5–1mg/kg).
- Aim for normotension during most procedures. Modest hypotension may infrequently be required to improve the surgical field. Mild hypocapnia is used in tumour surgery. Aim for $PaCO_2$ of 4.0–4.5kPa (30–34mmHg).
- Avoid hypotonic solutions for fluid maintenance. Replace blood loss with colloid or blood.
- Maintain normothermia. Hypothermia is rarely indicated.
- Use intermittent pneumatic compression device to the calves or feet.
- Closure of the dura, bone flap, and scalp takes at least half an hour. Administer IV morphine at this stage to provide analgesia when the remifentanil is stopped. Sudden hypertension on awakening may be treated with small boluses of labetalol. Avoid coughing, if possible.

Post-operative

- Further incremental doses of IV morphine may be required in the immediate post-operative period in the recovery area.
- Many routine craniotomies can be managed post-operatively on an adequately staffed neurosurgical ward. Continued monitoring of the patient's conscious level and neurological state is essential. Consider post-operative sedation and ventilation if there is continuing cerebral oedema or if the patient was severely obtunded preoperatively.
- On return to the ward, the majority of patients will experience pain in the mild to moderate range after craniotomy. At this stage, codeine phosphate (60–90mg), combined with regular paracetamol, is usually sufficient in >90% of patients. If not, PCA with morphine may be used.

Special considerations

- NSAIDs should be used only for post-operative analgesia after careful consideration. While they reduce opioid requirements and enhance opioid analgesia, they also increase bleeding time—a post-operative intracranial haematoma is potentially disastrous. Many patients will have also received diuretics and are potentially hypovolaemic.
- A central line is indicated for the majority of craniotomies to allow measurement of CVP, infusion of vasoactive drugs, and aspiration of air in the case of venous air embolism (VAE).

Ventriculo-peritoneal shunt

Procedure	CSF drainage for hydrocephalus
Time	45–120min
Pain	++
Position	Supine, head-up tilt
Blood loss	Minimal
Practical techniques	ETT, IPPV

Shunts are inserted for hydrocephalus. CSF is diverted from the cerebral ventricles to other body cavities, from where it is absorbed. Most commonly, a ventriculo-peritoneal shunt is created, more rarely a ventriculo-atrial or ventriculo-pleural shunt. An occipital burr hole enables a tube to be placed into the lateral ventricle. This is then tunnelled SC down the neck and trunk, and inserted into the peritoneal cavity through a small abdominal incision. A flushing device can be placed in the burr hole to keep the system clear, and a valve system is incorporated to prevent CSF draining too rapidly with changes in posture.

Preoperative

- As for craniotomy (see ➲ p. 393).
- Many patients requiring shunts are children, and the usual paediatric considerations apply.
- Patients often have raised ICP.
- Emergency cases may have a full stomach, requiring RSI.

Perioperative

- Shunt procedures are shorter and simpler than craniotomies. Use routine monitoring. Arterial and central venous lines are not required.
- Antibiotic treatment or prophylaxis is required, and strict antisepsis protocols are normally followed to reduce the incidence of shunt infection.
- Advancing the trocar to allow tunnelling of the shunt is particularly stimulating. Additional analgesia and/or muscle relaxation is often required at this stage.

Post-operative

- Any deterioration in conscious level is an indication for a CT scan to exclude shunt malfunction or a subdural haematoma.

Special considerations

- Patients are at risk of intracranial haemorrhage if CSF is drained too rapidly.
- Shunts often block or become infected, requiring revision.
- Watch for signs of a pneumothorax, as the trocar is placed subcutaneously.

Evacuation of traumatic intracranial haematoma

Procedure	Evacuation of extradural or subdural haematoma
Time	1.5–3hr
Pain	+/+++
Position	Supine, head-up
Blood loss	200–2000mL, X-match 2U
Practical techniques	ETT, IPPV, art line, CVP

Intracranial haematoma may be extradural, subdural, or intracerebral.
- Extradural: urgent evacuation is required, and certainly within an hour of pupillary dilation. The haematoma is usually the result of a tear in the middle meningeal artery. It is virtually always associated with a skull fracture, except in children when the fracture may be absent.
- Subdural haematoma: results from bleeding from the bridging veins between the cortex and dura. Early evacuation of an acute subdural haematoma improves outcome. Chronic subdural haematomas may occur in the elderly, often after trivial injury. They present insidiously with headaches and confusion and can be evacuated via a burr hole under LA.
- Intracerebral haematoma: occurs in hypertensive individuals, as a complication of treatment with warfarin or as a result of bleeding from an intracranial aneurysm.

Preoperative
- As for head injury (see p. 852).
- Most patients will have a reduced or deteriorating Glasgow coma score (GCS).
- ICP is usually raised.
- Patients may have associated injuries to the chest, pelvis, or abdomen, requiring resuscitation and treatment in their own right (see p. 856). Protect the C-spine, if necessary.
- Patients may have a full stomach, requiring RSI. Insert an orogastric tube after intubation.
- Check the blood clotting profile and the availability of blood products, prior to surgery.

Perioperative
- As for craniotomy (see p. 393).
- Patients require standard monitoring, including invasive BP and CVP monitoring.
- Ensure smooth induction and normotension. Maintain CPP using fluids and vasopressors if necessary. Assume that the ICP is 20mmHg—the

minimum acceptable MAP is therefore 80mmHg to achieve a CPP of 60mmHg.

- Ensure a head-up tilt; avoid N_2O; ventilate to an $ETCO_2$ of 4.0kPa (30mmHg), and give mannitol (0.5–1g/kg) or 5% saline (100mL) and furosemide (0.25–1mg/kg) as required.
- Once decompression has occurred, there may be a decrease in systemic BP, which can usually be treated with volume replacement.

Post-operative

- Most patients should be transferred to ICU. Further management should be guided by a protocol to maintain CPP and prevent 2° insults to the brain (see below).

Special considerations

- It is essential for the various teams to communicate and set priorities in the management of patients with multiple injuries. Priorities will vary from patient to patient (see ➔ p. 871).
- Hypotension in a head-injured patient is a medical emergency and must be treated promptly and aggressively.

Post-operative and intensive care unit management of the head-injured patient

- Management of head-injured patients is similar for post-operative patients and those not requiring surgery. Patients are best managed using a protocol designed primarily to maintain an adequate CPP/ cerebral oxygenation and control ICP. It involves preventing, identifying, and treating causes of 2° brain insults (Fig. 16.2).
- Causes of 2° insults are:
  - Intracranial—haematoma, oedema, convulsions, hydrocephalus, abscess, hyperaemia
  - Systemic—hypotension, hypoxia, hyponatraemia, pyrexia, anaemia, sepsis, hypercapnia, hyperglycaemia.
- Steroids should not be administered to patients following severe head injury.

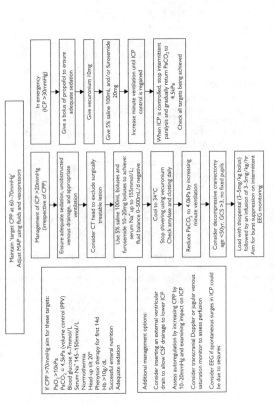

Maintain 'target CPP at 60–70mmHg'
Adjust MAP using fluids and vasopressors

Management of ICP >20mmHg
(irrespective of CPP)

Ensure adequate sedation, unobstructed venous drainage, and appropriate ventilation

Consider CT head to exclude surgically treatable lesion

Use 5% saline 100mL boluses and furosemide 10–20mg boluses to achieve: serum Na⁺ up to 155mmol/L; fluid balance 0–500mL/d negative

Cool to 34°C
Stop shivering using vecuronium
Check amylase and clotting daily

Reduce PaCO₂ to 4.0kPa by increasing minute ventilation

Consider decompressive craniectomy age <50yr, GCS >3, no fixed pupils

Load with thiopental (3–5mg/kg bolus) followed by an infusion of 3–5mg/kg/hr Aim for burst suppression on intermittent EEG monitoring

In emergency
(ICP >30mmHg)

Give a bolus of propofol to ensure adequate sedation

Give vecuronium 10mg

Give 5% saline 100mL and/or furosemide 20mg

Increase minute ventilation until ICP control is regained

When ICP is controlled, stop intermittent paralysis and gradually return PaCO₂ to 4.5kPa
Check all targets being achieved

If CPP >70mmHg aim for these targets:
PaO₂ >10kPa
PaCO₂ = 4.5kPa (volume control IPPV)
Blood glucose 4–7mmol/L
Serum Na⁺ 145–150mmol/L
Normothermia
Head-up tilt 20°
Phenytoin therapy for first 14d
Hb >10g/dL
Successful enteral nutrition
Adequate sedation

Additional management options:

Consider inserting an external ventricular drain to allow CSF drainage to lower ICP

Assess autoregulation by increasing CPP by 10–20mmHg and examining impact on ICP

Consider transcranial Doppler or jugular venous saturation monitor to assess perfusion

Consider EEG if spontaneous surges in ICP could be due to seizures

Fig. 16.2 Guidelines for managing adults with severe head injuries in ICU.

Pituitary surgery

Procedure	Trans-sphenoidal hypophysectomy
Time	90–180min
Pain	++
Position	Supine, head-up tilt
Blood loss	Nil usually, but large if venous sinus disrupted, G&S
Practical techniques	ETT, IPPV, art line

Pituitary tumours account for 15% of all intracranial tumours. They present with either hypersecretion of hormones (acromegaly/Cushing's syndrome) or mass effects (headaches, visual field defects, hydrocephalus, hypopituitarism). Hypophysectomy is undertaken urgently if the patient's sight is deteriorating rapidly.

Preoperative

Special considerations for acromegalic patients (see also ⮞ p. 156):
- Possible airway compromise due to macroglossia, prognathism, and hypertrophy of the epiglottis/vocal cords
- Hypertension and LV hypertrophy
- Sleep apnoea, diabetes mellitus.

Special considerations for Cushing's patients (see also ⮞ p. 167):
- Hypertension, truncal obesity
- Electrolyte abnormalities (hypokalaemia, hyperglycaemia)
- Steroid cover necessary pre- and post-operatively.

Perioperative

- As for craniotomy (see ⮞ p. 393).
- A throat pack should be inserted following intubation. Moffett's solution (see ⮞ p. 624) may be instilled into each nostril to improve surgical conditions.
- Surgical access is via the sphenoidal air sinuses.
- If there is suprasellar extension, a lumbar drain is inserted into the CSF. The anaesthetist may be required to instil a volume of sterile saline to advance the tumour into the operative field.
- Major haemorrhage may occur if there is disruption of the cavernous sinus/carotid arteries which lie lateral to the pituitary gland.

Post-operative

- Diabetes insipidus may occur in up to 50% of patients. It is managed initially with IV desmopressin (0.25–1 micrograms).
- Cerebrospinal rhinorrhoea may occur. It is usually self-limiting, but, if persistent, intermittent CSF drainage via a lumbar drain may be required.

Special considerations

Patients with preoperative pan-hypopituitarism or who develop post-operative endocrine disturbances should be referred to an endocrinologist for advice on hormone replacement. If a craniotomy is planned, rather than a trans-sphenoidal approach, refer to ➲ p. 393.

Posterior fossa surgery

Procedure	Excision or debulking of tumour, vascular procedures, foramen magnum decompression
Time	3–14hr
Pain	+/+++
Position	See below
Blood loss	100–2000mL, G&S
Practical techniques	ETT, IPPV, art line, CVP, consider monitoring for VAE

The posterior fossa lies below the tentorium cerebelli and contains the pons, medulla, and cerebellum. Within the brainstem lie the main motor and sensory pathways, the lower cranial nerve nuclei, and the centres that control respiration and CVS function. An increase in pressure in this area results in decreased consciousness, hypertension, bradycardia, respiratory depression, and loss of protective airway reflexes. The exit pathways for CSF from the ventricular system are also located here, and obstruction results in hydrocephalus. Space-occupying lesions and surgical disturbance in this area can therefore have a profound physiological impact (Table 16.1).

Table 16.1 Posterior fossa lesions

Tumour	Notes
Gliomas	Cerebellar astrocytomas, ependymomas, particularly arising from the 4th ventricle
Medulloblastoma	Often arising from the vermis of the cerebellum, usually in children
Acoustic neuroma	Arising from the 8th nerve in the cerebellopontine angle, usually benign
Haemangioblastoma	Young adults
Meningiomas	Less common in the posterior fossa
Metastatic tumours	
Abscesses and haematoma	
Vascular lesions	Aneurysms of the superior cerebellar, posterior inferior cerebellar, and vertebral arteries
Developmental lesions	Arnold–Chiari malformation

Preoperative

- Patients with posterior fossa lesions may have a reduced level of consciousness and impaired airway reflexes. Bulbar palsy may lead to silent aspiration. Pulmonary function must be assessed.
- Assess ICP—may be raised. If hydrocephalus is present, ventricular drainage may be required before the definitive procedure.
- Assess the fluid status—may be dehydrated if vomiting. A reduced intravascular volume will result in hypotension on induction or if placed in the sitting position.
- Check electrolytes and glucose, particularly if taking diuretics or steroids.
- Assess CVS function, particularly the presence of untreated hypertension, postural hypotension, and septal defects.

Perioperative

- As for craniotomy (see ⬆ p. 393).
- Insert an NGT if risk of post-operative bulbar dysfunction.
- Further specialized monitoring is required for posterior fossa surgery, including monitoring for VAE (see ⬆ p. 413) and nerve tract injury. The appropriate neurophysiological monitor used to detect a nerve tract injury depends upon the neural pathway at risk during the procedure. Spontaneous or evoked EMG activity, somatosensory evoked potentials, or brainstem auditory evoked potentials are frequently monitored. Lumbar CSF drainage is occasionally requested to improve surgical conditions and to reduce the incidence of post-operative CSF leaks.
- Avoid N_2O—it increases the cerebral metabolic rate and CBF, and may worsen the outcome of air embolism. Finally, there is a risk that any residual intracranial air will increase in volume and cause post-operative pneumocephalus.
- Surgical interference with vital centres may result in sudden and dramatic CVS changes. Inform the surgeon—gentler retraction or dissection usually resolves the problem. Use drugs, such as atropine and β-blockers, only if absolutely necessary, as they make the interpretation of further changes difficult.

Patient positioning

Surgical access to the posterior fossa requires the patient to be sitting, prone, or lateral. Careful attention is required in positioning the patient, as procedures are often prolonged.

- Sitting position: use of this position is uncommon. It provides optimum access to midline lesions, improves cerebral venous drainage, and lowers ICP. However, complications include haemodynamic instability, VAE, and the possibility of paradoxical air embolism, pneumocephalus, and quadriplegia. Absolute contraindications include cerebral ischaemia when upright and awake, and the presence of a patent ventriculo-atrial shunt or patent foramen ovale (should be screened preoperatively). Relative contraindications are uncontrolled hypertension, extremes of age, and COPD. To achieve this position, the head and shoulders are gradually elevated, with the neck partially flexed and the forehead resting on a horseshoe ring mounted on a frame. Avoid excessive head

flexion, since this can cause jugular compression, swelling of the tongue and face, and cervical cord ischaemia.
- Prone position: allows good surgical access without the risks associated with the sitting position. Abdominal compression should be avoided, as it results in increased cerebral VP. This is achieved by adequately supporting the chest and pelvis.
- Lateral position: the lateral or 'park bench' position is particularly suitable for lateral lesions such as acoustic neuroma and operations on a cerebellar hemisphere. The neck is flexed, and the head rotated towards the floor, ensuring that the jugular veins are not obstructed. Pressure points over the shoulder, greater trochanter, and peroneal nerves should be protected.

Post-operative

- Most patients can be safely extubated and managed on a properly staffed neurosurgical high dependency ward post-operatively.
- Airway obstruction can occur after posterior fossa surgery due to macroglossia, partial damage to the vagus, and excessive flexion of the cervical spine.
- Surgery on the medulla or high cervical lesions carries a significant risk of post-operative impairment of the respiratory drive.
- The patient should be admitted to ICU for ventilation if the preoperative state was poor, the surgical resection was extensive, there is significant cerebral oedema, or there are intraoperative complications.

Special considerations

- Acoustic neuroma: the facial nerve is particularly vulnerable and is monitored using EMG needles placed over the face. This allows the surgeon to identify when the nerve is at risk. NMB should be used only at induction to allow intubation. Often the 8th nerve function is also monitored to preserve any residual hearing. This requires a constant level of anaesthesia, so that neurophysiological changes can be attributed to surgery, rather than variations in anaesthetic depth. These requirements are best met using a remifentanil infusion, combined with a constant level of anaesthesia using a low concentration of an inhalation agent or a propofol infusion.
- VAE (see ➲ p. 413).
- Post-operative analgesia is managed as for craniotomy.

Awake craniotomy

Procedure	Epilepsy surgery, excision of tumours in eloquent cortical areas
Time	1.5–4hr
Pain	+/+++
Position	See below
Blood loss	100–2000mL, G&S
Practical techniques	LMA, art line, consider monitoring for VAE

Awake craniotomy allows intraoperative assessment of the patient's neurological status. It is mainly used to allow accurate mapping of the resection margins in epilepsy surgery, accurate location of electrodes in surgery for movement disorders, and excision of tumours from eloquent areas of the cortex (sensory, motor, speech areas). In tumour surgery, the aim is to achieve maximal tumour resection with minimal neurological deficit. It is used most effectively in combination with modern imaging techniques such as three-dimensional (3D) navigation systems. Awake craniotomy may be associated with a lower requirement for high dependency care, shorter length of stay, and reduced costs. In the past, a combination of LA and sedation was used, but the use of an asleep–awake–asleep technique with an LMA is gaining popularity, since it is associated with a lower incidence of complications such as oversedation, airway obstruction, hypoventilation, and an uncooperative patient.

Preoperative
- As for craniotomy (see ➋ p. 393).
- Both the neurosurgeon and neuro-anaesthetist must be experienced in awake craniotomy. Appropriate patient selection is essential. The patient must be well informed, motivated, and able to tolerate lying still for the duration of surgery. Confusion, anxiety, and difficulty in communication are contraindications. Obesity, oesophageal reflux, and highly vascular tumours may also cause problems.
- The patient should be given a full explanation of the procedures involved.
- Premedication is generally avoided, but routine medication should be administered on the day of surgery. Anticonvulsant prophylaxis should be prescribed routinely for all patients, and dexamethasone for those undergoing tumour surgery.

Perioperative
- Aims are to ensure adequate sedation, analgesia, cardiorespiratory stability, and to avoid hypercapnia and nausea and vomiting, as well as ensure an awake and cooperative patient when required for

intraoperative testing. Many techniques can be used to achieve this. Routine monitoring as for craniotomy should be used, including urinary catheterization if the procedure is expected to be prolonged.

- IV antiemetic prophylaxis is administered routinely (e.g. ondansetron 4mg IV). Anaesthesia is induced and maintained with a TCI of propofol and a remifentanil infusion (0.05–1 microgram/kg/min). The propofol dose is titrated against the patient's responses, haemodynamics, and possibly BIS monitoring. The patient's lungs are ventilated using an LMA, allowing monitoring and control of ventilation/$PaCO_2$. This minimizes the risks of hypoventilation and airway obstruction, providing good operative conditions. Adequate LA infiltration of the Mayfield fixator pin sites and the operative field is essential.
- When the tumour is exposed, the remifentanil is reduced to 0.005–0.01 microgram/kg/min to allow return of SV. When this occurs, the LMA is removed and the propofol stopped. Once the resection is complete, the patient is re-anaesthetized, and the LMA reinserted until the end of the procedure.
- Preoperative complications include: seizures, respiratory depression, restlessness, airway obstruction, air embolus, and brain swelling.

Post-operative

- Morphine should be administered at the end of the procedure.
- Other aspects of post-operative care are as for craniotomy (see ➲ p. 393).

Special considerations

- Ensure that a calm and quiet atmosphere is maintained in theatre. The patient should be draped in a fashion that allows constant access to the patient's airway and minimizes the feeling of claustrophobia.
- BIS monitoring may be useful in guiding the TCI.

Vascular lesions

Vascular lesions presenting for surgical management are usually either intra-cranial aneurysms or AVMs.

Intracranial aneurysms

- Berry aneurysms occur at vessel junctions, cerebral arteries having a weaker, less elastic muscle layer than systemic vessels. They may occur in association with atherosclerosis, polycystic kidneys, hereditary haemorrhagic telangiectasia, coarctation of the aorta, and Marfan's, Ehlers–Danlos, and Klinefelter's syndromes. The commonest sites are the internal carotid system (41%), the anterior cerebral artery (34%), and the middle cerebral artery (20%).
- They are commoner in ♀ and 40–60yr olds, and, in 25% of cases, they are multiple. In the UK, the incidence is 10–28/100 000 per year. The prevalence of aneurysms is 6% of the population in prospective angiographic studies.
- Aneurysms do not usually rupture until they are >5mm in diameter. They then present as a subarachnoid or an intracerebral haemorrhage. Classic symptoms include sudden onset of severe headache with loss of consciousness, which may be transient in mild cases. Occasionally, a patient presents with a focal neurological deficit due to the pressure of an enlarging aneurysm on surrounding structures.
- Grading of subarachnoid haemorrhage (SAH) (World Federation of Neurosurgeons): the grade of SAH influences morbidity and mortality (Table 16.2). It is also of value in deciding whether to operate or coil early (grades 1–3) or to delay intervention (grades 4–5).

Table 16.2 World Federation of Neurosurgeons grading of subarachnoid haemorrhage

Grade	GCS (see ➲ p. 852)	Motor deficit
1	15	−
2	13–14	−
3	13–14	+
4	7–12	±
>5	3–6	±

Arteriovenous malformations

- These are dilated arteries and veins with no intervening capillaries.
- They may present clinically with SAH or seizures.
- High blood flow through such lesions may 'steal' blood from surrounding tissue, leading to ischaemia.

Complications of aneurysmal subarachnoid haemorrhage

Neurological complications

Rebleeding

- The initial bleed and subsequent bleeds are the main cause of mortality. The highest risk period is in the first 24hr, during which there is a 4% risk of rebleeding, followed by a further risk of 1.5% per day for the next 4wk.
- There is a 60% risk of death with each episode of rebleeding. The main aim of management is to prevent rebleeding by securing the aneurysm either surgically by clipping it or angiographically by obliterating it endoluminally (see Interventional radiology, ➜ p. 411).
- Surgery was previously delayed for up to 10d to avoid the peak of vasospasm.
- The introduction of nimodipine has resulted in earlier surgery, ideally within 72hr. Grade 1–2 patients may be operated upon immediately.
- Most aneurysms are now secured by coiling. Craniotomy and clipping are much less common.

Delayed neurological deficit

- Delayed neurological deficit (DND) may present as focal or diffuse deficits and is a major cause of morbidity. It is the 2nd main cause of mortality.
- It is associated with vasospasm caused by substances released as the subarachnoid blood undergoes haemolysis. The most likely spasmogenic agent is oxyhaemoglobin.
- Although angiographic vasospasm occurs in up to 75% of studied patients, only half of these patients develop DND. Up to 20% of symptomatic patients will develop a stroke or die of vasospasm despite optimal management.
- DND peaks 3–14d after the initial bleed. With increasingly early surgery for aneurysms, it is now commonly seen post-operatively.

Treatment

- Calcium channel blockers: nimodipine is a relatively selective calcium channel antagonist with effective penetration of the blood–brain barrier. It is started at the time of diagnosis and continued for 3wk (60mg NG/PO 4-hourly). Alternatively, it can be administered IV (1mg/hr, increasing to 2mg/hr) either centrally or peripherally with a fast-flowing IV infusion (IVI). Nimodipine may cause systemic hypotension, which should be managed aggressively with fluids and, if necessary, vasopressors.
- Hypertensive, hypervolaemic therapy, with or without haemodilution ('triple H' therapy): this is based on the theory that vasospasm can be prevented or reversed by optimizing CBF. Goals are to increase cardiac output and BP using volume expansion and then vasoactive drugs. The resulting haemodilution may improve CBF by reducing viscosity. Disagreement exists as to the fluids/drugs that should be used and

which haemodynamic goals to aim for. Suggested values are normal MAP + 15%, CVP >12mmHg, and Hct 30–35%. Some centres advocate the use of cardiac output monitoring.
- Monitor therapy. Noradrenaline (0.025–0.3 micrograms/kg/min) and dobutamine (2–15 micrograms/kg/min) are used to increase MAP.
- In some centres, balloon angioplasty or intra-arterial papaverine is also used.

Hydrocephalus

Blood in the subarachnoid space may obstruct drainage of CSF and result in hydrocephalus and raised ICP. Sudden reduction in pressure with the insertion of a ventricular drain may increase the risk of rebleeding by reducing the transmural pressure across the aneurysm. Hydrocephalus must be ruled out by a CT scan before attributing neurological deterioration to DND/vasospasm.

Other neurological complication

These include seizures and cerebral oedema.

Medical complications

Life-threatening medical problems occur in nearly 40% of patients and account for about 23% of deaths. Many of the cardiorespiratory complications following SAH are related to the massive sympathetic surge and catecholamine release that follow SAH.
- Severe LV dysfunction/cardiogenic shock: nearly 45% of patients have an EF <50% or regional wall motion abnormalities. Treat with dobutamine.
- ECG abnormalities: up to 27% of patients will have ECG changes—T-wave inversion, ST-segment abnormalities, and Q waves. Strongly associated with a poor neurological grade, but not predictive of all causes of mortality.
- Neurogenic pulmonary oedema: initially hydrostatic pulmonary oedema resulting from an increase in PAP, followed by damage to the pulmonary microvasculature and an increase in pulmonary capillary permeability.
- Hyponatraemia: many patients are hypovolaemic and hyponatraemic as a result of excessive atrial natriuretic peptide release. Fluid restriction is inappropriate, and it should be managed with Na^+ repletion.
- Other complications include DVT, pneumonia, and hepatic, renal, and GI dysfunction.

Outcome following subarachnoid haemorrhage

~20% of patients will die from SAH at the time of the initial bleed. Of those who survive to reach hospital, a further 15% will die within 24hr, and 40% will make a good recovery.

Anaesthesia for vascular lesions

Procedure	Clipping of intracranial aneurysm, endovascular coiling of aneurysm
Time	>3hr
Pain	++/+++
Position	Supine, head-up, lateral, or prone
Blood loss	200–2000mL, X-match 2U
Practical techniques	ETT, IPPV, art line, CVP

Clipping an aneurysm involves the use of microsurgery to apply a spring clip across the neck of the aneurysm. Aneurysms arising from branches of the vertebral or basilar arteries require a posterior fossa craniotomy, whereas others may be reached from a frontal or fronto-parietal approach. There is often a need to control the aneurysm prior to clipping by applying a temporary clip to a proximal vessel.

Preoperative

- Assess the effects of the haemorrhage and any pre-existing arterial disease on the brain and other organs (see ➜ p. 407).
- Ensure adequate fluid intake and that fluid is not being unnecessarily restricted.
- Nimodipine treatment should be instituted.
- Ensure graduated compression stockings are fitted.
- Phenytoin (15mg/kg, followed by a single daily dose of 3–4mg/kg) should be prescribed prophylactically for the majority of patients.
- Discuss the anticipated difficulty of the surgical approach with the surgeon, as it influences the decision to use induced hypothermia, barbiturates, and other forms of cerebral protection.

Perioperative

As for craniotomy (see ➜ p. 393), but note the following:
- Standard monitoring, including invasive BP monitoring, should be instituted prior to induction. A CVP line can be inserted after induction. It will be useful not only intraoperatively, but also in the post-operative period to help guide 'triple H' therapy (see ➜ p. 407).
- Ensure adequate venous access with large-bore cannulae.
- Aim to avoid increases in arterial pressure that may result in aneurysm rupture, but maintain adequate CPP. Aim for pre-induction BP ± 10%.
- Hypocapnia can result in cerebral ischaemia after SAH and must be avoided. Ventilate to a normal $PaCO_2$.
- Maintain core temperature at 36–37°C for all grade 1–3 patients.
- Modern neurosurgical practice is to use temporary spring clips, rather than induced hypotension. The latter may still be required in difficult

cases or if rupture occurs. In this situation, aim for a systolic BP of 60–80mmHg. Moderate hypotension may be achieved using isoflurane (up to 1.5 MAC). Further hypotension is achieved using labetalol (5–10mg increments). Sodium nitroprusside is rarely used. Hypotension must not be induced in the presence of vasospasm.

- If rupture occurs:
  - Call for help
  - Increase IV infusions, and start blood transfusion
  - Inducing hypotension helps to reduce bleeding
  - Ipsilateral carotid compression
- Other cerebral protection measures should be considered electively if temporary clipping of a major cerebral vessel is planned or in case of aneurysm rupture. This includes the administration of thiopental (3–5mg/kg bolus, followed by 3–5mg/kg/hr), in which case EEG monitoring should ideally be used to allow titration of the dose to burst suppression. It may be necessary to use a vasopressor to support MAP when infusing thiopental. Inducing hypothermia to a temperature of 32°C is reserved for complex surgical vascular procedures. The patient is cooled, using surface devices, and rewarmed once the cerebral circulation is restored.

Post-operative

- ICU/HDU care is required post-operatively for patients with a poor grade preoperatively, those who had a stormy perioperative course, and those requiring treatment for vasospasm.
- Codeine phosphate and regular paracetamol may be prescribed for analgesia.
- A decrease in the GCS may indicate vasospasm, intracranial haematoma, or hydrocephalus—perform a CT scan.

Arteriovenous malformations

- Surgery is not urgent, unless the AVM or a resulting haematoma is causing pressure effects.
- The procedure may be associated with significant blood loss—cross-matched blood and adequate IV access are essential.
- Blood may be shunted through the AVM, resulting in relative ischaemia to the surrounding tissue. When the lesion is excised, a relative hyperperfusion of surrounding tissue may occur, resulting in cerebral oedema and increased ICP.
- There is no risk of vasospasm, and, when indicated, hypotension may be induced with relative safety. This is achieved using isoflurane ± labetalol, as outlined for SAH (see p. 409).
- In children, AVMs can cause high-output failure due to intracerebral shunt. CCF may be precipitated by excision of the lesion.

Interventional radiology

Intracranial aneurysms

Most intracranial aneurysms are currently treated by releasing Guglielmi detachable coils (GDCs) into the aneurysmal lumen via microcatheters inserted in the femoral artery, until occlusion of the aneurysm is achieved. This approach is associated with better independent survival at 1yr than after craniotomy and clipping of the aneurysm. The risk of death is significantly lower in the coiled than the clipped group at 5yr. The risk of late rebleeding is acceptable, but higher, after coiling than clipping.

- The procedure is undertaken in an angiography suite by a neuro-radiologist. Ensure a skilled anaesthetic assistant and monitoring facilities as for a GA clipping of aneurysm.
- A CVP line is not always necessary. It is preferable to monitor the arterial pressure before induction of anaesthesia, although the femoral artery introducer sheath inserted by the radiologist can be transduced. This provides a reliable mean but overestimates diastolic, and underestimates systolic, BP.
- The patient will need temperature monitoring and warming devices, and a wide-bore IV cannula.
- It is important to maintain a normal MAP and $PaCO_2$. This may be difficult, as coiling is not a particularly stimulating procedure.
- The induction and maintenance of anaesthesia is the same as for clipping of an aneurysm, although a normal ETT or a ProSeal LMA may be used, instead of an armoured tube.
- Recovery should be smooth and rapid. An incompletely secured aneurysm may require control of the MAP post-operatively. Patients who have had neurological complications need to be transferred to a neurological ICU for post-operative ventilation.

Special considerations

- Unfamiliar environment, remote site, radiation, radiology equipment, closed skull, contrast and flush, heparin, antiplatelet drugs, and thrombolysis.
- In patients with a high risk of a thrombotic event from a coil in the parent vessel, it may be necessary to administer aspirin (500mg IV) and to continue heparin into the post-operative period. Thrombotic events occurring during the procedure are often managed with abciximab.

Complications

- Intraoperative vasospasm can result from manipulation of the vessel and is managed by withdrawing the catheter from the vessel and allowing a few minutes for recovery. Alternatively, intra-arterial nimodipine may be administered.
- Rupture of the aneurysm or haemorrhage is identified by extravasation of contrast. The intracranial haemorrhage may increase ICP and MAP, with or without bradycardia. Aim to reverse the heparin, and reduce MAP to the level before the bleed. Measures to reduce ICP (see ➜ p. 392 and p. 398) may be required.

- Patients with a reduced post-operative GCS should have a CT scan to exclude hydrocephalus or vascular complications. It may be necessary to insert an external ventricular drain (EVD) and transfer to ICU for continued management.

Arteriovenous malformation: cerebral and spinal

Embolization may be used to obliterate an AVM or reduce its size before definitive surgery. This minimizes intraoperative bleeding, while preserving the arterial supply to the brain. Staged procedures are commonly undertaken due to rapid blood flow, multiple fistulae, feeding and draining vessels, and associated aneurysms. The material used is usually a liquid polymer (e.g. Onyx) or glue.

Anaesthesia is as for coiling of aneurysms. Hypotension can cause intracerebral steal, and raised ICP from recent intracranial haemorrhage may worsen hypertension. Controlled hypotension may be used for short periods to produce 'flow arrest' through the AVM and enable the embolic glue to set, rather than be carried straight through. This is achieved by using isoflurane ± labetalol, as outlined for SAH (see ➲ p. 409).

Special considerations
- The femoral artery may need cannulation on multiple occasions. An Angio-Seal™ (artificial collagen plug) is therefore not used; instead haemostasis is achieved by applying pressure manually which may take 15–20min. The patient should remain anaesthetized for this to avoid coughing or movement of the leg. Retroperitoneal haematoma may occur.
- If the nidus is suitable, the AVM may be treated by radiosurgery in a specialist centre.

Complications
- Inadvertent occlusion of normal vessels, causing cerebral ischaemia.
- PE from systemic shunting of particulate materials.
- Bleeding from incomplete embolization, perforation of arterial feeders, or rupture of an associated aneurysm. Subtle changes in the dynamics of the fistula may also increase the risk of haemorrhage.
- The sudden occlusion of the AVM can result in cerebral hyperperfusion if the AVM and normal brain share venous drainage. This will result in cerebral oedema and increased ICP.

Venous air embolism

- VAE can occur whenever the operative site is higher than the right atrium. Its incidence is particularly high during craniotomy in the sitting position and when the surgeon is dissecting tissues that do not allow veins to collapse despite a negative pressure within them (e.g. the emissary veins in the posterior fossa).
- VAE causes pulmonary microvascular occlusion, resulting in an increased physiological dead space. Bronchoconstriction may also develop. A large volume of air causes frothing within the right atrium, leading to obstruction of the RV outflow tract and a reduction in cardiac output.
- Signs of VAE include hypotension, arrhythmias, increased PAP, decreased $ETCO_2$, and hypoxia.
- N_2O does not increase the risk of VAE but may worsen its outcome.

Detection of venous air embolism

- $ETCO_2$ is generally the most useful monitor, as it is widely available and sensitive. Air embolism results in a sudden reduction in $ETCO_2$. Hyperventilation, low cardiac output, and other types of embolism will also result in reduction in $ETCO_2$.
- Doppler ultrasound is the most sensitive non-invasive monitor. It uses ultra-high-frequency sound waves to detect changes in blood flow velocity and density. Unfortunately, it is not quantitative and does not differentiate between a massive or physiologically insignificant air embolism. Positioning the probe and diathermy interference can prove problematic.
- TOE allows determination of the amount of air aspirated but is more invasive, is difficult to place, and needs expertise to interpret.
- Pulmonary artery catheters are invasive, but sensitive, monitors for VAE. However, an increase in PAP is not specific for air.
- The least sensitive monitor is a precordial or an oesophageal stethoscope to detect a 'millwheel' murmur. This is apparent only after massive VAE, which is usually clinically obvious.

Prevention

- Avoid the sitting position, unless essential.
- Elevate the head only as much as necessary.
- Ensure adequate blood volume to maintain a positive CVP.
- Small amounts of PEEP (5–10cmH$_2$O) may reduce the risk of air entrainment.
- A 'G-suit' or medical antishock trousers may be used to increase VP and reduce hypotensive episodes in patients in the sitting position.

Treatment

- Treatment is supportive.
- Inform the surgeon, who should flood the operative field with fluid. This stops further entrainment of air and allows the identification of open veins that can be cauterized or waxed if within bone.
- Stop N_2O if in use, and increase the FiO_2 to 1.0.

- If possible, position the operative site below the level of the heart to increase VP.
- Aspirate air from the CVP line. The tip should be placed close to the junction of the SVC and the right atrium.
- Support the BP with fluid and vasopressors.
- If a large volume of air has been entrained and surgical conditions permit, turn the patient into the left lateral position to attempt to keep the air in the right atrium.
- Commence CPR, if necessary.

Paradoxical air embolism

- Air emboli may enter the systemic circulation through the Thebesian veins in the heart, the bronchial vessels, or a patent foramen ovale. Such defects may be small and not picked up preoperatively.
- Small volumes of air in the systemic circulation can have disastrous consequences.
- Intracardiac septal defects are an absolute contraindication to surgery in the sitting position.

Neurological determination of death

The commonest causes of brainstem death are head injury, intracranial haemorrhage, cerebral tumours, and hypoxic brain injury. To diagnose brainstem death, the patient needs to fulfil certain preconditions and have absent brainstem reflexes.

Preconditions

- The patient is deeply comatose, apnoeic, and dependent on mechanical ventilation.
- The coma must be caused by a known and irreversible cause of brain injury.
- Reversible causes for brainstem depression have been excluded: sedatives, muscle relaxants, alcohol, hypothermia, and metabolic or endocrine disturbances.

Absence of brainstem responses

Tests of brainstem reflexes should be performed only when the preconditions are fulfilled.

- Pupils are fixed, and there is no direct or consensual response to light. The pupils are usually dilated, but this is not essential for the diagnosis.
- Corneal reflex is absent.
- There is no motor response within the cranial nerve distribution to painful stimuli applied centrally or peripherally. Spontaneous and reflex movements (spinal reflexes) may persist in brainstem-dead patients.
- Oculo-vestibular reflex is absent. There is no eye movement in response to the injection of 50mL of ice-cold water into the external auditory meatus—direct access to the tympanic membrane should be verified using an auroscope. The eyes should be observed for at least 1min after each injection.
- There is no gag or cough reflex in response to a suction catheter passed into the pharynx or down the ETT.
- Apnoea is present on disconnection from mechanical ventilation. This test is done last to avoid unnecessary hypercapnia should any of the other reflexes be present. The patient should be preoxygenated by ventilating with 100% O_2, and the minute ventilation reduced to achieve a $PaCO_2$ of 6kPa (45mmHg). The patient is then disconnected and observed continuously for any respiratory movement for 5min. The $PaCO_2$ should be measured and should be high enough to ensure an adequate stimulus to ventilation (>6.7kPa (50mmHg) in a previously normal individual). Hypoxia is avoided during apnoea by passing a suction catheter down the ETT and supplying 5–10L/min of O_2, while monitoring the SaO_2.

Other considerations

- The diagnosis of brainstem death should be made by two medical practitioners trained and experienced in the field. One must be a consultant, and the other could be a second consultant or a doctor who has been registered for a minimum of 5yr. Neither should be a member of the transplant team.

- The tests must be performed on two occasions, separated by an adequate time interval, to satisfy all concerned.
- The diagnosis should not normally be considered until at least 6hr after the onset of an apnoeic coma or 24hr after the restoration of circulation if the cause was a cardiac arrest. If therapeutic hypothermia was used, the tests should be performed at least 24hr after the restoration of normothermia.
- Death is confirmed after the 2nd set of tests, but the time of death is recorded as the completion of the 1st set of brainstem death criteria.
- No additional tests are required in the UK, but other countries may require EEG, cerebral angiography, or brainstem evoked potentials.
- The coroner (Procurator Fiscal in Scotland) needs to be informed of most of these patients due to the underlying diagnosis and if organ donation is contemplated.
- Care of the relatives is essential at this time, irrespective of whether the patient is to be an organ donor or not.

Organ retrieval from a donor after brain death

Procedure	Procurement of donor organs via long midline incision and median sternotomy
Time	Up to 6hr, depending on which organs are retrieved
Pain	N/A
Position	Supine
Blood loss	Large fluid losses likely, X-match 4U
Practical techniques	Usually from ICU IPPV, CVP, and art line

Demand for donor organs continues to exceed supply, and potential organ donors should be identified and discussed with a donor coordinator. The only absolute contraindications to donation are CJD, HIV, active tuberculosis (TB), and recent malignancy in the potential donor. The typical donor after brain death (DBD) is now older, has a higher BMI and more co-morbidities, and is more likely to have died from an intracranial haemorrhage than a head injury.

Pathophysiology of brainstem death

- Early, short-lived massive sympathetic outflow occurs during brainstem herniation, causing hypertension, tachycardia, myocardial dysfunction, impaired organ perfusion, and tissue ischaemia.
- Autonomic collapse results in a reduction in cardiac output, hypotension, and atropine-resistant bradycardia. Circulatory collapse follows, if left untreated.
- Deterioration in lung function is common due to neurogenic pulmonary oedema, acute lung injury, and pre-existing disease.
- Reduced circulating T_3 and T_4, with increased peripheral conversion of T_4 to reverse T_3, causes depletion of myocardial energy stores, myocardial dysfunction, and a global shift to anaerobic metabolism.
- Hyperglycaemia is due to reduced circulating insulin and insulin resistance.
- Reduced ADH secretion leads to neurogenic diabetes insipidus, with hypovolaemia and electrolyte disorders (hypernatraemia, hypermagnesaemia, hypokalaemia, hypophosphataemia, hypocalcaemia).
- Release of tissue fibrinolytic agents and plasminogen activators from the necrotic brain causes a coagulopathy.
- Temperature regulation is lost due to hypothalamic dysfunction, resulting in hypothermia.

Preoperative

- Check that brainstem death has been confirmed and that agreement to organ donation has been obtained from the relatives and the coroner.
- Emphasis in management changes from cerebral resuscitation to optimal organ perfusion and oxygenation.
- Ensure intravascular volume resuscitation using continuous CVP monitoring. Avoid fluid overload in potential lung donors where a CVP >6mmHg may increase the A–a O_2 gradient and reduce the number of donor lungs that can be retrieved successfully. If hypotension persists, despite fluid replacement, then an infusion of vasopressin should be started as the 1st-line vasopressor. PAFC and TOE are often requested for potential heart donors with high inotrope requirements. They allow assessment of the cardiac structure and function and prevent intravascular overload.
- Continue regular chest physiotherapy and suctioning.
- If desmopressin has been used to control diabetes insipidus, it should be changed to vasopressin (ADH)—restores vascular tone and arterial pressure without a direct myocardial effect.
- The use of hormone resuscitation (Table 16.3), using T_3 replacement, methylprednisolone, and vasopressin, varies among transplant centres. Their use should be guided by the local retrieval team or in-house protocols. High-dose methylprednisolone increases the successful retrieval of lungs for transplantation.
- Correct hypernatraemia with 5% glucose (Na^+ <155mmol/L). Glucose 4%/NaCl 0.18% with KCl should be used to replace normal urinary water and electrolyte losses. Clotting abnormalities should be corrected with clotting factors and platelets.
- Central venous access via the right internal jugular vein and left radial arterial access are preferred due to early ligation of the left innominate vein and right subclavian artery, respectively.
- Order CXR, ECG, echocardiography, and 4-hourly ABGs for potential heart/lung donors.
- Maintain physiological parameters outlined in Table 16.4.

Perioperative

- Standard monitoring plus CVP, arterial line, core temperature, and urine output. Maintain core temperature >35°C. Frequent analysis of ABGs, electrolytes, Hct, glucose, and clotting. Large-bore IV access (right upper limb) is mandatory for the replacement of fluid losses (up to 8L) with crystalloid, colloid, or red cells (keep Hct >30%).
- The need for GA is controversial. Many use up to 1 MAC isoflurane or fentanyl (5–7 micrograms/kg) to control reflex pressor responses during surgery. This can also be achieved using labetalol or GTN. Non-depolarizing neuromuscular-blocking agents are administered to obtund reflex muscular contractions due to the preserved spinal reflexes and to improve surgical access. Pancuronium and vecuronium are cardiostable and preferred.
- Large and frequent haemodynamic fluctuations occur due to compression of the IVC, manipulation of the adrenals, and blood/fluid

Table 16.3 Hormone resuscitation during organ retrieval

	Bolus	Infusion	Action
Liothyronine (tri-iodothyronine, T_3)	4 micrograms	3 micrograms/hr	Reverses myocardial dysfunction and reduces inotrope requirements
Vasopressin (ADH)	1U	0.5–2U/hr	Treats diabetes insipidus and restores vascular tone. Titrated to MAP >60mmHg or SVR 800–1200 dyn.s/cm^5
Insulin		Sliding scale	To maintain blood sugar 6–9 mmol/L
Methylprednisolone	15mg/kg	±	Improves oxygenation and increases donor lung procurement by reducing cytokine-mediated cellular injury

Table 16.4 Target parameters for organ retrieval

Target parameters	
CVP	4–10mmHg (<6mmHg for potential lung donors)
MAP	60–80mmHg
PAOP	10–15mmHg
Cardiac index	>2.2–2.5L/min/m^2
Hb	100g/L (Hct 30%)
SpO_2	>95% (with lowest FiO_2 and PEEP)
V_T	6–8mL/kg
$PaCO_2$	4.5–5.5kPa (34–41mmHg)
Urine output	1–3mL/kg/hr
Peak inspiratory pressure	<30cmH$_2$O

loss. Hypotension is treated with colloid titrated to the CVP, vasopressin infusion, and metaraminol (0.5mg increments).
- Broad-spectrum antibiotics are given as per local transplant protocol.
- Full heparinization (300IU/kg) should be administered centrally prior to surgical cannulation of the major vessels.
- Epoprostenol (5–20ng/kg/min) may be needed for 10min via the PA if the lungs are to be harvested.

- PAFC/CVC withdrawn before ligation of the SVC.
- Note the time of aortic cross-clamp as the beginning of organ ischaemic time.
- At the end, discontinue mechanical ventilation/monitoring, and remove the ETT after lung inflation and trachea cross-clamp.
- The abdominal surgical team continues to operate in circulatory arrest.

Special considerations

- Empathy and sensitivity in dealing with the donor's family are paramount throughout the management of the potential organ donor.
- The quality of care afforded to the multiorgan donor could affect the outcome of >6 recipients.
- In the event of a cardiac arrest, CPR should be commenced, as procurement of the liver and kidneys can still proceed rapidly with cross-clamping of the aorta at the diaphragm and infusion of cold preservation solution into the distal aorta and portal vein.

Further reading

Pasternak JJ, Lanier WL (2011). Neuroanesthesiology update 2010. *J Neurosurg Anesthesiol*, **23**, 67–99.

[Postgraduate issue on clinical neurosciences] (2007). *Br J Anaesth*, **99**, 1–138.

Vascular surgery

Mark Stoneham

General principles

Most vascular surgery involves operating on arteries diseased or damaged by atherosclerosis, causing poor peripheral blood flow (ischaemia) or emboli. Mortality is high; elective AAA surgery has a mortality of 7%,[1] while that of emergency AAA is >50%. This is markedly increased in the presence of uncontrolled CVS disease. Operations may be long and involve blood transfusion, marked fluid shifts, and significant impairment of lung function. All major vascular operations should now take place in one of the designated 'vascular centres'.

- Vascular patients are usually elderly arteriopaths with significant associated disease. Hypertension (66%), IHD (angina, MI), heart failure, diabetes mellitus, and COPD (50% are current or ex-smokers) are common. Many patients are taking aspirin, β-blockers, diuretics, heart failure medications, and perhaps insulin or oral hypoglycaemics.
- Some patients are anticoagulated; others will receive anticoagulants perioperatively, so consider the pros and cons of regional techniques carefully (see ➡ p. 1141). However, regional techniques can reduce morbidity and mortality (see ➡ p. 423).
- Vascular patients tend to have serial operations, so there may be several previous anaesthetic records to review. Thirty to 40% of vascular operations occur out of hours.
- Measure NIBP in both arms—there may be differences due to arteriopathy (use the higher of the two values clinically, or put your arterial line in this side).
- All patients receiving synthetic vascular grafts require prophylactic antibiotic cover.
- Develop a working relationship with your vascular surgeon—you will have a better chance of being warned of untoward events (e.g. aortic clamping/unclamping, sudden massive blood loss, etc.).

Preoperative assessment

- Quantify the extent of any cardiorespiratory disease, both in terms of the planned surgical procedure and the post-operative period. Carefully consider (and document) whether regional anaesthesia is appropriate.
- Include direct questions about exercise tolerance (walking distance on the flat, ability to climb stairs) and the ability to lie supine. Look for signs of cardiac failure.
- Investigations: FBC, U&Es, ECG, CXR, coagulation, and LFTs.
- A dynamic assessment of the cardiac function is required for all elective aortic surgery and for any patients with symptomatic/new cardiac disease. CPET is the 'gold standard' for all AAA patients—open or endovascular (see ➡ p. 15). Alternatives, however, include echocardiography, exercise ECG, stress echocardiography, radionuclide thallium scan, and multigated acquisition scan (MUGA). Refer patients with critically IHD to cardiology for angiography and possible coronary revascularization before aortic surgery.[2] Emergent vascular patients may have to undergo surgery before such dynamic investigations can be performed.

- Lung function tests (including ABG analysis while breathing air) should be performed in patients with significant respiratory disease presenting for AAA repair.

Premedication

Continue β-blockers and statins perioperatively. Anxiolytic premedication may be useful for major surgery.

Regional anaesthesia and analgesia in vascular surgical patients

Regional anaesthesia may be used alone for distal vascular surgery and is commonly used for carotid surgery, although no major differences in outcome between general and regional anaesthesia were shown by the GALA trial of 3500 patients undergoing carotid endarterectomy (CEA).[3] Epidural analgesia is commonly used to supplement GA for AAA. The advantages of regional techniques include:

- Improved patient monitoring (CEA)
- Reduced hospital stay and cost (CEA)
- Improved blood flow, reduced DVT, reduced reoperation (peripheral revascularization)
- Post-operative pain relief (AAA, distal revascularization, amputation)
- Reduced pulmonary complications (AAA surgery)
- Pre-emptive analgesia for amputations—possible reduction in phantom limb pain
- Treatment of proximal hypertension during aortic cross-clamp.

Epidural catheters and anticoagulation

See ➔ p. 1141.

References

1 Mani K, Lees T, Beiles B, et al. (2011). Treatment of abdominal aortic aneurysm in nine countries 2005–2009: a vascunet report. Eur J Vasc Endovasc Surg, 42, 598–607.

2 McFalls EO, Ward HB, Moritz TE (2004). Coronary artery revascularization before elective major vascular surgery. N Engl J Med, 352, 2795–804.

3 GALA Trial Collaborators Group (2008). General anaesthesia versus local anaesthesia for carotid surgery: a randomized, controlled trial. Lancet, 372, 2132–42.

Abdominal aortic aneurysm repair

Procedure	Excision of aortic aneurysmal sac and replacement with synthetic graft (tube/trouser graft)
Time	2–4h
Pain	++++
Position	Supine, arms out (crucifix)
Blood loss	500–2000+ mL, X-match 6U. Suitable for auto-transfusion
Practical techniques	ETT + IPPV, art + CVP lines. Epidural if possible

Preoperative

- The elderly often have multiple coexisting diseases.
- Mortality for elective surgery is ~5% (predominantly MI and multiorgan failure).
- Careful preoperative assessment is essential. Scrutinize the ECG for signs of ischaemia, and check for any renal impairment. The patient needs dynamic cardiac assessment preoperatively (see p. 37 and p. 15). Check access sites for CVP and arterial line.
- HDU/ICU for post-operative care. Alert the patient to this plan, especially if a period of post-operative IPPV is planned. Pre-optimization is performed in some units—patients are admitted to the HDU/ICU a few hours preoperatively to have lines, etc. inserted and to have the haemodynamic status 'optimized'. This is not widely adopted.
- Continue the usual cardiac medications perioperatively.

Perioperative

- Have available vasoconstrictors (ephedrine and metaraminol), vasodilators (GTN), and β-blockers (labetalol).
- Two 14G or greater IV access. A hot-air and IVI warmer are essential. Monitor intraoperative temperature.
- A Level-1® fluid warmer or equivalent is extremely useful.
- There is no good evidence supporting the use of isovolaemic haemodilution; however, cell salvage should be mandatory in every case, as there is good evidence that it reduces the usage of allogeneic blood in aortic surgery.
- Arterial line and thoracic epidural (T6–T11) pre-induction. Take a baseline blood gas some time before cross-clamping.
- Have at least two syringe drivers present—inotropes, vasodilators, and eventually the epidural will all need them.
- Use a 5-lead ECG (leads II and V_5)—this increases the sensitivity for detection of myocardial ischaemia.
- Triple-lumen CVP after induction. Consider inserting a PAFC introducer in complex cases, as this will allow rapid fluid administration and facilitate

PA catheter insertion if necessary (use the right internal jugular or left subclavian vein to facilitate easier insertion of a PA catheter, if required).

- Be obsessive about temperature control from the start. Avoid heat loss, as it is easier to keep a patient's temperature constant than to try to increase it.

- Continuous cardiac output monitoring is useful during the cross-clamp period for all patients, particularly those with impaired cardiac function. Possibilities include: PA catheter, LiDCO™, PiCCO™, and oesophageal Doppler; however, the latter is not accurate during aortic cross-clamping.

- Careful induction with monitoring of invasive arterial BP. Use moderate/high-dose opioid, e.g. remifentanil (0.1–0.2 micrograms/kg/min) or high-dose fentanyl (5–10 micrograms/kg). Treat hypotension with fluids at first and then cautious vasoconstriction (metaraminol 0.25–0.5mg). There is no difference in myocardial outcome between sevoflurane-based anaesthesia, compared with TIVA.[4]

- Hypothermia is likely, unless energetic efforts are made to maintain the temperature during induction, line insertion, and perioperatively. Warming blankets should not be placed on the lower limbs while the aortic cross-clamp is in place, as this may worsen lower limb ischaemia.

- Insert a urinary catheter for hourly measurements of urine output.

- Heparin will need to be given just before cross-clamp; 3000–5000U is usual. This may be reversed after unclamping with protamine 0.5–1mg per 100U of heparin IV slowly—hypotension results if given too quickly.

- Proximal hypertension may follow aortic cross-clamping and is due to a sudden increase in SVR, increased SVC flow, and sympatho-adrenal response. Treat by deepening the anaesthesia and/or a bolus of β-blocker (labetalol 5–10mg), GTN infusion, or epidural LA.

- While the aorta is clamped, metabolic acidosis will develop due to ischaemic lower limbs. Maintaining the minute ventilation will cause a respiratory alkalosis to develop, which will minimize the effects of this metabolic acidosis when the aorta is unclamped. Check ABGs to assess Hct, metabolic acidosis, respiratory compensation, and ionized Ca^{2+}.

- Cross-clamp time is usually 30–60min. During this time, start giving fluid, aiming for a moderately increased CVP (5cmH$_2$O greater than the baseline) by the time unclamping occurs. This helps CVS stability, reduces sudden hypotension, and may help preserve the renal function. Release of the cross-clamp one limb at a time also helps haemodynamic stability.

- Hypotension following aortic unclamping is caused by a decreased SVR, relative hypovolaemia, and myocardial 'stunning' due to the return of cold metabolic waste products from the legs. Treat with IV fluids and/or lighten the anaesthetic depth and/or small doses of inotropes, e.g. adrenaline 10 microgram aliquots (1mL of 1:100 000) and/or a bolus of calcium gluconate (up to 10mL of 10%). Inotropes may be needed post-operatively.

- For fluid replacement, give isotonic crystalloid or colloid to replace insensible, 3rd space, and initial blood loss. Give blood products when a deficiency is identified, e.g. Hct <25%, platelets <100 × 10^9/L. Check

the ACT (normal <140s) if you suspect coagulopathy. TEG will give you the whole coagulation picture.
- TOE may be used to give additional information during the cross-clamp period.[5]

Post-operative
- ICU/HDU is essential post-operatively. HDU may be appropriate for otherwise fit patients who can be extubated at the end of the case. Extubate if warm, haemodynamically stable, and with a working epidural. Otherwise transfer to ICU intubated.
- Opioid infusion and/or PCA if no epidural. Routine observations, including invasive arterial and CVP monitoring and urine output, should be continued post-operatively to assess haemodynamic stability. There is potential for large fluid shifts which need replacement. Assess distal pulses.

Special considerations
- Management of epidural: a bolus of epidural diamorphine 2–3mg at induction will last for 12–24hr. Use epidural LA sparingly, until the aorta is closed. It is easier to treat the hypotension of aortic unclamping with a functioning sympathetic nervous system.
- Renal failure occurs in 1–2% of cases and is multifactorial in origin—but is associated with a mortality of 50% following AAA repair. It is more likely if the cross-clamp is suprarenal. There is no evidence that dopamine prevents renal failure, merely acting as an inotrope. Mannitol is used routinely by some (0.5g/kg during cross-clamp) as a free radical scavenger and an osmotic diuretic. Avoid hypovolaemia, and monitor the urine output hourly.

References
4 Lindholm EE, Aune E, Norén CB, *et al.* (2013). The anesthesia in abdominal aortic surgery (ABSENT) study: a prospective, randomized, controlled trial comparing troponin T release with fentanyl-sevoflurane and propofol-remifentanil anesthesia in major vascular surgery. *Anesthesiology,* **119**, 802–12.
5 Matyal R, Hess PE, Asopa A, Zhao X, Panzica PJ, Mahmood F (2012). Monitoring the variation in myocardial function with the Doppler-derived myocardial performance index during aortic cross-clamping. *J Cardiothorac Vasc Anesth,* **26**, 204–8.

Emergency repair of abdominal aortic aneurysm

This is a true anaesthetic and surgical emergency. It may be:
- Acute: presents with CVS collapse. Death is likely, unless the rupture is contained in the retroperitoneal space
- Dissecting: dissects along the arterial intima—presents with back/abdominal pain.

Prehospital mortality for ruptured AAA is 50%, and half of those reaching hospital also do not survive. Management is as for elective AAA (see p. 424), with the following additional considerations.
- Where doubt exists (and the patient is haemodynamically stable), the diagnosis is confirmed by ultrasound or CT scan.
- If hypovolaemic shock is present, resuscitate to a systolic pressure of 90mmHg. Avoid hypertension, coughing, and straining, as this may precipitate a further bleed. Titrate IV morphine against pain.
- Pre-induction, insert two 14G peripheral cannulae and (ideally) an arterial line. Use of the brachial artery may be necessary, and sometimes an arterial 'cut-down' is indicated. Central venous access can wait, until after the cross-clamp is applied. If peripheral IV access is difficult, insert a PAFC introducer into the right internal jugular vein.
- Epidural analgesia is usually inappropriate.
- A urinary catheter can be placed before or after induction.
- Induction must be in theatre, with the surgeons scrubbed, surgical preparation completed, drapes on, and blood available in theatre and checked. RSI is usually required. Suitable induction agents include midazolam/remifentanil, etomidate (also give hydrocortisone 50–100mg), and ketamine. As soon as endotracheal intubation is confirmed, the surgeons can begin. Treat hypotension with IV fluids and small doses of vasopressors/inotropic agents.
- Hot-air warming and at least one warmed IVI are essential (a Level-1® blood warmer is invaluable).
- Use a colloid or crystalloid, depending on preference. Use a balanced crystalloid such as Hartmann's solution, rather than 0.9% NaCl (helps prevent metabolic acidosis).
- Have both IV lines running maximally at induction. One assistant should be dedicated to managing IV fluid and ensuring an uninterrupted supply. Once the cross-clamp is applied, some haemodynamic stability may be restored.
- Cell salvage, if available, is mandatory.
- Hypothermia, renal impairment, blood loss, and coagulopathy are common perioperative problems. Hypothermia is a particular hazard, as bleeding post-operatively is likely (platelet function is markedly reduced below 35°C). While there is no place for routine administration of platelets and FFP, consider early use when needed.

- Do not attempt to extubate at the conclusion of surgery—a post-operative period of ventilation on the ICU is essential to allow the correction of biochemical/haematological abnormalities.
- Use near-patient testing (Hb and TEG), if available, to guide blood product administration. If the patient is exsanguinating and cross-matched blood is not available, use type-specific.

Endovascular stenting of elective or emergency abdominal aortic aneurysm

Procedure	Placement and deployment of bifurcated stent by interventional radiologists into aortic aneurysmal sac via femoral arteries
Time	1–4hr
Pain	+
Position	Supine
Blood loss	0–2000+ mL, X-match 6U
Practical techniques	Epidural + sedation, art + CVP lines

This technique is associated with lower operative morbidity and mortality than standard open AAA repair,[6] but it is still unproven whether it lowers the risk of aneurysm rupture; thus, post-operatively, patients must be kept under CT surveillance for the rest of their lives. Significant complications, such as migration of the stent and endoleak, can develop, as well as frank rupture.

- The procedure is usually performed in the radiology/angio suite. The surgeons gain access to the aorta via the femoral arteries, and the stent is inserted by an interventional radiologist.
- If an aneurysm rupture does occur (incidence is around 2%), mortality rises to >50%.
- Pre-assessment, monitoring, and cross-matching are all exactly as for an open repair. However, since the patient will not undergo aortic cross-clamping, patients who have been refused open surgery because of significant LV impairment may tolerate endovascular repair. ICU is usually not needed post-operatively.
- General or regional anaesthesia is appropriate, depending on preference, although regional anaesthesia may shorten the procedure.[7] One regime is an epidural/sedation technique consisting of an epidural bolus of diamorphine 2–3mg, followed by a bupivacaine 0.25% infusion (4–8mL/hr), in conjunction with propofol TCI (0.5–1 microgram/kg/min).
- Post-operatively, the patient may go to the HDU or the vascular ward for overnight monitoring.
- Increasingly, patients with ruptured AAAs are being stented,[8] which may improve outcome once standardized protocols are established.

References

6 Prinssen M, Verhoeven EL, Buth J, et al.; Dutch Randomized Endovascular Aneurysm Management (DREAM) Trial Group (2004). A randomized trial comparing conventional and endovascular repair of abdominal aortic aneurysms. *N Engl J Med*, **351**, 1607–18.

7 Asakura Y, Ishibashi H, Ishiguchi T, Kandatsu N, Akashi M, Komatsu T (2009). General versus locoregional anesthesia for endovascular aortic aneurysm repair: influences of the type of anesthesia on its outcome. *J Anesth*, **23**, 158–61.

8 Rayt HS, Sutton AJ, London NJ, Sayers RD, Bown MJ (2008). A systematic review and meta-analysis of endovascular repair (EVAR) for ruptured abdominal aortic aneurysm. *Eur J Vasc Endovascul Surg*, **36**, 536–44.

Thoraco-abdominal aortic aneurysm repair

Procedure	Excision of aortic aneurysmal sac extending above the origin of the renal arteries and replacement with a synthetic graft. May involve thoracotomy and the need for OLV
Time	3–6hr
Pain	++++
Position	Supine, arms out (crucifix), may be right lateral if thoracotomy
Blood loss	1000mL–+++, X-match 8U, plus platelets and FFP
Practical techniques	DLT + IPPV, art + CVP lines. Thoracic epidural

Thoracic aneurysms of the ascending aorta require median sternotomy and CPB. Transverse aortic arch repair often requires hypothermic circulatory arrest as well.

Special considerations

As for infrarenal aortic aneurysm repair, with the following considerations:
- The aneurysm may compress the trachea and distort the anatomy of the upper vasculature.
- Intensive care is essential for post-operative ventilation and stabilization.
- The aortic cross-clamp will be much higher than for a simple AAA. This means that the kidneys, liver, and splanchnic circulation will be ischaemic for the duration of the cross-clamp.
- Access to the thoracic aorta may require OLV—thus, a left-sided DLT may be required (see p. 363). A Univent® tube is a possible alternative (see ➔ p. 364).
- Proximal hypertension following aortic cross-clamping is more pronounced. Use aggressive vasodilatation with GTN (infusion of 50mg/50mL run at 10mL/hr until it starts to work) or esmolol (2.5g/50mL at 3–15mL/hr).
- Hypotension following aortic unclamping is often severe, requiring inotropic support post-operatively—use adrenaline (5mg/50mL), starting at 5mL/hr.
- Acidosis is a particular problem—metabolic acidosis develops during cross-clamping and is potentially exacerbated by respiratory acidosis due to prolonged OLV. Use balanced crystalloids; consider using HCO_3^-, and ventilate post-operatively until it is resolved.
- Renal failure occurs in up to 25% of cases—principally related to the duration of cross-clamping. Monitor urine output; give mannitol 25g before cross-clamping, and maintain the circulating volume.

- Spinal cord ischaemia, leading to paralysis, may develop. This is related to the duration of cross-clamping and occurs because a branch of the thoracic aorta (artery of Adamkiewicz) reinforces the blood supply of the cord. Techniques used for prevention (none is infallible) include: CSF pressure measurement and drainage through a spinal drain; spinal cord cooling through an epidural catheter; intrathecal Mg^{2+}; distal perfusion techniques; CPB; and deep hypothermic circulatory arrest. Surgeons performing this surgery have their own preferred techniques.
- Fluid balance is as for infrarenal AAA, although blood loss will be more extreme, blood transfusion will almost certainly be required, and platelets and FFP are more commonly used. Cell salvage is mandatory.
- Patients require ventilation post-operatively, until acidosis and hypothermia are corrected and the lungs fully re-expanded.

Carotid endarterectomy

Procedure	Removal of atheromatous plaque from the internal carotid artery (ICA). The ICA is clamped and opened, the plaque stripped off, and then the artery closed either directly or with a Gore-Tex® vein patch
Time	1–3hr
Pain	++
Position	Supine, head-up. Contralateral arm board
Blood loss	Minimal, G&S
Practical techniques	Cervical plexus block + sedation, art line ETT + IPPV, arterial line

An operation to reduce the incidence of stroke in symptomatic (TIA or CVA) patients with >70% carotid stenosis. Combined perioperative mortality and major stroke incidence of 2–5%. Patients are usually elderly arteriopaths, but dynamic cardiac assessment is not usually required.

- Monitoring cerebral perfusion during carotid cross-clamping is an important, but controversial, area. Advocates of regional anaesthesia cite the advantages of having a conscious patient in whom neurological deficits are immediately detectable and treatable by the insertion of a carotid shunt or pharmacological augmentation of BP.
- Under GA, other techniques may be used for monitoring cerebral perfusion, including measurement of carotid artery stump pressure, EEG processing, monitoring somatosensory evoked potentials, transcranial Doppler of the middle cerebral artery, and, more recently, near-infrared spectroscopy. Individual units will have their own protocols.
- Considerable controversy exists as to whether to use general or regional anaesthesia.[9]

Preoperative

- Elderly patients, often with severe CVS disease. Most are hypertensive. BP control during CEA can be difficult.[10]
- Determine the normal range of BP from ward charts. Measure BP in both arms. Use the highest, and aim for 160/90.
- Document pre-existing neurological deficits, so that new deficits may be more easily assessed.
- Have available vasoconstrictors (ephedrine and metaraminol) and vasodilators (GTN, labetalol).
- Consider cerebral monitoring techniques—there will be protocols in your unit.
- Premedication: sedative/anxiolytic, particularly if using GA.

Perioperative

- 20G and 14G IV access plus an arterial line in the contralateral arm (out on an arm board).
- Monitoring: 5-lead ECG, arterial line, NIBP, SpO$_2$, ETCO$_2$.
- Maintain BP within 20% of baseline. During cross-clamping, maintain BP at or above baseline. If necessary, use vasoconstrictors, e.g. metaraminol (10mg diluted up to 20mL; give 0.5mL at a time).

General anaesthesia for carotid endarterectomy

- Careful IV induction. BP may be labile during induction and intubation. Give generous doses of short-acting opioids, and consider spraying the cords with lidocaine.
- Most anaesthetists use an ETT—the LMA cuff has been shown to reduce carotid blood flow, but this is of unknown significance. Secure the tube, and check connections very carefully (the head is inaccessible during surgery).
- Remifentanil infusion, combined with superficial cervical plexus block, gives ideal conditions, with rapid awakening. Otherwise isoflurane/opioid technique. Maintain normocapnia. Avoid N$_2$O.
- Extubate before excessive coughing develops. Close neurological monitoring in recovery until fully awake.

The 'awake carotid'

- Cervical dermatomes C2–C4 may be blocked by deep and/or superficial cervical plexus block or cervical epidural (rarely used in the UK) (see also ➔ p. 1106).
- Patient preparation and communication are vital. A thorough explanation of the awake technique is invaluable.
- The site for the injection is the cervical transverse processes, which may be palpated as a bony ridge under the posterior border of the sternocleidomastoid. For the deep block, use three 5mL injections of 0.5% bupivacaine at C2, C3, and C4 or a single injection of 10–15mL of 0.5% bupivacaine at C3. Reinforce this with 10mL of 0.5% bupivacaine injected along the posterior border of the sternocleidomastoid (superficial block). Avoid the deep block in patients with respiratory impairment, as they may not tolerate unilateral diaphragmatic paralysis. Infiltration along the jawline helps to reduce pain from the submandibular retractor.
- Ensure the patient's bladder is emptied preoperatively. Give IV fluids only to replace blood loss—a full bladder developing, while the carotid is cross-clamped, can be tricky to manage.
- Sedation (e.g. propofol TCI 0.5–1 microgram/mL, remifentanil 0.05–0.1 microgram/kg/min) may be carefully employed during block placement and dissection. Once dissection is complete, patient discomfort is much reduced. Avoidance of sedation during carotid cross-clamping will allow continuous neurological assessment. Give O$_2$ throughout.
- An L-bar angled over the patient's neck allows good access for both surgeon and anaesthetist.
- Despite an apparently perfect regional block, ~50% of patients will require LA supplementation by the surgeon, particularly around the carotid sheath. This is reduced using remifentanil sedation.

- Monitor the patient's speech, contralateral motor power, and cerebration.
- Neurological deficit presents in three ways:
  - Profound unconsciousness on cross-clamping
  - Subtle, but immediate, deficit following cross-clamping, e.g. confusion, dysphasia, delay in answering questions
  - Delayed deficit—usually related to relative hypotension.
- Attentive monitoring of the patient is vital, particularly during cross-clamping. If a neurological deficit develops, tell the surgeon who will place a shunt. Recovery should be rapid, once the shunt is in place—if it is not, convert to GA. Pharmacological augmentation of BP may improve cerebration by increasing the pressure gradient of the collateral circulation across the circle of Willis. Increase the inspired O_2 concentration. A small percentage of patients will require conversion to GA (use of an LMA is probably easiest).
- For patients who do not tolerate regional anaesthesia, GA is the best option.

Post-operative

- Careful observation in a well-staffed recovery room for 2–4hr is mandatory. HDU is optimal, if available, particularly for those patients who develop a neurological deficit.
- Airway oedema is common in both GA and regional cases, presumably due to dissection around the airway. Cervical haematoma occurs in 5–10% of cases. Immediate re-exploration is required for developing airway obstruction (the regional block should still be working). Remove skin sutures in recovery as soon as the diagnosis is made to allow drainage of the haematoma.
- Haemodynamic instability is common post-operatively. Hyperperfusion syndrome, consisting of headaches and ultimately haemorrhagic CVA, is caused by areas of the brain previously 'protected' by a tight carotid stenosis being suddenly exposed to hypertensive BP. Thus, BP must be controlled. Careful written instructions should be given to staff about haemodynamic management. An example is:
  - If systolic BP >160mmHg, give labetalol 5–10mg boluses IV or a hydralazine infusion
  - If systolic BP <100mmHg, give colloid 250mL stat.
- New neurological symptoms and signs require immediate surgical consultation.
- Carotid stenting is a developing procedure for symptomatic carotid patients performed in the radiology suite, in which a stent is placed under LA into the stenotic carotid artery. Anaesthetic supervision may be required because of the complications, which include perioperative stroke and haemodynamic disturbances.

References

9 GALA Trial Collaborators Group (2008). General anaesthesia versus local anaesthesia for carotid surgery: a randomized, controlled trial. *Lancet*, **372**, 2132–42.
10 Stoneham MD, Thompson JP (2009). Arterial pressure management and carotid endarterectomy. *Br J Anaesth*, **102**, 442–52.

Peripheral revascularization operations

Procedure	Bypass operations for patients with occlusive arterial disease of the legs. The long saphenous vein or a Gore-Tex® graft is used to bypass occluded arteries
Time	1–6hr
Pain	+++
Position	Supine
Blood loss	Usually 500–1000mL, X-match 2U
Practical techniques	Combined spinal/epidural with sedation, consider art line. ETT/IPPV, consider LMA

- Femoropopliteal bypass—femoral to above-knee popliteal artery.
- Femorodistal bypass—femoral to anterior or posterior tibial artery.
- Femorofemoral crossover graft—from one femoral artery to another.

Preoperative

- Constitute a large proportion of elective vascular surgery.
- Duration of surgery is unpredictable—overruns are not uncommon.
- Assess the CVS system. Usually better tolerated than aortic surgery. A dynamic assessment of the cardiac function is not usually necessary, unless there have been new developments, e.g. unstable angina.
- The choice between general and regional anaesthesia is up to the individual. There is a suggestion that regional anaesthesia is associated with lower reoperation rates. Long operations (>3hr) may make pure regional techniques impractical, but they are still possible.

Perioperative

- IV access: ensure at least one large (14 or 16G) IV cannula.
- Insert an arterial line for long cases (over 2hr) if haemodynamic instability is expected or in sicker patients. Otherwise use standard monitoring with 5-lead ECG. CVP monitoring is rarely necessary.
- GA techniques include ETT plus IPPV or LMA plus SV. The surgeon should be able to perform femoral nerve block perioperatively.
- Regional anaesthesia is an alternative, offering good operating conditions and post-operative pain relief. Single-shot spinal anaesthesia may not give enough time for some procedures, although adding intrathecal clonidine or diamorphine may help. Combined spinal/epidural anaesthesia is probably better. Consider epidural diamorphine (2–3mg), and start an infusion of 0.25% bupivacaine at 5–10mL/hr. Always give supplemental O_2. If the patient requests sedation, propofol TCI is ideal.
- Heparin (3000–5000U) should be given before clamping—reverse with protamine 0.5–1mg/100U of heparin slowly after unclamping.

Post-operative

- O_2 overnight.

Axillobifemoral bypass

Procedure	Extraperitoneal bypass (trouser graft) from axillary artery to femoral arteries
Time	2–4hr
Pain	++++
Position	Supine
Blood loss	<1000mL, X-match 2U
Practical techniques	GA—ETT, IPPV, art line, consider CVP

This operation is performed less commonly due to the rapid advance of stenting techniques; however, it is still occasionally performed on patients with completely occluded aorto-iliac vessels. It is a last-chance operation for patients with completely occluded aortic or iliac arteries. Some will already have had aortic surgery and have infected grafts. It is an extraperitoneal operation, so patients with severe cardiorespiratory disease who might be excluded from aortic surgery may tolerate it better. However, do not be misled—it is still a long operation which can involve significant blood loss, morbidity, and even mortality.

Preoperative

- Usual preoperative assessment of vascular patients (see ➲ p. 422). Try to obtain recent information about the cardiac function. An echocardiograph can easily be done at the bedside.
- Some of these patients will be very sick, either from pre-existing cardiorespiratory disease or from infected aortic grafts. Surgery may be their only hope of life, although it carries very high risk. Provided the patient understands this, the operation may be appropriate. These are not cases for inexperienced trainees to undertake alone.

Perioperative

- GA with ETT and IPPV is appropriate. An arterial line and large-gauge cannula are mandatory; CVP monitoring is optional.
- Heparin/protamine will be required at clamping/unclamping.

Post-operative

- Extubation at the end of surgery is usually possible, but a period of time on the HDU is recommended, if possible.
- PCA for post-operative analgesia.

Amputations

(Below/through/above knee, Syme's, digits, etc.)

Procedure	Removal of necrotic or infected tissue due to vascular ischaemia
Time	30–120min
Pain	++++
Position	Supine
Blood loss	Usually 200–500mL, G&S
Practical techniques	Spinal or epidural with sedation. Sciatic/femoral blocks ± GA

Preoperative

- Commonly sick, bed-bound diabetics with significant CVS disease who have had repeated revascularization attempts previously.
- Many will be in considerable discomfort preoperatively (less so the diabetics) and may be on large doses of enteral or parenteral opioids. Regional analgesia may give the more predictable post-operative relief.

Perioperative

- Spinal anaesthesia ± sedation offers excellent anaesthesia, which can be directed unilaterally. The duration of block (and post-operative pain relief) can be extended with intrathecal diamorphine (0.25–0.5mg) or intrathecal clonidine (15–30 micrograms).[11]
- Epidural analgesia offers better post-operative analgesia and can be sited preoperatively, if required (pre-emptive analgesia).
- GA is an option, but additional regional blockade is advisable (combined sciatic/femoral blocks will ensure analgesia for up to 24hr). An epidural catheter may be placed next to the sciatic nerve by the surgeon for the post-operative infusion of LA (e.g. bupivacaine 0.25% at 5mL/hr).
- Occasionally, these patients are septic due to the necrotic tissue. The only way they will improve is to have the affected part amputated, so cancellation may not be an option.

Post-operative

- Regional analgesia is the best option; otherwise PCA.
- Phantom limb pain is a problem for 60–70% of amputees at some time. It must be distinguished from surgical pain—get pain team input.
- Pre-emptive analgesia (preoperative siting of epidural) is believed by some to reduce the incidence and severity of chronic pain.
- Combined sciatic/femoral nerve blocks are an alternative to an epidural, particularly when the patient is receiving anticoagulation.
- Even with perfect regional analgesia, you may need to continue enteral opioids post-operatively.

Reference

11 Ypsilantis E, Tang TY (2010). Pre-emptive analgesia for chronic limb pain after amputation for peripheral vascular disease: a systematic review. *Ann Vasc Surg*, **24**, 1139–46.

Thoracoscopic sympathectomy

Procedure	For patients with sweaty palms/axillae. The sympathetic trunk is divided via a thoracoscope inserted through a small axillary incision
Time	30–60min
Pain	++
Position	Supine, affected arm on arm board
Blood loss	Minimal
Practical techniques	IPPV via DLT, SV via LMA

- Patients are usually young and fit with hyperhidrosis (sweaty palms and axillae).
- Surgical technique involves cutting the thoracic sympathetic trunk at T2 or T3 thoracoscopically.
- Traditionally, this is done using one-lung anaesthesia (DLT), with the patient in the reverse Trendelenburg position.
- A simpler technique involves the patient breathing spontaneously through an LMA. When the surgeon insufflates CO_2 into the pleural cavity, the lung is pushed away passively, allowing surgery to take place. The degree of shunt produced is less dramatic than with OLV. Assisted ventilation must be avoided, except to reinflate the lung manually at the end. The CO_2 insufflator machine regulates intrapleural pressures.
- With either technique, at the conclusion of the procedure, the lung must be re-expanded (under the surgeon's direct vision) to prevent a pneumothorax.
- LA can be deposited by the surgeon directly onto the sympathetic trunk and into the pleural cavity.
- A post-operative chest radiograph is required to confirm lung reinflation.
- Synchronous bilateral sympathectomy is a much more challenging operation. This can lead to profound hypoxia when the 2nd lung is collapsed, due to persistent atelectasis in the 1st lung. It is certainly inappropriate for all but the very fittest patients. The mortality of this procedure has been highlighted.[12]

Reference
12 Collin J (2004). Uncovering occult operative morbidity and mortality. *Br J Surg*, **91**, 262–3.

First rib resection

Procedure	Resection of the 1st/cervical rib in patients with thoracic outlet syndrome
Time	1–2hr
Pain	++
Position	Supine, affected arm on arm board
Blood loss	Minimal
Practical techniques	IPPV via ETT, avoid muscle relaxants

- Patients are usually young and fit.
- The position is similar to that for thoracoscopic sympathectomy.
- Muscle relaxants should be avoided, as the surgeon needs to be able to identify the brachial plexus perioperatively. Intubate under opioid/induction agent alone, or use mivacurium/opioid, and then hyperventilate with isoflurane/opioid or similar.
- At the conclusion of surgery, the wound is filled with saline, and manual ventilation performed with sustained inflation pressures >40cmH$_2$O. This is to check for a lung leak and exclude a pleural injury.
- A superficial cervical plexus block provides good post-operative analgesia (see ➲ p. 434 and p. 1106).
- A post-operative CXR is required in recovery.

Varicose vein surgery

Procedure	Removal of tortuous veins of the lower extremities: High tie and strip—long saphenous vein removal (sometimes bilateral) Short saphenous vein surgery—tied off in popliteal fossa
Time	30min to 3hr
Pain	++
Position	Supine or prone for short saphenous surgery
Blood loss	Up to 1000mL
Practical techniques	LMA/SV for most; ETT/IPPV for prone

- Patients are usually young and fit.
- The main operation is usually combined with multiple avulsions to remove varicosities. These are minute scars, which can, however, bleed profusely.
- Blood loss can be minimized by elevating the legs.
- Patients may need combined long and short saphenous surgery (i.e. two operative incisions on the same leg) and may require turning during the operation. In selected slim patients without aspiration risk, this can be done with the patient breathing spontaneously through an LMA.
- A combination of NSAIDs and LA into the groin wound gives good post-operative analgesia. Caudal anaesthesia is possible for prolonged re-explorations.
- Bilateral surgery is common and takes 30–60min per incision.
- Redo surgery is also common and can be very prolonged.

Further reading

Atkinson C, Ramaswamy KK, Stoneham MD (2013). Regional anesthesia for vascular surgery. *Semin Cardiothorac Vasc Anesth*, **17**, 92–104.

Levine WC, Lee JJ, Black JH, Cambria RP, Davison JK (2005). Thoracoabdominal aneurysm repair: anesthetic management. *Int Anesthesiol Clin*, **43**, 39–60.

Moores C, Nimmo A, eds. (2012). *Core topics in vascular anaesthesia*. Cambridge: Cambridge University Press.

Mukherjee D, Eagle KA (2003). Perioperative cardiac assessment for noncardiac surgery: eight steps to the best possible outcome. *Circulation*, **107**, 2771–4.

Shine TS, Murray MJ (2004). Intraoperative management of aortic aneurysm surgery. *Anesthesiol Clin North America*, **22**, 289–305, vii.

Stoneham MD, Stamou D, Mason J (2015). Regional anesthesia for carotid endarterectomy. *Br J Anaesth*, **114**, 372–83.

Orthopaedic surgery

Richard Griffiths and Ralph Leighton

General principles

Approximately 180 000 major joint replacements are performed annually in England and Wales.[1] Emphasis is now shifting to longer, more minimally invasive surgery permitting shorter hospital stays.[2] A diverse population of mostly elderly patients presents many challenges to the anaesthetist. Many operations are amenable to regional anaesthesia.

Frequent problems include arthritis, obesity, co-morbidity/polypharmacy, lengthy procedures, significant blood loss, and specific problems related to tourniquets, bone cement, and VTE.

Preoperative

- Liaison with the surgeon is essential, particularly if undertaking regional techniques.
- Arthritis often makes assessment of cardiorespiratory fitness difficult.
- Patients with rheumatoid disease are at risk of atlantoaxial instability (see ⭢ p. 184).
- If planning a regional technique (particularly a central block), it is important to consider factors affecting clotting (timing of the last dose of anticoagulant) and discuss specific risks and benefits with the patient (see ⭢ p. 1141).
- A high risk of VTE occurs with certain operations requiring antithromboembolic measures, e.g. LMWH, stockings, foot pumps (see ⭢ p. 11).

Perioperative

- Give IV antibiotic prophylaxis (see ⭢ p. 1211).
- Utmost care with positioning is essential to avoid soft tissue or nerve injuries. This is a shared responsibility between the anaesthetist and surgeon.
- Maintenance of normothermia with blood warmers and warm-air blankets can reduce both morbidity and mortality.[3]
- Consider invasive monitoring for those patients with CVS disease.
- Blood loss may be significant (use a large-bore cannula with an extension) and may be increased by certain pathologies, e.g. Paget's.
- Monitor blood loss accurately. Consider cell salvage, including drain salvage.
- A urinary catheter should be inserted for long procedures or when epidurals/spinal opioids are used.

Post-operative

- Good analgesia will have a positive effect on recovery, mobility, and discharge.
- Liaise with the surgeon if prescribing NSAIDs, but use with care in those over 75 (see ⭢ p. 707 and p. 1064).

Regional anaesthesia

- Regional anaesthesia may be used for most joint replacements (alone, with sedation, or as an adjuvant to GA). Central neuraxial blockade and major nerve blocks are commonly performed.

- In major orthopaedic surgery, blocks may provide post-operative pain relief and may reduce PONV.
- There is some evidence that regional anaesthesia, either alone or in combination with GA, may improve outcome in hip and knee arthroplasty, although these data are based on large observational studies.[4,5]
- Good fixation of cement and joint prosthesis requires a dry, bloodless surgical field. Regional anaesthetic (particularly spinal/epidural) reduces bleeding at the surgical site, without the need for other pharmacological hypotensive anaesthetic techniques.
- Surgeons often prefer the operating conditions produced by regional techniques.[6]

References

1 National Joint Registry (2013). *10th Annual report 2013. National Registry for England, Wales and Northern Ireland. Surgical data to 31 December 2012.* ℛ http://www.njrcentre.org.uk/njrcentre/Portals/0/Documents/England/Reports/10th_annual_report/NJR%2010th%20Annual%20Report%202013%20B.pdf.

2 Connolly D (2003). Orthopaedic anaesthesia. *Anaesthesia,* **58**, 1189–93.

3 Kirkbride DA (2003). Thermoregulation and mild perioperative hypothermia. *BJA CEPD Reviews,* **3**, 24–8.

4 Memtsoudis SG, Sun X, Chiu YL, *et al.* (2013). Perioperative comparative effectiveness of anesthetic technique in orthopedic patients. *Anesthesiology,* **118**, 1046–58.

5 Hunt LP, Ben-Shlomo Y, Clark EM, *et al.* (2013). 90 day mortality after 409,096 total hip replacements for osteoarthritis, from the NJR for England & Wales: a retrospective analysis. *Lancet,* **382**, 1097–104.

6 Oldman M, McCartney CJL, Leung A, *et al.* (2004). A survey of orthopedic surgeons' attitudes and knowledge regarding regional anesthesia. *Anesth Analg,* **98**, 1486–90.

Fat embolism syndrome

Fat embolism syndrome (FES)[7] is associated with trauma or surgery and has an extremely variable presentation—diagnosis is often made by exclusion. Although embolization of fat occurs frequently, the syndrome is comparatively rare (1%). Early surgery and avoidance of intramedullary fixation have both reduced the incidence. Current treatment is supportive (early mortality 1–20%), but serious long-term complications are uncommon.

FES is classically seen in patients with long bone fractures who develop sudden tachypnoea and hypoxia. Although sometimes a petechial rash is seen (check conjunctiva), firm diagnosis is frequently difficult.[8]

Features (as defined by Gurd)

Major
- Respiratory symptoms—tachypnoea, dyspnoea, bilateral crepitations, haemoptysis, diffuse shadowing on CXR.
- Neurological signs—confusion, drowsiness.
- Petechial rash.

Minor
- Tachycardia.
- Retinal change—fat or petechiae.
- Jaundice.
- Renal—oliguria or anuria.

Laboratory
- Thrombocytopenia.
- Sudden decrease in Hb by 20%.
- Raised ESR.
- Fat macroglobulaemia.

Treatment

- Early resuscitation and stabilization are vital.
- Early O_2 therapy may prevent onset of syndrome.
- May require mechanical ventilation (10–40% of patients).
- Steroid use is controversial.[9]
- FES usually resolves within 7d.

References

7 Mellor A, Soni N (2001). Fat embolism. *Anaesthesia*, **56**, 145–54.
8 Gurd AR, Wilson RL (1974). The fat embolism syndrome. *J Bone Joint Surg Br*, **56**, 408–16.
9 Sen RK, Tripathy SK, Krishnan V (2012). Role of corticosteroid as a prophylactic measure in fat embolism syndrome: a literature review. *Musculoskelet Surg*, **96**, 1–8.

Cement implantation syndrome

Methylmethacrylate bone cement is an acrylic polymer that has been used extensively in orthopaedic surgery for 30yr. Its use is associated with the potential for hypoxia, hypotension, and CVS collapse. Fatal cardiac arrest is a reported complication. There are many suggested aetiologies, of which fat embolization appears to be the most likely. Air embolization (Doppler evidence in 30% of patients) and direct effects of the cement are also possible. There is now a proposed classification of bone cement implantation syndrome (BCIS), ranging from grade 1, with mild hypotension and hypoxia, to grade 3, with CVS collapse.[10]

Severe embolic events (up to 85% of patients) and pulmonary dysfunction (mean reduction in SaO_2 of 7%) are commonest with femoral cement insertion.[11] The ability of the patient to withstand these should be considered before use.[12]

Problems typically occur shortly after cement insertion. Hypotension is common (10–30%), independent of the anaesthetic technique, and worsened if there is any degree of hypovolaemia.

Prevention and treatment

- Suction applied to the bone cavity to evacuate air and fat during cement insertion dramatically reduces the incidence of complications.
- Measure BP frequently during this time.
- Ensure adequate blood volume prior to cementing.
- Increase FiO_2 (hypoxia common).
- Stop N_2O.

It has been suggested that α-agonists might be superior to adrenaline when resuscitating these patients.[13]

References

10 Donaldson AJ, Thomson HE, Harper NJ, Kenny NW (2009). Bone cement implantation syndrome. *Br J Anaesth*, **102**, 12–22.
11 Pitto RP, Koessler M, Kuehle JW (1999). Comparison of fixation of the femoral component without cement and fixation with use of a bone-vacuum cementing technique for the prevention of fat embolism during total hip arthroplasty. *J Bone Joint Surg*, **81**, 831–43.
12 Parry G (2003). Sudden deaths during hip hemi-arthroplasty. *Anaesthesia*, **58**, 922–3.
13 McBrien ME, Breslin DS, Atkinson S, Johnston JR (2001). Use of methoxamine in the resuscitation of epinephrine-resistant electromechanical dissociation. *Anaesthesia*, **56**, 1085–9.

Tourniquets

Tourniquets[14] are commonly used to produce a bloodless field.

- Only pneumatic tourniquets should be used, as mechanical tourniquets can cause areas of unpredictably high pressure in the underlying tissues.
- Small tourniquets on fingers and toes are dangerous, because they are easily forgotten. It is best to use a rubber strip with artery forceps.
- Expressive exsanguination using an Esmarch bandage is contraindicated in cases of tumour or severe infection because of the risks of dissemination. It is also contraindicated if DVT is suspected—fatal PE has been reported.[15] It also represents a potential risk of LV failure from fluid overload if compression of both legs is carried out simultaneously (adds 15% to the circulating volume); therefore, limit to one leg only in patients at risk. Effective exsanguination can be achieved by arm or leg elevation for 5min at 90°, without mechanical compression.
- Peripheral arterial disease is a relative contraindication to use.
- Avoid in severe crush injuries.
- SCD: use of tourniquets is controversial. Sickling of red blood cells under anoxic conditions causes thrombosis, but some surgeons use limb tourniquets after full exsanguination. If employed, use for as short a time as possible (see also ➡ p. 198).

Site of application

The upper arm and thigh have sufficient muscle bulk to distribute the cuff pressure evenly and are the recommended sites. For short operations (<1hr) in fit patients, a calf tourniquet is preferred by some surgeons.

Cuff width

The American Heart Association concluded that, if a sphygmomanometer cuff has a width of 20% greater than the diameter of the upper arm or 40% of the circumference of the thigh (to a maximum of 20cm), then the pressure in the underlying central artery will be equal to that in the cuff. This avoids the need for excessively high cuff pressures. Modern silicone cuffs tend to be smaller than this, measuring 90mm in width (bladder 70mm) for the arm and 105mm (bladder 75mm) for the leg. Cuff length should exceed the circumference of the extremity by 7–15cm. The cuff should be positioned at the point of maximum circumference of the limb. The tissues immediately underlying the cuff should be protected with cotton wool. This is not necessary with a correctly applied modern silicone cuff.

Pressure

- Base on the unsedated patient's BP measured on the ward preoperatively.
- Upper limb: systolic BP + 50mmHg. Lower limb: twice systolic BP. This higher pressure is needed because there is often not enough room above the operating site for a full-sized cuff.
- The use of lower inflation pressures may minimize complications following the use of tourniquets and speed up post-operative recovery. In a normotensive patient, a pressure of 200mmHg should be ideal for the upper limb and 250mmHg for the lower limb.

Tourniquet time

The minimum time possible should be the aim. Notify the surgeon at 1hr, and remove as soon as possible after that. If the operation is difficult, the time can be extended to 1.5hr. Two hours should be regarded as a maximum, but this will not be safe for all patients. PEs can occur following tourniquet release. When monitored using TOE, the rate was higher with increased tourniquet time.[16]

Tourniquet pain

After 30–60min of cuff inflation, a patient may develop an increase in HR and diastolic BP. This response results from 'tourniquet pain'. This also occurs under anaesthesia, although the response is usually abolished by spinal or epidural techniques. In volunteers, when a tourniquet is inflated, a dull pain, associated with an increase in BP, occurs after 30min. Often the physiological changes are resistant to analgesic drugs and increased depth of anaesthesia. β-blockers, in particular labetalol, may be useful. Small doses of ketamine given IV (0.25mg/kg) before tourniquet inflation has been reported to attenuate these BP rises.[17,18]

References

14 Deloughry JL, Griffiths R (2009). Arterial tourniquets. *Contin Educ Anaesth Crit Care Pain*, **9**, 56–60.

15 Boogaerts JG (1999). Lower limb exsanguinations and embolism. *Acta Anaesthesiol Belg*, **50**, 95–8.

16 Hirota K, Hashimoto H, Kabara S, *et al.* (2001). The relationship between pneumatic tourniquet time and the amount of pulmonary emboli in patients undergoing knee arthroscopic surgeries. *Anesth Analg*, **93**, 776–8.

17 Satsumae T, Yamaguchi H, Sakaguchi M, *et al.* (2001). Preoperative small dose ketamine prevented tourniquet induced arterial pressure increase in orthopaedic patients under general anesthesia. *Anesth Analg*, **92**, 1286–9.

18 Kam PC, Kavanaugh R, Yoong FF (2001). The arterial tourniquet: pathophysiological consequences and anaesthetic implications. *Anaesthesia*, **56**, 534–6.

Total hip replacement

Procedure	Prosthetic replacement of femoral head and acetabulum
Time	90–120min
Pain	+++
Position	Lateral or supine
Blood loss	300–500mL, G&S
Practical techniques	Spinal with sedation or GA/LMA ± nerve block

Total hip replacement is one of the most frequently performed orthopaedic operations. The 10th annual report from the National Joint Registry (NJR)[19] shows that there were 76 488 1° hip operations in 2012. The average age of patients for 1° hip arthroplasty was almost 69yr. Cemented arthroplasties account for 33% of all operations, with uncemented procedures totalling another 48%. Hip resurfacing procedures are falling in popularity—<1% of all operations. Regional anaesthesia offers several advantages[20] and can be supplemented with sedation or GA. Prevention of thromboembolic complications is of the utmost importance.

Preoperative

- Careful preoperative evaluation of the patient is essential.
- It may be appropriate to avoid the use of cement in patients with severe cardiac disease, and this should be discussed with the surgeon beforehand.
- Antithrombotic measures should commence on admission to hospital.

Perioperative

- Place a 16G or larger cannula in the upper arm (if a lateral position is anticipated).
- Ensure adequate hydration prior to performing a spinal anaesthesia and during cement insertion.
- For single-shot spinal anaesthesia: ~3mL of bupivacaine 0.5%, depending on patient size. Diamorphine (0.25–0.5mg) may be added for more prolonged analgesia.
- When using spinal anaesthesia in the lateral position, intermittent doses of midazolam or TCI propofol are useful sedation techniques, with face mask supplemental O_2. Be careful using midazolam in the elderly, as it may lead to acute delirium. On occasions, induction of GA is required. For the supine position, consider an LMA with light GA.
- For longer cases, a combined spinal/epidural technique can be used. Post-operative analgesic requirements rarely require this approach for an uncomplicated 1° hip replacement.
- GA (rather than sedation) ± epidural or suitable block should be considered for any complex operation because of the prolonged surgical time.

- Using an epidural post-operatively will necessitate inserting a urinary catheter (which also helps monitor fluid balance) at some stage in the majority of patients. This is best performed at the time of surgery.
- If centroneuraxial blockade is contraindicated, a psoas lumbar plexus block (or a femoral 3-in-1 block) provides comparable analgesia and can be used to supplement GA.
- Aim to maintain BP at an adequate level, based on preoperative readings; hypotension is not indicated.
- Intraoperative antibiotic prophylaxis will be required.
- Actively warming the patient reduces intraoperative blood loss significantly[21] and reduces morbidity and mortality.
- Blood recovery and autologous transfusion should be considered for complex surgery.

Post-operative

- Surgeons usually prefer the patient to be placed on their bed in the supine position, with the legs abducted using a pillow, to prevent dislocation of the prosthesis.
- Antithromboembolic prophylaxis is important—at least 1% of patients develop DVT, even with measures in place (see ● p. 11).
- O_2 therapy for up to 24hr is advisable in most patients.
- Hb should be checked 24hr post-operatively and treated with either transfusion or iron supplements, as indicated (see ● Special considerations, p. 451).
- Patients are mobilized at 24–48hr, and simple oral opioids with regular paracetamol or NSAIDs are usually sufficient for post-operative analgesia. Caution with NSAIDs in the elderly. If an epidural has been inserted, a post-operative infusion is rarely necessary and needs to cease prior to mobilization.

Special considerations

- Blood loss varies significantly. It is also affected by the anaesthetic technique. The average loss is 300–500mL (reduced by centroneuraxial techniques). A similar amount may be lost in the drain and tissues post-operatively.
- The decision to transfuse is multifactorial and includes general fitness, continuing surgical losses, and local practice.
- The benefits of epidural analgesia may be limited to the early post-operative period (up to 6hr).[22]
- Use of bone cement is associated with a 3-fold higher risk for PE.[23] Unfractionated heparin is associated with a 6-fold higher risk for DVT, compared with LMWH.[24]

Bilateral total hip replacement

- Preferred by some surgeons in younger, fit patients.
- This is a major operation; careful patient selection is vital. Significant CVS disease increases mortality.
- GA with epidural is most practical.
- Consider invasive monitoring (arterial line ± CVP).

References

19 National Joint Registry (2013). *10th Annual report 2013. National Registry for England, Wales and Northern Ireland. Surgical data to 31 December 2012.* ℬ http://www.njrcentre.org.uk/njrcentre/Portals/0/Documents/England/Reports/10th_annual_report/NJR%2010th%20Annual%20Report%202013%20B.pdf.

20 Memtsoudis SG, Sun X, Chiu YL, *et al.* (2013). Perioperative comparative effectiveness of anesthetic technique in orthopedic patients. *Anesthesiology*, **118**, 1046–58.

21 Winkler M, Akca O, Birkenberg B, Hetz H, *et al.* (2000). Aggressive warming reduces blood loss during hip arthroplasty. *Anesth Analg*, **91**, 978–84.

22 Choi PT, Bhandari M, Scott J, Douketis J (2003). Epidural analgesia for pain relief following hip or knee replacement. *Cochrane Database Syst Rev*, **3**, CD003071.

23 Borghi B, Casati A (2002). Thromboembolic complications after total hip replacement. *Int Orthop*, **26**, 44–7.

24 Kirkbride DB (2003). Thermoregulation and mild perioperative hypothermia. *BJA CEPD Reviews*, **3**, 24–8.

Revision of total hip replacement

Procedure	Revision of previous total hip replacement Revision may include one or both components
Time	2–6hr, depending on complexity
Pain	++++
Position	Lateral or supine
Blood loss	1L, occasionally considerably more, X-match 2U
Practical techniques	GA ± epidural/nerve block

This is essentially the same as 1° hip replacement, except for increased length of surgery, blood loss, and post-operative pain. Twelve per cent of hip procedures in England and Wales are now revision arthroplasties. The complexity of surgery is very variable. These operations can be prolonged, with substantial blood loss, so discuss the anticipated operation with the surgeon.

Preoperative

General principles as for total hip replacement, except:
- Patients are more elderly and usually have more medical problems.
- The operation takes longer, at least 2–3hr, often more. This is too long for a single-shot spinal.
- Blood loss can be significant, with 1L or more commonly lost perioperatively.
- Post-operative pain can be a significant problem.

Perioperative

- Generally as for 1° hip replacement, including a urinary catheter.
- If significant blood loss is anticipated or the patient's CVS status indicates it, insert an arterial line, and consider a CVP line.
- Technique should be planned, according to the length of surgery, the operative position, and patient factors.
  - For complex revisions anticipated to take >3hr, an IPPV technique with epidural supplementation may be most appropriate.
  - If central neuraxial block is contraindicated, consider supplementing GA with nerve blocks (femoral 3-in-1 or psoas compartment lumbar plexus).
- Use blood recovery and autologous transfusion wherever possible.
- Perioperative blood transfusion is frequently required, and blood loss may be substantial. Two units of cross-matched blood should be available in theatre, with the ability to obtain more within 30min.

Post-operative
- Mobilization varies with the complexity of the revision and the strength of reconstruction.
- For pain relief, an epidural infusion is useful. PCA is a suitable alternative.
- Supplemental O_2 is required for 24hr or longer, particularly if significant blood loss or an underlying cardiorespiratory disease.
- Remember thromboembolic prophylaxis.

Total knee replacement

Procedure	Prosthetic replacement of the knee joint
Time	1–2hr
Pain	++++/+++++
Position	Supine
Blood loss	Minimal with tourniquet, 250–500mL without. G&S. Post-operative autologous blood salvage often used
Practical techniques	Spinal plus local infiltration. GA plus local infiltration Epidural or combined spinal/epidural ± LMA

Similar patient population to hip surgery. Generally a shorter operation with less blood loss and less chance of cement hypotension. A tourniquet is commonly used, so beware of tourniquet pain. Post-operatively, pain can be extreme and must be anticipated. There has been a move away from nerve blocks and a focus on spinal anaesthesia plus local infiltration to enable faster mobilization and early discharge. Nerve blocks may delay mobilization significantly.

Preoperative
As for hip surgery.

Perioperative
- The patient is always supine, and therefore airway control under sedation can be a problem.
- Spinal anaesthesia, with or without intrathecal opioids, is the preferred technique.[25] GA is often used.
- A tourniquet is commonly used; therefore, perioperative blood loss is not problematic, although expect to lose up to 500mL (and frequently more) from the drains in the 1st hour post-operatively. There is a trend to reduce the use of the tourniquet.
- If a tourniquet is used, one may see 'breakthrough' of tourniquet pain after about 1hr, causing CVS stimulation and hypertension. This is commoner with leg blocks and is treated by deepening anaesthesia or adding IV opioid. Ketamine (0.25mg/kg) is effective at preventing the associated rise in BP.[26] Ensure the patient is well preloaded before the tourniquet is released. A short-lived reperfusion event is common (fall in BP and SaO_2, rise in $ETCO_2$) and is usually best prevented by fluid loading before and during tourniquet release.

Post-operative
- Post-operative pain is usually the most significant problem, and this is the main determinant of the anaesthetic technique. Many patients are now already on opioids, and this makes the management of post-operative pain more difficult.
- When blood loss into the drains continues to be brisk after the 1st 500mL, the surgeon will often clamp the drains for a period of time.

Bilateral total knee replacement

- Bilateral knee replacements should only be considered in young, fit, motivated patients.[27] Elderly patients and those with significant CVS disease are high-risk.
- The advantage is that two admissions/operations are avoided.
- The disadvantage is that bilateral total knee replacement is a major CVS stress and is associated with unpredictable blood loss and fluid requirements.
- GA plus epidural is probably the most practical technique.
- Invasive monitoring should be considered (arterial line).

Revision of total knee replacement

Same as 1° knee replacement, except it takes longer, ≥2hr.

- The technique is as for 1° knee replacement.
- If done without a tourniquet, then 2U of blood should be cross-matched.

References

25 Andersen LO, Gaarn-Larsen L, Kristensen BB, Husted H, Otte KS, Kehlet H (2010). Analgesic efficacy of local anaesthetic in knee arthroplasty: volume v concentration. *Anaesthesia*, **65**, 984–90.

26 Satsumae T, Yamaguchi H, Sakaguchi M, *et al.* (2001). Preoperative small dose ketamine prevented tourniquet induced arterial pressure increase in orthopaedic patients under general anesthesia. *Anesth Analg*, **92**, 1286–9.

27 Oakes DA, Hanssen AD (2004). Bilateral total knee replacement using the same anesthetic is not justified by assessment of the risks. *Clin Orthop Relat Res*, **428**, 87–91.

Arthroscopic lower limb procedures

Procedure	Arthroscopy, EUA, and washout ± excision of torn cartilage, removal of loose body
Time	20–60min
Pain	++
Position	Supine, with leg over side of table
Blood loss	Nil
Practical techniques	GA/LMA or spinal

General principles

- The patient population is generally younger than those having joint replacements.
- Smaller procedures are done as day cases and therefore require a technique that allows early ambulation and discharge home. The main procedures undertaken are examination under anaesthesia (EUA), meniscal surgery/loose body removal, synovectomy, and ligament reconstruction.
- Virtually all are done on the knee, though arthroscopy is also performed on the ankle.
- Arthroscopy for knees with osteoarthritis is not supported by evidence of effectiveness.[28]

Technique

- Premedication with paracetamol and NSAID.
- GA/LMA is a 'standard' day-case anaesthetic with IV opioids such as fentanyl 1 microgram/kg.
- A tourniquet is often used.
- Prescribe NSAIDs and strong oral analgesics to take home.
- Many surgeons instil 10–20mL of 0.5% bupivacaine ± morphine (10mg) into the joint cavity for post-operative pain relief.
- Ketamine in low dosage (IV) has been suggested to enhance analgesia (0.15mg/kg).[29]
- Ideally, IV morphine should be avoided in day-case arthroscopic procedures due to the high incidence of PONV.
- EUA ± washout can be performed under intra-articular and infiltration LA alone. Nerve blocks have been used but are limited by the long duration of action of anaesthesia and the failure to block the site of the arterial tourniquet.

References

28 Bandolier. *Surgery for arthritic knees.* ℘ http://www.medicine.ox.ac.uk/bandolier/band102/b102-3.html.

29 Menigaux C, Guignard B, Fletcher D, et al. (2001). Intraoperative small-dose ketamine enhances analgesia after outpatient arthroscopy. *Anesth Analg*, **93**, 606–12.

Cruciate ligament repair

Procedure	Arthroscopic reconstruction of anterior cruciate ligament using patellar tendon ± hamstrings
Time	1.5–2hr
Pain	+++/++++
Position	Supine
Blood loss	Nil
Practical techniques	Patellar tendon and hamstring repair: LMA + GA or spinal

Technique

- These operations are of two main types: using the patellar tendon only for the repair, and using both the patellar tendon and hamstring ligaments.
- Usually 12hr of analgesia are required prior to mobilization.
- Nerve blocks have been used but hinder post-operative mobilization.
- Oral opioids, combined with paracetamol and NSAIDs, are the mainstay of analgesia.
- If the hamstrings are used, the operation takes longer, and there is more post-operative pain.

Ankle surgery

General principles

- Four main types of procedure: tendon transfers, open reduction and internal fixation (ORIF) of fractures, joint arthrodesis, and prosthetic joint replacement (Table 18.1).
- In 2012, there were over 500 ankle replacement procedures carried out in England and Wales.
- Ankle arthrodesis takes 1–2hr. Tendon transfer is generally quicker than this, and joint replacement may take longer.
- These operations are amenable to regional anaesthetic techniques, either alone or combined with GA.
- Tourniquets are often used, and tourniquet pain has to be considered (see ➲ p. 448).
- Patients may be supine, prone, or occasionally on their side.
- In the case of ORIF following trauma, surgery may need to be undertaken urgently if distal circulation is compromised. Beware of the risk of aspiration from a full stomach, and also take time to ensure that any other significant injury has been properly managed.
- If regional block is considered for ORIF, check that there is no concern about the development of compartment syndrome post-operatively, as the symptoms will be masked by the block (see ➲ p. 483).

Technique

- Local, regional, general, or a combination of techniques can be used for all procedures on the ankle.
- Nerve blocks are popular and, for ankle surgery, require sciatic (or popliteal) and femoral (or saphenous) nerve blockade—the saphenous nerve (terminal branch of the femoral nerve) supplies the skin down to the medial malleolus of the ankle.
- Nerve blocks following a spinal anaesthetic improve analgesia well into the 1st post-operative day. GA can also be combined with nerve blocks.
- Care must be taken in trauma cases with fractured ankles, as nerve blocks may mask compartment syndrome. Always discuss your proposed technique with the surgeon. The general rule is that nerve blocks are best avoided in trauma cases. Local infiltration is useful.
- Tendon transfer surgery takes up to 1hr and is not particularly painful post-operatively.
- ORIF may be an emergency if the vascular supply is compromised, and an RSI is the best anaesthetic option in this situation. A good alternative for ORIF is spinal anaesthesia. The addition of intrathecal opioid (e.g. diamorphine 0.25–0.5mg) prolongs the period of analgesia.
- Ankle joint replacement is a procedure that is increasing in popularity. Usually the procedure is accomplished within 2hr.

Table 18.1 Summary of ankle procedures

Procedure	Time (hr)	Pain (+ to +++++)	Position	Blood loss	Practical technique
Tendon transfer/repair	~1	++	Supine (ruptured tendo-achilles—prone)	Nil with tourniquet	GA + LMA with infiltration of LA by surgeon
					Spinal if supine. IPPV if prone
ORIF of ankle fracture	Variable 1.5–2	++/+++	Supine, occasionally on side or prone	Nil with tourniquet	GA (if in doubt, RSI) or spinal
					Generally avoid nerve blocks
Arthrodesis of ankle joint	1.5–2	+++	Supine	Nil with tourniquet	GA or spinal with nerve blocks
					PCA
					Spinal + nerve blocks
Prosthetic replacement of ankle joint	2+	++/+++	Supine	Nil with tourniquet	GA + nerve blocks
					Spinal + nerve blocks

Foot surgery

General principles

- Most operations are on the forefoot and toes, e.g. 1st metatarsal osteotomy, Keller's, excision of ingrowing toenails, and terminalization of toes. Other operations in the midfoot include tendon transfers and some osteotomies (Table 18.2).
- The patient population varies, and many are elderly. Those for terminalization of toes may well have concomitant problems such as diabetes and/or CVS disease.
- Osteotomies tend to be painful post-operatively.
- Surgical time is 30min to 1hr.
- Many are done as day cases and require early ambulation and discharge with adequate pain relief.
- Nerve blocks make a valuable contribution to post-operative analgesia, particularly in osteotomies and nail bed excision, and promote early ambulation. However, onset time is relatively long, and they need to be performed a full 40min prior to surgery, if planned without GA. With experience, this can work well, but, for the less experienced, it is best to undertake them primarily for post-operative pain relief in combination with LMA and GA.
- Adrenaline must not be used for 'ring' or 'web-space' blocks and is best avoided in ankle blocks if the peripheral circulation is poor.
- Breakthrough pain from the tourniquet can be a problem, especially if surgery is longer than 45min. Place the tourniquet as distally as possible to reduce this effect.

Technique

- Regional blocks useful for foot surgery include ring/web-space or ankle blocks for toe surgery, ankle block for forefoot surgery, and sciatic (or popliteal) nerve block for operations on the midfoot. Most commonly, these blocks are performed for post-operative pain relief and are combined with GA.
- An alternative in all cases is spinal anaesthesia.

Table 18.2 Summary of forefoot procedures

Site	Procedure	Time (min)	Pain (+ to +++++)	Position	Blood loss/ X-match	Technique
Toes	Excision of nail bed, terminalization	30	+++	Supine	Nil	Ring or toe web block with sedation or GA/LMA + ankle block
Forefoot	Tendon transfers	30–60	+/++	Supine	Nil	GA/LMA + local infiltration Ankle block with sedation or GA/LMA
Forefoot	1st metatarsal osteotomy, Keller's	30–60	+++	Supine	Nil	GA/LMA with ankle block or infiltration
Midfoot	Tendon transfers	30–60	+/++	Supine	Nil	GA/LMA + local infiltration
Midfoot	Osteotomy	30–60	+++	Supine	Nil	GA/LMA ± sciatic nerve block at knee

Spinal surgery

Definition

- Surgery on the spinal column between the atlanto-occipital junction and the coccyx.[30]
- Can be loosely divided into four categories (Table 18.3):
  - Decompression of the spinal cord and nerves
  - Stabilization and correction of spinal deformity
  - Excision of spinal tumours
  - Trauma.

General principles

Children present for scoliosis surgery, young and middle-aged adults for decompressive surgery, and older patients for stabilization.

- Most procedures are in the prone position, although anterior and lateral approaches are used. Some procedures will involve turning the patient during the operation.
- Airway access will be limited during surgery and must be secure.
- Prevent excessive abdominal or thoracic pressure due to incorrect patient positioning, which may compromise ventilation and circulation.
- Surgical blood loss can be considerable. Ensure good vascular access and accurate measurement of blood loss. Consider cell salvage.
- Long procedures necessitate active prevention of heat loss.
- Assessment of spinal function may be required during the procedure.

The prone position

A specially designed mattress, allowing unhindered movement of the abdomen and chest (e.g. a Montreal mattress), should be used to minimize complications, as outlined below:

- Turning the patient from prone to supine requires log rolling by a trained team to avoid applying twisting forces in the axial plane. This is especially important for the poorly supported cervical spine, which may be unstable due to fractures or degenerative disease. The surgeon should be present as part of the team for this manoeuvre. Specially designed mechanical hoists can be used to transfer patients from the trolley to the operating table.
- Pressure on the abdomen applies pressure to the diaphragm and increases the intrathoracic pressure, which, in turn, decreases thoracic compliance. This can lead to basal atelectasis and the need for higher lung inflation pressures, particularly in obese patients.
- Raised intra-abdominal pressure also compresses veins and decreases venous return, which may result in hypotension or increased venous bleeding from the surgical site.
- Accurate assessment of the circulation with invasive arterial monitoring and an indwelling urinary catheter is recommended for all major procedures. CVP may be difficult to interpret in the prone position and is rarely required.

Table 18.3 Summary of spinal surgery procedures

Operation	Description	Time (hr)	Position	Blood loss/ X-match	Pain (+ to +++++)	Notes
Discectomy or microdiscectomy	Excision of herniated intervertebral disc	1–2	Prone	Not significant	+/++	Microdiscectomy can be done as day case
Cervical discectomy	Excision of herniated cervical intervertebral disc	2	Prone/head on horseshoe or halo traction pins	Not significant	++/+++	May be an emergency with neurological deficit
Spinal fusion ± decompression	Correction of spondylolisthesis or spinal stenosis for pain or instability—often several levels	1–2 (then 1 per level)	Prone	500–2000mL, X-match 4U	+++/+++++	May take bone graft from pelvis. Metal implantation
Cervical fusion ± decompression	Fusion of unstable neck (e.g. arthritis, trauma)	2–3	Supine or prone. Cervical traction in place or applied at start	300–1000mL, G&S	++/+++	Neck can be very unstable and need awake fibreoptic intubation. Application of traction pins very stimulating
Excision of spinal tumour (e.g. vertebrectomy)	Tumours may be 1° or 2° from any part of the spine	2–6+	Supine, prone, or lateral tilt	Potentially massive, X-match 6U + clotting factors available	+++/+++++	Often difficult surgery with potential for major blood loss and neurological damage

| Kyphoscoliosis surgery | Correction of major spinal deformities in patients who may have severe physical disability | 3–6+ | Supine and/or prone | Potentially massive, X-match 6U + clotting factors available | +++/+++++ | Often in children with severe restrictive respiratory disease and coexisting abnormalities. May involve surgery in abdominal and thoracic cavities. Spinal nerve monitoring used in some centres. May need post-op ICU for IPPV |
| Repair of vertebral fracture | Repair for neurological deficit or instability | 2–6 | Supine and/or prone | 500–2000mL, X-match 4U | ++/++++ | Often associated with other major injury (esp. rib fracture). May be in ICU/IPPV. Neurological deficit often not reversible. Note: suxamethonium may be contraindicated |

- Peripheral pressure areas are at particular risk in the prone position. Pillows and silicone pads should be used judiciously to protect all areas. Ensure that the breasts and genitalia are not trapped. During long cases, it may be necessary to move the patient's limbs and head every hour to avoid stagnation of peripheral blood and the development of pressure necrosis. Pay particular attention to the nose, eyes, chin, elbows, knees, and ankles.
- The arms are usually placed 'above the head' which puts the brachial plexus at risk of stretching or being pressed against the mattress. Ensure that the axillae are not under tension after positioning.

Anaesthesia

- Plans for the recovery period should be made in advance and will be dictated by local experience. Long cases, those involving excessive blood loss, and major paediatric cases will need post-operative care in the HDU. Few patients require post-operative ventilatory support.
- Secure venous access is vital. It may be difficult to access the cannula, so an extension with a three-way tap is recommended.
- Choice of anaesthetic will be dictated by personal experience, but most will choose an IV induction with muscle relaxation and opioid supplementation. Both low-flow volatile anaesthesia and TIVA are frequently used. Remifentanil is useful perioperatively.
- If spinal cord integrity is at risk during surgery, it may be necessary to use spinal cord monitoring. This is a specialist service provided by a neurophysiologist but may require that muscle relaxation is allowed to wear off. It may be necessary to deepen the anaesthesia during this phase, but, in reality, this is rarely a problem. Somatosensory evoked potential monitoring is the most commonly employed technique. Intra-operative monitoring has superseded the 'wake-up test' when patients were woken in the middle of surgery and asked to perform simple motor functions before being re-anaesthetized.
- In patients with paraplegia or other large areas of muscle denervation (2d to 8 months), suxamethonium should be avoided (see ➔ p. 237).
- Airway access is likely to be limited once the procedure has started, so securing oral endotracheal intubation with a non-kinking tube is usual. Patients with unstable necks due to trauma or RA can be intubated using AFOI or with manual in-line stabilization, depending on the degree of instability and the anticipated difficulty of intubation (see ➔ p. 184). The tube should be moulded around the face, with no bulky joints adjacent to the skin. A throat pack may be used to decrease the flow of secretions onto the pillow, and the tube then secured with adhesive tape or film. Attention to detail and the use of padding are vital to protect pressure areas.
- Most patients will be paralysed and ventilated for these procedures, with positional considerations noted above.
- Check the position of the ETT when the patient has been turned. Check that ventilation is adequate, without excessive inflation pressures, before surgery starts, as the only recourse may be to return the patient to the supine position if problems develop.

- Blood loss may be significant, with venous oozing proving hard to control. The use of cell salvage techniques (see ➲ p. 1046) is advisable for long procedures involving instrumentation of multiple levels. All patients should have samples grouped and saved, and more major procedures should have blood cross-matched, even if cell salvage is employed (see below).
- Hypotensive anaesthesia may reduce blood loss during major spinal surgery. The MAP should be maintained at a safe level—for normotensive patients >60mmHg. Direct arterial monitoring is mandatory when the BP is being manipulated.
- The type of analgesia required will vary, depending on the magnitude of surgery. Minor procedures (e.g. microdiscectomy) may manage with NSAIDs alone, in association with infiltration of the operative site with LA. Most procedures will necessitate opioids. PCA morphine is effective after adequate IV loading. The use of regional analgesia is encouraged where there is no need to assess neurological function, and the use of epidural and paravertebral analgesia is growing in popularity for major procedures such as correction of scoliosis. The catheter is usually placed by the surgeon at the end of the procedure, and infusions of LA or opioids continued for several days post-operatively.
- Effective analgesia is particularly important for surgery to the thoracic spine where post-operative respiratory function will be compromised if analgesia is inadequate. Consider also using incentive spirometry and chest physiotherapy.

Reference

30 Raw DA, Beattie JK, Hunter JM (2003). Anaesthesia for spinal surgery in adults. *Br J Anaesth*, **91**, 886–904.

Shoulder surgery

General considerations

Soft tissue operations around the shoulder are frequently extremely painful. This pain is not predictable and may last for several days, although it is certainly worst within the first 48hr.

Anaesthesia

- The patient is usually positioned with the head distal to the anaesthetist, requiring particular attention to the security of the airway. It is often easier to intubate the patient (south-facing Ring, Adair, and Elwyn (RAE) or armoured tube), except for shorter procedures where an LMA may be suitable. Long ventilator and gas sampling tubes are required.
- Venous access should be placed in the opposite arm (with a long extension) or at the ankle/foot.
- The patient may be placed supine, with head-up tilt, lateral, or in a deck-chair position. When using steep head-up tilt in patients with compromised CVS function, change the posture slowly, and consider direct arterial pressure monitoring.
- There is the potential for air embolus, while in these positions.
- Although blood loss is rarely significant, patients may be unable to take oral fluids for some hours post-operatively.
- Regional anaesthesia is a useful adjunct in shoulder anaesthesia, and an interscalene block is the method of choice (see ➋ p. 1108). Although procedures may be performed under regional anaesthesia alone, it is more commonly used to supplement GA and to provide post-operative analgesia. When planning an interscalene block, inform the patient that their whole arm may go numb and that they may sense that full inspiration is not possible when they wake up (phrenic nerve blockade). Interscalene block is contraindicated in patients with contralateral phrenic nerve/diaphragmatic palsy or recurrent laryngeal nerve damage. Interscalene catheters can be used for prolonged post-operative analgesia.[31]
- When an interscalene block is impractical, infiltration of LA by the surgeon may also provide post-operative analgesia. A catheter can be placed in the subacromial space and used to instil further quantities of LA in the post-operative period.[32] This is particularly effective in Bankart's and capsular shift operations.
- For rotator cuff repairs, an epidural catheter placed surgically over the repair can be used to supplement post-operative analgesia. Regular boluses (10mL of 0.25% bupivacaine 2- to 4-hourly) are better than an infusion.
- Potent analgesia is often required for 1–2d. The combination of PCA opioid/NSAIDs/paracetamol is usually effective. Good posture (sitting up with the elbow supported on a pillow) is also important.

References

31 Denny NM, Barber N, Sildown DJ (2003). Evaluation of an insulated Tuohy needle system for the placement of interscalene brachial plexus catheters. *Anaesthesia*, **58**, 554–7.

32 Axelsson K, Nordenson U, Johanzon E, et al. (2003). Patient-controlled regional analgesia (PCRA) with ropivacaine after arthroscopic subacromial decompression. *Acta Anaesthesiol Scand*, **47**, 993–1000.

Total shoulder replacement

Procedure	Prosthetic shoulder replacement
Time	2–3hr
Pain	+++/++++
Position	Supine, head-up, or deck-chair
Blood loss	250–500mL
Practical techniques	ETT + IPPV, interscalene block

Preoperative
- Many patients are elderly; severe rheumatoid disease is common.
- Ask about respiratory function/reserve if planning an interscalene block (some diaphragmatic function will be lost for several hours).
- Check the airway (particularly in RA) and range of neck movement. Some patients will need fibreoptic intubation.

Perioperative
- Consider performing an interscalene block before inducing anaesthesia (see ⟳ p. 1108).
- Place IV infusion and BP cuff on the opposite arm with a long extension.
- Intubate with a preformed 'south-facing' ETT.
- Hypotension is common when changing to a head-up position.
- If interscalene block has been performed, anaesthesia is usually unremarkable. Sometimes breakthrough stimulation occurs during the glenoid phase (may receive fibres from T2 which are not always covered by the block).
- If no interscalene block, load the patient with morphine, and ask the surgeon to infiltrate with LA (20–30mL of 0.25% bupivacaine).
- Antibiotic prophylaxis.

Post-operative
- Pain is worst in the first 24hr post-operatively. PCA/intermittent morphine is usually satisfactory.
- NSAIDs are useful.

Special considerations
- Air/fat embolism is a rare event.
- In high-risk patients, direct arterial monitoring is advised.

Other shoulder operations
- Most shoulder surgery may be carried out using the anaesthetic guidelines on ⟳ p. 468. Arthroscopic surgery is generally less painful, and patients get effective post-operative analgesia if the surgeon injects 10–20mL of bupivacaine 0.5% within the joint space at the end of surgery.

- Bankart's and capsular shift operations for recurrent dislocations are more painful for larger, muscular patients, but not generally as painful as cuff repairs and open acromioplasties.
- Massive cuff repairs are often extremely painful, and an interscalene block is useful. PCA should be considered, and a loading dose of morphine should be administered during surgery. Consider an interscalene catheter with infusion of LA.
- Pain following any operation around the shoulder is unpredictable, and some patients who have had short procedures suffer severe pain for several days. A flexible approach is required for analgesia.
- Beware the pain-free patient following major shoulder surgery and connected to PCA morphine. When the regional block wears off, effective analgesia may take some time to establish.

Elbow replacement surgery

Procedure	Prosthetic elbow replacement
Time	Variable
Pain	+/++
Position	Supine, arm out on table
Blood loss	Minimal
Practical techniques	GA, tourniquet

Total elbow arthroplasty[33] is performed in patients with an ankylosed or a very stiff elbow (e.g. RA). This procedure is becoming commoner, but, in 2012, only 288 were performed in England and Wales. The operation aims to provide an increase in the range of motion of the joint and pain relief. Complications, including reoperation, are frequent.

Technique
- Assess the patient for other manifestations of rheumatoid disease (see ➲ p. 184).
- LMA/ETT GA and IV opioids.
- A tourniquet is often used.
- Ensure careful positioning to prevent tissue injury and to reduce post-operative pain from other arthritic areas.
- Regional techniques—vertical infraclavicular block (VIB; see ➲ p. 1110) is probably the block of choice.
- Post-operative ulnar nerve compression is common and may necessitate further surgery.

Reference
33 Mansat P, Morrey BF (2000). Semiconstrained total elbow arthroplasty for ankylosed and stiff elbows. *J Bone Joint Surg*, **82**, 1260–8.

Anaesthesia for hand surgery

Procedure	Various
Time	Variable
Pain	+/+++
Position	Supine, arm out on table
Blood loss	Minimal
Practical techniques	Regional analgesia ± GA, tourniquet

The majority of hand surgery procedures (Table 18.4) are suitable for local or regional anaesthesia as a day case. This can be combined with GA or additional sedation, if required. Some procedures, such as carpal tunnel release or trigger finger release, can be done under local infiltration alone. IV regional anaesthesia (IVRA) is suitable for procedures below the elbow of 30min or less, although it is now rarely performed.

An upper arm tourniquet is almost always used for any type of hand surgery. Positioning and duration of use will be an important determinant of whether the patient is able to tolerate regional or local anaesthesia alone. Patients with a good brachial plexus block will usually tolerate 60–90min of arm ischaemia.

An axillary brachial plexus block can provide excellent anaesthesia to the hand, arm, and forearm, although tourniquet pain may be a problem. Other approaches include infra- and supraclavicular approaches.

Preoperative

- Full assessment as for GA. The patient may request a GA, and regional anaesthesia may fail.
- Check that patients can lie flat for the proposed duration of operation if planned to be awake.
- Assess movement of the operative arm. Can the patient achieve the necessary position for regional block or the surgery planned?

Perioperative

- Make sure the patient's bladder is empty.
- Use full monitoring, whether or not GA/sedation is to be used.
- Perform a local block, with the patient awake or lightly sedated.
- Choose an appropriate and familiar block for the planned site of surgery ± tourniquet.
- Augment plexus anaesthesia with elbow or wrist blocks, as necessary, to improve success rates.
- Provide sedation or GA, depending on safety and the patient's wishes. Have equipment and drugs ready to convert to sedation or GA, if necessary, during the operation.

Post-operative

- Surgery involving soft tissues and the skin is generally less painful than surgery to the bones and joints.
- Simple analgesic combinations are usually adequate for the less painful procedures.
- Opioids or regional catheter techniques may be required for the more painful operations.
- Some patients dislike the post-operative 'dead arm' following brachial plexus block.

Special considerations

- Tourniquet pain can be reduced by blocking the intercostobrachial nerve SC on the medial aspect of the upper arm above the level of the tourniquet.
- Adrenaline-containing solutions should be avoided near digits.

Table 18.4 Surgical procedures on the hand

Operation	Description	Time (min)	Pain (+ to +++++)	Notes
Trigger finger release and carpal tunnel release	Tendon or nerve release	5–15	+	These procedures can usually be carried out under local-infiltration anaesthesia
Dupuytren's contractures (simple)	Usually confined to ulnar and median distribution. Usually <30min tourniquet time	<60	+	GA with wrist block or infiltration. Brachial plexus block with upper arm tourniquet ± GA. Quick procedure: wrist block with wrist tourniquet
Dupuytren's contracture (complex)	Severe disease or redo procedure may need skin grafting	60–120	+	Prolonged tourniquet time means that a brachial plexus block or a GA with local block is often required
MCP joint replacement (e.g. Swanson)	MCP joint replacement usually for rheumatoid	30 per joint	++/+++	Generally frailer patients with systemic disease
Tenolysis, capsulotomies, tendon grafts	These procedures may need patient participation to assess the adequacy of the procedure	15–60	+/++	If hand movement is required, then any block must be distal. A wrist block with sedation is usually adequate
Digit reimplantation	Microvascular surgery	Hours	++	A GA is usually required because of the prolonged procedure. Regional anaesthesia for the sympathectomy is helpful
Ulnar head excision or trapeziectomy	Surgery for wrist pain in rheumatoid disease	30–60	++/+++	As pain is severe, a single-shot brachial block or catheter technique is ideal, with or without a GA

Anaesthesia for major trauma

Major trauma presents many challenges to the anaesthetist. Multiple injuries can cause significant physiological disturbance and may require urgent and/ or prolonged surgery from different specialties. Significant injuries may be unrecognized or not present until surgery. All patients should be resuscitated, according to Advanced Trauma Life Support (ATLS®) guidelines. See also ➔ p. 844.

General considerations

- Major trauma cases often require a number of procedures. Lifesaving surgery clearly takes priority, but it may be possible to perform several procedures at once.
- The patient should be personally fully reviewed preoperatively. Major injuries are easily missed in A&E. Check the CXR for missed pathology.
- Immediately prior to anaesthesia, every patient should have a minimum of an ATLS® 1° survey. A high index of suspicion should exist for injuries that may not have been apparent at the initial assessment but may cause cardiorespiratory compromise—pneumothorax, spinal cord injury, cardiac tamponade, fat embolism, and occult haemorrhage.
- Hypothermia causes significant morbidity and should be rigorously avoided and treated.
- Lifesaving surgery should not be delayed by unnecessary investigations.

Management of anaesthesia

Teamwork

It is important to use all members of the medical staff efficiently. Effective communication is an important determinant of outcome.

Airway

- Endotracheal intubation is usual.
- Intubation is more likely to be difficult; all the usual equipment should be available before starting induction of anaesthesia.
- Always assume a full stomach. Place a gastric tube during surgery to attempt gastric decompression. The tube should be placed orally if there are associated nasal/mid-face or base-of-skull fractures.

Ventilation

- Ventilator settings may have to be adjusted from 'normal' values to take into account problems that are particular to trauma patients.
- Patients with actual or potentially raised ICP should have their $PaCO_2$ kept at 4.5–5kPa (35–38mmHg) to help maintain a stable ICP.
- Patients with chest trauma may require the use of special ventilator settings. It may be necessary to use an ICU ventilator.

Circulatory access

- Ensure adequate venous access—preferably two 14–16G cannulae. If venous access is difficult, consider a cut-down/femoral line/external jugular line, or an intraosseous access.
- Do not delay lifesaving surgery with attempts to fully resuscitate hypovolaemia.

- Continue resuscitation during transfer to theatre; 'permissive hypovolaemia' or 'hypotensive resuscitation' to a systolic BP of 80mmHg may be preferable for the trauma victim with ongoing uncontrolled haemorrhage.[34]
- Although not introduced into civilian practice as yet, aggressive treatment of blood loss in recent military campaigns has reduced the impact from the four hypos—hypothermia, hypoxaemia, hypovolaemia, and hypocoagulability.[35]
- Attach one IV line to a high-performance warming system, preferably with an automatic pressurization system. This line should be dedicated to fluid resuscitation, unless haemorrhage is massive; this ensures adequate heating of all infused fluid. Ideally, one person should be solely responsible for checking and dealing with all fluid on this line.
- An arterial line should be inserted when practical. They are not normally required immediately and should not delay surgery.
- Central venous access is not usually a priority and may be difficult due to injuries to the vasculature and hypovolaemia. It is best carried out after fluid resuscitation. A femoral line may be the most practical (and quickest) option if infusions of vasopressors/inotropes are required—however, avoid in abdominal trauma.

Temperature
- Use a temperature probe and peripheral nerve stimulator. Try to maintain body temperature.

Regional anaesthesia
- Regional anaesthesia may be considered as an adjunct, although preoperative urgency, haemodynamic instability, coagulopathy, and the possibility of compartment syndrome often make it impractical.

Problems
- Unexplained hypotension and tachycardia: consider hypovolaemia, pneumothorax, pericardial tamponade, and fat/air embolism.
- Unexplained hypoxia is often associated with a rise in inflation pressure: consider tension pneumothorax and fat embolism.
- Unexplained hypertension: consider pain, raised ICP (search for associated neurological signs; obtain brain CT scan), and rarely traumatic disruption of the thoracic aorta.

Changing anaesthetic teams
Major trauma cases often involve prolonged surgery by multiple teams; you may need to hand over the patient to different anaesthetist(s). This handover should be as detailed as possible. The anaesthetist should document the time and details of the handover on the anaesthetic record.

References

34 Stern SA (2001). Low-volume fluid resuscitation for presumed hemorrhagic shock: helpful or harmful? *Curr Opin Crit Care*, **7**, 422–30.
35 Moor P, Rew D, Midwinter MJ, Doughty H (2009). Transfusion for trauma: civilian lessons from the battlefield? *Anaesthesia*, **64**, 469–72.

Cervical spine fracture

Surgery for cervical spine fracture may comprise the application of stabilizing devices (halo traction, skull tongs, plaster jacket) or definitive fixation of the bony column (usually performed as a semi-elective procedure).

General considerations

- Patients have usually suffered major trauma, although fractures can occur following minor injury if pre-existing cervical spine disease.
- Controversy exists as to the best method of securing the airway. Awake intubation is considered safe in trained hands; however, it may result in coughing and can be difficult and unpleasant for the patient. Direct laryngoscopy under GA with manual in-line neck stabilization (MILNS) may be associated with more neck movement.

Anaesthesia

- Patients for halo traction, skull tong application, and other stabilizing procedures will usually be in full neck immobilization. This is removed following the application of the stabilizing device—usually under LA. Sedation may be required. GA is occasionally required for more complex stabilization or in confused/agitated patients. It should be performed as per anterior cervical stabilization (see ➔ p. 464 and p. 479).
- Patients for open cervical spine stabilization require either an anterior or a posterior approach, and, in a few patients, both.
- Perform a full neurological examination before anaesthesia to assess the level and extent of any spinal cord injury. This is particularly important for patients who are to be turned prone.
- Anterior approaches are usually performed in the supine head-up position, through an oblique incision across the anterior aspect of the neck. The posterior approach is performed in the prone position, using a longitudinal incision. Occasionally, fractures to C1/C2 may require an approach through the mouth.
- Arterial and venous lines should be placed and must be well secured to prevent kinking. A forced-air warming system should be used, and urinary catheterization is required. NG decompression is usual for prolonged surgery or those with pre-existing spinal cord injury.
- For prone positioning, extreme care is needed during turning (involve the surgeon). The surgeon should control the head/neck, while at least three people perform the turn. The anaesthetist should hold the ETT *in situ* and should be in charge of coordinating the turn. Some centres use awake intubation, followed by awake positioning, prior to induction of anaesthesia.
- Blood loss is rarely significant for these procedures, and so deliberate arterial hypotension is not usually required.

Anaesthesia for repair of cervical spine fracture

Procedure	Anterior/posterior repair of cervical fracture
Time	2–6hr
Pain	++/+++
Position	Supine head-up or prone for posterior approach
Blood loss	250–1000mL, X-match 4U
Practical techniques	GA, art line, AFOI

Preoperative

- Mostly trauma patients, often with other injuries. Sometimes older patients with fractures in a previously diseased cervical spine. Check for other manifestations of the underlying disease (e.g. rheumatoid).
- Check the presence/degree of cervical spine injury, level of lesion, and likely approach.
- Check the need for post-operative ventilation and HDU care. Commoner with high lesions, which may need aggressive chest physiotherapy.
- Consider the technique of intubation. The patient may be in skull traction, which does not limit mouth opening but does limit neck movement. Full neck immobilization (with a hard cervical collar and sandbags/tape) limits both neck movement and mouth opening.

Perioperative

- Insert arterial and venous lines, preferably in the same arm.
- Intubation: awake nasal intubation is commonest,[36] but a smaller tube size results. Awake oral intubation is harder to perform but gives a larger tube size. If the surgeon is planning an intraoral approach, check whether an oral or nasal ETT is preferred.
- Suxamethonium is contraindicated in patients with spinal cord lesions that are >72hr old. In practice, it is rare to need suxamethonium.
- Positioning should be in combination with the surgeon. Some request check of residual neurological function following awake intubation and after turning prone.
- Check all pressure areas before draping. Procedures are prolonged.
- Bone graft may be required and is usually taken from the iliac crest.

Post-operative

- PCA morphine is usually satisfactory.
- NSAIDs are useful.

Special considerations

- Patients with acute spinal cord lesions may demonstrate signs of neurogenic shock, including bradycardia and hypotension (see ➡ p. 237). This is best treated with judicious use of fluids and pressor agents, guided by CVP monitoring. Cervical spine surgery is rarely performed in the 1st few hours after injury, which makes these problems uncommon. However, spinal hyperreflexia may occur in patients with longer-standing lesions, and these should be treated symptomatically (see ➡ p. 237).
- Tracheostomy is not advisable in patients scheduled for anterior fusion. Discuss with the surgeon if this is a likely option.

Reference

36 Sidhu VS, Whitehead EM, Ainsworth QP, Smith M, Calder I (1993). A technique of awake fibre-optic intubation. Experience in patients with cervical spine disease. *Anaesthesia*, **48**, 910–13.

Anaesthesia for limb fractures

Procedure	Closed or open reduction of limb fractures
Time	5min to many hours
Pain	Variable
Position	Usually supine
Blood loss	Minimal, but can be up to 2000mL for open procedures
Practical techniques	GA ± block, regional block alone

Discuss with the surgeon the nature and duration of the likely repair (manipulation under anaesthesia (MUA) may become ORIF). If planning a regional block, you should also discuss the risk of compartment syndrome (see ➲ p. 448).

Preoperative
- Check that no additional surgery is likely.
- Ensure the absence of other significant chest/abdominal/head injuries.
- Patients with recent (<24hr) moderate or severe head injury require very careful consideration before proceeding to non-lifesaving surgery.
- Check the state of cervical spine clearance where relevant.
- Check the state of hydration of the patient and the time of the last food/drink in relation to the time of injury.
- In practice, the stomach may never empty in some patients, particularly children, and, if in doubt, consider the patient at risk of a full stomach.
- Check a chest radiograph for all major trauma patients.

Perioperative
- Ensure at least one large-gauge infusion/IVI warmer for all open reductions involving proximal limb fractures.
- Do not site IV on an injured limb.
- Blood loss is very variable. Proximal limb fractures (femur, humerus) and use of bone grafting cause considerable blood loss.
- The use of a tourniquet will reduce bleeding but may be contraindicated because of the fracture type/site.
- Give antibiotic prophylaxis prior to commencement of surgery/application of tourniquet.
- Patients are at risk of fat embolism (see ➲ p. 446).

Patients with pre-existing head injury may require ICP monitoring and post-operative ventilation. GA can obscure the signs of deterioration in conscious level, and anaesthesia may also contribute to a rise in ICP.

Post-operative

- Post-operative analgesia requirements depend on the nature of the surgery.
- Closed reductions can often be managed with a combination of perioperative opioid and NSAIDs/paracetamol/opioid orally.
- More complex repairs, including external fixation, may require the use of a PCA.

Special considerations

- Regional anaesthesia can be a useful addition for the provision of analgesia and may also be used as the sole anaesthetic for some fracture reductions. However, an LA block may obscure neurological signs of a developing compartment syndrome. The best strategy is to discuss the problem with the surgeon beforehand.
- In humeral fractures where surgical wire banding is planned, avoid regional blocks. The radial nerve is easily trapped during surgery, and the diagnosis is delayed with a regional block.
- If bone grafting is anticipated from the pelvis, then the donor site will be painful.

Compartment syndrome

Compartment syndrome[37] arises when the circulation and tissues within a closed space are compromised by increased pressure. Ischaemia, necrosis, and loss of function result, further increasing compartmental pressure. Damage can become irreversible after only 4hr.

Compartment syndrome is a serious limb-threatening condition, which may also lead to systemic organ dysfunction if incorrectly managed. It should be anticipated in any significant limb injury, with or without fracture, especially in crush situations. It can also be caused by tourniquets, malpositioning in theatre, systemic hypotension, haemorrhage, oedema, and direct injection of drugs. In obtunded patients, where clinical signs may be masked, or in the presence of spinal cord injuries, measurement of compartmental pressure may be indicated. Early diagnosis and treatment are vital. Urgent fasciotomy may be required.

Signs and symptoms of compartment syndrome include:
- Pain, mainly over the affected compartment, worsened by passive stretching of the muscles
- Tense swelling over the compartment, with drum-tight fascia/skin
- Paraesthesiae in the distribution of nerves traversing the compartment
- Weakness or paralysis of the limb is a late sign
- Distal pulses are usually present.

Measuring compartment pressures
- This can be undertaken using a pressure transducer (as in an arterial line) attached to a needle placed into the suspect compartment.
- If the compartmental pressure is within 30mmHg of the diastolic pressure, diagnosis is confirmed.

Special considerations
- Compartment syndrome can occur with open fractures—some compartments may not be able to decompress through the open wound.
- Keep the limb at the level of the heart. Avoid elevation, as this may decrease perfusion below critical levels.
- Release all constricting bandages, dressings, or casts encircling the limb. If this does not rapidly relieve symptoms, urgent surgical fasciotomy will be required to save the limb.
- After fasciotomy, the limb should be splinted to prevent contractures, and the fracture stabilized to prevent further bleeding.
- Ensure the patient is well hydrated and has a good urine output. Myoglobinuria is maximal after reperfusion.

Regional anaesthesia
Avoid local blocks or epidurals if the patient is at risk of developing compartment syndrome, as the analgesia will mask early signs. The cardinal symptom is pain, and this occurs early in the syndrome. Risk is especially high in tibial and forearm fractures, so avoid blocks in these situations.

Reference
37 Mar GJ, Barrington MJ, McGuirk BR (2009). Acute compartment syndrome of the lower limb and the effect of postoperative analgesia. *Br J Anaesth*, **109**, 3–11.

Anaesthesia for femoral neck fracture

Procedure	Cannulated screws, DHS, cemented/uncemented hemiarthroplasty
Time	10–120min
Pain	+/+++
Position	Supine (? on hip table), occasionally lateral
Blood loss	250–750mL
Practical techniques	SV LMA and regional block
	Spinal ± sedation
	ETT + IPPV

Hip fractures are common: ~80 000 per annum in the UK (80% ♀). Average age is 83yr, and 80% occur in those >75yr. In Western society, the lifetime risk is 18% (women) and 6% (men).[38] The 3-month mortality is ~12%, increasing to 21% at 1yr.[39]

Preoperative

- Physiological reserve is reduced, and co-morbidity is common. Ideally, resuscitation should start as soon as the patient is admitted to hospital. Thorough preoperative assessment must take place, and surgery should be scheduled for the earliest possible daytime session.
- Surgical treatment can be either fracture fixation or femoral head replacement, depending on the nature of fracture, surgical preference, previous mobility, and life expectancy.
- Determine which procedure is to be performed (Table 18.5). Cannulated hip screws are quick, largely non-invasive procedures with a small incision and little blood loss. Cemented/uncemented hemiarthroplasty is a longer procedure, similar to the femoral part of a 1° hip replacement. Dynamic hip screw (DHS)/Richards screw and plate are intermediate procedures.
- Any decision to delay surgery should be based on a realistic attempt to improve the patient's medical condition, rather than a fruitless pursuit of 'normal' values. A mild chest infection is unlikely to improve in a bed-bound elderly patient, whereas frank pneumonia with sepsis and dyspnoea may respond to rehydration, antibiotics, and chest physiotherapy. Good communication between the surgeons, orthogeriatricians, and anaesthetists is important.
- An attempt should be made to control AF preoperatively to prevent severe perioperative hypotension.
- Dehydration is common, as oral intake is often much reduced. IV fluids must be commenced as soon as the patient is admitted to a hospital.
- Analgesia should be commenced, as often the patient is in considerable pain. A fascia iliaca block instituted in an A&E setting can provide 'dynamic' analgesia and reduces the requirement for opioids.[40]

Table 18.5 Surgical procedures for fractured neck of femur

Operation	Description	Time (min)	Pain (+ to +++++)	Position	Blood loss/X-match	Notes
Cannulated screws	Screws across femoral neck (previously 'Garden screws')	20	+++	Supine, hip table	Nil	Minimally invasive, small thigh incision. Can be done with local/nerve block and sedation, if necessary. X-ray-guided
Richards screw and plate (RSP)	Plate along femur, with compression screw into femoral head	30–45	++	Supine, hip table	<400mL	Somewhat larger thigh incision/blood loss. X-ray-guided
Dynamic hip screw (DHS)	As RSP	30–45	++	Supine, hip table	<400mL	As RSP
Dynamic compression screw (DCS)	As RSP	30–45	++	Supine, hip table	<400mL	As RSP
Girdlestone osteotomy	Removal of femoral head. No prosthesis	30–45	++	Supine	<400mL	More extensive incision, but no prosthesis, hence quicker than below. Limited mobility afterwards
Austin Moore hemiarthroplasty	Replacement of femoral head. No cement	60–90	+++	Supine	400–600mL	Similar to total hip replacement, without acetabular component
Thompson's hemiarthroplasty	Replacement of femoral head. Cemented	60–90	+++	Supine	400–600mL	Similar to total hip replacement, without acetabular component
Exeter bipolar	Replacement of femoral head and acetabular component. Cemented	60–90	+++	Supine	400–800mL	Similar to total hip replacement, with acetabular component

Perioperative

- For fracture fixation, the patient is usually positioned supine on a 'hip table'. This involves placement of a groin prop, with the table supporting the upper body only. Feet are tied into shoe supports, and the table is then elevated to allow radiographic screening. For hemiarthroplasty, the patient is lateral or supine on an ordinary operating table.
- Blood loss is variable. Much of the measured loss is old haematoma, but significant haemorrhage may occur and necessitate transfusion.
- Choice of anaesthetic technique. Regional and general anaesthesia are both advocated, but there is emerging evidence that regional anaesthesia has advantages.[41,42] Options include:
  - Regional anaesthesia: epidural, spinal, psoas plexus (see ➔ p. 1135, p. 1126), and 3-in-1 nerve block (see ➔ p. 1128) have all been used for operative anaesthesia and post-operative analgesia. Sedation may be necessary, but any sedative can produce unpredictable effects in the elderly and should only be used when necessary
  - Spinal anaesthesia may decrease the incidence of post-operative confusion and DVT. A small dose of IV ketamine or alfentanil may be useful as analgesia when turning the patient before performing the block, but avoiding all sedatives is preferable.
  - GA with opioid supplementation
  - Regurgitation and aspiration occasionally occurs with LMAs in this group—if the patient is at risk, use endotracheal intubation.
- Check pressure points after placement on the 'hip table', as these patients are prone to pressure damage.
- Use some form of passive or active warming device to prevent hypothermia. Insulate the head, and secure a warming blanket/ polythene sheet around the chest and lower abdomen.
- Cemented hemiarthroplasty may be associated with a marked drop in arterial pressure, $ETCO_2$, and HR during cement insertion. Take the same precautions as with a total hip replacement (see ➔ p. 447).

Post-operative

- Pain is often only due to the incision, which is small for cannulated screws and DHS, but larger for hemiarthroplasty, although DHS procedures may carry a considerable amount of post-operative pain.[43]
- Fracture pain will be reduced but is still present on rolling and turning in bed.
- Post-operative analgesia can be provided by regular IV paracetamol; opioids should be used sparingly.[44] Most patients will require some post-operative analgesia, although some do not. Take care with NSAIDs because of the increased risk of GI and renal complications.

Special considerations

- In high-risk patients, procedures can be undertaken with LA alone. Morbidity and mortality risks should be understood by the patient and relatives, and, in some patients, the resuscitation status should be reviewed.
- A useful resource for all anaesthetists involved in the management of hip fracture patients is the NHS Hip Fracture Anaesthesia Network.[45]

References

38 Gillespie W (2001). Hip fracture. *BMJ*, **322**, 968–75.

39 Parker MJ, Pryor GA, Myles J (2000). 11 year results in 2,846 patients of the Peterborough hip fracture project: reduced morbidity, mortality and hospital stay. *Acta Anaesthesiol Scand*, **71**, 34–8.

40 Foss NB, Kristensen BB, Bundgaard M, et al. (2007). Fascia iliaca compartment blockade for acute pain control in hip fracture patients: a randomized, placebo-controlled trial. *Anesthesiology*, **106**, 773–8.

41 Neuman MD, Silber JH, Elkassabany NM, Ludwig JM, Fleisher LA (2012). Comparative effectiveness of regional versus general anesthesia for hip fracture surgery in adults. *Anesthesiology*, **117**, 72–92.

42 Association of Anaesthetists of Great Britain and Ireland, Griffiths R, Alper J, Beckingsale A, et al. (2012). Management of proximal femoral fractures 2011: Association of Anaesthetists of Great Britain and Ireland. *Anaesthesia*, **67**, 85–98.

43 Foss NB, Kristensen MT, Palm H, Kehlet H (2009). Postoperative pain after hip fracture is procedure specific. *Br J Anaesth*, **102**, 111–16.

44 Cuvillon P, Ripart J, Debureaux S, et al. (2007). [Analgesia after hip fracture repair in elderly patients: the effect of a continuous femoral nerve block: a prospective and randomised study]. *Ann Fr Anesth Réanim*, **26**, 2–9.

45 NHS Networks. ℘ http://www.networks.nhs.uk/nhs-networks/hip-fracture-anaesthesia.

Plastic surgery

Jonathan Warwick

General principles

The complexity of anaesthesia ranges from the routine to the challenging. Some extensive procedures (e.g. free flap repairs, craniofacial reconstruction) may involve invasive monitoring, extensive blood loss, and post-operative intensive care support.

Regional techniques

Minor body surface procedures may be performed under LA infiltration alone. Upper and lower limb surgery is especially suitable for regional or peripheral nerve block. Sedation to supplement a regional technique may be required in anxious patients or for longer procedures. Propofol (0.5–1.0 microgram/mL TCI, or 10–15mL/hr of 1% solution), supplemented with a small dose of midazolam (1–2mg), is effective. Significant body surface procedures (e.g. excision and grafting of skin tumours) can be accomplished in those unfit for GA, using extensive infiltration of LA and IV sedation. Incremental sedation with ketamine (10mg) and midazolam (1mg) is a safe and potent analgesic/sedative combination in the elderly.

The difficult airway

(See also ➔ p. 954.)

Patients with head and neck pathology causing airway difficulty are often encountered. Airway difficulty may arise from anatomical deformity due to tumour, trauma, infection, previous operation, or scarring. Competence in difficult airway techniques (e.g. fibreoptic intubation) is required. The 'shared airway' is regularly a feature of head and neck surgery. Discuss with the surgeon which tube you propose to use and by which route to achieve the best surgical access (oral, nasal, conversion to tracheostomy). How will the tube be secured (tied, taped, stitched)?

Poor access to patient

The operating site may be extensive (e.g. burns debridement) or multiple (e.g. free flap procedures). This may produce added difficulty with:
- Heat conservation. It may be difficult to achieve enough access to the patient's body surface area to maintain temperature. Heated under-blankets are useful.
- Monitoring. ECG leads, the pulse oximeter probe, and the BP cuff may all be difficult to position adequately.
- Vascular access. Position cannulae away from the operative field. Use femoral vessels or the foot, if necessary. Long extension sets may be required.

Smooth emergence

Avoid the patient coughing and straining at the end of the procedure. This will put tension on delicate suture lines and increase bleeding and haematoma formation, especially for facial procedures. The combination of propofol maintenance and the LMA produces a particularly smooth emergence.

Attention to detail

Successful anaesthesia for plastic surgery requires thoroughness and careful attention to detail. Patients for aesthetic surgery will have high expectations and will be well informed.

Analgesia

Pain relief is always a challenge—in practice, effective pain control may be more readily achievable in patients recovering from plastic surgery for several reasons.

- Most procedures are performed on the body surface. These tend to be less painful than procedures involving the body cavities and are usually amenable to LA infiltration. Continuous catheter techniques may be useful in limb procedures.
- Patients recovering from head and neck procedures are often surprisingly comfortable despite extensive surgery.
- Major body cavities and abdominal musculature are usually not involved. The pain experienced after an abdominoplasty is significantly less than pain following a laparotomy.
- Plastic surgery procedures seldom involve new fractures of long bones.
- The GI tract is usually unaffected. The oral route for drugs is frequently available which may make dosing and administration of analgesics simpler.

Long operations

Patients undergoing complicated reconstructive procedures may be in theatre for many hours. Give careful consideration to:

- **Vascular access**. Check that line placement will not interfere with the site of surgery. Invasive arterial monitoring is desirable. A central venous line will assist with estimations of the intravascular volume and provide dependable venous access in the post-operative period. Site at least one large-bore peripheral (14–16G) cannula for fluid administration and a small cannula (20–22G) for other infusions such as TCI and PCA
- **Blood loss**. Ensure blood has been cross-matched. The initial dissection is usually the period of most blood loss, and a moderate hypotensive technique may help to limit this. Thereafter, losses may be insidious and ongoing. Aim to keep track by swab weighing, visual estimation, regular Hb or Hct estimations. Non-invasive cardiac output monitoring can help optimize the fluid status. Assessment of stroke volume, flow time, or stroke volume variation, using devices such as the oesophageal Doppler monitor or LiDCO™, may give valuable information to the anaesthetist
- **Fluid balance**. Urinary catheterization is essential. Ensure careful monitoring of fluid balance, especially in children and patients with poor cardiorespiratory function
- **Body temperature**. Monitor the core temperature (e.g. rectal, nasopharyngeal, oesophageal). Maintain the temperature by using low fresh gas flows (FGFs), an HME filter, warmed IV fluids, a warm ambient theatre temperature (e.g. 24°C), a heated mattress, or external warming blankets (e.g. Bair Hugger®). Take care not to overheat.
- **Positioning**. Ensure that structures, such as the cervical spine and brachial plexus, are not in positions of stress. Take care with pressure

areas. Make liberal use of cotton wool padding (Gamgee) over bony prominences. Raise the heels off the table, using foam pads or boots.

- **DVT prophylaxis**. VTE is often initiated during surgery. All patients should receive daily LMWH, thromboembolism compression stockings, and intermittent calf compression, while in theatre.
- **NGT**. Consider emptying the stomach. Children are especially prone to gastric distension during prolonged procedures.
- **Eye care**. Lightly tape and pad the eyes for protection. Avoid excessive padding, since this may negate the natural protection afforded by the bony orbit. Prophylactic antibiotic ointment is unnecessary. Do not allow corneal abrasion to develop from surface drying. A simple eye ointment is helpful if the eyes are left uncovered.
- **ETT cuff pressure**. Cuff pressure will gradually increase if N_2O is used. Where possible, recheck the cuff pressure at intervals during the case, if possible.
- **Post-operative care**. Discuss the preferred site of post-operative care with the nursing staff and surgical team. Surgeons often prefer patients to return to the plastic surgery ward where wound care and nursing observation may be more attuned to the specifics of the operation. Closer patient observation, invasive monitoring, and regular blood gas estimation may be more achievable in an ICU/HDU. The site for immediate post-operative care is principally dictated by the general condition of the patient.

Miscellaneous plastic surgical procedures

Table 19.1 presents the important information for those procedures which are not covered in the individual topics within this chapter.

Table 19.1 Other plastic surgical procedures

Operation	Description	Time (min)	Pain (+ to +++++)	Position	Blood loss/ X-match	Notes
Abdominoplasty	Excision of redundant lower abdominal skin	120	++ to +++	Supine	G&S	LMA or ETT, IPPV
Carpal tunnel release	Release of flexor sheath at the wrist to relieve median nerve entrapment	30	+	Supine, arm board	Nil (tourniquet)	LA infiltration, brachial plexus block, or day-case GA
Dupuytren's contracture	Excision of contracted palmar fascia	60–90	+	Supine, arm board	Nil (tourniquet)	Brachial plexus block or day-case GA
External angular dermoid	Excision of congenital dermoid cyst, usually from lateral supraorbital ridge	30	Ns	Supine, head ring	Nil	LMA and SV
Flexor/extensor tendon repair	Repair of hand tendons following trauma. Often multiple. May be extensive. May involve nerve/vessel repairs	30–120	+ to ++	Supine, arm board	Nil (tourniquet)	Brachial plexus block ± GA, LMA and SV, IPPV for extensive repairs
Gynaecomastia	Excision or liposuction of excess ♂ breast tissue	45	+ to ++	Supine	Nil	LMA and SV

(Continued)

Table 19.1 (Contd.)

Operation	Description	Time (min)	Pain (+ to +++++)	Position	Blood loss/ X-match	Notes
Hypospadias repair	Correction of congenital abnormality of ♂ urethra. Usually infant	90	++	Supine	Nil	LMA and SV. Caudal or penile block
Insertion of tissue expander	SC insertion of saline-filled silastic bags, often scalp	45	+ to ++	Supine, head ring	Nil	LMA and SV
Neck, axilla, and groin dissection	Block dissection of regional lymph nodes to excise 2° malignant disease	90–120	++	Supine, head ring	2U	LMA or ETT, IPPV
Preauricular sinus	Excision of congenital sinus tract, often bilateral	45	+	Supine, head ring	Nil	LMA and SV
Pretibial laceration	Excision of pretibial wound and SSG	45	+ to ++	Supine	Nil	Spinal or GA
Syndactyly	Release of congenital fusion of two or more digits. May be bilateral. May require FTSG	60–180	++	Supine	Nil (tourniquet)	LMA and SV. ETT + IPPV for extensive repairs

Breast reduction

Procedure	Reduction of breast size by glandular resection. Usually bilateral
Time	3hr
Pain	++
Position	Supine, 30° head-up. Arms may be positioned on boards, or with elbows flexed and hands placed behind the upper part of the buttocks
Blood loss	500mL, G&S
Practical techniques	IPPV via ETT or LMA

Preoperative

- Bilateral breast reduction is not primarily an aesthetic procedure. These patients may suffer from severe neck and back pain. Participating in exercise and sport is not possible. There may be symptoms of emotional disturbance.
- Patients are usually fit—aged 20–40yr. Many surgeons exclude patients with a BMI >30 due to a higher incidence of wound breakdown, infection, and haematoma formation.
- A mastopexy is a surgical procedure for correcting breast ptosis when breast volume is adequate. Anaesthetic implications are similar. Blood loss is less.
- FBC and G&S. Cross-matching is generally unnecessary, except for larger reductions.
- Timing in relation to the menstrual cycle is unimportant.
- All patients should receive DVT prophylaxis (compression stockings, daily LMWH).

Perioperative

- Balanced GA—IPPV may be preferable, since the surgeon often puts pressure on the chest wall during surgery. IPPV will maintain satisfactory chest expansion with good aeration and control of $PaCO_2$, and help minimize blood loss. An LMA may be satisfactory for IPPV.
- Place ECG electrodes on the patient's back. Lie the patient on 'incontinence pads' to absorb blood loss.
- Take care to position the patient carefully on the operating table. The anaesthetic machine is usually at the head end. Ensure that the chest and arms are symmetrical. Confirm that cannulae are firmly positioned, and their plastic caps covered with cotton wool/'Gamgee' if the hands are to be positioned behind the buttocks. Local pressure damage to the skin may otherwise ensue. Drip extension sets are needed; ensure that the drip runs freely.
- Blood loss depends on the surgical technique. Use of cutting diathermy causes less bleeding than a scalpel. Infiltration with dilute

adrenaline-containing LA helps reduce blood loss. All surgeons have their own recipe. Check the dosage being used; in practice, this is seldom a concern (see Liposuction, ➋ p. 504).
- Fewer than 5% of patients require transfusion. Mild falls in Hb are well tolerated in this young patient group.
- Moderate reductions may involve removal of 500g of tissue per breast.

Post-operative
- Bilateral breast reduction does not cause significant post-operative pain. Following a dose of morphine towards the end of surgery, regular simple analgesics and NSAIDs are usually adequate. IV PCA is generally unnecessary. An occasional dose of IM opioid may be required.
- Haematoma formation is an early complication. Occasionally, nipple perfusion may be compromised and requires decompression of the pedicle. Return to theatre may be indicated. Later complications include wound infection, dehiscence, and fat necrosis.

Special considerations
Occasionally, patients for massive breast reduction are encountered (>1kg of tissue removal per breast). Two to 4U of blood should be cross-matched. The complication rate is higher. Older patients may have coexisting cardio-pulmonary disease and require further investigation. Intubation and IPPV are the preferred technique.

Breast augmentation

Procedure	Bilateral or unilateral augmentation of breast size
Time	90min
Pain	++/+++
Position	Supine, 30° head-up. Arms may be out on boards, or with elbows flexed and hands placed behind the upper part of the buttocks
Blood loss	Minimal
Practical techniques	SV or IPPV via LMA

Preoperative

- Breast augmentation may be performed for:
  - Reconstruction following mastectomy
  - Correction of breast asymmetry
  - Aesthetic bilateral augmentation.
- Patients are usually fit and well. Check FBC.

Perioperative

- Position on the operating table as for breast reduction.
- Conventional augmentation involves the creation of an SC pocket for a silicone implant via an inframammary incision.
- Alternative techniques involve pocket formation by the insertion of an inflatable capsule mounted on an introducer via a small incision in the anterior axillary line. This is then removed, and the implant inserted.

Post-operative

- Post-operative discomfort may be related to the size of the implants. Large implants cause more tissue stretching and post-operative pain.
- In general, breast augmentation appears to cause more discomfort than breast reduction. Give regular NSAIDs and simple analgesics. Opioid analgesia may be needed, but PCA techniques are seldom required.
- Haematoma formation may require early return to theatre. Later complications include infection, capsule formation, and rupture.

Special considerations

- An association between silicone breast implants and the development of systemic symptoms of connective tissue diseases has been suggested. This association has not been proven, following data from large studies.
- Soybean oil-filled implants have been withdrawn from use in the UK. There are insufficient data concerning the long-term consequences of soybean oil breakdown. Saline implants are not perceived as sufficiently realistic and are unpopular with many women.
- Breast reconstruction following mastectomy is common. Options include insertion of a breast implant, reconstruction with a pedicled myocutaneous flap (e.g. latissimus dorsi or transverse rectus abdominis muscle, TRAM), and a free flap repair (usually TRAM).

Correction of prominent ears

Procedure	Surgical correction of prominent ears, usually caused by the absence of an antehelical fold. May be unilateral
Time	1hr
Pain	+
Position	Supine, 30° head-up
Blood loss	Minimal
Practical techniques	Day-case anaesthesia, flexible LMA, and SV

Preoperative
- Patients are usually children (4–10yr) and fit. They may not present for surgery until teenage or early adulthood.
- Surgery is offered as the child grows older and is aware of prominent ears. Often precipitated by teasing at school. The child may be self-conscious and anxious.
- Obtain consent for suppositories.

Perioperative
- Day-case anaesthetic technique.
- Anaesthetic machine usually at the foot end.
- PONV is common. Propofol maintenance is well tolerated.
- Avoid morphine. Use shorter-acting opioids (fentanyl or alfentanil) and NSAIDs.
- Surgeons use extensive LA/adrenaline infiltration to aid surgery. This provides good analgesia.
- IV crystalloid 20mL/kg may improve the quality of early recovery.

Post-operative
- NSAIDs (e.g. ibuprofen syrup 20–30mg/kg/day) and paracetamol.
- Dressings should be firm without being excessively tight. Scalp discomfort and itching can be a source of irritation.
- Excessive pain may be due to haematoma formation and requires return to theatre for drainage.

Special considerations
Allow time for extensive bandaging at the end of the operation. If intubation is used, early reduction in the anaesthetic depth will lead to coughing when the head is manipulated for bandage application. An LMA is ideal.

Facelift (rhytidectomy)

Procedure	Surgical reduction of facial folds and wrinkles to create a more youthful appearance
Time	3–4hr. More extensive procedures 6–8hr
Pain	+
Position	Supine, 30° head-up
Blood loss	Minimal
Practical techniques	IPPV via LMA or ETT, hypotensive technique, facial nerve blocks

Preoperative

- Most patients are aged 45–65yr and fit and well. They may have high expectations of anaesthesia and surgery and may have undergone previous facelift procedures.
- NSAIDs should be discontinued for at least 2wk prior to surgery.

Perioperative

- Many surgeons in the US perform routine facelift procedures under LA infiltration alone. Cost constraints in patients who are self-funding have contributed to this practice. Standard practice in the UK is for GA. Facelifts should always be regarded as major procedures.
- Incisions are placed in concealed areas (e.g. preauricular, extending up to the temporal region within the hair). The skin is mobilized by SC undermining, and wrinkles/skinfolds are improved by traction. Redundant skin is excised. Surgery is adapted to suit the needs of the patient and may include forehead lift, upper and lower blepharoplasty, and removal of submental/submandibular fat. It is occasionally combined with septorhinoplasty.
- Discuss the choice of airway device with the surgeon. A nasal north-facing tube provides the surgeon with good access to the face. Consider using a throat pack if there is nasal surgery.
- The anaesthetic machine is usually at the patient's foot end. Long breathing system tubing and drip extension sets are required.
- A moderate hypotensive technique (70–80 systolic) and 30° head-up tilt will help minimize blood loss and improve surgical conditions. A propofol and remifentanil maintenance is ideal.
- Use routine antiemetics.
- LA infiltration and specific nerve blocks provide good post-operative pain relief.
- Use a warming blanket.

Post-operative

- A smooth emergence is important to avoid bleeding beneath delicate suture lines. Deep extubation and substitution with a flexible LMA is a useful technique. Clonidine (1–2 micrograms/kg) is helpful in creating smooth conditions for emergence. Avoid post-operative shivering (treat with pethidine 25mg IV). Bleeding and haematoma formation may require an early return to theatre.

- There is a requirement for morphine in the immediate recovery period and to facilitate a smooth emergence, but pain is not a prominent feature of facelift. Discomfort is attributed to platysma tightening. Regular post-operative NSAIDs and simple analgesics are required. Marked pain should raise the suspicion of haematoma formation.

Special considerations

- The observed benefits from facelift procedures may only last 3–5yr. Repeat operations are common. Some patients may undergo several facelifts during their lifetime.
- Recent advances have involved more extensive procedures with deeper tissue undermining. These are all performed under GA. The composite facelift mobilizes the platysma, cheek fat, and orbicularis oculi muscle. This flap is then repositioned en bloc with the overlying skin. Complications are more frequent.

Free flap surgery

Procedure	The transfer of tissue from a donor site and microvascular anastomosis to a distant recipient site
Time	Variable, depending on procedure. Minimum 4hr, often 6–8hr or longer
Pain	+++
Position	Variable. Usually supine. May require position change during surgery
Blood loss	Often 4–6U
Practical techniques	ETT + IPPV, art + CVP lines, flow monitoring (Oesophageal Doppler or LiDCO™), urinary catheter, epidural catheter for lower limb flaps

Preoperative

- Free flaps are most commonly used to provide tissue cover following trauma or resection for malignancy. This is a widely used reconstructive technique. Understand what operation is proposed and what the aims of surgery are. Typical procedures are:
  - Free TRAM myocutaneous flap to reconstruct a breast following mastectomy
  - Free gracilis muscle flap to cover an area of lower limb trauma with tissue loss
  - Free radial forearm fasciocutaneous flap to the oropharynx following tumour excision.
- The aim of anaesthesia is to produce a hyperdynamic circulation with high cardiac output, adequate vasodilatation, and wide pulse pressure. Patients with lower limb trauma are often young and fit. Patients with head and neck cancer are often smokers with IHD. The elderly or patients with a limited cardiorespiratory reserve may not be suitable for surgery.

Perioperative

- Be prepared for a long surgical procedure. All patients should receive a balanced GA. Regional anaesthesia alone is seldom appropriate for these long procedures.
- Isoflurane is the inhalational agent of choice due to its beneficial effects on SVR. Propofol maintenance is also ideal, since it lowers SVR, is rapidly metabolized, is antiemetic, and may avoid post-operative shivering (there is also some *in vitro* evidence that propofol may be more favourable for microvascular flow by avoiding the effect of volatiles on red cell membrane stiffness). Remifentanil is used by many.
- A regional block is helpful to supplement anaesthesia. The sympathetic block and dense analgesia produce excellent conditions for graft survival. Lower limb flaps are especially suitable. Surgery on multiple sites may

not all be covered by the block. Skin grafts are often taken from the leg to cover a muscle flap.

- Anaesthetic management requires a good practical knowledge of circulatory physiology. Blood flow through the microvasculature must be optimal to help ensure flap survival. Blood flow is primarily influenced by changes in perfusion pressure, calibre of the vessel, and blood viscosity (the Hagen–Poiseuille formula). We only have a superficial understanding of the physiology of the microcirculation. Much of our anaesthetic management is based on perceived wisdom, rather than on the results of RCTs.
- Monitor core (e.g. rectal, oesophageal) and peripheral **temperature**. Insulate the skin probe from any overlying warming blanket. Aim for a normal, or even supranormal, core temperature and a core–peripheral difference of <2°C. This must be achieved by the time that microvascular anastomosis is commenced. A widening of the core–peripheral temperature difference may herald vasoconstriction. Local vascular spasm may jeopardize the surgery.
- Flow monitoring, using an oesophageal doppler or LiDCO™, is now widely available and may be extremely helpful in judging the adequacy of intravascular filling, especially in patients with more limited CVS reserve.
- Correct any preoperative fluid deficit, and begin **volume loading**. Continue maintenance crystalloid, and add 10mL/kg colloid bolus (e.g. Gelofusine®, Isoplex®), as required, to expand the intravascular volume. Aim for CVP 12mmHg (or 2–4mmHg above baseline), urine output 2mL/kg/hr, widened pulse pressure, and low SVR. A colloid will expand the intravascular volume more effectively than a crystalloid. Transplanted tissue lacks intact lymphatics, and excess crystalloid may contribute to flap oedema. Avoid excessive volume loading in the elderly, who are more prone to develop pulmonary oedema.
- **Moderate hypotension** and haemodilution during the early phase of dissection may help limit blood loss. Thereafter, maintain systolic arterial pressure (SAP) at 100mmHg or higher, depending on preoperative BP recordings.
- Viscosity is closely related to Hct. Viscosity rises dramatically when Hct >40%. Aim for 30%, which, in theory, gives the best balance between blood viscosity, arterial O_2 content, and tissue O_2 delivery.
- **Dextran** reduces platelet adhesiveness and factor VIII concentration. It may help maintain graft patency. Depending on surgical preference, give 500mL of Dextran 40 during the procedure, and include 500mL in the daily IV fluid for 2–3d.
- Potent vasodilators (e.g. sodium nitroprusside, hydralazine, and phenoxybenzamine) are unnecessary. Sufficient vasodilatation can be produced by the anaesthetic agent, provided that the patient is warm, volume-loaded, pain-free, and normocarbic. Nifedipine 10mg, given with the premedication and continued three times a day for 5d, in high-risk patients, such as smokers, diabetics, and arteriopaths, may improve flap survival. Chlorpromazine 1–2mg IV (dilute a 50mg ampoule to give a 1mg/mL solution for injection) is useful to narrow a widened core–peripheral temperature difference when all other factors have

been corrected. The surgeon may use papaverine directly on the vessels to prevent local spasm.
- Prophylactic antibiotics are given at induction and may be repeated during the procedure.

Post-operative
- Aim for a smooth emergence.
- Continue meticulous care well into the post-operative period. Flap observation is a specialized nursing skill, and care is often best provided on the plastic surgical ward. The need for HDU/ICU may be dictated by patient factors.
- Vasoconstriction from cold, pain, low circulating volume, hypotension, and hypocarbia will put the flap at risk and needs prompt correction.
- Treat shivering with pethidine 25mg IV. Continue with a warming blanket in recovery.
- The health of the flap is monitored clinically. Hourly observations include a **'flap chart'** where the temperature, colour, and arterial pulses (using a Doppler probe, if possible) are monitored. A pale, pulseless flap with sluggish capillary filling may indicate problems with the arterial supply. A swollen, dusky flap, which blanches easily with a brisk capillary return, indicates a venous outflow problem. An early surgical decision needs to be made concerning re-exploration.
- Analgesia by continuous epidural is ideal for lower limb flaps.
- An axillary brachial plexus catheter (e.g. continuous infusion of 0.25% bupivacaine 5mL/hr for 2–3d) is useful for procedures on the forearm and hand.
- Careful consideration should be given as to whether more invasive analgesic techniques are justified for procedures on the upper torso (e.g. thoracic epidural or intrapleural analgesia). Potential risks may outweigh the benefits. These patients often do very well with IV PCA. For head and neck procedures, IV PCA is best.
- Attitudes vary, concerning perioperative NSAIDs. They are valuable analgesics and reduce platelet adhesiveness. They may produce increased oozing following lengthy and extensive surgery. Administration post-operatively when a clot is more established may be preferable.

Special considerations
- The reimplantation of severed digits or limbs should be managed as for a free flap.
- A 'pedicle flap' is constructed when AV connections remain intact, but the raised flap is rotated to fill a neighbouring defect. Examples include rotation of the rectus abdominis muscle to fill a sternal wound, rotation of the pectoral muscle to reconstruct a defect in the side of the neck following tumour excision, and pedicled latissimus dorsi breast reconstruction. While the procedure may be technically simpler than free tissue transfer, anaesthesia requires similar attention to detail.
- Overall free flap survival is >95%. Flap failure will result in further reconstructive procedures. Patients in a poor general condition with coexisting disease have the highest risk of flap failure.

Liposuction

Procedure	Vacuum aspiration of SC fat via a small skin incision and a specialized blunt-ended cannula
Time	Variable 30–90min
Pain	+
Position	Variable, depending on site. Usually supine
Blood loss	1–40% of the volume of fat aspirated, depending on infiltration technique
Practical techniques	Local infiltration with IV sedation/LMA and SV

Preoperative
- Procedure may be used for:
  - Lipoma removal
  - Gynaecomastia
  - Reducing the bulk of transplanted flaps to make them more closely contour the surrounding skin
  - Cosmetic removal of SC fat ('liposculpture') in the abdominal wall, thighs, buttocks, and arms.
- Patients presenting for aesthetic surgery are often fit and well.

Perioperative
- The total amount of fat aspirated depends on patient requirement and surgical judgement.
- Fat is infiltrated with dilute LA with adrenaline. Back and forth movement of the cannula disrupts fatty tissue which is then aspirated by either suction apparatus or syringe.
- Injection of fluid helps fat breakdown and aids aspiration. There are several recipes for SC infiltration solutions: 1000mL of warmed Hartmann's solution containing 50mL of 1% lidocaine and 1mL of 1:1000 adrenaline is popular; 1mL of infiltrate per 1mL of aspirate is commonly used (superwet technique).
- The tumescent technique refers to a large volume of LA/adrenaline infiltrate to produce tissue turgor. Developed as an outpatient technique and performed without additional anaesthesia or sedation. Three mL of infiltrate per 1mL of aspirate is often used. There is little evidence that this technique is superior to the superwet technique, and it may produce more complications. It may provide unsatisfactory anaesthesia when used alone. Additional sedation or GA may be necessary.
- Blood loss depends on the volume of LA/adrenaline infiltrate used and the extent of liposuction required. Loss is ~1% of the volume of the aspirate for the tumescent technique. This may increase to 40% without SC infiltration.
- Extensive liposuction physiologically resembles a burn injury, and large fluid shifts result. Replace aspirate 1:1 with IV crystalloid.

Post-operative
- Pressure dressings are usually applied.
- Encourage oral fluids, and monitor urine output.
- Check Hct following extensive liposuction (>2500mL of aspirate).
- Bruising can be considerable.
- Use NSAIDs and simple analgesics for pain relief.

Special considerations
- Dose safety limits for large-volume LA infiltration are controversial. Doses significantly higher than the conventional lidocaine/adrenaline toxic dose (5mg/kg) are often used, e.g. 30–70mg/kg. This may be possible due to the adrenaline producing slower drug absorption, the poor vascularity of fat, and the aspiration of much of the infused solution before the drug has been absorbed.
- Complications are associated with excessive liposuction. In the UK, aspiration is restricted to ~2L of fat. Considerably higher-volume procedures have been reported, especially in the US (in excess of 10L). Deaths have occurred from pulmonary oedema and lidocaine toxicity. Morbidity is related to high aspiration volume and high lidocaine dosage.

Skin grafting

Procedure	Free skin grafts applied to surgically created raw surfaces following debridement, or to granulating wounds
Time	Variable 30min–2hr
Pain	++/+++ (especially the donor site)
Position	Variable. Depends on the area to be grafted. Usually supine
Blood loss	Nil for simple grafts. Extensive debridement and grafting of burns may require 6–8U
Practical techniques	GA/LMA spontaneous respiration (with LCNT or femoral 3-in-1 block if thigh donor site). Spinal for lower limb surgery

Preoperative
- Patients for simple excision and grafting of isolated lesions may be otherwise well.
- Elderly patients for excision/grafting of skin lesions or pretibial lacerations may be in poor general health. A local or regional technique may be preferable to GA.
- Patients with extensive burns for debridement and grafting require careful assessment (see p. 507).

Perioperative
- **Full-thickness skin graft (FTSG)**. Consists of the epidermis and dermis. Used in small areas where the thickness, appearance, and texture of the skin are important. Usually harvested with a scalpel. FTSG can be harvested using SC LA infiltration with a 27G needle. Addition of hyaluronidase aids spread (e.g. 1500IU to 100mL of LA solution). The donor site needs to be closed directly:
  - Post-auricular skin for grafts to the face
  - Groin or antecubital fossa to the hand for management of flexion contractures.
- **Split skin graft (SSG)**. Consists of the epidermis and a variable portion of the dermis. Much wider usage than FTSG. Usually harvested with a skin graft knife or power-driven dermatome. Donor sites will heal spontaneously within 2wk. Donor sites are chosen according to the amount of skin required, colour and texture match, and local convenience. Meshing is used to expand the extent of the area that the graft is required to cover. Common donor sites are the thigh, flexor aspect of the forearm, upper arm, and abdomen. SSG can be harvested using LA cream. It should be applied at least 2hr in advance and covered with an occlusive dressing. Anaesthesia does not extend into the deeper dermis, so the technique is unsuitable for FTSG. The lateral cutaneous nerve of thigh (LCNT) or femoral 3-in-1 block provides useful analgesia of a thigh donor site. Excess harvested skin can be stored at 4°C for 2–3wk.

Post-operative

- The SSG donor site is a painful wound. Supplement with LA (LCNT or femoral block) where possible. The type of dressing is important for donor site comfort: alginate dressing impregnated with LA (e.g. 40mL of 0.25% bupivacaine) is commonly used. Dressings are difficult to secure on the thigh and frequently slip when the patient mobilizes. A thin adhesive fabric dressing is used by some surgeons and may afford better protection and donor site comfort. The dressing is soaked off after 2wk. NSAIDs and simple analgesics are usually required for 3–4d. Itching follows when the acute pain settles and healing is under way.

Special considerations

Burns patients

(See also ➔ p. 864.)

- Extensive debridement and grafting of burns are a major procedure. These patients should receive a balanced GA. Current management is to aim to debride burnt tissue and cover with SSG at the earliest opportunity (often within 48hr). This converts the burn to a healthy surgical wound. Potential sources of sepsis are eradicated; fluid shifts are less, and intensive care management tends to be more stable.
- Two anaesthetists may be required. Two surgical teams will considerably speed up the procedure and help minimize complications.
- Blood loss. Ensure 6–8U are cross-matched. Debrided tissue bleeds freely. Losses can be difficult to estimate, particularly in small children. Regularly check Hct, and maintain at ~30%.
- Temperature control. A large exposed body surface area will lose heat rapidly by radiation and evaporation. Measure core temperature. Use all methods available for heat conservation. Little body surface area may be available for warming blankets. Maintain the operating theatre at 25°C.
- Monitoring. Placement of non-invasive monitoring devices may be difficult. An arterial line facilitates measurement of BP and blood sampling. A central venous line is valuable to provide reliable venous access for this and future procedures, and helps in the management of intravascular volume. Maintain strict asepsis during line insertion. Cannulae may need to be stitched. Try to place through intact skin. A urinary catheter is essential.
- Suxamethonium is contraindicated, except in the first 24hr following burn. Massive K+ release may cause cardiac arrest.
- Post-operative care. Return to the burns unit. Large body surface area burns (e.g. >40%) or those with additional injury (e.g. smoke inhalation) may need continued ventilation on ICU until warm and stable.
- Analgesia is best provided by IV opioids, either as PCA or continuous infusion. Suggest early intervention of the acute pain team. Dressing changes may be helped by Entonox® or ketamine/midazolam sedation.
- Antibiotics and early nutrition are important to increase survival.

General surgery

Matt Rucklidge

Andrew McLeod and Tim Wigmore

Matt Rucklidge

See also:

Major colorectal surgery

General considerations

Major surgery generates a neuroendocrine, metabolic, and inflammatory response which may result in adverse physiological changes, including: pulmonary dysfunction, increased cardiac demand, pain, nausea, and vomiting. This may result in delayed mobilization, prolonged hospital stay, and increased morbidity and mortality.

Fast-track surgery and enhanced recovery after surgery

Fast-track surgery and enhanced recovery after surgery (ERAS) programmes use a collection of strategies to decrease post-operative surgical complications and improve patient recovery. Pioneered by the Danish surgeon Henrik Kehlet in the 1990s, enhanced recovery programmes for major colorectal surgery are now commonplace, and the strategies of ERAS are applicable to many other surgical specialties.[1]

Key aspects of ERAS include:
- A multiprofessional approach to the planning and perioperative management of surgery, anaesthesia, and recovery.
- Detailed preoperative patient education, information, and risk assessment.
- Avoidance of prolonged starvation and preoperative dehydration. Clear fluids up to 2hr before surgery should be routine, and preoperative carbohydrate drinks may be beneficial.
- No sedative premedication.
- No bowel preparation—may cause dehydration and difficulty in perioperative fluid management.
- Avoid routine use of NGTs and surgical drains.
- Prophylactic antibiotics administered within 30min before surgical incision to reduce the risk of surgical site infection.
- Minimally invasive surgical approaches (small incisions or laparoscopic techniques) may reduce pain and length of hospital stay.
- Avoidance of perioperative hypothermia (see ➜ p. 515).
- Appropriate fluid management using a goal-directed approach, e.g. oesophageal Doppler management.
- Close attention to the prevention of nausea and vomiting.
- Multimodal analgesia, including simple analgesics (paracetamol, NSAIDs), and LA techniques (thoracic epidural, rectus sheath block, TAP block) or intrathecal opioids, which reduce parenteral opioid use and opioid complications. Close involvement of the acute pain team post-operatively.
- Early removal of urinary catheter.
- Early enteral feeding—may reduce muscle loss, length of stay, and possibly infection.
- Early mobilization and input from physiotherapy.

Preoperative preparation
- History, examination, ECG if indicated, FBC, U&Es. Other blood tests, as indicated.

- Assessment of exercise function (e.g. CPET) (see ➊ p. 15).
- Optimize nutrition and cardiac and respiratory function.
- Discuss analgesia strategies.
- Discuss invasive monitoring, if planned.
- Consider premedication with H_2 antagonist or PPI if risk of regurgitation, and discuss RSI.
- Consider whether post-operative HDU/ICU care is indicated (e.g. poor preoperative respiratory and/or cardiac function, anticipated prolonged and complex procedure), and ensure a bed is booked before surgery.
- Ensure clear fluids (including clear carbohydrate drinks) are taken up to 2hr prior to surgery to reduce dehydration.

Perioperative

- Large-bore IV access, with long extension if access to arms restricted. Arms are commonly placed by the sides in laparoscopic colorectal surgery.
- Site low thoracic epidural, if planned, and administer test dose (see ➊ p. 513).
- RSI if evidence of abdominal obstruction or risk of regurgitation.
- Prophylactic antibiotics before skin incision (see ➊ p. 1211).
- Avoid prolonged exposure during preparation for surgery, and establish active patient warming (fluid warmer, hot-air blanket, warming mattress/blanket) as soon as possible. Monitor central temperature, and aim for normothermia (see ➊ p. 515).
- Urinary catheter with urimeter.
- Several studies have shown that excess perioperative fluid is detrimental. Appropriate (goal-directed) fluid management (see ➊ p. 517).
- PONV is common after GI surgery. Reduce risk through adequate hydration, multimodal analgesia to avoid or limit opioids, avoidance of N_2O, and administration of different classes of antiemetic.
- Procedures may be prolonged; pay special attention to pressure areas. Be prepared for lithotomy or the Lloyd–Davies position with steep head-down tilt. Prolonged surgery in this position may require higher FiO_2 and PEEP to maintain oxygenation due to reduction in FRC.
- If no epidural, consider single-shot spinal with long-acting opioid, insertion of a wound catheter or rectus sheath catheters to provide post-operative LA.
- There are conflicting reports of the role of intraoperative high FiO_2 on patient outcomes. A systematic review and meta-analysis found that a high FiO_2 has a weak beneficial effect on nausea, decreases the risk of surgical site infection in patients receiving prophylactic antibiotics, and does not increase the risk of atelectasis.[2]

Post-operative

- Prescribe overnight O_2, and continue, as required, to maintain SpO_2 >95%. Supplemental O_2 should be prescribed if using an opioid-based analgesic technique (e.g. PCA, opioid infusion).
- Treat nausea and vomiting aggressively.
- Early oral fluids wherever possible.

- Monitor fluid balance closely. Consider ongoing losses from abdominal drains, ileostomy, and NG aspirate. Following major surgery, measure urine output hourly for at least 24hr.
- Arrange a chest radiograph if CVP line sited.
- If epidural sited, continue post-operatively.
- Prescribe regular simple analgesia, e.g. paracetamol (IV or oral) or NSAIDs, if not contraindicated. Other agents, including clonidine, gabapentin, and ketamine, may further reduce post-operative opioid use and opioid side effects.
- Referral to acute pain team for post-operative review.
- Worsening post-operative pain may indicate a complication of surgery.
- Consider daily FBC/U&Es until return of normal bowel function.

Intraoperative monitoring

- Balance the health of the patient with the complexity and duration of the surgical procedure, and consider the additional information invasive monitoring will provide against risks involved in placement and interpretation (Table 20.1).
- Fluid administration, guided by minimally invasive cardiac output monitoring, to optimize stroke volume and cardiac output has been shown to improve outcomes in patients undergoing colorectal surgery.[3] Several minimally invasive cardiac output monitors are now available (see ➲ p. 1016).

Table 20.1 Suggested indications for additional monitoring

Minimally invasive cardiac output monitoring	Abdominal surgery with potential fluid shifts, CVS compromise, likely requirement for perioperative inotropes
Arterial line	CVS, respiratory compromise, major blood loss, need for blood gas sampling
CVP	Need for vasopressors and/or inotropes. Requirement for post-operative total parenteral nutrition

References

1 Kehelet H (2009). Fast-track colorectal surgery. *Lancet*, **371**, 791–3.
2 Hovaguimian F, Lysakowski C, Elia N, Tramèr MR (2013). Effect of intraoperative high inspired oxygen fraction on surgical site infection, postoperative nausea and vomiting, and pulmonary function. Systematic review and meta-analysis of randomized controlled trials. *Anesthesiology*, **119**, 303–16.
3 Hamilton MA, Cecconi M, Rhodes A (2011). A systematic review and meta-analysis of the use of pre-emptive hemodynamic intervention to improve postoperative outcomes in moderate and high-risk surgical patients. *Anesth Analg*, **112**, 1392–402.

Analgesia

Laparoscopic techniques are increasingly used in colorectal surgery, which reduces post-operative pain and enhances recovery. However, abdominal incisions are painful, and whatever surgical technique is used, high-quality multimodal analgesia is essential to limit opioid-related side effects (nausea, vomiting, sedation, ileus, urinary retention) and encourage early mobilization. This can include:

- Local infiltration of small wounds.
- Intraperitoneal infiltration in laparoscopic surgery.
- TAP block (see ➲ p. 1123).
- Rectus sheath infiltration (see ➲ p. 1125).
- Insertion of wound catheter.
- Spinal (± intrathecal opioid) injection.
- Epidural analgesia.
- Simple IM/SC opioids for less invasive procedures, e.g. appendicectomy, reversal of colostomy.
- Parenteral opioids by PCA, e.g. lower abdominal procedures, open cholecystectomy following failed laparoscopy, and for laparotomy when an epidural is contraindicated or refused. Ensure additional O_2 therapy and hourly sedation/pain scoring.
- Regular paracetamol should be administered to reduce opioid or epidural requirements. Prescribe NSAIDs, with caution in the elderly; this group may be susceptible to side effects.

Epidural analgesia

Advantages include

- Improved pain relief. Thoracic epidurals provide superior analgesia to systemic opioids for laparotomy.
- Improved post-operative respiratory function, resulting in reduced incidence of respiratory failure.
- Improved post-operative GI motility.
- Improved myocardial function. By providing superior analgesia, stress-induced increases in HR, coronary vasoconstriction, and myocardial workload are reduced.
- Potentially improved post-operative patient mobilization.
- Reduction in thromboembolism.
- Reduced sedation and PONV.

Disadvantages include

- Risks related to insertion, including post-dural puncture headache (PDPH), epidural haematoma, and abscess (see ➲ p. 729).
- Risk related to misplaced catheter, e.g. intrathecal, intravascular.
- Perioperative hypotension which may lead to excessive administration of post-operative fluids.
- Epidural failure.
- Post-operative motor blockade, delaying patient mobilization.
- Itch associated with epidural opioids. Urinary retention.

Epidural analgesia and outcome after abdominal surgery

While improved analgesia is well established, the influence of epidural analgesia on mortality/morbidity following major abdominal surgery is less clear. A meta-analysis of RCTs found neuraxial block was associated with significantly decreased perioperative morbidity and mortality.[4] However a large RCT, the MASTER Anaesthesia Trial, found that mortality and most adverse morbid outcomes in high-risk patients undergoing major surgery were not reduced by the use of an epidural, and this was also found in selected subgroups at increased risk of respiratory and cardiac complications.[5,6]

Practical considerations for epidural analgesia

- The catheter should be sited at an appropriate level. A useful guide is to place the catheter at a level corresponding to the dermatome innervating the middle of the planned abdominal incision. In general, site at T10–T11 for lower abdominal procedures, and T8–T9 for upper abdominal procedures.
- Placement while awake or anaesthetized is controversial. Inserting the epidural awake is probably safer in adults (especially if thoracic), since it enables patient feedback during insertion and test dosing.
- Epidural test dose, e.g. 3mL of 0.5% bupivacaine.
- Give an intraoperative epidural loading dose of 8–10mL of 0.25–0.5% bupivacaine/levobupivacaine with 50–100 micrograms of fentanyl (divide into 3–4mL boluses), and assess response.
- Bupivacaine/levobupivacaine takes 15–20min to achieve its maximum effect, and top-ups should be performed cautiously. An extensive sympathetic block may develop with relatively low volumes of LA in thoracic epidurals.
- If extensive bleeding is expected, or in cardiovascularly unstable patients, it is often wise to avoid epidural LA until bleeding is controlled and the patient has stabilized.
- Effective epidural block for AP resection (which requires analgesia and anaesthesia across thoracic, lumbar, and sacral dermatomes) can be difficult. Effectiveness may be improved by the addition of an epidural opioid and larger volumes of a weaker anaesthetic solution, e.g. 0.125% bupivacaine.

An appropriate regime for post-operative analgesia consists of a mix of LA and opioid, e.g. bupivacaine 0.125% plus fentanyl 4 micrograms/mL (2–10mL/hr).

References

4 Rodgers A, Walker N, Schug S, et al. (2000). Reduction of post-operative mortality and morbidity with epidural or spinal anaesthesia: results of overview of randomized trials. BMJ, **321**, 1493–7.

5 Rigg JR, Jamrozik K, Myles PS, et al.; MASTER Anaethesia Trial Study Group (2002). Epidural anesthesia and analgesia and outcome of major surgery: a randomized trial. Lancet, **359**, 1276–82.

6 Peyton P, Myles PS, Silbert BS, Rigg JA, Jamrozik K, Parsons R (2003). Perioperative epidural analgesia and outcome after major abdominal surgery in high risk patients. Anesth Analg, **96**, 548–54.

Temperature control

Patients under anaesthesia may become hypothermic due to loss of the behavioural response to cold, impairment of thermoregulatory heat-preserving mechanisms, anaesthetic-induced peripheral vasodilatation, exposure during surgery, and the use of unwarmed IV or irrigation fluids. In addition, fluid depletion prior to anaesthesia may result in poor peripheral perfusion and impaired heat distribution.

Patients undergoing laparotomy are at high risk of inadvertent hypothermia due to prolonged procedures, an open abdomen, and limited access for external body warming. Even mild hypothermia is associated with a number of adverse outcomes:
- Myocardial ischaemia or arrhythmias.
- Increased perioperative blood loss.
- Increased risk of surgical site infection.
- Prolonged duration of action of neuromuscular antagonists.
- Increased duration of recovery and possible increased hospital stay.

Inadvertent perioperative hypothermia has been identified by NICE as a common, but preventable, complication of surgery and anaesthesia which may be associated with poor patient outcome.[7]

NICE recommends the following:
- Maintaining patient thermal comfort preoperatively by encouraging the wearing of warm clothing.
- Assessment of risk of perioperative hypothermia.
- Maintaining ambient temperature in wards and theatre suites.
- Recording core temperature immediately prior to leaving the ward, every 30min intraoperatively, and every 15min in recovery until a temperature of 36°C is recorded.
- Only commencing induction of anaesthesia if the patient's core temperature is above 36°C.
- Active warming of all patients having anaesthesia for longer than 30min, and warming of IV fluids if >500mL used.

Hypothermia develops in a characteristic three-phase pattern.
- Phase 1: rapid reduction in core temperature of 1–1.5°C within the 1st 30–45min, as the tonic vasoconstriction that normally maintains core to periphery temperature gradient is inhibited.
- Phase 2: more gradual reduction in core temperature of a further 1°C over the next 2–3hr due to heat loss by radiation, convection, and evaporation exceeding heat gain determined by metabolic rate. Evaporative heat loss is exacerbated during major abdominal surgery.
- Phase 3: a plateau phase where heat loss is matched by metabolic heat production. Occurs when anaesthetized patients become sufficiently hypothermic that vasoconstriction is triggered. If a thoracic epidural is used, compensatory vasoconstriction is lost.

Cutaneous warming

- **Passive insulation.** A single layer of insulation (e.g. space blanket) traps a layer of air and may reduce cutaneous heat loss by 30%. Insulation to exposed areas, e.g. wrapping the head, may further reduce heat loss.

- **Active warming**. Forced-air warming devices are more effective than passive insulation. They reduce heat loss through radiation and may increase heat gain if forced air is warmer than the skin. Active warming by a circulating water mattress, or an electric mattress, pad, or blankets can also be used, though evidence for their superiority over forced-air warming devices is limited.

Internal warming

- **Airway humidification**. An HME filter humidifies and warms inhaled gases; however, <10% of heat loss occurs via the respiratory tract.
- **Fluid warming**. Prevents conductive heat loss associated with the administration of cold fluids. IV fluids should be prewarmed by storage in a thermostatically controlled cabinet or warmed to 37°C by an active warming device. Unwarmed irrigation fluids in the bladder or abdomen may induce significant heat loss.
- **Invasive internal warming techniques**. Internal warming CPB and peritoneal dialysis are very effective at transferring significant heat but are not relevant for the management of mild perioperative hypothermia.

Reference

7 National Institute for Health and Care Excellence (2008). *Inadvertent perioperative hypothermia: the management of inadvertent perioperative hypothermia in adults.* ℘ http://www.nice.org.uk/nice-media/pdf/CG65NICEGuidance.pdf.

Fluid management

Patients undergoing major colorectal surgery are at risk of significant fluid loss. Appropriate fluid administration throughout the perioperative period helps maintain cardiac output and O_2 delivery. There is evidence that outcome following major surgery can be improved by optimizing fluid therapy, and goal-directed fluid therapy should be used where possible (see ➔ p. 1016).

A recent Cochrane review concluded that, while mortality is not reduced, goal-directed therapy can reduce post-operative complications and length of stay.[8] The optimum type of fluid for performing goal-directed therapy is unknown. An RCT found no clinical benefit of using hydroxyethyl starch (HES) for goal-directed fluid therapy in colorectal surgery, compared with crystalloid, despite HES patients requiring less fluid than those in the crystalloid group.[9] The UK Medicines and Healthcare Products Regulatory Agency (MHRA) recently suspended the use of HES products in the UK because of concerns they may be associated with an increased risk of renal injury and death, compared to crystalloids.[10] Using a balanced crystalloid (e.g. Hartmann's) and blood/blood products, where necessary, is probably the best approach.

Causes of fluid loss

- **Preoperative**: reduced fluid intake due to underlying disease process and preoperative fasting. Increased fluid losses due to vomiting, bowel preparation, and sequestration into an obstructed bowel.
- **Intraoperative**: large evaporative losses from an open abdomen, sequestration of fluid into the omentum and bowel lumen (3rd space loss), blood loss, and NG loss.
- **Post-operative**: ongoing sequestration of fluid into the omentum and bowel (paralytic ileus), ongoing blood and NG loss.

Losses must be replaced with an individualized fluid regime that reflects both fluid and electrolyte requirements. Those with large preoperative fluid deficits should have IV fluids instigated well before surgery. A balanced crystalloid solution (e.g. Hartmann's solution) is usually appropriate. Significant fluid shifts may affect serum electrolyte concentrations, and these should be monitored throughout the perioperative period.

Post-operative paralytic ileus

- Bowel function begins to return 24–36hr post-operatively but may not return to normal until 72hr or longer. Prolonged ileus leads to collection of fluid and gas in the bowel, resulting in distension, pain, nausea, vomiting, and delayed mobilization/discharge. The aetiology of the ileus is multifactorial and includes manipulation of the bowel at surgery, hormonal stress response, increased sympathetic activity, post-operative pain, immobility, opioids, hypokalaemia, and other electrolyte imbalances.

References

8 Grocott MP, Dushianthan A, Hamilton MA, Mythen MG, Harrison D, Rowan K; Optimisation Systematic Review Steering Group (2013). Perioperative increase in global blood flow to explicit defined goals and outcomes after surgery: a Cochrane Systematic Review. *Br J Anaesth*, **111**, 535–48.

9 Yates DRA, Davies SJ, Milner HE, Wilson RJT (2014). Crystalloid or colloid for goal-directed fluid therapy in colorectal surgery. *Br J Anaesth*, **112**, 281–9.

10 Medicines and Healthcare Products Regulatory Agency (2013). *MHRA suspends use of hydroxy-ethyl starch (HES) drips.* http://webarchive.nationalarchives.gov.uk/20141205150130/http://www.mhra.gov.uk/NewsCentre/Pressreleases/CON287028.

Summary of general surgical 'open' procedures

If performed laparoscopically, procedures will be less painful but may be of longer duration (Table 20.2).

Table 20.2 General surgical open procedures

Operation	Description	Time (min)	Pain (+ to ++++)	Position	Blood loss (L)	Notes
Hemicolectomy	Resection of right or left hemicolon	1–3	++++	Supine	0.5	Low thoracic epidural or opioid infusion/PCA ± rectus block
Sigmoid colectomy	Resection of sigmoid colon with bowel anastomosis	1–3	++++	Supine. Head-down. May need Lloyd-Davies	0.5–1.0	Low thoracic epidural or opioid infusion/PCA ± rectus block
Hartmann's procedure	Resection of sigmoid colon with colostomy	1–3	++++	Supine. Head down. May need Lloyd-Davies	0.5–1.0	Low thoracic epidural or opioid infusion/PCA± rectus block
Anterior resection	Resection of rectum	2–3	++++	Head down. Lloyd-Davies	0.5–1.5	Low thoracic epidural ± rectus block
AP resection	Resection of rectum and anus	2–4	+++++	Head-down. Lloyd-Davies	0.5–2.0	Low thoracic epidural. Can be difficult to block sacral nerve roots. ± rectus block
Gastrectomy	Resection of stomach	2–3	+++++	Supine	0.5–1.0	Thoracic epidural, consider CVP/art line
Cholecystectomy (open)	Resection of gall bladder	1	+++/ ++++	Supine	0.5	Right upper quadrant incision. PCA
Closure of loop colostomy or loop ileostomy	Local closure of colostomy or loop ileostomy	0.5–1	++	Supine	Nil	Still requires muscle relaxation. May need PCA ± TAP block
Reversal of Hartmann's	Laparotomy. Bowel ends re-anastomosed	1–2	++++	Supine. Head-down. May need Lloyd-Davies	0.5–1.5	Low thoracic epidural ± rectus block

Oncological considerations

General considerations

- **Cardiac injury** may be induced by drugs (anthracyclines, fluorouracil, trastuzumab) or the stress of chemotherapy on a compromised heart. Anthracycline-induced cardiac failure may be irreversible and has a mortality of above 30%.
- **Pulmonary toxicity** occurs in 10% of patients exposed to bleomycin, consisting of acute, followed by chronic, fibrosing alveolitis. FiO_2 should be limited, as O_2 free radicals may be mediators.
- **Hepatic veno-occlusive disease** (HVOD) is a progressive obliteration of venous channels in the liver.
- **Tumour lysis syndrome** can follow initial chemotherapy (typically for lymphoma and high-count leukaemias). Mass cell death leads to acute renal impairment, with hyperkalaemia, hyperuricaemia, hyperphosphataemia, and hypocalcaemia.
- **Mediastinal masses** (particularly in leukaemia or lymphoma patients) can cause complete airway collapse under anaesthesia, even in the asymptomatic. Warning signs include stridor, wheeze, orthopnoea, and SVC obstruction.
- **SVC obstruction** can arise from compression by a tumour or lymph nodes (usually bronchogenic carcinoma) or direct vessel invasion. Pleural effusions and ascites are common in ovarian cancer, metastatic disease, and mesothelioma.
- **Paraneoplastic syndromes** occur in 10% of cancer patients (especially lung, lymphoma, breast, prostate, ovarian, and pancreatic tumours). Anaesthetic considerations:
  - Eaton–Lambert myasthenic syndrome is common in small cell lung cancer (SCLC) and breast, thymus, and GI tract tumours (see ❯ p. 242)
  - Cushing's syndrome occurs in tumours of the lung, pancreas, thymus, and ovary (see ❯ p. 167)
  - Hypercalcaemia is caused by bony metastases or parathyroid-like compounds (see ❯ p. 160)
  - Hyponatraemia and SIADH-like syndromes may be caused by SCLC and also lymphoma, leukaemia, and pancreatic/carcinoid tumours (see ❯ p. 167 and p. 178)
  - Cachexia can be caused by vomiting, loss of appetite, or other GI disturbances. Hypoalbuminaemia (<35g/L) is a risk factor for poor outcomes.
- **Radiotherapy** may cause fever and nausea/vomiting, and patients may be dehydrated. Previous radiotherapy causes ongoing localized fibrosis, which may impede laryngoscopy and airway management.
- **Chemotherapy** commonly causes immunosuppression and myelosuppression.
- **VTE** affects at least 15% of cancer patients.
- Do Not Attempt Resuscitation (DNAR) orders may be present in cancer patients. Where these conflict with safe anaesthetic principles, it is reasonable to modify or suspend the order perioperatively.

Anaesthesia for oncology procedures

- Dexamethasone as an antiemetic should be avoided, as it may have a cytotoxic effect and risks precipitation of tumour lysis.
- Inspired O_2 concentration should be considered in patients who have been previously treated with bleomycin because of potential risk of causing rapidly progressive pulmonary toxicity.
- Brachytherapy places a radioactive source close to the tumour via an applicator. It is often used in patients unfit for surgery and may involve single or multiple treatments. Procedures usually last 1.5–3hr but may be longer. Blood loss is usually minimal, but post-operative pain may be an issue. Post-operative radioactivity can require patients to be recovered in an isolated environment. Anaesthetic options are:
  - Light GA
  - Sedation (although this may not produce reliable immobility)
  - Epidural or spinal anaesthesia (some procedures may outlast spinal block, requiring the insertion of catheters).

Further reading

Allan N, Siller C, Breen A (2012). Anaesthetic implications of chemotherapy. *Contin Educ Anaesth Crit Care Pain*, **12**, 52–6.

Farquhar-Smith P, Wigmore T, eds. (2011). *Anaesthesia, intensive care and pain management for the cancer patient.* Oxford: Oxford University Press.

Hack HA, Wright NB, Wynn RF (2008). The anaesthetic management of children with anterior mediastinal masses. *Anaesthesia*, **63**, 837–46.

The emergency laparotomy

(See also septic shock, ➔ p. 875; ICU patient, p. 879.)

Outcomes following emergency laparotomy, especially in elderly patients, are poor. The UK Emergency Laparotomy Network reported a direct relationship between age and mortality. Mortality was ~10% for patients in their 50s, increasing by ~5% each decade, such that those in their 80s had a 30-day mortality of almost 25%.[11] There are many other factors associated with poorer outcome, including urgency of surgery, surgical pathology, experience of medical personnel, and provision of post-operative critical care.[12] The time available for preparation is often limited, and it is important to balance the benefits of preoperative resuscitation with those of timely surgery. Whatever the underlying pathology, disordered cellular metabolism results in generalized organ system dysfunction, including:

- CVS—widespread vasodilatation, loss of reactivity to catecholamines, depressed myocardial function, arrhythmias.
- Pulmonary—acute lung injury or ARDS, fluid extravasation into pulmonary interstitium, alveolar collapse, hypoxaemia, shunting, reduced compliance and FRC, and increased work of breathing.
- Haematological—DIC with low platelets, hypofibrinogenaemia, prolonged clotting times.
- Renal—hypoperfusion due to relative hypovolaemia and systemic vasodilatation may result in renal failure and altered drug clearance.
- Metabolic—impaired glucose tolerance, altered drug metabolism.
- Hepatic—impaired hepatic O_2 delivery at a time of increased hepatic O_2 consumption, resulting in liver dysfunction.

Outcomes following emergency laparotomy are likely to be improved by following a defined pathway of care. The key components are: early antibiotics, timely surgery with an experienced medical team, goal-directed fluid therapy, and appropriate level of post-operative care (Table 20.3).

Preoperative assessment

- Sepsis is common. Prompt antibiotic administration is associated with improvements in survival. Provide cover in line with local guidelines.
- O_2 should be administered preoperatively to all sick patients.
- An NGT should be inserted in patients presenting with intestinal obstruction.
- While a period of preoperative resuscitation may benefit some patients, this should not delay surgery which should be performed by an experienced team.
- Assess the risks and benefits of surgery. This can be challenging in the elderly patient where risks are high. Liaise with HDU/ICU to organize a post-operative bed, if required.
- Investigations: FBC, electrolytes (including Mg^{2+}), LFTs, amylase, clotting, ECG, chest radiograph where appropriate, lactate, and blood G&S.
- In general, balanced salt solutions (e.g. Hartmann's solution) should be used, in place of 0.9% NaCl, to reduce the risk of inducing hyperchloraemic acidosis.[13]

Table 20.3 National Emergency Laparotomy Audit standards of care for patients undergoing emergency laparotomy

Risk assessment	High-risk patients (predicted mortality >10%, age >65yr, shock) should receive surgery under the direct care of consultants in anaesthesia and surgery

Preoperative	• Prompt surgical review with assessment of risk (P-POSSUM)
	• If sepsis present—sepsis bundle with early antibiotics <1–3hr
	• Appropriate imaging to define pathology (CT recommended)
	• Communication between consultant surgeon and anaesthetist
	• Access to theatres according to surgical urgency:
	  • Ongoing haemorrhage—immediate surgery
	  • Septic shock—surgery within 3hr of the decision to operate
	  • Severe sepsis (with organ dysfunction)—surgery within 6hr to minimize deterioration into septic shock

Intraoperative	• Antibiotic therapy in line with specific hospital policy • Goal-directed fluid therapy • Ensure normothermia • Assessment of base excess and serum lactate • Effective analgesia

End-of-surgery care bundle	• Reassess risk in light of operative findings
	• Within 30min of end of surgery, assess:
	  • Lactate/base ratio
	  • PaO_2/FiO_2 ratio
	• Admission to critical care if:
	  • High-risk patient (e.g. any elderly patient)
	  • >10% predicted mortality (P-POSSUM)
	  • Lactate >4mmol/L
	  • PaO_2/FiO_2 ratio <40
	  • Hypothermia <36°C

- Electrolytes will often be deranged and should be corrected as far as possible prior to surgery.
- Monitor blood sugar; control will likely deteriorate in diabetic patients, and non-diabetics may develop impaired glucose tolerance.
- Metabolic acidosis should improve with aggressive fluid and CVS manipulation. Tissue hypoxia is the likely cause of acidosis if blood lactate is high. If acidotic with normal lactate, exclude renal failure and underlying metabolic disorders, e.g. diabetic ketoacidosis. If surgery is indicated and the pH is unresponsive, 1mmol/kg (1mL/kg) of 8.4% sodium bicarbonate IV should be considered.

- Thrombocytopenia and coagulopathy should be anticipated and treated appropriately, especially in the septic patient and following transfusion of large volumes of stored blood. Liaise with haematologists to optimally manage the transfusion of blood products. Increased INR may require the administration of vitamin K (5–10mg slow IV).
- Use IV morphine for pain control prior to surgery, and avoid NSAIDs due to risk of renal damage, decreased platelet function, and gastroduodenal ulceration.

Monitoring

- Invasive arterial BP monitoring should be used and established pre-induction. Not only does it enable close haemodynamic monitoring, but it also facilitates near-patient testing of Hb, coagulation, and acid/base status.
- A CVC may be required for perioperative vasopressor and inotrope infusion. Central access also allows monitoring of central venous O_2 saturation ($ScvO_2$) which may help identify an imbalance between O_2 delivery and consumption. A low perioperative $ScvO_2$ has been shown to be related to increased risk of post-operative complications in high-risk surgery. Aim for $ScvO_2 \geq 70\%$.[14]
- Use a minimally invasive cardiac output monitor to enable goal-directed fluid therapy (see ➲ p. 1016).
- Measure core temperature throughout, and maintain normothermia.

Perioperative care

- Consider anaesthetizing all sick patients on the operating table in theatre, and, in some cases, insist the theatre team are scrubbed and prepared for surgery.
- Aspirate the NGT prior to induction.
- Have a large-bore IV infusion running.
- Anticipate hypotension following induction. Have vasopressors (ephedrine and metaraminol/phenylephrine) and vagolytics (atropine, glycopyrronium) drawn up and to hand.
- Preoxygenate, and perform RSI.
- Choice of induction agent and dose depend on CVS stability. Thiopental and propofol are commonly used for RSI. Etomidate causes less hypotension on induction; however, it may temporarily interfere with steroid synthesis, so its use in critically ill patients (already at risk of adrenocortical insufficiency) is controversial.[14] Ketamine (1–2mg/kg IV) may be useful in the severely compromised patient, but avoid in those with pre-existing CVS disease.
- Relaxants. Suxamethonium for rapid sequence, then use drugs metabolized independently of liver and renal function, e.g. atracurium.
- Fluids. There is limited evidence that goal-directed therapy in patients undergoing emergency surgery improves outcomes. However, studies of high-risk patients undergoing non-emergency abdominal surgery suggest a benefit. Use a balanced crystalloid (e.g. Hartmann's) and blood/blood products where necessary.
- Analgesia. Centroneuraxial blockade should be used cautiously in this group of patients due to risks of infective complications, excessive

hypotension, and potential coagulopathy. If an epidural is used, LA agents should be restricted until CVS stability is achieved. In some patients, this may be post-operatively on the ICU.
* Fentanyl/morphine for intraoperative analgesia. Give with induction, and supplement, as needed. Caution with remifentanil; may cause significant hypotension if hypovolaemic.
* Rectus sheath catheters can be inserted at the end of the procedure, and LA administered post-operatively (see ➲ p. 1125).
* Active warming should be undertaken, with the aim of maintaining normothermia (see ➲ p. 515).
* Patients who require repeated bolus doses of vasopressors, despite an adequately restored circulating volume, should be commenced on an infusion of vasopressor/inotrope early. Noradrenaline is the 1st choice for the vasodilated septic patient. Dopamine may be useful in patients with compromised systolic function but causes more tachycardia and may be more arrhythmogenic. Dobutamine may be useful in patients with measured or suspected low cardiac output in the presence of adequate fluid resuscitation but may worsen hypotension if fluid resuscitation is inadequate. The influence of dopexamine on patients undergoing major abdominal surgery has been widely examined, but results are conflicting.[15] Dopexamine stimulates dopamine receptors and is a potent β_2-agonist. It inhibits noradrenaline reuptake but has no direct α activity. These actions result in positive inotropism, afterload reduction, and renal and splanchnic dilatation.
* Monitor lactate and ABGs throughout the case to help guide perioperative management and aid decision-making in the post-operative destination.

Post-operative
* Wherever possible, patients who have undergone major surgery should be nursed in HDU/ICU. Elderly patients have a high mortality, and all should be admitted post-operatively to a critical care facility. Patients who are cold, cardiovascularly unstable, acidotic, or hypoxic should be kept intubated and ventilated until stable. If inotropes/vasopressors have been needed in theatre, they should be continued post-operatively, and measures of cardiac output and O_2 delivery continued. If an ICU/HDU bed is unavailable, patients should be kept in recovery for ongoing observation, and the same level of ICU/HDU care provided.
* Urine output should be measured hourly throughout the perioperative period, maintaining an output >0.5mL/kg/hr. In patients with persistently low urine output, assess whether acute tubular necrosis (ATN) is developing, and reconsider fluid balance.
* Post-operative CXR to check CVP line position.
* Administer O_2 for a minimum of 72hr post-operatively.
* Regular chest physiotherapy.
* In the elderly, ongoing post-operative care should include input from a specialist in elderly medicine.

References

11 Saunders DI, Murray D, Pichel AC, Varley S, Peden CJ; UK Emergency Laparotomy Network (2012). Variations in mortality after emergency laparotomy: the first report of the UK Emergency Laparotomy Network. *Br J Anaesth*, **109**, 368–75.

12 Stoneham M, Murray D, Foss N (2014). Emergency surgery: the big three—abdominal aortic aneurysm, laparotomy and hip fracture. *Anaesthesia*, **69** (Suppl. 1), 70–80.

13 Powell-Tuck J, Gosling P, Lobo DN, et al. (2011). *British consensus guidelines on intravenous fluid therapy for adult surgical patients.* ℘ http://www.bapen.org.uk/pdfs/bapen_pubs/giftasup.pdf.

14 Collaborative Study Group on Perioperative ScvO2 Monitoring (2006). Multicentre study on peri- and postoperative central venous oxygen saturation in high-risk surgical patients. *Crit Care*, **10**, R158. ℘ http://www.ncbi.nlm.nih.gov/pmc/articles/pmc1794462/.

15 Davies SJ, Yates D, Wilson RJ (2011). Dopexamine has no additional benefit in high-risk patients receiving goal-directed fluid therapy undergoing major abdominal surgery. *Anesth Analg*, **112**, 130–8.

Laparoscopic surgery

Laparoscopic surgery is well established for a range of procedures, including cholecystectomy, hernia repair, and appendicectomy. It is increasingly used for more complex procedures, including major colorectal resection, prostatectomy, and nephrectomy. Benefits of laparoscopy over laparotomy include:

- Reduced tissue trauma, wound size, and post-operative pain
- Improved post-operative respiratory function, reduced post-operative ileus
- Earlier mobilization, shorter hospital stays
- Improved cosmetic results.

Surgical requirements

- Insufflation of gas (usually CO_2) into the peritoneal cavity creates a pneumoperitoneum and separates the abdominal wall from the viscera.
- CO_2 is the most frequently used gas, being non-combustible (which allows the use of diathermy or laser), as well as colourless, non-toxic, and highly soluble.
- CO_2 is insufflated at a rate of 4–6L/min to a pressure of 10–15mmHg.
- The pneumoperitoneum is maintained by a constant gas flow of 200–400mL/min.

Patient positioning

- Upper abdominal procedures—place head-up (reverse Trendelenburg). Lower abdominal procedures—place head-down (Trendelenburg). Some left tilt is usual with cholecystectomy.
- Patients placed head-down are at greater risk of reduction in FRC, V/Q mismatch, and atelectasis. Cephalad movement of the lungs and carina, in relation to a fixed ETT, increases the risk of endobronchial intubation.
- Patients placed head-up are at increased risk of reduced BP and cardiac output due to decreased venous return. Those most at risk include the hypovolaemic patient, the elderly, and patients with pre-existing CVS disease.

Effects of gas insufflation

- The physiological effects of pneumoperitoneum are summarized in Table 20.4.
- Stretching of the peritoneum may cause vagal stimulation, resulting in sinus bradycardia, nodal rhythm, and occasional asystole. Anticipate and treat with vagolytics, e.g. atropine, glycopyrronium.
- Gas insufflation may result in sympathetic response, leading to hypertension and tachycardia.
- CO_2 is readily absorbed from the peritoneum and may cause hypercapnia and acidosis.
- Extraperitoneal gas insufflation may occur through a misplaced trocar or insufflation needle, via an anatomical defect (e.g. between the pleura and peritoneum), or when gas under pressure within the abdomen dissects through tissue planes. This may result in SC emphysema, pneumomediastinum, pneumopericardium, or pneumothorax.

- Passage of CO_2 from the abdomen can be anticipated in laparoscopic procedures around the diaphragm (e.g. see Hiatus hernia repair, ⮞ p. 359) where a communication is made between the abdomen and chest. Pneumomediastinum and pneumothorax may occur, and suggestive signs include a rapidly rising $ETCO_2$, rising airway pressures, and falling O_2 saturations. Evacuating the CO_2 from the abdomen will often rapidly resolve the problem, and recommencing surgery under reduced insufflation of CO_2 will usually enable completion of surgery. If there is significant cardiac or respiratory compromise, manage like a tension pneumothorax by needle decompression.
- During prolonged procedures with a rising $ETCO_2$, a 'CO_2 break' may be required (see ⮞ p. 530).
- Venous gas embolism may rarely occur when gas is inadvertently insufflated directly into a blood vessel. Physiological effects are less with CO_2 than air due to its greater plasma solubility; however, a significant embolism may be fatal. Signs of a significant venous gas embolism include reduced $ETCO_2$, desaturation, arrhythmias, myocardial ischaemia, hypotension, and elevated CVP (see ⮞ p. 413).
- CVS depression with a fall in cardiac output. Treat with fluids, vasodilators, and inotropes.

Table 20.4 Physiological effects of pneumoperitoneum

Respiratory	
Airway pressure	↑
FRC	↓
Pulmonary compliance	↓
V/Q mismatch	↑
CVS	
Venous return	↓
SVR	↑
Cardiac output	↔ ↓
Risk of arrhythmias	↑
GI	
Risk of regurgitation	↑
Neurological	
ICP	↔ ↑
CPP	↔ ↑

Trauma

- Introduction of trocars may cause damage to organs (e.g. spleen, bladder, liver, bowel, stomach). Organ damage may not always be apparent at the time of injury.
- Damage to blood vessels may result in massive haemorrhage, necessitating rapid conversion to an open procedure.

Preoperative

- Contraindications to laparoscopic surgery are relative; risks are increased with IHD, valvular heart disease, increased ICP, and hypovolaemia.
- All patients scheduled must be considered at risk of conversion to an open procedure, and a plan for analgesia discussed.
- Laparoscopic procedures are increasingly performed in obese patients due to improved post-operative recovery when compared to an open procedure.
- Premedication with H_2 antagonists or PPIs if at risk of regurgitation (e.g. obesity, hiatus hernia). Simple analgesics (paracetamol, NSAIDs) may be beneficial.

Perioperative

- GA with endotracheal intubation, muscle relaxation, and controlled ventilation is considered the safest technique, as it protects against pulmonary aspiration, enables the control of $PaCO_2$, and aids surgical exposure.
- Avoid gastric distension during bag–mask ventilation which may increase the risk of gastric injury during trocar insertion.
- For lower abdominal procedures, a urinary catheter may be required to decompress the bladder and reduce the risk of injury.
- Systemic absorption of CO_2 and raised intra-abdominal pressure will require increased minute volume and result in higher intrathoracic pressure.
- Aim for normocapnia, but beware of adverse effects of high intrathoracic pressure. Controlling $ETCO_2$ during prolonged procedures, especially in the obese and head-down position, can be difficult and may occasionally necessitate intermittent release of intraperitoneal gas or tolerance of a degree of hypercapnia. With high peak inspiratory pressures, check the position of the ETT, and try a change to pressure-controlled ventilation, I:E ratio of 1:1, and 5cm H_2O PEEP. When the patient is levelled out, remember to check the $\dot{V}_T$ or alter ventilation mode/pressures.
- N_2O is controversial due to possible associations with bowel distension and increased PONV.
- Analgesia: dictated by the procedure. Pain may be intense, but short-lived and short-acting opioids, e.g. fentanyl and alfentanil, may be effective for short procedures. Remifentanil infusion can be useful for longer procedures and may help counter the haemodynamic changes due to the pneumoperitoneum. Longer-acting opioids may be required for extensive laparoscopic operations. In extensive laparoscopic surgery,

epidural analgesia or spinal anaesthesia ($\pm$ intrathecal opioid) may be beneficial.
- Fluids: avoid hypovolaemia, as this exaggerates the deleterious CVS effects of laparoscopy.
- Antiemetics: high incidence of nausea and vomiting following laparoscopic surgery. Give prophylactic antiemetic, and prescribe post-operatively.
- Monitoring: pay close attention to $ETCO_2$ and airway pressure. Invasive arterial BP and CVP monitoring may be required for extensive procedures or for patients with CVS or respiratory compromise.

If hypoxia occurs, consider:
- Hypoventilation—inadequate ventilation due to pneumoperitoneum, head-down position, etc.
- Reduced cardiac output—IVC compression, arrhythmias, haemorrhage, myocardial depression, venous gas embolism, extraperitoneal gas
- V/Q mismatch—reduced FRC, atelectasis, endobronchial intubation, venous gas embolism, pulmonary aspiration, and rarely pneumothorax
- SC emphysema during the procedure should arouse suspicion—stop gas insufflation immediately, and check for the source of the problem.

Post-operative
- At the end of the operation, encourage the surgeon to expel as much intraperitoneal gas as possible to reduce post-operative pain.
- Intraperitoneal LA infiltration of port sites may reduce post-operative analgesia requirements. Twenty to 30mL of 0.25% bupivacaine on the gall bladder bed may reduce post-operative analgesic requirements for laparoscopic cholecystectomy.
- Pain varies and is often worst in the 1st few hours. Shoulder tip pain due to diaphragmatic irritation may be troublesome but is usually short-lived. Significant pain extending beyond the 1st day raises the possibility of intra-abdominal complications.
- Prescribe regular paracetamol and NSAIDs, with opioid, as required, for more extensive procedures. Consider post-operative antiemetic.

Special considerations
- LMA: some anaesthetists use an LMA for laparoscopic procedures. This is an individual choice but should be avoided if the patient has a history of reflux or obesity, with an anticipated difficult or prolonged procedure (especially in the 'head-down' position), or with an inexperienced surgeon. An LMA may be useful for short procedures (e.g. laparoscopic sterilization), provided that the anaesthetist is experienced and patient selection appropriate. Third-generation supraglottic airway devices (SADs) (e.g. LMA Proseal, LMA Supreme, i-Gel, etc.) may be advantageous because of their gastric drain tubes.
- Regional anaesthesia is not generally used as the sole anaesthetic technique because of the high level of block required to cover the pneumoperitoneum.

Laparoscopic cholecystectomy

Procedure	Laparoscopic removal of gall bladder
Time	40–80min
Pain	++/+++
Position	Supine, 15–20° head-up, table tilted towards surgeon
Blood loss	Not significant
Practical techniques	GA, ETT, IPPV

Preoperative

- Patients are classically, though not always, '♀, forty, fair, fat, and fertile'.
- Complications of gallstone disease (e.g. pancreatitis) may make surgery more difficult and increase the risk of conversion to an open procedure.
- With appropriate patient selection and perioperative techniques, the procedure can be performed as a day case. Procedures for managing unanticipated admissions must be in place.
- If planned as a day case, list early in the day.
- Consider NSAID and paracetamol premedication.

Perioperative

- Ensure effective face mask ventilation following induction to avoid inflating the stomach which increases the risk of injury during trocar insertion. Insert a naso-/orogastric tube following intubation, and remove at the end of surgery to deflate the stomach, if necessary.
- Ensure adequate IV access—haemodynamic changes may be profound and potential for sudden blood loss.
- Combination of pneumoperitoneum and obesity may make ventilation difficult.
- Paracetamol and NSAIDs IV, if not administered preoperatively.
- High risk for PONV. Consider prophylactic antiemetics (e.g. dexamethasone and ondansetron).
- IV fluids improve the speed of recovery.
- Short-acting opioids (remifentanil, fentanyl) may counter the haemodynamic fluctuations and limit post-operative opioid-related side effects.
- Ask the surgeon to infiltrate the port sites with LA at the end.
- Conversion to an open procedure is typically about 5%. This is usually due to difficulty identifying the cystic duct, suspected common bile duct injury, uncontrolled bleeding from the cystic artery, stones present in the common bile duct, or acute inflammatory changes.

Post-operative

- IV opioids may be required. Avoid/limit morphine to encourage early mobilization and recovery. Fentanyl is usually adequate.

Special considerations

- This can be a very stimulating procedure, particularly during diathermy around the liver.
- LA applied to the gall bladder bed may reduce post-operative analgesic requirements (20mL of 0.25% bupivacaine).
- If conversion to open cholecystectomy, pain can be significant, and a morphine/fentanyl PCA may be required. LA should be infiltrated by surgeons, and a wound catheter for post-operative LA may be beneficial.

Laparoscopic hemicolectomy/anterior resection

Procedure	Laparoscopic removal of colon
Time	90–180min
Pain	+++/++++
Position	Supine, steep head-down, table tilted towards/away from surgeon
Blood loss	<500mL (increases if converted to laparotomy)
Practical techniques	GA, ETT, IPPV

Preoperative

- Laparoscopic colorectal surgery involves small incisions, extreme positioning, and less post-operative pain but may be prolonged, particularly while surgeons are learning the skills. Conversion to open surgery is commoner than with cholecystectomy and is influenced by surgical experience and complexity of the procedure.
- Patients may be anaemic due to malignancy—check Hb and G&S.
- Many patients are elderly and have significant co-morbidity.
- Surgery will involve prolonged steep head-down tilt—beware of patients at risk from raised ICP (recent head injury) or intracranial haemorrhage (venous malformations, aneurysms).

Perioperative

- Careful face mask ventilation following induction to avoid inflating the stomach.
- Some surgeons will request a naso-/orogastric tube during surgery. Check, as it is easier to place before surgery starts.
- An arterial line is useful, with the transducer fixed in position to ensure it does not become dislodged during patient positioning.
- Endotracheal intubation and adequate muscle relaxation throughout the case—always use a peripheral nerve stimulator (PNS). Remifentanil infusion is useful to moderate the stimulating effects of the pneumoperitoneum.
- Multimodal analgesia. Rectus sheath catheters, TAP block, or wound catheters with PCA usually work well.
- Monitor the temperature, and warm actively.
- Ensure all fixings are firmly tightened down and the shoulders padded.
- Antibiotic prophylaxis.
- CVP or minimally invasive cardiac output monitoring for high-risk patients.
- Avoid letting the surgeon persist for too long in the steep head-down position if progress is not being made—time passes quickly for them!

- Restrict IV crystalloid during surgery, as fluid losses are small and the head-down positioning causes venous engorgement. Ensure the head is in a neutral position and that ETT fixation does not restrict venous blood flow.
- Ventilation is described on ➲ p. 530.
- Careful eye protection is advised, as gastric secretions may reflux in the steep head-down position.

Post-operative

- Conjunctival oedema is common, and some anaesthetists have reported restlessness after prolonged head-down.
- PCA morphine or fentanyl. Other analgesics, as indicated.

Appendicectomy

Procedure	Resection of appendix
Time	20–40min
Pain	++/+++
Position	Supine
Blood loss	Not significant
Practical techniques	RSI, ETT, IPPV, ilioinguinal block, TAP block

Preoperative
- Patients are usually aged 5–20yr and are often fit unless appendix ruptured, in which case patients may be unwell.
- Occasionally presents in the elderly. May be the presenting condition of caecal adenocarcinoma requiring right hemicolectomy.
- Check fluid status, and replace deficit prior to surgery, if possible.
- Obtain consent for suppositories.
- Obtain consent for any regional block, e.g. TAP block, ilioinguinal block.

Perioperative
- Prophylactic antibiotics.
- RSI.
- Muscle relaxation required for surgery.
- Consider NSAID and paracetamol IV.
- Ask the surgeon to infiltrate locally or perform right ilioinguinal nerve block or right-sided TAP block.
- Extubate awake on the left side.

Post-operative
- Prescribe regular simple analgesics, opioid as required (PRN), antiemetic, and IV fluids until tolerating oral fluids.

Inguinal hernia repair

Procedure	Repair of inguinal muscular canal defect through which bowel protrudes
Time	30–60min
Pain	++/+++
Position	Supine
Blood loss	Not significant
Practical techniques	GA, SV, LMA, inguinal field block. Spinal. Local infiltration and/or sedation

Preoperative

- Patients are usually adult ♂ or young children.
- Can usually be performed as a day-case procedure

Perioperative

- Inguinal field block may be used as sole technique for surgery or to complement GA (see ➔ p. 1122).
- The iliohypogastric and ilioinguinal nerves are easily blocked, 2cm caudal and medial to the anterior superior iliac spine (ASIS) (see ➔ p. 1122). The genitofemoral nerve is located 1–2cm above the midpoint of the inguinal ligament, deep to the aponeurosis of the external oblique. This may be left to the surgeon to block, reducing the risk of vascular or peritoneal puncture.

Special considerations

- If day case, prescribe adequate analgesia to take home, e.g. NSAID, paracetamol, tramadol 50–100mg qds.
- Repair using inguinal hernia field block is probably the technique of choice in the high-risk patient if the operator is experienced in LA techniques. Low-dose propofol infusion may be a useful adjunct in cases performed solely under LA.

Haemorrhoidectomy

Procedure	Excision of haemorrhoids
Time	20min
Pain	++/+++
Position	Supine, lithotomy, head-down
Blood loss	Not significant
Practical techniques	GA, SV, LMA ± caudal. Spinal ('saddle block')

Preoperative
- Assess suitability for LMA/lithotomy/head-down position.
- Consider ETT if the patient is obese or history of reflux.

Perioperative
- Opioid analgesia (fentanyl or alfentanil)—short, but intensely painful, stimulus.
- LA infiltration by the surgeon during the procedure usually provides effective pain relief.
- Potential for bradycardia/asystole, as surgery starts. Anticipate and have vagolytics to hand.

Post-operative
- Avoid PR route of drug administration.

Special considerations
- Avoid spinal anaesthesia followed by immediate head-down tilt.
- Anal stretch is an intense stimulus. There is a risk of laryngospasm and coughing if anaesthesia is too light. Anticipate and deepen the anaesthetic, e.g. increase the volatile, and give a bolus of short-acting opioid, e.g. alfentanil (500 micrograms). The anal stretch can also produce an increase in vagal tone.
- A sacral-only spinal block ('saddle block') using heavy bupivacaine is a useful alternative, with little effect on CVS dynamics.

Testicular surgery

Procedure	Removal/biopsy of testis, marsupialization of hydrocele, vasectomy, testicular torsion
Time	30min–1hr
Pain	++/+++
Position	Supine
Blood loss	Not significant
Practical techniques	GA, LMA, spermatic cord block. RSI/ETT if emergency (e.g. torsion). Spinal LA infiltration

Preoperative
- Often suitable for day surgery.

Perioperative
- Beware vagal responses—have atropine ready.

Special considerations
- Innervation of testes and scrotum: somatic innervation is via the ilioinguinal, genitofemoral, pudendal, and posterior scrotal nerves (branches of the posterior cutaneous nerve of the thigh) with nerve root contributions from L1 to S3. Autonomic innervation is from the sympathetic chain T10–L4 and the parasympathetic plexus S1–S3. Local techniques therefore need to cover T10–S3.
- A spermatic cord block can be used as an adjunct to GA or as part of a local technique for scrotal surgery. The block covers all nerves, except the pudendal and posterior scrotal branches. If used as part of an LA technique, supplemental infiltration of the scrotal skin is also required.
- Spermatic cord is best blocked under direct vision by the surgeon. However, if a local technique is planned, feel for the spermatic cord, as it enters the top of the scrotum, and infiltrate 5–10mL of LA around it.

Breast surgery

(See also Breast reduction, ◑ p. 495; and Breast augmentation, p. 497.)

General considerations

Breast cancer is now the commonest cancer in the UK, and the incidence has increased by 50% over the last 25yr. Mortality from breast cancer, however, has fallen steadily since 1990, probably because of earlier detection and improved treatment. Over this time, there have been significant advances in more extensive combined procedures of breast resection and reconstruction. Patients are often anxious, and management of post-operative pain and nausea/vomiting may be difficult.

Preoperative

- Anxiety is often high. It is important to gain the patient's confidence at the preoperative visit, discuss analgesia, and prescribe anxiolysis (e.g. temazepam 10–20mg) if necessary.
- Patients who have recently undergone chemotherapy may be immunocompromised. Check FBC for evidence of bone marrow suppression and anticipate potentially difficult venous access.
- Reconstructive procedures, mastectomy following radiotherapy, mastectomy where breasts are large, and breast reduction surgery increase the risk of blood loss. Check Hb and ensure blood is grouped and screened.

Perioperative

- Standard monitoring is appropriate for most procedures. Longer procedures will require active warming and temperature measurement.
- Avoid venous access on the side of surgery.
- Additional invasive monitoring may be required for prolonged reconstructive procedures, including free flap surgery (see ◑ p. 501).
- LMA and SV are often appropriate for short- to medium-length procedures. Use intubation and mechanical ventilation for prolonged procedures, the obese, and patients at risk of aspiration.
- Give balanced analgesia, including NSAID, if tolerated, systemic opioid, and regional techniques, if necessary (see ◑ p. 1122).
- Breast surgery patients are at high risk of PONV. Avoid causative agents, and administer prophylactic antiemetics.

Regional analgesia

- Regional techniques may offer advantages in some cases; however, the risks in healthy women undergoing minor procedures may outweigh the benefits.
- Consider for more radical procedures, e.g. radical mastectomy/axillary clearance and breast reconstruction.
- Regional techniques include: paravertebral block, thoracic epidural, intercostal blocks, and intrapleural block. Beware of the complications of each technique. Ultrasound may be beneficial in paravertebral block.

- A retrospective study found that breast surgery supplemented by a paravertebral block may reduce the risk of cancer recurrence; however, further prospective studies are required.[16]

Post-operative

- HDU may be required after extensive procedures.
- If a paravertebral catheter or thoracic epidural is sited, continue infusion post-operatively.

Special considerations

- Patients may present with previous breast surgery and axillary clearance. Cannulation should be avoided in the arm on the affected side due to the risk of infection and potential development of lymphoedema. There is limited evidence of the risk of short-term cannulation on the affected side, and, if venous access is limited, it may be appropriate to use the affected side and remove at the end of the case.
- Chronic pain, typically presenting in the affected anterior chest wall, ipsilateral axilla, or upper arm, may occur following breast surgery. Intensity of the pain following extensive surgery, post-operative radiotherapy, and chemotherapy are risk factors.

Reference

16 Exadaktylos AK, Buggy DJ, Moriarty DC, Mascha E, Sessler DI (2006). Can anesthetic technique for primary breast cancer surgery affect recurrence or metastasis? *Anesthesiology*, **105**, 660–4.

Anaesthesia for obesity

Nick Kennedy and Mark Abou-Samra

Introduction

The prevalence of morbid obesity is increasing in the UK. Recent UK government statistics, published in 2013, suggest that the proportion of adults with a normal BMI decreased between 1993 and 2011, from 41% to 34% among men and from 50% to 39% among women.[1]

The data also showed that there was a marked increase in the proportion of adults that were obese, from 13% in 1993 to 24% in 2011 for men and from 16% to 26% for women over the same time period. This trend does not only apply to adults.[1]

In 2011, around three in ten boys and girls (aged 2–15) were classed as either overweight or obese (31% and 28%, respectively), which is very similar to the 2010 findings (31% for boys and 29% for girls).[1]

Anaesthesia and surgery may entail considerable risk for obese patients. Obesity is a multisystem disorder, particularly involving the respiratory and CVS systems; therefore, a multidisciplinary approach is required.

Reference

1 Health and Social Care Information Centre, Lifestyles Statistics. *Statistics on obesity, physical activity and diet: England, 2013.* ⅈ http://www.hscic.gov.uk/catalogue/PUB10364/obes-phys-acti-diet-eng-2013-rep.pdf.

Definitions

Obesity is classified by the BMI. BMI is defined as weight (in kg) divided by height (in m) squared (Box 21.1).

Box 21.1 BMI definitions

BMI (in kg/m^2)
- <19.9: underweight
- 20–24.9: normal
- 25–29.9: overweight
- 30–39.9: obese
- 40–49.9: morbidly obese (35–49.9 with co-morbidities)
- 50–59.9: super obese
- 60–69.9: super super obese
- >70: hyper obese

Indications for surgery

In the UK, NICE has issued guidance on when bariatric surgery should be offered.

All of the following criteria should be fulfilled:[2]

- BMI of 40kg/m^2 or more
- BMI between 35kg/m^2 and 40kg/m^2 with other significant co-morbidities that could be improved if the patient lost weight
- All appropriate non-surgical measures have been tried but have failed to achieve or maintain adequate, clinically beneficial weight loss for at least 6 months
- Bariatric surgery is also recommended as a 1st-line option for adults with a BMI of >50kg/m^2 in whom surgical intervention is considered appropriate.

UK guidelines for all patients having bariatric surgery stipulate all patients must have been through a formal bariatric surgery multidisciplinary team assessment. Mortality is very low in bariatric surgery in experienced hands.

Reference

2 National Institute for Health and Care Excellence (2006). *Obesity: guidance on the prevention of overweight and obesity in adults and children. Clinical guideline 43.* http://www.nice.org.uk/guidance/cg43.

Common co-morbidities

Respiratory system

- OSA (see also ➲ p. 112):
  - This is defined as apnoeic episodes (defined as excursion for >10s) during sleep and can be obstructive (pharyngeal wall collapse), centrally driven, or mixed
  - Several tools are available to assess OSA. Commonly used are the Epworth Sleepiness Scale and STOP BANG OSA assessment score (<5 low risk of OSA, ≥5 high risk of OSA):
    — Snore loudly
    — Tired: daytime somnolence
    — Observed apnoeic episodes
    — Pressure: hypertension
    — BMI >35kg/m²
    — Age >50
    — Neck circumference >15.75in
    — Gender: ♂
- Referral to a sleep service should be considered preoperatively. Formally, a diagnosis of OSA is made using overnight PSG (sleep study), but overnight oximetry is a convenient and cheap alternative.
- Hypopnoea: is defined as reduced airflow through the airways, which disturbs sleep, the frequency of which is measured over the total sleep time.
- Apnoea–hypopnoea index (AHI): this is a reflection of the severity of the OSA:
  - <5 normal
  - 5–15 mild
  - 15–30 moderate
  - >30 severe.
- OSA is usually treated with face mask CPAP overnight.
- Generally, patients with significant sleep apnoea should be treated with CPAP, but whether to treat patients with a new diagnosis of OSA pre-bariatric surgery and delay surgery is less clear. There is not much evidence that treating OSA for a period of time (1–3 months) prior to surgery changes surgical or longer-term outcomes. However, many patients benefit from CPAP treatment, and their general well-being, functional status, and alertness are rapidly much improved.
- Obesity hypoventilation syndrome (OHS):
  - OHS is at the severe end-stage of OSA in obese patients, characterized by diurnal variation in ventilation and a $PaCO_2$ >5.9. Sensitivity to CO_2 is reduced due to loss of central drive, leading to hypoventilation
  - O_2 consumption is increased by metabolically active adipose tissue and the workload of supporting muscles, with associated increase in CO_2 production.
- FRC is reduced in the awake obese patient and decreases significantly following induction, which may encroach upon the closing capacity. Pulmonary compliance is decreased due to heavy chest wall and

splinted diaphragm. O_2 desaturation occurs rapidly in the obese apnoeic patient.

- Obesity and asthma—obese patients may have clinical signs that appear to be asthma. In many cases, the bronchoconstrictive symptoms experienced by the obese are often due to airway closure without affecting the calibre of the airways.[3] This increase in airway closure is a direct effect of obesity and is not due to any intrinsic lung disease. It is not improved by bronchodilator therapy.

Cardiovascular system

- The excess adipose tissue exerts increasing metabolic demands on the CVS system, leading to increased cardiac output, myocardial demand, arterial pressure, and increased blood volume.
- Hypertension is much more prevalent in obesity. This results in LV dilatation and hypertrophy, which causes a reduction in ventricular compliance, leading to diastolic dysfunction, impaired ventricular filling, and elevated LVEDP.
- Blood volume is increased 2° to increased activity of the renin–angiotensin system and 2° polycythaemia.
- The increase in blood volume, coupled with elevation of LVEDP, increases the risk of developing heart failure.
- LV failure and pulmonary vasoconstriction, 2° to chronic hypercapnia, result in pulmonary hypertension, dilatation of the right heart, and resultant cor pulmonale.
- The increased level of circulating catecholamines (2° to OSA), ventricular hypertrophy, and fat infiltration of the pacing and conducting systems, coupled with potential hypokalaemia from diuretic therapy, increase the risk of arrhythmias.[4]
- In addition to all these factors, the increased incidence of diabetes mellitus and reduced level of activity increases the risk of developing IHD in the obese population.

Endocrine system

Insulin resistance and diabetes

- Insulin resistance with hyperinsulinaemia is characteristic of obesity and is present before the onset of hyperglycaemia. After the onset of obesity, the first demonstrable changes are impairment in glucose removal and increased insulin resistance, which result in hyperinsulinaemia. This increases hepatic very low density lipoprotein (VLDL) synthesis, plasminogen activator inhibitor-1 synthesis, sympathetic nervous system activity, and sodium reabsorption. These changes contribute to hyperlipidaemia and hypertension in obese subjects.[5]
- Peripheral resistance to the effects of insulin on glucose and fatty acid utilization leads to type 2 diabetes. A curvilinear relationship between BMI and the risk of type 2 diabetes was found in women in the Nurses Health Study, at a BMI >35kg/m².[6]
- Many obese patients will be on complex antidiabetic drug regimens. Normal protocols may not work in the obese, and their insulin requirements appear to be greater than the non-obese.

- Bariatric surgery, particularly gastric bypass, often has a profound effect on type 2 diabetes control immediately post-operatively, before any weight loss occurs. Complete resolution of type 2 diabetes occurs within a year in up to 80% of patients post-gastric bypass.

Metabolic syndrome
- This is defined as the occurrence of several metabolic risk factors for both type 2 diabetes and CVS disease (abdominal obesity, hyperglycaemia, dyslipidaemia, and hypertension). The National Cholesterol Education Program (NCEP/ATP III) is the most widely used, and its criteria include the presence of any three of the following five traits:
  - Abdominal obesity, defined as a waist circumference in men ≥102cm and in women ≥88cm
  - Serum triglycerides ≥1.7mmol/L or drug treatment for elevated triglycerides
  - Serum HDL cholesterol <1mmol/L in men and <1.3mmol/L in women, or drug treatment for low HDL cholesterol
  - BP ≥130/85mmHg or drug treatment for elevated BP
  - Fasting plasma glucose (FPG) ≥5.6mmol/L or drug treatment for elevated blood glucose.
- The hyperinsulinaemia and hyperglycaemia associated with obesity, along with adipokines, may lead to vascular endothelial dysfunction, an abnormal lipid profile, hypertension, and vascular inflammation, all of which promote the development of atherosclerotic CVS disease.[7]
- CRP and IL-6 levels rise with increasing obesity and lead to a pro-inflammatory process associated with it, whereas adiponectin levels, a biomarker of insulin sensitivity, decreased.
- The prevalence of obese patients admitted to critical care is increasing. Outcome data show predominantly either equal or lower mortality in obese than in normal-weight critically ill patients.[8] This phenomenon, the obesity paradox,[9] has been observed in obese patients with heart failure and sepsis too. There is also no evidence that surgical outcomes in obese are worse than normal-weight patients.

Gastrointestinal
- These patients are more likely to have raised intra-abdominal pressures and are at greater risk of developing a hiatus hernia, contributing to an increased risk of reflux and aspiration.

Venous thromboembolic disease
(See also ➲ p. 11.)
- A number of studies have found a significantly increased risk for DVT and PE in obese subjects;[10–12] in addition, there is an increased risk of recurrent VTE once anticoagulation treatment has been withdrawn.[13]
- Obesity also appears to contribute to further increasing the risk of VTE in a number of other settings:
  - Smoking and age in patients with factor V Leiden mutation[14]
  - Long-duration air travel.
  - Women taking oral contraceptives.[15]

References

3 Chapman DG, Irvin CG, Kaminsky DA, Dixon AE (2013). Weight loss reduces airway closure during bronchoconstriction in obese asthmatics. *Am J Resp Crit Care Med*, **187**, A3791.

4 Shenkman Z, Shir Y, Brodsky JB (1993). Perioperative management of the obese patient. *Br J Anaesth*, **70**, 349–59.

5 Kaplan NM (2015). Obesity and weight reduction in hypertension. ℘ http://www.uptodate.com/contents/obesity-and-weight-reduction-in-hypertension?source=search_result&search=obesity+and+weight+reduction+in+hyperten+si+on&selectedTitle=5~150.

6 Willett WC, Dietz WH, Colditz GA (1999). Guidelines for healthy weight. *N Engl J Med*, **341**, 427–34.

7 Lindsay RS, Howard BV (2004). Cardiovascular risk associated with the metabolic syndrome. *Curr Diab Rep*, **4**, 63–8.

8 Arabi YM, Dara SI, Tamim HM, *et al.*; Cooperative Antimicrobial Therapy of Septic Shock (CATSS) Database Research Group (2013). Clinical characteristics, sepsis interventions and outcomes in the obese patients with septic shock: an international multicenter cohort study. *Crit Care*, **17**, R72.

9 Habbu A, Lakkis NM, Dokainish H (2006). The obesity paradox: fact or fiction? *Am J Cardiol*, **98**, 944–8.

10 Goldhaber SZ, Savage DD, Garrison RJ, *et al.* (1983). Risk factors for pulmonary embolism. The Framingham Study. *Am J Med*, **74**, 1023–8.

11 Hansson PO, Eriksson H, Welin L, *et al.* (1999). Smoking and abdominal obesity: risk factors for venous thromboembolism among middle-aged men: 'the study of men born in 1913'. *Arch Intern Med*, **159**, 1886–90.

12 Kucher N, Tapson VF, Goldhaber SZ, DVT FREE Steering Committee (2005). Risk factors associated with symptomatic pulmonary embolism in a large cohort of deep vein thrombosis patients. *Thromb Haemost*, **93**, 494–8.

13 Eichinger S, Hron G, Bialonczyk C, *et al.* (2008). Overweight, obesity, and the risk of recurrent venous thromboembolism. *Arch Intern Med*, **168**, 1678.

14 Severinsen MT, Overvad K, Johnsen SP, *et al.* (2010). Genetic susceptibility, smoking, obesity and risk of venous thromboembolism. *Br J Haematol*, **149**, 273–9.

15 Pomp ER, le Cessie S, Rosendaal FR, Doggen CJ (2007). Risk of venous thrombosis: obesity and its joint effect with oral contraceptive use and prothrombotic mutations. *Br J Haematol*, **139**, 289–96.

Risk scoring

The Obesity Surgery Mortality Risk Score (OSMRS) represents the 1st validated scoring system for risk stratification in bariatric surgery, and it aims to aid informed consent discussions, guide surgical decision-making, and allow standardization of outcome comparisons between treatment centres (Table 21.1).

Table 21.1 Obesity Surgery Mortality Risk Score[16]

Risk factor	Points
Age >45yr	1
Hypertension	1
♂ sex	1
Risk factors for PE*	1
BMI ≥50kg/m²	1
Total:	
Risk group (score)	Post-operative mortality risk (deaths/total number of patients)
Class A (0 or 1 points)	0.2%
Class B (2 or 3 points)	1.2%
Class C (4 or 5 points)	2.4%

* Previous VTE, pulmonary hypertension, preoperative vena cava filter, or hypoventilation due to obesity.

Reference

16 Demaria EJ, Murr M, Byrne TK, et al. (2007). Validation of the Obesity Surgery Mortality Risk Score in a multicenter study proves it stratifies mortality risk in patients undergoing gastric bypass for morbid obesity. Ann Surg, 246, 578–82.

Perioperative practicalities

Patients, if able, can walk directly into theatre, and anaesthesia is induced on the operating table, reducing manual handling risk. Operating tables with the appropriate maximum weight allowance must be used.

- A Hover mattress underneath the patient is very helpful to facilitate patient transfer post-surgery.
- There must be enough trained and experienced staff in theatre to assist with moving the patient, should it become necessary.
- Standard monitoring should include a correct-sized BP cuff. This may be impossible in the normal upper arm position in many patients. Using a forearm cuff is virtually always possible instead and, although not validated, is effective and used by many bariatric anaesthetists as standard.
- Invasive arterial catheters are rarely needed, unless for CVS indications.
- Venous cannulation is often difficult. CVCs may be necessary. Anterior chest wall veins are sometimes useful in the obese patient.
- Calf compression devices should be used, and particular care given to pressure areas to prevent sores and nerve injury. If arm boards are used, over-abduction must be avoided as this risks brachial plexus injury.

Patient positioning is very important. 'Sniffing the morning air' position may be difficult to achieve due to the large soft tissue mass of the neck and chest wall. A ramped position is ideal, and many adjuncts to achieve this are commercially available.

- Preoxygenation in the head-up position will slow the rapid desaturation that can occur when supine.
- Generally, obese patients do not have difficult airways. AFOI should be considered in any patients who have a history or clinical signs suggestive of airway problems. If the patient is preoxygenated to an end-tidal O_2 (ETO_2) >80%, then minimal bagging will be needed while waiting for the muscle relaxant to take effect.
- The use of short-acting anaesthetic agents, such as remifentanil and desflurane, or a TIVA technique with propofol and remifentanil aid rapid recovery from anaesthesia and minimize post-operative hypoventilation and hypoxaemia.
- Monitoring of NMB is essential, as incomplete reversal of neuromuscular-blocking agents is problematic in the obese.

Airway considerations in the obese

The Royal College of Anaesthetists National Audit Project 4 (NAP4) report in 2011 refers to airway difficulties in the obese patient being twice that in the general population, and higher in the morbidly obese. Particular complications included an increased frequency of aspiration and other complications during the use of SADs, difficulty at tracheal intubation, and airway obstruction during emergence or recovery. When rescue techniques were necessary in obese patients, they failed more often than in the non-obese. Obesity needs to be recognized as a risk factor for airway difficulty, and plans modified accordingly.[17]

In response to this publication, the Society for Obesity and Bariatric Anaesthesia (SOBA) produced a document providing some guidance on how to manage these patients; this included:[18]

- Preoxygenation and intubation in the obese patient should be performed with the patient in the head-up or ramped position. This improves the efficacy of preoxygenation, maximizes the time before desaturation, reduces the risk of reflux, and reduces the incidence of difficult intubation close to that of the non-obese population.
- Obesity is a weak risk factor for difficult intubation, and the predictors of difficulty are generally the same as for normal-weight patients.
- Increased work of breathing and early airway closure occurring during tidal ventilation suggests that obese patients should not be allowed to breathe spontaneously for anything other than the shortest procedure. These patients will desaturate rapidly, so the time interval from induction of anaesthesia to assisted ventilation of the lungs should be minimized.
- Caution should be taken with the use of SADs in patients with a BMI of >35kg/m^2.
- Tracheal extubation in an obese patient should likewise be performed in the head-up position, with the patient awake.
- In the event of a failed intubation during RSI, the advice is to follow the Difficult Airway Society (DAS) guidelines by allowing the patient to wake up.
- Problems usually occur because of poor planning, choice of technique, or inadequate preparation. Morbidly obese patients should be managed by an experienced anaesthetist as part of an experienced team.

References

17 Cook T, Woodall N, Frerk C (2011). *Major complications of airway management in the UK: results of the Fourth National Audit Project of the Royal College of Anaesthetists and the Difficult Airway Society.* ℘ http://www.rcoa.ac.uk/nap4.
18 Nightingale CE, Cousins J, Fox WTA, et al. (2011). Comment on Fourth National Audit Project from the Society for Obesity and Bariatric Surgery. *Br J Anaesth*, **107**, 272–3.

Pharmacology

- Recommendations on which weight to use for calculating drug doses in various classes of drug are found on the SOBA one-page guideline (Fig. 21.1).
- The IBW in kg can be calculated via the Broca formula:
  - Men: height in cm minus 100
  - Woman: height in cm minus 105.
- Volume of distribution for drugs is altered due to a smaller proportion of TBW, greater proportion of adipose tissue, increased lean body mass, and increased blood volume and cardiac output.
- Hydrophilic drugs (e.g. competitive neuromuscular blockers such as rocuronium, vecuronium, and atracurium) have similar absolute volumes of distribution, clearance, and elimination half-lives. Base the dose on the ideal body mass.
- Lipophilic drugs (e.g. thiopental, propofol, opioids, and benzodiazepines) have increased volumes of distribution, normal clearance, and increased elimination half-lives. Titrate to cardiac output, which equates to the lean body weight in a fit patient.
- Increased plasma cholinesterase activity. Suxamethonium dose should be based on the total body weight to a maximum of 200mg.

Suxamethonium may seem to be the neuromuscular-blocking agent of choice for induction of anaesthesia in obese patients,[19] as they have a reduced safe apnoea time; it has a rapid onset and allows rapid tracheal intubation. In addition, its short duration of action allows earlier resumption of SV, should difficulty in securing the airway be encountered. However, it has been demonstrated in one study that the use of suxamethonium was associated with more rapid desaturation when compared to rocuronium for an RSI.[20]

References

19 Ingrande J, Lemmens HMJ (2010). Dose adjustment of anaesthetics in the morbidly obese. *Br J Anaesth*, **105** (suppl 1), i16–23.
20 Taha SK, El-Khatib MF, Baraka AS, *et al.* (2010). Effect of suxamethonium vs rocuronium on onset of oxygen desaturation during apnoea following rapid sequence induction. *Anaesthesia*, **65**, 358–61.

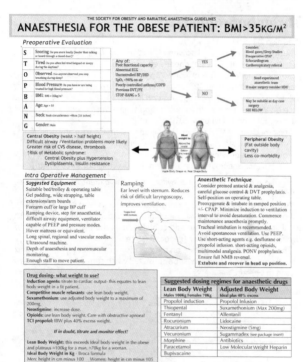

Fig. 21.1 SOBA guidelines for the patient with BMI >35.

Reproduced with kind permission of Society for Obesity and Bariatric Anaesthesia. ℘ http://www.sobauk.com.

Thromboprophylaxis

(See also ➔ p. 11.)

Obesity and surgery are known risk factors for VTE, but there is limited information about the independent effects of obesity on the incidence of post-operative VTE. The Million Women Study[21] concluded that VTE risk increases with increasing BMI, and the associated excess risk is much greater following surgery than without surgery. In the UK, NICE has offered guidance on VTE prophylaxis in its publication *Venous thromboembolism: reducing the risk*, published in January 2010:[22]

Start mechanical VTE prophylaxis at admission. Choose any one of:

- Antiembolism stockings (thigh or knee length).
- Foot impulse devices.
- Intermittent pneumatic compression devices (thigh or knee length).

Continue mechanical VTE prophylaxis, until the patient no longer has significantly reduced mobility.

Add pharmacological VTE prophylaxis for patients who have a low risk of major bleeding, taking into account individual patient factors and according to clinical judgement. This should continue, until the patient no longer has significantly reduced mobility (generally 5–7d).

There has been no guidance on the duration or the dosing for the obese. Therefore, local guidelines must be consulted when considering VTE prophylaxis in this group.

References

21 Parkin L, Sweetland S, Balkwill A, Green J, Reeves G, Beral V; Million Women Study Collaborators (2012). Body mass index, surgery, and risk of venous thromboembolism in middle-aged women: a cohort study. *Circulation*, **125**, 1897–904.

22 National Institute for Health and Care Excellence (2010). *Venous thromboembolism: reducing the risk: reducing the risk of venous thromboembolism (deep vein thrombosis and pulmonary embolism) in patients admitted to hospital. Clinical guideline 92.* ℞ http://www.nice.org.uk/guidance/cg92.

Intragastric balloon insertion and removal

Procedure	Placement of 700mL silicone balloon into stomach via gastroscope which is inflated with 700mL of saline dyed with methylthioninium chloride (methylene blue). Balloons are removed after a maximum of 6 months via gastroscopy
Time	15–30min
Pain	None
Position	Left lateral or sitting up
Blood loss	None
Practical techniques	IV sedation, topical anaesthesia or GA with intubation

Preoperative

Intragastric balloons are typically inserted in:
- Patients with BMI 25–35, as a weight loss adjunct in those patients who do not qualify for bariatric surgery. These patients are usually very low risk.
- Very high-BMI patients often >60–70, usually with many significant co-morbidities, in whom invasive surgical procedures are deemed too risky.

Perioperative

- Topical anaesthesia is possible in cooperative patients.
- Low-risk patients are usually suitable for IV sedation, and often an anaesthetist is not required. Left lateral position is usual for insertion of the balloon. Balloon removal can be done in a similar fashion.
- High-risk patients—IV sedation may be poorly tolerated and risky, due to hypoventilation, hypoxia, and airway obstruction. A GA with intubation and ventilation may be indicated.
- Very large patients tolerate lying on their side very poorly and are better dealt with sitting up.

Special considerations

- Intragastric ballloon insertion is associated with considerable nausea immediately post-operatively. Antiemetic should be given perioperatively and prescribed for the patient to take home. There is no nausea associated with balloon removal.
- Both insertion and removal of balloons can usually be done as day-case procedures, even in high-risk patients.

Gastric banding

Procedure	Placement of silicone adjustable band around the top of the stomach to create a small pouch above it. A small injection port is placed SC and connected to the band with tubing to allow the band to be inflated with saline to control passage of food past it
Time	45–90min
Pain	+
Position	Supine, head-up
Blood loss	Minimal
Practical techniques	GA, ETT, IPPV (with PEEP)

Preoperative

Gastric banding is a relatively straightforward laparoscopic procedure with a very low mortality rate.

Gastric banding is commonly used for the lower-BMI and lower-risk bariatric surgical patients, but some centres use gastric banding for most of their cases, and some patients choose banding, so some very high-BMI and high-risk patients present for banding.

Preoperative analgesia with paracetamol is recommended.

Perioperative

- Ensure equipment appropriate for weight and adequate staff numbers are available.
- Insert two IV cannulae.
- Extreme care in positioning the patient to avoid damage due to pressure or overhanging tissue.
- Take precautions to ensure the patient does not slide down the table when head-up.
- Standard perioperative monitoring. Use forearm BP cuff if upper arm too large or wrong shape to place a cuff.
- Preoxygenate fully in head-up position.
- Intubation and ventilation are mandatory. Use V_T appropriate for IBW or lean body mass.
- Face mask ventilation can be difficult. Expect rapid desaturation during apnoea, and have a plan for airway management. RSI is not mandatory.
- Use short-acting anaesthetic agents, sevoflurane, or desflurane. TIVA with propofol is a good technique, but correct dosing may be difficult.
- Good NMB is important.
- Antiemetics are important immediately post-operatively to prevent strain on the band sutures. Give two drugs perioperatively.

- Opioid analgesia is usually required post-operatively—fentanyl or morphine. Limit intra-operative opioids—titrate dosage upwards in recovery.
- Patients should be woken up and extubated sitting up. Plan for an electric bed.
- Ensure the surgeon infiltrates all port sites with LA.

Post-operatively

- Ensure patients are nursed sitting up in recovery.
- Titrate opioids in recovery.
- Most patients can be safely managed without HDU but this should be considered for patients with significant OSA.
- Encourage early mobilization.
- Thromboprophylaxis as per local protocol.

Gastric bypass

Procedure	Roux-en-Y gastric bypass. Almost always laparoscopic
Time	90–200min
Pain	++
Position	Supine, head-up
Blood loss	>500mL, occasionally more due to ooze from splenic injury or stomach. G&S required
Practical techniques	GA, ETT, IPPV (with PEEP)

Preoperative

- Gastric bypass involves a small bowel anastomosis, formation of a Roux limb, creation of a gastric pouch, and a gastrojejunal anastomosis. Surgical techniques differ, and it is important to establish in what order the surgeon will do the procedure.
- Many surgeons ask for a large (typically 34 French gauge) bougie (or large NGT or dilator) to be passed orogastrically by the anaesthetist during pouch formation. This identifies the pouch and prevents stapling of the oesophagus. The bougie is then pushed distally into the Roux limb during gastrojejunal anastomosis to allow suturing around it. There are other techniques involving circular staplers, so ensure you understand what is used, how it works, and when it is needed. Discuss with the surgeon preoperatively.

Perioperative

- See Gastric banding, ❢ p. 558.
- Antiemetics immediately post-operatively to prevent strain on the anastomosis. Two agents are recommended perioperatively.

Post-operatively

- Post-operative CPAP is quite safe. No evidence of damage to the gastric anastomosis.

Special considerations

- Sometimes surgeons ask for an NGT to be inserted to decompress the stomach prior to pouch formation. If so, insert it orogastrically, and remove as soon as the stomach is decompressed. Leaving an NGT *in situ* runs the risk of stapling it into the pouch, an avoidable disaster.
- Many surgeons test the gastrojejunal anastomosis for leaks by asking for an orogastric tube to be passed into the pouch after the anastomosis is complete. Leak testing is achieved by either injecting air down the NGT or commonly by injecting ~60mL of dilute methylthioninium

chloride (methylene blue) (or food dye) into the pouch. Leaks are usually obvious to see. Beware of the dyed fluid refluxing back into the mouth. Inserting a sucker into the mouth during this procedure helps prevent the dye from being either aspirated or refluxing out and onto the patient's face and hair!

Post-operative complications to watch for:
- Anastomotic leak. Tachycardia (a post-operative tachycardia is a leak until proven otherwise), excessive pain. Pain on drinking.
- Bleeding. Signs of severe bleeding similar to any other procedure. Staple line bleeding can present as melaena or haematemesis in the 1st 24hr. Unless the patient is shocked, conservative management is warranted.
- In the event of a suspected leak, the best investigation is usually to re-laparoscope the patient as soon as possible.

Sleeve gastrectomy

Procedure	Stomach divided by stapling to reduce it to about 25% of its original size. A large portion of the stomach along the greater curvature is removed through a small incision. The result is a sleeve or tube-like structure. Almost always laparoscopic
Time	90–150min
Pain	++
Position	Supine, head-up
Blood loss	>500mL, occasionally more due to ooze from stomach staple line. G&S required
Practical techniques	GA, ETT, IPPV (with PEEP)

Preoperative
- Sleeve gastrectomy often performed in high-risk patients, instead of a gastric bypass, as it is an easier and quicker procedure. Increasingly the weight loss procedure of choice.
- Some surgeons ask for a large (typically 34 French gauge) bougie (or large NGT or dilator) to be passed orogastrically by the anaesthetist during the procedure. This allows the surgeon to staple alongside the bougie, identify the anatomy, and prevent stapling of the oesophagus. Ensure you understand what is used, how it works, and when it is needed. Discuss with the surgeon preoperatively.

Perioperative
- See Gastric banding, ⮞ p. 558.
- Antiemetics immediately post-operatively to prevent strain on the anastomosis. Two agents are recommended perioperatively.

Post-operatively
- Post-operative CPAP is safe.

Special considerations
- As gastric bypass.

Liver transplantation and resection

Mark Bellamy

General principles

The majority of patients who present for liver transplantation have either acute hepatic failure or end-stage liver disease. A small proportion undergo transplantation for other conditions, including polycystic liver disease, hepatoma, and metabolic liver disease which could give rise to future liver failure or catastrophic systemic illness (e.g. Wilson's disease). Most transplants are performed semi-electively in those with end-stage disease. Worldwide, the commonest indication for hepatic transplantation is post-hepatitis C cirrhosis. This is likely to change in the future, as more effective antiviral therapies become available.

Preoperative assessment includes investigation/treatment of:

- Jaundice, hyponatraemia, ascites, pleural effusions
- Diabetes (a common co-morbidity with hepatitis C)
- Renal failure
- Systemic vasodilatation with hypotension and cardiac failure
- Poor nutritional state and reduced muscle mass
- Portopulmonary syndromes (associated severe portal and pulmonary hypertension, leading to RV failure and potential cardiac arrest intraoperatively)
- Hepatopulmonary syndromes (hypoxia and intrapulmonary shunting occurs in 0.5–4% of patients with cirrhotic liver disease)
- Varices (oesophageal, gastric, rectal, abdominal wall)
- Coagulopathy (prolonged PT, low platelet count, fibrinolysis).

Haemodynamic instability can result from cardiac consequences of the underlying pathology (e.g. alcoholic cardiomyopathy), from pericardial effusions, and from circulatory failure due to vasodilatation and low SVR. Anaemia resulting in a low plasma viscosity further reduces effective tissue perfusion.

Surgical techniques vary, but there are a number of common features.

- **Stage 1** of the operation is dissection (which involves laparotomy) and haemostasis (including ligation of varices). The liver is exposed, its anatomy defined, and slings placed around the major vessels.
- **Stage 2** of the operation is the **anhepatic** phase, during which the hepatic artery, portal vein, hepatic veins, and bile duct are divided.
- Two main techniques are used for hepatectomy and the implantation of the donor liver:
  - Division of the hepatic veins with caval preservation, followed by a 'piggy back' implant where the new liver, with its own attached vena cava, is anastomosed, cava-to-cava, with the recipient's native vena cava. This can be done side-to-side or end-to-side. Surgery is usually performed with the native vena cava side-clamped, so that surgery can be completed while preserving venous return from the lower part of the body. Some surgeons additionally create a temporary portocaval shunt to maintain gut venous return during the anhepatic phase of the procedure.
  - Removal of the liver with its included portion of the vena cava, followed by implantation of the new liver by anastomosis of the donor vena cava (above and below the liver) into the position of the

original cava. The 2nd technique is used less commonly, as the native vena cava has to be cross-clamped at both points of the division. Venous return during this phase is severely compromised, leading to haemodynamic instability.

- Venovenous bypass is employed in some centres to facilitate venous return from the lower part of the body (femoral vein to right internal jugular or brachiocephalic vein).

- Anastomoses are then made between the donor and recipient portal vein. During this stage, patients with acute liver failure may become profoundly hypoglycaemic, although this is less common in patients being transplanted for chronic liver disease.

- Stage 3 of the procedure is the post-reperfusion phase, beginning with the re-establishment of blood flow through the liver (portal vein to vena cava). This may be accompanied by a massive reperfusion syndrome, comprising the release of cytokines, complement activation, transient reduction in core temperature, arrhythmias, and hypotension. Immediately after reperfusion, there is a rapid elevation in plasma K^+, as it is washed out of the liver graft (although usually minor, this can sometimes reach 8–9mmol/L with poorer-quality grafts). Preservation solution constituents, including adenosine, may also have clinically important, if transient, effects (bradycardia, hypotension).

As the cell membranes of the graft begin to function normally, electrolyte gradients are restored, and a fall in plasma K^+ ensues (sometimes producing ventricular arrhythmias). Hypotension at this stage results from myocardial depression and subsequently vasodilatation. Myocardial depression usually resolves within 2 or 3min, but vasodilatation may persist for several hours. Following reperfusion, the hepatic artery is re-anastomosed, and finally the bile duct reconstructed, either by direct duct-to-duct anastomosis or by construction of a Roux loop.

Liver transplantation

Procedure	Transplantation of entire liver
Time	4–10hr
Pain	Variable, but less than other comparable procedures (e.g. gastrectomy, thoracotomy). Back pain/shoulder pain may be a feature. PCA; avoid NSAIDs
Position	Supine, one or both arms out
Blood loss	Extremely variable. 0–4000mL, X-match 6U (initially, then use uncross-matched blood, if necessary) and FFP 0–12U. Cell saver mandatory (typically reinfuse 2000mL)
Practical techniques	ET, IPPV (details in ➋ Perioperative, p. 566)

Preoperative

- Includes investigation and correction of the factors mentioned on
  ➋ p. 564.
- Usual tests include: FBC, U&Es, clotting, ECG, echocardiogram, chest radiograph, liver/chest CT, spirometry, immunology, virology, and hepatic angiographic MRI scan. High-risk cases may benefit from CPET, stress ECG/dobutamine stress echocardiography.
- Preoperative fluids are not routinely administered, except in patients with renal impairment and hyperacute liver failure (dextrose-based solutions).

Perioperative

- Establish peripheral venous and arterial access before induction.
- Induce anaesthesia (propofol, thiopental, etomidate) and relaxant (atracurium, vecuronium, rocuronium). Vasopressors may be required.
- Ventilate to normocapnia, using O_2-enriched air and volatile agent (isoflurane, sevoflurane, desflurane). Establish infusion of an opioid agent (alfentanil, remifentanil, fentanyl). Patients undergoing transplantation for fulminant liver failure are at risk of raised ICP. In this patient group, volatile agents must be avoided, and TCI propofol may be used. ICP monitoring may be used, depending upon the jaundice–encephalopathy interval (0–7d always—raised ICP in 70% of cases; 7–28d occasionally—raised ICP in 20%; 28–90d seldom—raised ICP in 4%).
- Establish central venous monitoring. TOE is used in some centres. Insert a large-bore NGT. In patients with suspected pulmonary hypertension, there may be a role for PA catheterization.
- Lines for venovenous bypass (10–20% of cases; not used at all in some centres) can either be placed by the surgical team, using femoral cut-downs, or be inserted percutaneously, using extracorporeal

membrane oxygenation lines (21Fr in the right internal jugular and right femoral veins). These are used for both venovenous bypass and large vascular access. Venovenous bypass uses heparin-bonded circuitry, so systemic anticoagulation is unnecessary.

- The patient's temperature must be rigorously maintained, as hypothermia quickly develops, especially during the anhepatic phase or with massive transfusion. A forced warm air blanket should be placed over the patient's head, upper chest, and arms, and another over the legs.
- Fluids are administered by a rapid infusion system and are warmed through a countercurrent heating mechanism (e.g. Level-1® system with high-flow disposables and high-flow taps, allowing transfusion of 600mL/min at body temperature). Perioperatively and post-operatively, the Hct is maintained between 0.26 and 0.32 by infusion of blood, and the RV end-diastolic volume index maintained at 140mL/m² by infusion of other colloidal fluids, as appropriate.
- FFP is transfused, ~2U per unit of blood transfused. Clotting is monitored and fine-tuned by TEG.
- Antifibrinolytic agents are commonly administered—tranexamic acid (15mg/kg bolus, then 5mg/kg/hr by infusion) is given during the anhepatic phase. Aprotinin is no longer used routinely because of concerns over pulmonary thromboembolism.
- A glucose-containing solution is infused continuously to maintain blood sugar.
- Induction immunosuppression (e.g. methylprednisolone 0.5–1g) may be administered before graft reperfusion.
- K^+ and Ca^{2+} should be monitored regularly during surgery and supplemented, when required, to maintain normal values. Hypocalcaemia is common during the anhepatic phase as a result of chelation with unmetabolized citrate. This can lead to cardiac depression and poor clotting. Recheck electrolytes immediately prior to graft reperfusion.
- Severe metabolic acidosis is common but rarely needs correction. At the start of reperfusion, a bolus dose of 10mmol Ca^{2+} is administered to protect the patient against the cardiac effects of K^+ released from the liver graft. Progressive hypotension follows reperfusion. This may be severe and requires small incremental IV doses of adrenaline (50 micrograms) to maintain MAP at a clinically acceptable value (above 70mmHg). In severely ill patients, an infusion of noradrenaline may subsequently be required.
- Some centres use a prophylactic vasopressin analogue, such as terlipressin, before reperfusion.
- Coagulopathy with defibrination and thrombocytopenia may also occur at graft reperfusion. Treatment includes bolus doses of antifibrinolytic drugs and platelets, as guided by the TEG. The haemodynamic and biochemical mayhem of graft reperfusion should resolve rapidly in the event of a functioning liver graft. Persisting acidosis or hypocalcaemia are suggestive of graft 1° non-function, which represents a transplantation emergency. This may necessitate urgent retransplantation.

- There is no proven strategy for avoiding renal failure, other than optimizing fluid balance and avoiding nephrotoxins. In patients at particularly high risk, avoidance of nephrotoxic immunosuppressants (such as ciclosporin, tacrolimus) in the early post-operative period may have a role.

Post-operative

- Patients should be managed on ICU. Early extubation is often feasible. As a result of improved techniques, the mean intensive care stay post-transplant can be reduced to 6hr.
- Analgesia: PCA/epidural/paravertebral blocks have all been used to good effect. Epidural analgesia is possible in only a minority of cases because of coagulopathy. Avoid NSAIDs (interaction with calcineurin inhibitors to induce renal failure).
- Post-operative fluids: maintenance fluid/NG feed at 1.5mL/kg/hr.
- Give blood/HAS/FFP to maintain optimal stroke volume, CVP not above 12mmHg (risk of hepatic venous congestion), Hct at 0.26–0.32, and PT <23s.
- Bleeding post-operatively is relatively uncommon (5–10%).
- Graft 1° non-function occurs in up to 5% of cases, requiring retransplantation.
- Hepatic artery thrombosis occurs in 0.5–5% of cases. Thrombectomy may be attempted, but superurgent retransplantation may be necessary.
- Other post-operative problems include sepsis (10–20%) and acute rejection (up to 40%). These are managed medically with good results.
- Immunosuppression is usually started with standard triple therapy (steroid/azathioprine/tacrolimus) and then tailored to the individual. Other drugs in current use include ciclosporin, mycophenolate mofetil, sirolimus, and basiliximab.
- Long-term results of liver transplantation are encouraging. One-year survival figures in major centres now run between 85% and 95%, with a good long-term quality of life.

Hepatic resection

Procedure	Resection of liver tissue
Time	2–6hr
Pain	As for transplantation. Epidural commoner
Position	Supine, arms out
Blood loss	1000mL, X-match 10U
Practical techniques	ET, IPPV (details on ➜ p. 564 and p. 566)

The major indication for hepatic resection is metastatic colorectal adeno-carcinoma. Most patients presenting for hepatic resection are otherwise relatively fit. Stigmata of liver disease and significant jaundice are unusual, except in those presenting for radical hepatic resection for cholangiocarcinoma where some patients require biliary stenting or drainage preoperatively to reduce jaundice prior to major surgery. The principles underlying anaesthesia for this group of patients are similar to those for any patient undergoing a major laparotomy.

- Major liver resection usually results in 30–75% of functional hepatic tissue being removed. As the remaining hepatocytes function poorly for some days following surgery, short-acting drugs should be used.
- Increasingly, surgeons are exploring the use of minimally invasive techniques.
- Drugs that might compound post-operative hepatic encephalopathy, or which rely on hepatic metabolism, should be avoided (e.g. benzodiazepines).
- Most resections are accomplished with minimal blood loss, but unexpected catastrophic haemorrhage may occur.
- Resection commences with perihepatic dissection and identification of vascular anatomy.
- Intraoperative diagnostic ultrasound is often used to pinpoint lesions requiring resection.
- Bleeding occurs from either vascular inflow (portal vein, hepatic artery) or venous back bleeding. Branches of the hepatic artery and portal vein to the segment of the liver to be resected have usually been ligated, so inflow bleeding should not be a major problem. In practice, the line of resection often passes through a watershed area between vital and devitalized tissue, and remaining inflow bleeding may require additional control by intermittent cross-clamping of vascular inflow to the rest of the liver (the so-called Pringle manoeuvre). This results in a degree of ischaemia–reperfusion injury to the remaining liver tissue, and potentially poor post-operative liver function. This can be minimized by ischaemic preconditioning and the use of intermittent, rather than continuous, clamping.

- Very radical liver resections are now possible where the liver is totally excised and dissected *ex vivo* following perfusion with an ice-cold preservation solution. Healthy parts of the liver are then attached to a Gore-Tex® vena cava graft and reimplanted. This is a prolonged and difficult procedure and anaesthetically similar to a liver transplantation.

Preoperative

- As for any major abdominal surgery, but including screening of liver function and coagulation.

Perioperative

- Patients undergoing major liver resection should have large venous access. Arterial pressure monitoring is common, but no longer universal as surgical techniques have improved. CVP monitoring, at one time universal, is now used on the basis of clinical need—in major centres, the surgeon and anaesthetist can predict those cases where it is likely to be unnecessary.
- Thoracic epidural analgesia is utilized to good effect post-operatively, though there is controversy (but few data) on the risks posed by post-operative coagulopathy.
- The anaesthetic technique employed should be aimed at preserving the hepatic blood flow and minimizing liver injury. Artificial ventilation of the lungs with O_2-enriched air and a volatile agent is the commonest way of achieving this. Isoflurane and sevoflurane may enhance ischaemic preconditioning and help preserve hepatic function where the Pringle manoeuvre is used (intermittent vascular inflow clamping).

Fluid management

- Maintenance of a high CVP used to be common to reduce the risk of air embolism, but it is associated with an increased risk of venous back bleeding. The evidence for clinically significant bubble embolism is mixed, most data deriving from pig studies.
- A reduced CVP substantially reduces bleeding. This approach has dramatically reduced transfusion requirements, with no reported adverse consequences, despite the theoretically increased risk of an air embolus. Techniques for reducing the CVP include epidural boluses and either head-up (reverse Trendelenburg) or head-down (Trendelenburg) tilt. Tilt in either direction can potentially reduce the pressure in the cava at the level of the hepatic veins. It is the author's own practice to use head-up tilt, aiming for CVP of 0–2mmHg.
- Intraoperative blood sampling allows accurate transfusion replacement. FFP is occasionally also required in cases of massive haemorrhage, in cases where there is a prolonged hepatic inflow cross-clamp time, or where very little hepatic tissue remains. However, intraoperative coagulopathy is relatively uncommon. Peak disturbances in clotting are seen on post-operative days 2–3. As with patients undergoing liver transplantation, active warming measures should be taken to maintain the patient's temperature and minimize any coagulopathy.

Post-operative

• Patients should initially be managed in an HDU. Coagulopathy and encephalopathy may develop post-operatively in those who have undergone very major resections. This has practical implications for the timing of removal of epidural catheters, etc.—which may require FFP cover.

• The overall results of radical hepatic resection are very encouraging, with many cases treated that were previously considered inoperable. Many remain disease-free 5yr following resection. In those cases where recurrences arise, further hepatic resection is often possible.

Further reading

Abu Hilal M, Lodge JP (2008). Pushing back the frontiers of resectability in liver cancer surgery. *Eur J Surg Oncol*, **34**, 272–80.

Dalmau A, Sabaté A, Aparicio I (2009). Hemostasis and coagulation monitoring and management during liver transplantation. *Curr Opin Organ Transplant*, **14**, 286–90.

Della Rocca G, Brondani A, Costa MG (2009). Intraoperative hemodynamic monitoring during organ transplantation: what is new? *Curr Opin Organ Transplant*, **14**, 291–6.

Fors D, Eiriksson K, Arvidsson D, Rubertsson S (2012). Elevated PEEP without effect upon gas embolism frequency or severity in experimental laparoscopic liver resection. *Br J Anaesth*, **109**, 272–8.

Lentschener C, Ozier Y (2002). Anaesthesia for elective liver resection: some points should be revisited. *Eur J Anaesthesiol*, **19**, 780–8.

Mandell MS, Tsou MY (2008). The development of perioperative practices for liver transplantation: advances and current trends. *J Chin Med Assoc*, **71**, 435–41.

Park GR, Kang Y, eds. (1995). *Anesthesia and intensive care for patients with liver disease*. London: Butterworth Heinemann.

Endocrine surgery

Pete Ford

Thyroidectomy

Procedure	Removal of all or part of the thyroid gland
Time	1–2hr, depending on complexity
Pain	+/++
Position	Bolster between shoulders with head ring. Head-up tilt
Blood loss	Usually minimal. Potentially major if retrosternal extension
Practical techniques	IPPV + reinforced ETT

General considerations
(See also ➲ p. 157.)
- Complexity can vary from removal of a thyroid nodule to removal of a long-standing retrosternal goitre to relieve tracheal compression.
- Retrosternal goitre is usually excised through a standard incision, but occasionally a sternal split is required.
- Recurrent laryngeal nerves and parathyroid glands may be damaged or removed.
- Straightforward unilateral surgery can be performed under superficial and deep cervical plexus block, but GA is usual (see ➲ p. 1106).

Preoperative
- Ensure that the patient is as near euthyroid as possible (see ➲ p. 157).
- Check for complications associated with hyperthyroidism: AF, tachycardia, proptosis.
- Acute preparation of thyrotoxic patients involves iodine and corticosteroids—both inhibit the conversion of T_4 to T_3 and narrow the window (7–10d) for surgery, necessitating joint management with the surgeon and endocrinologist.
- Check biopsy histology for malignancy.
- Ask about duration of goitre. Long-standing compression of the trachea may be associated with tracheomalacia.
- Ask about positional breathlessness. Assess the airway.
- Examine the neck. How big is the goitre? Consistency?—malignant goitres are hard. Can you feel below the gland (retrosternal spread)? Is there evidence of tracheal deviation (check the radiograph)?
- Look for signs of SVC obstruction—distended neck veins that do not vary with the respiratory cycle.
- Listen for stridor.
- Check the range of neck movements preoperatively, and do not extend them outside of their normal range during surgery.
- Preoperative paracetamol/NSAIDs (PO or PR) help post-operative pain control.

Investigations

- FBC, U&Es, Ca^{2+}, and thyroid function tests are routine.
- Chest radiograph. Check for tracheal deviation and narrowing. Thoracic inlet views may be necessary if retrosternal extension is suspected, and to detect tracheal compression in the anterior–posterior plane (retrosternal enlargement may be asymptomatic).
- CT scan accurately delineates the site and degree of airway encroachment or intraluminal spread. Advisable if there are symptoms of narrowing (e.g. stridor, positional breathlessness) or >50% narrowing on the radiograph. Plain radiographs overestimate diameters, due to magnification effects, and cannot be relied on when predicting ETT diameter and length. Furthermore, a CT scan will help assess the degree of retrosternal extension.
- ENT consultation to document cord function for medico-legal purposes is not routine in all units, unless an abnormality is likely, e.g. previous surgery and malignancy. Pre-existing cord dysfunction may be asymptomatic. Fibreoptic examination also defines any possible laryngeal displacement (useful in airway planning).

Airway planning

- The majority of cases are straightforward, even when there is some tracheal deviation or compression. A reinforced ETT will negotiate most distorted tracheas and permit optimal head positioning. Tracheal compression by a benign goitre will often accommodate an ETT beyond the predicted size, as the gland is soft. Preoxygenation should be followed by IV induction and a neuromuscular-blocking drug (after checking that the lungs can be inflated manually).
- The following features should lead to a more considered approach and may require discussion with the surgeon and radiologist:
  - Malignancy. Cord palsies are likely. Distortion and rigidity of surrounding structures. Possibility of intraluminal spread. The larynx may be displaced. The tumour can produce obstruction anywhere from the glottis to the carina
  - Significant respiratory symptoms or >50% narrowing on chest radiograph or lateral thoracic inlet view
  - Coexisting predictors of difficult intubation.

Options to secure the airway for complicated thyroid surgery

- Teamwork between the anaesthetist and surgeon is the key to successful and safe airway management.
- Inhalational induction with sevoflurane or halothane in patients with stridor and a suspected difficult upper airway. Stridor and decreased minute ventilation delay the onset of sufficiently deep anaesthesia for intubation. Topical LA may be useful.
- Fibreoptic intubation (see ➔ p. 969). Attempts to pass a fibreoptic bronchoscope in an awake patient with stridor are difficult, as the narrowed airway may become obstructed by the instrument. May be useful where there is marked displacement of the larynx or coexisting difficulties with intubation, e.g. ankylosing spondylitis.

- **LMA** may be difficult to place in patients with laryngeal displacement.
- **Tracheostomy** under LA. This will only be possible if the tracheostomy can be easily performed below the level of obstruction.
- Ventilation through **a rigid bronchoscope** is a backup option when attempts to pass an ETT fail. The surgeon and necessary equipment should be immediately available for complex cases, particularly those involving significant mid- to lower tracheal narrowing.
- 'Plan C' of the difficult airway algorithm (perform a cricothyroid puncture) may not be an option.

Perioperative

- Eye padding, lubrication, and tape are important, especially if the patient has exophthalmos.
- Full relaxation is required to accommodate tube movements. LA spray on the ETT reduces the stimulation produced by tracheal manipulation during surgery.
- Electrophysiological monitoring of the recurrent laryngeal nerves is now possible intraoperatively, using specialized reinforced ETTs.
- Securely fix the ETT with tape, avoiding ties around the neck. Access to check the tube is difficult during the procedure.
- Head and neck extension with slight head-up tilt.
- Consider a superficial cervical plexus block for post-operative analgesia. Some surgeons infiltrate SC with LA and adrenaline before starting. LA at the end can produce spurious nerve palsies (see p. 1106).
- Arms to sides, IV extension.
- Communicate with the surgeon if there are excessive airway pressures during manipulation of the trachea. Obstruction may be due to airway manipulation distal to the tube or the bevel of the tube abutting on the trachea.
- Monitor muscle relaxation on the leg.
- In cases of long-standing goitre, some surgeons like to feel the trachea before closing to assess tracheomalacia. They may ask for partial withdrawal of the ETT, so that the tip is just proximal to the operative site.
- At the end of surgery, reverse the muscle relaxant, and extubate with the patient sitting up to reduce venous compression. Use an extubation technique that minimizes coughing to reduce early 2° haemorrhage. Any respiratory difficulty should lead to immediate reintubation. The traditional practice of inspecting the cords immediately following extubation is difficult and unreliable. Possible cord dysfunction and post-operative tracheomalacia are better assessed with the patient awake and sitting up in the recovery room.

Post-operative

- Intermittent opioids with oral/rectal paracetamol and NSAIDs.
- The opioid requirement is reduced with SC infiltration and superficial cervical plexus blocks.
- Use fibreoptic nasendoscopy if there is doubt about recurrent laryngeal nerve injury.

Post-operative stridor

- **Haemorrhage** with tense swelling of the neck. Remove clips from the skin, and sutures from the platysma/strap muscles to remove the clot. *In extremis*, this should be done at the bedside. Otherwise return to theatre without delay. A haematoma will affect lymphatic and venous drainage of the upper airway, causing laryngeal and pharyngeal oedema. Removing the haematoma will not always restore airway patency immediately.
- **Tracheomalacia.** Long-standing large goitres may cause tracheal collapse. This is a very rare complication. Immediate reintubation, followed by tracheostomy, may be necessary.
- **Bilateral recurrent laryngeal nerve palsies.** This may present with respiratory difficulty immediately post-operatively or after a variable period. Stridor may only occur when the patient becomes agitated. Assess by fibreoptic nasendoscopy. May require tracheostomy.

Other post-operative complications

Hypocalcaemia

- Hypocalcaemia from parathyroid removal is rare. Serum Ca^{2+} should be checked at 24hr, and again daily if low.
- Presentation—may present with signs of neuromuscular excitability, tingling around the mouth, or tetany. May progress to fits or ventricular arrhythmias.
- Diagnosis—carpopedal spasm (flexed wrists, fingers drawn together) may be precipitated by cuff inflation (Trousseau's sign). Tapping over the facial nerve at the parotid may cause facial twitching (Chvostek's sign). Prolonged QT interval on ECG.
- Treatment: serum Ca^{2+} below 2mmol/L should be treated urgently with 10mL of 10% calcium gluconate over 3min plus alfacalcidol 1–5g orally (calcium gluconate is preferable, as calcium chloride will cause tissue necrosis if extravasation occurs). Check the level after 4hr, and consider Ca^{2+} infusion if still low. If hypocalcaemic, but level above 2mmol/L, treat with oral Ca^{2+} supplements (see also ⮕ p. 161).

Thyroid crisis

- This is rare, as hyperthyroidism is usually controlled beforehand with antithyroid drugs and β-blockers. May be triggered in uncontrolled or undiagnosed cases by surgery or infection.
- Diagnosis: increasing HR and temperature. May be difficult to distinguish from MH. Higher mixed venous $PvCO_2$ and higher creatinine phosphokinase in MH.
- Treatment: see ⮕ p. 158.

Pneumothorax

Pneumothorax is possible if there has been retrosternal dissection.

Further reading

Cook TM, Morgan PJ, Hersch PE (2011). Equal and opposite expert opinion. Airway obstruction caused by a retrosternal thyroid mass: management and prospective international expert opinion. *Anaesthesia*, **66**, 828–36.

Dempsey GA, Snell JA, Coathup R, Jones TM (2013). Anaesthesia for massive retrosternal thyroidectomy in a tertiary referral centre. *Br J Anaesth*, **111**, 594–9.

Farling PA (2000). Thyroid disease. *Br J Anaesth*, **85**, 15–28.

Parathyroidectomy

Procedure	Removal of solitary adenoma or four glands for hyperplasia
Time	1–3hr
Pain	+/++
Position	Bolster between shoulders with head ring. Head-up tilt
Blood loss	Usually minimal
Practical techniques	IPPV + ETT

General considerations

(See also ➲ p. 160.)

- Usual indication for operation is 1° hyperparathyroidism from parathyroid adenoma.
- With preoperative localization, removal of simple adenoma has been described using sedation and LA. GA is more usual.
- Carcinoma may require *en bloc* dissection.
- Total parathyroidectomy may also be performed in 2° hyperparathyroidism associated with CRF.
- Hypercalcaemia may produce significant debility, particularly in the elderly.

Preoperative

Hypercalcaemia is usual. With moderate elevation, ensure adequate hydration with 0.9% NaCl. Levels over 3mmol/L should be corrected before surgery, as follows:

- Urinary catheter.
- One litre of 0.9% NaCl in the 1st hour, then 4–6L over 24hr.
- Pamidronate 60mg in 500mL of saline over 4hr.
- Watch for fluid overload. CVP measurement may be necessary in some patients. Monitor electrolytes, including Mg^{2+}, phosphate, and K^+.

Severe hypercalcaemia may occasionally necessitate emergency surgery. It may cause arrhythmias and may antagonize the effects of NDMRs.

- Preoperative imaging using ultrasound and technetium-99m sestamibi scanning may be used to localize parathyroid adenomas, allowing a minimal access or targeted approach with a 2cm incision over the suspected gland.
- 2° hyperparathyroidism occurs 2° to low serum Ca^{2+} in CRF. In this situation:
  - Total parathyroidectomy may be required. Control afterwards is easier if no functioning parathyroid tissue is left
  - Dialysis will be required preoperatively
  - The risk of bleeding is increased
  - Alfacalcidol is usually started preoperatively

- 1° hyperparathyroidism has been associated with an increased risk of death from CVS disease, hypertension, LV hypertrophy, valvular and myocardial calcifications, impaired vascular reactivity, alterations in cardiac conduction, impaired glucose metabolism, and dyslipidaemia. PTH has serious consequences on cardiac function in renal failure
- A less utilized technique these days is to use methylthioninium chloride (methylene blue) to highlight the parathyroid glands. Most useful in four-gland hyperplasia; parathyroids are highly vascular and take up the dye faster than surrounding tissues. If given too early, however, the effect is lost, as the surrounding tissue colours. The usual dose is 5mg/kg, diluted in 500mL, given over 1hr prior to surgery. Complications of methylthioninium chloride (methylene blue) use include restlessness, paraesthesiae, burning sensation, chest pain, dizziness, headache, and mental confusion. Pulse oximetry will not be accurate if the infusion is too fast.

Perioperative

- Similar anaesthetic considerations as for thyroid surgery, using either a reinforced ETT or LMA.
- Airway encroachment is not usually a problem.
- Operation times may be unpredictable, especially if frozen section or parathyroid assays are performed.
- Consider active heat conservation.
- Point-of-care PTH assays are available, making intraoperative measurement of PTH possible in minimally invasive or targeted surgery, thereby allowing a rapid assessment of success intraoperatively.
- Extubation requires a cough-free technique, reducing the incidence of early 2° haemorrhage.

Post-operative

- Serum Ca^{2+} checked at 6hr and 24hr. Hypocalcaemia may occur (for diagnosis and treatment, see Thyroidectomy, → p. 574 and also → p. 577). Continuation of alfacalcidol in 2° hyperparathyroidism lessens the chance of hypocalcaemia post-operatively.
- Perform fibreoptic nasendoscopy if recurrent laryngeal nerve damage is suspected.
- Pain not usually severe, especially with LA infiltration or superficial cervical plexus blocks. Rectal paracetamol is useful. Avoid NSAIDs in patients with poor renal function.

Further reading

Mihai R, Farndon JR (2000). Parathyroid disease and calcium metabolism. *Br J Anaesth*, **85**, 29–43.

Phaeochromocytoma

Procedure	Removal of one or two adrenals or extra-adrenal tumour
Time	1–2hr open, possibly longer if laparoscopic
Pain	+/++ (depending if open or laparoscopic)
Position	Lateral or supine for open, lateral for laparoscopic
Blood loss	Variable
Practical techniques	IPPV + ETT, art and CVP lines, ± cardiac output monitor

- Tumours of chromaffin cells secreting noradrenaline (commonest), adrenaline, or dopamine (least common). May secrete >1 amine.
- May secrete other substances, e.g. VIP, ACTH.
- Ninety-nine per cent occur in adrenals; 10% bilateral; may be anywhere along the sympathetic chain from the base of the skull to the pelvis.
- Most are benign; a few are malignant.
- Occur in all age groups, less commonly in children.
- Can occur in association with MEN2A (medullary thyroid carcinoma, parathyroid adenomas) and MEN2B (medullary thyroid carcinoma and marfanoid features). Both have abnormalities of the *RET* oncogene on chromosome 10 (see ⊃ p. 577).
- Also found in patients with neurofibromatosis and von Hippel–Lindau syndrome (see ⊃ p. 308).

Presentation

- Hypertension can be constant, intermittent, or insignificant.
- Association of palpitations, sweating, and headache with hypertension has a high predictive value.
- Anxiety, nausea and vomiting, weakness, and lethargy are also common features.
- Acute presentations include pulmonary oedema, MI, and cerebrovascular episodes.
- Can present perioperatively. Unless the diagnosis is considered and appropriate treatment instituted, the mortality rate is high—up to 50%.

Diagnosis

- Clinical suspicion.
- With increased genetic testing of families, more patients are being diagnosed before they become symptomatic.
- Urinary catecholamines or their metabolites (metadrenaline and normetadrenaline) measured either over 24hr or overnight.
- CT radiocontrast may provoke phaeo crises, and its use must be avoided in unblocked patients. Modern contrast agents may be used.

- MIBG (*meta*-iodobenzylguanidine) scan—a radiolabelled isotope of iodine taken up by chromaffin tissue.
- MRI.
- Search in the abdomen first, and widen the search if tumour not located. MIBG is particularly helpful in revealing unusual sites.

Investigations relevant to anaesthesia

- Echocardiography—patients with a history of ischaemia or signs of heart failure require a cardiac echocardiography. Rarely, patients can present with a catecholamine cardiomyopathy.
- Blood glucose—excess catecholamines result in glycogenolysis and insulin resistance; some patients become frankly diabetic.

Preoperative

- Refer the patient to an experienced team. It is not acceptable to manage on an occasional basis.
- Usual management is sympathetic blockade with first α- and then β-blocker, if required, for tachycardia (**phenoxybenzamine**—a non-competitive, non-selective α-blocker and then **atenolol/ propranolol/metoprolol**).
- Phenoxybenzamine causes postural hypotension, lethargy, and nasal congestion.
- Whereas α-blockade is generally considered a necessity, the use of β-blockade is more controversial, and some anaesthetists will actively avoid them at the time of surgery.
- Preoperative blockade:
  - Allows safe anaesthesia for the removal of the tumour
  - Prevents hypertensive response to induction of anaesthesia
  - Limits surges in BP seen during tumour handling.
- Avoid unopposed β-blockade—theoretical risk of increasing vasoconstriction and precipitating a crisis. Although this has been reported, many patients will already have received β-blockers for hypertension before presentation, without adverse effects.
- Prazosin and doxazosin have been used. These are competitive, selective $α_1$-blockers. They do not inhibit presynaptic noradrenaline reuptake and thus avoid the tachycardia seen with non-selective α-blockade. The literature contains reports both in favour and against the use of selective blockade.
- Calcium channel blockers (particularly nicardipine) have been used. This inhibits noradrenaline-mediated Ca^{2+} influx into smooth muscle but does not affect catecholamine secretion by the tumour.
- Metirosine is an inhibitor of catecholamine synthesis. It is toxic and not widely used.
- There are no absolute criteria for fitness for surgery.

Assessment of sympathetic blockade

- Patients will often be admitted a few days prior to surgery to observe BP control and/or have had outpatient 24hr ambulatory BP monitoring.
- Aim for BP <140/90, with HR <100bpm.

- Erect and supine BP and HR. Should exhibit a marked postural drop >20mmHg, with a compensatory tachycardia.
- The duration of blockade is determined by the practicalities of tumour localization and scheduling of surgery.
- Blockade is started to treat symptoms, as well as to prepare for surgery.

Perioperative

- Laparoscopic or open adrenalectomy through a midline, transverse, or flank incision (introduction of gas for laparoscopic resection can result in hypertension in normal subjects, and this may be exaggerated in patients with phaeochromocytomas).
- Premedication, as required (e.g. temazepam 20–30mg).
- Monitoring to include direct BP and CVP (triple lumen to allow drug infusions). Consider cardiac output monitoring in patients with CVS disease and catecholamine cardiomyopathy.
- Large-bore IV access.
- Monitor and maintain temperature, particularly during laparoscopic resection which can be prolonged.
- Induction: avoid agents that release histamine, and thus catecholamines (use propofol, alfentanil or remifentanil, and vecuronium or rocuronium).
- Hypotension is unlikely at induction and can be treated with either ephedrine, metaraminol, or phenylephrine. Due to preoperative α-blockade, doses will likely need to be increased. Rarely, dilute adrenaline may be required.
- Maintenance: use isoflurane or sevoflurane. Desflurane should be avoided, as it can cause sympathetic nervous system activation.
- Consider epidural with opioid and LA for open procedures (sympathetic blockade will not prevent catecholamine-induced vasoconstriction); otherwise fentanyl/alfentanil/remifentanil until tumour removal, when morphine (10–20mg) can be substituted.
- Nicardipine and Mg^{2+} are also useful (block catecholamine release, block receptors, provide direct vasodilator, and possibly myocardial protection).
- Mg^{2+} is started prior to induction, given as a bolus of 2–4g, and then continued at a rate of 1–2g/hr. It is normal for the patient to feel nauseated with the Mg^{2+} bolus.
- Surges in BP can occur at induction, formation of the pneumoperitoneum, and with tumour handling. The fluctuations in BP tend to be transient, and medication needs to respond in a similar fashion. Hypertension can be treated in a number of ways: intermittent 2g boluses of Mg^{2+}, boluses of remifentanil, phentolamine, sodium nitroprusside, or labetalol (if associated with a tachycardia).
- Control HR at <100bpm with the β-blocker of choice.
- Once the tumour is resected, BP takes several minutes to decline. Prevent hypotension by ensuring an adequate preload. Maintain a high CVP of 10–15mmHg. Several litres of a crystalloid may be needed.
- Hypotension following resection can be due to low cardiac output or a low SVR. Treat the former with low-dose adrenaline, and the latter with metaraminol or phenylephrine. Vasopressin has been used in

resistant hypotension. Terlipressin 1mg bolus, followed, if required, by vasopressin, starting at 0.04U/min, then titrated to effect.
- It is unusual to require inotropic support by the time the patient is ready to leave theatre, unless there are coexisting medical problems.

Post-operative
- Patient should be nursed in ICU/HDU for 12hr.
- Monitor blood glucose. The withdrawal of catecholamine excess can lead to severe hypoglycaemia.
- If both adrenals are resected, the patient will require steroid support immediately. Hydrocortisone 100mg bolus in theatre, decreasing to maintenance dose after surgical stress. Fludrocortisone 0.1mg daily may be commenced with oral intake.
- Even when only one adrenal is removed, patients may occasionally be relatively hypoadrenal and require support. If this is suspected (e.g. unexpectedly low BP), a small dose of hydrocortisone (50mg) will do no harm, while the result of cortisol estimation is awaited.

Special considerations
Pregnancy
- There are many reports of the combination of a newly diagnosed phaeochromocytoma and pregnancy. Overall mortality is up to 17%.
- Phenoxybenzamine and metoprolol are safe.
- If phaeochromocytoma is diagnosed before mid trimester, it should be resected at this stage.
- There is a high mortality associated with normal delivery; consider lower-segment Caesarean section (LSCS), with or without resection of the phaeochromocytoma, at the same procedure.

Management of an unexpected phaeochromocytoma
- Any patient who has unexplained pulmonary oedema, hypertension, or severe unexpected hypotension should prompt consideration of the diagnosis; however, it can be very difficult. There is no quick available test to support the diagnosis in the acute situation.
- Once the diagnosis has been considered, if possible, surgery should be discontinued to allow acute treatment, investigation, and blockade prior to definitive surgery. Attempts to remove the tumour during a crisis may result in significant morbidity, or even mortality.
- Treatment acutely should consist of vasodilators and IV fluid; this may be counterintuitive in a patient with severe pulmonary oedema. The circulating volume in patients with phaeochromocytoma may be markedly reduced, and vasodilatation will result in a profound drop in BP. GTN can usually be successfully titrated in this situation.
- Patients who present with hypotension have an acutely failing heart due to profound vasoconstriction. These are the most difficult patients in whom to make the diagnosis and to treat. Additional catecholamines in this situation merely fuel the fire but are difficult to resist. The mortality rate is very high.

Further reading

James MFM (2010). Adrenal medulla: the anaesthetic management of phaeochromocytoma. In: James MFM, ed. *Anaesthesia for patients with endocrine disease*. Oxford: Oxford University Press, pp. 149–69.

O'Riordan JA (1997). Pheochromocytomas and anesthesia. *Int Anesthesiol Clin*, **35**, 99–127.

Prys-Roberts C (2000). Phaeochromocytoma—recent progress in its management. *Br J Anaesth*, **85**, 44–57.

Subramaniam R (2011). Phaeochromocytomas—current concepts in diagnosis and management. *Trends Anaesth Crit Care*, **1**, 104–10.

Urological surgery

Mark Daugherty

Cystoscopic procedures

- Includes cystoscopy, TURP, bladder neck incision, transurethral resection of bladder tumour, ureteroscopy, and/or stone removal or stent insertion.
- The majority of patients are undergoing procedures for benign prostatic hypertrophy or carcinoma of the bladder. The incidence of both these conditions increases markedly over 60yr, and bladder cancer is smoking-related, so patients frequently have CAD and COPD.
- FBC, creatinine, and electrolytes should be checked preoperatively, because bladder cancers can bleed insidiously. Both bladder cancer and benign prostatic hypertrophy can cause an obstructive uropathy/renal impairment, and drugs and the technique should be chosen accordingly.
- **Flexible cystoscopy** is largely used for diagnostic purposes, does not require full bladder distension, and can normally be performed under LA. Biopsies can be taken this way, with only a small amount of discomfort, and skilled surgeons can perform retrograde ureteric catheterizations. Occasional patients insist on sedation/GA for flexible cystoscopy. Midazolam or propofol is ideal.
- Rigid cystoscopy requires GA, due to the scope diameter and the use of an irrigating solution to distend the bladder and allow visualization of the surgical field. If large volumes of irrigant are absorbed, systemic complications due to fluid overload can result (see TURP syndrome, → p. 593).
- Spinal anaesthesia works well for rigid cystoscopic procedures and is commonly used for TURP. Sensory supply to the urethra, prostate, bladder neck, and bladder mucosa is from S2 to S4. Pain from bladder distension, however, is carried by T10–L2, so a higher block is required. Many patients will request sedation. In the elderly population, 1–2mg of midazolam is usually adequate. Higher doses may result in loss of airway control, confusion, and restlessness. A low-dose propofol infusion is an alternative. Spinal anaesthesia is advantageous for patients with severe COPD, as long as the patient can lie flat without coughing.
- Either hyperbaric or isobaric bupivacaine can be used. Hyperbaric bupivacaine usually produces a higher block than the isobaric solution, especially when the injection is performed with the patient in the lateral position and then turned supine; 2.5–3mL of 'heavy bupivacaine' 0.5% usually gives a block to T10. Do not tilt the patient head-down, unless the block is not sufficiently high.
- Patients with chronic chest disease tend to cough on lying flat. During surgery under regional block, coughing can seriously impair surgical access. Sedation can help to reduce the cough impulse.
- Patients with spinal cord injuries (see → p. 237) often require repeated urological procedures. Bladder distension during cystoscopy is very stimulating and prone to cause autonomic hyperreflexia, so a GA or spinal is advisable—check previous anaesthetic charts.
- Take particular care positioning elderly patients in lithotomy, especially those with joint replacements.

- **Permanent pacemakers** are not normally a problem, even with the almost continuous diathermy required for TURP, as long as the diathermy plate is positioned caudally, usually on the thigh.
- **Implantable defibrillators** can be triggered by the diathermy so need to be switched off preoperatively (see ➲ p. 81).
- **Penile erection** can make cystoscopy difficult and surgery hazardous. It usually occurs due to surgical stimulation when the depth of anaesthesia is inadequate, and can usually be managed by deepening anaesthesia. If the erection still persists, small doses of ketamine can be useful.
- **Antibiotic prophylaxis** (single dose of an agent with Gram-negative cover) is often required, particularly if the patient has an indwelling urinary catheter, an obstructed ureter, and positive results on preoperative midstream urine (MSU). Gentamicin 3mg/kg is popular.
- **DVT prophylaxis**: graduated compression stockings are generally considered adequate in low-risk patients undergoing cystoscopic procedures, as most will mobilize rapidly following surgery. However, low-dose heparin should also be used in patients with additional risk factors or those who have recently undergone other surgery and a period of immobility (see ➲ p. 11).

Post-operative complications of rigid cystoscopic procedures

- **Perforation of the bladder** can occur and can be difficult to recognize, especially in the presence of a spinal block, which may mask abdominal pain. Perforations are classified as extraperitoneal, when pain is said to be maximal in the suprapubic region, and intraperitoneal when there is generalized abdominal pain, shoulder tip pain due to fluid tracking up to the diaphragm, and signs of peritonism. Intraperitoneal perforations need fluid resuscitation and urgent surgery to prevent progressive shock.
- **Bacteraemia** can have a very dramatic onset with signs of profound septic shock. If the diagnosis is made quickly, there is usually a rapid response to IV fluids and appropriate antibiotics (e.g. gentamicin—single dose of 3–5mg/kg, followed by cefuroxime 750–1500mg 8-hourly; modify according to sensitivities on preoperative MSU). Always suspect this diagnosis with unexplained hypotension after a seemingly straightforward urinary tract instrumentation.
- **Bladder spasm** is a painful involuntary contraction of the bladder occurring after any cystoscopic technique, most commonly in patients who did not have an indwelling catheter preoperatively. Diagnosis is supported by the failure of irrigation fluid to flow freely in and out of the bladder. It responds poorly to conventional analgesics but is often eased by small doses of IV benzodiazepine, e.g. diazepam 2.5–5mg or hyoscine butylbromide 20mg slow IV or IM.
- **Bleeding and fluid overload** are dealt with under anaesthesia for TURP (see ➲ p. 590).

Miscellaneous urological procedures

Table 24.1 presents the important information for those procedures which are not covered in the individual topics within this chapter.

Table 24.1 Other urological procedures

Operation	Description	Time (min)	Pain (+ to ++++)	Position	Blood loss/X-match	Notes
Ureteroscopy	Investigate obstruction, remove stones	20–60	+	Lithotomy	Nil	LMA + SV. Check renal function. Possible antibiotic prophylaxis
Insert ureteric stent	To relieve ureteric obstruction, using image intensifier	20	+	Lithotomy	Nil	LM + SV. Possible antibiotic prophylaxis
Remove ureteric stents	Cystoscopy to retrieve stent	10–20	+	Lithotomy	Nil	Awake or LMA + SV. Often possible with flexi scope and LA
Insert suprapubic catheter	Transcutaneous insertion of catheter into full bladder	15	+	Lithotomy or supine	Nil	Sedation + LA or LMA + SV. Often frail patients with advanced neurological disease
Bladder neck incision	Transurethral diathermy incision of prostate at narrowed bladder neck	15–30	++	Lithotomy	Nil	LMA + SV. Younger patients than TURP
Urethroplasty	Reconstruction of urethra narrowed by trauma or infection—very variable procedure	90–240	++++	Lithotomy	300–2000mL	ETT + IPPV ± epidural. Beware prolonged lithotomy. Consider epidural for post-operative pain

Procedure	Description	Time (min)		Position	Blood loss	Anaesthetic considerations
Nesbitt's procedure	Straightening of penile deformation from Peyronie's disease	60–120	+++	Supine	Nil	LMA + SV. Consider caudal or penile block
Circumcision	Excision of foreskin	20	++	Supine	Nil	LMA + SV + LA. Penile block or caudal useful. Topical lidocaine gel to take home. LA alone possible in frail elderly
Urethral dilatation	Stretching of narrowed urethra with serial dilators	10	+	Lithotomy or supine	Nil	LMA or spinal. Possible antibiotic prophylaxis
Urethral meatotomy	Incision to widen urethral meatus	10	+	Supine	Nil	LMA + SV
Orchidectomy	Removal of testis—through groin or scrotum, depending on pathology	20–45	++	Supine	Nil	LMA + SV + ilioinguinal block. Need to block to T9/10 if using regional technique due to embryological origins
Vasectomy	Division of vas deferens via scrotal incision	20–40	++	Supine	Nil	LMA + SV. Often under LA
Pyeloplasty	Refashioning of obstructed renal pelvis via loin incision. Children and young adults	90–120	++++	Lateral 'kidney position'	300–500mL	ETT + IPPV + epidural/PCA. Similar considerations as nephrectomy. May be significant blood loss in children

Transurethral resection of the prostate

Procedure	Cystoscopic resection of the prostate using diathermy wire—monopolar/glycine irrigation being replaced by bipolar resectoscopes with saline irrigation
Time	30–90min, depending on size of the prostate
Pain	+
Position	Lithotomy ± head-down
Blood loss	Very variable (200–2000mL), can be profuse and continue post-op. G&S
Practical techniques	Spinal ± sedation is method of choice GA, LMA, and SV GA, ETT, and IPPV

Preoperative
- Patients are frequently elderly with coexistent disease and multiple medications.
- Check creatinine and serum Na^+; suggest postponing surgery if Na^+ is significantly low, as this is likely to fall further with absorption of irrigant.
- Heart failure or uncontrolled AF is a particular risk due to fluid absorption. Aim for optimal medical control preoperatively.
- Assess the mental state and communication—spinal anaesthesia is difficult if the patient is confused or deaf.

Perioperative
- Insert a large cannula, and use warmed IV fluids.
- **Spinal anaesthesia**: in theory, it is easier to detect changes in the mental state and signs of fluid overload (see p. 593); shown in some, but not all, studies to reduce blood loss; 2.5–3mL of bupivacaine (plain or hyperbaric) is usually adequate; frequent BP check—hypotension unusual with the above doses but can occur suddenly; check BP at the end when the legs are down (unmasks hypotension).
- **GA**: consider intubation if the patient is very obese or has a history of reflux; intraoperative fentanyl or morphine plus multimodal analgesia (paracetamol, NSAID, and tramadol/codeine) is usually adequate; unusual to need opioids post-operatively.
- **Blood loss** can be difficult to assess. In theory, can be calculated from measuring Hb and the volume of discarded irrigation fluid. In practice, it is commoner to visually assess the volume and colour, but this can be misleading. Checking the patient's Hb with a bedside device (e.g. HemoCue®) is useful. Blood loss is generally related to the size and weight of prostatic tissue excised (normally 15–60g), the duration of resection, and the expertise of the operator.
- Antibiotic prophylaxis usually required.

- Obturator spasm (see ➔ p. 595).
- Fluid therapy: crystalloid can be used initially. Bear in mind that a significant volume of hypotonic irrigating fluid may be absorbed, so do not give excessive volumes, and never use glucose. Consider switching to a colloid if hypotension results from the spinal anaesthesia. Replace blood loss with a colloid, and be ready to transfuse if the Hb falls below the transfusion trigger.

Post-operative

- Bladder irrigation with saline via a three-way catheter continues for ~24hr, until bleeding is reduced—inadvertent slowing of irrigation can lead to clot retention.
- There is generally little pain, but discomfort from the catheter or bladder spasm may be a problem (see ➔ p. 587).
- Severe pain suggests clot retention, bladder spasm (see ➔ p. 587), or bladder perforation (see ➔ p. 587).
- Clot retention can give a very distended painful bladder and vagal symptoms. It requires washout, sometimes under anaesthetic.
- Bleeding can continue and require further surgery—resuscitation may be necessary.
- Measure FBC, creatinine, and electrolytes the day following surgery.

Special considerations

- Hypothermia may result when large volumes of irrigation fluid are used (the fluid should be warmed to 37°C).
- If the prostate is very large (>100g), a simple open prostatectomy may carry fewer complications.
- The risk of complications increases with resection times of >1hr. If a resection is likely to take longer than an hour, consider limiting the resection to one lobe only, leaving the other to be done at a later date.
- Bipolar TURP has been shown to reduce the overall complication rate, transfusion rate, and TURP syndrome.

Laser TURP and transurethral vaporization of the prostate (TUVP)

- Several 'minimally invasive' techniques using lasers and other forms of heat have been developed which reduce the prostate size. These generally cause less bleeding and absorption of fluid so are sometimes chosen for patients perceived to be at higher risk from conventional TURP.
- The few RCTs show a reduction in the need for transfusion with minimal blood loss, reduced absorption of bladder irrigation, and reduced length of stay in hospital, with potential for day surgery. However, no clear difference in the complication rate or long-term urological outcome has yet been demonstrated.
- Anaesthetic requirements and the duration of surgery are similar to TURP, although the perceived benefits of spinals are no longer significant.

Brachytherapy for localized prostate carcinoma

- This consists of insertion of radioactive pellets through rods positioned in the prostate under ultrasound control. This is usually done outside of theatre in the radiotherapy department.
- The patient may require two or more procedures in the same day. Repeated GAs are possible, but a spinal catheter topped up before each procedure works well. Consider risks of remote site anaesthesia.
- For a single treatment, a spinal, using 0.5% bupivacaine with fentanyl 15 micrograms, is effective and allows safe transfer to radiotherapy.

TURP syndrome

- A combination of fluid overload and hyponatraemia,[1,2] which occurs when large volumes of irrigation fluid are absorbed via open venous sinuses. This syndrome is far less likely with the use of bipolar resectoscopes and saline irrigation. Laser enucleation has virtually eliminated the risk.
- Irrigation fluid must be non-conductive (so that the diathermy current is concentrated at the cutting point) and non-haemolytic (so that haemolysis does not occur if it enters the circulation), and must have neutral visual density, so that the surgeon's view is not distorted. For these reasons, it cannot contain electrolytes but cannot be pure water. The most commonly used irrigant is glycine 1.5% in water, which is hypotonic (osmolality 220mmol/L).
- Some irrigation fluid is normally absorbed, at about 20mL/min, and, on average, patients absorb a total of 1–1.5L, but absorption of up to 4–5L has been recorded. In clinical practice, it is almost impossible to accurately assess the volume absorbed.
- The amount of absorption depends upon the following factors:
  - Pressure of infusion—the bag must be kept as low as possible to achieve an adequate flow of irrigant at minimum pressure, usually 60–70cm above bladder, never >100cm. Higher pressures increase absorption
  - CVP—more fluid is absorbed if the patient is hypovolaemic or hypotensive
  - Long duration of surgery and large prostate—problems are commoner with surgery lasting >1hr or with a prostate weighing >50g
  - Blood loss—large blood loss implies a large number of open veins.
- TURP syndrome is more likely to occur in patients with poorly controlled heart failure. Do not increase the risks of fluid overload by giving an unnecessarily large volume of IV fluid.
- Glycine is a non-essential amino acid which functions as an inhibitory neurotransmitter, and it is unclear whether glycine toxicity plays a part in the syndrome. Ammonia is a metabolite of glycine and may also contribute to CNS disturbance.
- Ensure that the irrigation fluid is changed to saline in recovery to prevent further absorption of hypotonic glycine.
- Signs of **pulmonary oedema**, **cerebral oedema**, and **hyponatraemia** are the usual presenting features. They will be detected earlier in the awake patient. Mortality is high, unless recognized and treated promptly.
- **Early symptoms** include restlessness, headache, and tachypnoea, and these may progress to respiratory distress, hypoxia, frank pulmonary oedema, nausea, vomiting, visual disturbances, confusion, convulsions, and coma. In the anaesthetized patient, the only evidence may be tachycardia and hypertension. Rapid absorption of a large volume can lead to reflex bradycardia. Hypotension can also occur. The diagnosis can be confirmed by low serum Na^+. An acute fall to <120mmol/L is always symptomatic. A quick check of Na^+ is often possible by checking an ABG (use venous blood, unless concerned about acid/base balance).

- If detected intraoperatively, bleeding points should be coagulated, surgery terminated as soon as possible, and IV fluids stopped. Give furosemide 40mg, and check serum Na^+ and Hb. Support respiration with O_2 or intubation and ventilation, if required. Administer IV anticonvulsants, if fitting.
- Both severe acute hyponatraemia and over-rapid correction of chronic hyponatraemia can result in permanent neurological damage (most commonly central pontine myelinolysis).
- If serum Na^+ has fallen acutely to <120mmol/L and is associated with neurological signs, consider giving hypertonic saline (NaCl 1.8–3%) to restore Na^+ to around 125mmol/L (see ➲ p. 178).
- The volume of 3% saline (in mL) which will raise serum Na^+ by 1mmol/L is twice the TBW (in L). TBW in men is about 60% of body weight, i.e. for a 70kg man:
  - Calculate TBW = 70 × 0.6 = 42L
  - Therefore, 84mL of 3% saline will raise serum Na^+ by 1mmol/L
  - A volume of 1008mL of 3% saline over 24hr will raise serum Na^+ by 12mmol/L.
- In practice, give 1.2–2.4mL/kg/hr of 3% saline until symptomatic improvement. This should produce a rise in serum Na^+ of 1–2mmol/L/hr.
- Correction should ideally not be faster than 1.5–2mmol/L/hr for 3–4hr, then 1mmol/L/hr until symptomatic improvement or Na^+ >125mmol/L. Maximum rise should not exceed 12mmol/L in 24hr.
- Beware of compounding effects on Na^+ by other simultaneous treatments (diuretics, colloids, etc.).
- Admit to ICU/HDU for management, including regular measurements of Na^+.[1,2]

References

1 Adrogué HJ, Madias NE (2000). Hyponatremia. *N Engl J Med*, **342**, 1581–9.
2 Gravenstein D (1997). TURP syndrome: a review of the pathophysiology and management. *Anesth Analg*, **84**, 438–46.

Transurethral resection of bladder tumour

Procedure	Cystoscopic diathermy resection of bladder tumour
Time	10–40min
Pain	+/++ and bladder spasm
Position	Lithotomy
Blood loss	0 to >500mL
Practical techniques	GA with LMA; spinal ± sedation

Preoperative

- Commonest in smokers—check for CAD and COPD.
- Check Hb—chronic blood loss is common.
- Check renal function.
- Refer to previous anaesthetic charts—many patients have repeated surgery.

Perioperative

- Obturator spasm occurs when the obturator nerve, which runs adjacent to the lateral walls of the bladder, is directly stimulated by the diathermy current. It causes adduction of the leg and can seriously impair surgical access and increase the risk of bladder perforation. It can usually be controlled by reducing the diathermy current.
- Antibiotic prophylaxis (see p. 1211).

Post-operative

- Pain can be a problem with extensive resections—NSAIDs are useful (check renal function), and oral opioids may be needed.
- Bladder spasm is common (see p. 587).

Special considerations

- If using a spinal anaesthetic, ensure block to above T10 (see p. 586).

Open simple prostatectomy and radical prostatectomy

Procedure	Simple retropubic (Millen procedure): open excision of grossly hypertrophied benign prostate shelled out of capsule; radical retropubic: open complete excision of malignant prostate and pelvic lymph nodes with anastomosis
Time	60–120min (simple), 120–180min (radical)
Pain	+++/++++
Position	Supine
Blood loss	300–1000mL (simple); 500–2000mL (radical) X-match 2U, and use cell salvage if available
Practical techniques	ETT, IPPV, remifentanil ± rectus sheath catheters ± PCA

Preoperative
- Simple—elderly men, as for TURP.
- Radical—patients are selected if relatively young and medically fit.
- Check renal function.
- Consider HDU bed for radical prostatectomy, depending on local practice and medical factors.

Perioperative
- Prepare for major blood loss with a large IV cannula, blood warmer, heated blankets, etc.
- A Pfannenstiel-type incision is used for simple, and lower midline for radical prostatectomy.
- Consider using an arterial line and CVP line or cardiac output monitoring, particularly in patients with CVS disease.
- Ensure blood is available, and reorder intraoperatively, as necessary.
- Cell salvage techniques can be useful where blood loss is expected to be substantial (radical prostatectomy).
- Air embolism is a possible complication.
- Epidural should be used cautiously intraoperatively to avoid exacerbating hypotension due to blood loss.
- Consider using remifentanil infusion intraoperatively.

Post-operative
- Epidural or rectus sheath catheters, and possibly PCA.

Nephrectomy and partial nephrectomy

Procedure	Excision of kidney for tumour, other pathologies, or live donor
Time	1–2.5hr
Pain	+++/++++
Position	Supine or lateral (kidney position)
Blood loss	Depends on pathology, 300 to >3000mL. G&S/X-match, as required
Practical techniques	ETT + IPPV ± thoracic epidural or wound infiltration catheter

Preoperative

- Ascertain the pathology and surgical incision planned before deciding on the technique and monitoring.
- Check Hb—renal tumours can cause anaemia without blood loss.
- Check BP and renal function—'non-functioning' kidney or renovascular disease is associated with renal impairment and hypertension.
- Consider cell salvage intraoperatively.
- Check serum electrolytes—renal tumour can cause inappropriate ADH secretion.
- Check the chest radiograph if there is a tumour—there may be metastases, pleural effusions, etc.
- Radiofrequency ablation (RFA) is being developed for some tumours and avoids the need for open surgery. Laparoscopic nephrectomy is also becoming commoner (see ⊃ p. 528).

Perioperative

- Increasingly, nephrectomy and partial nephrectomy are being performed laparoscopically if the tumour size and location permit.
- For large tumours and polycystic kidneys, surgical practice in the UK is an open laparotomy via a paramedian or transverse incision for a tumour, and a loin incision with a retroperitoneal approach for other pathologies or donor nephrectomy.
- Loin incision requires the 'kidney position', i.e. lateral with the patient extended over a break in the table—a marked fall in BP is common on assuming this position due to reduced venous return from the legs and possible IVC compression. Further compression during surgery may result in a severe reduction in venous return and cardiac output.
- Ask the surgeon about the predicted extent of surgery—a large tumour may necessitate extensive dissection, possibly via a thoracotomy, or opening of the IVC to resect tumour margins, in which case sudden, torrential blood loss is possible. Occasionally, the IVC is temporarily clamped to allow dissection and to control haemorrhage; this gives a sudden fall in cardiac output. Inform the surgeon if BP falls suddenly,

have colloid and blood checked and available to infuse immediately under pressure, and have a vasoconstrictor or inotrope, such as metaraminol or ephedrine, prepared.
- Use large IV cannulae, blood warmer, CVP, and arterial line if the procedure is anything other than an uncomplicated, non-malignant nephrectomy or a small isolated tumour.
- If an epidural is used, a high block will be required post-operatively, but use it cautiously intraoperatively until bleeding is under control.

Post-operative
- All approaches are painful—epidurals are useful but need to cover up to T7/8 for a loin incision. Rectus sheath catheters may be useful for the anterior approach. PCA or an opioid infusion is an alternative.
- Intercostal blocks will give analgesia for several hours after a loin incision.
- Wound infiltration catheters have also proved very effective.
- NSAIDs are useful if renal function is good post-operatively and the patient is not hypovolaemic. Use cautiously.
- Monitor hourly urine output.

Partial nephrectomy
- Increasingly performed for a well-localized tumour or in a patient with only one kidney (beware precarious renal function).
- Blood loss can be large, as vessels are more difficult to control.
- Some surgeons suggest the administration of mannitol 12.5g, furosemide 10mg, and/or heparin 3000IU before clamping of the renal artery in an attempt to maintain renal perfusion and minimize ischaemia. Cooling with ice can also be used.
- If the renal function is markedly impaired preoperatively, optimization of fluid balance throughout the perioperative period is extremely important. Admission to HDU post-operatively should be considered.

Radical cystectomy

Procedure	Excision of bladder plus urinary diversion procedure (e.g. ileal conduit) or neo-bladder reconstruction (orthotopic bladder formation)
Time	3–5hr (longer with bladder reconstruction)
Pain	++++
Position	Lithotomy plus head-down
Blood loss	700 to >3000mL, X-match 4U, use cell salvage
Practical techniques	ETT, IPPV, art line ± oesophageal Doppler/CVP ± rectus sheath catheters/PCA/epidural

Preoperative

- Consider the use of an 'enhanced recovery pathway'.
- Check for IHD/COPD, plus renal function/FBC.
- Book an HDU bed, depending on local practice/coexisting problems.
- Ensure thromboprophylaxis is prescribed.

Perioperative

- The commonest post-operative problem is prolonged ileus, which contributes significantly to morbidity and mortality, and several of the measures recommended are thought to reduce its incidence.
- Prepare for major blood loss; large IV cannulae, blood warmer, CVP or oesophageal Doppler cardiac output, and direct arterial monitoring are routine. Ensure blood is available, and reorder intraoperatively, as necessary. Consider auto-transfusion intraoperatively. If blood salvage is used, discontinue it when the bowel is opened.
- If rectus sheath catheters are to be used, insert after induction. Surgical incision is subumbilical midline and does not permit easy placement of catheters during surgery.
- Remifentanil infusion gives stable anaesthesia and controllable BP; mild hypotension can aid surgery by reducing blood loss.
- Epidurals are now used infrequently, but, if placed, use cautiously intraoperatively; there will be plenty of time after the main blood-losing episode to establish an adequate block.
- Take measures to prevent heat loss, e.g. warm-air blanket.
- Antibiotic prophylaxis as for bowel resection.
- Use of NGTs is now rare—ask the surgeon if specifically required.
- Blood loss can be insidious from pelvic venous plexuses; consider weighing swabs.
- Air embolism is a possible complication, as in any major pelvic surgery.

Post-operative

- Rectus sheath catheters (for up to 5d), with or without a PCA, have proven very effective. Visceral pain tends to last for 24–36hr post-operatively, requiring parenteral opioids. This technique enables early mobilization, return of bowel function, and decreased post-operative ileus/length of hospital stay. There is some evidence that anastomotic leak is increased with the use of NSAIDs, so use cautiously after checking the renal function.
- Use CVP/urine output to guide fluid replacement—requirements are usually large due to intraperitoneal loss and ileus.
- Urine output via a new ileal conduit is difficult to monitor, as drainage tends to be positional. Following orthotopic reconstruction, urine drains from a number of different catheters so needs to be calculated each hour to monitor output.
- Early feeding, as part of enhanced recovery, may be associated with a reduced incidence of certain post-operative complications.
- Leakage from a ureteric anastomosis may present as urine in the abdominal drain—confirm by comparing biochemistry of the drainage fluid and urine from the conduit.

Robot-assisted laparoscopic prostatectomy

Procedure	Robotically assisted laparoscopic prostatectomy
Time	120–180min
Pain	+/++
Position	Lithotomy with steep Trendelenburg
Blood loss	Minimal
Practical techniques	ETT, IPPV, remifentanil, art line

Preoperative

- The commonest use of surgical robots to date is in urology, mostly for radical prostatectomy (robot-assisted laparoscopic prostatectomy, RALP).
- Advantages to the surgeon over conventional laparoscopy includes provision of 3D vision, filtration of any hand tremor, scaling of hand movements, greater range of movements within the patient, and a comfortable and stable position.
- Advantages to the patient may include a reduction in blood loss, pain, and length of stay ± a reduced incidence of incontinence and erectile dysfunction.
- Positioning will include a steep head-down tilt, so premedicate with a PPI (omeprazole 40mg) to reduce risk of gastric regurgitation.

Perioperative

- Positioning of the patient is important.
- Long operative times with steep head-down tilt has been associated with:
  - Neurapraxia (especially brachial). Take care with positioning, and use shoulder brace. Do not hyperextend the legs in lithotomy
  - Facial/airway oedema and stridor
  - Acid burns to eyes and oral ulceration due to reflux of gastric acid. Consider an oral gastric tube (not NG due to epistaxis risk), throat pack, and protect the eyes with lubricating ophthalmic ointment/pads
  - Increased ICP (exacerbated by hypercapnia) and increased intraocular pressure (beware patients with glaucoma).
- Ensure ETT is inserted as short as possible (risk of endobronchial intubation), and tape in position to minimize cerebral venous obstruction.
- Access to the patient is poor, so ensure reliable, large-bore venous access on the left side because of robot arm positioning.
- Robotic equipment is locked in position once inserted into the abdomen, so any inadvertent patient movement can cause grave surgical complications—use infusions of muscle relaxant or remifentanil.

- Avoid using N_2O. A remifentanil infusion works well and allows intermittent boluses of muscle relaxant only as required.
- Communicating with the surgeon may be difficult due to the bulk and space required for the equipment—the team needs to be familiar with the audio equipment and also able to undock and remove the robot quickly in case of an emergency requiring resuscitation.
- Large urine output can interfere with the surgical field—suggest minimal IV fluid (<1000mL) until anastomosis is complete (may also reduce the risk of airway oedema).

Post-operative

- Perform leak test prior to extubation to assess airway swelling.
- Cerebral oedema may be problematic. A short-acting volatile agent with remifentanil allows rapid assessment of the conscious level post-operatively. Most patients experience a degree of cerebral irritation or agitation initially on wakening.
- Post-operative pain is considerably less than for open procedures but can still be severe enough to require opioid analgesia for a short period, in addition to simple analgesics.

Percutaneous stone removal

Procedure	Endoscopic excision of renal stone via nephrostomy
Time	60–90min
Pain	++/+++
Position	Prone oblique
Blood loss	Variable, 0–1000mL
Practical techniques	ETT and IPPV

Preoperative

- Usually healthy young and middle-aged adults, but stones may be due to an underlying metabolic problem or due to bladder dysfunction from a neurological disability.
- Check renal function.

Perioperative

- Patient initially in the lithotomy position to insert ureteric stents, then turned semi-prone to place nephrostomy posterolaterally below the 12th rib, under radiographic control—potential to dislodge lines and for pressure area damage.
- Consider an armoured ETT to prevent kinking, and secure well. Need to turn the head towards the operative side, so best to position the ETT in the same side of the mouth.
- Support the chest and pelvis to allow abdominal excursion with ventilation.
- Support and pad the head, arms, and lower legs, and pad the eyes.
- Check ventilation during and after position changes.
- May need to temporarily interrupt ventilation for radiographs.
- Antibiotic prophylaxis may be required.

Post-operative

- Pain from nephrostomy is variable.
- Multimodal—paracetamol, NSAIDs (check renal function), PCA morphine, or oral tramadol.

Special considerations

- Hypothermia can occur if large volumes of irrigation fluid are used.
- Insertion of nephrostomy is often close to the diaphragm, with the possibility of breaching the pleura, causing a pneumothorax or hydrothorax—if in doubt, perform a CXR post-operatively.
- Rupture of the renal pelvis is a recognized complication when large volumes of irrigant may enter the retroperitoneal space.
- Post-operative Gram-negative septicaemia is a significant risk after any urinary tract surgery for stones (see ● p. 587).

Extracorporeal shock wave lithotripsy

Procedure	Non-invasive fragmentation of renal stones using pulsed ultrasound
Time	20–40min
Pain	+/++
Blood loss	Nil
Practical techniques	Sedation for adults. GA/LMA for children

In the early days of extracorporeal shock wave lithotripsy, patients were suspended in a water bath in a semi-sitting position, which produced a number of problems for the anaesthetist. Developments in the 1980s meant that a water bath was no longer required, and more recent refinements of the ultrasound beam have made it less uncomfortable, so that, with most current lithotripters, only a few patients need anaesthesia or sedation.

Preoperative
- Patients often undergo repeated lithotripsy, so refer to previous treatment records where possible.
- Premedication with paracetamol/NSAID (note renal function) is usually effective for treatment.

Perioperative
- Lateral position with arms above the head.
- Renal stones are located using ultrasound or an image intensifier, and the shock wave focused on the stones.
- Antibiotic prophylaxis may be required.

Post-operative
Mild discomfort only—oral analgesics or NSAIDs are adequate.

Special considerations
- Shock wave can cause occasional dysrhythmias, which are usually self-limiting. If persistent, the shock waves can be delivered in time with the ECG (refractory period). Judicious use of anticholinergics (glycopyrronium 200 micrograms) will increase the HR and increase the frequency of delivered shock.
- Pacemakers can be deprogrammed by the shock wave—seek advice from a pacemaker technician.
- Energy from shock waves is released when they meet an air/water interface. It is advisable to use saline, rather than air, for 'loss of resistance' if siting an epidural.

Renal transplant

Procedure	Transplantation of cadaveric or live donor organ
Time	90–180min
Pain	++/+++
Position	Supine
Blood loss	Not significant—500mL
Practical techniques	ETT and IPPV, CVP

Preoperative
- Usual problems related to CRF and uraemia (see ➋ p. 121).
- Chronic anaemia is common (Hb usually around 8g/dL). Do not transfuse to normal levels.
- There has usually been recent haemo- or peritoneal dialysis, therefore some degree of hypovolaemia and possibly residual anticoagulation.
- Check post-dialysis K^+. The patient's normal value may be quite high.
- Avoid A–V fistulae when placing the IV cannula. Avoid using a large forearm or antecubital veins, if possible (may be needed for future fistulae).

Perioperative
- Fluid load prior to induction—wide swings in arterial pressure are not uncommon.
- Commonly used agents that can be used in renal failure include sevoflurane, atracurium, remifentanil, and fentanyl.
- Consider a central line with strict aseptic technique, and monitor CVP—many units have protocols.
- Prior to graft insertion, gradually increase CVP to 10–12mmHg (using colloids or crystalloids) to maintain optimal graft perfusion and promote urine production.
- Maintain normothermia.
- Most centres use a cocktail of drugs, once the graft is perfused, to enhance survival (e.g. hydrocortisone 100mg, mannitol 20% 60mL, furosemide 80mg or more). Have these prepared.

Post-operative
- PCA is usually adequate; if using morphine, beware of much reduced clearance. A fentanyl PCA is preferable. An epidural is also possible, but not usually necessary. There is a danger of bleeding on insertion (residual anticoagulation from haemodialysis, poor platelet function, etc.) and problems with fluid loading and maintaining BP post-operatively.
- Avoid NSAIDs.
- Monitor CVP and urine output hourly. Maintain mild hypervolaemia to promote diuresis. Many units have protocols for fluid balance, e.g. previous hour's urine output plus 50mL of saline per hour.

Further reading

Berger JS, Alshaeri T, Lukula D, Dangerfield P (2013). Anesthetic considerations for robot assisted gynecologic and urology surgery. *J Anesth Clin Res*, **4**, 1–7.

Conacher ID, Soomro NA, Rix D (2004). Anaesthesia for laparoscopic urological surgery. *Br J Anaesth*, **93**, 859–64.

Dutton TJ, Daugherty MQ, Mason RG, McGrath JS (2014). Implementation of the Exeter enhanced recovery programme for patients undergoing radical cystectomy. *BJU Int*, **113**, 719–25.

Hanson R, Zornow M, Conlin M, Brambrink A (2007). Laser resection of the prostate: implications for anesthesia. *Anesth Analg*, **105**, 475–9.

Irvine M, Patil V (2009). Anaesthesia for robot-assisted laparoscopic surgery. *Contin Educ Anaesth Crit Care Pain*, **9**, 125–9.

Maffezzini M, Campodonico F, Canepa G, Gerbi G, Parodi D (2008). Current perioperative management of radical cystectomy with intestinal urinary reconstruction for muscle-invasive bladder cancer and reduction of the incidence of postoperative ileus. *Surg Oncol*, **17**, 41–8.

O'Donnell AM, Foo ITH (2009). Anaesthesia for transurethral resection of the prostate. *Contin Educ Anaesth Crit Care Pain*, **9**, 92–6.

SarinKapoor H, Kaur R, Kaur H (2007). Anaesthesia for renal transplant surgery. *Acta Anaesthesiol Scand*, **51**, 1354–67.

Gynaecological surgery

John Saddler

General principles

Many gynaecological patients are fit and undergo relatively minor procedures as day cases. Others are inpatients undergoing more major surgery. Elderly patients often require operations to relieve pelvic floor prolapse.

- Many patients are apprehensive, even for relatively minor surgery.
- PONV is a particular problem. With high-risk patients, use appropriate techniques; avoid N_2O, and give prophylactic antiemetics.
- Pelvic surgery is associated with DVT—ensure that adequate prophylactic measures have been taken.
- Prophylactic antibiotics reduce post-operative wound infection rates for certain operations—check your hospital protocol.
- Patients on the OCP should be managed according to local protocol; guidelines are suggested on ➲ p. 11.
- Vagal stimulation may occur during cervical dilatation, traction on the pelvic organs or the mesentery, or during laparoscopic procedures.
- Take care during patient positioning. Patients are often moved up or down the table, when airway devices can be dislodged and disconnections can occur. Pre-existing back or joint pain may be worsened in the lithotomy position, and, if the legs are supported in stirrups, there is a potential for common peroneal nerve injury.
- It may be reasonable to ask the gynaecologist to administer analgesic drugs rectally during anaesthesia—ensure that you have the patient's permission to do so.
- During laparotomies, ensure that patients are kept warm.
- During major gynaecological surgery, considerable blood loss may occur, and surgery may be prolonged.
- Many gynaecological operations formerly done through an open approach (e.g. hysterectomy, tubal pregnancy repair) are now done primarily using laparoscopic techniques.

Miscellaneous gynaecological procedures

Table 25.1 presents the important information for those procedures which are not covered in the individual topics within this chapter.

Table 25.1 Other gynaecological procedures

Operation	Description	Time (min)	Pain (+ to +++++)	Position	Blood loss/X-match	Notes
Colposuspension	Abdominal procedure for stress incontinence	40	+++	Supine	G&S	ETT, IPPV
Cone biopsy/ LLETZ	Removal of the terminal part of the cervix through the vagina	30	++	Supine	G&S	May bleed post-operatively. LMA, SV
Laparotomy, investigative	Abdominal assessment of pelvic mass	120	++++	Supine	2U	Ovarian tumours may be adherent to adjacent structures. Potentially large blood loss
Myomectomy	Abdominal excision of fibroids from uterus	60	+++	Supine	G&S	Blood loss may be greater than expected. ETT, IPPV
Oophorectomy	Removal of ovaries	40	+++	Supine	G&S	ETT, IPPV
Repair, anterior	Repair of anterior vaginal wall	20	++	Lithotomy	Nil	Often combined with vaginal hysterectomy. LMA ± caudal
Repair, posterior	Repair of posterior vaginal wall	20	++	Lithotomy	Nil	Often combined with vaginal hysterectomy. LMA ± caudal
Sacrocolpopexy	Abdominal repair of vault prolapse	60	+++	Supine	G&S	ETT, IPPV
Sacrospinous fixation	Vaginal operation for vault prolapse	40	++	Lithotomy	Nil	

(Continued)

Table 25.1 (Contd.)

Operation	Description	Time (min)	Pain (+ to +++++)	Position	Blood loss/X-match	Notes
Shirodkar suture	Insertion of suture around cervix to prevent recurrent miscarriage	20	++	Lithotomy	Nil	May need antacid prophylaxis (see ◑ p. 750)
Thermoablation	Thermal obliteration of endometrium	20	++	Lithotomy	Nil	May require opioids
TCRE	Endoscopic resection of endometrium	30	+	Lithotomy	Nil	Systemic absorption of water may occur from the glycine solution Treat as for TURP syndrome
Vulvectomy, simple	Excision of vulva	90	+++	Lithotomy	G&S	
Vulvectomy, radical	Excision of vulva and lymph nodes	150	++++	Lithotomy	2U	Epidural analgesia recommended

TCRE, transcervical resection of endometrium.

Minor gynaecological procedures

Procedure	D&C, hysteroscopy, oocyte retrieval
Time	20–30min
Pain	+
Position	Supine, lithotomy
Blood loss	Nil
Practical techniques	LMA, SV, day case

Minor operations that enable access to the endometrial cavity through the cervix include:
- **Dilatation and curettage (D&C):** largely superseded now by hysteroscopic examination.
- **Hysteroscopy:** the surgeon is able to visualize the endometrial cavity using a rigid scope. The hysteroscope is flushed with crystalloid to enable better visualization. Fluid volume is measured to ensure there is no uterine perforation (suspect if the volume recovered is less than the volume infused).
- A brief GA may be requested for an oocyte retrieval procedure. Patients will have received prior hormonal stimulation to induce the production of oocytes in the ovaries. These are removed, with the aid of ultrasound, through a transvaginal approach. This may also be performed with sedation.

Preoperative
- Many patients will be treated as day cases.
- Consider prescribing paracetamol and NSAIDs ± ranitidine/PPI.

Perioperative
SV using a face mask or LMA, propofol (infusion or intermittent bolus), or volatile.

Post-operative
Simple oral analgesics, plus antiemetic of choice.

Special considerations
- Vagal stimulation may occur with cervical dilatation; anticholinergic drugs should be immediately available.
- Stimulation may also induce laryngospasm—ensure adequate depth of anaesthesia.
- There is a risk of uterine perforation through the fundus whenever surgical instruments are introduced through the cervix and into the endometrial cavity. Antibiotics are usually prescribed if this is thought to have occurred. A small perforation can be treated expectantly; larger perforations may require a laparoscopy to evaluate the extent of the perforation.

Evacuation of retained products of conception, suction or vaginal termination of pregnancy

Procedure	ERPC; STOP/VTOP
Time	10–20min
Pain	+
Position	Supine, lithotomy
Blood loss	Usually minimal
Practical techniques	LMA, SV, day case

Preoperative
- Evacuation of retained products of conception (ERPC): remaining products of conception may have to be surgically removed after an incomplete miscarriage. This usually occurs between 6 and 12wk gestation. Substantial blood loss may have occurred preoperatively and may continue perioperatively. IV access and crystalloid/colloid infusion are required if the haemorrhage appears anything more than trivial.
- Suction or vaginal termination of pregnancy (STOP/VTOP) is a procedure undertaken at up to 12wk gestation.

Perioperative
- LMA or face mask. Intubate unfasted emergency patients.
- Avoid high concentrations of volatile agents due to the relaxant effect on the uterus. Propofol induction followed by intermittent boluses or TIVA and an opioid (fentanyl) is appropriate.
- A drug to help contract the uterus and reduce bleeding is usually requested. Oxytocin 5U is usually given. This may cause an increase in HR. The use of ergometrine, a vasoconstrictor, is declining, because it raises arterial pressure.

Post-operative
Oral analgesics and antiemetic.

Special considerations
- Pregnancies beyond 12wk can be terminated surgically by dilatation and evacuation (D&E). The procedure is similar to a STOP/VTOP, but there is greater potential for blood loss. Larger doses of oxytocin may be required.
- If there are symptoms of reflux oesophagitis, ranitidine or PPI premedication and intubation are indicated.
- If a pregnancy has gone beyond 16wk, it may be terminated medically with prostaglandin. These patients may still require an ERPC and should be managed similarly to a retained placenta (see ➜ p. 752).

Laparoscopy/laparoscopic sterilization

Procedure	Intra-abdominal examination of gynaecological organs through a rigid scope ± clips to Fallopian tubes
Time	15–30min
Pain	+/++
Position	Supine, lithotomy, head-down tilt
Blood loss	Nil
Practical techniques	ETT/IPPV, LMA/SV, day case

Preoperative

• Usually young and fit. Give oral analgesics preoperatively.

Perioperative

• Use a short-acting NDMR. 'Top-ups' may be required. Monitor with a nerve stimulator, and use reversal agents, if necessary, at the end.
• Endotracheal intubation.
• Give a short-acting opioid (e.g. fentanyl).
• Encourage infiltration of the skin incisions with local analgesia.
• An alternative technique for uncomplicated short procedures is to use SV and an LMA. This is only suitable for non-obese patients—the potential for gastric regurgitation and aspiration must be assessed carefully. If gas insufflation is hampered by abdominal muscle tone, deepen anaesthesia or use a small dose of mivacurium, and assist ventilation until return of SV.

Post-operative

Further opioids (e.g. morphine) may be required.

Special considerations

• As many of these procedures are short and may only take 10–15min, mivacurium may be useful.
• Bradycardias are common due to vagal stimulation. Atropine should be readily available. Many anaesthetists administer glycopyrronium prophylactically at induction.
• Shoulder pain is common post-operatively due to diaphragmatic irritation. Although self-limiting, it can be difficult to treat and is reduced by expelling as much CO_2 from the abdomen as possible at the end of the procedure.
• Occasionally, surgical instruments damage abdominal contents, and a laparotomy is required.
• Very rarely, CO_2 gas may be inadvertently injected intravascularly, resulting in gas embolus (see ➲ p. 413). This results in V/Q mismatch, with a fall in $ETCO_2$, impaired cardiac output, hypotension, arrhythmias,

and tachycardia. If this is thought to have occurred, the surgeon should be alerted; N_2O should be discontinued, and the patient should be resuscitated.
- If an LMA is used, consider premedication with oral ranitidine or a PPI, and the use of a device with a gastric channel (e.g. ProSeal).

Tension-free vaginal tape

Procedure	Tape insertion for stress incontinence
Time	20min
Pain	+
Position	Lithotomy
Blood loss	Minimal
Practical techniques	Various (see ➲ Perioperative, p. 615)

Preoperative
- Give oral analgesics preoperatively.

Perioperative
- Several anaesthetic techniques are currently employed.
- Some surgeons are happy with a spontaneous breathing technique with an LMA.
- Many require the patient to cough, so that the tension in the tapes can be adjusted. Here, a spinal or an LA technique can be employed, usually with sedation and/or TCI.
- Take care with positioning (lithotomy position).

Post-operative
- Patients may be day cases, but some stay overnight.
- Opioids (e.g. morphine) are only rarely required.

Special considerations
- Anaesthetic technique is largely determined by the surgical approach. Liaise carefully with the surgeon before induction of anaesthesia.

Abdominal hysterectomy

Procedure	Removal of uterus through abdominal incision (may also include ovaries as bilateral salpingo-oophorectomy)
Time	1hr, often longer
Pain	+++
Position	Supine, head-down
Blood loss	250–500mL, G&S
Practical techniques	ETT, IPPV, PCA

Preoperative
- Patients may be anaemic if they have had menorrhagia or post-menopausal bleeding.
- Renal function may be abnormal if an abdominal mass has been compressing the ureters.
- Many patients are anxious and may require premedication.
- PONV is common.
- Ensure prophylaxis for DVT has been initiated.

Perioperative
- Oral intubation and ventilation.
- If a Pfannenstiel ('bikini line') incision is anticipated, consider bilateral ilioinguinal blocks with bupivacaine (see ➲ p. 1122). The patient should be warned about the possibility of femoral nerve involvement. 'TAP' blocks are an alternative (see ➲ p. 1123).
- Deep muscle relaxation is required to enable the surgeon to gain optimal access.
- Antibiotic prophylaxis is usually required.
- Head-down positioning is often requested, which may cause ventilation pressures to rise with diaphragmatic compression. CVP will increase, and gastric regurgitation is also more likely.
- Blood loss is variable; some hysterectomies bleed more than expected. Cross-match blood early if bleeding appears to be a problem.
- Heat loss through the abdominal incision can be significant. Use a warm-air blanket over the upper body during the operation.

Post-operative
- Pain is usually reasonably well controlled with a PCA. This can be supplemented with LA blocks or wound infiltration, regular paracetamol, and NSAIDs. Regular administration of antiemetics may be required.
- O_2 therapy is indicated for 24hr post-operatively or longer. Patients usually tolerate nasal cannulae better than face masks.

Special considerations

- **Epidurals** provide useful analgesia in patients who have had midline ('up-and-down') incisions. **Rectus sheath catheters** are increasingly being used as an alternative to epidurals, usually in combination with a PCA.
- **Wertheim's hysterectomy** is undertaken in patients who have cervical and uterine malignancies. The uterus, Fallopian tubes, and often the ovaries are removed, but, in addition, the pelvic lymph nodes are dissected out. These operations take much longer, and there is a potential for substantial blood loss. An arterial line and goal-directed therapy should be considered. Epidural analgesia is useful for post-operative pain.

Vaginal hysterectomy

Procedure	Removal of the uterus through the vagina
Time	50min
Pain	+/++
Position	Lithotomy
Blood loss	Variable, usually <500mL
Practical techniques	LMA, SV, caudal. Spinal

Preoperative

A degree of uterine prolapse enables the operation to be performed more easily. Patients are often older and may be frail with underlying cardiac or respiratory problems.

Perioperative

- A spontaneously breathing technique with LMA is usual. Give a longer-acting IV opioid (e.g. morphine 5–10mg), and supplement with NSAIDs, if appropriate.
- A caudal with 20mL of bupivacaine 0.25% improves post-operative analgesia, but beware toxic levels (see below).
- Spinal anaesthesia (3mL of bupivacaine 0.5%), with or without supplemental sedation, is a satisfactory alternative.
- The surgeon usually infiltrates the operative field with a vasoconstrictor to reduce bleeding. Local analgesia infiltration at the same time will aid post-operative analgesia. Monitor the CVS system carefully during this period, and ensure that safe doses of these drugs are not exceeded.
- Take care with positioning. Many patients will have hip and/or knee arthritis and may have had surgery to these joints. Lloyd–Davies leg slings may be preferable to leg stirrups if leg joints articulate poorly. The common peroneal nerve may be compressed in leg stirrups.
- Keep the patient warm, preferably with a warm-air blanket.

Post-operative

- This operation is less painful than an abdominal hysterectomy. If opioids, NSAIDs, and local analgesia infiltration/caudal have been given intraoperatively, further analgesia needs are often very modest (IM/oral opioids).
- Elderly patients may require supplemental O_2 post-operatively.

Special considerations

- The procedure is often supplemented by either an anterior or a posterior repair which reduces bladder and bowel prolapse through the vagina.
- It is usually not possible to remove the Fallopian tubes and ovaries during a vaginal hysterectomy because of the restricted surgical field.

- Laparoscopically assisted vaginal hysterectomy (LAVH) is designed to enable the uterus, Fallopian tubes, and ovaries to be removed through the vagina. The operation begins with a laparoscopy, at which the broad ligament is identified and detached. There is a risk of haemorrhage and ureteric damage at this stage. Once satisfactory mobility of the gynaecological organs has been achieved at laparoscopy, they are then removed through a vaginal incision. Total laparoscopic hysterectomy (TLH) is becoming commoner where the gynaecological organs are removed abdominally. The anaesthetic principles for laparoscopy apply, except that a longer-acting muscle relaxant and an ETT should be used. PCA analgesia should be considered post-operatively.

Ectopic pregnancy

Procedure	Laparotomy to stop bleeding from ruptured tubal pregnancy
Time	40min
Pain	++/+++
Position	Supine
Blood loss	Can be massive, X-match 2U
Practical techniques	ETT, IPPV, PCA

Preoperative
- The presentation is variable. A stable patient may have ill-defined abdominal pain and amenorrhoea; others may present with life-threatening abdominal haemorrhage. At least one large-bore IV cannula should be inserted prior to theatre, and crystalloids, colloids, or blood products infused, according to the clinical picture.
- FBC, cross-match, and possibly a clotting screen should be requested on admission.
- Seek help from a 2nd anaesthetist if the patient is unstable.

Perioperative
- RSI.
- Careful IV induction if blood loss is suspected. Consider using ketamine if shocked.
- Continue IV fluid resuscitation.

Post-operative
- Clotting abnormalities are not uncommon if large volumes of blood have been lost. Send a clotting screen for analysis, if necessary, and organize FFP and platelet infusions, if indicated.
- Actively warm the patient in the recovery room with heated blankets, if possible.
- PCA for post-operative analgesia.

Special considerations
- Stable patients may undergo a diagnostic laparoscopy. Be aware that the pneumoperitoneum may impede venous return, resulting in hypotension.
- In most centres now, the operation is performed laparoscopically, and only converted to a laparotomy if there are any complications.

Ear, nose, and throat surgery

Fred Roberts

General principles

Airway problems are the major concern in ENT surgery, related to both the underlying clinical problem and the shared airway.

Presenting pathology may:
- Produce airway obstruction
- Make access difficult or impossible.

Surgeons working in, or close to, the airway can:
- Displace, obstruct, or damage airway equipment
- Obscure the anaesthetist's view of the patient
- Limit access for the anaesthetist during operation
- Produce bleeding into the airway (intra- and post-operatively).

The surgeon and anaesthetist should plan together to use techniques/equipment that provide good conditions for surgery, while maintaining a safe, secure airway. Whenever an airway problem is suspected intraoperatively, correcting it is the first priority, stopping the surgery, if necessary. Other structures around the head are inaccessible during surgery and need protection—especially the eyes. Ensure they are kept closed with appropriate tape, padded as necessary, and that pressure from equipment is prevented, especially for long cases.

Airway/ventilation management

Tracheal tube or laryngeal mask airway
- Traditionally, an ETT has been used for airway protection for the majority of ENT work.
- Preformed RAE tubes provide excellent protection with minimal intrusion into the surgical field.
- An oral (south-facing) RAE tube is used for nasal and much oral surgery, although a nasal tube (north-facing) allows better surgical access to the oral cavity.
- An LMA or equivalent supraglottic airway, usually of the reinforced flexible type, is the alternative approach. It offers adequate protection against aspiration of blood or surgical debris and reduces complications of tracheal intubation/extubation. It restricts surgical access to a greater degree, however, and is more prone to displacement during surgery (with potentially catastrophic results).

Spontaneous ventilation or intermittent positive pressure ventilation
- Continuous NMB is not required for most ENT surgery.
- Many ENT anaesthetists still favour SV, regarding movement of the reservoir bag as a valuable sign of airway integrity.
- If SV is used via an ETT, mivacurium is preferable to succinylcholine for intubation, as myalgia is particularly troublesome in a population where early mobilization is likely. Alternatives include combinations of high-dose propofol and alfentanil/remifentanil, or deep inhalational anaesthesia.
- IPPV enables faster recovery and return of airway reflexes.

Deep or light extubation

- Many ENT procedures create bleeding into the airway. Suction (and pack removal) under direct vision before extubation is essential in such cases, taking care not to traumatize any surgical sites.
- One particular danger site for blood accumulation is the nasopharynx behind the soft palate, an area not readily visible. Blood pooling here can be aspirated following extubation, with fatal results ('**coroner's clot**'). It is best cleared using either a nasal suction catheter or a Yankauer sucker rotated so its angled tip is placed behind the uvula.
- Laryngospasm can follow extubation, particularly in children, from recent instrumentation of the larynx or irritation by blood. The risk is minimized by extubating either deep or light (not in between).
- Deep extubation is best suited to SV. At the end of surgery, continue, or even increase, the volatile agent concentration, but change gases to 100% O_2 (to increase the FRC store). After careful suction, insert a Guedel airway; turn the patient left lateral/head-down (**tonsil position**); check respiration is regular (turning can produce transient coughing/ breath-holding), then extubate.
- Check airway/respiration are fine, and keep the patient in this position until airway reflexes return. Since the patient remains unconscious initially in recovery, care from appropriately skilled recovery staff is essential, with an anaesthetist immediately available in case of airway complications.
- In the early recovery period, continuous low suction can be done via a catheter just protruding from the Guedel airway.
- Light extubation is best suited to IPPV. After careful suctioning, any residual NMB is reversed, inhalational agents discontinued, and the trachea extubated after laryngeal reflexes have returned.
- Light extubation often produces a brief period of coughing/restlessness initially. This is less frequent with the use of opioids.
- Light extubation is recommended in all patients with a difficult airway or significant respiratory compromise.

Throat packs

- A throat pack[1] (wet gauze or tampons) is often used around the ETT/ LMA to absorb blood that might otherwise pool in the upper airway.
- It is particularly useful during nasal operations where bleeding can be substantial and is not cleared during surgery.
- The pack must be removed before extubation, as it can lead to catastrophic airway obstruction if left. Systems to ensure removal include:
  - Tie or tape the pack to the ETT
  - Place an identification sticker on the ETT or patient's forehead
  - Include the pack in the scrub nurse's count
  - *Always perform laryngoscopy prior to extubation.*

Nasal vasoconstrictors

- Topical vasoconstrictors are normally used to reduce bleeding in nasal surgery, administered by spray, gel, or soaked swabs. Moffett (1947) described a topical mixture which is still used (with assorted modifications), consisting of:
  - 2mL of cocaine 8%
  - 1mL of adrenaline 1:1000
  - 2mL of sodium bicarbonate 1%.
- Proprietary decongestants are a commonly used alternative such as pseudoephedrine or phenylephrine.
- Systemic absorption can result in a transient sympathomimetic response.
- Infiltration with adrenaline-containing solutions may be used in addition, with greater risk of systemic effects.

Remifentanil

- The intense opioid action of remifentanil, combined with its rapid recovery profile, has led to its widespread use in ENT, particularly for major cases.
- Normally given by infusion, clinical applications include:
  - Middle ear surgery/major head and neck resections (controlled arterial pressure reduces bleeding)
  - Parotidectomy (facilitates IPPV without relaxant)
  - Laryngoscopy/pharyngoscopy (attenuates hypertensive response).
- Beware of bradycardia/hypotension when used at induction, particularly in the elderly.
- Inter-patient variability greatly limits the value of predetermined infusion schemes.
- For major surgery, to prevent post-operative rebound hypertension/ agitation in recovery, continue remifentanil at a low infusion rate, or give morphine 15–20min before the end of surgery; clonidine up to 2 micrograms/kg IV is also useful.

Miscellaneous ear, nose, and throat procedures

Table 26.1 presents the important information for those procedures which are not covered in the individual topics within this chapter.

Reference

1 National Patient Safety Agency. *Throat packs.* Ⓜ http://www.nrls.npsa.nhs.uk/resources/?entr yid45=59853.

Table 26.1 Other ENT procedures

Operation	Description	Time (min)	Pain	Position	Blood loss	Notes
Mastoidectomy	Clearance of cholesteatoma from mastoid cavity	90–120	++	Head-up tilt, head tilted to side on ring	Minimal	RAE tube or LMA, SV, or IPPV. Bloodless field needed (see stapedectomy). If disease close to facial nerve, surgeon may request no relaxant used (see parotidectomy)
Drilling of ear exostoses	Excision of external auditory ('swimmer's') exostoses	60–90	++	Head-up tilt, head tilted to side on ring	Minimal	RAE tube or LMA, SV, or IPPV
BAHA	Application of bone-anchored hearing aid	90–120	++	Head-up tilt, head tilted to side on ring	Minimal	LA plus sedation or GA with RAE tube or LMA, SV, or IPPV
MUA nose	Correction of nasal fracture	1–15	+	Supine	Small	If quick, preoxygenate plus propofol only. If longer, RAE tube or reinforced LMA plus throat pack. Occasionally bleeds dramatically
Removal of foreign body from nose	Removal of foreign body from nose, usually in child	5–10	Nil	Supine, head ring	Nil	Gas induction, RAE tube or LMA, throat pack, SV. Avoid face mask ventilation if possible (risk of pushing foreign body down into lower airway)
Rhinoplasty	Cosmetic alteration or reconstruction of nose using bone/cartilage graft	60–90	++	Head-up tilt, head ring	Small	RAE tube or reinforced LMA, SV, or IPPV, throat pack. Moderate hypotension useful to decrease bleeding; remifentanil ideal

(Continued)

Table 26.1 (Contd.)

Operation	Description	Time (min)	Pain	Position	Blood loss	Notes
Lateral rhinotomy	Resection of nasal tumour via lateral rhinotomy	90	++	Head-up tilt, head ring	Moderate	RAE tube or reinforced LMA, SV, or IPPV, throat pack. Moderate hypotension useful to decrease bleeding
Uvulopalato-pharyngoplasty (UPPP)	Excision of uvula and lax tissue from soft palate, sometimes using laser	20–30	+++	Supine, pad under shoulders	Small	RAE tube or reinforced LMA, SV, or IPPV. Laser-proof tube if needed. Regular post-op NSAID plus paracetamol. OSA precautions if indicated
Submandibular gland excision	Excision of blocked/ diseased submandibular gland	45–60	++	Supine, pad under shoulders, head ring	Small	RAE tube or reinforced LMA on opposite side, SV or IPPV
Tracheobronchial foreign body removal	Removal of inhaled foreign body using rigid bronchoscope, usually in child (see also ⊙ p. 834)	20–30	NS	Supine, pad under shoulders	Nil	Deep inhalational anaesthesia using O_2 and sevoflurane, allowing surgeon intermittent access. LA spray. Glycopyrronium useful to prevent bradycardia
Laryngoscopy in child	Examination of larynx in child, usually for recurrent stridor or aspiration	15–20	NS	Supine, pad under shoulders	Nil	Inhalational induction, LA spray to larynx. Either SV via rigid surgical laryngoscope (circuit connected to scope) or LMA and fibreoptic laryngoscopy through it (ideal for small child and enables larynx to be viewed during emergence)
Direct pharyngoscopy	Examination of pharynx using rigid pharyngoscope	10–15	+	Supine, pad under shoulders	Nil	Check for reflux. Small (6–7) oral RAE tube secured on left, IPPV, mivacurium or intermittent suxamethonium. Risk of bleeding if biopsies done

Procedure	Description	Time		Position	Blood loss	Notes
Endoscopic stapling of pharyngeal pouch	Division of opening to pharyngeal pouch using staple gun endoscopically	15–20	+	Supine, pad under shoulders	Nil	Preoxygenate, avoid face mask ventilation, small (6–7) oral RAE tube secured on opposite side, IPPV. NGT at end and IV fluids as nil by mouth post-op
Excision of pharyngeal pouch	Excision of pharyngeal pouch via external approach	45–60	+	Supine, pad under shoulders, head ring	Nil	Preoxygenate, avoid face mask ventilation, small (6–7) oral RAE tube secured on opposite side, IPPV. Surgeon may want oesophageal bougie inserted to help recognize anatomy. Antibiotic cover, NGT at end, and IV fluids as nil by mouth post-op
Insertion of speaking valve (e.g. Provox®)	Insertion of speaking valve via tracheo-oesophageal puncture, following laryngectomy	15	+	Supine, pad under shoulders, head ring	Nil	Microlaryngoscopy tube inserted via tracheostomy, IPPV, mivacurium or intermittent succinylcholine, remifentanil or alfentanil to reduce CVS response
Pharyngo-laryngectomy	Extended resection of larynx and pharynx for tumour of hypopharynx, using oesophagectomy and stomach pull-up or free jejunum transfer. Involves laparotomy ± thoracotomy	6–10hr	++++	Supine, pad under shoulders, head ring	Major, X-match 4–6U	No access to patient whatsoever! Prepare as for laryngectomy with all lines, plus double-lumen tube if doing thoracotomy. Consider epidural analgesia for laparotomy/thoracotomy (using plain LA) with PCA morphine to cover remaining surgical sites. ICU mandatory post-op (see also ⊕ p. 383)

Preoperative airway obstruction

(See also ➲ p. 960.)

Assessment

- Patients with preoperative airway obstruction usually present for surgery either to establish the diagnosis or to relieve the obstruction.
- Obstructions may be supraglottic, glottic or subglottic. The commonest level for obstruction is the larynx, which classically produces stridor (high-pitched, inspiratory).
- In adults, tumours are the commonest cause of upper airway obstruction, though a haematoma or an infection (including epiglottitis) is also possible. In children, an infection (croup) or a foreign body is more likely; in the UK, Hib vaccination has virtually eliminated childhood epiglottitis.
- Extreme airway obstruction will cause obvious signs of respiratory distress at rest. Exhaustion or an obtunded conscious level indicate the need for immediate intervention.
- If the obstruction has a gradual onset, patients can compensate very effectively, and moderately severe obstruction can develop without gross physical signs. Features to help recognize a substantial degree of upper airway obstruction include:
  - Long, slow inspirations, with pauses during speech
  - Recent marked deterioration in exercise tolerance
  - Worsening stridor during sleep (history from spouse/night nursing staff).
- Oropharyngeal lesions rarely present with airway obstruction, and assessment is normally straightforward on preoperative examination. Important features are limitation of mouth opening and tongue protrusion, and identification of any masses compromising the airway.
- Useful information may come from radiographs (plain films, CT/MRI) or ENT clinic flexible or indirect laryngoscopy.

Management

- For life-threatening airway obstruction, emergency intervention may be needed, but usually surgery will be a planned procedure.
- For emergencies, avoid undue delays. While preparing theatre, helium by face mask can improve the flow past the obstruction (low density favourable for turbulent flow), though this must not delay definitive management. Medical helium comes premixed (79%) with O_2 (21%); additional O_2 should be added via a Y connector.
- The main problems in securing airway access are:
  - Airway obstruction likely to be worsened by lying the patient flat, GA (all techniques), or instrumenting the airway (laryngospasm, bleeding)
  - Identifying the laryngeal inlet may be difficult because of anatomical distortion (especially supraglottic lesions)
  - Severe stenosis may make passage of the tube difficult (particularly glottic or subglottic tumours).

There is little evidence to support any one particular anaesthetic technique. However, the use of IV induction agents or NMB carries the catastrophic risk of 'cannot intubate/cannot ventilate' (CICV) in a patient unable to breathe spontaneously.

- The three main options for establishing secure airway access are:
  - Direct laryngoscopy and intubation under deep inhalational anaesthesia
  - Awake intubation using fibreoptic laryngoscopy under LA
  - Tracheostomy under LA (or deep inhalational GA with face mask or LMA in less severe cases).
- Whichever technique is used, a full range of equipment should be prepared, including different laryngoscopes, cricothyroidotomy kit, and tubes in various sizes. A small ETT kept in ice will be stiffer, useful to get past a tight stenotic lesion.
- Fibreoptic intubation under LA is generally most useful for supraglottic lesions where anatomical orientation is the main problem; for stenotic lesions of the glottis/subglottis, the scope may block the airway completely.
- Deep inhalational anaesthesia, best with sevoflurane in O_2, may be slow because of reduced minute ventilation. A moderate degree of CPAP is effective at keeping the airway patent, as anaesthesia deepens. Once deep, LA spray to the larynx extends the available time for laryngoscopy before reflexes return.
- In children, deep inhalational anaesthesia is the only realistic option—best undertaken with the child sitting, comforted by a parent, and may be safer to site IV cannula after induction in small children to minimize upset. Avoid delays because of rapid and unpredictable decline in condition.
- In childhood epiglottitis, distortion of the epiglottis can make recognition of the glottis very difficult; a useful tip is to press on the child's chest and watch for a bubble of gas emerging from the larynx.
- Mason and Fielder[2] reviewed the merits of each technique for airway obstruction at different levels but concluded none is universally certain, safe, and easy, and the final decision in each case will be strongly influenced by the particular skills and experience of the anaesthetist and surgeon concerned.
- If complete airway obstruction occurs and all conventional attempts to secure the airway fail, emergency surgical access to the airway is the only option. Cricothyroidotomy is preferable to tracheostomy for emergency airway access, as it is quicker to perform, more superficial, and less likely to bleed (above the thyroid gland) (see ➲ p. 957).

Reference

2 Mason RA, Fielder CP (1999). The obstructed airway in head and neck surgery. *Anaesthesia*, 54, 625–8.

Obstructive sleep apnoea

(See also → p. 112.)

- OSA[3] is the commonest form of sleep apnoea syndrome. The airway obstructs intermittently because of inadequate muscle tone/coordination in the pharynx. The problem usually occurs in association with other factors such as obesity; several scoring systems[4] have been described to quantify these.
- In adults, surgery for OSA may include nasal operations and uvulopalatopharyngoplasty (UPPP), although the role of UPPP in OSA is controversial, as it may render nasal CPAP less effective in the long term.
- In children, OSA usually results from extreme adenotonsillar hypertrophy, and adenotonsillectomy is performed to relieve this.[5]
- OSA produces total obstruction, with repeated episodes of hypoxia leading to arousal (though not awakening). Multiple episodes can occur each night, with O_2 saturation falling repeatedly to as low as 50%.
- Repeated interruptions to sleep produce daytime lethargy and somnolence, while extensive nocturnal hypoxia can lead to pulmonary or systemic hypertension with ventricular hypertrophy and cardiac failure.
- A careful history (from the partner or parent) is the most valuable information initially. In OSA, snoring is interrupted by periods of silent apnoea broken by a 'heroic' deep breath.
- Sleep studies reveal the extent of apnoea. If a history unexpectedly gives a clear picture of OSA, consider patient referral.
- In children with suspected OSA, features of chronic hypoxaemia should be sought. These include polycythaemia and RV strain (large P wave in leads II and V_1, large R wave in V_1, deep S wave in V_6). If features exist, echocardiography and referral for sleep studies should be considered. In severe cases, corrective otolaryngological surgery should be undertaken before unrelated elective surgery.
- Perioperatively, the biggest danger is impairment of the respiratory drive and hypoxic arousal mechanisms by the sedative action of drugs.
- Anaesthetic management is aimed at minimizing periods of sedation and ensuring that ventilation and oxygenation are maintained until the patient is adequately recovered. Specific points include:
  - Avoidance of preoperative sedative drugs
  - Intubation is usually not a problem, unless other factors are present
  - Long-acting opioids should be avoided, if possible. Use NSAID, paracetamol, tramadol, or local infiltration where feasible
  - When needed, long-acting opioids should be given IV and titrated carefully against response (around 50% of normal dose requirement)
  - Close overnight monitoring (including pulse oximetry). Admission to HDU, or even ICU, may be necessary
  - For nasal surgery, a nasopharyngeal airway can be incorporated into the nasal pack and left in place overnight.

References

3 Loadsman JA, Hillman DR (2001). Anaesthesia and sleep apnoea. *Br J Anaesth*, **86**, 254–66.

4 Silva GE, Vana KD, Goodwin JL, Sherrill DL, Quan SF (2011). Identification of patients with sleep disordered breathing: comparing the four-variable screening tool, STOP, STOP-Bang, and Epworth Sleepiness Scales. *J Clin Sleep Med*, **15**, 467–72.

5 Warwick JP, Mason DG (1998). Obstructive sleep apnoea syndrome in children. *Anaesthesia*, **53**, 571–9.

Grommet insertion

Procedure	Myringotomy and grommet insertion, usually bilateral
Time	5–15min
Pain	+
Position	Supine, head tilted to side, head ring
Blood loss	Nil
Practical techniques	Face mask or LMA SV using T-piece or paediatric circle

Preoperative
- Usually children (1–8yr), normally day case.
- Repeated ear infections; check for recent URTI.
- Paracetamol/NSAID orally.

Perioperative
- LMA commonly used.
- Face mask suitable if surgeon happy to work round it, but assistant needed to adjust vaporizer, etc. Insert Guedel airway before draping, and ensure reservoir bag visible throughout (T-piece ideal if face mask used).

Post-operative
- Need for additional analgesia unlikely.

Special considerations
- If face mask airway difficult, change early to LMA.
- Reflex bradycardia occasionally seen related to partial vagal innervation of tympanic membrane.

Tonsillectomy/adenoidectomy: child

Procedure	Excision of lymphoid tissue from oropharynx (tonsils) or nasopharynx (adenoids)
Time	20–30min
Pain	+++
Position	Supine, pad under shoulders
Blood loss	Usually small, can bleed post-op
Practical techniques	South-facing uncuffed RAE tube or reinforced LMA, placed in groove of split blade of Boyle–Davis gag; SV or IPPV

Preoperative

- Careful history to exclude OSA (see ➋ p. 112) or active infection.
- Topical LA on hands (mark sites of veins).
- Paracetamol/NSAID PO (see ➋ p. 634).
- Consent for PR analgesia if to be used.

Perioperative

- IV or inhalational induction (sevoflurane)—Guedel airway useful if nasopharynx blocked by large adenoids.
- Intubate (uncuffed RAE) using relaxant or deep inhalational anaesthesia, or insert LMA using propofol/opioid or deep inhalational anaesthesia.
- Secure in midline, no pack (obscures surgical field).
- Beware surgeon displacing/obstructing tube intraoperatively, particularly after insertion or opening of Boyle–Davis gag.
- T-piece ideal for SV, but ensure reservoir bag always visible.
- Reliable IV access essential, though IV fluids not routine.
- Analgesia with morphine or fentanyl titrated IV plus paracetamol/ NSAID PR if not given preoperatively.
- Antiemetic: at least one recommended—dexamethasone or ondansetron.
- Careful suction of oropharynx and nasopharynx at end under direct vision (generally done by surgeon).
- Extubate left lateral/head-down (tonsil position), with Guedel airway.

Post-operative

- Keep patient in tonsil position until airway reflexes return.
- High-quality recovery care essential.
- Analgesia with IV morphine/fentanyl initially, then oral paracetamol/ NSAID/morphine. Dexmedetomidine has been used.
- Leave IV cannula (flushed) in place in case of bleeding.

Special considerations

- In small children, a pillow under the chest can be used to provide the necessary tilt.
- Avoid blind pharyngeal suction with a rigid sucker, as this may start bleeding from the tonsil bed.
- NSAIDs increase bleeding slightly (especially if given preoperatively);[6] needs to be balanced against benefits.
- LA infiltration of the tonsil bed is not recommended.
- Beware continual swallowing in recovery, a sign of bleeding from the tonsil/adenoid bed.
- Adenoidectomy/tonsillectomy now widely done as a day case with an extended (5–6hr) post-operative stay; morphine still suitable for analgesia. Concern about possible transmission of variant Creutzfeldt–Jakob disease (vCJD) via contaminated equipment used in adenotonsillectomy led to a single-use only policy in the UK in 2001. This was subsequently lifted in the light of further data.

Bleeding after adenotonsillectomy

- May be detected in recovery or many hours later.
- Loss may be much greater than readily apparent (swallowed blood).
- Senior anaesthetist must be involved.
- Problems include:
  - Hypovolaemia
  - Risk of aspiration (fresh bleeding and blood in stomach)
  - Difficult laryngoscopy because of blood in the airway or oedema
  - Residual anaesthetic effect.
- Resuscitate preoperatively; check Hb (HemoCue® ideal); cross-match, and give blood, as needed. Note: Hb will fall as IV fluids administered (dilution).
- Options:
  - RSI: enables rapid airway protection, but laryngoscopy may be difficult (blood, swelling)—generally preferred
  - Inhalational induction left lateral/head-down: allows time for laryngoscopy but takes longer, and unfamiliar technique to many.
- Use wide-bore gastric tube to empty stomach after bleeding stopped.
- Extubate fully awake.
- Extended stay in recovery for close monitoring.
- Nasopharyngeal pack occasionally needed (secured via tapes through nose) if bleeding from adenoids cannot be controlled. Usually very uncomfortable—patient may need midazolam/morphine to tolerate.
- Check post-operative Hb.

Reference

6 Møiniche S, Rømsing J, Dahl JB, Tramèr MR (2003). Nonsteroidal antiinflammatory drugs and the risk of operative site bleeding after tonsillectomy: a quantitative systematic review. *Anesth Analg*, **96**, 68–77.

Tonsillectomy in adults

As for child, except:
- Usually more painful post-operatively in adult—give morphine in theatre
- IPPV–relaxant technique used more commonly. Mivacurium useful with quick surgeon
- Preoperative oral NSAID avoids suppository use, though may increase bleeding risk.
- Occasionally, patients present with peritonsillar abscess (quinsy). Now normally treated with antibiotics, and tonsillectomy performed later. If drainage essential because of airway swelling, pus usually aspirated with syringe and large needle under LA infiltration.

Myringoplasty

Procedure	Reconstruction of perforated tympanic membrane with autograft (usually temporalis fascia)
Time	60–90min
Pain	++
Position	Supine, head tilted to side, head ring, head-up tilt
Blood loss	Minimal
Practical techniques	South-facing RAE tube or LMA (usually reinforced); SV or IPPV

Preoperative

Usually young, fit patients.

Perioperative

- Ensure coughing avoided during surgery; LA spray to larynx; monitor NMB if IPPV–relaxant technique used.
- Dry field improves the surgical view, though not as important as for stapedectomy—head-up tilt and avoiding hypertension/tachycardia normally sufficient.
- Remifentanil infusion suitable.
- Routine antiemetic useful.

Post-operative

- PRN paracetamol or NSAID PO/IV; may need morphine.
- PRN antiemetic.

Special considerations

Using N_2O may produce diffusion into the middle ear and risk the graft lifting off; either avoid or discontinue 20min before the end of the case.

Stapedectomy/tympanoplasty

Procedure	Excision/reconstruction of damaged middle ear structures
Time	2–4hr
Pain	++/+++
Position	Supine, head tilted to side, head ring, head-up tilt
Blood loss	Minimal
Practical techniques	South-facing RAE tube or LMA (usually reinforced). IPPV normally. Arterial line often used

Preoperative

- Check for CVS disease, as this will limit the degree of hypotension possible.
- Oral premedication options include benzodiazepines, β-blockers, and clonidine.

Perioperative

- Monitor to ensure adequate NMB.
- Bloodless field enables greater surgical accuracy—simple measures include: potent opioid pre-induction; ensure coughing avoided at intubation (LA spray to larynx helpful); head-up tilt to reduce VP.
- Further benefit achieved by lowering arterial BP (mean of 50–60mmHg in healthy patients) and HR (<60bpm).
- Remifentanil infusion ideal to achieve this. Alternatively, use IV labetalol (combined α-/β-blocker, 5mg increments) or IV β-blocker (metoprolol 1mg increments, esmolol infusion) plus vasodilator (isoflurane, hydralazine 5mg increments). Arterial line strongly advised with CVS disease or if potent vasodilators used; head-up tilt further reduces perfusion pressure to the brain.
- Give at least one antiemetic routinely.

Post-operative

- Regular antiemetic for 24–48hr.
- PRN paracetamol or NSAID PO/IV/PR; may need morphine.

Special considerations

- N_2O diffusion into the middle ear may disrupt surgery, though less important than in myringoplasty. Either avoid or discontinue 20min before the end of the case.

Nasal cavity surgery

Procedure	Submucous resection of septum, septoplasty, turbinectomy, polypectomy, functional endoscopic sinus surgery
Time	20–60min
Pain	++
Position	Supine, head ring, head-up tilt
Blood loss	Usually minor
Practical techniques	South-facing RAE tube or LMA (usually reinforced); SV or IPPV. Throat pack

Preoperative
- Obstructive airways disease often associated with nasal polyps.
- Combination of procedures mentioned in the box above frequently performed.

Perioperative
- Face mask ventilation often needs Guedel airway due to blocked nose.
- Nasal vasoconstrictor usually applied (topical or infiltration).
- Leave eyes untaped for polypectomy (the optic nerve can be close, and the surgeon needs to check for eye movement).
- Suck out pharynx (particularly behind soft palate—'coroner's clot'; see p. 623) before extubation; less easy with LMA.

Post-operative
- Left lateral/head-down with Guedel airway in place until airway reflexes return.
- Analgesia with PRN paracetamol or NSAID PO/IV/PR.
- Nose usually packed, producing obstruction of nasal airway—if disturbing to patient, or in cases of OSA, nasopharyngeal airway(s) can be incorporated into the pack.
- Sit patient up as soon as awake to reduce bleeding.

Special considerations
- Leave IV cannula in overnight, as can bleed post-operatively.

Microlaryngoscopy

Procedure	Examination of larynx using operating microscope (plus excision/biopsy; may use laser)
Time	10–30min
Pain	+/++
Position	Supine, pad under shoulders, head extended
Blood loss	Nil
Practical techniques	Microlaryngeal tube and conventional IPPV. TIVA and jet ventilation using injector system (O_2 plus entrained air) via: • Injector needle on the operating laryngoscope • Semi-rigid tracheal catheter • Cricothyroidotomy needle/cannula

Ventilation during microlaryngoscopy

Microlaryngeal tube and conventional intermittent positive pressure ventilation

- Microlaryngeal tube is a long 5.0mm ETT with a high-volume/ low-pressure cuff.
- Enables maintenance of anaesthesia with inhalational agents.
- Protects against aspiration of blood/surgical debris but restricts surgeon's view.
- Use long, slow inspiration for IPPV because of high resistance of tube. Measured inflation pressure will be high, but the patient's airway pressures distal to tube will be lower.
- Cannot be used for laser work, as tube will be ignited; jet ventilation used instead.

Jet ventilation

- Ventilation achieved using an injector system, such as the adjustable-flow Manujet®, delivering O_2 and entrained air via:
  - Injector needle attached to the proximal end of the operating laryngoscope, and ventilation started when correctly aligned with larynx. Various needle sizes available with different flow rates. Technique not suitable if good view of larynx is unobtainable and has disadvantage of blowing debris/smoke into trachea with ventilation
  - Semi-rigid tracheal catheter (ordinary suction catheter not suitable), with the tip placed midway down the trachea. Special catheters available with gas sampling port or made from laser-proof material
  - Cricothyroidotomy needle/cannula placed through the cricothyroid membrane under LA before induction and aimed towards the carina. Commercial versions available or a Tuohy needle can be used; beware gas injected into tissues if needle misplaced/displaced.
- Induce in theatre, or use a microlaryngeal tube initially, then remove and change to jet ventilation when all ready in theatre (not with cricothyroidotomy needle).

- Ensure the anaesthetic machine in theatre is situated close to enable easy face mask ventilation at induction/recovery.
- TIVA needed for maintenance (propofol/remifentanil infusion).
- Ventilate using normal respiratory rate, and adjust inspiratory flow (alter injector settings, or change needle size) to produce appropriate degree of chest expansion.
- Accurate flow/pressure measurement not easy; barotrauma a potential risk.
- Stop ventilation intermittently during surgical work (clear communication essential).
- Provides minimal obstruction to surgical view.
- At end of the case, either continue jet ventilation until SV re-established or discontinue and ventilate by face mask until SV recommences.

Preoperative

- Patients often elderly and usually smokers; CVS/respiratory system problems common.
- Carefully assess the airway for evidence of obstruction. History, examination, ENT clinic assessment, plain films, and CT scan may all help, but, if any degree of stridor present, obstruction must be substantial (see ➔ p. 628).
- Ensure all equipment is ready before induction, including cricothyroidotomy kit, and that surgeon is available for emergency tracheostomy, if required.

Perioperative

- If airway obstruction suspected, secure airway initially, using principles on ➔ p. 628. Inserting a cricothyroid cannula under LA pre-induction provides a route for ventilation in the event of total obstruction.
- Give short-acting opioid (alfentanil, remifentanil) to attenuate hypertensive response.
- Muscle relaxation is usually essential: mivacurium or intermittent suxamethonium (plus glycopyrronium/atropine to prevent bradycardia).
- Use of rocuronium and reversal with sugammadex may be an option.
- LA spray to larynx reduces risk of laryngospasm, though this impairs airway protection, so recover left lateral, head-down.

Post-operative

- Analgesia with PRN paracetamol or NSAID PO/IV/PR.
- May develop stridor post-operatively from oedema of an already compromised airway—dexamethasone 8–12mg IV sometimes used to prevent this.

Special considerations

- Jet ventilation essential if laser work planned.
- Microlaryngoscopy can be used to inject inert material (e.g. silicone) into paralysed vocal cords to improve phonation, though this can lead to airway obstruction if overdone.
- High-frequency jet ventilation has been used, though complex and assessment of ventilation difficult.

Tracheostomy

Procedure	Insertion of a ETT via neck incision
Time	30min
Pain	++
Position	Supine, pad under shoulders, head ring, head-up tilt
Blood loss	Normally small, though can bleed from thyroid vessels
Practical techniques	IPPV, ETT with tubing going 'north', changed to tracheostomy tube during case. LMA if airway not a problem, IPPV or SV. Can be done under LA

Preoperative

- Normally done for long-term ICU ventilation or airway obstruction.
- ICU patients almost certainly already intubated. If ventilation difficult and oxygenation critical, set up ICU ventilator in theatre, using TIVA, rather than inhalational agents.
- Stop NG feeds, if applicable.
- If tracheostomy is for airway obstruction, secure airway initially, using principles on **➲** p. 628.
- Before induction, ensure all equipment prepared (including cricothyroidotomy kit) and the surgeon ready for emergency tracheostomy, if required.

Perioperative

- Secure ETT with tape to allow easy removal during case, with pilot cuff readily accessible.
- Aspirate NGT (if present), and clear oropharynx of secretions before draping.
- Drape patient to allow anaesthetist access to ETT for tube change.
- Long tubing needed for breathing circuit and gas sampling.
- Before changing to tracheostomy tube, preoxygenate for 3–4min (increasing volatile agent as necessary), and check NMB is adequate.
- Ensure scrub nurse has correct tracheostomy tube and sterile catheter mount.
- Deflate ETT cuff before surgeons incise trachea, so it can be reinflated and ventilation continued if problems occur.
- Withdraw ETT slowly into upper trachea (do not remove from trachea until tracheostomy secure and certain), and connect breathing circuit and capnograph to new tracheostomy tube via sterile catheter mount.
- Beware false passage created during tracheostomy tube insertion, especially in the obese; check position with fibreoptic endoscopy, if any doubt.
- If problems occur, remove tracheostomy tube, and advance ETT back down trachea.

Post-operative

- Regular suction to new tracheostomy (blood, secretions).
- Humidify inspired gases.
- Analgesia in recovery with paracetamol or NSAID IV/PR or morphine IV. Usually little analgesia required thereafter.
- A new tracheostomy often produces protracted coughing—morphine, benzodiazepines, or low-dose propofol useful for control.
- Antiemetic, as required.
- If tracheostomy tube comes out, reinsertion can very difficult in first few days—orotracheal intubation often more practical. Two retraction sutures left in tracheal incision are useful for identifying and opening the stoma.

Special considerations

- Can be done under LA, though difficult in a dyspnoeic, struggling patient.
- In ICU, tracheostomy is now usually done percutaneously, using dilatational technique; theatre cases are likely to be the difficult ones.
- Tracheostomy is not the ideal route of approach for emergency airway access; cricothyroidotomy is more accessible and less likely to bleed.
- LMA can be used if tracheostomy is done at start of larger procedure and upper airway normal.

Tracheostomy tubes

- Specific features available include:
  - Fenestration: allows speech by patient occluding the lumen with a finger and exhaling through hole in back wall of tube.
  - Inner tube (e.g. Shiley®): permits removal for cleaning.
  - Adjustable flange: length can be modified for short trachea or deep stoma.
  - Channel in obturator for guide-wire.
- Tube change:
  - New tube must be inserted with obturator in place to prevent stomal damage.
  - May be difficult to find trachea in new tracheostomy; guide-wire may be useful.
  - Prepare for orotracheal intubation in case of problems
  - Cannot be left in place longer than 28d (classified as an implant thereafter).

Laryngectomy

Procedure	Excision of larynx (epiglottis and glottis) with creation of an end-stomal tracheostomy
Time	3–4hr
Pain	+++
Position	Supine, pad under shoulders, head ring, head-up tilt
Blood loss	Moderate to substantial; X-match 2U
Practical techniques	IPPV, ETT with tubing going 'north', changed to tracheostomy during case
	Art line, urinary catheter, CVP line if surgery likely to be long/complicated or if indicated by cardiac disease

Preoperative

- Some degree of airway obstruction likely. Patient likely to have had recent GA (for diagnosis) to guide airway management; beware if some time has elapsed.
- If no recent GA, assess the airway as for microlaryngoscopy (see Ⓓ p. 639).
- Usually smokers; CVS/respiratory system problems and malnutrition common.
- Discuss implications of tracheostomy preoperatively (communication, secretions, coughing produced by tube). Speech therapist will do much of this.

Perioperative

- Insert fine-bore NG feeding tube at induction, and fix securely (can be sutured to nasal septum).
- Warming blanket and fluid warmer.
- Long tubing needed for breathing circuit and gas sampling tube.
- Remifentanil infusion ideal.
- Substantial blood loss can accumulate under drapes at back of neck and may not be apparent until end of case.
- For CVP access, all neck lines hinder surgery; femoral best, though antecubital fossa (ACF) or subclavian can be used.
- Antibiotic prophylaxis for at least 24hr.
- When changing to tracheostomy tube, see precautions for tracheostomy (see Ⓓ p. 641), though end-stoma makes tracheal access safer and easier.
- During surgery, long tube (armoured or special preformed) via tracheostomy is useful to enable surgical access round stoma, then changed for standard tracheostomy tube at end.

Post-operative

- HDU ideal.
- Humidification and regular suction essential (blood, secretions).
- New tracheostomy produces protracted coughing—morphine, benzodiazepines, or low-dose propofol useful for control.
- Analgesia with PRN morphine IV/NG, plus PRN paracetamol or NSAID NG/IV/PR. Analgesic requirements usually surprisingly low.
- Antiemetic, as required.

Special considerations

- Beware of air emboli (see ➔ p. 413) during dissection—early detection by sudden fall in ETCO$_2$.
- For previous laryngectomy patients presenting for surgery, to ventilate via stoma, use paediatric face mask turned through 180°, LMA applied to neck, or intubate awake after LA spray to stoma. Tracheostomy tube insertion is usually easy, though check stoma for stenosis or tumour recurrence, and always preoxygenate.
- Partial laryngectomy, with laryngeal reconstruction and temporary tracheostomy, favoured by some as alternative to radiotherapy in early laryngeal tumours.

Pharyngectomy

Procedure	Excision of pharynx (includes glossectomy and radical tonsillectomy); can involve mandibular split for surgical access and tissue transfer (flap) Extended resection also involving laryngectomy usually requires reconstruction using distant flap (see ➔ p. 501)
Time	6–8hr
Pain	++++
Position	Supine, pad under shoulders, head ring, head-up tilt
Blood loss	Major, X-match 4U initially
Practical techniques	IPPV, ETT (nasal may be best) with tubing going 'north' initially, changed to tracheostomy during case. Art line, CVP line, urinary catheter

Preoperative

- Discuss plans with surgeons to ensure what needs to be left untouched, e.g. forearm flap.
- Assess airway carefully; patient likely to have had recent GA (for diagnosis) to guide airway management.
- CVS/respiratory system problems and malnutrition common.
- Inform patient about lines, tracheostomy, etc.
- Ensure ICU bed available.

Perioperative

- Insert fine-bore NG feeding tube at induction, and fix securely (can be sutured to nasal septum).
- Femoral route best for CVP access.
- Long tubing needed for breathing circuit and gas sampling tube.
- Warming blanket and fluid warmer.
- Access to patient severely restricted; ensure all lines/tubes secure at start.
- Remifentanil infusion ideal.
- Substantial blood loss may be hidden under drapes; check regular HemoCue®.
- Ensure patient is well filled, especially if free flap used (aim for Hb of 100g/L) (see ➔ p. 501).
- Antibiotic prophylaxis for at least 24hr.

Post-operative
- ICU essential.
- Keep sedated and ventilated until stable and warm.
- Regular flap observations.
- Avoid tracheostomy ties round neck (may compromise flap blood supply).
- Humidification and regular suction (blood, secretions) to tracheostomy.
- Analgesia with PCA morphine once awake and PRN diclofenac/paracetamol NG/IV/PR.
- Antiemetic, as required.

Radical neck dissection

Procedure	Excision of sternomastoid, internal and external jugular veins, and associated lymph nodes. Modified or selective neck dissection preserves some of these structures (notably internal jugular vein)
Time	2–4hr
Pain	+++
Position	Supine, pad under shoulders, head on ring tilted to side, head-up tilt
Blood loss	Moderate to substantial, X-match 2–4U
Practical techniques	IPPV, ETT with tubing going 'north' or south-facing RAE tube on opposite side. Art line, urinary catheter, CVP line if surgery likely to be long/complicated or with cardiac disease

Preoperative
- Assess airway carefully, as may be an associated head and neck tumour or previous major surgery.
- May be performed with another procedure, e.g. laryngectomy.

Perioperative
- Warming blanket and fluid warmer.
- Long tubing is needed for the breathing circuit and gas sampling.
- Remifentanil infusion ideal.
- Can bleed briskly from large neck vessels, with substantial accumulation of blood under drapes (may not be apparent until end of case).
- For CVP access, femoral is best. Must avoid remaining jugulars, as head and neck venous drainage dependent on them.

Post-operative
- Head and neck oedema likely for several days (impaired venous drainage). Keep head up as much as possible, and avoid excessive IV fluids.
- To reduce chance of agitation/rebound hypertension and wound haematoma in recovery, continue remifentanil at a low infusion rate, or give morphine 15–20min before end of surgery; clonidine up to 2 micrograms/kg IV also very useful. Treat any hypertension early.
- Analgesia with PRN paracetamol or NSAID PO/IV/PR, morphine PO/IV. Surprisingly low analgesic requirements normally.
- Antiemetic, as required.

Special considerations
- Beware of air emboli during dissection—early detection by sudden fall in ETCO$_2$ (see ➔ p. 413).
- Surgical manipulation of carotid sinus can produce marked bradycardia.
- If neck dissection previously done on other side, oedema is usually worse and can raise ICP. Dexamethasone 8–12mg IV preoperatively (then 4mg IV 6-hourly) is used by many to reduce this.

Parotidectomy

Procedure	Excision of parotid gland, usually preserving facial nerve
Time	2–5hr
Pain	++/+++
Position	Supine, head ring, head tilted to side and moderately extended, head-up tilt
Blood loss	Usually small/moderate, G&S. Greater for malignancy
Practical techniques	South-facing RAE tube and IPPV normally used, though SV possible for suitable patients. Reinforced LMA and IPPV or SV also possible. No NMB during dissection around facial nerve

Preoperative
- Check if suitable for SV—not if elderly, obese, or respiratory disease.
- Check mouth opening, especially if malignant.

Perioperative
- Warming blanket and fluid warmer, plus urinary catheter if prolonged.
- Avoid NMB after initial dose (check recovery with PNS) to allow surgical testing for facial nerve.
- Remifentanil infusion ideal to allow IPPV without NMB and also reduce blood loss.
- Alternatively, suppress respiratory drive with other opioid, volatile agent, or propofol infusion, combined with moderate hyperventilation.
- LA spray to larynx useful to prevent coughing.
- If SV used, ensure patient settled initially using high level of volatile agent.

Post-operative
- To reduce chance of agitation/rebound hypertension and wound haematoma in recovery, continue remifentanil at a low infusion rate, or give morphine 15–20min before end of surgery; keep head up, and treat hypertension early; clonidine up to 2 micrograms/kg IV is very useful.
- Antiemetic, as required.
- Analgesia with PRN morphine IV/PO, paracetamol or NSAID PO/IV/PR.

Special considerations
- Surgeon normally uses nerve stimulator to identify facial nerve during dissection and may wish to leave ipsilateral eye exposed to monitor response.
- Large-bore IV access at start, as occasionally bleeds substantially (especially malignant tumours).

Maxillofacial and dental surgery

Alastair Martin and John Bowden

Sedation for dentistry

Patients who are unable to tolerate dental treatment under LA can often be managed by a combination technique using sedation. These procedures are usually performed by the dentist in the dental clinic. PO or IV sedation can be provided by short-acting benzodiazepines such as midazolam. Inhalational sedation can be provided by sub-anaesthetic concentrations of N_2O (up to 50%) in O_2 using a nasal mask—termed 'relative analgesia.' Whichever route of administration is used, it is important to ensure that the patient *remains conscious throughout*. The patient must be monitored by a trained member of staff (and not the dentist who may be distracted by the procedure).

General considerations

- Patients should be ASA 1 or 2. (Patients with significant co-morbidities should have their procedures in the hospital setting with an anaesthetist present.)
- Patients will require an escort for the procedure and to care for them afterwards.
- Written instructions should be provided regarding limitations on driving (as for GA) and operating machinery post-operatively. The patient should be told to avoid a heavy meal/alcohol prior to treatment. Patients should follow standard starvation guidelines when an anaesthetist is present and conversion to GA is a possibility.
- Inhalational sedation cannot be used in patients with nasal obstruction or those unable to cooperate with breathing through a nasal mask.
- LA is used in all patients after sedation has been established.
- The patient should be able to communicate throughout the procedure.
- Resuscitation equipment must be available

Suitable regimes

- Single-agent regimes are safer.
- For adults, midazolam 2mg IV; wait 90s, then give 1mg every 30s until sedated. Expect to give 6–10 mg (Society for Advancement of Anaesthesia in Dentistry (SAAD) guidelines).
- Low-dose propofol infusion (only with suitable training).
- O_2 (100%) via nasal mask; add 10% N_2O for 1min, then 20% for 1min. Continue increments of 5% until sedated (up to 50%).

Special considerations

- Have flumazenil available for reversal of midazolam.
- Allow at least 1hr for recovery following IV sedation.
- Following N_2O sedation, 100% O_2 must be administered to prevent diffusion hypoxia.
- The patient can be discharged once they are able to stand and walk unaided.

Anaesthesia for dentistry

General considerations

- GA for dental procedures should be undertaken in hospital and reserved for patients unable to tolerate LA (i.e. young children and adults with learning difficulties).
- Patients with learning difficulties may have trouble understanding the procedure and are often anxious. A short-acting anxiolytic agent, such as midazolam, and a topical anaesthetic cream may help.
- Patients may have a more complex medical disorder, such as Down's syndrome, or other congenital abnormality. It is important to exclude any significant cardiac pathology. Routine antibiotics for endocarditis prophylaxis are no longer recommended.
- Patients requiring extensive work can be treated in a day-case unit but may require overnight stay if they have major co-morbidities.
- **Positioning.** There is no longer a place for 'dental chair' anaesthesia. Postural hypotension can easily be overlooked, and it is now standard practice to keep patients supine or slight head-up.
- **LA infiltration** should be used whenever possible—be careful in very young children where it may lead to accidental biting/laceration.
- **Dental labelling.** Deciduous teeth are assigned letters A–E in each quadrant, and adult teeth are numbered 1–8. Roots are indicated by 'x', supernumerary (extra) teeth by '$', and buried or unerupted teeth by a circle around the letter/number. These are drawn with the patient 'facing you' and may be written as a complete mouth grid (as shown in Fig. 27.1) or as quadrants.
- **Simple extractions** may be very quick procedures, lasting a few minutes. LMAs (flexible) are preferable for multiple extractions. A prop/gag is inserted by the surgeon to facilitate surgical access—ensure that it does not obstruct the airway. During extractions, airway patency must be maintained and may require jaw support. When extractions are complete, a pack is positioned over the dental sockets to absorb any oozing blood.
- **Restoration work** can take over an hour and often requires intubation and ventilation.

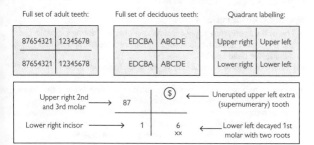

Fig. 27.1 Dentition labelling.

Dental extractions

(See also ➔ p. 781.)

Procedure	Dental extractions
Time	2–10min
Pain	+/++
Position	Supine
Blood loss	Nil
Practical techniques	LMA/nasal mask

Preoperative

- Usually children 3–12yr, dental phobics, or patients with learning difficulties.
- Beware of undiagnosed pathology, e.g. heart murmurs.
- Obtain consent for analgesic suppositories, if required.

Perioperative

- Give pre-emptive oral analgesia, e.g. paracetamol and ibuprofen.
- If a sedative premedication is needed, consider buccal or nasal midazolam.
- Apply a topical anaesthetic for cannulation if IV induction planned.
- Give propofol for induction, sevoflurane for gas induction.
- Tape the eyes closed.
- Maintenance with volatile agent or IV agent.
- Use LA infiltration (by dentist/oral surgeon); opioids are not usually needed for short day cases.
- Simple extractions do not require antibiotic cover.
- Stabilize the head and neck manually during the procedure.
- Place young children in the lateral position, slightly head-down at the end.

Post-operative

- Regular paracetamol and ibuprofen.

Special considerations

- The oral surgeon may apply considerable pressure during extraction, and the anaesthetist should apply counterpressure to support and stabilize the head and jaw.
- Beware of potential hypoxia. Give 100% O_2 for maintenance, if necessary.
- When using a nasal mask, mouth breathing can occur around the dental pack, resulting in decreased uptake of the anaesthetic agent and the patient becoming light. This can be a problem when using short-acting agents such as sevoflurane—use isoflurane for maintenance, or give small increments of propofol (if oxygenation is adequate).
- Children with blocked noses can be safely anaesthetized using an LMA (provided there is no URTI).

Oral/maxillofacial surgery

General principles

Anaesthesia for intraoral/maxillofacial procedures requires management of a shared airway and potentially difficult intubation. Nasal intubation is frequently used to improve surgical access to the mouth. At the preoperative visit, check nostril patency, and ask about epistaxis and the use of anticoagulants. Discuss the choice of airway with the surgeon.

- Simple intraoral procedures are often possible, using a reinforced LMA. For unilateral intraoral procedures, an oral ETT (e.g. RAE tube) placed on the opposite side of the mouth may be acceptable. Oral airways may be dislodged, and vigilance is required (particularly when using LMAs).
- If the nasal route is chosen for intubation, use an LA and/or a **vasoconstrictor** mixture (lidocaine 5%/phenylephrine 0.5%, or xylometazoline). There are many varieties of nasal tube—the 'Polar Preformed North Nasal' from Portex® is ideal. These 'north-facing' tubes are made of soft material and cause little nasal trauma. Sizes of 6.0, 6.5, and 7.0mm should be available. Place in warm water before use to soften the material even further. The tube should be padded with gauze to protect the patient's forehead. Consider fixing with clear adhesive film. Avoid excessive tension/pressure on the anterior nares which risks causing necrosis.
- Patients who have had previous surgery and/or radiotherapy may have thick fixed ('woody') soft tissues and poor neck mobility. Intubation may be harder than predicted by bedside tests. Consider indirect laryngoscopy techniques (e.g. CMAC®/Glidescope® or fibreoptic intubation)
- **Protect the eyes** with tape and eye pads or surgically positioned plastic contact lenses (e.g. the Crouch Corneal Protector®).
- Position the patient with the head at the opposite end to the anaesthetic machine—a long breathing circuit and gas analysis/spirometry lines are normally required. Secure the breathing circuit with a tube holder. Ensure the pilot cuff is accessible.
- Stabilize the head with a horseshoe or head ring. For operations on the roof of the mouth, use a bolster under the shoulders to extend the neck further. Positioning the patient slightly head-up will reduce bleeding.
- **Throat packs** are used to minimize contamination of the airway with blood and debris. Ribbon gauze or tampons may be used.
- A robust system should be in place to ensure that throat packs are not inadvertently left *in situ*. This should include discussion at 'Time Out', a visual reminder (e.g. throat pack sticker and an entry on the swab/sharps board), confirmation of removal in the 'Sign Out' swab count (see p. 623), and clear documentation.

Extubation

- There is a risk of aspiration of blood, pus, and debris. The oropharynx and larynx should be suctioned at the end of the case (preferably under direct vision). Patients should be extubated sitting at 30-45° to reduce bleeding from venous congestion (or in the left lateral position with head-down tilt if there is a high risk of airway soiling).
- Some anaesthetists extubate the patient using a 'deep', spontaneous breathing technique. Some exchange the ETT for an LMA and allow the patient to wake slowly in recovery. Others prefer to extubate awake.
- Whichever technique is used, the aim is to avoid bleeding and swelling caused by coughing and straining. The use of a nasotracheal tube or LMA, which do not stimulate the gag reflex as much as an oral tube, facilitates a smoother extubation. Consider also spraying the vocal cords with lidocaine at intubation.
- If a nasal tube has been used, it is possible to convert it into a nasopharyngeal airway by withdrawing it until the tip lies in the oropharynx, inserting a safety pin (to prevent the tube from slipping back into the nostril) and cutting at the 15cm mark.

Free flap surgery

- Major maxillofacial reconstructions are performed using tissue/bone free flaps (particularly from the radial forearm/fibula).
- These operations may be lengthy, 6–10+ hr.
- The same principles apply as for plastic surgery free flaps (see ➲ p. 501), with the added complication of a potentially difficult airway, both pre- and post-surgery.
- HDU or ICU care is usually indicated post-operatively.
- Traditionally, surgical tracheostomies were often performed because of the risk of post-operative airway compromise. Sedation and overnight ventilation on the ICU with a nasal ETT is becoming increasingly common and may avoid tracheostomy. Nasal tubes may be left in the short term (12–24hr).
- Ensure throat packs are removed before transfer to the ICU.
- Sedation should be titrated down to minimize the need for vasopressors.
- The patient should be nursed with the head and neck in a neutral position to avoid tension on newly anastomosed vessels, and head-up to minimize venous congestion.

Extraction of impacted/buried teeth

Procedure	Removal of teeth
Time	3–45min
Pain	+
Position	Supine, head ring, bolster under shoulders if teeth to be extracted in roof of mouth
Blood loss	Minimal
Practical techniques	Nasal tube, throat pack, and IPPV—extubate awake or deep LMA and SV

Preoperative

- Careful assessment of the airway. Check nostrils for patency.
- If the patient has a dental abscess there may be marked swelling of the face and severe trismus. AFOI may be necessary (see ➋ p. 969).

Perioperative

- Consider an LMA/oral tube for simple/unilateral extractions.
- Intubate with a warmed, preformed nasal tube after applying a vasoconstrictor to the nasal mucosa (see ➋ p. 653).
- Protect the eyes with tape and pads.
- The surgeon should anaesthetize the appropriate terminal branches of the maxillary division (infraorbital, greater palatine, nasopalatine) and mandibular division (inferior alveolar, lingual, buccal, mental) of the trigeminal nerve with a long-acting LA (bupivacaine 0.25% or 0.5% with adrenaline 1:200 000).
- Give an intraoperative opioid and NSAID/paracetamol, if not given preoperatively.
- IV antibiotics may be administered to minimize the risk of infection (e.g. co-amoxiclav 1.2g or clindamycin 600mg for patients with penicillin allergy). Check your local antibiotic policy.
- Steroids (e.g. dexamethasone 8mg IV) may be given for antiemesis and to minimize swelling.

Post-operative

- Balanced analgesia with regular paracetamol and NSAIDs. Prescribe rescue analgesia with PRN tramadol or codeine phosphate. (Codeine is no longer advised for children.)

Special considerations

- Talk to the surgeon to ascertain the likely length of surgery. Remember that some patients require GA only because they are 'dental-phobic.' The surgical extractions may be simple, and the operative time consequently very short. A short-acting muscle relaxant may be required.

Fractures of the orbito-zygomatic complex

Procedure	Elevation of fractured zygomatic complex ± fixation
Time	10–180min
Pain	+/++
Position	Supine, with head-up tilt, head ring
Blood loss	Minor (may be more with internal fixation)
Practical techniques	Oral RAE tube and IPPV. LMA/SV for simple elevation

These fractures may occur in isolation or may be associated with damage to other parts of the facial skeleton. There may be limitation of mouth opening due to interference with movement of the coronoid process of the mandible by the depressed zygomatic complex. Following elevation, the fracture may be stable or unstable and require internal fixation. Most surgery is carried out via a temporal approach. The intraoral route is also used. Unstable fractures require plating or wiring via skin or intraoral incisions.

Preoperative
- Assess the patient carefully for associated injuries, particularly head and neck injuries. Treatment of these fractures does not have high clinical priority. The operation is often easier if a period of time elapses (5–7d) to allow the associated facial swelling to disperse.
- Make a careful airway assessment.

Perioperative
- Intubate the patient with an oral RAE tube. For simple fracture elevations, a flexible LMA may be used, but discuss with the surgeon whether open fixation of the fracture is planned.
- Insert a throat pack if the intraoral approach is planned.
- Lubricate and protect the eye on the non-operative side.
- Give antibiotics if metalwork is to be inserted (e.g. co-amoxiclav 1.2g or clindamycin 600mg), and steroids (e.g. dexamethasone 8mg IV) as requested.
- Be prepared for potential bradycardia (vagally mediated), as the zygoma fracture is reduced (Gillies lift).
- Extubate with the patient breathing spontaneously, and do not apply excessive pressure over the zygoma with the face mask post-extubation.

Post-operative
- IV opioids may be required in recovery.
- Prescribe oral analgesia for the ward.
- Eye observations in recovery to detect retrobulbar haemorrhage (which would require a return to theatre).

Mandibular fractures

Procedure	Reduction and fixation of a fractured mandible
Time	2–3hr
Pain	+
Position	Supine, with head-up tilt, head ring
Blood loss	Variable. Consider G&S
Practical techniques	Nasal tube, throat pack, and IPPV. Fibreoptic intubation may be required

Mandibular fractures can be treated by either closed reduction and indirect skeletal fixation (using interdental wires, arch bars, or splints) or open reduction and direct skeletal fixation using bone plates. Direct skeletal fixation (using plates) is commoner. Rarely, indirect skeletal fixation is used, and the patient's teeth may be wired together at the completion of surgery.

Preoperative

- Ensure careful assessment for associated injuries.
- Make a meticulous assessment of the airway. There may be severe trismus and marked soft tissue swelling.
- Assess nostril patency. Check for evidence of basal skull fracture and CSF leak, as these contraindicate nasal intubation.

Perioperative

- Nasal intubation (or tracheostomy). The surgeons cannot work around an oral airway.
- Acute trismus makes intubation look potentially difficult preoperatively, as mouth opening may be markedly limited, but this tends to relax following induction. Patients with older fractures and those complicated by infection tend not to relax as much.
- Marked swelling may make intubation more difficult, and an AFOI may occasionally be required.
- Bilateral mandibular fractures also allow increased anterior jaw displacement after induction, but airway maintenance by face mask may not always be easy due to increased jaw movement/swelling. An RSI with suxamethonium may be appropriate.
- Gas induction and effective pre-oxygenation may be more difficult due to pain when applying the face mask.

Post-operative

As for patients having maxillary/mandibular osteotomies.

Maxillary/mandibular osteotomy

Procedure	Surgical realignment of facial skeleton
Time	3–6hr
Pain	++
Position	Supine, with head-up tilt, head ring
Blood loss	Variable. Occasionally can be severe. G&S
Practical techniques	Nasal tube, throat pack, and IPPV. Consider art line

Patients presenting for orthognathic surgery may have malformations isolated to one jaw or have multiple craniofacial deformities as part of a syndrome. They have often had prior dental extractions and preoperative orthodontic work. There are many surgical procedures performed to correct facial deformities. Patients are usually in their late teens or early twenties and are generally fit and healthy. When a mandibular osteotomy is performed, the bone is plated and often transiently stabilized by wiring the maxilla and mandible together. Rarely the patient remains 'wired' at the end of the case. If vomiting occurs post-operatively or intraoral bleeding occurs, fatal airway obstruction may occur, unless the fixation can be instantly removed. This requires expert trained staff and adequate facilities post-operatively.

Preoperative
- Assess the airway carefully. Check the nostrils for patency.
- Check Hb and G&S (as per local guidelines).
- Thromboembolic prophylaxis (compression stockings, LMWH). Consider the use of intermittent pneumatic compression boots in theatre.

Perioperative
- Intubate nasally using a preformed nasal tube (see ➲ p. 653). Spraying the cords and larynx with lidocaine may reduce coughing on extubation.
- Good venous access. Consider invasive pressure monitoring due to the length of surgery.
- Put lubricating ophthalmic ointment into the eyes, and protect them with pads and tape or plastic contact lenses.
- Position the patient carefully on the operating table. Place the head on a ring, and tilt the table head-up.
- Preventing hypertension or mild induced hypotension is useful to help minimize blood loss. Remifentanil infusion (0.1–0.75 micrograms/kg/min, or TCI 2–6ng/mL, although >12ng/mL may occasionally be needed), as part of a balanced anaesthetic, may help control BP. Other choices include GTN infusion (2–10mg/hr) and β-blockade (e.g. labetalol 5–10mg boluses or by infusion). As a general guide, maintain the MAP at 60mmHg or above.

- Give IV antibiotics (e.g. co-amoxiclav 1.2g or clindamycin 600mg) and steroids (e.g. dexamethasone 8mg IV) to minimize swelling.
- Keep the patient warm. Measure the core temperature; warm IV fluids, and use a heating mattress and/or hot air blower. These may need to be reduced after 2–3hr, as patients tend to overheat.
- Monitor blood loss carefully. HemoCue® is a useful way of tracking Hb concentration in theatre.
- The patient's jaws will rarely be wired together on completion of surgery. Ensure that throat packs are removed and that the oropharynx is cleared of blood and debris before this is done.
- Administer prophylactic antiemetics (ondansetron plus cyclizine) to minimize the risk of nausea and vomiting. Dexamethasone 8mg is also effective and reduces swelling.
- Extubate the patient once fully awake. Withdraw the nasal tube and cut, and safety pin (15cm mark at the nostril) to leave as a nasopharyngeal airway.
- Prescribe small doses of IV opioid to be administered in recovery.
- Ensure that you and the nursing staff are familiar with the position of any wires that hold the jaws together. Make sure wire cutters are with the patient at all times if the patient remains wired.

Post-operative

- Some units send these patients to HDU. Others send them to the ward after a lengthy period in recovery.
- Administer humidified O_2.
- Ensure all oral analgesics are prescribed in a soluble form. PCA or IM opioids should also be prescribed.
- Continue prophylactic antibiotics and steroids post-operatively, as per your unit's protocol (usually 24–48hr).
- Prescribe IV fluids. Encourage the patient to take fluid by the oral route as soon as possible.

Further reading

Coulthard P (2006). Conscious sedation guidance. *Evid Based Dent*, **7**, 90–1.

Coyle M, Tyrrell R, Godden A, et al. (2013). Replacing tracheostomy with overnight intubation to manage the airway in head and neck oncology patients: towards an improved recovery. *Br J Oral Maxillofac Surg*, **51**, 493–6.

Royal College of Anaesthetists (1999). *Standards and guidelines for general anaesthesia for dentistry.* ℘ http://www.rcoa.ac.uk.

Standing Dental Advisory Committee (1990). *General anaesthesia, sedation and resuscitation in dentistry. Report of an expert working party (the Poswillo report).* London: Department of Health.

The Society for the Advancement of Anaesthesia in Dentistry (SAAD). ℘ http://www.saad.org.uk/.

Ophthalmic surgery

Steve Gayer

General principles

Intraocular pressure

IOP normally ranges between 10 and 20mmHg, but transient changes occur with posture, coughing, vomiting, and Valsalva manoeuvres. These are normal and have no bearing on the intact eye. However, IOP approaches atmospheric pressure when the globe is opened during surgery, so force generated from such changes may cause vitreous extrusion, haemorrhage, or lens prolapse. Anaesthesia should strive to ensure a smooth intraoperative course by preventing coughing, retching, and vomiting, lest harmful elevations of IOP occur (Table 28.1).

Factors affecting IOP (analogous to factors affecting ICP) are as follows:
- Aqueous humour volume (balance of production and drainage)
- Choroidal blood volume (balance of arterial flow and venous drainage)
- Head-up position (via its effect on the above)
- Tone in extraocular muscles
- Mannitol and acetazolamide: mannitol (0.5g/kg IV) reduces IOP by withdrawing fluid from the vitreous. Acetazolamide (500mg IV) reduces IOP by decreasing ciliary body aqueous production. Both can be used in the medical management of glaucoma, but the anaesthetist may be required to administer them intraoperatively to reduce IOP acutely. Both are mild diuretics; urinary catheterization may be indicated.
- Anaesthetic factors.

Table 28.1 Anaesthesia and intraocular pressure

Anaesthetic factors increasing IOP	Anaesthetic factors decreasing IOP
External compression of the globe by tightly applied face mask	Induction agents principally by reduction in arterial and venous pressure
Laryngoscopy—either pressor response or straining in an inadequately relaxed patient	Non-depolarizing muscle relaxants by reduction in tone of extraocular muscles
Suxamethonium increases IOP transiently by contracting extraocular muscles	Head-up tilt at 15°, assists venous drainage
Large volumes of LA solution placed in the orbit. This effect is transient (2–3min)	Moderate hypocapnia: 3.5–4.0kPa (26–30mmHg) reduces choroidal blood volume by vasoconstriction of choroidal vessels

Oculomedullary reflexes

(Oculocardiac, oculorespiratory, and oculoemetic reflexes)
- Incidence: 20–80%. Commonly seen in paediatric squint surgery.
- Triggers: traction on extraocular muscles, pressure on globe.
- Afferent arc: long and short ciliary nerve fibres, via ciliary ganglion to trigeminal ganglion near floor of 4th ventricle.
- Efferent arc: vagus, fibres to respiratory and vomiting centre.
- Effects: bradycardia, junctional rhythm, sinus arrest, VT, respiratory arrest, nausea, and vomiting.
- Prevention: bradycardia, respiratory arrest, and nausea moderated to some extent by the use of LA (to abolish the afferent arc), avoiding hypercapnia (which appears to sensitize the reflex) and prophylactic glycopyrronium (200–400 micrograms) or atropine (300 micrograms).
- Atropine is fractionally absorbed by the eye, so it is not contraindicated for the glaucoma patient.

Preoperative assessment

The majority of ophthalmic operations are day cases under LA. Most patients are elderly and may have one or more serious systemic diseases. Patients scheduled for GA should have routine investigations performed. Patients having cataract extraction under LA, however, do not warrant routine investigation. Many centres do not routinely fast such patients, and a light meal, 2–3hr preoperatively, may be less disruptive for this elderly population and facilitate better diabetic control. Light sedation in these unfasted patients is not uncommon.

Preoperative assessment for LA eye surgery includes:
- Axial length
- INR/APTT if on warfarin or heparin
- Blood glucose if diabetic
- Ability to lie flat for 1hr (cough, sleep apnoea, heart failure, arthritis, etc.)
- Hearing/comprehension—will they be able to hear and understand instructions?
- Anxiety level—will sedation be required?
- Ability to tolerate supplemental O_2—is there a risk of CO_2 retention, requiring the delivery of a precise concentration of O_2?

General anaesthesia versus local anaesthesia

There are a number of advantages to avoiding GA in this population. These include:
- Minimization of physiological disturbance
- Economic factors—increased patient throughput (ward admissions and theatre throughput), less demand on nursing resources, portering, etc.

There are situations when GA is preferable:
- Patients who refuse the operation under LA. Unless there are overwhelming risks, such patients should be offered GA, provided they are fully informed about the risks and accept them
- Children and patients with learning disabilities/movement disorders

- Major and lengthy operations (oculoplastics and vitreoretinal) are commonly performed under GA, since it may be unrealistic to expect patients to tolerate them otherwise.
- Patients unable to lie flat and remain motionless for up to 1hr (although some surgeons can operate in a 'deck-chair' position, rather than true supine for LA).

Miscellaneous ophthalmic procedures

Table 28.2 presents the important information for those procedures which are not covered in the individual topics within this chapter.

Table 28.2 Other ophthalmic procedures

Operation	Description	Time (min)	Pain (+ to +++++)	Position	Blood loss	Notes
Trabeculectomy	Surgical correction of glaucoma	50–80	+	Supine	Nil	Usually performed under LA block—peribulbar may be preferred to sub-Tenon's. Axial length may not have been checked
Moh's reconstruction	Plastics procedure on eyelids after excision of basal cell carcinoma	45–60	+	Supine	Nil	May be under LA but may require use of fat or fascia taken from the thigh, so GA may be preferred
Enucleation	Removal of globe for tumour or chronic infection	60–90	++	Supine	0–200mL	Anaesthetic technique as for vitreoretinal surgery. Local techniques not appropriate
Evisceration	Removal of globe contents for later replacement with prosthesis	60–90	+	Supine	Nil	Anaesthetic technique as for vitreoretinal surgery. Local techniques not appropriate
Syringing of tear ducts in babies		30	+	Supine		Straightforward technique. SV via LMA. Throat pack to absorb any 'wash'
EUA of eyes in babies		10–20	+	Supine		Beware oculocardiac reflex. Have atropine 10 micrograms/kg prepared

Basic anatomy
for ophthalmic anaesthesia

- The **orbit** is 40–50mm deep and pyramidal in shape, with its base at the orbital opening and its apex pointing to the optic foramen. Its volume is ~30mL, of which 7mL is occupied by the globe and its muscle cone, and the remainder by loose connective tissue through which LA solutions can spread. The lateral walls of both orbits form an angle of 90°—the angle between the medial and lateral wall of each orbit is 45°. The medial wall is parallel to the sagittal plane.

- The **globe** lies in the anterior part of the orbit and sits high and lateral (i.e. nearer the roof than the floor, and nearer the lateral than the medial wall). This is important when considering needle access, which is usually achieved either medially or inferolaterally where the gap between the globe and orbital wall is greatest. The **sclera** forms the fibrous bulk of the globe. It is 1mm thick and, although tough, can be penetrated by a sharp needle. Deep to the sclera is the uveal tract which comprises the ciliary body, iris, and choroid layer. Superficial to and enclosing the sclera is the membranous **Tenon's capsule**, lying directly underneath the conjunctiva. It is easily recognized, being white and avascular. The **four recti and two oblique muscles** control eye movement and influence IOP. The lateral rectus is innervated by the abducens nerve (VIth), the superior oblique by the trochlear nerve (IVth), and the rest by the oculomotor nerve (IIIrd) (LR_6SO_4)$_3$. The recti form the muscle 'cone' which encloses the sensory nerves, ciliary ganglion, optic nerve, and retinal artery and vein. It is through this cone that peribulbar LA drugs must diffuse to effect their action.

- The cranial nerves enter the cone and pierce the muscles on their intraconal surface. These are motor only. The sensory supply is via branches of the trigeminal (Vth) cranial nerve. The 1st division of the trigeminal (**ophthalmic nerve**, V_1) enters the orbit via the superior orbital fissure and supplies branches intraconally to the sclera/cornea, and extraconally to the upper lid and conjunctiva after leaving the orbit via the superior orbital notch. The 2nd division (**maxillary nerve**, V_2) enters the orbit via the inferior orbital fissure. Branches of this nerve are entirely extraconal and supply the lower lid and inferior conjunctiva after leaving the orbit via the inferior orbital foramen.

- The **ciliary ganglion**, lying within the cone, relays sensory fibres from the globe to V_1 and receives a parasympathetic branch from the (motor) IIIrd cranial nerve and sympathetic fibres from the carotid plexus.

Ophthalmic anaesthesia options

Ophthalmic anaesthesia can be divided into two classes.

Akinetic anaesthesia
- Needle injection of LA:
  - Into the extraocular muscle cone (retrobulbar or intraconal block)
  - External to the muscle cone (peribulbar or extraconal block).
- Cannula infusion of LA beneath the Tenon's capsule.
- GA.

Kinetic analgesia
- Topical LA drops or lidocaine gel.
- Supplemental intracameral injection of preservative-free LA.
- Subconjunctival injection.

Needle-based blocks

Retrobulbar (or intraconal)
(See Fig. 28.1.)
- Steeply angled and deeply placed.
- Low volume (1–3mL of agent).
- Rapid akinesia and analgesia.
- May require separate facial nerve block for lid akinesia.
- Greater potential for complications:
  - Globe perforation—posterior or inferior pole of the eye
  - Optic nerve sheath injection—brainstem anaesthesia, trauma
  - Intravascular injection—convulsions, apnoea, loss of consciousness
  - Retrobulbar haemorrhage.
- Not recommended without training and experience. Globe penetration or perforation may lead to permanent visual loss. Brainstem anaesthesia may cause apnoea, dysrhythmias, and cardiac arrest.

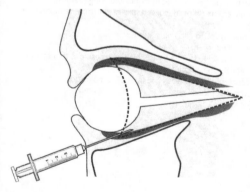

Fig. 28.1 Retrobulbar (intraconal) block.

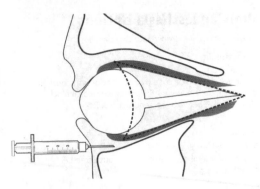

Fig. 28.2 Peribulbar (extraconal) block.

Peribulbar (or extraconal)
(See Fig. 28.2.)
- Minimally angled, parallel to the globe, with shallow placement.
- High volume (4–10mL of agent).
- More gradual onset of akinesia and analgesia.
- Facial nerve block not required.
- Lesser potential for significant complications. Retrobulbar haemorrhage and globe penetration less likely if use single inferolateral injection technique and avoid superior aspect of orbit.
- May be supplemented with a medial canthus block.

Cannula-based (sub-Tenon's) block

(See Fig. 28.3.)
- Cannula may be rigid (usually metal) or flexible, long (32mm), short (25mm), or ultrashort (10mm), curved or straight (may be tapered or have stops).
- Lesser potential for serious complications:
  - Vortex vein haemorrhage
  - Globe perforation (extremely rare; high myopes have thin sclera)
  - Central retinal artery occlusion.
- Higher incidence of minor (mostly cosmetic) complications:
  - Conjunctival haemorrhage
  - Chemosis.

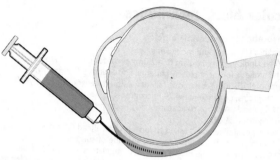

Fig. 28.3 Sub-Tenon's block.

Ocular block techniques

Peribulbar (extraconal) block

- Establish IV access and monitoring.
- When indicated, midazolam 0.5–2.0mg provides effective anxiolysis and amnesia for most elderly patients. For deeper sedation, use propofol 10–30mg ± narcotic (alfentanil 250 micrograms, fentanyl 50 micrograms, or remifentanil 20 micrograms).
- Instil topical LA drops to anaesthetize the conjunctiva (proxymetacaine 0.5%).
- Patient lies supine and is asked to look straight ahead (1° gaze).
- Confirm proper patient, procedure, and side of surgery.
- Palpate junction of the medial two-thirds and lateral one-third of the inferior orbital rim with the non-dominant hand where a groove is felt at the junction of the maxilla and zygoma (Fig. 28.4).
- Slightly lateral to this point and just above the rim (Fig. 28.4), insert a 20–32mm 23–25G needle mounted on a 10mL syringe, and pass slowly backwards, parallel to the globe and perpendicular to all planes. The insertion point is derived in this manner to prevent injection of LA into the inferior rectus and inferior oblique muscles. Needle entry can be either transcutaneous or, by retraction of the lower lid, transconjunctival.
- If the needle tip contacts the bone, it is redirected slightly superiorly to follow the orbit floor.
- The needle does not need to be placed deeply. Trainees and those with little experience should not hesitate to keep the tip shallow in the orbit. The globe should be observed carefully for any sign of rotation during insertion, indicating scleral contact.
- Consider aspiration, and then slowly inject 4–10mL of LA. Stop injecting if globe becomes tense/proptosed or if the upper eyelid fills, as this is likely to indicate retrobulbar injection, requiring a smaller volume of agent.

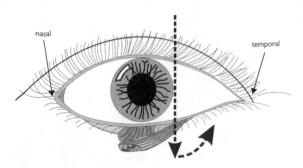

Fig. 28.4 Needle insertion site.

- Following injection, some employ digital massage or a compression device (Honan balloon) to dissipate LA and normalize IOP.
- If a further 'top-up' is needed, use a medial canthus injection. This is an advanced technique. At a point, just medial to the caruncle, the needle is passed backward, with the bevel facing the globe, at an angle of 10° to the sagittal plane, directed towards the medial wall of the orbit. If the medial wall is contacted, the needle is withdrawn slightly and redirected laterally. Inject 3–4mL of LA.

The larger volumes of solution required for a peribulbar block tend to cause proptosis and a temporary increase in IOP. In the intact globe, this has no consequence but can be problematic when the globe is opened for surgery. Hyaluronidase mixed into the LA is useful. The raised IOP usually disappears when the solution has dissipated; alternatively, a compression device can be applied over the eye at a set pressure (25mmHg), which reduces the volume of blood and aqueous in the eye. Upon release, the eye becomes hypotonic and remains so for about 5min until blood and aqueous volumes are re-established.

Relative contraindications to peribulbar (extraconal) block
- **Axial length >26mm.** In severely myopic patients, the globe often has a long anteroposterior diameter or may have an abnormal hernial outpouched structure (staphyloma) which can increase the potential of globe perforation. Where the axial length is >26mm, consider a sub-Tenon's approach, topical anaesthesia, or GA.
- Perforated or infected eye.
- Inability to lie flat and still.

Complications
- **Globe perforation:** <0.01%. Not always obvious. May be painless or associated with sudden pain on injection. It may be noted at the time of surgery if the eye becomes hypotonic, in which case there is a serious risk of retinal haemorrhage and detachment which may require laser retinopexy or vitrectomy.
- **Retrobulbar haemorrhage:** incidence 0.07%. Often innocuous. Rarely severe bleeding is recognized by rapid orbital swelling and proptosis. The surgeon should be informed immediately, and the pulsation of the central retinal artery assessed. If this is compromised, a lateral canthotomy may be required to relieve IOP.
- 'Systemic complications' (oculocardiac reflex, neurogenic syncope, epileptic seizure) are rare, but monitoring is key. Most are self-limiting.

Sub-Tenon's block
- Apply topical proxymetacaine 0.5% to the conjunctiva, and retract the lower lid, either with the help of an assistant or using a lid speculum.
- Confirm proper patient, procedure, and side of surgery.
- In the inferonasal quadrant, the conjunctiva is lifted with Moorfield's forceps at a point 5–7mm from the limbus (cooperative patients are asked to look superotemporally).
- A small incision is made in the conjunctiva with blunt-tipped Westcott's scissors which are then used to dissect inferonasally in a plane between

the sclera and Tenon's capsule. The Tenon's capsule is recognized as white and avascular, which distinguishes it from the vascular sclera.
- Once in this plane, a blunt cannula (Stevens cannula or similar) is inserted, and 3–8mL of LA is deposited. Care must be taken to dissect in the correct plane. If the cannula is placed subconjunctivally, the LA solution will reflux out or may cause considerable chemosis.
- Sub-Tenon's block can be used safely in patients with axial lengths >26mm, although there are rare reports of scleral penetration. It is the block of choice in anticoagulated patients, since any bleeding point can be cauterized directly, but be aware that vortex vein haemorrhage has been reported. This is commoner with long, rigid cannulae.

Topical/infiltration anaesthesia
- Reserved for anterior segment surgery such as cataract extraction.
- Topical LA drops can be used to provide up to 15min of anaesthesia. Proxymetacaine 0.5% (proparacaine in the US) is the agent of choice. Note that topical LAs are toxic to the corneal epithelium—prolonged administration may cause clouding/irritation.
- Topical LA gels (lidocaine) have a longer duration of action. Gels act as barriers to antiseptics, so the correct order of administration is: drops–antiseptic–gel.
- Note that anaesthesia is not as complete as with a formal ophthalmic block. The iris and ciliary body retain their sensitivity, and akinesia is not a feature. Proper patient selection is key, otherwise one may find oneself involved in a '**vocal local**' session. The surgeon and staff need to ensure that good communication is maintained with the patient at all times. Anxiolytic agents may be useful.
- Intracameral injection by the surgeon (0.1mL of isotonic preservative-free lidocaine) to the anterior chamber may be used to provide anaesthesia to the iris and ciliary body.

Local anaesthetic solutions
- The commonest solution is a 1:1 mixture of lidocaine 2% and bupivacaine 0.5% (or levobupivacaine 0.75%). For routine cataract extraction, lidocaine 2% alone gives sufficient duration, but, for more prolonged vitreoretinal surgery, levobupivacaine 0.75% is more suitable.
- Hyaluronidase can be added to promote spread and reduce IOP.[1] Concentrations between 1 and 30U/mL are used. The drug data sheet suggests 15U/mL. A recombinant form of hyaluronidase is now available.
- Adrenaline may produce an untoward tachycardia if absorbed systemically via the punctum and nasal mucosa. Unless vasoconstriction is needed, it should be avoided in elderly patients.
- Alkalinization and warming of the LA (to 37°C) may reduce latency and decrease pain on injection.

Reference
1 Schulenburg HE, Sri-Chandana C, Lyons G, Columb MO, McLure HA (2007). Hyaluronidase reduces local anaesthetic volumes for sub-Tenon's anaesthesia. *Br J Anaesth*, **99**, 717–20.

General anaesthetic techniques

The aim is to minimize increases in IOP, while maintaining CVS stability and avoiding overly deep anaesthesia in a population that is likely to be elderly and have several co-morbidities.

Indications

- Patient preference.
- Paediatric patients.
- Other patient factors (e.g. movement disorders, marked cough, dementia, claustrophobia).
- Long operations (e.g. vitreoretinal, corneal transplantation).
- Orbital involvement (e.g. blowout fracture, optic nerve fenestration).
- Multiple operation sites (e.g. oculoplastics with distant graft site).

Preoperative

In addition to routine consultation and investigations (see ➔ p. 7), the preoperative visit should identify patients with co-morbidities such as diabetes and CVS disease. Pacemakers and internal defibrillators should be evaluated in a suitable time frame prior to surgery. Consider temporarily disabling automated internal defibrillators. Insulin-dependent diabetics will often have reduced their morning dose of insulin and will be fasted. Such patients will require close monitoring of blood glucose and the institution of a euglycaemic control regimen.

Endotracheal tube or laryngeal mask airway?

Unless contraindicated, the LMA is ideal. It obviates laryngoscopy and the possible adverse effects on IOP. It produces minimal stimulation once in place and permits lighter anaesthesia. The quality of emergence is also superior (see ➔ p. 674).

Ventilation or spontaneous respiration?

For extraocular and minor surgery (including cataract extraction), SV is acceptable. Controlled ventilation has a number of advantages in intraocular and more major surgery. It allows control of CO_2 (reducing IOP and desensitizing the oculomedullary reflex) and permits the other benefits of a balanced technique.

- Ventilating via an LMA is usually uneventful. Pressure control or pressure support allows avoidance of high airway pressures (>15cmH$_2$O, with the risk of gastric insufflation). Volume-based positive pressure ventilation, by adjusting the V_T to an appropriate airway pressure and using a more symmetrical I:E ratio (1:1.5), is also acceptable.
- Always monitor the CO_2 waveform. Any change usually heralds a change in ventilation before it is clinically apparent (malpositioned LMA, inadequate muscle relaxation).
- Use spirometry, if available. An open flow–volume loop graphically demonstrates the presence of a leak and potential LMA displacement.
- Use a nerve stimulator routinely when electing to paralyse patients. Coughing and gagging are less well tolerated by ophthalmic surgeons than by their orthopaedic colleagues.

Nitrous oxide?

N_2O should be avoided in vitreoretinal surgery if intraocular gas bubbles, such as sulphur hexafluoride (SF_6), octafluoropropane (C_3F_8), air, or similar, are planned. Discuss this with the surgeon in advance, or simply make it a routine habit to use an O_2/air combination.

Supplementary local block?

A local block, in addition to GA, is a key strategy for post-operative pain management. It is particularly useful for vitreoretinal surgery, corneal transplantations, and paediatric and oculoplastic procedures. A sub-Tenon's block (with negligible risk) is the preferred technique and can be administered following induction.

Emergence without coughing

With an LMA, emergence is usually smooth. If an ETT is used, spray the cords with lidocaine at intubation; however, the effect is short-lived and may no longer be effective at extubation. Other techniques include extubating in a deep plane of anaesthesia or administering a bolus of IV lidocaine (1mg/kg) or propofol (30–40mg) just prior to extubation.

It is best not to lighten anaesthesia until surgery is complete and the 'sticky drapes' removed (if a block has been used, drape removal may be the most stimulating part of the operation). Emergence hypertension (and the concomitant raised IOP), if it occurs, can be moderated by the use of IV lidocaine (up to 1mg/kg) a few minutes before emergence.

A standard technique: summary

- IV induction: propofol bolus or TCI.
- Airway: reinforced or ProSeal LMA, if appropriate.
- Consider controlled ventilation.
- Maintenance: propofol infusion (~5mg/kg/hr or 2.5 micrograms/mL if TCI) or volatile agent.
- Use an O_2/air mixture. Avoid N_2O.
- Analgesia provided ideally with an LA block, if indicated, or with short-acting narcotics (alfentanil/remifentanil) for stimulating procedures.

General points

- Tape the non-operative eye. Participate in the 'timeout' to ensure the correct eye is exposed and not draped.
- Access to the airway may be limited—have a low threshold for moving everyone out of the way if you suspect difficulties.
- Glycopyrronium may reduce the incidence/severity of bradycardia.

Do not allow the surgeon to extubate the patient. Be sure to have the LMA/ETT securely in hand prior to removal of the sticky drapes.

Post-operative

Analgesia requirements are usually modest, especially if supplemental LA is administered intraoperatively. Nausea and vomiting are common in squint surgery, but less so in the majority of other cases. It is reasonable to use PONV prophylaxis (ondansetron 100 micrograms/kg) in squint surgery, although it is only modestly effective.

Cataract extraction and intraocular lens

Procedure	Phacoemulsification of opacified lens, removal and replacement with artificial intraocular implant
Time	20–40min
Pain	Minimal
Position	Supine
Blood loss	Nil
Practical techniques	Local technique, sub-Tenon's or needle block, LMA (armoured), SV/IPPV; ETT (RAE, armoured), IPPV

Preoperative

- Check the axial length (<26mm for peribulbar block).
- For operations under LA, the patient must be able to lie flat and still. Active cough is a relative contraindication.
- Patient cooperation may be necessary with laser capsulotomy. No block. Minimal or no sedation prior to the laser portion of the procedure.
- Men with benign prostatic hypertrophy may take tamsulosin and have **'floppy iris'** syndrome. They may require increased surgical manipulation, warranting a solid block.
- Consider INR if excessive warfarin anticoagulation suspected.
- Most commonly day case.

Perioperative

- Use supplemental O_2 (via nasal cannulae).
- Monitor BP, SpO_2, and nasal expired CO_2, if possible. The latter serves as an apnoea indicator and is useful if sedation is used. Be aware that sedation may serve to disinhibit, rather than sedate, some patients.
- If sedation is required, use midazolam (0.25–1mg) with fentanyl (25–50 micrograms), remifentanil (20–50 micrograms), or propofol (20mg). This is best employed during block insertion. The patient should then be allowed to awaken when in theatre to gain cooperation and avoid sleeping, snoring, and airway problems.
- Glaucoma patients' chronic miotic drop therapy may make surgical access difficult and require the use of an iris retractor. Ensure a dense regional block to minimize discomfort from surgical manipulation.

Post-operative

- Simple oral analgesics only required.

Strabismus surgery

(See also ➔ p. 781.)

Procedure	Extraocular surgery for correction of squint—may be unilateral or bilateral
Time	60–90min
Pain	+
Position	Supine
Blood loss	Nil
Practical techniques	LMA (armoured), IPPV/SV, ETT (RAE, armoured), IPPV

Preoperative

- Patient population mainly children (commonest ophthalmic operation in children); GA.
- Older teenagers and adults may often have surgery via regional anesthesia.
- Adjustable sutures are fine-tuned, only after all LAs have fully dissipated. Use short-acting agents (i.e. lidocaine).
- There may be a higher incidence of MH than in the general population (controversial).
- May be day case.
- Preoperative analgesia (20mg/kg of soluble paracetamol).

Perioperative

- Higher incidence of oculocardiac reflex; have atropine prepared. Prophylaxis with glycopyrronium is not proven.
- Maintain normocapnia to reduce incidence and severity of the oculocardiac reflex. Consider controlled ventilation via an LMA or tracheal tube.
- Suxamethonium should be avoided, because the tone in the ocular muscles remains abnormal for up to 20min, making surgical assessment and correction difficult.
- Suspect MH if hypertension, tachycardia, hypercapnia, and increasing temperature.
- All anaesthetics affect eye movement and the position of neutral gaze (Guedel's signs). Propofol may affect this the least, and the rapid recovery it affords allows early assessment of the correction in recovery. Anaesthesia with volatile agents should be of sufficient depth to ensure neutral gaze.
- High incidence of PONV. Consider multimodal PONV prophylaxis with serotonin antagonist (ondansetron 100 micrograms/kg), metoclopramide, or dexamethasone. Avoid opioids. Consider total IV technique with propofol.
- Consider paracetamol or rectal diclofenac (1mg/kg).

Post-operative
- Post-operative pain is mild and can be treated with oral analgesics and topical proxymetacaine eye drops.
- PONV rescue with repeat dose of serotonin antagonist is minimally effective. Consider a different class of antiemetic.

Vitreoretinal surgery

Procedure	Intraocular surgery. Vitrectomy, cryotherapy, laser, plombage, insertion of oil and/or gas, scleral banding ('explant')
Time	90–180min
Pain	++/+++
Position	Supine
Blood loss	Nil
Practical techniques	LMA (armoured), IPPV; ETT (RAE, armoured), IPPV. Sub-Tenon's or needle block ± GA

Preoperative

- Patient population generally aged 60–70yr. May have coexisting morbidities, e.g. hypertension, IHD, and diabetes.
- Severe myopes, at risk for retinal detachment, are generally younger.
- Retinal detachments may be semi-urgent, particularly if 'macula on'.
- Note if recent retinal surgery on the other eye (see ◆ Perioperative, p. 678).

Perioperative

- Often prolonged operations, performed largely in the dark.
- Surgery is characterized by alternating periods of intense and minimal stimulation. Achieving a depth of anaesthesia and analgesia to accommodate these extremes is not easy without concurrent local block. Use long-acting LA.
- Retinal detachment patients with myopia will be at increased risk of globe puncture (staphyloma, long axial length). Retro/peribulbar blocks are relatively contraindicated. Consider sub-Tenon's with light-handed dissection, as even blunt scissors may cut the typically thinner sclera.
- Consider GA—LMA/propofol/remifentanil/O_2/air.
- Avoid N_2O. Intraocular tamponade with gas (SF_6 or C_3F_8) may be used, usually towards the end of the case. It is recommended that N_2O be discontinued 20min beforehand. It is probably better to omit altogether, as surgeons seldom give notice. If a supplementary block is not used, remifentanil or a deeper plane of inhalational anaesthesia should be considered, since cryotherapy and scleral indentation can be very stimulating.
- Oculocardiac reflex may be encountered upon surgical rotation of the globe and traction on the extraocular muscles.
- Beware of premature emergence, as the other eye is often examined, and possibly cryocauterized.
- Consider deep extubation and other manoeuvres to prevent bucking and associated increase in IOP with emergence from GA.

Post-operative

- With block, the post-operative analgesic requirement is minimal.
- Otherwise, simple oral analgesics.

Other anterior segment procedures

Procedure	Penetrating keratoplasty (cornea transplantation), glaucoma drainage, intracapsular cataract extraction
Time	30–180min
Pain	+/++
Position	Supine
Blood loss	Nil
Practical techniques	LMA (armoured), IPPV; ETT (RAE, armoured), IPPV; sub-Tenon's or needle block ± GA

Preoperative

- Glaucoma patient population varied, but generally geriatric. May have coexisting morbidities, e.g. hypertension, IHD, and diabetes.
- Check glaucoma patients' medication list. Non-selective β-blocker drops can cause bradycardic rhythms. Ecothiopate may prolong the effects of suxamethonium.
- Cornea transplant patients are of all ages. Be wary of drug allergies, particularly for Stevens–Johnson patients.

Perioperative

- As with vitreoretinal surgery, these are characterized by alternating periods of intense and minimal stimulation. Achieving a depth of anaesthesia and analgesia to accommodate these extremes is not easy without concurrent local block.
- Control of IOP is crucial. Scleral incision of a tense eye can result in sudden decompression and iris/lens prolapse, vitreous loss, or expulsive choroidal haemorrhage.
- Controlled ventilation and $ETCO_2$ monitoring to ensure avoiding hypercapnia and elevated IOP.
- Consider agents to lower pre-existent or persistent high IOP (mannitol, acetazolamide).
- Complete akinesia is indicated for cornea transplantation. Ensure a good solid block and/or deep level of GA.
- Oculocardiac reflex: IV atropine is not contraindicated for glaucoma patients, as it is only fractionally absorbed by the eye.
- A supplementary sub-Tenon's block improves intraoperative stability, obviates the need for opioids, and reduces post-operative pain and nausea. Place after induction, or ask the surgeon to perform.

Post-operative

- With block, post-operative analgesic requirement is minimal.
- PONV may be due to elevated post-operative IOP. Consider re-evaluation by the ophthalmologist.
- Otherwise, simple oral analgesics.

Dacrocystorhinostomy

Procedure	Probing of tear duct, insertion of drainage tube, formation of stoma between tear duct and nasopharynx
Time	30–45min
Pain	+
Position	Supine, slight head-up
Blood loss	Can be relatively bloody, with soiling of nasopharynx
Practical techniques	ETT (RAE, armoured), IPPV; LMA (armoured), IPPV

Preoperative

- Lacrimal surgery can range from simple probing of the tear ducts to insertion of tubes or formal dacrocystorhinostomy (DCR). The latter is usually done under GA, although block and sedation are feasible.
- DCR may be bloody. Blood will pass into the nasopharynx/oropharynx. Topical vasoconstrictor solutions (cocaine/Moffett's soaked pledgets) placed intranasally after induction may reduce this. Infiltrate the surgical field with LA containing a vasoconstrictor to further reduce bleeding. Beware of ensuing tachyarrhythmias.
- Slight head-up tilt and deliberate moderate hypotension (or avoidance of hypertension) further improve the operative field.
- Intubation (oral RAE or reinforced) protects the lower airway definitively, but a reinforced LMA may be used where topical vasoconstriction, moderate hypotension, and surgical cooperation are available. Consider placing a throat pack.
- Controlled ventilation, by facilitating moderate hypocapnia, may also contribute to mucosal vasoconstriction and improved operative field.
- If using an LMA, positive pressure ventilation may reduce the likelihood of blood soiling the lower airway.

Post-operative

- Post-operative analgesia provided by oral NSAIDs and paracetamol/codeine.
- Ask the surgeon to irrigate the ducts with topical LA.

Special considerations

- DCR can be performed under LA alone, with suitable surgical experience.

Penetrating eye injury

(See also ⊃ p. 781.)

Procedure	EUA, debridement, closure of punctum
Time	30–90 min
Pain	+/+++
Position	Supine
Blood loss	–
Practical techniques	ETT (RAE, armoured), IPPV; LMA (armoured), IPPV; needle block

Preoperative

- Although relatively straightforward in adults, this can be difficult to manage in children (in whom it is a common injury, representing more than a third of paediatric trauma cases). The essential danger is that elevation of IOP, either pre- or perioperatively, risks extrusion of the vitreous, haemorrhage, and lens prolapse.
- Pain, eye rubbing, crying, breath-holding, and screaming will elevate IOP. IV sedation may be required to control such a child.
- Give analgesia (PO/PR paracetamol/NSAIDs). Opioids should be avoided, if possible (or at least used cautiously and with an antiemetic), since vomiting will also affect IOP adversely.
- Patients may have a full stomach. Traumatized children may still have a full stomach several hours post-injury.

Perioperative

- Suxamethonium causes a transient increase in IOP. However, induction agents *reduce* IOP and so moderate its effects. The risks imposed by suxamethonium should be balanced against the risks (specific to each case) imposed by a full stomach. If in doubt, use suxamethonium following a large dose of induction agent.
- Practical alternatives to suxamethonium:
  - Wait. If immediate operative repair is not imperative (and it seldom is), the case can be deferred until the stomach is considered safe. Prokinetic agents may be of use
  - If no airway problems are anticipated, use a rapid sequence technique with rocuronium (1mg/kg) or 'high'-dose vecuronium (0.15mg/kg). Sugammadex, if available, can rapidly reverse these agents if airway difficulty is encountered.
- The pressor response to intubation can be moderated by IV lidocaine (1mg/kg), IV esmolol, or pre-priming with induction agent immediately prior to intubation.
- Opioids may be used as part of a balanced technique.
- An LA technique can be considered in certain patients at marked risk from GA.

Post-operative

- Paracetamol/codeine preparations and PO/PR diclofenac.

Further reading

Gayer S (2006). Rethinking anesthesia strategies for patients with traumatic eye injuries: alternatives to general anesthesia. *Curr Anesth Crit Care*, **17**, 191.

Gayer S, Kumar CM (2008). Ophthalmic regional anesthesia techniques. *Minerva Anestesiol*, **74** (1–2), 23–33.

Guise P (2003). Sub-Tenon's anesthesia: a prospective study of 6000 blocks. *Anesthesiology*, **98**, 964–8.

Kumar CM, Dodds C, Gayer S (2012). *Ophthalmic anaesthesia*. Oxford: Oxford University Press.

Kumar CM, Dodds C, McLure H, Chabria R (2004). A comparison of three sub-Tenon's cannulae. *Eye*, **18**, 873–6.

Ruschen H, Bremner FD, Carr C (2003). Complications after sub-Tenon's eye block. *Anesth Analg*, **96**, 273–7.

The Royal College of Ophthalmologists (2010). *Cataract surgery guidelines September 2010*. London: The Royal College of Ophthalmologists. ℜ http://www.rcophth.ac.uk/core/core_picker/download.asp?id=544.

Vohra SB, Good PA (2000). Altered globe dimensions of axial myopia as risk factors for penetrating ocular injury during peribulbar anesthesia. *Br J Anaesth*, **85**, 242–3.

Day surgery

Mary Stocker

Day surgery

- A surgical day case is a patient who is admitted, operated upon, and discharged on the same calendar day. The surgery must have been planned as day surgery. In the UK (unlike the US), a 24hr stay is not classed as day surgery, as this requires overnight admission. Organization is the key to efficient good-quality day surgery and requires close cooperation between all agencies involved, including surgeons, anaesthetists, day unit staff, GPs, patients, and their carers.
- Facilities: an efficient organization requires 'ring-fenced' theatres and ward space. Day surgery can be managed successfully in a variety of hospital configurations; however, day cases on inpatient wards and theatres have a higher admission rate and will suffer cancellation when there are bed shortages. Self-contained units with their own facilities, but within an acute hospital, offer the best option.
- Staff: senior staff should perform day-case anaesthesia and surgery. Increasingly complex patients and procedures are being transferred to day surgery, and anaesthesia must be performed to a high standard to minimize unplanned admissions. The day surgery environment provides many opportunities for training of junior staff, but supervision and guidance from senior clinicians with day surgery expertise is essential.

Patient preparation and optimization

Patients should follow a sequential pathway and undergo preoperative assessment by experienced day surgery nursing staff, according to set day-case criteria. Nurses should have the support of a consultant anaesthetist who they can approach for advice.

- Ideal practice is where patients attend assessment at the hospital on the day of their surgical outpatient appointment. This ensures time to complete any investigations and to review difficult patients.
- Some patient groups can undergo telephone assessment, in particular those who are young, fit, on no medication, and undergoing a procedure that does not require specific tests.
- Successful day surgery requires anaesthetic departments to consider patients who fall outside traditional guidelines and judge if they can be made fit for day surgery.
- Protocols can be used for preoperative investigations, but these should be kept to those absolutely essential for the surgery, as very few investigations in a day surgery pathway alter management.
- Clear instructions must be given to the patient regarding what will happen on the day of surgery, what they need to bring on the day, and the organization of someone to take them home and care for them post-operatively. These instructions should be reinforced with clear written information.
- Most cancellations on the day of surgery can be avoided by careful preoperative assessment by experienced staff. Those due to acute illness, however, may still occur.

Day-case selection criteria

Criteria need to be agreed with the local anaesthetic department and will vary, according to the day surgery unit setting, e.g. more challenging patients and procedures can be undertaken where the unit is integrated into a hospital with all support services. Stand-alone units on isolated sites will need more conservative criteria.

- *Health status*: day surgery is no longer reserved purely for the fit and healthy. Most patients with stable medical conditions are appropriate for day surgery, and many complex patients will do better in a day-case environment if they are managed appropriately, e.g. insulin-dependent diabetics, severe COPD patients, patients on dialysis, epileptics. Always try to remember these two questions:
    1. What can we do to enable this patient to be managed as a day case?
    2. Would anything be done differently if the patient were to be treated as an inpatient? If the answer is no, then day surgery is probably the optimal pathway.
- *Age*: there is no upper age limit; physiological fitness should be considered, rather than the chronological age, remembering that the elderly are usually better managed in their home environment. Babies as young as 6 weeks can be managed on a day-case basis (excluding premature infants <60 weeks post-gestational age due to the risk of sudden infant death syndrome, SIDS).
- *Obesity*: with appropriately skilled staff and equipment, even the morbidly obese can be successfully managed as day cases. It can be the ideal option, as early mobilization reduces the risk of complications. Assessment should include questions about OSA.
- *Complexity of surgery*: there is no time limit for surgical duration. Procedures associated with significant post-operative pain (that cannot be controlled with oral analgesia supplemented by regional anaesthetic techniques), inability to eat and drink, or prolonged immobility should not be performed.
- *Transport*: all patients must be escorted home by a responsible, informed adult and be adequately supervised during their recovery at home for a minimum of 24hr. Some units now employ carers for patients with no home support to enable them to be treated as day cases.
- *Social support*: patients must have suitable home conditions with adequate toilet facilities, and a telephone should be readily available for advice in an emergency. Patients must agree/understand that they should not drive, cycle, operate machinery, or consume alcohol for 24hr after their anaesthetic. This advice must be contained in the preoperative verbal and written instructions given to the patient and reinforced prior to discharge.
- *Geography*: though it is procedure-dependent, as a rule, the patient should live within 1hr of travelling distance from the hospital.

Conduct of anaesthesia

Use LA or short-acting GA drugs that have few residual psychomotor effects and a low incidence of PONV.

Preoperative

- Avoid sedative premedication, if at all possible. If necessary (usually only for patients with special needs), use oral midazolam (up to 0.5mg/kg) in a little undiluted sweet fruit cordial (as it tastes awful).
- Routine use of antacid drugs is unnecessary; however, in those with a history of regurgitation, ranitidine (300mg PO) or omeprazole (40mg PO) is appropriate.
- Oral analgesics—paracetamol 1g and NSAIDs reach peak effect after 1–2hr and are a useful adjunct to anaesthesia, with very few side effects. Slow-release ibuprofen (1600mg) preoperatively is very effective and provides long-acting post-operative pain relief.

Perioperative

- TIVA with propofol (without N_2O) is widely used. Propofol induction with sevoflurane maintenance is an alternative.
- For larger procedures, incremental fentanyl, often 2–4 micrograms/kg in divided doses. IV morphine should be avoided.
- Consider NSAIDs, if not already given, and LA for every suitable patient/operation.
- Give IV fluids in a dose of 15mL/kg. This reduces the incidence of dizziness and aids recovery.
- Whenever possible, use an LMA, avoiding intubation, muscle relaxants, and reversal agents. Laryngeal masks for gynaecological laparoscopy and armoured laryngeal masks for wisdom tooth extraction can be used safely in most circumstances.
- Antiemetics are not indicated routinely but should be reserved for treatment of any PONV or prophylaxis in those with a significant history of PONV or surgical procedures with a high incidence of PONV (e.g. ovarian/tubal surgery, squints, scrotal surgery).

Post-operative

- Balanced analgesia with paracetamol, NSAIDs, LA, and short-acting opioids is usually adequate. If more analgesia is needed, it is imperative to use it early—consider IV fentanyl 50–100 micrograms.
- Give oral morphine if stronger analgesia is required. Remember that morphine in doses above 0.1mg/kg increases the admission rate.
- Antispasmodic agents, such as hyoscine, and physical therapies, such as hot water bottles, may help, particularly for cramping lower abdominal pain following gynaecological surgery.

Post-operative nausea and vomiting

(See also ➜ p. 1085.)
- A multifactorial approach to the prevention of PONV should be used. The Steward scoring system is more useful for day surgery patients. Patients experiencing PONV must be actively managed before discharge home.

- For high-risk patients, LA techniques or GA using TIVA, avoidance of N_2O or opioids, multimodal analgesic therapy, good hydration (IV fluids), and minimal (2hr) fluid fast are appropriate. Dexamethasone 8mg, in combination with cyclizine 50mg, are effective prophylactic agents. This is an approach that works well and leaves a small number of patients requiring treatment, for which a 5-HT$_3$ antagonist, such as granisetron, is suitable.

Regional anaesthesia

Regional anaesthesia is widely used in Europe and North America for day-case anaesthesia. PONV is reduced. Timing and planning are important, as blocks take longer to set up or wear off, compared with GA. The increased use of ultrasound enables many procedures to be undertaken under purely regional anaesthesia with huge efficiency gains, particularly if entire lists are undertaken this way. Spinals should be performed early on the list, as they must have worn off completely before discharge to allow safe ambulation. However, it is reasonable to discharge patients with working plexus blocks, thus allowing the benefit of prolonged post-operative analgesia. Remember that patients need special instructions on the care of the anaesthetized part so as to avoid inadvertent damage. This would include a sling for patients with brachial plexus blocks.

Local anaesthesia and sedation

With increased use of LA, short-acting sedative drugs will inevitably be used to increase tolerability. It must be noted that sedation is a poor adjunct to an imperfect LA block. However, judicious use of propofol infusions (TCI 1–1.5 micrograms/mL) or remifentanil (0.05mg/kg/min) can provide good amnesia with few post-operative effects. If sedation is to be used, it must be provided and monitored by someone other than the operating surgeon.

Specific blocks

- **Field block**: excellent for LA hernia repair, as provides post-operative analgesia and obviates the need for GA. LA for inguinal surgery is best placed by the surgeon under direct vision. Attempt at ilioinguinal nerve block by anaesthetists has a high incidence of blockade of the femoral nerve, with subsequent unplanned admission due to difficulty mobilizing.
- **Spinals**: use 25/26G pencil-point needles, and consider using either shorter-acting agents, such as hyperbaric prilocaine, or 2-chloroprocaine to reduce the duration of spinal anaesthesia to 90 and 40min, respectively. Alternatively, consider reduced-dose spinals (5–7.5mg of bupivacaine with 10–25 micrograms of fentanyl). This gives a similar onset of anaesthesia with less motor block and a shorter discharge time, compared with standard doses (4hr versus 6hr).
- **Epidurals** are less suitable due to the time factor in achieving a block.
- **Caudals**: use dilute solutions (0.125% bupivacaine). Preservative-free ketamine 0.5mg/kg or clonidine 1 microgram/kg can be added to prolong the block for up to 24hr. Warn patients about ambulation difficulties.

- **Femoral blocks**: these are usually inappropriate due to difficulty mobilizing post-operatively; however, subsartorial blocks which block the sensory, but not the motor, branch of the femoral nerve are ideal for procedures such as anterior cruciate ligament repair or unicondylar knee replacement.

Specific discharge criteria for regional techniques

Spinals
- Full recovery of motor power and proprioception.
- Passed urine.

Regional blocks
- Understanding of protection of partially blocked limb.
- Instructions regarding when the block should have regressed and whom to contact if it has not.
- Adequate mobility on crutches, if required

Discharge drugs

All patients should have a supply of suitable oral post-operative analgesics at home or be given them on discharge. There should be procedure-specific analgesic protocols, e.g. cases of inguinal hernia repair or laparoscopic surgery should be given at least 5d supply of analgesics (e.g. ibuprofen 400mg qds plus co-codamol 30/500 two tablets qds).

Discharge criteria

- Stable vital signs.
- Fully awake and orientated.
- Has at least taken oral fluids.
- Passed urine following urological surgery or spinal/caudal anaesthesia.
- Ambulant.
- Pain and nausea well controlled.
- Minimal bleeding or wound drainage.

Discharge organization

- IV cannula removed, and wound checked.
- Written and verbal discharge information.
- Discharge drugs.
- Suture removal organized, if required.
- GP letter.
- Contact telephone number.
- Collected by responsible adult.

Post-operative admission

Reasons for overnight admission:
- Patient does not fulfil discharge criteria before unit closes.
- Observation after surgical or anaesthetic complications.
- Unexpected more extensive surgery.
- Uncontrolled pain or PONV.

Overall, unanticipated admission occurs in 0.5–2.0% of cases, depending on the mix of surgery. However, with increasingly complex procedures, this becomes more challenging to achieve, and consideration to the development of a procedure-specific anaesthetic guideline is required. Examples of procedures where this has been found useful include laparoscopic cholecystectomy and tonsillectomy. Common anaesthetic reasons for hospital admission are inadequate recovery, nausea/vomiting, and pain. Anaesthesia-related complications are more frequent with GA than with local or regional anaesthesia. Surgical reasons include bleeding, extensive surgery, perforated viscus, and the need for further treatment.

Further reading

Association of Anaesthetists of Great Britain and Ireland (2010). *Pre-operative assessment and patient preparation—the role of the anaesthetist.* London: Association of Anaesthetists of Great Britain and Ireland.

Association of Anaesthetists of Great Britain and Ireland (2011). *Day case and short stay surgery.* London: Association of Anaesthetists of Great Britain and Ireland.

British Association of Day Surgery. ℘ http://www.bads.co.uk [for updates, a series of handbooks on topics referred to in this chapter, and new day surgery links].

Chung F, Mezei G (1999). Adverse outcomes in ambulatory anesthesia. *Can J Anaesth*, **46**, RI8–26.

Jackson I, McWhinnie D, Skues M (2012). *The pathway to success—management of the day surgical patient.* ℘ http://daysurgeryuk.net/en/shop/handbooks/the-pathway-to-success-management-of-the-day-surgical-patient/.

Smith I, McWhinnie D, Jackson I, eds. (2012). *Day case surgery (Oxford Specialist Handbooks).* Oxford: Oxford University Press.

Society for Ambulatory Anesthesia. ℘ http://www.sambahq.org.

Watson B, Allen J (2013). *Spinal anaesthesia for day surgery patients. A practical guide*, 3rd edn. ℘ http://daysurgeryuk.net/en/shop/handbooks/spinal-anaesthesia-for-day-surgery-patients-a-practical-guide-3rd-edition/.

Laser surgery

John Saddler

General principles

- Laser is an acronym for light amplification by stimulated emission of radiation. Laser light is an intense beam of energy capable of vaporizing tissues. Lasers have numerous medical and surgical applications, but also create unique hazards to patients and staff.
- Light is a form of radiant energy that spans the mid range of the electromagnetic spectrum. It is released as photons and travels as a wave.
- In a laser tube, the application of an energy source on a lasing medium creates stimulated emissions of photons. These bounce back and forth between carefully aligned mirrors and are focused into a high-intensity beam. The light produced is monochromatic (all the same wavelength) and coherent (all the wave peaks moving synchronously at the same amplitude).
- Lasers are defined by their wavelengths, which also determine their colour. Some lasers are outside the visible spectrum and require a light guide to direct the laser beam to the surgical site (Table 30.1).
- Fibreoptic bundles can be used to transmit visible and near-infrared wavelength lasers. Wavelengths out of this range usually require an articulated arm.

Table 30.1 Types of surgical laser in common use

Laser type	Wavelength (nm)	Colour
Dye laser	360–670	Blue to red
Argon	488–515	Blue/green
Helium–neon	633	Red
Ruby	694	Red
Nd–YAG	1064	Near-infrared
CO_2	10 600	Far-infrared

Laser wavelength and colour

Laser light striking a tissue surface may be:
- **Reflected**. Reflection off shiny surfaces may damage the eyes of staff in the vicinity.
- **Transmitted** to deeper layers. Lasers pass through tissues to a variable depth, which is partially determined by the wavelength.
- **Scattered**. Shorter wavelengths induce greater scattering.
- **Absorbed**. This produces the clinical effect when the absorbed light is converted to heat. Organic tissue contains various substances capable of absorbing light. These are termed chromophores and include Hb, collagen, and melanin. Each substance has a particular absorption spectrum, which is determined by its chemical structure. For example, oxyhaemoglobin, which is targeted in vascular lesions, has absorption peaks at 418, 542, and 577nm. Laser light at, or close to, these frequencies will be the most effective.

Safety aspects

- A designated laser safety officer should be present at all times when a laser is in use. Signs should be displayed outside all theatre doors which should be locked from the inside when lasers are being used.
- Laser light can be reflected off mirrored surfaces. Medical instruments used with lasers should have matt, rather than shiny, surfaces.
- Eyes are very susceptible to injury. Retinal and corneal damage can occur, depending on the frequency of the beam. All operating room personnel must wear safety glasses appropriate for the laser in use. These should have side shields to protect the lateral aspect of the eye. If an anaesthetized patient is receiving laser radiation near the eyes, protective matt metallic eye covers can be applied.
- Damage to the skin can occur, depending on the type of laser in use. Anaesthetized patients must have all exposed skin covered with drapes. These should be made of absorbable material, and not plastic which is potentially combustible. Tissue adjacent to the lesion can be protected with moistened pads or swabs. In all cases, the eyes should be taped closed and covered with moist swabs. Plastic tape is combustible and should be avoided.
- Some skin preparation fluids are flammable and should not be used during laser surgery.
- Laser light can ignite plastic and rubber materials. Carefully consider the optimum method of airway maintenance if lasers are employed within the airway. The simplest approach is to use a Venturi system (Sanders injector). This uses a high-pressure O_2 source and entrainment of atmospheric air. The injector is placed in the lumen of a rigid laryngoscope or bronchoscope which is open at both ends and permits entrainment of O_2-enriched air during inspiration and escape of CO_2 exhaust gases during expiration. This system of a 'tube within a tube' is safe and reduces the chances of barotrauma-induced pneumothorax or pneumomediastinum. IV anaesthesia is usually employed to ensure an adequate depth of anaesthesia. It is also important to prevent the patient from moving or coughing, so a suitable muscle relaxant should be administered, and neuromuscular transmission monitored with a nerve stimulator.
- If the use of an ETT is required, unmodified conventional tubes cannot be used, because they support combustion and can potentially cause airway fires. Various laser tubes are available, e.g. Laser-Trach™ (Sheridan), Laser-Shield™ (Xomed), and Laser-flex™ (Covidien). The cuffs of these tubes are vulnerable and can be protected by damp pledgets. The cuff should be filled with saline, which can be mixed with methylthioninium chloride (methylene blue) so that a cuff puncture is obvious.
- Both N_2O and O_2 support combustion. If using a circuit, rather than an O_2 injector, 30% O_2 and air are a sensible choice.
- If air is not available, O_2 and N_2O can be used, but take special care to protect the tube cuff.

- A laser plume is created at the site of contact with human tissue. This contains fine particulates which are potentially hazardous to health workers. Smoke evacuation systems must be used to remove laser plume contaminants. Aerosolization of viruses can occur during laser surgery for papillomata—special masks are worn to reduce the risk.
- If a fire occurs in an airway during laser surgery, the source should be removed, and mask ventilation with 100% O_2 should be initiated. Reintubation and bronchoscopy with lavage may be required. Severe damage may require a tracheostomy.

Examples of medical lasers

Pulsed dye laser

This uses light at a wavelength that targets red blood cells within blood vessels. The energy is dissipated within the dermis and causes only minimal epidermal scarring. This is used mainly for treating port wine skin lesions. Children requiring laser therapy to these lesions will often be subjected to multiple treatments, usually under GA. Post-operative pain may be a problem, particularly if large areas are treated. Combinations of paracetamol and NSAIDs may be effective, but occasionally opioid analgesics are required.

Carbon dioxide laser

These lasers have a long wavelength (10 600nm, outside the visible spectrum) and are preferentially absorbed by water. Target cells are heated to the point of vaporization by the beam. They penetrate to only a very shallow depth, so tissue damage can be directly observed. They are used in aesthetic facial surgery to reduce the wrinkling associated with ageing, and in ENT practice to vaporize vocal cord and airway lesions. Care must be taken to avoid eye and airway injury (see → p. 693).

Nd–YAG laser

This laser is also outside the visible range and, unlike the CO_2 laser, is transmitted through clear fluids and absorbed by dark matter. It can penetrate to a depth of 1cm. It has multiple applications, including airway neoplasms, vascular malformations, and ophthalmic surgery.

Further reading

English J, Norris A, Bedforth N (2006). Anaesthesia for airway surgery. *Contin Educ Anaesth Crit Care Pain*, **6**, 28–31.
Kitching AJ, Edge CJ (2003). Lasers and surgery. *Contin Educ Anaesth Crit Care Pain*, **3**, 143–6.

Anaesthesia for radiology

Philippa Dix

Anaesthesia for computed tomography and magnetic resonance imaging scanning

The anaesthetist working in the medical imaging department may be expected to use unfamiliar equipment in a potentially hazardous environment. Ensure that trained assistance, monitoring, etc. are available, and familiarize yourself with the surroundings. Locate the nearest resuscitation facilities (self-inflating bag/mask, portable O_2, 'crash' trolley, and defibrillator)—confirm that your assistant and the radiographers also know where these are!

Indications for anaesthesia

- Infants and uncooperative children. Small babies (under 2 months) will often sleep through a scan if given a feed and wrapped up well.
- Older children or adults with psychological, behavioural, or movement disorders.
- Intubated patients such as acute trauma victims and patients receiving intensive care.
- Analgesia, sedation, or anaesthesia may also be required for interventional procedures performed under CT or possibly MRI guidance.
- Patients for elective scans commonly have a range of problems. Check the indications for scan and nature of the underlying pathology—developmental delay, epilepsy, malignancy, and psychiatric and movement disorders. Significant CVS and respiratory problems are uncommon, but beware of 'syndromes' with CVS manifestations.

Anaesthesia—general points

- Choice of sedation or GA and type of GA depends upon the needs of the patient, the nature of the investigation, and the skills and experience of the anaesthetist (see later).
- Check whether the anaesthetic machines are using piped gases or cylinders. If using cylinders, confirm that a full spare O_2 cylinder is immediately available.
- Plan the location of the anaesthetic machine, suction and monitoring, and the configuration and routing of the breathing system in advance.
- Decide where to induce the patient—a dedicated induction area may not be available or may be very small. It is usual to induce on a tilting trolley, then transfer to the scanner when anaesthetized.
- Certain equipment configurations (e.g. the anaesthetic machine in the scan room and monitors in the control room) may require two anaesthetists to manage the patient safely.
- Ensure satisfactory recovery facilities are available, i.e. appropriately equipped recovery bay and an experienced recovery nurse near the scanner, or arrangements for safe transfer of the patient to an operating department recovery room.

Anaesthesia for computed tomography

- The CT scanning environment does not restrict the type of equipment used, but space is often limited, so compact anaesthetic machines and monitors are more practical.
- The patient, anaesthetic machine, and monitors must all be visible from the control room.
- The patient's head is usually accessible during CT scanning, so an LMA may be used if the patient does not require IPPV or airway protection.
- A variety of anaesthetic (and sedation) techniques can be used. The final choice should be determined by the equipment available and the patient's needs.
- Only 'light' anaesthesia to produce immobility and lack of awareness is required.

Hazards

- CT scanning generates potentially harmful ionizing radiation, so it is preferable for the anaesthetist to monitor the patient from outside the scan room. If it is necessary to remain near the patient, wear appropriate radiation protection.
- Cannulae, catheters, drains, and ETTs can be pulled out during transfers and by movement of the patient through the scanner—ask the radiographer how far the table will move, and check that lines and the breathing system do not snag other equipment.

Contrast media

- Modern intravascular contrast media for X-ray imaging utilize highly iodinated, non-ionic, water-soluble compounds.
- Common agents are iohexol (Omnipaque™), iopromide (Ultravist™), and iopamidol (Niopam™) which are monomeric, and the dimeric compound iodixanol (Visipaque™). Concentrations equivalent to 300–320mg of iodine/mL are typically used.
- You may be asked to administer IV contrast to anaesthetized patients. The volume required varies with the preparation, investigation, age, and body weight but may be up to 150mL (Table 31.1).
- Check the timing of injection with the radiographer, because some 'dynamic' investigations (e.g. aortography) require contrast to be administered as the scan is occurring.
- Contrast is viscous and can be difficult to inject through small cannulae or injection ports (take the bung off, and inject via the hub of the cannula).
- Automated contrast injectors should not be connected to central venous lines. The high pressure developed by the rapid injection of viscous medium down a long, narrow lumen can burst the line.
- IV iodine-containing contrast media occasionally trigger allergic reactions (ask about iodine sensitivity).

Table 31.1 Typical volumes of contrast media for CT scanning

Investigation	Adult volume (mL)	Child volume (mL)
CT head	50–100	10 plus 2mL/kg
CT body	100–150	(Up to adult dose)
Aortography	100	–
Urography	2–3mL/kg	2–3mL/kg

• These agents may cause renal failure in patients who are dehydrated or who have impaired renal function, so ensure adequate hydration in patients who have been starved for GA. Lactic acidosis can be precipitated in patients taking biguanides (metformin), and these should ideally be avoided for 48hr before and after the scan.

Practical considerations

• Metal-containing objects (such as ECG leads, pressure transducer cables, and clips) lying in the X-ray beam can cause artefacts, so route them away from the area to be scanned.
• Thoracic or abdominal scans may require 'breath-holds' to reduce respiratory movement artefacts. Both paralysed and spontaneously breathing patients can be ventilated manually, and their lungs held in inspiration for the few seconds needed to perform each individual scan.
• The patient's arms usually need to be positioned above the head during thoracic or abdominal scans. Wide adhesive tape is useful for securing the limbs (keep a roll on the anaesthetic machine).
• Intensive care patients requiring CT scans should be managed like any inter-ICU transfer, with full transport monitoring and ventilatory support. Ideally, the ICU resident or consultant should supervise the patient and review the scan with the reporting radiologist. Getting such patients into and out of the scanner can be a slow process.

Anaesthesia for magnetic resonance imaging

MRI is a versatile imaging tool free from the dangers of ionizing radiation. A computer creates cross-sectional or 3D images from minute radiofrequency signals generated as hydrogen nuclei are flipped in and out of alignment with a powerful magnetic field by high-frequency magnetic pulses.

- Non-invasive but can be unpleasant—the subject has to lie motionless in a narrow, noisy tunnel, with the part of the body to be imaged closely surrounded by an 'aerial coil' (a very claustrophobic environment).
- Typical sequence of scans lasts 15–25min, but complex scans may take much longer.
- Up to 3% of adults cannot tolerate scanning without sedation or anaesthesia.
- Provision of safe anaesthesia for MRI requires specialized equipment and careful organization—unlike CT, you cannot simply take a standard machine and monitor to the MRI scanner.

Hazards

- Most scanners use a super-conducting magnet to generate a high-density static magnetic field, which is always present. Field strength is measured in tesla (T)—most scanners use 0.5–1.5T magnets (about 10 000 times the Earth's magnetic field).
- Near the scanner (>5mT field strength), the static field exerts a powerful attraction on ferromagnetic materials (e.g. scissors, gas cylinders, laryngoscopes) which can become projectiles. Electric motors (e.g. in syringe drivers) may run erratically, and any information stored on magnetic media (credit cards, cassette tapes, or floppy disks) will be erased. The magnetic field decreases as the distance from the scanner increases—beyond the 0.5mT boundary or outside the scan room can be considered safe.
- Devices (e.g. hypodermic needles) made from non-ferromagnetic stainless steel can be taken into the scan room. If you are unsure about an object, do not risk it!
- Oscillating magnetic fields induce eddy currents in electrical conductors (e.g. ECG leads, metallic implants). These currents may disrupt or damage electronic equipment (including pacemakers) and cause heating effects that can result in burns.
- Large masses of metal (e.g. anaesthetic machines, gas cylinders) near the scanner or small amounts of non-ferrous metals within the 3D volume being scanned can distort the magnetic fields, causing poor-quality images.
- The scan room is usually shielded to prevent external electrical interference from swamping the magnetic resonance signals. All electrical equipment within the scan room must also be fully shielded, and electrical conductors entering the room (e.g. monitoring cables) require special radiofrequency filters.
- Rapidly changing magnetic fields cause mechanical vibrations and extremely loud 'knocking' noises, which can potentially damage hearing.

Equipment

Two alternative approaches are feasible:
- Specialized 'MRI-compatible' equipment within the scan room, or
- Conventional equipment outside the scanner's magnetic field in the control room.

Standardizing on one option keeps the anaesthetist, anaesthetic machine, and monitors together. Choice depends upon the space, funds, frequency of GA, and individual preference. Using conventional equipment at a distance avoids crowding the scanner, is less expensive, and allows faulty monitors to be substituted. The anaesthetist can regulate the anaesthetic and monitor the patient without being in the scan room, and hazards can be reduced by applying the simple rule that 'nothing enters the scan room, except the patient and the trolley'.

A typical set-up is as follows:
- Induction area adjacent to, but outside, the scan room (beyond the 0.5mT boundary), equipped with a compact conventional anaesthetic machine and monitoring.
- Piped gases, scavenging, and suction in both the induction area and control room.
- Non-magnetic tipping trolley for patient transfer into the scanner.
- Compact (e.g. wall-mounted) anaesthetic machine and ventilator in the control room with a 10m coaxial (Bain) breathing system.
- Respiratory gas/agent side-stream analyser with capnograph display fitted with an extended sampling tube (increases the response time by 5–10s).
- MRI-compatible pulse oximeter (fibreoptic patient probe and shielded cable).
- ECG with MRI-compatible (carbon fibre) patient leads and electrodes.
- NIBP machine with an extended hose, non-metallic connectors, and a range of cuffs.
- Recent technology allows a monitor unit within the scan room, with a slave unit in the control room, improving patient monitoring during transfers.
- Equipment may be MRI-conditional, which must not be taken beyond the 5mT line, or MRI-safe, which can be taken right into the scanner.

Practical considerations and techniques

- Physically and 'magnetically' restricted access makes patient observation and treatment difficult, so a secure airway is a priority.
- Neonates and young babies (<2 months)—will often sleep through a short scan, if fed, wrapped up, and placed on their side in the scanner.
- Babies and small children (<15kg), and any patient with an intracranial space-occupying lesion, suspicion of raised ICP, or needing a protected airway—use intubation and IPPV.
- Larger children and adults (if no risk of raised ICP)—use SV and a standard LMA (*not* a flexible one with a wire spiral).
- If intubating a patient for a head scan, use an RAE tube—it keeps the connectors and breathing system clear of the head coil.

- Tape the valve on the pilot tube of a cuffed ETT or LMA outside the aerial coil, or the metal of the spring will distort the images.
- Be careful with MRI-conditional equipment (e.g. ICU ventilator, monitor unit). Do not place it on the moving table, as it might be moved inside the 5mT line, at which point it will be strongly attracted to the magnet. Similarly, be aware of the position of all MRI-conditional equipment.
- Sedation with oral or IV benzodiazepines may be used by radiologists for healthy, but claustrophobic, adults. Patients with severe back or root compression pain may also require strong analgesia to tolerate positioning for a scan.
- The role of sedation for MRI scanning in children is unclear. Some children's centres have reported successes with structured sedation programmes run by dedicated sedationists. However, the safety of having heavily sedated children in the medical imaging department without direct anaesthetic supervision has been questioned.

Tips for intermittent positive pressure ventilation through a 10m breathing system

- Use a system that functions as a 'T-piece' (Mapleson D or E), so dead space is unaffected by the length.[1] Ayre's T-piece and coaxial Bain systems work well and are both suitable for ventilating babies and small children.
- Airway pressures measured near the ventilator may not accurately represent distal pressures at the ETT.
- V_T delivered to the lungs will be reduced by 'compression losses' of the gas within the system and by expansion of the tubing during inspiration, making it difficult to compensate for significant leaks round uncuffed ETTs—change to a slightly larger tube, so the leak is minimal.
- As a result of these effects, IPPV using a simple pressure generator (e.g. Penlon Nuffield 200 with a Newton valve) may not be effective in children weighing >15kg.
- Increased expiratory resistance of some long systems (e.g. Ayre's T-piece) generates a positive expiratory pressure which increases with the FGF.

Intensive care patients

- Same considerations apply as for CT scanning (see p. 697), but potential hazards are greater, so the risk/benefit balance should be assessed carefully.
- Do not scan patients who are haemodynamically or otherwise unstable.
- Electronic pressure transducers, metal-containing ICP 'bolts', temporary pacing wires, and conventional ECG leads must be removed before the patient enters the scan room.
- Full checks (and, if necessary, plain radiographs) must be performed to confirm there are no hazardous metallic implants or foreign bodies present.
- Patients who are stable on inotrope infusions can be scanned, but infusion pumps must remain at a safe distance from the magnet—ideally outside the scan room. Prepare duplicate pumps in the control room, with extended infusion lines threaded with the breathing system into the

scan room. Connect the patient to the running infusions, while outside the room; check they are stable, then move into the scanner.

Patient and staff safety

- To avoid accidental injury, all patients having an MRI scan must complete a screening/consent form. In cases of children or sedated ICU patients, these must be completed on their behalf by relatives or staff.
- To prevent injury and property damage, all staff must similarly complete a screening questionnaire and leave metallic objects, pagers, credit cards, etc. outside the room.
- Greatest dangers arise from ferromagnetic implants and foreign bodies—certain types of artificial heart valves, old cerebral aneurysm clips, steel splinters in the eye, where movement could disrupt valve function or precipitate intracranial or vitreous haemorrhage, respectively.
- Patients and staff with cardiac pacemakers must remain outside the 0.5mT boundary.
- Anaesthetized and sedated patients should have their ears protected to prevent noise-induced auditory damage.
- IV MRI contrast media are paramagnetic but do not contain iodine, and have a narrow therapeutic index. Side effects include headache, nausea and vomiting, local burning, and wheals (2.4%). Severe hypotension/anaphylactoid reactions are rare (~1:100 000).
- Commonly used agents are gadopentetic acid (Magnevist™) at a dose of 0.2–0.4mL/kg and gadodiamide (Omniscan™) at 0.2mL/kg. More recently, gadobutrol (Gadovist™) at 0.1mL/kg and gadoteric acid (Dotarem™) at 0.2mL/kg have been used in patients with a reduced GFR or an unknown GFR (most children). These agents are associated with a lower risk of nephrogenic systemic fibrosis.

Cardiac arrest

- Do not attempt ALS in the scan room.
- Do not allow the cardiac arrest team into the scan room.
- Start basic life support (BLS) with non-metallic, self-inflating bag and chest compressions.
- Remove the patient from the scan room on a non-magnetic trolley, and continue resuscitation outside the 0.5mT boundary.

Reference

1 Sweeting CJ, Thomas PW, Sanders DJ (2002). The long Bain breathing system: an investigation into the implications of remote ventilation. *Anaesthesia*, **57**, 1183–6.

Further reading

Association of Anaesthetists of Great Britain and Ireland (2002). *Provision of anaesthetic services in magnetic resonance units*. London: Association of Anaesthetists of Great Britain and Ireland.

Hatch DJ, Sury MRJ (2000). Sedation of children by non-anaesthetists. *Br J Anaesth*, **84**, 713–14.

Menon DK, Peden CJ, Hall AS, Sargentoni J, Whitwam JG (1992). Magnetic resonance for the anaesthetist. Part I: physical principles, applications, safety aspects. *Anaesthesia*, **47**, 240–55.

Peden CJ, Menon DK, Hall AS, Sargentoni J, Whitwam JG (1992). Magnetic resonance for the anaesthetist. Part II: anaesthesia and monitoring in MR units. *Anaesthesia*, **47**, 508–17.

Shellock FG (2001). *Pocket guide to MR procedures and metallic objects: update 2001*. Baltimore: Lippincott Williams & Wilkins.

Anaesthesia for interventional radiology

In this subspecialty, minimally invasive procedures are performed under image guidance, usually in the X-ray department. Procedures are often performed to avoid open surgical procedures to reduce post-procedure pain and recovery time. They may be diagnostic or therapeutic. The imaging utilized may involve radiation exposure, e.g. fluoroscopy and CT, or may be ultrasound or MRI.

Common interventional procedures

- Angioplasty/stenting/coiling: vascular, neuro, and cardiac.
- Embolizations: blocking vessels to reduce bleeding in a planned surgical operation, to stop bleeding post-surgically following trauma, or stopping tumour growth.
- Chemo-embolization: combination of delivering cancer treatment directly to a tumour and then blocking its blood supply.
- RFA: local destruction of tissue by heating.
- Cryoablation: local destruction of tissue by freezing.
- Thrombolysis.
- Biopsies.
- Vertebroplasty/cementoplasty: injection of cement into bone to reduce pain in tumours and fractures.

Indications for anaesthesia

- Patient may be required to be very still for long periods of time.
- Procedure may be very painful.
- Paediatric patients.

Anaesthesia for interventional radiology: general points

- As previously described for CT and MRI (see ➐ p. 697 and p. 699), it is vital for the anaesthetist and their assistant to familiarize themselves with the equipment available in this 'isolated' environment. Monitoring and the anaesthetic machine must be fully checked, and the location of the resuscitation equipment checked. Scavenging is often not possible, so TIVA may be useful or an Aldasorber may be used. Depending on the patient and procedure, you may be in or outside the scan room. Induction generally occurs within the radiology suite. Before starting, check you have all the drugs drawn up that you anticipate using for anaesthesia and those you may want in an emergency (metaraminol, ephedrine, atropine). After the procedure, the patient is woken up in radiology and then generally transferred to main theatre recovery. The procedure table usually does not tilt, so it is recommended to induce anaesthesia on an anaesthetic trolley and transfer the patient after induction

Angioplasty/stenting/coiling

- A balloon-tipped catheter is inserted into a narrow or blocked vessel, and the balloon inflated. A stent may be placed to keep it open. Vascular and cardiac procedures often do not require GA.

- Endovascular repair of AAA (see ➲ p. 429) is associated with a lower mortality and is favoured in those patients with poor LV function. This may be done under regional (epidural and sedation) or general anaesthesia.
- Intracranial angioplasty and stenting are used for the treatment of intracranial aneurysms. GA is required, because the patient must be completely still. A similar anaesthetic technique should be used as for craniotomy (see ➲ p. 393 and p. 411). Induction should be cardiovascularly stable, avoiding any drop in CPP, and the airway secured with an ETT. Invasive monitoring should be used. Care should be taken to ensure normocapnia and normothermia.

Embolizations
- Procedures that are superficial, involve an AVM, or involve the use of alcohol for embolization are very painful and require sedation or GA.
- Depending on the position of the patient, choose an ETT or LMA.
- In obstetrics, uterine artery embolization is now included in the NICE guidelines for massive obstetric haemorrhage. Balloon catheters can be placed in the uterine artery and inflated to stop the pelvic bleeding. This can be done in an emergency or can be inserted before a Caesarean section in a case that is anticipated to bleed.

Radiofrequency ablations
- In this procedure, the tumour is destroyed by heating. Depending on the size of the tumour, it may take as long as 40min, is painful, and requires a GA.
- RFA is commonly used to treat hepatic and renal tumours—either metastases, difficult-to-reach tumours, or tumours in those patients who are too frail for an open procedure.
- Depending on the position of the tumour, the patient may need to be prone and so requires an ETT; otherwise, a laryngeal mask is often sufficient.

Cryoablation
- These procedures tend not to be painful, and often sedation is all that is required.

Thrombolysis
- Minimally invasive treatment that dissolves blood clots and improves blood supply. This can be used to treat arteries in diseased vascular beds, DVT, coronary emboli, PEs, and thrombosis in fistulae.
- Contrast media help define the clot. This is then dissolved by either medication delivered directly to it or a mechanical device.
- GA is rarely required.

Anaesthesia for the elderly

Stu White and Jeffrey Handel

General considerations

'Elderly' arbitrarily refers to patients >65yr, who are the most rapidly expanding demographic of the surgical population. Age-related physiological and cognitive decline, co-morbidity, and frailty contribute to the higher risk of perioperative morbidity and mortality among older patients. Polypharmacy is common.

Ageing is associated with progressive deterioration of function in all systems, the effect of which may be compounded by organ-specific co-morbidity.

Cardiovascular

- Significant CVS disease is present in 50–65% of patients.
- Myocardial fibrosis and ventricular wall thickening occur, reducing ventricular compliance. Small changes in filling may have major effects upon cardiac output and BP.
- AF is common and reduces stroke volume through loss of the atrial component of ventricular filling.
- Maximal cardiac output with exercise decreases by ~1% per year from the 5th decade.
- Reduced arterial compliance causes systolic hypertension and widened pulse pressure.
- Reduced autonomic responsiveness impairs CVS responses to hypotension. The hypotensive effect of anaesthetic agents is likely to be more pronounced.
- Capillary permeability is increased, leading to a greater risk of pulmonary oedema.

Respiratory

- Ventilatory responses to hypoxia and hypercapnia decline. Post-operative apnoea is commoner. Ventilatory reserve declines.
- O_2 consumption and CO_2 production fall by 10–15% by the 7th decade. Patients are able to tolerate a longer period of apnoea following preoxygenation, and minute volume requirement is reduced.
- Loss of elastic recoil increases pulmonary compliance, but chest wall compliance falls due to degenerative changes in joints. Therefore, total thoracic compliance may fall.
- Loss of septa increases the alveolar dead space. Closing volume increases to exceed the FRC in the upright posture at 66yr, resulting in venous admixture. Thus, normal PaO_2 falls steadily [(13.3 − age/30) kPa, or (100 − age/4) mmHg].
- Airway protective reflexes decline, increasing the risk of post-operative pulmonary aspiration.
- In edentulous patients, maintenance of a patent airway and face mask seal may be difficult. Leaving false teeth *in situ* may help.

Renal

- Renal mass and number of glomeruli fall progressively (by 30% in the 8th decade), resulting in reduced GFR. Creatinine clearance falls comparably, although serum creatinine may not rise because of decreased production from a reduced muscle mass (see p. 120).

- Tubular function deteriorates, leading to reduced renin–aldosterone response, ADH sensitivity, and concentrating ability. As a result, all renal homeostatic functions deteriorate, so that elderly patients are more susceptible to fluid overload and hypovolaemia. Hypo- and hypernatraemia are more likely to occur.
- Reduced clearance of renally excreted drugs necessitates dose adjustment. Particular care must be taken with potentially nephrotoxic drugs such as aminoglycosides.

Hepatic

- Hepatic mass and blood flow fall by up to 40% by the 9th decade. Although cellular function is relatively well preserved in healthy patients, the reduction in size reduces clearance and prolongs the effect of drugs that are metabolized and excreted by the liver. These include opioids, propofol, benzodiazepines, and NDMRs.

Central nervous system

- Brain size and neuronal mass decrease. The average brain weight falls by 18% between the ages of 30 and 80yr. Dementia affects 10% of patients over 65yr of age, and 20% over 80yr. However, it is important to distinguish between dementia and reversible confusional states due to hypoxia, sepsis, pain, metabolic derangement, and depression. The hospital environment may precipitate anxiety and confusion.
- The elderly have lower requirements for opioid analgesics and sedatives and are more susceptible to depression of the conscious level and respiration. This is likely to be due to a pharmacodynamic, as well as a pharmacokinetic, effect. Pain threshold may be increased.
- Post-operative delirium (POD) and cognitive dysfunction (POCD) are common in the elderly, occurring in >10% of patients. Disturbances of cerebral perfusion and cellular oxygenation are likely to be contributory factors. Potentially reversible risk factors for POD include severe pain, infection, malnutrition, electrolyte imbalance, dehydration, environmental disturbances, and substance withdrawal (alcohol, medication).
- The thirst response to reduced ECF volume and increased plasma osmolality is reduced in the elderly, increasing susceptibility to fluid depletion.

Pharmacology

- TBW is reduced, while fat percentage is increased. The volume of distribution of water-soluble drugs is reduced, reducing dose requirements, while that of lipid-soluble drugs is increased which may prolong clearance. The initial volume of distribution falls because of reduced cardiac output. This reduces the dose requirement and is particularly relevant for induction agents. Arm–brain circulation time is prolonged, increasing the time taken for induction agents to take effect.
- Reduced plasma albumin concentration decreases the dose requirement of drugs, such as barbiturate induction agents, which are bound to albumin.

- MAC of inhaled agents decreases steadily with age (6% reduction per decade) and is reduced by around 40% by the age of 80yr (see ➲ p. 1209). This may be related to a reduction in neuronal mass. Reductions in blood/gas partition coefficient and cardiac output in the elderly result in shorter onset time.
- The risk of GI bleeding due to NSAIDs is increased. These agents may also contribute to the development of ARF in the presence of impaired renal perfusion. ACE inhibitors exacerbate this risk. Fluid retention due to NSAIDs may precipitate heart failure in susceptible patients.

Thermoregulation

- Temperature regulation is impaired, increasing the risk of hypothermia.
- Post-operative shivering increases skeletal muscle O_2 consumption, while vasoconstriction increases myocardial work and O_2 demand.

Endocrine

- Glucose loading is increasingly poorly tolerated in elderly patients. The incidence of diabetes rises and may reach 25% in patients above 80yr of age.

Nutrition

- Nutritional status is frequently poor in the elderly, under-recognized by clinicians, and compounded by a lack of appetite resulting from surgery, pain, and nausea.
- Perioperative complications and length of hospital stay may be reduced by nutritional supplementation prior to major surgery.

Haematology and the immune system

- Hypercoagulability and DVT become commoner with advancing age.
- Disorders causing anaemia are commoner, and the response of the marrow to anaemia is impaired.
- Immune responses are reduced in the elderly, putting them at increased risk of infection. This is due to reduced bone marrow and splenic mass with loss of the thymus.

Anaesthetic management of the elderly

Perioperative mortality increases with age, ASA status, and the type and urgency of surgery. The 30-day mortality after hip fracture surgery is ~8% in the UK (see also ➔ p. 484), and after emergency laparotomy ~10% aged 50, rising by ~5% per decade. Outcome is improved by thorough multi-disciplinary preoperative assessment, choice of an anaesthetic technique appropriate to the patient's condition, and meticulous perioperative care aimed at minimizing physiological disturbance.

Preoperative assessment and management

- A systematic review is vital. In patients who have sustained a fracture, an underlying medical cause for a fall should be sought.
- Day surgery is particularly appropriate for fit patients undergoing minor surgery, as the disorientation associated with a change of environment is minimized.
- The level of physical activity that can be sustained is a useful indicator of CVS and respiratory fitness but is often limited by joint disease.
- The mental state should be evaluated. The abbreviated mental test or mini-mental state examination may be useful in differentiating dementia from acute confusional states.
- Consideration should be given to pre-optimization of medical conditions. This may require cross-specialty involvement and high dependency care. The benefits from delaying surgery, while this takes place, should be balanced against the risks, particularly in non-elective surgery. In patients with lower limb fractures, delay in mobilization may increase the risk of pressure sores, DVT, and pneumonia.
- With the exception of oral hypoglycaemics, regular medications should be continued until the time of surgery. Alcohol should not be withheld the day before surgery, and nicotine patches may be helpful in smokers. Sedative premedications should generally be avoided, particularly benzodiazepines, centrally acting anticholinergics, and pethidine. Antacid prophylaxis should be considered. Maintaining β-blockade may reduce the risk of MI.

Perioperative management

- The type of anaesthesia appears less important than the care with which it is given with regard to the patient's physiological condition. However, regional anaesthesia may reduce bleeding, risk of DVT, respiratory infection, and cognitive dysfunction (particularly if given without/with minimal sedation). MAC or minimum inhibitory concentration (MIC) if using TIVA, should be age-adjusted.
- Careful monitoring is necessary to detect hypotension during GA induction and shortly after spinal anaesthesia administration. Consideration should be given to invasive BP and depth of anaesthesia monitoring. Prolonged arm–brain circulation time delays the onset of IV induction agents; flush the drugs with saline, and remain patient to avoid an inadvertent overdose.

- Temperature should be measured, and hypothermia prevented using fluid warmers, active body-warming devices, and elevation of ambient temperature.
- Prolonged surgery and periods of hypotension increase the risk of pressure sores. Care should be taken to reduce pressure with soft padding. During long procedures, it is advisable to relieve pressure and massage vulnerable areas intermittently.

Post-operative management

- High dependency facilities should be considered if this is likely to reduce morbidity or mortality significantly or if an identifiable organ support is required.
- Fluid balance, vital signs, serum electrolytes, and haematology must be carefully monitored and treated appropriately. Patients with CVS disease may need to have an Hb of >9–10g/dL.
- Reversible factors should be sought if the patient exhibits delirium.
- Pain is common but undertreated in elderly surgical patients, particularly if cognitively impaired. Regular paracetamol prescription and regional analgesia should always be considered and are preferable to opioids and NSAIDs.
- Anaesthetists should facilitate post-operative patient 're-enablement' through age-appropriate anaesthesia, fluid therapy, thermoregulation, analgesia, and communication.

Post-operative cognitive dysfunction

POCD is the persistent impairment of cognitive function (e.g. memory loss and concentration) after surgery, without a clear precipitating event or CNS pathology, and is distinct from POD and dementia. The severity is variable but may have a significant impact upon the quality of life and independence. The cause is likely to be multifactorial and may relate to inflammatory reactions, altered hormonal homeostasis, and/or direct anaesthetic agent toxicity. POCD is commoner after major surgery, cardiac surgery, and emergency surgery. There are no generally agreed criteria for the assessment of POCD. The incidence of POCD is similar after general and regional (with sedation) anaesthesia. The 1-week and 1-year incidence of POCD may be reduced, using focused anaesthesia intervention (treatment of hypoxaemia and hypotension), guided by the depth of anaesthesia and cerebral saturation monitoring.

When not to operate

Heroic curative surgery may not be appropriate if the chance of benefiting the patient is felt to be very low. Decisions regarding futility of surgery are difficult and should be multidisciplinary and taken at consultant level, with the involvement of the patient and their family. Palliative procedures to improve the quality of life should be considered if the patient is adequately prepared. These decisions must be carefully documented.

Key points

- Older patients must be assumed to have the mental capacity to make decisions about their treatment.
- Access to surgical or critical care should not be rationed on the basis of age. Patients must be involved in discussions about the utility/futility of surgery and/or resuscitation.
- Avoid sedative premedications, and use regional analgesic techniques, where possible, to minimize the requirement for opioids.
- Monitor the temperature, and use active warming devices to prevent hypothermia.
- Always consider invasive BP and depth of anaesthesia monitoring.
- Drug/MAC requirements are reduced. Use opioids and NSAIDs with caution, particularly if there is co-morbid renal disease.
- Take care with positioning, and intermittently relieve pressure during long procedures to reduce the risk of pressure sores.
- Reversible factors should be sought if the patient exhibits delirium (pain, hypoxaemia, distended bladder, myocardial/cerebral ischaemia, electrolyte disorder, drugs).
- Facilitate early mobilization, and consider thromboprophylaxis if mobilization will not be rapid.

Further reading

American College of Surgeons (2012). ACS NSQIP®/AGS best practice guidelines: optimal preoperative assessment of the geriatric surgical patient. http://site.acsnsqip.org/wp-content/uploads/2011/12/ACS-NSQIP-AGS-Geriatric-2012-Guidelines.pdf.

Association of Anaesthetists of Great Britain and Ireland, Griffiths R, Alper J, Beckingsale A, et al. Management of proximal femoral fractures 2011: Association of Anaesthetists of Great Britain and Ireland. Anaesthesia, 67, 85–98.

Ballard C, Jones E, Gauge N, et al. (2012). Optimized anaesthesia to reduce post operative cognitive decline (POCD) in older patients undergoing elective surgery, a randomized controlled trial. PLoS One, 7, e37410.

Corcoran TB, Hillyard S (2011). Cardiopulmonary aspects of anaesthesia for the elderly. Best Pract Res Clin Anaesthesiol, 25, 329–54.

Dodds C, Kumar C, Veering B (2014). Oxford textbook of anaesthesia for the elderly patient. Oxford: Oxford University Press.

Griffiths R, Beech F, Brown A, et al.; Association of Anaesthetists of Great Britain and Ireland. Peri-operative care of the elderly 2014: Association of Anaesthetists of Great Britain and Ireland. Anaesthesia, 69, 81–98.

Schofield P (2014). The assessment and management of peri-operative pain in older people. Anaesthesia, 69, 54–60.

Stoneham M, Murray D, Foss N (2014). Emergency surgery: the big three—abdominal aortic aneurysm, laparotomy and hip fracture. Anaesthesia, 69, 70–80.

Strom C, Rasmussen LS, Sieber FE (2014). Should general anaesthesia be avoided in the elderly? Anaesthesia, 69, 35–44.

Obstetric anaesthesia and analgesia

James Eldridge and Maq Jaffer

Physiology and pharmacology

- From early in the 1st trimester of pregnancy, a woman's physiology changes rapidly, under the influence of increasing progesterone and oestrogen production. The effects are widespread.
- Cardiac output increases by ~50%. Diastolic BP falls in early to mid trimester and returns to pre-pregnant levels by term. Systolic pressure, although following the same pattern, is less affected. CVP and PAOP are not altered.
- Cardiac output increases further in labour, even with effective epidural analgesia, peaking immediately after delivery. It is in this period, when the preload and afterload of the heart are changing rapidly, that women with impaired myocardial function are at greatest risk.
- Uteroplacental blood flow is not autoregulated and so is dependent on uterine BP.
- Aortocaval occlusion occurs when the gravid uterus rests on the aorta or the IVC. Near term, complete caval occlusion in the supine position is almost universal, although only 10% of women have overt supine hypotensive syndrome because there is sufficient collateral circulation. Even in the absence of maternal hypotension, placental blood supply may be compromised in the supine position. After the 20th week of gestation, a left lateral tilt should always be employed. If either mother or fetus is symptomatic, the degree of tilt should be increased.
- Plasma volume increases by 50% by term, while the red cell mass only increases by 30%, resulting in physiological anaemia of pregnancy.
- Pregnant women become hypercoagulable early in the 1st trimester. Antepartum maternal deaths from PE occur most commonly in the 1st trimester.[1] Plasma concentrations of factors I, VII, VIII, IX, X, and XII are all increased. Antithrombin III levels are depressed. *All pregnant women should be risk assessed for appropriate antenatal and post-natal thromboprophylaxis.*
- $PaCO_2$ falls to ~4.0kPa (30mmHg). FRC is reduced by 20%, resulting in airway closure in 50% of supine women at term. This, in combination with a 60% increase in O_2 consumption, renders pregnant women at term vulnerable to hypoxia, especially when supine.
- In labour, painful contractions and excessive breathing of Entonox® can result in further hyperventilation, and marked alkalosis may occur. Arterial pH in excess of 7.5 is common.
- Gastric emptying and acidity are little changed by pregnancy. However, gastric emptying is slowed in established labour and almost halted if systemic opioids are administered for analgesia. Barrier pressure (the difference in pressure between the stomach and lower oesophageal 'sphincter') is reduced, but the incidence of regurgitation into the upper oesophagus during anaesthesia, in otherwise asymptomatic individuals, is not significantly different in the 1st and 2nd trimesters.

- By 48hr post-partum, intra-abdominal pressure, gastric emptying, volume, and acidity are all similar to non-pregnant controls. Although the lower oesophageal sphincter tone may take longer to recover, mask anaesthesia is acceptable 48hr after delivery in the absence of other specific indications for intubation.[2]
- Renal blood flow increases by 75% at term, and GFR by 50%. Both urea and creatinine plasma concentrations fall.
- Neurological tissue has a greater susceptibility to the action of LAs during pregnancy—MAC is also reduced.
- The volume of distribution increases by 5L, affecting predominantly polar (water-soluble) agents. Lipid-soluble drugs are more affected by changes in protein binding. The fall in albumin concentration increases the free active portion of acidic agents, while basic drugs are more dominantly bound to α-1 glycoprotein. Some specific binding proteins, such as thyroxine-binding protein, increase in pregnancy.
- Although plasma cholinesterase concentration falls by about 25% in pregnancy, this is counteracted by an increase in the volume of distribution, so the actual duration of action of agents, such as suxamethonium, is little changed.

Pharmacology tables

- See Table 33.1 for dosing regimes.
- See Table 33.2 for commonly used uterotonics.

References

1 Cantwell R, Clutton-Brock T, Cooper G, et al. (2011). Centre for Maternal and Child Enquiries (CMACE). Saving Mothers' Lives: reviewing maternal deaths to make motherhood safer: 2006–08. The Eighth Report on Confidential Enquiries into Maternal Deaths in the United Kingdom. *BJOG*, 118 (Suppl 1), 1–203.

2 Bogod DG (1994). The postpartum stomach—when is it safe? *Anaesthesia*, 49, 1–2.

Table 33.1 Summary of dosing regimes for obstetric anaesthesia

Procedure	Technique	Suggested dose
Labour	Epidural loading dose	20mL of 0.1% bupivacaine with 2 micrograms/mL of fentanyl
	Epidural infusion	10mL/hr of 0.1% bupivacaine with 2 micrograms/mL of fentanyl
	Top-ups	10–20mL of 0.1% bupivacaine with 2 micrograms/mL of fentanyl
	CSE	Intrathecal: 0.5–1mL of 0.25% bupivacaine with 5–25 micrograms/mL of fentanyl
		Epidural: as above
	PCEA	5–10mL boluses of 0.1% bupivacaine with 2 micrograms/mL of fentanyl with a 10–20min lockout
LSCS	Spinal	2.5mL of 0.5% bupivacaine in 8% glucose ('heavy') plus 300 micrograms of diamorphine
	Epidural	15–20mL of 2% lidocaine with 1:200 000 adrenaline
		(± 0.5–2mL of preservative-free 8.4% sodium bicarbonate)
	CSE	Normal spinal dose (reduce if slow onset of block is required)
		If needed, top up the epidural with 5mL aliquots of 2% lidocaine with 1:200 000 adrenaline
Post-LSCS analgesia	GA	Bilateral ilioinguinal nerve blocks, rectus sheath/TAP blocks
		IV aliquots of morphine until comfortable
		Parenteral opioid (oral or PCA)
		75mg of diclofenac IV and 1g of paracetamol IV, followed by 50mg of diclofenac PO 8-hourly
	Regional and GA	Regular paracetamol. Other analgesics PRN
	Regional	100mg of diclofenac PR, followed by 50mg of diclofenac PO 8-hourly
		Epidural diamorphine (2.5mg) in 10mL of 0.9% NaCl 4-hourly, as required

CSE, combined spinal/epidural; LSCS, lower-segment Caesarean section; PCA, patient-controlled analgesia; PRN, as required; TAP, transversus abdominis plane.

Table 33.2 Commonly used uterotonics

Drug	Dose	Comment
Oxytocin	2–5IU bolus 30–50IU in 500mL of crystalloid and titrated, as indicated	Synthetically produced hormone, causing uterine contraction and peripheral vasodilatation. A 5IU bolus can cause a temporary drop in systolic BP of 30%, and tachycardia is common. Has mild ADH actions. Early preparations made from animal extracts had significant ADH activity
Carbetocin	100 micrograms IV over 1min	Long-acting analogue of oxytocin (half-life 40min vs 5–10min). Although manufacturer suggests to avoid in pre-eclampsia, eclampsia, and epilepsy, it has been used in studies in pre-eclamptic women. However, experience still limited. Relatively expensive
Ergometrine	0.5mg IM or slow IV injection	An ergot alkaloid derivative. Produces effective uterine constriction, but nausea and vomiting are very common. Systemic vasoconstriction may produce dangerous hypertension in at-risk groups (e.g. pre-eclampsia, specific cardiac disease)
Carboprost (15-methyl prostaglandin F2α)	0.25mg IM every 15min to a max of 2mg	Effective uterine constrictor. Also causes nausea, vomiting, and diarrhoea. May produce pyrexia, severe bronchospasm; may alter pulmonary shunt fraction and induce hypoxia (caution in asthmatics)
Misoprostol	0.8–1mg PR	Effective uterine constrictor. As with carboprost, can also cause nausea, vomiting, and diarrhoea. May also cause pyrexia, bronchospasm, and alter shunt fraction, but not usually as severe as with carboprost

Analgesia for labour

- The three most commonly used types of analgesic agents in labour are inhaled N_2O, opioids, and regional techniques.
- However, there are numerous techniques that help mothers in labour. These include prepared childbirth, massage, warm water baths, and transcutaneous electrical nerve stimulation (TENS). Although the evidence that these alter pain scores is weak, they are all useful techniques that many women find very beneficial.
- N_2O/O_2 (Entonox®) is the most commonly used inhalational agent and may be slightly more efficacious than pethidine, but complete analgesia is never attained.
- Worldwide, pethidine remains one of the most popular opioids for labour analgesia. However, its efficacy has been questioned; it has a long half-life in the fetus (18–23hr), is known to reduce fetal heart rate variability in labour, and is associated with changes in neonatal neurobehaviour, including an effect on breastfeeding. When regional analgesia is contraindicated, fentanyl or remifentanil PCA may be more beneficial (see remifentanil PCA, ➋ p. 736). Diamorphine has also been advocated, although it may prolong labour by >1hr.[3]
- Regional analgesia remains the most effective form of pain relief for labour.
- Uterine pain is transmitted in sensory fibres, which accompany sympathetic nerves and end in the dorsal horns of T10–L1. Vaginal pain is transmitted via the S2–S4 nerve roots (the pudendal nerve). Spinal, combined spinal/epidural (CSE), and epidural analgesia have largely replaced other regional techniques (paracervical, pudendal, caudal block). Neuraxial techniques can be expected to provide effective analgesia in over 85% of women. A meta-analysis of randomized studies, comparing regional techniques with opioid or no analgesia, confirmed improved analgesia. However, neuraxial analgesia was associated with hypotension, increased oxytocin use, an increased incidence of maternal pyrexia, and a 40% increase in the incidence of instrumental deliveries,[4] although techniques, such as using low concentrations of LA, can reduce this effect[5] (see ➋ p. 726). Fetal umbilical pH was marginally improved with epidural analgesia.
- Remember that acceptable analgesia for women in labour does not mean a complete absence of sensation.
- Using 'low-dose' epidural techniques can reduce the incidence of hypotension and motor blockade, decrease the incidence of assisted delivery, while increasing maternal satisfaction. The instrumental delivery rate can be reduced by:
  - Using synergistic agents, such as opioids, to reduce the total dose of LA administered
  - Establishing, as well as maintaining, the regional analgesia with low-dose epidural LA and opioid or low-dose intrathecal LA and opioid

- Using patient-controlled epidural analgesia (PCEA) or intermittent top-ups to maintain analgesia. In general, infusions deliver a greater total dose of LA than intermittent top-ups, while PCEA delivers the smallest total dose.
- The choice of LA may also affect motor block. At equimolar doses, ropivacaine produces less motor block than bupivacaine, but it is not as potent as bupivacaine, and the relative motor block at equipotent doses remains controversial.

References

3 Wee M, Tuckey J, Thomas PW, Burnard S (2014). A comparison of intramuscular diamorphine and intramuscular pethidine for labour analgesia: a two-centre randomised blinded controlled trial. *BJOG*, **121**, 447–56.

4 Anim-Somuah M, Smyth RM, Jones L (2011). Epidural versus non-epidural or no analgesia in labour. *Cochrane Database Syst Rev*, **7**, CD000331.

5 Sultan P, Murphy C, Halpern S, Carvalho B (2012). Comparison of ultra-low and higher-concentration epidural local anaesthetic solutions in labour: a meta-analysis. In: Abstracts of free papers presented at the Annual Meeting of the Obstetric Anaesthetists' Association, Liverpool, 24–25 May 2013. *Int J Obstet Anesth*, **21**, S11.

Regional labour analgesia

Indications

- Maternal request.
- Expectation of operative delivery (e.g. multiple pregnancy, malpresentation).
- Maternal disease—in particular, conditions in which sympathetic stimulation may cause deterioration in maternal or fetal condition.
- Specific CVS disease (e.g. regurgitant valvular lesions).
- Severe respiratory disease (e.g. CF).
- Specific neurological disease (intracranial A–V malformations, spinal cord injury etc.).
- Obstetric disease (e.g. pre-eclampsia).
- Conditions in which GA may be life-threatening (e.g. morbid obesity).

Contraindications

- Maternal refusal.
- Allergy (true allergy to amide LAs is rare).
- Local infection.
- Uncorrected hypovolaemia.
- Coagulopathy. The acceptable cut-off points which determine when neuraxial analgesia can be used are largely decided by expert opinion, in conjunction with an understanding of the pathology and pharmacology. The AAGBI guidelines can be accessed online[6] and are reproduced in Table 42.4. Remember that spinal analgesia is probably safer than epidural analgesia. It is always important to consider the risk and benefit for individual patients. Generally, in the absence of pharmacological agents that affect clotting, a platelet count above 75×10^9/L, together with a normal clotting screen, is considered to be acceptable. However, a slightly lower platelet count may be acceptable in patients with idiopathic thrombocytopenia. In most circumstances, tests of coagulation and the platelet count should be within 6hr of the time of the procedure, but, especially with pre-eclampsia, it is also important to consider the rate at which the platelet count is falling.
- Raised ICP (excluding the majority of individuals with idiopathic intracranial hypertension)

Relative contraindications

- Expectation of significant haemorrhage.
- Untreated systemic infection (provided systemic infection has been treated with antibiotics, the risk of 'seeding' infection into the epidural space with neuraxial procedures is minimal).
- Specific cardiac disease (e.g. severe valvular stenosis, Eisenmenger's syndrome, peripartum cardiomyopathy). Although regional analgesia has been used for many of these conditions, extreme care must be taken to avoid rapid changes in BP, preload, and afterload of the heart. Intrathecal opioid without LA may be advantageous for these patients.

- 'Bad backs' and previous back surgery do not contraindicate regional analgesia/anaesthesia, but scarring of the epidural space may limit the effectiveness of epidural analgesia and increase the risk of inadvertent dural puncture. Intrathecal techniques can be expected to work normally.

Consent

Most UK anaesthetists do not take written consent before inserting an epidural for labour analgesia, but 'appropriate' explanation must be given. The information offered varies according to local guidelines and with the degree of distress of each individual woman. The Obstetric Anaesthetists' Association has produced an information leaflet for mothers[7] which includes a quantitative estimate of the incidence of a variety of potential complications, including neurological injury. It is available in a number of languages. The explanation and, in particular, the possible hazards discussed must be documented, as many women do not accurately recall information given in labour. Information about labour analgesia should always be available antenatally.

References

6 Association of Anaesthetists of Great Britain and Ireland, Obstetric Anaesthetists' Association, and Regional Anaesthesia UK (2013). Regional anaesthesia and patients with abnormalities of coagulation. *Anaesthesia*, **68**, 966–72. http://www.aagbi.org/sites/default/files/rapac_2013_web.pdf.

7 Obstetric Anaesthetists' Association. *LabourPains.com*. http://www.labourpains.com/UI/Content/Content.aspx?ID=5.

Epidural analgesia for labour

- Make sure a trained midwife is available to provide one-to-one care.
- Scrupulous attention to sterile technique is required. A mask, hat, gown, and gloves should be worn.
- Establish IV access. In the absence of previous haemorrhage or dehydration, when low-dose LA techniques are used, large fluid co-loads are unnecessary.
- Position in either a full lateral or sitting position. Finding the midline in the obese may be easier in the sitting position. Accidental dural puncture may be slightly lower in the lateral position.
- Fetal HR should be recorded before and during the establishment of analgesia.
- Skin sterilization with 0.5% chlorhexidine is common in the UK. However, most sterilizing solutions, including chlorhexidine, are neurotoxic, so great care must be taken to avoid contamination of the neuraxial equipment or the anaesthetist's gloves. It is recommended that chlorhexidine is never on the sterile work surface, and it is sensible to complete skin sterilization before the neuraxial equipment is unwrapped. Chlorhexidine must be allowed to dry before the skin is touched.
- Locate the epidural space (loss of resistance to saline may have slight advantages in both the reduced incidence of accidental dural puncture and reduced incidence of 'missed segments', compared with loss of resistance to air).
- The incidence of puncturing a blood vessel with the epidural catheter is reduced if 10mL of saline is flushed into the epidural space before the catheter is inserted. Always insert the catheter as gently as possible.
- Introduce 4–5cm of the catheter into the epidural space. (Longer has an increased incidence of unilateral block, and shorter increases the chance that the catheter pulls out of the space.) Multihole catheters have a lower incidence of unsatisfactory blocks.
- Check for blood/CSF.
- If blood is aspirated, see if the catheter can be withdrawn further (leave a minimum of 3cm in the space). If blood is still present, remove the catheter, and reinsert.
- Give an appropriate test dose. An 'appropriate' test remains controversial. Using 0.5% bupivacaine significantly increases motor block. Using 1:200 000 adrenaline to detect IV placement of a catheter has both high false positive and false negative rates. Many anaesthetists will use 8–15mL of 0.1% bupivacaine with a dilute opioid (2 micrograms/mL fentanyl) as both the test and main doses. This will exclude intrathecal placement but may not exclude intravascular placement. However, the complete absence of a detectable block after a normal labour analgesia loading dose is a warning sign of possible IV cannulation. Remember every dose is a 'test dose'!
- If required, give further LA to establish analgesia. There should be no need to use concentrations >0.25% bupivacaine.
- Measure maternal BP every 5min for at least 20min after every bolus dose of LA.

- Once the epidural is functioning, it can be maintained by one of three methods:
  - Intermittent top-ups of LA administered by a PCEA. A variety of regimens have been proposed. In general, larger volumes of low-concentration bupivacaine with opioid produce more effective analgesia. However, it is important to use a dose that will not create a dangerously high block if the dose was to be accidentally given intrathecally. A common regimen would be 5–10mL boluses of 0.0625–0.1% bupivacaine with 2 micrograms/mL fentanyl and a 15–20min lockout period
  - A continuous infusion of LA (5–12mL/hr of 0.0625–0.1% bupivacaine with 2 micrograms/mL fentanyl)
  - Intermittent top-ups of LA administered by midwives (this is now rare in the UK). Historically, boluses of 5–10mL of 0.25% bupivacaine were used, but a more modern approach would be to use a larger volume of a lower concentration such as 10–15mL of 0.1% bupivacaine with 2 micrograms/mL fentanyl.

Combined spinal/epidural analgesia for labour

A combination of low-dose subarachnoid LA and/or opioid, together with subsequent top-ups of weak epidural LA, produces a rapid onset of analgesia with minimal motor block. An epidural technique alone can produce a similar degree of analgesia and motor block but may take 10–15min longer to establish.

- Indications for CSEs include establishing rapid analgesia in women who are unable to cope with labour pain, re-establishing analgesia for women who have had a failed epidural, and preservation of leg strength for women who want to walk in labour.
- In some centres, CSEs are used routinely because of the rapid speed of onset, the reliable initial analgesia, together with some evidence of improved epidural analgesia after the initial spinal analgesia has receded.[8,9]
- CSE can be performed as a needle-through-needle technique or as separate injections in the same, or in different, intervertebral spaces:

Either:

- Locate the epidural space at the L3/4 interspace or below with a Tuohy needle. (The level of the iliac crests usually corresponds to the spinous process of L4 (Tuffier's line), although there is variation between individuals.) Pass a 25–27G pencil-point needle through the Tuohy needle to locate the subarachnoid space
- Inject the subarachnoid solution (e.g. 0.5–1.0mL of 0.25% bupivacaine with 5–25 micrograms of fentanyl or the equivalent dose in mg)
- Without rotating the epidural needle, insert an epidural catheter.

Or:

- Perform the spinal at L3/4 or below with a 25–27G pencil-point needle
- Inject the spinal solution
- Insert an epidural catheter at a different interspace
- This technique is particularly helpful when women are unable to stay still because of pain. The spinal is usually quick and relatively easy, and, once analgesia has been established, an epidural can be performed with a more cooperative patient.

After 15min, once the analgesia from the spinal solution is established, check the degree of motor and sensory block, and then administer an epidural test dose. If this dose is given accidentally intrathecally, the block would be expected to change significantly within 5min.

Further management of the epidural is the same as for epidural analgesia alone.

'Walking' epidurals

Effective analgesia with minimal motor block of the lower limbs can be readily produced with low doses of an epidural or intrathecal LA, usually in combination with an opioid, e.g. subarachnoid injection of 1–2.5mg of bupivacaine with 10–25micrograms of fentanyl or an epidural bolus of 15–20mL of 0.1% bupivacaine with 2 micrograms/mL fentanyl, and subsequent epidural top-ups of 15mL of the same solution, as required.

In some centres, women with minimal motor blockade are encouraged to mobilize. The possible advantages of these techniques include:

- Minimal motor block associated with these techniques increases maternal satisfaction scores
- Intrathecal, as opposed to epidural, techniques produce a more rapid onset of analgesia.

Mobilization

Mobilization has been criticized, because:

- Leg strength may be compromised, and this becomes increasingly likely with repeated doses of epidural LA
- Impaired proprioception may make walking dangerous, even when leg strength has been maintained. While dynamic posturography suggests that, following an initial intrathecal dose of 2.5mg of bupivacaine and 10 micrograms of fentanyl, proprioception is adequate for safe walking, this may no longer be true after repeated epidural top-ups
- Intrathecal opioid may cause temporary fetal bradycardia, probably by altering uterine blood flow through a change in maternal spinal reflexes
- Assessing the fetal condition is difficult when the mother is mobile.

In practice, even when a technique is used that could allow walking, only ~50% of women actually choose to do so. Despite this, most women prefer the added sense of control engendered by retaining leg strength.

If women are to be allowed to walk, always wait at least 30min from the initiation of the block before attempting mobilization. Then:

- Check the strength of straight leg-raising in bed
- Ask the woman if she feels able to stand
- When the woman first stands, have two assistants ready to offer support, if required
- Perform a knee bend
- Ask the woman if she feels safe
- Allow full mobilization
- After each top-up, the same sequence must be repeated.

References

8 Cappiello E, O'Rourke N, Segal S, Tsen LC (2008). A randomized trial of dural puncture epidural technique compared with the standard epidural technique for labor analgesia. *Anesth Analg*, **107**, 1646–51.

9 Simmons SW, Taghizadeh N, Dennis AT, Hughes D, Cyna AM (2012). Combined spinal-epidural versus epidural analgesia in labour. *Cochrane Database Syst Rev*, **10**, CD003401.

The poorly functioning epidural

Look for the pattern of failure (Table 33.3). Remember that a full bladder may cause breakthrough pain. Ask the midwife if a full bladder is likely. Carefully assess the spread of the block. It is important to be confident that the epidural could be topped up for a Caesarean section, if required. Therefore, if in doubt, re-site the epidural.

Table 33.3 How to handle a poorly functioning epidural

Pattern of failure	Remedy
Global failure: No detectable block despite at least 10mL of 0.25% bupivacaine (or equivalent)	Re-site the epidural
Partial failure	
Unilateral block: Assess the block	Top-up epidural, with the painful side in a dependent position (use LA and 50–100 micrograms of fentanyl)
Feel both feet to assess whether they are symmetrically warm and dry	Withdraw the catheter 2–3cm, and give a further top-up
Is the pattern consistent with where the pain is felt?	Re-site the epidural
Missed segment: True missed segments are rare. Commonly, a 'missed segment' felt in the groin is a partial unilateral block	Top-up with opioid (i.e. 50–100 micrograms of fentanyl). The intrathecal mode of action will minimize segmental effects
	Continue as per unilateral block
Back pain: Severe back pain is associated with an occipito-posterior position of the fetus and may require a dense block to establish analgesia	Top up with more LA and opioid
Perineal pain	Check sacral block and that the bladder is empty
	Top up with more LA in the sitting position
	Continue as per unilateral block

Complications of epidural analgesia

Hypotension

In the absence of fetal distress, a fall in systolic BP of 20% or to 100mmHg (whichever is higher) is acceptable. However, uterine blood flow is not autoregulated, and prolonged or severe hypotension will cause fetal compromise. IV fluid loading is not routinely required when using low doses of LA, but patients should not be hypovolaemic before instituting regional analgesia. When hypotension or fetal distress is detected, it should be treated quickly.

- Avoid aortocaval occlusion—make sure that the patient is in the full lateral position. (Remember that, in the lateral position, BP should be measured in the dependent arm—there is often a 10mmHg difference between the upper and lower limbs.)
- Give an IV fluid bolus of crystalloid solution and, if the fetus is distressed, mask O_2 supplementation.
- Give 6mg IV ephedrine, and repeat as necessary.
- If the fetus is distressed, call the obstetricians.
- Remember that brachial artery pressure may not reflect uterine artery blood flow. If fetal distress is detected and is chronologically related to a regional anaesthetic procedure, treat as above, even in the absence of overt hypotension.

Subdural block

Subdural block occurs when the epidural catheter is misplaced between the dura mater and arachnoid mater. In obstetric practice, the incidence of clinically recognized subdural block is <1:1000 epidurals. However, subdural blocks may be clinically indistinguishable from epidural blocks. Definitive diagnosis is radiological. The classical characteristics of a subdural block are:

- A slow onset (20–30min) of a block that is inappropriately extensive for the volume of LA injected. The block may extend to the cervical dermatomes, and Horner's syndrome may develop
- The block is often patchy and asymmetrical. Sparing of motor fibres to the lower limbs may occur
- A total spinal may occur with top-up doses. This is probably due to an increase in volume, causing the arachnoid mater to rupture.

If a subdural is suspected, re-site the epidural catheter.

Total spinal

The incidence of unexpected high or total spinal is variously reported to be 1:1500 to 1:4500 epidurals. Usually the onset is rapid, although delays of 30min or more have been reported. Delayed onset may be related to a change in the maternal position or a subdural catheter placement.

Symptoms are of a rapidly rising block. Initially, difficulty in coughing may be noted (which is commonly seen during regional anaesthesia for a Caesarean section), then loss of hand and arm strength, followed by difficulty with talking, breathing, and swallowing.

If the block is rising to a concerning height, think about the likely cause.
- If the block is likely to be due to a correctly sited epidural LA, but excess dose, position the patient head-up.
- If the block is due to subarachnoid plain LA (which is hypobaric, compared to CSF), a head-up position may actually encourage the block to spread further. So gently position the mother in a left lateral position, which should minimize dural compression through epidural vein engorgement (which occurs with caval occlusion), and observe very closely. Sudden movements may cause CSF to move further.
- Make sure that the equipment for ventilatory and CVS support are immediately available. Respiratory paralysis, CVS depression, unconsciousness, and finally fixed dilated pupils may ensue.

Unsurprisingly, total spinals are reported more often after epidural anaesthesia than epidural analgesia, as larger doses of LA are employed.

Management of total spinal
- Maintain airway and ventilation; avoid aortocaval compression, and provide CVS support.
- Even if consciousness is not lost, intubation may be required to protect the airway.
- Careful maternal and fetal monitoring is essential and, if appropriate, delivery of the fetus. In the absence of fetal distress, a Caesarean section is not an immediate requirement.
- Ventilation is usually necessary for 1–2hr.

Accidental intravenous injection of local anaesthetic

'Every dose is a test dose.' The maxim is to avoid injecting any single large bolus of LA IV. Remember that initial placement of a catheter IV or partial IV positioning of epidural catheters occurs in 5% of siting. The risk can be minimized by:
- Meticulous attention to the technique during placement. Always check for blood in the catheter
- Always being alert to symptoms of IV injection with every dose of LA, even when previous doses have been uncomplicated
- Dividing all large doses of LA into aliquots
- Using appropriate LAs.

If neurological or cardiovascular symptoms occur
- Stop injecting the LA.
- Treat according to BLS and ALS protocols.
- Administer 20% lipid emulsion (see Management of local anaesthetic toxicity, ➲ p. 1148).

Neurological damage

Neurological damage does occur after childbirth, but establishing cause and effect is difficult. Neurological sequelae following delivery under GA is as common as delivery under regional anaesthesia, suggesting that obstetric causes of neurological problems are probably commoner than any effects from the regional technique. Prolonged neurological deficit after epidural anaesthesia occurs in ~1:10 000 to 1:15 000. Major neurological damage probably occurs in <1:80 000 neuraxial procedures in the obstetric population, and this group of patients probably has the lowest risk of any patient population.[10]

Reference

10 Cook TM, Counsell D, Wildsmith JA; Royal College of Anaesthetists Third National Audit Project (2009). Major complications of central neuraxial block: report on the Third National Audit Project of the Royal College of Anaesthetists. *Br J Anaesth*, **102**, 179–90.

Dural puncture

When loss of CSF is greater than production, as might occur through a dural tear, CSF pressure falls, and the brain sinks, stretching the meninges. This stretching is thought to cause headache. Compensatory vasodilatation of intracranial vessels may further worsen symptoms.

The incidence of dural puncture should be <1% of epidurals. All midwives, as well as obstetric and anaesthetic staff, should be alert to the signs of PDPH, as symptoms may not develop for several days. If untreated, headaches are not only unpleasant, but also can very rarely be life-threatening, usually as a result of intracranial haemorrhage or coning of the brainstem.

Management of an accidental dural puncture can be divided into immediate and late.

Immediate management

The initial aim is to achieve effective analgesia without causing further complication.

Either:
- If a dural puncture occurs, pass the 'epidural' catheter into the subarachnoid space
- Label the catheter clearly as an intrathecal catheter, and only allow anaesthetists to perform top-ups
- Give intermittent top-ups through the catheter (1.0–2.5mg of bupivacaine ± 5–25 micrograms of fentanyl. Tachyphylaxis may occur with prolonged labour)
- Advantages:
  - The analgesia produced is likely to be excellent
  - There is no possibility of performing another dural puncture on reinsertion of the epidural
  - The unpredictable spread of the epidural solution through the dural tear is eliminated
  - The need for an epidural blood patch (although not the incidence of PDPH) may be reduced[11]
- Disadvantages:
  - There is a theoretical risk of introducing infection
  - The catheter may be mistaken for an epidural catheter

Or:
- Remove the epidural catheter
- Reinsert the epidural at a different interspace—usually one interspace higher. If the reason for the dural puncture was difficult anatomy, a senior colleague should take over
- Run the epidural as normal, but beware of intrathecal spread of LA. Be particularly cautious if the epidural catheter is topped up with a large dose of anaesthetic for a Caesarean section. All top-ups should be given by an anaesthetist.

With either technique, the patient should be informed, at the earliest opportunity, that a dural puncture has occurred and of the likely sequelae. Labour itself may be allowed to continue normally. Arrange daily post-natal follow-up.

Late management

Following a dural puncture with a 16G Tuohy needle, the incidence of PDPH is ~90%. In only 40% of dural punctures is CSF recognized flowing from the Tuohy needle. In >30% of individuals who develop PDPH, a dural puncture was not recognized in labour.

Headaches in the post-natal period are common. The key differentiating factor between a 'normal' post-natal headache and PDPH is the positional nature of the latter.

Common features of PDPH include:

- Typically, the onset is 24–48hr post-dural puncture. Untreated, they are said to last 7–10d, but the evidence is poor.
- Characteristically, PDPH is worse on standing. Headache is often absent after overnight bed rest but returns after mobilizing.
- The headache is usually fronto-occipital and may be associated with neck stiffness.
- The headache may be relieved by tight abdominal compression—while abdominal binders are no longer used as a treatment, this can be a useful diagnostic tool.
- Photophobia and difficulty in accommodation are common. Hearing loss, tinnitus, and VIth nerve palsy with diplopia are possible. If these signs develop, women should be encouraged to have a blood patch sooner rather than later, as these signs are an indication of a more severe headache, and the risk of more serious complications—seizures, subdural haematoma, and cerebral herniation—may be increased
- Nausea in up to 60% of women.

Treatment is either to alleviate symptoms, while waiting for the dural tear to heal itself, or to seal the puncture. Epidural blood patching is the only commonly used method of sealing dural tears, although neurosurgical closure has been reported.

Prophylactic treatment

- There is a high incidence of bacteraemia shortly after delivery. This, combined with the poor efficacy of prophylactic blood patching, means that the use of prophylactic blood patching has fallen out of favour.
- Although bed rest alleviates symptoms, the incidence of PDPH after 48hr is the same for those cases that mobilized throughout. Because of the risk of thromboembolism, bed rest should not be routinely encouraged in asymptomatic women.

Symptomatic treatment

Although there is no well-established mechanism for preventing PDPH, once a dural puncture has occurred, various treatments have been proposed to alleviate symptoms, while waiting for the dural puncture to seal itself.

- Simple analgesics (paracetamol and NSAIDs) are the mainstays of symptomatic treatment. They should always be offered, even though they are unlikely to completely relieve severe PDPH.
- Adequate fluid intake should be encouraged, although there is no evidence that hydration reduces the incidence of PDPH.

- Caffeine/theophyllines act by reducing intracranial vasodilatation, which is partially responsible for the headache. IV aminophylline has been shown to reduce the incidence of headache. However, concern has been expressed that the incidence of seizures following dural puncture may be increased in the presence of caffeine.
- Epidural infusion of saline is no longer recommended. Although compression of the dural sac with epidural saline can alleviate symptoms, after 24hr of continuous infusion, the incidence of PDPH is only marginally reduced. However, radicular pain in the lower limbs may occur, and patients are immobilized.
- In relatively small RCT studies, ACTH analogues reduced the incidence of headache after a known dural puncture, while IV dexamethasone increased the incidence. However, the studies are small, and the results need to be treated with caution.[12,13]
- A number of case series have also supported the use of gabapentin or pregabalin. However, again the numbers are small, and the results need to be treated with caution.[14]

Definitive treatment is with epidural blood patching.

Epidural blood patch

Epidural blood patch performed around 48hr post-partum has a 60–90% cure rate at the 1st attempt (with a lower success rate if performed between 24 and 48hr post-partum, and lower still if performed at <24hr post-partum). The proposed mechanism of action is 2-fold:

- Blood injected into the epidural space compresses the dural sac and raises the ICP. This produces an almost instantaneous improvement in pain
- The injected blood forms a clot over the site of the dural tear, and this seals the CSF leak.

Blood injected into the epidural space predominantly spreads cephalad, so blood patches should be performed at the same or lower interspace as the dural puncture.

- Consent must be obtained. The patient should be apyrexial and not have a raised WCC.
- Two operators are required. One should be an experienced 'epiduralist'; the other is required to take blood in a sterile manner.
- The patient should have a period of bed rest before performing the patch to reduce the CSF volume in the epidural space.
- Aseptic technique must be meticulous both at the epidural site and the site of blood letting (usually the antecubital fossa).
- An epidural should be performed at the same or a lower vertebral interspace as the dural puncture, with the woman in the lateral position to minimize CSF pressure in the lumbar dural sac.
- Once the epidural space has been identified, 20mL of blood is obtained.
- Inject the blood slowly through the epidural needle, until either a maximum of 20mL has been given or pain develops (commonly in the back or legs). If pain occurs, pause, and, if the pain resolves, try continuing with a slow injection. If the pain does not resolve or recurs, then stop.

- To allow the clot to form, maintain bed rest for at least 2hr, and then allow slow mobilization.
- As far as possible, the patient should avoid straining, lifting, or excessive bending for 48hr, although there are obvious limitations when a woman has a newborn infant to care for.
- Follow-up is still required. Every woman should have clear instructions to contact the anaesthetists again if symptoms recur, even after discharge home.

Serious complications of blood patching are rare. However, backache is common, with 35% of women experiencing some discomfort 48hr post-epidural blood patch and 16% of women having prolonged backache (mean duration 27d). Other reported complications include repeated dural puncture, neurological deficits, epileptiform fits, and cranial nerve damage. Suggestions that labour epidurals after blood patching may be less effective have not been confirmed.

References

11 Heesen M, Klöhr S, Rossaint R, Walters M, Straube S, van de Velde M (2013). Insertion of an intrathecal catheter following accidental dural puncture: a meta-analysis. *Int J Obstet Anesth,* **22,** 26–30.

12 Basurto Ona X, Uriona Tuma SM, Martínez García L, Solà I, Bonfill Cosp X (2013). Drug therapy for preventing post-dural puncture headache. *Cochrane Database Syst Rev,* **2,** CD001792.

13 Bradbury CL, Singh SI, Badder SR, Wakely LJ, Jones PM (2013). Prevention of post-dural puncture headache in parturients: a systematic review and meta-analysis. *Acta Anaesthesiol Scand,* **57,** 417–30.

14 Wagner Y (2012) Gabapentin in the treatment of post-dural puncture headache: a case series. *Anaesth Intensive Care,* **40,** 714–18.

Remifentanil for labour analgesia

Remifentanil is an ultrashort-acting mu-agonist opioid, which is broken down by tissue and plasma esterases. It has an analgesia half-life of about 6min and a rapid onset time of 30–60s. Although remifentanil readily crosses the placenta, it is also rapidly metabolized in the fetus. These features make remifentanil a potentially useful analgesic agent in labour. Like all opioids, it does not produce complete analgesia but appears to be more effective than IM pethidine. When compared with a fentanyl PCA, the analgesic effect may be little different, but, as might be expected, remifentanil is associated with less need for fetal resuscitation, which is good, and an increased incidence of maternal respiratory depression, which is potentially worrying.[15]

Up to 40% of women who use remifentanil PCA for pain relief in labour will develop respiratory depression. So remifentanil must only be used with direct (in the room) supervision and careful training of all the staff involved in its administration. There have been numerous case reports of maternal respiratory arrests with remifentanil.

The ideal PCA regimen has not been established. Many proposed techniques are based on body weight, but the technique below is based on a fixed dose which has the advantage of simplicity. The addition of N_2O may improve analgesia further but may increase the risk of hypoxaemia.[16]

Technique

- Of critical importance is establishing one-to-one care with a trained individual (midwife) who must be continuously present in the labour room.
- No opioid should have been used in the previous 4hr.
- Establish dedicated IV access.
- PCA bolus dose of 20–40 micrograms and lockout of 2min.
- Monitor with continuous pulse oximetry.
- Give O_2 if SpO_2 <94% on air.
- Thirty-minute observations of respiratory rate, sedation score, and pain scores.
- Always flush the cannula when PCA is discontinued.

Call the anaesthetist if:
- The patient is not rousable to voice.
- Respiratory rate <8 breaths/min.
- SpO_2 <94% despite O_2 supplementation.

References

15 Marwah R, Hassan S, Carvalho JC, Balki M (2012). Remifentanil versus fentanyl for intravenous patient-controlled labour analgesia: an observational study. *Can J Anaesth*, **59**, 246–54.
16 Hinova A, Fernando R (2009). Systemic remifentanil for labor analgesia. *Anesth Analg*, **109**, 1925–9.

Caesarean section

With all Caesarean sections, it is vital that the obstetrician clearly communicates the degree of urgency to all staff. The four-point classification[17] in Table 33.4 is a modification of a system originally proposed by Lucas.

Table 33.4 Categories of urgency of Caesarean section

Category 1	Maternal or fetal compromise with immediate threat to the life of mother or fetus
Category 2	Maternal or fetal compromise that is not immediately life-threatening
Category 3	No maternal or fetal compromise, but requires early delivery
Category 4	No maternal or fetal compromise. Delivery timed to suit mother and maternity services

- For all emergency Caesarean sections, the patient must be transferred to theatre as rapidly as possible. Fetal monitoring should be continued until abdominal skin preparation starts.
- For category 1 (emergency) sections, the objective should be to deliver the fetus as quickly as possible, while not compromising maternal safety. It is the obstetrician's responsibility to call the urgency of the Caesarean section, but it is the anaesthetist's responsibility to choose a method of anaesthesia that is safe. While, in many centres, GA is commonly used for category 1 sections, do not be pressured into choosing a form of anaesthetic that is inappropriate for the mother.
- Categories 2–4 Caesarean sections are usually performed under regional anaesthesia.
- Remember that the classification of urgency should be continuously reviewed. Category 1 sections can become category 2, and vice versa.

Regional anaesthesia for Caesarean section

Regional anaesthesia for Caesarean section was initially driven by maternal preference. It was subsequently found that regional anaesthesia is also safer than GA, although, with good-quality training, and modern anaesthetic standards and equipment, the difference in maternal mortality appears to be less than it was in the past.[18]

Advantages of regional anaesthesia

- Both mother and partner can be present at the delivery. Usually, the perioperative experience for the family is much more affirmative.
- Minimal risk of aspiration and lower risk of anaphylaxis.
- The neonate is more alert, which promotes early bonding and breastfeeding.
- Fewer drugs are administered, with less 'hangover' than after GA.
- Better post-operative analgesia and earlier mobilization.

Mothers who are nervous about having a Caesarean section under regional anaesthesia should be given a clear explanation of the advantages and disadvantages of regional anaesthesia and GA but should never be coerced into having a regional technique.

There are three techniques for neuraxial anaesthesia—epidural, spinal, and CSE. Epidural anaesthesia is most commonly used for women who already have labour epidural analgesia. Spinal anaesthesia is the most popular technique for an elective Caesarean section, although, in some centres, CSEs are preferred.

The speed of onset of sympathectomy that occurs with spinal anaesthesia (as opposed to epidural) results in a greater fall in maternal cardiac output and BP and may be associated with a more acidotic neonate at delivery. This can be minimized by using a prophylactic phenylephrine infusion (see p. 746) and careful positioning of the mother. When there is particular concern about the speed of onset of a block, a CSE approach can be used, injecting only a small dose of intrathecal LA and extending the block, if required, using the epidural catheter. Spinal anaesthesia generally provides a better quality of analgesia than epidural anaesthesia.

Whatever technique is chosen, a careful history and an appropriate examination should be performed. This should include checking:

- Blood group and antibody screen. Routine cross-matching of blood is not required, unless haemorrhage is expected or if antibodies that interfere with cross-matching are present.
- Ultrasound reports to establish the position of the placenta. A low-lying anterior placenta puts a woman at risk of major haemorrhage, particularly if associated with a scar from a previous Caesarean section (see Placenta praevia, p. 765).

An explanation of the technique must be offered. Although a Caesarean section under regional anaesthesia becomes routine for the anaesthetist, it can be an intimidating prospect for the mother. Reassurance and support are important. However, the possibility of complications must also be mentioned, including the possibility of intraoperative discomfort and its management. Pain during regional anaesthesia remains a leading obstetric anaesthetic cause of maternal litigation. Document all complications that are discussed.

References

17 Royal College of Obstetricians and Gynaecologists, Royal College of Anaesthetists (2010). *Classification of urgency of Caesarean section—a continuum of risk. Good practice No. 11.* https://www.rcoa.ac.uk/system/files/PUB-GoodPracticeNo11.pdf.

18 Hawkins JL, Chang J, Palmer SK, Gibbs CP, Callaghan WM (2011). Anesthesia-related maternal mortality in the United States: 1979–2002. *Obstet Gynecol*, **117**, 69–74.

Caesarean section: epidural

- Indications for a Caesarean section under epidural anaesthesia include:
  - Women who already have epidural analgesia established for labour
  - Specific maternal disease (e.g. cardiac disease) where rapid changes in SVR might be problematic, although, more commonly, these individuals will have a careful CSE.
- Advantages and disadvantages of epidural anaesthesia for a Caesarean section are described in Table 33.5.

Table 33.5 Epidural anaesthesia for Caesarean section

Advantages	Disadvantages
A functioning labour epidural is easy to top up	Slow onset
Stable BP	Large doses of LA
Intraoperative top-up possible	Poorer quality of block than spinal anaesthesia
Epidural can be used for post-operative analgesia	

Technique

- History/examination/explanation and consent.
- Ensure that antacid prophylaxis has been given.
- Establish 16G or larger IV access. Start crystalloid co-load.
- Insert epidural catheter at the L2/3 or L3/4 vertebral interspace.
- Position the patient in the supine position with a left lateral tilt or wedge.
- Give supplemental O_2 by face mask if SpO_2 <95% on air. (This is very important in obese patients, who may become hypoxic when supine, and may also be beneficial for a compromised fetus.)
- Test the dose, then incrementally top up the epidural with LA and opioid:
  - Five to 8mL boluses of 2% lidocaine with 1:200 000 adrenaline every 2–3min, up to a maximum of 7mg/kg (~20mL), or
  - Five mL of 0.5% bupivacaine/levobupivacaine/ropivacaine every 4–5min, up to a maximum of 2mg/kg in any 4hr period. (The single-enantiomer LAs may offer some safety advantage; however, lidocaine is still safer than either ropivacaine or levobupivacaine.)
- Opioid (e.g. 100 micrograms of fentanyl or 2.5mg of diamorphine) improves the quality of the analgesia, and a slightly lower dermatomal block height may be accepted before starting surgery (i.e. T6 to light touch).
- Establish an S4–T4 block (nipple level). Always check the sacral dermatomes, as epidural LA occasionally does not spread caudally. Anaesthesia to light touch is more reliable at predicting adequacy of block than loss of cold sensation.[19] Document the level of block obtained and the adequacy of perioperative analgesia.

- Hypotension is much less common than with intrathecal techniques. However, if hypotension does occur, treat hypotension with (also see ➜ p. 746):
  - Boluses of 500 mL of crystalloid
  - Fifty to 100 micrograms of phenylephrine IV bolus (expect a reflex bradycardia) or 6mg of ephedrine IV. α-agonists may be more effective and may be associated with less fetal acidosis than ephedrine (see ➜ p. 746)
  - Increasing the left uterine displacement.
- At delivery, give 2–5IU of oxytocin as a slow IV bolus. If tachycardia must be avoided, then an IV infusion of 30–50IU of oxytocin in 500mL of crystalloid, given over 4hr, is an acceptable alternative.
- At the end of the procedure, give NSAID, unless contraindicated (100mg of diclofenac PR).
- Epidural diamorphine given at the time of surgery improves post-operative analgesia, while epidural fentanyl has little post-operative analgesic benefit.

Reference

19 Russell IF (1995). Levels of anaesthesia and intraoperative pain at Caesarean section under regional block. *Int J Obstet Anesth*, 4, 71–7.

Caesarean section: spinal

Spinal anaesthesia is the most commonly used technique for elective Caesarean sections. It is rapid in onset, produces a dense block, and, with intrathecal opioids, can produce long-acting post-operative analgesia. However, hypotension is much commoner than with epidural anaesthesia (Table 33.6).

Table 33.6 Spinal anaesthesia for Caesarean section

Advantages	Disadvantages
Quick onset	Single shot
Good-quality analgesia	Limited duration
Easy to perform	Inadequate analgesia is difficult to correct
	Rapid changes in BP and cardiac output

Technique

- History/examination/explanation and consent.
- Ensure that antacid prophylaxis has been given.
- Establish 16G or larger IV access. Start crystalloid co-load.
- Position the patient. A sitting position usually makes finding the midline easier, which may be helpful with obese patients, and may be associated with a faster onset, although the height of block is less predictable. A lateral position is associated with a slower onset of block, particularly if a full lateral position is maintained until the block has fully developed. The block height may be slightly more consistent, and the women may sometimes find it more comfortable than sitting if the fetal head is very low.
- Perform spinal anaesthetic at L3/4 interspace, using a 25G or smaller pencil-point needle. (The level of the iliac crests usually corresponds to the spinous process of L4 (Tuffier's line), although there is variation between individuals.)
- With the orifice pointing cephalad, inject the anaesthetic solution, e.g. 2.5mL of 0.5% hyperbaric bupivacaine with 300 micrograms of diamorphine or 15 micrograms of fentanyl. Intrathecal diamorphine improves post-operative analgesia, while intrathecal fentanyl has little post-operative analgesic benefit. (A total of 100 micrograms of preservative-free morphine is also used and can produce prolonged post-operative analgesia. However, there is a high incidence of PONV and an increased risk of late respiratory depression.)
- After injection of the solution, move the woman to a supine position with a left lateral tilt or wedge. When hyperbaric LA solutions are used, it is important that the cervical spine is kept elevated (pillow) to prevent LA from spreading to the cervical dermatomes. If supine hypotension occurs, increase the tilt, or, if severe, temporarily move the woman to a full lateral position.

- Start pressor infusion. Hypotension is commoner with spinal anaesthesia than epidural anaesthesia. Try to prevent hypotension, rather than treat it after it has occurred. When possible, a continuous infusion of the pressor agent should be started at the time of the injection of spinal LA (see prevention and treatment of hypotension, p. 746).
- Continue as for epidural anaesthesia for Caesarean section (see p. 739).

Caesarean section: combined spinal/epidural

In some centres, CSE is the technique of choice. Indications include:
- Limiting the speed of onset of a block. A small initial intrathecal dose of LA can be supplemented through the epidural catheter, as required.
- Expectation of prolonged surgery.
- Ability to use the epidural catheter for post-operative analgesia.

Advantages and disadvantages of this technique are summarized in Table 33.7.

Table 33.7 Combined spinal/epidural anaesthesia for Caesarean section

Advantages	Disadvantages
Quick onset	Rapid change in BP and cardiac output
Good-quality analgesia	Technically more difficult, with higher failure rate of spinal injection
Intraoperative top-up possible	
Epidural can be used for post-operative analgesia	Untested epidural catheter

Technique
- History/examination/explanation and consent.
- Ensure that antacid prophylaxis has been given.
- Establish 16G or larger IV access. Start crystalloid co-load.
- The intrathecal injection may be performed by passing the spinal needle through the epidural needle (needle-through-needle technique) or by performing the intrathecal injection completely separately from the epidural placement in either the same or a different interspace. The needle-through-needle technique is associated with an increased incidence of failure to locate CSF with the spinal needle but only involves one injection. If a two-injection technique is used, the epidural is sited at a higher interspace and usually inserted first because of the time delay that may occur in trying to locate the epidural space after the spinal injection. There is a theoretical risk of damaging the epidural catheter with the spinal needle.
- With either technique, perform the spinal injection at L3/4 or below. (The level of the iliac crests usually corresponds to the spinous process of L4 (Tuffier's line), although there is variation between individuals.)

Needle-through-needle technique
- Either use a dedicated CSE set or locate the epidural space at L3/4 or below with a Tuohy needle and then pass a long 25G or smaller pencil-point needle through the Tuohy needle into the intrathecal space. Inject the anaesthetic solution, with the needle orifice pointing cephalad (e.g. 2.5mL of 0.5% hyperbaric bupivacaine with 300 micrograms of diamorphine or 15 micrograms of fentanyl).
- Insert the epidural catheter. Aspirate the catheter carefully for CSF.

Two-needle technique
- Position the patient, and perform an epidural. After the catheter is in position, perform a spinal injection at L3/4 or below with a 25G or smaller pencil-point needle.
- With either technique, testing the catheter with LA before the intrathecal dose has receded may be unreliable. However, using the catheter intraoperatively is reasonable, as the anaesthetist is continuously present to deal with the consequences of an intrathecal injection. This may not be true if opioids are given through the catheter for post-operative analgesia at the end of the procedure before the block has receded.

If the spinal block is inadequate, inject LA, or 10mL of 0.9% NaCl, through the epidural catheter; 0.9% NaCl works by compressing the dural sac, causing a cephalad spread of intrathecal LA.

Continue as for spinal anaesthesia for Caesarean section (see → p. 741).

Special considerations
- Although the incidence of major complications of a central neuraxial block, as identified by the national audit project of The Royal College of Anaesthetists, was higher when a CSE technique was used, the numbers were very small (two or four patients, depending on whether an optimistic or pessimistic analysis was used), and the study cautions against over-interpretation of these results.[20]

Reference
20 Cook TM, Counsell D, Wildsmith JA; Royal College of Anaesthetists Third National Audit Project (2009). Major complications of central neuraxial block: report on the Third National Audit Project of the Royal College of Anaesthetists. *Br J Anaesth*, **102**, 179–90.

Inadequate anaesthesia

Every patient should be warned of the possibility of intraoperative discomfort, and this should be documented. Between 1% and 5% of attempted regional anaesthesia for Caesarean section are inadequate for surgery. The majority should be identified before operation commences.

Preoperative inadequate block

Epidural

- If no block develops, then the catheter is incorrectly positioned. It may be reinserted, or a spinal performed.
- If a partial, but inadequate, block has developed, the epidural may be resited or withdrawn slightly. Should the toxic limit for the LA agent have been reached, elective procedures can be abandoned, but, for urgent procedures, a GA or a spinal anaesthetic will be required. If a spinal is chosen, exceptional care with positioning and observation of the block level is required, as a 'high' or 'total' spinal can occur. Use a normal spinal dose of hyperbaric LA, as this should ensure adequate anaesthesia, but control the spread with careful positioning.

Spinal

- If no block develops, a repeat spinal may be performed.
- If a partial, but inadequate, block develops, an epidural may be inserted and slowly topped up.
- Use a GA, if required.

Intraoperative inadequate block

In this situation, good communication with the mother and surgeon is essential. If possible, stop surgery. Identify the likely cause of pain (e.g. inadequately blocked sacral nerve roots, peritoneal pain). Try to give the mother a realistic expectation of the continued duration and severity of the pain. If the pain has occurred before the delivery of the fetus, it is very likely that a GA is required.

- If patient requests GA, comply in all but exceptional circumstances. If the anaesthetist feels that the severity of the pain is not acceptable, persuade the patient that GA is required.

Spinal

- Reassure, and treat with:
  - Inhaled N_2O
  - IV opioid (e.g. 25–50 micrograms of fentanyl, repeated as necessary). Inform the neonatologists that opioid has been given
  - Surgical infiltration of LA (care with total dose)
  - GA.

Epidural and combined spinal/epidural

- Treat as per spinal anaesthesia, but, in addition, epidural opioid (e.g. 100 micrograms of fentanyl) and/or more epidural LA can be given.

Hypotension

Preventing maternal hypotension, rather than treating BP after hypotension has occurred, is associated with better fetal outcome and less maternal nausea. There are two principal methods of treating hypotension—pressor agents and fluid.

Pressor agents

Using prophylactic pressor agents is beneficial for both mother and fetus. Ephedrine was used to treat hypotension in obstetric neuraxial anaesthesia for many years. However, in the last decade, it has been established that treatment to normotension with phenylephrine is associated with better fetal umbilical pH than when ephedrine is used, although the difference is marginal. If phenylephrine is used, bolus doses of 50–100 micrograms can cause profound reflex bradycardias, so, if possible, use a phenylephrine infusion instead.

- A simple regime is to use a syringe driver with a solution of 100 micrograms/mL of phenylephrine (i.e. make up 10mg in 100mL of saline, and decant 20mL into a syringe).
- Start infusing at 30mL/hr, as the spinal solution is injected.
- Titrate to response, adjusting the rate of infusion up or down in increments of 10mL/hr.
- During the infusion, expect the HR to gradually slow, so give anticholinergic agents, as required.
- Reduce and stop the infusion post-delivery.
- Be careful with this technique in hypertensive individuals. Start at a lower infusion rate.
- Metaraminol can be used as an alternative to phenylephrine.

Fluid

A fluid preload was a traditional part of the anaesthetic technique for regional anaesthesia. It had two functions:
- To maintain the intravascular volume in a patient who is likely to lose 500–1000mL of blood
- To reduce the incidence of hypotension associated with regional anaesthesia.

However, crystalloid preloading is very ineffective at preventing hypotension. In addition, in women with severe pre-eclampsia, large preloads are harmful, as the rise in filling pressures and the reduced colloid osmotic pressure will predispose to pulmonary oedema. Using colloids as a preload is more effective, but colloids may be associated with significant problems such as anaphylaxis. There is evidence that co-loading with crystalloid (giving fluid as the block is establishing) is more effective than preloading.

A co-load should be:
- Timely (given immediately before or during the onset of the regional technique to minimize redistribution)
- Limited to 10–15mL/kg of crystalloid. Larger volumes should be avoided, as they offer little advantage and may be harmful
- More fluid should only be given as clinically indicated
- Emergency Caesarean section should not be delayed to allow a fluid preload to be administered.

Caesarean section: general anaesthesia

Elective GA is now uncommon in the UK, limiting opportunities for training. The majority of complications relate to the airway. Failed intubation is much more frequent in obstetric than non-obstetric anaesthesia (see ➔ p. 749). All obstetric theatres should have equipment to help with the difficult airway, and all obstetric anaesthetists should be familiar with a failed intubation drill.

Indications for GA include:

- Maternal request.
- Urgent surgery (in experienced hands and with a team that is familiar with rapid regional anaesthesia, a spinal or epidural top-up can be performed almost as rapidly as a GA).
- Regional anaesthesia contraindicated (e.g. coagulopathy, maternal hypovolaemia).
- Failed regional anaesthesia.
- Additional surgery planned at the same time as a Caesarean section.

Technique

- History and examination. In particular, assess the maternal airway—mouth opening, Mallampati score, thyromental distance, neck mobility (see ➔ p. 942).
- Antacid prophylaxis, including 30mL of 0.3M sodium citrate (see ➔ p. 750).
- Start appropriate monitoring.
- Position supine with a left lateral tilt or wedge.
- Preoxygenate for 3–5min or, in an emergency, with 4–8 VC breaths with a high flow through the circuit. Ensure a seal with the face mask. At term, women have a reduced FRC and a higher respiratory rate and O_2 consumption. This reduces the time required for denitrogenation, but also reduces the time from apnoea to arterial O_2 desaturation.
- Perform RSI with an adequate dose of induction agent (e.g. 5–7mg/kg of thiopental). Isolated forearm techniques suggest that awareness without recall may be common when the dose of the induction agent is reduced.
- A 7.0mm ETT is adequate for ventilation and may make intubation easier.
- Propofol has also been used for Caesarean section, without any major reported complications, although, at present, thiopental is still the most commonly used agent in the UK.
- Ventilate with 50% O_2 in N_2O. If severe fetal distress is suspected, then 75% O_2 or higher may be appropriate. Maintain $ETCO_2$ at 4.0–4.5kPa (30–34 mmHg).
- Use 'overpressure' of the inhalational agent to rapidly increase the end-tidal concentration of the anaesthetic agent to at least 0.75 MAC (e.g. 2% isoflurane for 5min, then reduce to 1.5% for a further 5min).
- At delivery:
  - Give 2–5IU of oxytocin IV bolus. If tachycardia must be avoided, then an IV infusion of 30–50IU of oxytocin in 500mL of crystalloid, infused over 4hr, is effective

- • Administer opioid (e.g. 10–15mg of morphine ± 100 micrograms of fentanyl), IV paracetamol, and IV diclofenac (unless contraindicated)
- • Ventilate with 35% inspired O_2 concentration in N_2O. The inhalational agent can be reduced to 0.75 MAC to reduce uterine relaxation.
- At the end of the procedure, consider performing bilateral ilioinguinal nerve blocks, rectus sheath, or TAP blocks (see ➔ p. 1125 and p. 1123) which can all improve post-operative analgesia.
- If a woman has eaten shortly before surgery, consider passing a large-bore orogastric tube to empty the stomach before extubation.
- Extubate awake. Be aware that extubation is a high-risk time.
- Give additional IV analgesia, as required.

Recovery

- Be aware that recovery units are potentially dangerous places for mothers after GAs, particularly if the recovery is staffed by midwives who may be less familiar with airway care. The same standard of recovery staff should be available to women on labour wards as in a normal theatre recovery unit.

Effect of general anaesthesia on the fetus

- Lower fetal 1min and 5min Apgar scores are commoner when GA is used for Caesarean section. Most anaesthetic agents, except for muscle relaxants, rapidly cross the placenta. Thiopental can be detected in the fetus within 30s of administration, with peak umbilical vein concentration occurring around 1min. Umbilical artery to umbilical vein concentrations approach unity at 8min. Opioids administered before delivery may cause fetal depression. Although rarely required, neonatal respiratory depression can be rapidly reversed with naloxone (e.g. 200 micrograms IM or 10 micrograms/kg IV). If there is a specific indication for opioids before delivery, they should be given, and the neonatologist informed. Hypotension, hypoxia, hypocapnia, and excessive maternal catecholamine secretion may all be harmful to the fetus.

Failed intubation

Failed intubation is ten times commoner in the obstetric population (~1:300, compared to 1:3000). Causes of failed intubation include obesity, increased fatty tissue, pharyngeal/laryngeal oedema, large tongue, large breasts, incorrect cricoid pressure, complete dentition, and the experience and training of anaesthetic staff.[21]

For failed intubation drill, see **➔** p. 913 and p. 952.

When intubation fails, but mask ventilation succeeds, a decision on whether to continue with the Caesarean section must be made. A suggested grading system is shown in Box 33.1.[22]

> ### Box 33.1 Grades of urgency in Caesarean section
> - Grade 1: mother's life dependent on surgery.
> - Grade 2: regional anaesthetic unsuitable (e.g. coagulopathy/ haemorrhage).
> - Grade 3: severe fetal distress (e.g. prolapsed cord).
> - Grade 4: varying severity of fetal distress with recovery.
> - Grade 5: elective procedure.

For grade 1 cases, surgery should continue, and for grade 5 the mother should be woken. The action between these extremes must take account of additional factors, including the ease of maintaining the airway, the likely difficulty of performing a regional anaesthetic, and the experience of the anaesthetist. Once a failed intubation has occurred and an airway has been established, while waiting for the muscle relaxant to wear off, reapply fetal monitoring as this may give useful additional information to guide management.

If the surgery continues, decisions will have to be made on whether to use 1st- or 2nd-generation laryngeal masks and whether to use muscle paralysis (if yes, then rocuronium with an availability of sugammadex may be useful). Ask the obstetricians to avoid fundal pressure at delivery, if possible, because fundal pressure can increase intragastric pressure to >70 mmHg.

References

21 McGlennan A, Mustafa A (2009). General anaesthesia for Caesarean section. *Contin Educ Anaesth Crit Care Pain*, **9**, 148–51.
22 Harmer M (1997). Difficult and failed intubation in obstetrics. *Int J Obstet Anaesth*, **6**, 25–31.

Antacid prophylaxis

Aspiration of particulate matter, blood, or bile is associated with worse outcome than aspiration of gastric fluid. Fluid aspiration is commonly associated with chemical pneumonitis, and the severity of this is, in turn, dependent on the volume and acidity of the aspirated fluid. Use of antacids and prokinetic agents can elevate the gastric pH and reduce the intragastric volume. A suggested regime is as follows.

Elective surgery

* Ranitidine 150mg orally, 2hr and 12hr before surgery.
* Metoclopramide 10mg orally, 2hr before surgery.
* A total of 30mL of 0.3M sodium citrate immediately before induction of GA. (Gastric pH >2.5 is maintained for only 30min after 30mL of 0.3M sodium citrate. If a GA is required after this, a further dose of citrate is required.)

Emergency surgery (if prophylaxis has not already been given)

* Ranitidine 50mg by slow IV injection immediately before surgery (PPIs are an alternative). Remember this will not alter the risk of aspiration during induction but may offer benefit by the time of extubation.
* Metoclopramide 10mg IV injection immediately before surgery.
* A total of 30mL of 0.3M sodium citrate orally immediately before induction of GA.

Post-operative analgesia

Most post-partum women are very well motivated and mobilize quickly. However, effective analgesia does allow earlier mobilization. The mainstays of post-operative analgesia are opioids, NSAIDs, and paracetamol.

Opioids

Intrathecal/epidural opioid

- When given as a bolus at the beginning of surgery, fentanyl lasts little longer than the LA and provides almost no post-operative analgesia. Epidural fentanyl may be given as an infusion or as intermittent post-operative boluses (50–100 micrograms up to 2-hourly for two or three doses) if the epidural catheter is left *in situ*.
- Intrathecal diamorphine (300 micrograms) can be expected to provide 6–18hr of analgesia. More than 40% of women will require no other post-operative opioid. Higher doses have been recommended but are associated with an increased incidence of side effects. Pruritus is very common (60–80% of cases), although only 1–2% have severe pruritus. Oral chlorphenamine may help, although, for severe pruritus, 20–200 micrograms of naloxone IM may also be considered (but this is likely to reduce the analgesic effect).
- Epidural diamorphine (2.5mg in 10mL of saline) provides 6–10hr of analgesia after a single dose. Intermittent doses may be given if the epidural catheter is left *in situ*. Preservative-free pethidine may also be used (10–50mg epidurally).
- Intrathecal preservative-free morphine (100 micrograms) provides long-lasting analgesia (12–18hr). Doses above 150 micrograms are associated with increased side effects without improved analgesia. However, pruritus and nausea are common. The low lipophilicity of morphine may increase the risk of late respiratory depression. Epidural morphine (2–3mg) provides analgesia for 6–24hr, but pruritus is again common, and nausea occurs in 20–40% of cases. Diamorphine is used much more commonly in the UK than morphine.

Intravenous patient-controlled analgesia or oral opioids

- IV PCA or oral opioids can be used, although these are not as effective as neuraxial analgesia.

Neonatal effects of maternal opioids

- A small quantity of opioid may be transferred to the neonate through breast milk (see Breastfeeding and drug transfer, → p. 753).

Non-steroidal anti-inflammatory drugs

- NSAIDs are very effective post-operative analgesics, reducing opioid requirements. They should be administered regularly, whenever possible, but beware renal impairment in severe pre-eclampsia, and care with significant haemorrhage.

Retained placenta

- IV access with a 16G or larger cannula.
- Assess the total amount and rate of blood loss and CVS stability. Blood loss may be difficult to accurately assess. If rapid blood loss is continuing, then urgent cross-match and evacuation of the placenta under GA are required.
- Regional anaesthesia is safe, provided the estimated blood loss is <1000mL, but, if there are signs suggesting hypovolaemia, a GA may be required.
- Remember antacid prophylaxis.
- For GA, use an RSI technique with a cuffed ETT.
- Regional anaesthesia can be performed either by topping up an existing epidural or with a spinal (e.g. 2mL of 0.5% hyperbaric bupivacaine plus 15 micrograms of fentanyl or 300 micrograms of diamorphine intrathecally). A T7 block reliably ensures analgesia.
- Occasionally, uterine relaxation is required. Under GA, this can be produced by increasing the halogenated vapour concentration. Under regional anaesthesia, a sublingual GTN spray is usually effective, although expect transient hypotension.
- On delivery of the placenta, give 5IU of oxytocin ± an infusion of oxytocin (e.g. 30–50IU in 500mL of crystalloid over 4hr).
- At the end of the procedure, give an NSAID, unless contraindicated.

Breastfeeding and drug transfer

For drugs to be transferred to a neonate through breastfeeding, they must be secreted in the milk, absorbed in the neonatal GI tract, and not undergo extensive first-pass metabolism in the neonatal liver. In general, for breastfed infants, the neonatal serum concentration of a drug is <2% of the maternal serum concentration, resulting in a sub-therapeutic dose. Most drugs are therefore safe. However, there are some exceptions to this rule—either because transfer is much higher or because transfer of even minute quantities of a drug is unacceptable. Drugs with high protein-binding may displace bilirubin and precipitate kernicterus in a jaundiced neonate.

Factors that make significant transfer more likely include:

• Low maternal protein-binding
• Lipophilicity or, with hydrophilic drugs, a molecular weight of <200Da.
• Weak bases (which increase the proportion of ionized drug in the weakly acidic breast milk, leading to 'trapping').

Timing of drug administration can reduce drug transfer. For instance, breastfeed just before drug administration, or, if the neonate has a consistent sleep period, give the drug at the beginning of this.

Remember, breastfeeding constitutes a metabolic and fluid stress for the mother, so, if surgery is contemplated, keep the mother well hydrated and avoid long periods of starvation. Try to minimize nausea and vomiting.

Codeine, oxycodone, dihydrocodeine, and oral morphine, and breastfeeding

Although small quantities of opioid are transferred in breast milk, the risk of neonatal respiratory depression is very small. However, one neonatal death was reported following prolonged use of post-operative codeine analgesia. There have also been case reports of neonatal respiratory depression after maternal administration of oral morphine, oxycodone, and dihydrocodeine. So post-natal women taking opioids should be observed, and, if they, or their offspring, appear excessively drowsy, the opioid should be stopped. Breastfeeding women should not be discharged with opioid analgesia.

Table 33.8 gives information on some agents; a full list of drug compatibility with breastfeeding is beyond the scope of this book.[23]

Reference

23 Hale TW (2012). *Medications and mothers' milk 2012*, 15th edn. Plano, TX: Hale Publishing.

Table 33.8 Some important drugs and breastfeeding

Drug	Comment
Opioids	Minimal amount delivered to neonatal serum. Minor concern about the long duration of action of pethidine metabolite—norpethidine. Care with codeine and other oral opioids if mother or neonate excessively drowsy
NSAIDs	Most NSAIDs are considered safe in breastfeeding. Some would advise caution with aspirin because of unsubstantiated concerns about causing Reye's syndrome in the neonate
Antibiotics	Penicillins and cephalosporins are safe, although trace amounts may be passed to the neonate
	Tetracycline should be avoided (although absorption is probably minimal because of chelation with Ca^{2+} in milk)
	Chloramphenicol may cause bone marrow suppression in the neonate and should be avoided
	Ciprofloxacin is present in high concentrations in breast milk and should be avoided
Antipsychotics	Generally suggested that these should be avoided, although the amount excreted in milk is probably too small to be harmful. Chlorpromazine and clozapine cause neonate drowsiness
Cardiac drugs	Amiodarone is present in milk in significant amounts, and breastfeeding should be discontinued
	Most β-blockers are secreted in minimal amounts. Sotalol is present in larger amounts. Avoid celiprolol
	While enalapril and captopril have no known adverse effects, other ACE inhibitors, ARBs, and amlodipine should be avoided
Anticonvulsants	While carbamazepine does not accumulate in the neonate, phenobarbital and diazepam may. Neonates should be observed for evidence of sedation

Fetal death *in utero*

Death *in utero* of a formed fetus is emotionally devastating for a family. The delivery can also be very traumatic, and it is important to be as supportive as possible during this period. The cause of the fetal loss is varied, and often uncertain. Remember that deaths *in utero* can be associated with a concealed abruption, sepsis, and DIC.

Sometimes, women will have to be delivered by Caesarean section, but the majority undergo a vaginal delivery.

Analgesia for labour includes all the normal techniques. Patient-controlled IV opioids are often used, as is neuraxial analgesia. However, before any neuraxial techniques are performed, check that maternal clotting is normal. Clotting derangement can occur, even when the fetal death is thought to have occurred very recently.

Delivery by Caesarean section can be performed under regional anaesthesia or GA. This should be guided by maternal preference, as well as maternal safety.

Pregnancy-induced hypertension, pre-eclampsia, and eclampsia

Pre-eclampsia remains a leading cause of maternal death. It is a systemic disorder. The precise aetiology is complex and incompletely understood. Immunological factors, genetic factors, endothelial dysfunction, as well as abnormalities in placental implantation, fatty acid metabolism, coagulation, and platelet factors, have all been implicated. The earlier in gestation that pre-eclampsia manifests itself, the more severe the disease. Developing hypertension in pregnancy is a risk factor for developing hypertension and CVS disease in later life.

Definitions

- Hypertension: a sustained systolic BP >140mmHg or diastolic BP >90mmHg.
- Chronic hypertension: hypertension that existed before the 20th week of pregnancy.
- Pregnancy-induced hypertension: hypertension that develops in pregnancy.
- Pre-eclampsia: pregnancy-induced hypertension in association with proteinuria (spot urinary protein:creatinine ratio (PCR) >30mg/mmol, or proteinuria >300mg/24hr or 1+ on urine dipstick). Incidence is 6–8% of all gestations.
- Severe pre-eclampsia: pre-eclampsia in association with any of the following: a sustained BP >160/110; PCR >250mg/mmol, proteinuria >5g/24hr, or 3+ on urine dipstick; urine output <400mL/24hr; pulmonary oedema or evidence of respiratory compromise; epigastric or right upper quadrant pain; hepatic rupture, platelet count <100 × 10^9/L; evidence of cerebral complications. Incidence is 0.25–0.5% of all gestations.
- Eclampsia: convulsions occurring in pregnancy or puerperium in the absence of other causes. Signs of pre-eclampsia may not be manifest until after a fit.

Pathophysiology

Cardiorespiratory

- Hypertension and increased sensitivity to catecholamine and exogenous vasopressors.
- Reduced circulating volume, but increased TBW.
- In severe pre-eclampsia, SVR is increased and cardiac output reduced. However, some women have elevated cardiac output, with normal or only marginally increased SVR. Fetal prognosis is improved in this group.
- Poor correlation between CVP and PAOP.
- Increased capillary permeability which may result in:
  - Pulmonary oedema. Be very careful to avoid fluid overload
  - Laryngeal and pharyngeal oedema. Stridor may result.

Haematological

- Reduced platelet count with increased platelet consumption, and hypercoagulability with increased fibrin activation and breakdown. DIC may result.
- Increased Hct, consequent on the reduced circulating volume.

Renal function
- Reduced GFR.
- Increased permeability to large molecules, resulting in proteinuria.
- Decreased urate clearance, with rising serum uric acid level.
- Oliguria in severe disease.

Cerebral function
- Headache, visual disturbance, and generalized hyperreflexia.
- Cerebrovascular haemorrhage.
- Eclampsia (resulting from cerebral oedema or cerebrovascular vasoconstriction).

Fetoplacental unit
- Reduced fetal growth, with associated oligohydramnios.
- Poor placental perfusion and increased sensitivity to changes in maternal BP.
- Reduction of umbilical arterial diastolic blood flow and particularly reverse diastolic flow are indicative of poor fetal outcome and an indication for early intervention.

Management of pre-eclampsia

- 1° prevention: unfortunately, there remains no effective prophylactic treatment to prevent pre-eclampsia. Some obstetricians may use low-dose aspirin or calcium supplementation in selected high-risk pregnancies, but benefit is marginal.
- 2° prevention relies on detecting disease at an early stage, and then slowing or stopping its progression. However, while there are a variety of CVS and biochemical markers that can predict pre-eclampsia, as yet, there are no methods for preventing disease progression.
- Tertiary prevention is the concept of controlling the symptoms of pre-eclampsia, preventing major harm, until the placenta is delivered. Symptoms will usually start to resolve within 24–48hr of delivery. When pre-eclampsia develops at term, there is no advantage to delaying delivery. However, if pre-eclampsia develops before term, a compromise has to be made between maternal and fetal health. Maternal symptoms are controlled for as long as possible to allow fetal growth to be optimized. If fetal or maternal condition deteriorates, delivery should be expedited. If the fetus is preterm, when possible, delivery is delayed to allow the administration of steroids to promote fetal lung maturation.
- Antihypertensive therapy:
  - BP should be controlled to below 160/110 to prevent maternal morbidity, particularly from intracranial haemorrhage, encephalopathy, and myocardial ischaemia/failure. Elevation of systolic pressure, in particular, is associated with intracranial haemorrhage. Systolic BP of 180 mmHg should be treated as a medical emergency
  - In the UK, the 1° antihypertensive agent is the combined α- and β-blocker labetalol. If contraindicated or additional agents are required, methyldopa or nifedipine can be used.

- ACE inhibitors are associated with oligohydramnios, stillbirth, and neonatal renal failure. They should be avoided.
- Rapid control of severe hypertension can be achieved with:
  - Labetalol (5–10mg IV every 10min)
  - Hydralazine (5mg IV aliquots to a maximum of 20mg). The 1st IV dose of hydralazine is sometimes given with a 500mL crystalloid fluid bolus
  - Oral nifedipine (10mg). Sublingual nifedipine should be avoided because of rapid changes in placental circulation, which may compromise the fetal condition.
- Magnesium prophylaxis in pre-eclampsia effectively reduces the incidence of eclampsia. Magnesium is used for patients with severe hypertension and proteinuria, or mild/moderate hypertension with severe headache, visual disturbance, epigastric pain, papilloedema, ≥3 beats of clonus, liver tenderness, HELLP syndrome, ALT/AST ≥70IU/L, or platelet count <100 × 10^9/L.
  - For magnesium dosing, see Eclampsia, ➔ p. 760.
- Fluid management in severe pre-eclampsia is critical. Intravascular volume is depleted, but TBW is increased. Excessive fluid load may result in pulmonary oedema, but underfilling may compromise the fetal circulation and renal function. General principles are:
  - Units should follow a fluid management protocol
  - A named individual should have overall responsibility for fluid therapy
  - Measure the hourly urine output
  - Usually the total fluid intake is limited to 80mL/hr. Beware of fluid loads being delivered with drugs. It may be necessary to increase the concentrations of agents, such as oxytocin or magnesium, to stay within the 80mL/hr limit.
- Avoid fluid loading before regional analgesia.
- Be cautious with fluid during Caesarean section—aim to be fluid-neutral at the end of surgery.
- Invasive arterial pressure monitoring is indicated in severe pre-eclampsia for:
  - Monitoring the response to laryngoscopy and surgery during GA
  - Taking repeated ABGs
  - Monitoring rapidly acting hypotensive agents.
- CVP monitoring is rarely indicated, even in severe pre-eclampsia. CVP often does not correlate with PAOP.

Analgesia for vaginal delivery
- Effective epidural analgesia controls excessive surges in BP during labour and is recommended.
- Check platelet count before performing an epidural. The 'acceptable' level of platelet count is debatable and based on little evidence. However, common general guidelines are:
  - If the platelet count is <100 × 10^9/L, a clotting screen is required
  - If the platelet count is >75 × 10^9/L and the clotting screen is normal, then regional techniques are acceptable
  - With a platelet count of <75 × 10^9/L, a careful assessment from a senior individual is required, and the potential risks and benefits should be discussed with the patient

- Usually, a platelet count within 6hr of insertion is adequate, but, if the maternal condition is deteriorating or if the platelet numbers are rapidly falling, then a count must be performed immediately before placement.
- Fluid loading before regional analgesia is not required, but monitor the BP and fetus carefully, and treat changes in BP promptly with cautious doses of ephedrine or phenylephrine.

Anaesthesia for Caesarean section in pre-eclamptic patients

GA or regional anaesthesia may be used. GA is indicated if significant thrombocytopenia (see ➋ p. 756) or coagulopathy has developed.

General anaesthesia

- Assess the airway carefully. Sometimes, partners may be better able to assess the onset of facial oedema. A history of stridor is of major concern. A selection of small tube sizes must be available. Consider AFOI in severe cases.
- Obtund the hypertensive response to laryngoscopy, e.g. alfentanil 1–2mg (inform the paediatrician that opioids have been used) and/or labetalol 10–20mg before induction. A remifentanil infusion or bolus may be useful if the anaesthetist is familiar with its use. In very severe pre-eclampsia, intra-arterial pressure monitoring is required before induction.
- If magnesium has been used, expect a prolongation of action of NDMRs. Use a reduced dose, and assess the neuromuscular function with a nerve stimulator.
- Magnesium can also cause uterine relaxation, so, particularly with GA, an oxytocin infusion may be helpful.
- Ensure adequate analgesia before extubation. The hypertensive response to extubation may also need to be controlled with antihypertensive agents (e.g. labetalol 10–20mg).

Regional anaesthesia

Despite the depleted intravascular volume that occurs with severe pre-eclampsia, pre-eclamptic patients are actually less prone to the hypotensive consequences of regional anaesthesia than normal individuals. Spinal anaesthesia consistently produces better analgesia than epidural anaesthesia and should not be avoided.

- As with regional analgesia, the platelet count, and, if necessary, a clotting screen, needs to be assessed (see ➋ p. 757).
- A reduced volume of fluid co-load should be used. By the end of the procedure, aim to have given no more crystalloid than the measured blood loss.
- Use ephedrine or phenylephrine, as indicated. However, be cautious, because they may have an increased effect.

Effective post-operative analgesia is required, but avoid NSAIDs, as these patients are prone to renal impairment and may have an impaired platelet count or function. When the proteinuria has resolved, which is often within 48hr, NSAIDs may be introduced.

Continue care in the HDU or ICU.

Eclampsia

- Eclampsia:[24] incidence 1:3500 pregnancies in the UK, but there are wide international variations. Remember most seizures in pregnancy are not due to eclampsia. Always be alert to the differential diagnosis.
- Eclamptic fits occur most commonly in the 3rd trimester or within 12hr of delivery.
- Eclampsia is a life-threatening event.
- Management is aimed at immediate control of the fit and 2° prevention of further fits.

Management

- Airway (left lateral position with jaw thrust), breathing (bag-and-mask ventilation, and measure O_2 saturation), and circulation (obtain IV access, and measure BP, when possible; avoid aortocaval compression).
- Control fits with magnesium:
  - Load with 4g IV over 5min, followed by 1g/hr for 24hr
  - Recurrent seizures should be treated with 2–4g bolus over 5min.
- Therapeutic level: 2–4mmol/L. Magnesium levels may be monitored clinically (loss of reflexes (>5.0mmol/L), reduced respiratory rate (6.0–7.0mmol/L)) or with laboratory monitoring. Reduce the infusion rate with oliguria (cardiac arrest may occur at >12.0mmol/L).
  - Patients on calcium channel antagonists are at particular risk of toxicity.
  - Toxicity can be treated with IV calcium (e.g. 10mL of 10% calcium chloride or calcium gluconate).
- If eclampsia occurred before delivery, once the fit has been controlled, think about the urgency of the delivery. In general, provided the fetus is not distressed, eclampsia is not an indication for an emergency Caesarean section. The patient should be stabilized on magnesium, and then consideration given to vaginal or operative delivery. Care should be continued on the HDU or ICU.

Reference

24 Cantwell R, Clutton-Brock T, Cooper G, et al. Centre for Maternal and Child Enquiries (CMACE) (2011). Saving Mothers' Lives: reviewing maternal deaths to make motherhood safer: 2006–08. The Eighth Report on Confidential Enquiries into Maternal Deaths in the United Kingdom. *BJOG*, **118** (Suppl 1), 1–203.

HELLP syndrome

Haemolysis, elevated liver enzymes, and low platelets comprise the HELLP syndrome. It is usually associated with pre-eclampsia or eclampsia, but these are not a prerequisite for diagnosis. Severe HELLP syndrome has a 5% maternal mortality. HELLP rarely presents before the 20th week of gestation, but one-sixth of cases present before the 3rd trimester, and a further third present post-natally (usually within 48hr of delivery). Symptoms are sometimes of a vague flu-like illness, which may delay the diagnosis. Maintain a high index of suspicion.

Features of HELLP

- Evidence of haemolysis (a falling Hb concentration without evidence of overt bleeding, haemoglobinuria, elevated bilirubin in serum and urine, elevated lactate dehydrogenase (LDH)).
- Elevated LFTs—AST, ALT. Epigastric or right upper quadrant abdominal pain is present in 90% of women with HELLP. Liver failure and hepatic rupture may occur. Extreme elevation in AST is associated with poor maternal outcome. (Consider the differential diagnosis of acute fatty liver of pregnancy—remember the potential for hypoglycaemia.) Most women with right upper quadrant pain and a platelet count of <20 × 10^9/L have had an intrahepatic or subcapsular bleed.
- A falling platelet count. Counts of <100 × 10^9/L are of concern, while a count of <50 × 10^9/L is indicative of severe disease.
- Hypertension and proteinuria are present in 80% of women with HELLP, and 50% suffer from nausea and vomiting. Convulsions and GI haemorrhage are occasional presenting features.

The only definitive treatment is delivery of the placenta. Although steroids do not alter disease progression, if the maternal condition is not deteriorating rapidly and the fetus is premature, delivery may be delayed to allow the administration of steroids to promote fetal lung maturity.

- The method of delivery depends on the maternal condition and the likelihood of successfully inducing labour. Severe HELLP syndrome may require an urgent Caesarean section.
- Coagulation abnormalities may preclude the use of regional analgesia/anaesthesia. Consideration must be given to both the absolute platelet number as well as its rate of fall. All patients require a clotting screen.
- Be prepared for a major haemorrhage.

Further management is supportive, with appropriate replacement of blood products, as required.
- Invasive monitoring is dictated entirely by the clinical condition of the patient.
- ARDS, renal failure, and DIC may develop.
- After delivery of the placenta, recovery can be expected to start within 24–48hr. These patients should be managed on the HDU or ICU.

Massive obstetric haemorrhage

(See also ➔ p. 1049, p. 847, p. 1001.)

- At term, the gravid uterus receives 10–20% of the cardiac output, and, when haemorrhage occurs, blood loss can be rapid.[25,26] In the developing world, haemorrhage is the leading cause of maternal death.
- Estimates of 'normal' blood loss after vaginal delivery are of the order of 250–400mL, and, after Caesarean section, around 500–1000mL. Blood loss is usually underestimated.
- Although various definitions have been proposed for massive haemorrhage, acute blood loss of >1000mL should prompt full resuscitation measures.
- Protocols for major haemorrhage should be available in every delivery suite.

Aetiology of obstetric haemorrhage

Antenatal

- Placental abruption. Bleeding is often associated with pain. Blood loss may be concealed with retroplacental bleeding. Fetal compromise is common. While small bleeds may be treated conservatively, significant bleeds have a fetal mortality as high as 35%.
- Placenta praevia/accreta (see ➔ p. 765). Usually a small painless bleed. May be catastrophic.
- Uterine rupture. Fetal distress is almost universal. Usually happens in the presence of a previous uterine scar and is classically said to be painful, but painless dehiscence is not uncommon.

Post-natal

- The mnemonic of the four 'Ts' is commonly used—tone, tissue, trauma, and thrombin.
- Tone: uterine atony is associated with chorioamnionitis, prolonged labour, and uterine distension (e.g. polyhydramnios, macrosomia, multiple gestation).
  - Uterine inversion. This is a rare complication. It is associated with uterine atony, and further relaxation may be required to enable replacement. After replacement, uterotonics should be administered.
- Tissue: retained placenta. Haemorrhage may be massive but is usually <1L, and occasionally minimal.
- Tissue: retained products of conception. This is the leading cause of late haemorrhage but is rarely massive.
- Trauma: trauma to the genital tract can cause significant blood loss. While vaginal and vulval haematomas are usually self-limiting, retroperitoneal haematomas may be extensive and life-threatening.
- Thrombin: lack of clotting factors of various causes, including massive haemorrhage itself, increases the risk of further bleeding.

Diagnosis

Diagnosis of haemorrhage is usually self-evident, although concealed bleeding can occur, especially with placental abruptions. In addition, signs of CVS decompensation may be delayed, as women are usually young and fit and start with a pregnancy-induced expansion of their intravascular volume.

Beware of the woman with cold peripheries—this is abnormal in pregnancy. Hypotension is a late and worrying sign.

Management

- In the event of a major haemorrhage requiring surgery, do not delay operation until cross-matched blood is available.
- Call for help.[25,26] Senior anaesthetic and surgical staff should be present. Blood transfusion services should be alerted.
- Follow ABC principles.
- Give supplemental O_2. If laryngeal reflexes are obtunded, intubate and ventilate.
- In antenatal patients, avoid aortocaval compression.
- Insert two 14G cannulae, and take blood for cross-matching. If needed urgently, request type-specific blood (this can be retrospectively cross-matched).
- Fluid-resuscitate initially with crystalloid.
- If required, give group O Rh-negative blood (i.e. blood loss of 2–3L and ongoing, without the imminent prospect of cross-matched blood being available, and/or the presence of ECG abnormalities). Bedside Hb measurements are useful.
- Start appropriate monitoring. Urine output and invasive monitoring of central venous and arterial pressures may be indicated, depending on the rate of blood loss and maternal condition. However, early monitoring of CVP is not essential, as hypotension is almost always due to hypovolaemia. Increasingly, cardiac output monitoring (oesophageal Doppler or arterial waveform analysis) is being used.
- Treat the cause of haemorrhage (see ➲ p. 762).
- If surgery is required:
  - Do not perform a regional technique if the patient is hypovolaemic
  - Beware of coagulopathies in the presence of concealed abruption
- With continuing haemorrhage, further equipment, including warming devices and rapid transfusion devices and lines, should be available.
- Correct coagulopathy with platelets, FFP, and cryoprecipitate, as indicated. Fibrinogen levels of <2g/dL after 1L of blood loss is associated with major haemorrhage. It is currently unclear whether this is causative or associative. Aim to maintain fibrinogen >1.5g/dL.
- Using empiric ratios of red cells, FFP, and platelets (such as '1:1:1') has been advocated, as has goal-directed therapy using bedside monitoring of coagulation (TEG/thromboelastometry).
- The antifibrinolytic agent tranexamic acid is also being investigated. In the relatively small studies conducted so far, there has been a minimal reduction in blood loss, but importantly no increase in DVTs or embolic events. Based on trauma studies, many anaesthetists would give 1g of tranexamic acid during major haemorrhage.
- Cell salvage use is now well established in obstetric practice. To reduce the reinfusion of fetal tissue, do not collect fluid that is rich in amniotic fluid, and, after processing, reinfuse through a leucocyte depletion filter. The process of collection, washing, and reinfusion through a filter is slow, so, while the total amount of allogenic blood needed is reduced, with major rapid blood loss, allogenic blood will still be needed.

- Remember, during massive transfusion, calcium supplementation may be needed.
- Once blood loss has been controlled, continue care on HDU or ICU.

Specific treatment for haemorrhage

Think of the cause of the bleeding. Often treatment is surgical, either removing tissue or repairing trauma. Uterine atony can be treated with uterotonics and, in some circumstances, can also be treated surgically with uterine brace sutures. Applying direct pressure to the bleeding site can be done manually, or with balloons or packs. Pressure on, or occlusion or ligation of, blood vessels supplying the bleeding site also has a role. Ultimately, hysterectomy may be required to control bleeding.

- Firm bimanual pressure can temporarily control post-partum haemorrhage due to uterine atony.
- Manual or mechanical, external or internal pressure on the aorta may be lifesaving.
- Uterotonics can only be used in the post-natal period. A common sequence is 2–5IU of oxytocin bolus, oxytocin infusion, ergometrine 500 micrograms slow IV or IM, and carboprost 250 micrograms IM repeated every 15min (max 2mg). There are contraindications to all of these agents, so consider the appropriate uterotonic on an individual basis (see chart, ➔ p. 719).
- Uterine compression brace sutures (e.g. B-Lynch suture) may be helpful.
- Intrauterine balloon tamponade (Bakri balloons, Rusch balloons, condom catheters, Sengstaken–Blakemore, or Foley catheters have all been advocated). Usually they are left *in situ* for up to 24hr and then deflated over a period of hours.
- Surgical ligation of blood vessels, direct pressure on bleeding points, and firm manual pressure can all help control blood loss, while a circulating volume is re-established and/or coagulopathy is corrected. Consider leaving packs *in situ* and then re-exploring the abdomen 6–24hr later.
- Interventional radiology is especially useful when a major haemorrhage is anticipated. It may not reduce the incidence of a Caesarean hysterectomy but probably reduces blood loss.[25] Balloon catheters can be prophylactically placed in the anterior division of the internal iliac vessels before delivery (but only inflated at the moment of delivery!). Interventional radiology can also be used during an unexpected major bleed, but be very cautious of moving a patient to a radiology suite if they are cardiovascularly unstable.
- Ultimately, hysterectomy may be required. The decision to perform a hysterectomy should not be delayed until the patient is *in extremis*.

References

25 Ballas J, Hull AD, Saenz C, *et al.* (2012). Preoperative intravascular balloon catheters and surgical outcomes in pregnancies complicated by placenta accreta: a management paradox. *Am J Obstet Gynecol,* **207**, 216.e1–57.
26 Cantwell R, Clutton-Brock T, Cooper G, *et al.* Centre for Maternal and Child Enquiries (CMACE) (2011). Saving Mothers' Lives: reviewing maternal deaths to make motherhood safer: 2006–08. The Eighth Report on Confidential Enquiries into Maternal Deaths in the United Kingdom. *BJOG,* **118** (Suppl 1), 1–203.

Placenta praevia and accreta

Placenta praevia

- Placenta praevia occurs when the placenta implants between the fetus and cervical os. The incidence is about one in 200 pregnancies but is higher with previous uterine scars and multiparity.
- Three questions can be used to evaluate the implications of placenta praevia:
  - Is a vaginal delivery possible? (Unlikely if the placenta extends to within 2cm of the os, especially if the fetal head is not engaged in the pelvis.)
  - If not, does the placenta cover the anterior lower segment of the uterus? (If it does, the obstetrician may have to divide the placenta to deliver the fetus, and blood loss is likely to be increased.)
  - Is there a uterine scar from previous surgery? (Placenta accreta is commoner if the placenta overlies a uterine scar, and the risk of significant haemorrhage increases further.)
- Diagnosis is usually made by ultrasound. Obstetric management is usually to try to preserve the pregnancy until the 37th gestational week. Premature labour, excessive bleeding, or fetal distress may necessitate delivery. If, at 37wk gestation, a vaginal delivery is not possible, a Caesarean section is performed.

Placenta accreta, increta, and percreta

- Placenta accreta occurs with an abnormal implantation of the placenta. Usually the endometrium produces a cleavage plane between the placenta and myometrium. In placenta accreta, the placenta grows through the endometrium to the myometrium. In placenta increta, the placenta grows into the myometrium, and, in placenta percreta, the placenta grows through the myometrium to the uterine serosa and into the surrounding structures. Because the normal cleavage plane is absent, following delivery, the placenta fails to separate from the uterus, which can result in life-threatening haemorrhage.
- Incidence is rising, possibly as a result of the increasing numbers of Caesarean sections performed. Placenta accreta is much commoner when the placenta implants over a previous scar. The more scars on the uterus, the greater the risk of placenta accreta and Caesarean hysterectomy. The presence of uterine fibroids and previous uterine compression sutures also increases the risk of placenta accreta. Diagnosis of percreta may be made by ultrasound ± MRI scan or the presence of haematuria. However, placenta accreta and increta are often diagnosed at surgery.

Anaesthetic management

- Anaesthetic management is dictated by the likelihood of major haemorrhage, maternal preference, and the obstetric/anaesthetic experience levels. Patients with placenta praevia are at risk of haemorrhage because:
  - The placenta may have to be divided to facilitate delivery
  - The lower uterine segment does not contract as effectively as the body of the uterus, so the placental bed may continue to bleed following delivery

- With accreta, the placenta may not separate from the uterus, and uterine contraction is impaired. Further increase in risk occurs sequentially with placenta increta and percreta.
- Although the sympathectomy that occurs with regional anaesthesia may make the control of BP more difficult, practical experience shows that regional anaesthesia can be safely used for placenta praevia, provided the patient is normovolaemic before the neuraxial technique is performed. Even in Caesarean hysterectomy, the degree of hypotension and blood loss is the same with regional anaesthetic and GA techniques. However, if significant haemorrhage does occur, hypotensive and bleeding patients will require reassurance which may divert the anaesthetist's attention from volume resuscitation, and the experience is unlikely to be pleasant for the mother.
- Regional anaesthesia should therefore only be undertaken by experienced anaesthetists, with additional help available. If regional anaesthesia is considered appropriate, mothers and their partners should be warned that GA may be required usually in the 1st 10min after delivery.
- If intubation is anticipated to be difficult, it should be undertaken at the start of the operation, so that the anaesthetist is not dealing with bleeding and difficult intubation at the same time.

Technique
- Experienced obstetricians and anaesthetists are essential.
- All patients admitted with placenta praevia should be seen and assessed by an anaesthetist.
- Interventional radiology should be considered (see ➡ p. 764).
- When a Caesarean section is to be performed, 2–8U of blood should be cross-matched, depending on the anticipated risk of haemorrhage.
- Cell salvage should be used, if available (see ➡ p. 1047).
- Obstetric staff experienced in Caesarean hysterectomy should be immediately available.
- Two 14G cannulae should be inserted, and equipment for massive haemorrhage must be present.
- If regional anaesthesia is used, a CSE may offer advantages, as the surgery may be prolonged.
- For bleeding patients, a GA is the preferred choice.
- Have a selection of uterotonics to hand. Even if massive haemorrhage is not encountered, an oxytocin infusion is advantageous (see ➡ p. 719).
- The lower segment of the uterus does not contract as effectively at delivery, so, even when the placenta is posterior and separates normally, there is still increased potential for bleeding.
- If massive bleeding does occur, follow the massive obstetric haemorrhage guidelines (see ➡ p. 762). Remember a hysterectomy may be the only method of controlling bleeding. Excessive delay in making this decision may jeopardize the maternal life.
- Even if no significant bleeding occurred intraoperatively, continue to observe closely in the post-natal period, as haemorrhage may still occur.

Amniotic fluid embolism

- AFE remains the fourth commonest direct cause of maternal death in the UK (CEMACH 2006–2008).[27]
- Incidence: ~1:12 000 live births.[28]
- Effects are probably due to an anaphylactic response to fetal tissue.
- Within the first 30min after AFE, intense pulmonary vasoconstriction occurs and can be associated with right heart failure, hypoxia, hypercapnia, and acidosis.
- This is followed by left heart failure and pulmonary oedema.
- Expect a coagulopathy.
- Incidence of AFE is increased with:
  - Age >35yr
  - Multiparous women
  - Obstructed labour, particularly in association with uterine stimulants
  - Multiple pregnancies
  - Short labours.
- AFE is often a diagnosis of exclusion, but clinical features include:
  - Sudden collapse with acute hypotension and fetal distress
  - Pulmonary oedema (>90% of cases) and cyanosis (80%)
  - Coagulopathy (80%). Haemorrhage may be concealed
  - Fits (50%)
  - Cardiac arrest (occurs in nearly 90% of severe cases).

Little advance has been made in treating this devastating condition, although care with the use of uterine stimulants and timely diagnosis of obstructed labour may help to reduce the incidence.

Once AFE has occurred, treatment is purely supportive:

- Airway, breathing, and circulation.
- Senior staff should be present (obstetric, anaesthetic, paediatric, and midwifery).
- Haematology services should be alerted, as large quantities of blood products may be required.
- Early delivery of the fetus is vital for both maternal and fetal survival.
- Measure the coagulation profile regularly. Platelets, FFP, and cryoprecipitate may all be required.
- Intensive care will be required for those who survive the initial insult.

Early mortality is high (50% within the 1st hour). Even in those who survive, long-term neurological problems are common.

References

27 Cantwell R, Clutton-Brock T, Cooper G, *et al.* Centre for Maternal and Child Enquiries (CMACE) (2011). Saving Mothers' Lives: reviewing maternal deaths to make motherhood safer: 2006–08. The Eighth Report of Confidential Enquiries into Maternal Deaths in the United Kingdom. *BJOG,* **118** (Suppl 1), 1–203.

28 Abenhaim HA, Azoulay L, Kramer MS, Leduc L (2008). Incidence and risk factors of amniotic fluid embolism: a population-based study on 3 million births in the United States. *Am J Obstet Gynecol,* **199**, e1–8.

Obesity in pregnancy

(See also ➲ p. 543.)
In the developed world, obesity is increasing. In the UK 2010–2012 Health Survey, >25% of women have a BMI >30, and 3.5% have a BMI >40.

Maternal obesity[29] is a major risk factor for death from thromboembolic disease and cardiac disease. It is also associated with gestational diabetes, pre-eclampsia, post-partum haemorrhage, wound infections, operative deliveries (in 2010, the UK Obstetric Surveillance System (UKOSS) reported that the Caesarean section rate in the UK was 50% for women with a BMI of 50), and shoulder dystocia. Fetal effects include an increased incidence of miscarriage, neural tube defects, macrosomia, and admission to neonatal intensive care.

Obese women are often folate- and vitamin D-deficient, and they should have oral supplements in pregnancy.

Anaesthetic concerns include difficult IV access, difficulty in performing neuraxial techniques, a propensity for desaturation due to a combination of reduced FRC and increased O_2 consumption, an increased difficulty in intubation, and high inflation pressures. OSA can develop or be made worse by pregnancy.

Management is geared to reviewing women in the antenatal period, making an assessment of the level of risk, especially if GA is required, and having a plan documented in the patient's notes.

In many units, a BMI of 40 at booking is the cut-off for reviewing women in an anaesthetic antenatal clinic, although internationally recommendations vary from BMI >30 to BMI >45.

Key points to consider

- Is intubation or GA likely to be problematic (see ➲ p. 553)?
  - If yes, women should be encouraged to have an epidural early in labour, and they should be warned that, in the event of a GA, there may be a delay to ensure that a senior anaesthetic team is present. This delay may have implications for the fetal health if fetal distress is present.
  - There should be a written plan documenting who needs to be present for an anaesthetic. In the UK, the joint Centre for Maternal and Child Enquiries (CMACE)/Royal College of Obstetricians and Gynaecologists (RCOG) guideline has recommended a specialty trainee year 6 or above should be available, but individual assessment should be made, as one, or even two, consultants may be required for some individuals.
- Are the lumbar spinous processes palpable?
  - It is harder to site epidurals in larger women, with failure of epidural analgesia reported to be up to 25%. There is also an increased risk of dural puncture if the depth to the epidural space is >6cm. When the spinous processes are difficult to palpate, it is more likely that neuraxial or spinal anaesthesia will be difficult.
  - Advise women of the advantage of an early epidural. This allows time for senior anaesthetists to be summoned and for re-siting if the epidural fails.

- There should be written guidance as to who should site the epidural.
- Some centres recommend ultrasound to assist in siting epidurals. However, experience is needed. If ultrasound is used, having the probe in a longitudinal orientation gives a more accurate prediction of the depth to the epidural space than when the probe is transverse.
- Do patients suffer from sleep apnoea?
  - If so, are they using CPAP machines? If they do, remind patients to bring their CPAP machine to the delivery suite.
  - Look for signs of right heart failure (ECG/echocardiography, as indicated).
  - Remember these patients may be very sedated by opioids. Especially in the event of a GA, think about whether HDU care is needed post-operatively.
- Is venous access likely to be difficult?
  - If so, early venous access should be obtained. Ultrasound may be of assistance. Very rarely, central venous lines may be needed.
- At the antenatal visit, some discussion about limiting weight gain in pregnancy and weight loss after pregnancy may be helpful but needs to be done diplomatically.

Consideration should also go into the equipment available in the delivery suite, maternity theatres, and maternity wards. Most units have the appropriate BP cuffs, theatre tables, lateral transfer equipment, such as hover mattresses, and a selection of airway devices. Some units use ramps to position patients on theatre tables. Many units do not have the appropriate hoists, wide wheelchairs, and seated scales for the super-morbidly obese. When admitted in labour, make sure that all members of the team (anaesthetists, obstetricians, midwives, theatre, and recovery staff) are aware of the plan and that appropriate equipment is to hand.

Remember that recovery for these individuals, especially those with sleep apnoea, is potentially dangerous. Think about the appropriate site and the level of observation required.

Reference

29 Cantwell R, Clutton-Brock T, Cooper G, *et al*. Centre for Maternal and Child Enquiries (CMACE) (2011). Saving Mothers' Lives: reviewing maternal deaths to make motherhood safer: 2006–08. The Eighth Report on Confidential Enquiries into Maternal Deaths in the United Kingdom. *BJOG*, **118** (Suppl 1), 1–203.

Maternal sepsis

> 'Be aware of sepsis—beware of sepsis.'[30]

In 2006–2008, sepsis was the leading cause of direct maternal deaths in the UK. The most frequent pathogen was β-haemolytic *Streptococcus* Lancefield group A, but *Escherichia coli* and *Staphylococcus aureus* are also common.

Maternal deaths are often associated with a failure to recognize sepsis quickly and inadequate or inappropriate early treatment. Early recognition and treatment of the signs and symptoms of maternal sepsis are crucial.

Recognition of sepsis (= systemic inflammatory response syndrome in the presence of infection)

The use of a 'track-and-trigger' system, such as Modified Early Obstetric Warning Scoring (MEOWS) charts, are recommended.

If a patient has two or more features of the SIRS criteria, they should be reviewed urgently. If they have SIRS and any risks or signs of infection, they should be reviewed by a senior doctor, and initial management/resuscitation should be instigated, with monitoring for severe sepsis.

Risks/signs of infection

- Temperature >38°C or <36°C. Hypothermia is a significant finding that may indicate severe infection.
- Persistent HR >100bpm.
- Tachypnoea (respiratory rate >20 breaths/min)—think sepsis until proven otherwise.
- Abnormal WCC (<4 × 10⁹/L or >12 × 10⁹/L).
- Sore throat or flu-like symptoms. Productive cough.
- Diarrhoea and/or vomiting.
- Abdominal, pelvic, or loin pain.
- Premature rupture of membranes ± offensive vaginal discharge (offensive suggests anaerobes; serosanguinous suggests streptococcal infection).
- Abnormal or absent fetal heart beat.
- Rash.
- Impaired mental state/confusion/lethargy.
- Headache/neck stiffness.
- Urinary symptoms.
- Wound infection—spreading cellulitis or discharge.

Signs and symptoms of severe sepsis (sepsis with end-organ dysfunction)

- Hypotension.
- Arterial hypoxaemia.
- Raised lactate.
- Acute oliguria (urinary output <0.5mL/kg/hr).
- Deranged renal function.
- Deranged liver function.
- Altered mental status.
- Coagulation abnormalities.
- Hyperglycaemia in absence of diabetes.

Management of patients with suspected/confirmed sepsis

Management of sepsis[30] is aimed at stabilizing the patient, while diagnosing and treating the underlying cause. Treatment is more likely to be effective if appropriate therapy is started early.

A multidisciplinary team approach is required and should include obstetricians, midwives, anaesthetists, microbiologists, and critical care staff. Critically ill patients should be cared for in level II or III facilities with the capability for invasive techniques of monitoring and experienced nursing/midwifery staff.

A protocoled approach is recommended for the early resuscitation with goal-directed treatment.

Within 1hr, aim to achieve:

- O_2 therapy (maintain O_2 saturation >94%)
- Bloods, blood cultures, and septic screen
- IV antibiotics
- Fluid therapy
- ABG (monitor pH and lactate)
- Continuous monitoring, including urine output.

Reassess the patient regularly; involve critical care as necessary, and ensure the consultant obstetrician and anaesthetists are informed and updated.

Reference

30 Cantwell R, Clutton-Brock T, Cooper G, et al. Centre for Maternal and Child Enquiries (CMACE) (2011). Saving Mothers' Lives: reviewing maternal deaths to make motherhood safer: 2006–08. The Eighth Report on Confidential Enquiries into Maternal Deaths in the United Kingdom. *BJOG*, **118** (Suppl 1), 1–203.

Cardiac disease and pregnancy

Between 2006 and 2008, cardiac disease[31] was the leading cause of maternal death in the UK. Obesity and increasing maternal age are associated with the increased incidence of cardiac disease. Causes of death include arrhythmias, cardiomyopathies (peripartum and other causes), aortic dissection, IHD, and CHD.[31] With the increased survival into childbearing years of patients with complex congenital cardiac malformations, and the movement of populations across the world, the incidence of structural cardiac lesions is increasing.

Pregnancy and labour present a severe stress test to these women. As a generality, if women are symptomatic with minimal activity before pregnancy, particularly if symptomatic at rest (New York Heart Association classes III and IV), the course of pregnancy is likely to be stormy, and mortality is of the order of 20–30%.

It is beyond the scope of this book to give anything but the broadest plans of how to manage women with cardiac disease during pregnancy.

- Assess early, and involve a multidisciplinary team consisting of a combination of obstetricians, anaesthetists, cardiologists, midwives, and neonatologists.
- Have a written plan for the delivery. Consider the site (ranging from a normal delivery suite to a cardiac theatre in a tertiary centre) and modality of delivery. Is vaginal delivery acceptable? Is epidural analgesia indicated? Should pushing in the 2nd stage be limited?
- Investigations should be performed, as indicated. The risk to the fetus from procedures, such as chest radiographs, is minimal.
- With each condition, in consultation with the cardiologists, consider the effects of vasodilatation, vasoconstriction, and positive and negative inotropic and chronotropic agents. This will help with the planning of the delivery and can allow written guidance on the acceptability of regional analgesia/anaesthesia or GA, as well as the use of oxytocin (potent vasodilator) and ergometrine (potent vasoconstrictor). It can also allow planning of the appropriate treatment for hypotension. Consider anticoagulation.
- Some centres use a form where all of these elements are documented. The form remains with the mother throughout her pregnancy.
- In most situations, rapid changes in pre- or afterload should be avoided, so always use oxytocin with extreme caution, and preferably only as an infusion.
- Expect the period of highest risk to be in the 1–2hr post-delivery (vasoactive uterotonics are given; there is unpredictable blood loss and unpredictable volume of autotransfusion, and cardiac output usually peaks).
- Continue management on ICU, if appropriate.

Specific points to consider

- Pulmonary hypertension has a very high mortality in pregnancy (>70%).
- Extreme caution is required to avoid sudden changes in afterload for patients with fixed cardiac output.

- Cyanotic heart lesions (i.e. right-to-left shunts) will not tolerate reductions in SVR. Nevertheless, epidural analgesia is sometimes used to minimize the stress of labour, but onset of analgesia must be slow, and use phenylephrine to maintain afterload. GA is probably the technique of choice for Caesarean section.
- Aortic stenosis may become symptomatic during pregnancy. Serial echocardiography is often used. Tachycardia and reduction in afterload should be avoided. Loss of sinus rhythm should be treated promptly. GA or slow-onset regional anaesthesia have both been advocated for Caesarean section. The technique is probably less important than the skill with which it is applied.
- Valvular insufficiencies are usually well tolerated during pregnancy.
- Women with symptomatic Marfan's disease (see ➔ p. 52 and p. 304), particularly if the aortic root is dilated, or type IV (vascular) Ehlers–Danlos syndrome have a high risk of aortic dissection. They are usually maintained on β-blockers. Unexplained severe chest pain is an indication for a CXR and an echocardiogram.
- MI during pregnancy has 20% mortality. Infarction occurs most commonly in the 3rd trimester. If possible, delivery should be delayed at least 3wk after infarction. Both elective Caesarean section and vaginal delivery have been advocated. In either case, cardiac stress should be minimized with effective analgesia.
- Peripartum cardiomyopathy is a dilated cardiomyopathy that occurs between the last month of pregnancy and 5 months post-partum. The diagnosis is based on echocardiography and is a diagnosis of exclusion. The incidence has marked geographic variation, ranging from 1:100 in parts of Nigeria to 1:4000 in the US. Estimates of mortality range from 7% to 50%. The treatment should be multidisciplinary, with the expectation of severe LV dysfunction. If the cardiomyopathy does not completely resolve, mortality in subsequent pregnancies is very high. Pre-conceptual counselling is crucial.

Reference

31 Cantwell R, Clutton-Brock T, Cooper G, et al. Centre for Maternal and Child Enquiries (CMACE) (2011). Saving Mothers' Lives: reviewing maternal deaths to make motherhood safer: 2006–08. The Eighth Report on Confidential Enquiries into Maternal Deaths in the United Kingdom. BJOG, 118 (Suppl 1), 1–203.

Surgery during pregnancy

One to 2% of women require incidental surgery during pregnancy. Surgery is associated with increased fetal loss and premature delivery, although this probably reflects the underlying condition that necessitated the surgery, rather than the anaesthetic or the surgery itself. The risk of teratogenicity is very small.

General considerations

- When possible, delay surgery until the post-natal period, or alternatively into the 2nd trimester when teratogenic risks to the fetus are reduced (the fetus is at greatest risk of major teratogenesis during the first 12 weeks of gestation).
- Make sure that the obstetric team are aware that surgery is planned.
- Remember gastric acid prophylaxis.
- Remember DVT prophylaxis. Pregnant women are hypercoagulable from the 1st trimester.
- Consider regional anaesthesia. The combination of a mother maintaining her own airway together with a minimal fetal drug exposure is desirable. However, data demonstrating that regional anaesthesia is safer than GA are lacking.
- Airway management in the 1st and early 2nd trimesters remains controversial. In asymptomatic women with no other indication for intubation, it is acceptable not to perform an RSI up to 18wk of gestation. However, be aware that the lower oesophageal sphincter tone is reduced within the first few weeks of pregnancy, and intra-abdominal pressure rises in the 2nd trimester. If patients have additional risk factors for regurgitation (e.g. symptomatic reflux, obesity), use an RSI.
- Every effort must be made to maintain normal maternal physiological parameters for the gestational age of the fetus throughout the perioperative period.
- Treat haemorrhage aggressively. Avoid hypovolaemia and anaemia, as both impact on fetal oxygenation.
- From the 20th week of gestation, use the left lateral tilt to reduce aortocaval compression. Remember that, although upper limb BP may be normal, uterine blood flow may still be compromised in the supine position.
- If GA is employed, use adequate doses of inhalational agents. Light anaesthesia is associated with increased catecholamine release, which reduces placental blood flow. The tocolytic effect of inhalational agents is advantageous.
- Fetal monitoring may be beneficial, although its value remains unproven. If fetal distress is detected, maternal physiology can be manipulated to optimize the uterine blood flow.
- The 1° risk to the fetus is premature labour in the post-operative period. Detection and suppression of premature labour are vital. Women should be told to report sensations of uterine contractions, so that appropriate tocolytic therapy can be instituted.

- Effective post-operative analgesia is required to reduce maternal catecholamine secretion. Although opioids can be used, they may result in maternal hypercapnia. Regional analgesia with LA agents may be preferential. If this would prevent the mother from detecting uterine contractions, consider external uterine pressure transduction—'tocodynamometry'. For minor surgery, LA and simple analgesics, such as paracetamol and codeine, may be used. Chronic dosage with NSAIDs should be avoided (see ➔ p. 776).

Teratogenicity

The fetus is at greatest risk of major teratogenesis during the period of organogenesis, predominantly in the first 12wk of gestation. However, minor abnormalities may occur after this. Causes of teratogenicity are diverse, including infection, pyrexia, hypoxia, and acidosis, as well as the better recognized hazards of drugs and radiation. Establishing whether drugs are teratogens can be difficult. Epidemiological studies have to be large to demonstrate associations, while animal experiments may not reflect either an appropriate dose exposure or human physiology. Although none of the commonly used anaesthetic agents are proven teratogens, specific concerns are addressed below.

Premedication

- Benzodiazepines. Case reports have associated benzodiazepines with cleft lip formation, but this has not been substantiated. A single dose has never been associated with teratogenicity. Long-term administration may lead to neonatal withdrawal symptoms following delivery, and exposure just before delivery may cause neonatal drowsiness and hypotonia.
- Ranitidine and cimetidine are not known to be harmful, but caution is advised with chronic exposure to cimetidine because of known androgenic effects in adults.

Induction agents

- Thiopental. Clinical experience with thiopental suggests that this is a very safe drug to use, although formal studies have not been conducted.
- Propofol is not teratogenic in animal studies. Its use in early human pregnancy has not been formally investigated. Propofol is safe to use during Caesarean section at term.
- Etomidate is also not teratogenic in animal studies. It is a potent inhibitor of cortisol synthesis, and, when used for Caesarean section, neonates have reduced cortisol concentrations.
- Ketamine should be avoided in early pregnancy, as it increases intrauterine pressure, resulting in fetal asphyxia. This increase in intrauterine pressure is not apparent in the 3rd trimester.

Inhalational agents

- Halothane and isoflurane have been used extensively in pregnancy and are safe. At high concentrations, maternal BP and cardiac output fall, resulting in a significant reduction in uterine blood flow. The halogenated vapours also cause uterine relaxation, which may be beneficial for surgery during pregnancy.

- Despite early concerns, epidemiological studies suggest that N_2O is safe. However, N_2O is consistently teratogenic in Sprague Dawley rats if they are exposed to 50–75% concentrations for 24hr during their peak organogenic period. Given that anaesthesia can be safely delivered without N_2O, it is sensible to avoid this agent.
- Muscle relaxants: because these agents are not lipophilic, only very small quantities cross the placenta, and so fetal exposure is limited. These agents are safe to use.
- Anticholinesterase inhibitors: these agents are highly ionized and so, like muscle relaxants, do not readily cross the placenta and are safe to use. Chronic use of pyridostigmine to treat myasthenia gravis may cause premature labour.

Analgesics
- Opioids readily cross the placenta, but brief exposure is safe. Long-term exposure will cause symptoms of withdrawal when the fetus is delivered. Animal studies suggest possible fetal teratogenicity if prolonged hypercapnia or impaired feeding develop as side effects of opioid exposure.
- Chronic exposure to NSAIDs in early pregnancy may be associated with increased fetal loss and, in the 3rd trimester, may cause premature closure of the ductus arteriosus and persistent pulmonary hypertension of the newborn. Single doses are unlikely to be harmful. These agents have been used to suppress labour, particularly in the 2nd trimester.
- Bupivacaine and lidocaine are safe. When used near delivery, bupivacaine has no significant neonatal neurobehavioural effects, while lidocaine may have a mild effect. Cocaine abuse during pregnancy increases fetal loss and may increase the incidence of abnormalities in the genitourinary tract.

Cervical cerclage

Procedure	Surgical treatment of incompetent cervical os
Time	20min
Pain	+
Position	Lithotomy
Blood loss	Nil
Practical techniques	Spinal/epidural. GA with RSI/cuffed ETT if >18wk gestation or reflux

An incompetent cervix may be caused by congenital abnormalities, cervical scarring, or hormonal imbalance. Premature dilation of the cervix and fetal loss may result, usually in the 2nd trimester. Cervical cerclage is performed to prevent this premature dilation and is one of the commonest surgical procedures undertaken in pregnancy. Although occasionally inserted before conception, it is usually performed between the 14th and 26th week. Emergency cerclage may be required in the face of a dilating cervix and bulging membranes. Not surprisingly, emergency treatment is less successful in maintaining a pregnancy than prophylactic cerclage.

Preoperative

- The risks of cerclage include membrane rupture (commoner if the membranes are already bulging), infection, haemorrhage, and inducing premature labour.
- Careful assessment of the airway, gestation, symptoms of reflux, and supine hypotension.
- Remember antacid prophylaxis.
- Explain the risks of teratogenicity/spontaneous miscarriage (see ➔ p. 775).

Perioperative

- Both regional anaesthesia and GA may be used.
- If GA is used and uterine relaxation is required to allow bulging membranes to be reduced, the halogenated vapour concentration can be increased.
- For regional anaesthesia, a T8–T10 level is required for intraoperative comfort. If uterine relaxation is required, 2–3 puffs of sublingual GTN spray may be used, and repeated as necessary, although transient hypotension is to be expected.

Post-operative

- In the post-operative period, women should be observed closely for premature labour.

Vaginal cervical cerclage sutures are usually removed at the 38th week of gestation.

Special considerations

Various permutations on cervical cerclage are available. These are broadly divided into transvaginal procedures and transabdominal procedures.

- The transabdominal procedure requires two operations—one for insertion, and another for a Caesarean section for delivery and removal of the suture. It also carries a greater risk of ureteric involvement.
- Transvaginal procedures are much commoner. Shirodkar and McDonald procedures are the two commonest methods. They both require anaesthesia for insertion but can be removed without anaesthetic.

Maternal resuscitation

Maternal cardiac arrest is fortunately rare. The basic algorithms for adult resuscitation (see ➔ p. 889) are appropriate for maternal resuscitation, with several important differences.

After 20wk gestation, attempts must be made to minimize vena caval obstruction, while performing effective cardiac compressions. The fetus can be displaced with firm lateral pressure (manual uterine displacement) or by using a tilt. Firm manual displacement is as good as tilting. If a wedge is used, the wedge must be non-compressible and support the trunk from the pelvis to the occiput, or the effectiveness of chest compressions may be compromised.

- After 4min, if cardiac output has not been established, the fetus should be delivered. This improves the chance of maternal, as well as fetal, survival.
- Remember that pregnant women have reduced oesophageal sphincter tone and that cricoid pressure and intubation should both be performed as rapidly as possible.
- Normal resuscitation drugs should be used. Adrenaline is the drug of choice, despite its effect on uterine circulation.
- Adrenaline is also the drug of choice in major anaphylactic reactions. Severe hypotension associated with anaphylaxis results in very poor fetal outcome.

Consideration should be given to the diagnosis and treatment of obstetric causes of maternal arrest. Common causes of maternal arrest include:
- Cardiac events
- Intracranial events
- Sepsis
- Haemorrhage
- PE
- AFE
- Iatrogenic events:
  - Hypermagnesaemia—treat with 10mL of 10% calcium chloride or gluconate
  - High or total spinal—supportive treatment (see ➔ p. 1138)
  - LA-induced arrhythmia—treat with 20% lipid emulsion (see ➔ p. 1148).

Paediatric and neonatal anaesthesia

Simon Berg

See also:

Neonatal/infant physiology

Paediatric anaesthesia embraces patients from the premature neonate to the adolescent. Major differences exist between the anatomy, physiology, and pharmacological response of children and adults (Tables 34.1, 34.2, and 34.3). In anaesthetic terms, special considerations apply to the neonate.

Definitions
- Neonate: first 44wk of post-conceptual age
- Premature infant: <37wk gestational age
- Infant: from 1 to 12 months of age
- SGA: small for gestational age
- Low birthweight (LBW): ≤2.5kg

Respiratory considerations
- At birth, each terminal bronchiole opens into a single alveolus, instead of fully developed alveolar clustering. The alveoli are thick-walled and constitute only 10% of the adult total. Alveolar growth continues by multiplication until 6–8yr.
- Cartilaginous ribs are horizontally aligned, so that the 'bucket handle' action of the adult thorax is not possible. Intercostal muscles are poorly developed, with a lower proportion of type 1 muscle fibres and fatigue more easily. The diaphragm has a more horizontal attachment, reducing mechanical advantage.
- Ventilation is essentially diaphragmatic and rate-dependent. Abdominal distension may cause splinting of the diaphragm, leading to respiratory failure.
- Chest wall compliance is high because of the cartilaginous thorax; intercostal or sternal recession is common with increased work of breathing or airway obstruction
- Closing volume occurs within tidal breathing in the neonate. Minor decreases in FRC increase the pulmonary shunt and lead to lung collapse. The application of CPAP improves oxygenation and reduces the work of breathing.
- Narrow airways result in increased resistance, up to the age of 8yr. Nasal resistance represents almost 50% of total airway resistance, accentuating the problem of children with nasal congestion who are obligate nasal breathers. An NGT can increase resistance by 50% in neonates.
- Apnoea is a common post-operative problem in preterm neonates. It is significant if the episode exceeds 15s or induces cyanosis or bradycardia. CPAP may be helpful, with the distending pressure triggering stretch receptors on the chest wall.
- Due to the higher metabolic rate and alveolar minute volume, volatile agents achieve a more rapid induction and emergence than with adults. They are profound respiratory depressants; most anaesthetized neonates require intubation and controlled ventilation.
- Respiratory parameters of the neonate are summarized in Table 34.1.

Table 34.1 Respiratory parameters in the neonate and adult

Parameter	Neonate	Adult
Tidal volume (spontaneous) (mL/kg)	7	7–10
Tidal volume (IPPV) (mL/kg)	7–10	10
Dead space (mL/kg)	2.2	2.2
V_D:V_T ratio	0.3	0.3
Respiratory rate (breaths/min)	30–40	15
Compliance (mL/cmH$_2$O)	5	100
Resistance (cmH$_2$O/L/s)	25	5
Time constant (s)	0.5	1.1
O$_2$ consumption (mL/kg/min)	7	3

Parameters for children over 2yr approximate to adult values. Estimate respiratory rate from the formula = 24 − age/2.

Cardiovascular considerations

- PVR falls at birth, in response to a rise in PaO$_2$/pH and a fall in PaCO$_2$. Subsequent closure of the foramen ovale and ductus arteriosus may reverse with hypoxia and acidosis, leading to pulmonary hypertension and right-to-left shunt (transitional circulation).
- The neonate has small ventricles with reduced contractile mass and poor ventricular compliance. Cardiac output is higher than in adults (200mL/kg/min) and rate-dependent. Normal systolic pressure is 70–90mmHg with low SVR.
- HRs up to 200 bpm can be tolerated. Bradycardia occurs in response to hypoxia and should be treated with O$_2$, rather than atropine. Neonatal and infant HRs <60 bpm require external cardiac compression.
- Autonomic and baroreceptor control is fully functional at term, but vagally mediated parasympathetic tone predominates.
- Incidence of CHD is 7–8 per 1000 live births—10–15% have associated non-cardiac pathology. All neonates with midline defects should be assessed for related cardiac lesions.
- CVS parameters in children are summarized in Table 34.2.

Gastrointestinal considerations

- The liver is immature. Enzyme systems have matured by 12wk, but some drugs are metabolized more slowly and others by different enzyme pathways from adults. The action of barbiturates and opioids in the neonate is prolonged and enhanced.
- Bilirubin metabolism is affected by a poorly developed glucuronyl transferase system. Rises in unconjugated bilirubin may lead to neonatal jaundice and kernicterus by crossing the blood–brain barrier. Some drugs (e.g. sulphonamides, diazepam, vitamin K) displace bilirubin from plasma proteins and exacerbate jaundice.
- Carbohydrate reserves are low in neonates. The premature baby and stressed neonate are vulnerable to hypoglycaemia.

Table 34.2 Cardiovascular parameters in children

Age (yr)	Heart rate (bpm)	Mean systolic BP (mmHg)	Mean diastolic BP (mmHg)
Neonate	80–200	50–90	25–60
1	80–160	85–105	50–65
2	80–130	95–105	50–65
4	80–120	95–110	55–70
6	75–115	95–110	55–70
8	70–110	95–110	55–70
10	70–110	100–120	60–75
12	60–110	110–130	65–80

Mean systolic BP over 1yr = 80 + (age in yr × 2).

- Vitamin K-dependent factors are low at term. The routine administration of vitamin K 1mg IM may prevent haemorrhagic disease of the newborn and is recommended before surgery in the 1st week of life.

Renal considerations
- Nephron formation is complete at term, but renal function is immature. Renal blood flow is reduced due to high renal vascular resistance. The GFR achieves adult values by 2yr, and tubular function by 6–8 months.
- Glucose and sodium reabsorption is less efficient in premature infants.
- Initially, neonates cannot excrete a large solvent or sodium load.
- It may be necessary to reduce drug dosages or extend frequency intervals.

Haematological considerations
Circulating blood volume is estimated as shown in Table 34.3.

Table 34.3 Estimating paediatric circulating blood volume

Neonate	90mL/kg
Infant	85mL/kg
Child	80mL/kg

- Post-delivery Hb concentrations range from 13 to 20g/dL (average 18g/dL), depending on the degree of placental transfusion. Subsequently, Hb concentration falls, as the increase in circulating volume exceeds growth in bone marrow activity, the 'physiological anaemia of infancy' which varies from 10 to 12g/dL.
- The predominant Hb type at term is HbF (80–90%). By 4 months, this has fallen to 10–15% and been replaced by HbA. HbF has a higher O_2 affinity due to reduced 2,3-diphosphoglycerate levels.
- Preoperative Hb <10g/dL is abnormal and should be investigated.

Central nervous system

- Neurons are complete at term, but the total number of brain cells is reduced. Dendritic proliferation, myelination, and synaptic connections develop in the 3rd trimester and 1st 2yr of life.
- The blood–brain barrier is more permeable in neonates—barbiturates, opioids, antibiotics, and bilirubin all cross more readily.
- Autoregulation of the cerebral circulation is present from birth.
- The brain contains a higher proportion of fat, which may allow volatile agents to reach higher concentrations more rapidly.
- All neonates, however immature, feel pain. The premature neonate may even be hypersensitive due to a relative increase of transmitters mediating nociception with the later development of descending inhibitory pathways.
- Dose requirements of volatile agents vary with age. The neonatal MAC is comparable to adult values and decreases with prematurity. MAC peaks at 1yr (~50% greater than adult values), then declines to reach adult levels by the onset of puberty (see ➲ p. 1209).

Weight

Approximate weights can be determined from the formulae in Table 34.4.

Table 34.4 Estimating the ideal weight of paediatric patients

Birth	3–3.5kg
3–12 months	Weight (kg) = [age (month) + 9]/2
1–6yr	Weight (kg) = [age (yr) + 4] × 2

All paediatric patients should be weighed preoperatively.

Thermoregulation

- Poorly developed thermoregulatory mechanism. High surface area to volume ratio with minimal SC fat and poor insulation. Vasoconstrictor response is limited, and the neonate is unable to shiver.
- *Non-shivering thermogenesis* is achieved by metabolism in brown fat found in the back, shoulders, and legs, and around the thoracic vessels. This considerably increases O_2 consumption and may worsen pre-existing hypoxia. Brown fat is deficient in premature infants.
- Neonates lose heat during surgery by conduction, convection, and evaporation, but predominantly by radiation. A *neutral thermal environment* is one in which O_2 demand, heat loss, and energy expenditure are minimal. This optimal ambient temperature depends on the age, maturity, and weight. Average temperatures are 34°C for the premature baby, 32°C for the neonate, and 28°C in the adult.
- GA depresses the thermoregulatory response. Heat is lost from the core to the cooler peripheral tissues. Prolonged hypothermia can lead to a profound acidosis, with impaired perfusion. Platelet function is impaired, but clotting factors are unaffected above 32°C. The duration of opioids and muscle relaxants is prolonged.

Measures to conserve heat loss

- Theatres should be heated before surgery to warm the walls and raise the ambient temperature (21°C is adequate for larger children, but infants and neonates may require 26°C). In practice, this is too hot; theatre temperature of 21°C is an adequate compromise if active measures are taken to reduce heat loss and maintain the 'microclimate' around the patient. Doors should stay closed to avoid draughts.
- Avoid exposure of the child; this applies particularly in the anaesthetic room. The head is relatively large in infants and should be covered with a bonnet, Gamgee, or even polythene. The rest of the body can also be insulated with warm Gamgee.
- Use an active warming device. These include a warming mattress or convective warm-air blanket. Overhead radiant heaters may be suitable for neonates.
- Humidify and warm anaesthetic gases. Heated water vapour humidifiers are available, but disposable heat and moisture exchangers are usually satisfactory. Use of a circle breathing system also provides a means of warming and humidifying anaesthetic gases.
- All perioperative fluids, especially blood, should be warmed.
- Cleaning fluids should be kept warm.
- Temperature measurement is essential in neonatal surgery, paediatric surgery of intermediate to long duration, and where major fluid and blood loss is expected.

Fluid balance

- Eighty per cent of neonatal total body weight is water; the value is higher in the preterm infant and reaches an adult level of 60% by 2yr. Extracellular water constitutes 45% of TBW at term (over 50% in the preterm) but attains an adult value of 35% by early childhood. Plasma volume tends to stay constant at 5% of total body weight, independent of age.
- Turnover of water is over double that of the adult; 40% of extracellular water is lost daily in infants as urine, faeces, sweat, and insensible losses. A small increase in loss or reduction in intake can rapidly lead to dehydration.
- Daily fluid maintenance is calculated from the calorie requirement—100kcal/kg for the infant, with older children requiring 75kcal/kg, and adults 35kcal/kg. Each kcal requires 1mL of water for metabolism.

Table 34.5 First 5d neonatal fluid requirement (mL/kg/d)

	Term	Preterm
Day 1	60	60
Day 2	90	90
Day 3	120	120
Day 4	150	150
Day 5	150	180

Neonatal fluid requirements

- Fluid is initially given cautiously, as the kidneys cannot easily excrete a water or sodium load. If under a radiant heater or undergoing phototherapy, 30mL/kg/d is added to the regime.
- The fluid of choice is 10% glucose. This is adjusted in increments of 2.5% to achieve normoglycaemia. A blood sugar below 2.6mmol/L is treated with 2mL/kg of 10% glucose.
- Routinely added electrolytes are sodium 3mmol/kg/d and potassium 2mmol/kg/d. Other electrolytes, including calcium, are added as indicated.
- The 1st 5d of neonatal fluid requirements are given in Table 34.5.

Paediatric fluid requirements

- Maintenance is calculated, using the '4–2–1' regime.
- The fluid of choice is 0.45% saline/5% glucose:
  - 4mL/kg/hr (100mL/kg/d) for each of the 1st 10kg
  - 2mL/kg/hr (50mL/kg/d) for each of the 2nd 10kg
  - 1mL/kg/hr (25mL/kg/d) for each subsequent kg.

- Maintenance requirement makes no allowance for extra losses from gastroenteritis, intestinal obstruction, and insensible loss from pyrexia. Additional sodium and potassium may also be required.
- Perioperative fluids comprise the basic maintenance requirement plus replacement of other observed fluid losses. These are replaced by isotonic crystalloid, i.e. 0.9% NaCl, Hartmann's solution, colloid, or blood, according to the clinical need. Glucose 1% or 2.5%/Hartmann's solution (add 10mL or 25mL of 50% glucose to 500mL of Hartmann's solution) is a useful perioperative fluid for infants. Regular blood glucose measurement is essential in neonatal surgery.
- Colloid solutions, including albumin and gelatin solutions, are routinely used.
- Transfusion is required after 15% of blood loss. Blood volume should be calculated prior to surgery (Table 34.3). Swabs should be carefully weighed, and suction volumes recorded.
- Post-operatively, use 0.45% NaCl/5% glucose (or Hartmann's solution for children >8–10 years) at two-thirds of maintenance.
- Glucose 4%/0.18% NaCl is no longer recommended due to the risk of hyponatraemia.

Fluid resuscitation

- Assessment of dehydration and hypovolaemia is made predominantly on clinical grounds (Table 34.6). Increased capillary refill time ≥2s, cold and blue peripheries, and an increasing core–peripheral temperature gap with a thready pulse are early signs of hypovolaemia. Rising HR is not always helpful and may reflect pain, anxiety, or fever. Oliguria and a reduced level of consciousness are late signs. Hypotension does not occur until >35% of blood volume is lost (Table 34.7).
- Administer fluid boluses of 20mL/kg crystalloid or 10mL/kg colloid, and then reassess.
- Give blood when 15% of the circulating volume is lost (Table 34.3), and aim for Hb of 8g/dL or packed cell volume (PCV) of 25% (*4mL/kg of blood raises the Hb concentration by 1g/dL*). Transfused blood should be fresh, if possible, warm, filtered, and CMV-negative. It can be rapidly transfused, using a syringe and a three-way tap.
- The 'swing' of the arterial or pulse oximeter trace is a valuable aid in assessing intravascular loss. CVP may be less sensitive in smaller children because of the greater venous capacitance.

Table 34.6 Clinical assessment of dehydration in paediatrics

Sign	5% dehydration	10% dehydration
Skin	Loss of turgor	Mottled, poor capillary return
Fontanelle	Depressed	Deeply depressed
Eyes	Sunken	Deeply sunken
Peripheral pulses	Normal	Tachycardia, weak pulse
Mental state	Lethargic	Unresponsive

Replacement volume (mL) = Weight (kg) × % loss, e.g. a 10% loss in a 5kg infant requires a replacement volume of 50mL.

Table 34.7 Clinical assessment of hypovolaemia in paediatrics

Sign	Compensated	Uncompensated	Irreversible
HR	↑	↑↑	↑↓
Systolic BP	Normal/↑	Normal/↓	↑↓
Pulse volume	Normal/↓	↓	↓↓
Capillary refill	Normal/↑	↑	↑↑
Skin colour	Pale	Mottled	White/grey
Skin temperature	Cool	Cold	Cold
Mental status	Agitated	Lethargic	Unresponsive
Respiratory rate	Normal/↑	↑↑	Sighing
Fluid loss	<25%	25–40%	>40%

Resuscitation

Clinical assessment of dehydration
See Table 34.6.

Clinical assessment of hypovolaemia
- Shock is the clinical state in which delivery of O_2 and metabolic substrates is inadequate for cellular demand.
- In compensated shock, oxygenation of the vital structures (brain and heart) is maintained by sympathetic reflexes at the expense of non-essential tissues. BP remains normal, with an increase in SVR.
- In decompensated shock, hypotension develops, and vital organ perfusion is compromised.
- With irreversible shock, there is cyanosis, bradycardia, and gasping respiration. This is a pre-terminal event.
- Hypovolaemia is the commonest cause of circulatory failure in children. Other causes of shock include pump failure (cardiogenic), distributive (sepsis, anaphylaxis, neurogenic), and obstructive (cardiac tamponade, tension pneumothorax).
- The immediate treatment is administration of 100% O_2 and transfusion of 20mL/kg crystalloid or colloid as often as required. Give blood if no improvement after 40mL/kg.

Post-operative hyponatraemia

- Post-operative hyponatraemia (serum sodium <135mmol/L) is uncommon. It can follow any fluid regime but is more likely with the administration of hypotonic fluids.
- Symptoms are often non-specific, including nausea, vomiting, and headache (a common early sign). It may also present as seizure or respiratory arrest.
- Hyponatraemic seizures respond poorly to anticonvulsants, and initial management should be to administer an infusion of 3% NaCl. Plan to increase serum sodium to >125mmol/L or until symptoms improve (1mL/kg of 3% NaCl should raise serum sodium by 1mmol/L).
- Asymptomatic hyponatraemia can be managed with 0.9% NaCl. If hypervolaemic, restrict fluids to 50% of maintenance.

Further reading

Association of Paediatric Anaesthetists (2007). *Consensus guideline on perioperative fluid management in children v1.1.* http://www.apagbi.org.uk/sites/default/files/Perioperative_Fluid_Management_2007.pdf.

Anaesthetic equipment

Oropharyngeal airway

- Ranges in size from 000 to 4 (4–10cm in length).
- Rarely useful in neonates who are obligate nasal breathers but may be advantageous in older children or in mask ventilation to prevent gastric distension.
- Estimating the size of the airway is crucial. Incorrect size will worsen the airway obstruction. Correct length is equal to the distance from the incisors to the angle of the jaw.
- The airway should not be inverted during insertion in infants, as this may damage the palate.

Nasopharyngeal airway

- Limited application in paediatric practice. Tolerated at lighter levels of anaesthesia than an oropharyngeal airway and may be of use during induction/recovery of some congenital airway problems or OSA.
- Well lubricated prior to insertion; bleeding is possible from mucosal or adenoidal trauma, especially in younger children.
- Appropriate length is equal to the distance from the tip of the nostril to the tragus of the ear.
- If an ETT is used as a modified nasopharyngeal airway, then the size is calculated by: age/4 + 3.5.

Face masks

- Clear plastic masks with an inflatable rim provide an excellent seal for spontaneous and assisted ventilation.
- Greater dead space than the traditional black rubber Rendell–Baker masks, but less threatening and easier to position.
- Manufactured in a round or teardrop shape; the round shape is suitable only for neonates and infants. Also available as 'flavoured' masks.
- Transparent design allows for observation of cyanosis/regurgitation and the presence of breathing.
- Size is estimated to fit an area from the bridge of the nose to the cleft of the chin.

Supraglottic airway devices

- Table 34.8 describes how to choose the appropriate size of LMA.
- Indications and insertion techniques are similar to adult use. An alternative method of insertion for the LMA is to advance it upside down and partially inflated behind the tongue before rotating through 180°.
- Smaller sizes have increased complication rates. The effectiveness of these smaller masks is not established for resuscitation.
- ILMA available in size 3 which is potentially useful for older children.
- Both the ProSeal LMA and i-Gel are available in a full range of paediatric sizes.[1]

Table 34.8 Estimating the size of LMA in paediatrics

Size of LMA	Weight (kg)	Cuff volume (mL)
1	0–5	2–5
1.5	5–10	5–7
2	10–20	7–10
2.5	20–30	12–14
3	>30	15–20

Laryngoscopes

- Laryngoscope blades available in different lengths from size 0 to 3.
- Curved Macintosh blade or straight-bladed Magill for infants (especially ≤6 months—high anterior larynx).
- Polio and McCoy blades are also available.

Tracheal tubes

- Paediatric ETTs are commonly uncuffed until ~8yr of age.
- Uncuffed tubes are available from 2mm to 7mm.
- Table 34.9 describes how to choose an appropriate size of tube.
- Standard cuffed tubes start from 5.0mm. New Microcuff tubes have been trialled successfully from birth to 5yr, reducing the tube exchange rate without increasing the incidence of post-extubation stridor.[2] Specific indications include children with poor lung compliance and high risk of aspiration. Cuff pressure should be limited to 20cmH$_2$O and continuously monitored. Paediatric versions of the RAE, armoured, and laser tubes all exist. A north-facing uncuffed preformed tube has been developed for routine paediatric surgery.
- The paediatric trachea is conical. The narrowest part is at the level of the cricoid ring, the only part of the airway completely surrounded by cartilage. If the ETT is too large, it will compress the tracheal epithelium at this level, leading to ischaemia with consequent scarring and the risk of subglottic stenosis.
- A correctly sized tube is one in which ventilation is adequate, but a small audible leak of air is present when positive pressure is applied at 20cmH$_2$O.
- Paediatric 8.5mm connectors can be used as an alternative to the standard 15mm connector. Catheter mounts should be avoided because of the large dead space involved.
- Tube length in cm can be calculated as:
  - Age/2 + 12 (or tube size × 3)—oral tube
  - Age/2 + 15—nasal tube.
- Tube size may also approximate to the size of the little finger or diameter of the nostril.
- Tube placement needs to be meticulous to avoid endobronchial intubation or inadvertent extubation.
- To assess the length of tube to be passed below the vocal cords, use the black guide line at the distal end of the tube or the tube size in cm. Ultimately, the position must be confirmed clinically.

Table 34.9 Paediatric endotracheal tube sizes

Weight or age	Tube size (mm)
>2kg	2.5
2–4kg	3.0
Term neonate	3.5
3 months–1yr	4.0
Over 2yr	Tube size = Age/4 + 4

Anaesthetic breathing systems

Ayre's T-piece with Jackson–Rees modification

- Jackson–Rees' modification of the Ayre's T-piece (Mapleson F) is the most commonly used circuit in paediatric anaesthetic practice. Suitable for all children up to 20kg, beyond which it becomes inefficient. Low-resistance, valveless, lightweight circuit. The expiratory limb exceeds the V_T to prevent entrainment of room air during SV. The open-ended 500mL reservoir bag or Jackson–Rees modification allows:
  - Assessment of the V_T
  - Ability to partially occlude the bag for CPAP or PEEP
  - Potential for assisted or controlled ventilation
  - Qualitative appreciation of lung compliance
  - Reduction in dead space during spontaneous ventilation (FGF washes out expired gas during the expiratory pause).
- Scavenging is limited. However, newer versions of the T-piece incorporate a closed bag with an expiratory valve and scavenging attachment. Requirements for FGF are higher in spontaneous than controlled ventilation. Recommendations are 2–3 times the alveolar minute volume for spontaneous breathing, or 1000mL plus 200mL/kg in controlled ventilation. FGF is dependent on the respiratory pattern. A rapid respiratory rate requires a higher FGF. Conversely, an end-expiratory pause during controlled ventilation will help reduce the FGF.
- Most children require a minimum FGF of 3L, which can then be adjusted to achieve normocapnia and an inspired CO_2 concentration of <0.6kPa (4.5mmHg). Partial rebreathing allows conservation of heat and humidification.
- $ETCO_2$ concentration may be underestimated in children below 10kg from dilution of expired gases. Sampling should be distal in the circuit.
- A Bain system (coaxial Mapleson D) can be used above 20kg.

Humphrey ADE system

- This hybrid system incorporates the Mapleson A, D, and E circuits in one breathing system.
- Studies indicate that the E mode behaves similarly to the T-piece and that the A mode is efficient in children over 10kg. Both the D and E modes are suitable for controlled ventilation.

- The expiratory valves are of low resistance and do not add appreciably to the work of breathing.

Circle absorption systems

- Low-flow anaesthesia is cost-efficient, reduces atmospheric pollution, and conserves warmth and moisture. The reaction of CO_2 with soda lime is exothermic, producing heat and water.
- Monitoring of inspiratory and expiratory levels of O_2, N_2O, CO_2, and volatile agent is mandatory.
- Paediatric circle systems using 15mm lightweight hose are suitable for children over 5kg. The unidirectional valves may increase resistance to breathing and should not be allowed to become damp.
- During controlled ventilation, the leak around the ETT may require gas flows to be increased.

Bain system

The coaxial Mapleson D system is unsuitable for children under 20kg due to the resistance of the expiratory valve.

Mechanical ventilation

- Standard adult ventilators are suitable down to 20kg.
- Below 20kg, a paediatric ventilator should be able to deliver small V_T, rapid respiratory rates, variable inspiratory flow rates, and different I:E ratios.
- Calculation of small V_T is meaningless because of compression of gases in the ventilator tubing and a variable leak around the ETT. More sophisticated ventilators may, however, be capable of measuring expired V_T, which is of more practical value.
- Some ventilators are designed to work with specific breathing systems. The Newton valve converts the Nuffield Penlon 200 ventilator from a time-cycled flow generator to a time-cycled pressure generator and can be attached directly to the expiratory limb of the Ayre's T-piece. It is suitable for neonates and children up to 20kg. Many new anaesthetic workstations incorporate integral ventilators attached to circle systems suitable for paediatric practice.
- Pressure-controlled ventilation is commonly used and reduces the risk of barotrauma/pneumothorax. This mode will compensate for a leak around the ETT, but not for changes in lung compliance, partial or complete tube obstruction, or bronchospasm.
- Volume control can make an allowance for changes in lung compliance, but at a potential cost of high peak airway pressures.
- Ultimately, setting ventilator parameters is based on clinical observation. Inspiratory flow, pressure, or volume is gradually increased until adequate chest movement is observed. Measurement of capnography and pulse oximetry confirms normocapnia and adequate oxygenation. The peak airway pressure is kept to a minimum. A ventilator alarm is mandatory.
- Most children can be ventilated adequately with inspiratory pressures of 16–20cmH$_2$O and a respiratory rate between 16 and 24 breaths/min.

Normally, inspiratory pressure should not exceed $30cmH_2O$. The rate can be adjusted accordingly to achieve normocapnia. A minimum PEEP of $4cmH_2O$ is advisable for infants and neonates to maintain the FRC.

• The ability to hand-ventilate using the Ayre's T-piece is essential. It should always be available in the event of ventilator failure or unexpected desaturation. Mechanical ventilation may be unsuitable for the small premature neonate. With gastroschisis and exomphalos, hand ventilation can assess changes in lung compliance and determine how much of the abdominal contents should be reduced back into the abdominal cavity. Hand ventilation during repair of a tracheo-oesophageal fistula can allow the surgeon maximum exposure and time to effect the repair.

References

1 Hughes C, Place K, Mason D (2012). A clinical evaluation of the i-gel supraglottic airway device in children. *Pediatr Anesth*, **22**, 765–71.

2 Weiss M, Dullenkopf A, Fisher JE, Keller C, Gerber AC (2009). Prospective randomised controlled multi-centre trial of cuffed or uncuffed tracheal tubes in small children. *Br J Anaesth*, **103**, 867–73.

Conduct of anaesthesia

Preoperative assessment

The preoperative visit is essential in establishing a rapport with both parents and children and in helping to dissipate anxiety. Communication should be simple, informative, and truthful.

- Avoid wearing a white coat. Involve the parents; try to question the child directly, when appropriate, and stay at eye level, if possible.
- A pre-admission visit reduces parental anxiety and is beneficial to children over 6yr. Play therapists can help provide an informal setting and informatively prepare the child by describing the course of events from the ward to induction of anaesthesia. A collection of photographs or a video may be helpful.

Preoperative investigations

Routine preoperative Hb is indicated for:

- Neonates and ex-premature infants under 1yr
- Children at risk of SCD (see ➔ p. 198)
- Children for whom intraoperative transfusion may be necessary
- Children with systemic disease.

A preoperative Hb of <10g/dL is abnormal and needs to be investigated. It does not necessarily entail cancellation if the child is haemodynamically stable and otherwise well.

Routine biochemistry is required for:

- Children with metabolic, endocrine, or renal disease
- Children receiving IV fluids.

The child with an upper respiratory tract infection

- The preschool child develops 6–8 URTIs per year. Almost 25% of children have a chronic runny nose due to seasonal rhinitis or adenoidal infection.
- Anaesthesia in the presence of an intercurrent URTI is associated with a higher risk of complications in younger children. There is an increased incidence of excess secretions, airway obstruction, laryngospasm, and bronchoconstriction. This risk is increased 5-fold using an LMA, and by a factor of ten if the child is intubated.
- Children with moderate to severe chest infections should be postponed. This will include those with productive cough, purulent chest or nasal secretions, pyrexia, and signs of viraemia or constitutional illness, including diarrhoea and vomiting.
- The child with a mild URTI is a difficult problem.[3] The history in these cases is crucial. It is important to decide whether the child is at the beginning or end of the URTI. Other members of the family or children at school may have already experienced the same infection, and this can provide useful information.
- A child deemed to be post-viral, apyrexial, with no chest signs, and constitutionally well is probably fit for surgery, even if they have a runny nose.

- Significant URTI requires postponement for 2wk, but this should be 4wk if lower respiratory tract involvement is suspected. Bronchiolitis warrants a delay of at least 6wk.

The child with a murmur

- The majority of pathological murmurs are diagnosed perinatally, and these children will already be under the care of a paediatric cardiologist.
- Previously unreported murmurs are commonly heard at 2–4yr. The majority are functional.
- A systolic murmur with normal heart sounds and palpable peripheral pulses in a child with normal O_2 saturation and no limitation in exercise tolerance can be assumed to be innocent. If there are any doubts, surgery should be deferred until a formal assessment has been made.
- NICE guidelines no longer recommend routine antibiotic prophylaxis for surgery in patients at risk of infectious endocarditis. However, if a child requires prophylactic antibiotics for a GI or genitourinary procedure, these should also include sensitivities to organisms that cause infectious endocarditis.

The anxious or uncooperative child

- Two-thirds of children have significant anxiety at induction. This may be due to fear of pain, e.g. cannulation, or general anxiety about anaesthesia and the operation.[4]
- Children with behavioural issues, such as autism or attention-deficit/hyperactivity disorder (ADHD), may cause particular problems. If the problem can be anticipated, a multidisciplinary approach should be adopted, and a plan instituted for the anaesthetic room.
- Some general tips:
  - Agree a plan with the parents beforehand, and involve the parents as much as possible
  - Medical equipment can be frightening. Keep to a minimum the amount on display. Drugs drawn up in advance
  - Minimize the number of people in the anaesthetic room. Maintain a calm, quiet atmosphere
  - Only one person at a time should speak to the child, at eye level if possible
  - Adapt the technique to the child's personality and developmental level
  - Support coping strategies or distraction techniques, e.g. book, bubbles. Consider the use of an electronic tablet with a favourite film or game.
- Premedication can be useful, and older children may choose this option. Oral midazolam is commonly used, with ketamine as an alternative, either alone or in combination with midazolam (see ➲ p. 798). Clonidine may be a useful option for autistic children.
- A decision on whether to proceed should centre on the best interests of the child.
- There should be a clinical holding policy as a guideline to facilitate clinical procedures.
- A Gillick competent child can consent to treatment against parental wishes but cannot refuse it (see ➲ p. 797).

Child protection

- Child protection training is mandatory for all hospital staff who work with children.[5]
- Anaesthetists may become suspicious of child abuse during resuscitation, on PICU, in the anaesthetic room, during the course of a surgical procedure, or rarely by direct disclosure.
- In these situations, it is essential to act in the best interests of the child.
- If there is concern about suspected abuse, the 1st point of contact should be the named clinical lead for safeguarding children or the consultant paediatrician on call.

Consent

- Allow time at the end of the preoperative assessment for parents to ask questions. Discuss the options of IV or inhalational induction and plans for post-operative pain relief. Obtain consent for suppository, neuraxial blockade, or regional/peripheral nerve block, if indicated, including attendant risks and benefits. Discuss the risks associated with GA.
- A young person is deemed competent to consent from 16yr. Children under 16yr may have the capacity to decide, depending on their ability to understand what is involved (Gillick competence).[6]
- Signed written consent is the preferred option.

Preoperative fasting

(See also ➋ p. 9.)
- Fasting instructions (Table 34.10) are designed to minimize the risk of regurgitation of gastric contents and consequent pulmonary aspiration.
- Fasting reduces the gastric volume but does not guarantee an empty stomach. Prolonged fasting does not further reduce the risk of aspiration and, in infants, can lead to dehydration and hypoglycaemia.
- Infants may be at greater risk of regurgitation due to reduced lower oesophageal sphincter tone and a tendency to distend the stomach during mask ventilation. However, the incidence of pneumonitis following aspiration in children is much lower than in adults.
- Clear fluids can be given safely up to 2hr preoperatively, and the intake of fluids (either water or a fruit squash drink) should be encouraged. Children are less irritable at induction, and there may be a reduction in PONV.
- The data for milk and solid food are less clear. Breast milk is cleared from the stomach more rapidly than formula milk in infants.
- Every unit should have fasting guidelines. Close liaison with ward staff ensures that children receive adequate clear fluid preoperatively and that milk feeds for neonates and infants are appropriately timed.

Table 34.10 Guidelines for preoperative fasting periods

Ingested material	Minimum fast (hr)
Clear liquids	2
Breast milk	4
Light meal, infant formula, and other milk	6

Topical anaesthetics

- Topical LA preparations reduce the pain of venepuncture and facilitate IV induction.
- EMLA® cream is a eutectic mixture of 2.5% lidocaine and 2.5% prilocaine in a 1:1 ratio. It should be applied for at least 45min and can produce vasoconstriction. The duration of action is 30–60min. EMLA® should be avoided in premature infants <37wk and used with caution in children <1yr receiving medication that may predispose to methaemoglobinaemia.
- Ametop® is a 4% gel formulation of tetracaine. The onset time is 30min for venesection and 45min for cannulation. There is a prolonged duration of action (4hr) after the cream has been removed. It is licensed from 4wk of age and has vasodilating properties. There may be a higher incidence of allergic reactions. The gel should be applied for no longer than 90min and removed earlier if a rash or itchiness develops.
- It is important to identify the veins to be anaesthetized and not blindly apply the cream to the dorsum of each hand. Keep the area bandaged to prevent removal or licking of the cream!
- Ethyl chloride is a cryoanalgesic. It is useful when topical creams are either contraindicated or forgotten.

Premedication

- Routine sedative premedication is unnecessary. ('Parents are often the best premedication.')
- Some children will require preoperative sedation. They include the excessively upset child, children with previous unpleasant experiences of anaesthesia and surgery, and certain children with developmental delay. Older children or adolescents may request premedication.
- Infants have not yet developed a fear of strangers and appear relatively undisturbed when separated from their mothers. The preschool child is most at risk. They are vulnerable to separation anxiety in a strange environment, but without the ability to reason.
- Even when anaesthesia and surgery are uneventful, there may be a disturbingly high incidence of post-operative psychological problems. Sleep disturbance, nightmares, bed-wetting, eating disorders, and behavioural changes have all been reported. Some authors suggest that sedative premedication, especially in the preschool age group, may reduce parental anxiety, improve patient compliance, and reduce the incidence of some of these post-operative behavioural changes.[4]
- Oral midazolam (0.5mg/kg) is a commonly used premedicant.[7] It acts within 15–30min to reduce anxiety, leading to a more cooperative child, but with minimal delay in recovery. The IV formulation is used but is extremely bitter and should be diluted in fruit juice or paracetamol syrup. Midazolam (0.2mg/kg) can also be given intranasally where it has a rapid onset of action within 5–15min but is poorly tolerated because of the burning sensation in the nasal mucosa.
- Ketamine can be given orally (2–5mg/kg) as a sole drug or in combination with midazolam. Its action starts within 15min, but it may

be associated with excess salivation and emergence delirium. Ketamine 2mg/kg IM may assist in anaesthesia of the uncooperative child who refuses to accept oral premedication.

- Clonidine given orally (4 micrograms/kg) produces good conditions for induction and may reduce post-operative analgesic requirements but is associated with hypotension and a delayed recovery.
- Alternative premedicants include temazepam (0.5–1mg/kg), alimemazine (2mg/kg), and promethazine (1mg/kg). They tend to be less predictable and longer-lasting.
- Modern anaesthetic agents do not require the routine use of anticholinergic agents. Antisialogogues are reserved for patients with excessive secretions, e.g. Down's syndrome and cerebral palsy, the suspected difficult airway, and co-administration with ketamine. Some anaesthetists still routinely give drying agents for neonates and the smaller child.
- Absorption of orally administered atropine (40 micrograms/kg) is variable. To be certain of the efficacy, administer 20 micrograms/ kg IM 30min preoperatively or 10 micrograms/kg IV at induction. Glycopyrronium (5 micrograms/kg IM or IV) is a suitable alternative. Atropine should also precede the administration of suxamethonium to protect against possible bradycardia which, in younger children, can occur following the 1st dose.
- Children undergoing cardiac surgery are traditionally heavily premedicated. Choices include morphine, which may prevent RV infundibular spasm in uncorrected Fallot's tetralogy, or a combination of drugs, e.g. PethCo®, which comprises a mixture of pethidine, promethazine, and chlorpromazine.

Parents in the anaesthetic room

- In the UK, a parent is routinely allowed into the anaesthetic room, while their child is anaesthetized. It is now accepted that enforced separation disempowers the parent and is an emotionally traumatic experience for both parent and child.
- Parents are naturally anxious over the loss of control, a strange environment, and the possibility of adverse events. Unfortunately, this parental anxiety may communicate itself to the child.
- Parental presence should not be compulsory. It is not always beneficial and may even be counterproductive with a very anxious parent. Evidence of benefit has only been demonstrated for children older than 4yr with a calm parent attending the induction.
- Preschool children are especially at risk of behavioural disturbance, probably because of difficulties in reasoning. In contrast, some adolescents may not wish their parents to accompany them.
- Anaesthetic induction appears to be the most distressing event experienced by parents. Separation from the child after induction, watching the child become unconscious, and the degree of stress experienced by the child before induction are all important factors.
- The parent should always be accompanied by a nurse who can comfort them and escort them out of the anaesthetic room once the child is asleep. It is extremely unusual to allow >1 parent into the anaesthetic

room. There may rarely be extenuating circumstances, but these should be discussed beforehand with the anaesthetist.

Induction of anaesthesia

- Induction should occur in a child-friendly environment.
- A dedicated paediatric theatre is not always an option. An alternative is a customized paediatric anaesthetic trolley incorporating a comprehensive range of airway and vascular equipment.
- Prepare drugs and equipment before the child arrives. Recheck the weight (Table 34.4):

  $$\text{Weight (kg)} = (\text{Age} + 4) \times 2$$

- Online calculators or smartphone apps can be useful to check doses.
- Precalculate the dose of atropine and suxamethonium in prepared syringes (Table 34.15).
- Pulse oximetry is the minimum monitoring acceptable in the anaesthetic room, although it will not read accurately on the agitated child. Many children will tolerate an ECG and BP cuff prior to induction.

Inhalational induction

(See also ➔ p. 967)

- It is important to learn >1 method. Not all children are susceptible to the same technique.
- Sevoflurane is the volatile agent of choice. It is rapidly acting, giving a smooth induction, with less CVS depression than halothane. It is not odourless but is relatively non-irritant. For the suspected difficult airway, use sevoflurane in 100% O_2; otherwise 50% N_2O/O_2 is satisfactory, and anecdotally N_2O may obtund the patient's sense of smell, facilitating induction. Emergence delirium is commoner with sevoflurane than halothane. There is a strong association with rapid awakening, particularly in the preschool age group, increased preoperative anxiety, and inadequate analgesia.
- Halothane is an alternative but is less available. Induction should proceed through incremental increases in concentration. Start with 100% O_2, and add in N_2O once the airway is secure.
- Involve the parent as much as possible. This may involve holding the child or even participating in the induction.
- Position the child either supine on the trolley or across the lap of the parent, so that the parent or anaesthetic assistant can gently restrain the arms, if necessary. Warn the parent that the child's head will become floppy and need support.
- For smaller children, a cupped hand method is useful. Occlude the end of the bag to direct all the FGF towards the patient's mouth and nose.
- A face mask is often tolerated by older children. This can be held by the parent, child, or anaesthetist, and the child can be encouraged to blow up the bag 'like a balloon'. A flavoured face mask may be useful initially, but the volatile agent rapidly becomes the dominant smell.
- The parent should be warned of abnormal movements when the child is nearly anaesthetized.
- Once anaesthesia is achieved and the eyelash reflex is absent, anaesthesia can be maintained with another volatile agent, if desired.

Intravenous induction

- The smaller child sits across the parent's lap, and the arm is placed under the parent's axilla, thereby obstructing the child's view. The older child will usually lie on the trolley, with the parent on one side holding the child's hand, while the other is cannulated.
- The induction agent of choice is propofol 3–5mg/kg, with 1% lidocaine (1mL/10mL propofol) added to reduce pain on injection. It is licensed for children over 1 month.
- The Paedfusor TCI system is approved for >1 month or >5kg.[8] The dose is age-dependent and proportionally greater than the adult dose due to the higher volume of distribution and clearance in children.
- If using a small vein, the dilution of propofol with an equal volume of saline significantly reduces pain on injection.
- Thiopental 4–6mg/kg is a suitable alternative and is licensed for neonates (2mg/kg).
- Ketamine 2mg/kg is reserved for haemodynamically compromised patients or those with severe CVS disease, usually in conjunction with fentanyl 1–2 micrograms/kg. Emergence phenomena are less common in children, especially in combination with midazolam, but the incidence of PONV and salivation is higher.

Comparison of intravenous and inhalational induction

- IV induction is simple and safer but is associated with more hypoxia—possibly because children are rarely preoxygenated.
- Inhalational induction produces more coughing and laryngospasm.
- Psychological studies suggest that inhalational induction may be more traumatic to the child.[9]
- In practice, it seems prudent to opt for IV induction, if possible, unless the child actively chooses an inhalational method.

Tips for cannulation

- Securing IV access can be difficult, even for paediatric anaesthetists! It is important to realize this; relax, and send for help, if necessary. Good lighting, competent anaesthetic assistance, and a selection of cannulae with prepared saline flush syringes are all essential.
- Neonates often have surprisingly good superficial veins on the hand and wrist. Conversely, healthy children between 3 months and 2yr can be notoriously difficult because of the fat pads over hands and feet.
- Compression of a limb by the assistant should be gentle to act as a venous, rather than arterial, tourniquet. The skin is often mobile and should be gently stretched. In neonates, it may be easier for the anaesthetist to flex and squeeze the wrist with the non-cannulating hand.
- Examine the wrists and dorsum of the feet for superficial veins. Scalp veins are possible in neonates. Long saphenous and cephalic veins may be palpated.
- In some children, most commonly in the feet, the skin is surprisingly tough, and a small nick in the skin with a 21G needle may be necessary. Loosening the cap of the cannula or priming with saline will permit flashback of blood in small veins.

- Transfixion is possible in smaller children. It is potentially useful for all veins, but especially in 'blind' long saphenous and femoral vein cannulation. Slowly pull back the cannula until in the vein, and then gently advance.
- If cannulating the femoral vein, a small support under the pelvis and slight external rotation may be useful.
- A cold light source can be used to locate the veins in neonates and infants.
- The use of ultrasound is becoming commoner. A small 'footprint' probe of 7–10MHz is suitable for most ages. It is particularly useful for central access, but veins in the antecubital fossa and the long saphenous vein can also be visualized. Transfixion is a common technique because of compression of the vessel.[10]
- If all else fails, intraosseous access can be an invaluable alternative. Observing aseptic precautions, prepare an area of the skin over the anteromedial aspect of the tibia, 1cm below and medial to the tibial tuberosity. The intraosseous needle is inserted perpendicularly to the skin and advanced in a twisting, pushing movement against the bone, until there is a sudden loss of resistance. The position is confirmed if the needle remains upright without support, marrow can be aspirated, and fluid can be administered without SC swelling around the entry site. Children can be successfully anaesthetized via this route, although thiopental should be avoided because of its irritant properties. The intraosseous route is particularly useful in fluid resuscitation of the shocked child before definitive IV access can be gained. Routine blood samples, including cross-match, can be taken from this site before induction. Battery-powered devices are available (EZ-IO).
- Surgical cut-down is rarely needed, often technically difficult, and should be reserved as a last resort.

Airway management

- Airway complications, including coughing, laryngospasm, and upper airways obstruction, are commoner in children.
- Key to airway management is the triple manoeuvre of *head tilt*, *chin lift*, and *jaw thrust*.
- Hyperextension of the neck in the neonate often occludes the airway, and a neutral position is usually more successful. For older children, the adult 'sniffing the morning air' position should be adopted.
- Smaller children do not require a pillow; this may lead to unwanted head flexion.
- The paediatric face mask should be accurately sized and held gently, but firmly, on the face with the thumb and forefinger. The other fingers should curl around and grip the mandible. It is important to avoid pressing on the floor of the mouth, which will push the tongue forward and obstruct the airway.
- Early use of an oropharyngeal airway may be useful in older children.
- A nasopharyngeal airway may be attempted. This should be well lubricated. It is indicated in cases of micrognathia and can be inserted at lighter levels of anaesthesia.

- The most important technique in the management of the airway is judicious use of CPAP. Ensure a good seal with the face mask, and then partially occlude the bag of the Ayre's T-piece.

Laryngospasm
(See also **➲** p. 903.)
- Laryngospasm is commoner in children than adults. Additional risk factors include inhalational induction, asthma, URTI, and chronic lung disease. Children become cyanotic more rapidly than adults because of increased metabolic rate/O_2 consumption and reduced FRC.
- Contrary to the old adage, children do not 'always take a final breath'. Bradycardia is a premorbid event, indicating an inadequate cardiac output and a significant risk of cerebral hypoxia.

  - Partial laryngospasm management:
    - 100% O_2
    - CPAP
    - Gentle assisted ventilation
    - Propofol 1–2mg/kg bolus.
  - Complete laryngospasm management:
    - 100% O_2
    - CPAP
    - Assisted ventilation may exacerbate the condition by inflating the stomach and forcing the arytenoids and false cords against the true vocal cords
    - Early administration of suxamethonium (1–2mg/kg) and atropine (10 micrograms/kg) may be necessary.

Intubation
For tube size, see **➲** p. 792.
- Neonatal intubation is not normally difficult, only different. The neonate has:
  - Proportionately larger head, shorter neck, larger tongue, smaller mandible
  - Larynx is more anterior/superior (C3–C4, compared with C5–C6)
  - Epiglottis is large, floppy, V-shaped, with obliquely angled vocal cords.
- Awake intubation for neonates is rarely practised. In the absence of recognized medical conditions with associated airway complications, paediatric intubation is usually straightforward. Below 6 months of age, use a straight-bladed laryngoscope. The head should be in a neutral position, and the shoulders supported, if necessary. Advance the laryngoscope blade past the larynx, then withdraw slowly until the larynx becomes visible, i.e. the blade is posterior to the epiglottis. Gentle cricoid pressure is often helpful. If nasal intubation is required, use a laryngoscope blade with minimal guttering to allow more room for instrumentation in the oropharynx. Over 6 months of age, a curved blade is usually easier. Intubation can be performed in the conventional adult position, with the blade resting in the vallecula.

- Most intubated neonates will also require an NGT (8–10FG).
- Always have a range of ETTs available, including a half size above and below the original estimation.
- Complications are common in children. Oesophageal and endobronchial intubation, extubation, kinking of the tube, and disconnection should all be anticipated. Secretions are far more likely to cause obstruction because of the smaller tube sizes involved, and periodic suction may be necessary.
- Intubation increases the work of breathing. The reduction in the cross-sectional area of the neonatal trachea with a size 3.5 tube *in situ* increases airway resistance by a factor of 16. Most intubated infants should undergo controlled ventilation as part of the anaesthetic technique.

Tube fixation
- Tube fixation is crucial. The neonatal trachea is only 4cm in length. Inadvertent extubation and endobronchial intubation are common.
- Secure with a '*three-point fixation*' to prevent movement of the tube in all three planes.
- Two pieces of trouser-shaped Elastoplast® may be used, with one 'leg' across the upper lip while the other 'leg' is wrapped around the tube. An oropharyngeal airway helps splint the tube.
- There are numerous other methods of fixation, all equally valid. The tube should be secured to the maxilla, rather than the more mobile mandible.
- The Portex Polar preformed ETT is a north-facing uncuffed tube which is easy to use, facilitates tube fixation, and reduces the incidence of endobronchial intubation.

Difficult intubation
- The key to difficult intubation is to identify the at-risk patient and plan accordingly with appropriate help, assistance, and equipment. Some conditions are well known to be associated with airway problems (e.g. Pierre–Robin, Treacher–Collins, and Goldenhar syndromes). Other patients can be identified by assessment of the airway preoperatively, specifically the presence of micrognathia and retrognathia.
- Premedicate with atropine 20 micrograms/kg IM or glycopyrronium 5 micrograms/kg IM 30min preoperatively to dry secretions. Give pseudoephedrine or oxymetazoline nose drops. Sedative premedication should be avoided.
- Airway management may be difficult. The traditional method is deep inhalational anaesthesia with CPAP and an IV *in situ*. Laryngoscopy and intubation are attempted, with the patient breathing spontaneously. Halothane is now rarely available, and sevoflurane is the agent of choice; a propofol infusion can be used to supplement this technique.
- The McCoy version of both Seward and Macintosh blades is available in paediatric sizes.
- A blind nasal approach to intubation is possible, but experience in the technique is declining, and there is a risk of trauma.

- An LMA will often secure the airway adequately, without the need for intubation. Other supraglottic airway devices (ProSeal LMA, cuffed oropharyngeal airway (COPA), and i-Gel) may be potentially useful.
- If intubation is still necessary, it may be possible to pass a bougie through the LMA into the trachea and then railroad a ETT. A size 3 ILMA is available and may be suitable for a larger child. A fibreoptic bronchoscope can also be used via the LMA.
- Videolaryngoscopy allows a magnified, high-resolution view of the airway, with visual confirmation of intubation. The blade is usually inserted in the midline without a tongue sweep.[11] The Airtraq, Glidescope, and C-Mac are all available in a range of neonatal and paediatric sizes.[4,5] The Bullard laryngoscope and paediatric Bonfils fibrescope are also potential alternatives.
- Fibreoptic intubation is rarely necessary. Children need to be anaesthetized, but a propofol infusion is an alternative method to volatile anaesthesia. Smaller-size neonatal and paediatric bronchoscopes do not all have a suction channel and should be checked to confirm that the selected ETT will fit over them.
- Conventional tubes may present problems in railroading, and armoured tubes should be used. Alternatively, a guide-wire can be inserted into the trachea, using the suction channel. An exchange catheter is passed over the wire, and then the tube railroaded over the exchange catheter.[12]
- A tracheostomy is rarely required. It is exceedingly difficult as an emergency procedure. Paediatric cricothyroidotomy cannulae are available in 18G and 16G sizes and should be present in the anaesthetic room.

Rapid sequence induction
(See also ➲ p. 963.)
- Ranitidine and metoclopramide are not routinely prescribed.
- Preoxygenation does not usually present problems with infants and older children but may be more difficult in preschool children.
- Inhalational induction may be necessary, after which cricoid pressure can be applied while breathing spontaneously.
- Suxamethonium should be preceded by atropine to prevent bradycardia. Rocuronium is not recommended for paediatric patients.
- Cricoid pressure often facilitates intubation. If intubation cannot be achieved initially, mask ventilation should gently recommence while cricoid pressure is maintained.
- There should be a low threshold for using an NGT in neonates and small infants. If already *in situ* in the neonate, it should remain in place, rather than being removed. There is no consensus for older children.
- Since the TT is uncuffed, a throat pack may help prevent intraoperative aspiration but has no application in the higher-risk periods of induction and reversal.
- The child should be extubated awake in the left lateral position.

Maintenance
- Position the infant and smaller child with both arms raised at the level of the head. Exposure of the hand allows assessment of the pulse,

- peripheral temperature, colour, and capillary refill. A blocked IV may be more easily cleared, and a new cannula may be easier to site.
- The pulse oximeter probe should be sited on the same arm as the IV infusion, and the contralateral arm to the BP cuff. Avoid oximeter probes on the feet, as the trace is usually lost once abdominal surgery commences.
- Check that the ETT is still *in situ* and securely fixed, and the lungs are ventilating adequately and equally. The connections should all be secure, and the tube and breathing circuit supported, if necessary.
- Confirm that cannulae are secure, working, and accessible; extension tubing may be necessary. Three-way taps allow the administration of drugs and fluid volume when necessary. Neonatal surgery requires a minimum of two cannulae (maintenance and volume).
- Blood sugar should be checked regularly.
- Even small air bubbles in IV fluids can be potentially harmful to infants, especially in the presence of an ASD or VSD. A bubble trap should be routinely included in the tubing for these patients.
- Theatre temperature should be 21°C and preheated. The child's head should be covered, and body exposure reduced to a minimum. It is easier to prevent hypothermia than to treat it. Both IV and cleaning fluid should be warmed.
- Routine monitoring should include ECG, BP (with appropriate sized cuff), pulse oximeter, capnography, and full gas monitoring with a ventilator alarm when indicated. Temperature measurement is important, and, for the neonate, routine use of a precordial or oesophageal stethoscope is recommended. The width of the BP cuff should be 20% greater than the diameter of the arm to avoid artefactually raised BP.
- Electronic monitoring is often unreliable with the sick or shocked neonate. It should support, but not replace, clinical observation. The oesophageal or precordial stethoscope permits a continuous qualitative assessment of heart sounds and ventilation. More importantly, it 'ties' the anaesthetist to the patient.
- Do not let the surgeon start operating until you are ready.
- Anaesthetic complications in paediatric practice are as common during maintenance as at induction or in the post-operative period.

Reversal

- Following surgery, the child should be warm, well saturated, normocarbic, and pain-free. A cold acidotic neonate will not breathe post-operatively.
- LMA can be removed, either deep or awake. If an armoured LMA is *in situ*, a bite block will be needed. There is often a stage shortly before waking when the mouth opens slightly to mimic a small yawn; this is an ideal opportunity to deftly remove the LMA.
- Most children should be extubated awake. If warm and with adequate analgesia, this is tolerated well. Exceptions include tonsillectomy and other procedures when coughing is to be avoided. In these cases, deep extubation is preferable.
- Neonates should be extubated awake, preceded by an assisted ventilation to preoxygenate the lungs.

Post-operative nausea and vomiting

- PONV is uncommon under the age of 2yr. Predictors of risk include high-risk procedures (adenotonsillectomy, squint surgery), travel sickness, and previous PONV.
- Opioids increase the risk of PONV by 30%. Regional anaesthesia and other opioid-sparing techniques should be encouraged.
- There is some evidence of reduced PONV with TIVA in children. N_2O does not appear to be associated with an increased risk of PONV in children.[13]
- Combinations of antiemetics and the use of 5-HT$_3$ antagonists with dexamethasone 0.1mg/kg may be more efficacious than simple monotherapy.
- Children considered high-risk should receive ondansetron 0.15mg/kg at induction.
- Cyclizine 1mg/kg can be used as a second-line rescue therapy.

References

3 Tait A, Malviya S (2005). Anaesthesia for children with an upper respiratory tract infection: still a dilemma. *Anesth Analg*, **100**, 59–65.

4 Hearst D (2009). The runaway child: managing anticipatory fear, resistance and distress in children undergoing surgery. *Paediatr Anaesth*, **19**, 1014.

5 Royal College of Anaesthetists, Association of Anaesthetists of Great Britain and Ireland, Association of Paediatric Anaesthetists of Great Britain and Ireland, Royal College of Paediatrics and Child Health (2014). *Child protection and the anaesthetist: safeguarding children in the operating theatre, July 2014.* ℘ http://www.apagbi.org.uk/sites/default/files/images/CHILD-PROTECTION-2014.pdf.

6 Gillick v West Norfolk and Wisbech AHA (1985). **3** ALL ER 402.

7 McCluskey A, Martin GH (1994). Oral administration of midazolam as a premedicant for paediatric day case anaesthesia. *Anaesthesia*, **49**, 782–5.

8 Mani V, Morton N (2010). Overview of total intravenous anesthesia in children. *Paediatr Anaesth*, **20**, 211–22.

9 Kotiniemi LH, Ryhanen PT (1996). Behavioural changes and children's memories after intravenous, inhalation and rectal induction of anaesthesia. *Paediatr Anaesth*, **6**, 201–7.

10 Murphy P, Arnold P (2011). Ultrasound-assisted vascular access in children. *Contin Educ Anaesth Crit Care Pain*, **11**, 44–9.

11 Gooden C (2009). Videolaryngoscopy and the pediatric airway. *Anesthesiology News*, 47–51.

12 Walker RWM, Ellwood J (2009). The management of difficult intubation in children. *Paediatr Anaesth*, **19**, 77–87.

13 Association of Paediatric Anaesthetists of Great Britain and Ireland (2009). *Guidelines on the prevention of post-operative vomiting in children.* ℘ http://www.apagbi.org.uk/sites/default/files/APA_Guidelines_on_the_Prevention_of_Postoperative_Vomiting_in_Children.pdf.

Further reading

Airtraq. *Intubating with Airtraq.* ℘ http://www.airtraq.com/index.php?option=com_content&task=view&id=231&Itemid=334.

Verathon. ℘ http://verathon.com/contact-us/glidescope-pediatric-airway-rounds.

Vidacare (EZ-IO). ℘ http://www.vidacare.com.

Post-operative pain relief

Children feel pain as much as adults. Underdosage is common due to inadequate knowledge and fear of side effects. Poor-quality pain relief can lead to prolonged hospital stay, maladaptive behaviour (temper tantrums, bed-wetting, and nightmares), and chronic pain issues.

Similar principles to adult practice apply (see ➲ p. 1061), including the application of multimodal analgesia and specialized pain charts.

- Pain assessment can be challenging with infants and neonates. Use physiological/behavioural pain scales, e.g. FLACC, CRIES.
- Older children may be able to self-report using faces charts, e.g. Wong–Baker or visual analogue scales.[14]
- Non-pharmacological methods: explanation, reassurance, distraction (stories, play, music).
- Simple analgesics (Table 34.11): paracetamol and NSAIDs are widely prescribed for minor cases/day surgery and for their morphine-sparing effects. Drugs should be given regularly. Single doses of IV perioperative analgesics should be documented on the front of the drug chart to avoid multiple doses being given post-operatively.
- Codeine is no longer recommended for children under 12 years.[15]
- Opioids: morphine infusions can be administered cautiously to neonates, and as nurse-controlled analgesia (NCA) for smaller children with a background infusion. PCA can be used effectively in children as young as 6yr, some with a low background infusion. Bolus function must not be activated by parents (Table 34.12).
- Caudal analgesia and peripheral nerve blocks (PNBs) are extremely useful for day cases. Epidural blockade is of proven benefit in abdominal and orthopaedic surgery. Below 6 months, it is technically easier, and possibly safer, to insert the catheter via the caudal route (see ➲ p. 810).
- Liaison with the ward staff is crucial, and a standardized pain management approach, preferably with an acute pain service, is the ideal.

Regional anaesthesia

- Successful regional blockade provides conditions for light and haemodynamically stable GA. The stress response is attenuated, and early pain-free emergence is possible, leading to a smooth post-operative recovery.
- Unlike adults, few children tolerate these techniques awake, and the majority of regional blocks are performed on anaesthetized patients.
- Motor blockade is unnecessary, and low concentrations of LA can be used. The most widely used solutions are 0.25% bupivacaine/levobupivacaine and 0.2% ropivacaine.

References

14 My Child Is In Pain. *Information for parents whose child has had day case surgery.* http://mychildisinpain.org.uk/.

15 Medicines and Healthcare Products Regulatory Agency (2013). *Drug safety update July 2013.* http://www.elmmb.nhs.uk/newsletters-minutes/mhra-drug-safety-updates/?assetdetesctl545367=53339.

Table 34.11 Mild to moderate post-operative pain in children

Codeine phosphate (over 12 years only)[15]	1mg/kg	IM, PO, PR	6-hourly
Diclofenac	1mg/kg (over 6 months)	PO, PR	8-hourly
	1mg/kg (over 2 years)	IV	12-hourly max 2 days
Ibuprofen	5mg/kg (1–3 months)	PO	8-hourly
	10mg/kg (over 3 months)	PO	8-hourly
Paracetamol (over 1 month)	7.5mg/kg (preterm)	PO	8-hourly
	10mg/kg (neonate)	PO	8-hourly
	20mg/kg (child <50kg)	PO	6-hourly
	1g (child >50kg)	PO	6-hourly
	20mg/kg (infant 1–3 months) (loading dose: 30mg/kg)	PR	6-hourly
	20mg/kg (child >3 months) (loading dose: 40mg/kg)	PR	6-hourly
	7.5mg/kg (preterm)	IV	8-hourly
	10mg/kg (neonate)	IV	8-hourly
	15mg/kg (child >1 month)	IV	6-hourly
	1g (child >50kg)	IV	6-hourly
Morphine sulfate solution	300–500 micrograms/kg	PO	4-hourly

Table 34.12 Severe post-operative pain in children

Morphine	50–100 micrograms/kg IV incremental boluses
Morphine infusion	Morphine 1mg/kg in 50mL of saline, i.e. 20 micrograms/kg/mL
	Rate: 1–2mL/hr (20–40 micrograms/kg/hr)
Morphine NCA	Morphine 1mg/kg in 50mL of saline, i.e. 20 micrograms/kg/mL
	Rate: 1mL/hr. Bolus: 1mL. Lockout: 20min
Morphine PCA	Morphine 1mg/kg in 50mL of saline, i.e. 20 micrograms/kg/mL
	Bolus: 1mL. Lockout: 5min

Caudal block

Caudal extradural analgesia (CEA) has a wide application in children. It is suitable for all surgery below the umbilicus, including general surgery, urology, and orthopaedics. The technique is easier than with adults, with a higher success rate of ~95%. CEA can achieve a higher dermatomal block than adults. Epidural fat is less dense and less tightly packed, with the result that LA can spread more easily.

Technique

- Position the patient in the left lateral position, with the legs flexed at the hip. Aseptic technique is a prerequisite.
- Identify the sacral hiatus as the apex of an equilateral triangle with the base formed by a line joining the posterior superior iliac spines (Fig. 34.1).
- Alternatively, with the hips flexed at 90°, a line extended from the midline of the femur will intersect with the sacral hiatus. The natal cleft does not always correspond to bony midline structures.
- Define the boundaries of the sacral hiatus. This is again a triangle with the base formed by a line joining the sacral cornua and the apex representing the lower part of the 4th sacral vertebra. The sacral hiatus is covered by the sacrococcygeal membrane.
- Make a small nick in the skin with a needle to reduce the possibility of a dermoid. Direct a blunt, short-bevel (regional block) needle at 60° to the skin from the midpoint of the line joining the sacral cornua. Alternatively, use a 22G or 20G cannula, depending on the size of the child. A small 'give' indicates penetration of the sacrococcygeal membrane. Flatten the cannula or needle slightly, then advance. If using a cannula, withdraw the stylet to just behind the cannula before advancing the cannula into the caudal space. Do not advance the needle or cannula any more than is necessary. Advancement of a cannula, rather than a needle, may reduce the incidence of inadvertent dural or vascular puncture. Easy progression of the cannula is a good prognostic indicator of success.
- Test aspiration should be gentle; vessel walls can collapse, producing a false negative result. Aspiration should be repeated during injection of the LA. The 'whoosh' test using air should be avoided because of the risk of air embolism, but the 'swoosh' test with saline may be helpful. The commonest reason for a failed attempt is positioning the needle too caudally.
- Bupivacaine 0.25% is commonly administered—if the planned volume of LA is >1mL/kg, use 0.19% bupivacaine (three parts of 0.25% bupivacaine to one part of saline). Duration of the block averages 4–8hr. For doses, see Table 34.13.
- Ultrasound can be used to assess the caudal anatomy and to confirm the spread of the injectate in the caudal extradural space.
- Caudal blockade can be extended with:
  - Clonidine 1 microgram/kg
  - Diamorphine 30 micrograms/kg
  - Morphine 50 micrograms/kg (preservative-free).
- Adrenaline has been implicated in cases of spinal ischaemia and should be avoided.

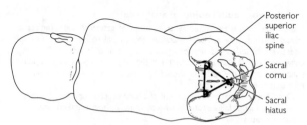

Fig. 34.1 Anatomy for caudal block.

Table 34.13 Regional analgesia doses in children

Caudal extradural blockade	Sacral: 0.5mL/kg of 0.25% bupivacaine
	Lumbar: 1mL/kg of 0.25% bupivacaine
	Thoracolumbar: 1.25mL/kg of 0.19% bupivacaine
Supplements to extend duration of caudal	Clonidine 1–2 micrograms/kg
	Diamorphine 30 micrograms/kg
	Morphine 50 micrograms/kg (preservative-free)
Lumbar epidural (intraoperative)	0.75mL/kg of 0.25% bupivacaine
Thoracic epidural (intraoperative)	0.5mL/kg of 0.25% bupivacaine
Epidural infusion	0.1% bupivacaine + fentanyl 2 micrograms/mL (sterile premixed bag)
	Rate: 0.1–0.4mL/kg/hr
Spinal block	0.1mL/kg of 0.5% 'heavy' bupivacaine + 0.06mL for needle dead space
Wound infiltration	1mL/kg of 0.25% bupivacaine

Clonidine causes post-operative sedation. Morphine and diamorphine increase the incidence of urinary retention and should be reserved for surgery in which catheterization is required. Ketamine is no longer recommended, especially in younger children, because of the potential risk of neuronal apoptosis.[16]

Advantages/complications of caudal analgesia

- Simple, safe, successful, with a wide range of indications.
- Motor block, paraesthesiae, hypotension, urinary retention, inadvertent dural puncture, and intravascular injection can all occur. All these complications are rare using a single-shot caudal technique.

Continuous caudal epidural analgesia

Caudal injection is restricted in its duration of action. A catheter can be introduced into the epidural space via the caudal route. It is a safe and effective method of administering epidural analgesia in infants. The single curve of the back allows the catheter to thread predictably into the epidural space; the tip of the catheter should be close to the level of the dermatomes that need to be blocked.

- Over 2yr of age, the development of a lumbosacral curvature tends to lead to a higher failure rate. However, some authors claim comparable success rates.
- Because of the proximity of the perineum, a caudal catheter should not be left *in situ* for longer than 36hr.

Reference

16 Lonnqvist PA, Walker SM (2012). Ketamine as an adjunct to caudal block in neonates and infants: is it time to re-evaluate? *Br J Anaesth*, **109**, 138–40.

Epidural/subarachnoid block

Epidural block

(See also ➲ p. 513 and p. 724.)

Epidural blockade is technically more difficult in children and requires experience. The ligamentum flavum is less well developed, and the intervertebral spaces are narrower. In infants, the epidural space is rarely located at a depth >15mm and often as superficially as 10mm from the skin. The technique is similar to that used in adults. Either a midline or paramedian approach is acceptable. The NAP3 study demonstrated that paediatric epidurals resulted in fewer complications than adults.[17] Severe neurological complications, including fatalities, have been reported in association with using air to find the epidural space in neonates. The caudal route may represent a safer alternative with this group.[18]

- Epidural needle: 18G for infants/children, 19G for neonates/infants (catheter 'end-hole' only).
- For suitable doses, see Table 34.13.

Subarachnoid block

Spinal anaesthesia is rarely performed in children. One of the few indications is for herniotomy in the high-risk neonate, e.g. the O_2-dependent premature or ex-premature infant with chronic lung disease.

- Expert assistance is crucial. The infant needs to be firmly gripped in the lateral or sitting position. The technique needs to be precise. The needle should be directed at right angles to the skin in the midline below L3, with L5–S1 reported as the safest approach. Prior infiltration of LA into the skin will help prevent patient movement.
- The block has a rapid onset, but duration rarely >40min. If sedation is required during the surgery, the incidence of post-operative apnoea is comparable with a GA technique.
- Spinal needle: 5cm 21G.
- For suitable doses, see Table 34.13.

References

17 Royal College of Anaesthetists (2009). *National Audit Project 3 (NAP3). National audit of major complications of central neuraxial blockade in the United Kingdom. Brief summary of results.* ℘ http://www.rcoa.ac.uk/nap3-brief-summary-of-major-results.

18 Lonnqvist PA, Morton NS (2005). Postoperative analgesia in infants and children. *Br J Anaesth,* **95**, 59–68.

Peripheral nerve blocks

- Ultrasound guidance is gaining popularity.[19] It is associated with shorter procedure time, higher success rates, and longer duration and less volume of LA. 'Real-time' assessment of the needle position may reduce the chance of inadvertent puncture of the abdominal viscera during performance of blocks of the abdominal wall.[20] Children can be imaged with high-frequency (10MHz) linear ultrasound probes; nerves tend to be more superficial.
- Many online resources exist to assist education.[21]
- If not skilled at a particular block, infiltration by the surgeon is often very effective. Advice about maximum doses is often useful!

Ilioinguinal and iliohypogastric nerve block

(See also ⮕ p. 1122.)
- Useful alternative to caudal blockade in herniotomy, hydrocele, and orchidopexy, especially for children >20kg. It should be avoided for neonatal herniotomy, as the LA may obscure the operating field. The block can be performed easily under direct vision by the surgeon.
- At a point 1cm medial to the ASIS, direct a regional block needle or a blunted 21G needle at right angles to the skin. There is resistance at the aponeurosis of the external oblique. At this point, 'bounce' the needle until a loss of resistance is encountered. Ultrasound-guided technique may be technically difficult in smaller children.
- Dosage: 0.75mL/kg of 0.25% bupivacaine. Retain 1–2mL for an SC fan injection laterally, medially, and inferiorly.
- Advantages: it is an easy block to perform. It decreases the level of anaesthesia and reduces post-operative analgesic requirement.
- Disadvantages: it does not block visceral pain from traction of the spermatic cord or peritoneum and is unsuitable for a high undescended testis. There is a 10% incidence of femoral nerve block.

Dorsal nerve block of penis

(See also ⮕ p. 1122.)
This block is indicated for distal surgery to the penis, including circumcision, meatoplasty, and simple hypospadias repair.
- Raise two SC swellings of LA on either side of the midline, each 5mm from the pubic symphysis at the dorsal base of the penis. Use a 23G or 21G needle.
- Alternatively, a simple ring block at the base of the penis can be performed using a 25G or 27G needle.
- Dosage: 4–10mL of 0.25% bupivacaine. Avoid adrenaline.
- Advantages: these techniques are safe, simple, and predictable. They avoid the need for injection deep to the Buck's fascia close to the corpora cavernosa and penile vessels.
- Disadvantages: does not always block the ventral surface of the penis. Theoretical complications, including haematoma and ischaemia, are unlikely using the superficial technique.

Transversus abdominis plane block

(See also ➲ p. 1123.)
- Indicated for lower abdominal surgery, including herniotomy, appendicectomy, and some laparoscopic surgery.
- Identify the triangle of Petit in the mid-axillary line at the midpoint between the costal margin and the iliac crest.
- Direct a blunt 21G needle or regional block needle perpendicular to the skin to elicit a 'double pop'.
- For the ultrasound-guided approach, see References[20] (see also ➲ p. 1124).
- Dosage: 1mL/kg of 0.25% bupivacaine.
- Advantages: safe, simple, and effective.
- Disadvantages: potential for intraperitoneal injection, bowel perforation, and LA toxicity.

Rectus sheath block

(See also ➲ p. 1125.)
- Indicated for midline hernias and single-port laparoscopic surgery.
- Identify the midpoint of the rectus sheath. Making a small nick in the skin, advance a blunted or regional block needle until a 'pop' is elicited.
- Ultrasound-guided technique[20] is probably a safer option, especially in younger children.
- Bilateral block. Total dose: 1mL/kg of 0.25% bupivacaine.

Femoral nerve block

(See also ➲ p. 1128.)
- This block is indicated for surgery to the knee or femur.
- Position the patient supine, with the leg slightly externally rotated.
- Direct the regional block needle just lateral to the femoral artery below the inguinal ligament. There may be two 'pops', as the needle passes through the fascia lata and fascia iliaca.
- Confirmation by a nerve stimulator or ultrasound.
- Dosage: 0.5mL/kg of 0.25% bupivacaine.

Sciatic nerve block

(See also ➲ p. 1129.)
This block is indicated for ankle surgery or lower limb procedures, in combination with a femoral nerve block (take care with the total dose of LA used).
- Proximal block: leg flexed at the hip. Identify the midpoint of a line joining the greater trochanter and ischial tuberosity; the nerve here lies deep to the biceps femoris. Needle insertion perpendicular to the skin; confirm with a nerve stimulator or ultrasound.
- Popliteal block: lateral position. The popliteal triangle is bordered by the biceps femoris laterally, the semimembranosus and semitendinosus medially, and at the base by the popliteal crease. The nerve is superficial to the artery and vein. Direct the needle just laterally to the apex of the popliteal triangle in a cephalad direction, using a nerve stimulator. Alternatively, use ultrasound to identify the bifurcation of the sciatic nerve near this point, and surround with LA.
- Dosage: 0.5mL/kg of 0.25% bupivacaine.

Axillary block

(See also ➲ p. 1111.)

This block is indicated for hand and lower arm surgery—ultrasound is useful.

- Position the patient supine, with the arm abducted to 90° and the elbow flexed.
- Direct a 23G or 25G needle with the attached extension tubing just above and parallel to the axillary artery. The needle is advanced until it pulsates, or the position can be confirmed with a nerve stimulator. A click or loss of resistance is not always elicited in children. Alternatively, ultrasound is used to identify the nerves clustering around the axillary artery. Aim to surround each with a 'halo' of LA.
- Dosage: 0.5mL/kg of 0.25% bupivacaine.
- Advantages: safe and effective.
- Disadvantages: upper arm and shoulder surgery cannot be performed. The axillary artery may be difficult to palpate.

References

19 Rubin K, Sullivan D, Senthilkumar S (2009). Are peripheral and neuraxial blocks with ultrasound guidance more effective and safe in children? *Paediatr Anaesth*, **19**, 92–6.
20 Suresh S, Chan WS (2009). Ultrasound guided transversus abdominis plane block in infants, children and adolescents: a simple procedural guidance for their performance. *Paediatr Anaesth*, **19**, 296–9.
21 Blockjocks.com. *Ultrasound-guided regional anaesthesia education forum*. ➲ http://www.blockjocks.com/.

Diaphragmatic hernia

Procedure	Repair of defect in diaphragm either by suturing to abdominal wall or with a synthetic graft
Time	1–2hr
Pain	+++
Position	Supine
Blood loss	Usually minimal to moderate
Practical techniques	GA plus IPPV, art line

Preoperative
- Incidence of 1:3000–4000 deliveries, affecting the left side in 85% of cases. Associated with other anomalies (cardiac 20%).
- Characteristically present in respiratory distress with tachypnoea, cyanosis, and a scaphoid abdomen. The chest radiograph is diagnostic. The diagnosis is usually made antenatally on ultrasound.
- Overall mortality of 50% from lung hypoplasia, abnormal pulmonary vasculature, and pulmonary hypertension.
- Never an emergency. Gas exchange should be optimized, preferably with FiO_2 <0.5, before surgery. This is not always possible.
- Usually already intubated and ventilated. Ventilatory support can include high-frequency oscillation (HFO) and NO.
- An NGT essential preoperatively to prevent the stomach and small bowel in the chest cavity from compressing the lung.

Perioperative
- Cautious ventilation via a face mask, and avoid N_2O to prevent distension of air in the bowel and stomach causing mediastinal displacement.
- An NGT, two IV cannulae, an arterial line, preferably in the right radial artery for preductal sampling. Oesophageal stethoscope with temperature probe.
- Avoid excessive airway pressures (preferably <25cmH$_2$O) because of pulmonary hypoplasia and consequent risk of pneumothorax. Use rate in first instance to improve gas exchange.
- High-dose fentanyl (25 micrograms/kg) to reduce pulmonary vasoconstriction response to surgical stress.
- High-risk babies will need the operation on special care baby unit if conventional ventilation not possible.

Post-operative
- Post-operative ventilation for at least 24hr, then attempt to wean.
- Infant may deteriorate within 12hr due to pulmonary hypertensive crises. Pulmonary vasculature is reduced and abnormal. Smooth

muscle in the media fails to regress; therefore, there is an exaggerated vasoconstrictive response to hypoxaemia and acidosis.
- Rarely, if minimal defect, extubate immediately.

Special considerations
- Pulmonary hypertension is treated by assisted hyperventilation with 100% O_2 and fluid boluses, if necessary. Epoprostenol or N_2O can be used for surgery. Extracorporeal membrane oxygenation (ECMO) is a last resort but has been used.
- To assist weaning, a thoracic epidural may be of benefit, inserted either conventionally or via the caudal route.

Gastroschisis/exomphalos

Procedure	Replacement of abdominal contents into the abdominal cavity
Time	2hr
Pain	++/+++
Position	Supine
Blood loss	Moderate
Practical techniques	GA + IPPV

Preoperative

- Obvious neonatal diagnosis from birth, but usually diagnosed *in utero*. Overall incidence is 1:3000–4000.
- Gastroschisis is a defect in the anterior abdominal wall usually on the right, causing herniation of abdominal contents without a covering sac. Repair is an urgent procedure.
- In exomphalos, there is a failure of the gut to return to the abdominal cavity during fetal development, resulting in persistent herniation through the extra embryonal part of the umbilical cord, which covers it. This may include other abdominal organs.
- There is an increased incidence of associated anomalies, including cardiac disease in exomphalos. A full cardiology assessment should be performed.
- Gastroschisis is associated with low birthweight and thickened bowel wall due to exposure to amniotic fluid.
- Exposed abdominal contents result in large evaporative heat and water losses and predispose to infection. They should initially be covered with cling film or equivalent.

Perioperative

- May already be intubated and ventilated. Otherwise intubate conventionally.
- NGT and oesophageal temperature/stethoscope.
- Two IV cannulae for maintenance and volume.
- Arterial monitoring may be useful.
- Heat conservation is important. Warm the theatre, and use a warming mattress, hot air mattress, or radiant heater. Keep the patient's head covered. Use warmed fluids.
- Fluid losses may be considerable.
- Intraoperative analgesia: fentanyl 1.5–10 micrograms/kg or epidural if extubation within 48hr is contemplated.

Post-operative

- Post-operative ventilation, especially if the abdomen is tense, should be in the head-up position.

- Assiduous attention to fluid balance. There may be large abdominal losses of crystalloid and protein.

Special considerations
- Lines should be sited in the arms, as abdominal distension may impair venous return from the lower body.
- Simpler to insert a percutaneous long line or central line at this stage for parenteral feeding. Post-operatively, progressive oedema makes cannulation more difficult.
- Manual ventilation is useful to assess the effect of replacement of abdominal contents on lung compliance to determine the correct degree of abdominal reduction.
- Complete reduction is not always possible. A silo is then created around the extra-abdominal contents to be gradually reduced on the ICU. Fluid loss and infection are major issues.

Tracheo-oesophageal fistula

Procedure	Ligation of fistula plus anastomotic repair of oesophageal atresia
Time	2hr
Pain	+++
Position	Left lateral for right thoracotomy
Blood loss	Moderate
Practical techniques	GA + IPPV ± manual ventilation

Preoperative

- Incidence: 1:3500. The commonest type (85%) is oesophageal atresia with a distal fistula. The majority of cases are now diagnosed *in utero*. It should always be excluded in cases of hydramnios.
- High incidence of prematurity (30%) and cardiac disease (25%).
- Presents clinically with choking and cyanotic episodes on feeding, with an inability to pass an NGT.
- Constant risk of pulmonary aspiration. A double-lumen Replogle tube in the oesophagus allows irrigation and suction.

Perioperative

- Inhalational or IV induction. Gentle mask ventilation to minimize gastric distension via a fistula.
- Careful ETT placement. Confirm symmetrical ventilation with the tube distal to the fistula.
- Two IV cannulae for maintenance and volume. Arterial line is useful.
- Intraoperative access will be needed to pass the transanastomotic tube nasally to facilitate oesophageal repair.
- Manual ventilation may be necessary to assess lung compliance after ligation of the fistula, to assist in repair of the oesophagus and to periodically reinflate the left lung. Surgical retraction may impede ventilation.
- Intraoperative analgesia: fentanyl (5–10 micrograms/kg) or epidural either by the thoracic or caudal route, if early weaning is anticipated.
- The operation is usually performed via a right thoracotomy, using an extrapleural approach. Thoracoscopic repair is becoming popular.

Post-operative

- The majority of cases are ventilated post-operatively, especially if the oesophageal repair is under tension. It is critical to secure the NGT or transanastomotic tube.

Special considerations

- Attention to the positioning of the ETT to avoid ventilating the stomach via the fistula. Preoperative bronchoscopy may be useful. The fistula is normally situated on the posterior aspect of the trachea, just proximal to the carina. The tube may need to be advanced or withdrawn, or the bevel rotated.

Patent ductus arteriosus

Procedure	Ligation or clipping of ductus arteriosus
Time	1hr
Pain	+
Position	Left thoracotomy
Blood loss	Usually minimal. Occasionally massive if the vessel is torn
Practical techniques	IPPV, fentanyl

Preoperative
- Small premature babies: 25% of premature infants <1.5kg recovering from hyaline membrane disease have a patent ductus arteriosus. Associated with other cardiac anomalies.
- Indications are for failure of medical treatment, ventilator dependence, and risk of developing bronchopulmonary dysplasia.

Perioperative
- High-risk group. Operation may be undertaken on the special care baby unit.
- Patient is usually already ventilated with full monitoring.
- Adequate IV access for transfusion. Arterial monitoring.
- IPPV with O_2, N_2O, and fentanyl up to 10 micrograms/kg with a low dose of volatile agent. Replace N_2O with air if frail.
- Active heat conservation.
- Avoid saturations >96% because of retinopathy of prematurity.
- Local infiltration for analgesia, interpleural block by surgeon, or thoracic epidural if early weaning considered.

Post-operative
- Post-operative ventilation until stable, then attempt to wean.

Special considerations
- Sudden ligation of the ductus may precipitate an acute rise in systemic BP and increase the risk of intraventricular haemorrhage. The duct should be clamped gently, or alternatively the concentration of the volatile agent can be temporarily increased.
- Older children requiring patent ductus arteriosus occlusion tend to be fit, although some present with cardiac failure. Procedure can be performed radiologically as a day case using a coil device.

Pyloric stenosis

Procedure	Splitting the pylorus muscle longitudinally down to the mucosa
Time	30min
Pain	+
Position	Supine
Blood loss	Minimal
Practical techniques	GA + IPPV, ? RSI

Preoperative

- Incidence of 1:350 births; commoner in first-born ♂; 80% are ♂, 10% are premature.
- Present with biochemical abnormalities, notably hypochloraemic alkalosis. Operation is never urgent, and full resuscitation should occur.
- Electrolytes, particularly Cl^- and HCO_3^-, and pH should be within normal limits, with $Cl^- \geq 100mmol/L$.

Perioperative

- No complete agreement, but there is a risk of pulmonary aspiration from gastric outflow obstruction.
- An NGT is mandatory and will be *in situ*. Aspirate, and do not remove. It does not reduce the effect of cricoid pressure and may act as an escape valve if mask ventilation increases intragastric pressure.
- IV is usually in place. Induction may be rapid sequence or non-depolarizing relaxant, for which some anaesthetists use cricoid pressure. Consider rapid sequence if there is excessive NG loss (>2mL/kg/hr).
- Fentanyl (1 microgram/kg) plus paracetamol IV/PR. Local infiltration (up to 1mL/kg of 0.25% bupivacaine ± adrenaline). If locally given pre-incision, fentanyl can be omitted.
- Can be performed laparoscopically, in which case a rectus sheath block may be useful.
- Extubate awake in the left lateral position.

Post-operative

- Remove the NGT at the end of the procedure.
- Give paracetamol PO/PR, as required.
- Feed within 6hr, but maintain IV fluids until feeding is established.
- Apnoea alarm overnight.

Special considerations

- Resuscitate with 5% glucose/0.45% NaCl plus 20mmol/L KCl (HCO_3^- <32mmol/L). More severe cases will require 0.9% NaCl. Use colloid initially if hypovolaemia is present. Replace NG loss with 0.9% NaCl.

Intussusception

Procedure	Reduction of invaginated bowel
Time	1–2hr
Pain	+++
Position	Supine
Blood loss	Moderate, may be large
Practical techniques	RSI + IPPV

Preoperative
- Intussusception is the commonest cause of obstruction in infants over 2 months of age; incidence is 2:1000 births.
- Invagination of the bowel into an adjacent lower segment, usually at the terminal ileum or ileocaecal valve. Rarely caused by a polyp or Meckel's diverticulum (5% of cases).
- Presents with paroxysmal pain, blood, and mucus in stool (redcurrant jelly stool), and a sausage-shaped mass in the right abdomen.
- Seventy per cent of cases are reduced by air or barium enema.
- Child may be profoundly shocked. Urgent fluid resuscitation with gastric decompression and electrolyte correction will be needed. Colloid and blood may be required. Delay can result in perforated or necrotic bowel. Fluid loss may be greater than expected.

Perioperative
- RSI. Retain the NGT *in situ*.
- Fentanyl 2–5 micrograms/kg plus volatile agent. Consider an epidural if stable.
- Two cannulae of adequate size. CVP line in severe cases.
- Routine monitoring, temperature measurement, and urinary catheter.
- Prolonged intussusception with ischaemic gut requiring resection often leads to metabolic acidosis and septic shock. Admission to a paediatric ICU will be required.

Post-operative
- Epidural, TAP block, or local wound infiltration, and morphine NCA.

Special considerations
No consensus as to whether the child should receive surgery at the base hospital or be transferred to a regional centre. If transferred, this should not delay resuscitation or blood cross-match, which can be sent with the patient.

Herniotomy

Procedure	Excision of patent processus vaginalis
Time	20min
Pain	++
Position	Supine
Blood loss	Minimal
Practical techniques	SV + LMA, caudal or regional block. IPPV, caudal or local infiltration. Spinal or caudal block

Preoperative

- Otherwise fit ASA 1 child. Commoner in boys.
- Twenty per cent of preterm babies present for surgery at ~40wk post-conceptual age or when ready to leave the special care baby unit.

Perioperative

- Inhalational or IV induction with laryngeal mask, then caudal or ilioinguinal block and intraoperative opioids if necessary.
- For infants, intubate with controlled ventilation. With neonates, avoid ilioinguinal block, as spread of LA may obscure the surgical field. Use either caudal or post-operative infiltration.
- Diclofenac or paracetamol suppository. Alternatively paracetamol IV.

Post-operative

- Day case: regular paracetamol and ibuprofen.
- Term babies in the 1st 4wk of life and ex-premature infants up to 60wk post-conceptual age should be admitted overnight for pulse oximetry and apnoea alarm monitoring.

Special considerations

- The majority of herniotomy repairs are in healthy children and suitable as day cases.
- There is no consensus as to the most appropriate regional block. Caudal blockade is indicated for bilateral herniotomy repair and children up to 20kg. Ilioinguinal block is effective in children over 5kg (see p. 810 and p. 814).
- Laparoscopic repair is becoming commoner. Local infiltration provides adequate analgesia.
- The ex-premature baby may be small for dates and O_2-dependent with chronic lung disease. Post-operative apnoea and bradycardia are documented risks associated with GA for this group. Hypocarbia and hypothermia should be avoided, and O_2 saturation between 90% and 95% is acceptable. Caffeine (10mg/kg IV) given at induction reduces the risk of apnoea by 70%.

- To avoid GA, a spinal technique may be used (see ➲ p. 813). This may be technically difficult and complicated by a bloody or dry tap. It is too short-acting for bilateral repair. A single-shot caudal is an alternative method. Supplementary sedation results in the same risk of post-operative apnoea as with GA.
- A strangulated hernia that does not reduce is an emergency and requires fluid resuscitation and an NGT. Precautions should be taken against regurgitation and aspiration.

Further reading

Craven PD, Badawi N, Henderson-Smart DJ, O'Brien M (2003). Regional (spinal, epidural, caudal) versus general anaesthesia in preterm infants undergoing inguinal herniorrhaphy in early infancy. *Cochrane Database Syst Rev*, **3**, CD003669.

Circumcision

Procedure	Removal of prepuce (foreskin)
Time	20min
Pain	++
Position	Supine
Blood loss	Minimal
Practical techniques	SV, LMA, caudal/penile block/ring block

Preoperative
- Common day-case procedure, but move towards more conservative management, including simple stretch or preputioplasty.
- Obtain consent for a suppository and regional block.

Perioperative
- Inhalational or IV induction. Laryngeal mask.
- Regional block: caudal, penile block, or ring block (see ➲ p. 810, p. 814, and p. 1122).
- Diclofenac or paracetamol suppository. Alternatively paracetamol IV.

Post-operative
- Regular paracetamol and ibuprofen.
- Topical lidocaine gel can be applied frequently, without exceeding the toxic dose.

Special considerations
- A regional block must be performed prior to the surgery.
- There is no consensus as to the optimal strategy for pain relief. Caudal is technically easier in infants, and penile block may be more suitable in children over 10kg. Ring block is easier in boys >5kg, producing excellent and consistent analgesia. All methods are effective.
- Circumcision is one of the most painful day-case procedures; parents should be warned and advised to apply topical gel regularly and continue paracetamol for several days.

Orchidopexy

Procedure	Release of undescended testis into scrotum
Time	30min
Pain	++
Position	Supine
Blood loss	Minimal
Practical techniques	SV, LMA + regional block

Preoperative

- Boys, usually over 2yr (2% of population).
- Common day-case procedure.
- Obtain consent for a suppository and regional block.

Perioperative

- Inhalational or IV induction. Laryngeal mask.
- Regional technique: caudal, ilioinguinal block, or local infiltration.
- Diclofenac or paracetamol suppository. Alternatively paracetamol IV.
- Give supplementary opioids, if indicated.

Post-operative

- Regular paracetamol and ibuprofen. Morphine sulfate solution, if necessary.

Special considerations

- Adequate analgesia is difficult if the testis is high. In this case, aim for a high-volume, low-concentration mid-thoracic caudal block. Use 1.25mL/kg of 0.19% bupivacaine (three parts of 0.25% bupivacaine, one part of normal saline) (see ➲ p. 810 and p. 811).
- If an ilioinguinal block is used, only the anterior of the scrotum is anaesthetized; use local infiltration for the scrotal incision (see ➲ p. 814 and p. 1122).
- Testicular traction, even with a seemingly adequate blockade, may lead to intraoperative bradycardia or laryngospasm, especially with an ilioinguinal block. Surgery should be stopped, and anaesthesia deepened; supplementary opioids may be required.
- Suspected torsion of the testis is a surgical emergency, and the need for an RSI will have to be considered. Analgesic techniques are as before.
- A high testis may need surgery in two stages. The 1st procedure is to identify the testis and, if possible, bring it down to the inguinal ring. This is usually performed laparoscopically and will require intubation, controlled ventilation with intraoperative opioids, and PR diclofenac or IV/PR paracetamol.

Hypospadias

Procedure	Restoration of urethral opening to the tip of the penis
Time	1–3hr
Pain	++
Position	Supine
Blood loss	Minimal
Practical techniques	SV/IPPV + regional block

Preoperative

- Usually an isolated problem, but there may be an association with certain rare dysmorphic syndromes.
- Obtain consent for a suppository and regional block.

Perioperative

- Inhalational or IV induction.
- If procedure <1hr, use LMA plus SV.
- If procedure >1hr, use LMA or ETT plus IPPV.
- Extended caudal: 1mL/kg of 0.25% bupivacaine with clonidine/ morphine.
- Diclofenac or paracetamol suppository. Alternatively paracetamol IV.
- Employ heat conservation measures.

Post-operative

- Regular NSAIDs/paracetamol. Consider morphine NCA (not always necessary).
- Opioids can be used in the caudal block, because the patient will be catheterized, but they must be admitted overnight (see ⮕ p. 810 and p. 811).

Special considerations

- May be a simple procedure, e.g. meatal advancement and glanduloplasty (MAGPI), or extensive involving a buccal mucosa graft. The anaesthetic technique can be adjusted accordingly.
- Avoid erection with a regional block plus an adequate depth of anaesthesia.

Cleft lip and palate

Procedure	Repair of defect in upper lip and palate
Time	1–2hr
Pain	++
Position	Supine, head ring, shoulder support
Blood loss	Minimal for cleft lip. Moderate for cleft palate
Practical techniques	IPPV. Armoured or RAE tube

Preoperative

- Incidence of 1:300–600 births but can be 1:25 where there is a family history.
- Both the lip and palate are involved together in 50% of cases.
- Isolated cleft palate incidence is 1:2000 live births. Increased incidence of congenital abnormalities.
- Associated syndromes often involve a difficult airway, e.g. Pierre–Robin, Treacher–Collins, and Goldenhar syndromes. Therefore, make a careful assessment of the airway.
- Discuss risks and complications. Obtain consent for suppository.
- Administer IM atropine 20 micrograms/kg 30min preoperatively if a difficult airway is suspected.

Perioperative

- Inhalational or IV induction. When there is a suspected airway problem, perform inhalational induction with sevoflurane and CPAP (see ⮕ p. 800 and p. 804). Intubate deep with the child breathing spontaneously or following muscle relaxant once a safe airway has been established. Videolaryngoscopy or a Bullard laryngoscope may be useful.
- A preformed RAE tube may be obstructed or kinked by the gag, especially the smaller sizes. A reinforced tube will resist compression but needs to be carefully secured at the correct length.
- IPPV preferable.
- Use a throat pack, and make sure the eyes are protected.
- The surgeon usually places the gag. Encourage LA infiltration to improve analgesia and reduce blood loss.
- Fentanyl (2–4 micrograms/kg) and paracetamol IV/PR or diclofenac PR plus local infiltration. Clonidine or ketamine can be used as part of an opioid-sparing technique.
- Dexamethasone 0.1mg/kg may prevent post-operative swelling.
- Consider an infraorbital nerve block for cleft lip repair and a nasopalatine plus palatine block for palatal surgery.
- Morphine 0.1 mg/kg prior to reversal or ketamine 0.5mg/kg IM if the infant is floppy or hypotonic.

Post-operative

- Extubate awake. Suction the pharynx early and carefully to prevent damage to the repair.
- Nasal stents may be inserted to maintain patency of the airway. A tongue stitch is rarely used.
- Routine post-operative analgesia to include regular paracetamol and ibuprofen, and morphine sulfate solution PRN. IV morphine may be required initially.

Special considerations

- Intubation is usually uncomplicated.
- The laryngoscope blade rarely lodges in the cleft. If there is a problem, a roll of gauze can fill the gap.
- Prolonged surgery may cause a swollen tongue from pressure of the mouth gag.
- Cleft palate repair can produce upper airways obstruction, and extreme care is needed for extubation.
- With airway problems, opioids should be given cautiously. Post-operative monitoring should include pulse oximetry and apnoea alarm.
- Cleft lip is usually repaired at 3 months, and cleft palate at 6–9 months. The lip may be repaired at the neonatal stage to improve the scar and assist maternal bonding. There is little evidence to support this.

Congenital talipes equinovarus

Procedure	Correction of club foot abnormality
Time	45min–1hr
Pain	++
Position	Supine, sometimes prone for posterior release
Blood loss	Minimal
Practical techniques	SV, LMA, caudal. If prone, then ETT + IPPV, caudal

Preoperative
- Occurs in 1:1000 births.
- Usually an isolated anomaly but may occur in association with some myopathic diseases, hence increased theoretical risk of malignant hyperthermia.
- Obtain consent for a suppository and regional block.

Perioperative
- Inhalational or IV induction with LMA. If prone, intubate and ventilate. Give additional opioids, if indicated.
- Extended caudal blockade: 1mL/kg of 0.25% bupivacaine (see ➲ p. 810 and p. 811).
- PR diclofenac or paracetamol PR/IV.

Post-operative
Give regular paracetamol and ibuprofen plus morphine sulfate solution PRN and antiemetic, if required.

Special considerations
For prolonged pain relief, either top up the caudal at the end of the procedure by using an indwelling 22G or 20G cannula or extend the duration of the block by adding clonidine (1–2 micrograms/kg) to the initial dose of bupivacaine.

Femoral osteotomy

Procedure	Stabilizing the hip in congenital dislocation by realigning the proximal femur
Time	2hr
Pain	+++
Position	Supine
Blood loss	Moderate/potentially large
Practical techniques	SV + LMA or ETT + IPPV + caudal/epidural

Preoperative

- Usually an isolated defect. Commoner in girls or where there is a family history.
- Obtain consent for a suppository and regional block.

Perioperative

- Inhalational or IV induction. SV plus LMA or ETT plus IPPV.
- Adequate IV access.
- Caudal block plus clonidine (see ➲ p. 810 and p. 811). Avoid caudal opioids because of risk of urinary retention. Alternatively lumbar epidural or intraoperative opioids (see ➲ p. 813 and p. 808).
- Paracetamol IV/PR or diclofenac PR.
- Employ heat conservation measures.
- Attention to blood loss.

Post-operative

- Epidural infusion (Table 34.13).
- Extended caudal or morphine NCA, with regular NSAIDs and paracetamol (see ➲ p. 808).
- A hip spica provides support and helps with pain relief.

Special considerations

- Blood loss may be extensive if revision surgery.
- A hip spica complicates urinary retention in girls.

Inhaled foreign body

Procedure	Removal of foreign body from bronchial tree
Time	30–60min
Pain	+
Position	Supine
Blood loss	Nil
Practical techniques	SV or IPPV

Preoperative
- Commonest reason for bronchoscopy in the 1–3yr age group.
- A foreign body in the upper airways may present as an emergency acute airway obstruction.
- Obstruction of lower airways follows several days after a history of coughing. Peanut oil is an irritant and leads to mucosal oedema and chemical pneumonitis. Chest radiograph shows characteristic hyperinflation during expiration, but a foreign body is often not visible.
- Treat symptoms as indicated, e.g. dehydration, pneumonia, wheeze.

Perioperative
- Inhalational induction is usual to avoid displacing the object further. Use 100% O_2 with sevoflurane.
- Deep inhalational maintenance with sevoflurane. TIVA is becoming a more popular technique, usually supplementing the volatile agent.
- Apply topical anaesthesia to the vocal cords (4% lidocaine, up to 3mg/kg), and consider a drying agent (atropine 20 micrograms/kg IM 30min preoperatively or 10 micrograms/kg IV at induction, or glycopyrronium 5 micrograms/kg IM or IV).
- Prior to bronchoscopy, maintain the airway with a face mask or LMA.
- Rigid bronchoscopy: the Storz bronchoscope has an attachment for a T-piece. Check compatibility before the procedure.
- For foreign objects in the upper airways, maintain SV.
- If the foreign body is in the lower airway, then IPPV with a muscle relaxant is acceptable, since the object will be pushed distally by the bronchoscope until it can be grasped by forceps. Give assisted ventilation via a T-piece or high-frequency jet ventilation. Intubation will then be required once the scope is removed.
- This may be a difficult surgical procedure.

Post-operative

- If bronchoscopy is traumatic, give dexamethasone 0.25mg/kg IV, then two doses 8-hourly of 0.125mg/kg.
- Consider physiotherapy, bronchodilators, and antibiotics, as indicated.

Special considerations

- If tracheal/ball–valve obstruction suspected, IPPV is contraindicated.
- Intubation may assist lung ventilation and sizing of the bronchoscope if a tracheal foreign body is excluded.

Medical problems

Acute laryngotracheobronchitis (croup)

- Croup occurs predominantly in epidemics in autumn and early spring. The peak age of incidence is 6 months to 2yr. It is viral in aetiology. The majority of cases are due to parainfluenza, but influenza and respiratory syncytial virus are possible.
- Symptoms are coryzal for the 1st few days but then progress to a characteristic barking cough/hoarseness, with profuse secretions and occasional dysphagia. Pyrexia is mild or absent.
- The larynx, trachea, and bronchi are all involved and become more oedematous, leading to the onset of stridor. An anxious child will exacerbate the condition, as the trachea will tend to collapse on inspiration.
- The majority of children respond to conservative measures and reassurance. There is no evidence to support the use of humidified steam tents. In severe cases, steroids (dexamethasone 0.25mg/kg IV, followed by two further doses 8-hourly of 0.125mg/kg) and nebulized adrenaline (0.5mg/kg, up to a maximum of 5mg) are required.
- Ten per cent of children are admitted, and 1% will require intubation.
- The majority of children have a single isolated episode.

Acute epiglottitis

- This is an acute life-threatening infection caused by Hib. It most commonly presents at 2–3yr.
- There is a rapid onset of oedema of the epiglottis and aryepiglottic folds. The child has a high temperature, usually >39.5°C, and presents sitting or leaning forwards, with drooling saliva, and unable to swallow, with the tongue pushed forwards. Inspiratory and expiratory stridor is rapidly progressive and a late sign.
- Acute epiglottitis is a medical emergency. The antibiotic of choice is ceftriaxone (50mg/kg IV once daily). Intubation is indicated in 60% of cases; in some centres, all children are routinely intubated.
- Following the introduction of the Hib vaccine, this condition is now rare.

Anaesthetic management

- The differential diagnosis between croup and epiglottitis is not always obvious. If epiglottitis is even remotely suspected, there must be liaison with an ENT surgeon at consultant level.
- Induction occurs in the anaesthetic room or operating theatre, with the full range of appropriate equipment and monitoring available.
- During anaesthesia, the ENT surgeon should be scrubbed in theatre, with the tracheostomy set open.
- Traditionally, IV access has been contraindicated prior to induction because of the risk of acute glottic closure. However, the use of a topical cream facilitates an atraumatic venepuncture. Unless access is obviously difficult, cannulation should proceed before anaesthesia.

- Inhalational induction is performed in the sitting position, with sevoflurane in 100% O_2. Once anaesthetized, the child can be moved to a more recumbent position and maintained with sevoflurane, up to concentrations of 8%, if needed. CPAP should be routinely applied, but the airway is not usually difficult to maintain.
- In croup, laryngoscopy is usually straightforward, but the ETT required may be surprisingly narrow. Start with one size smaller than normal. Older children may require a tube that has been cut to a longer length. If possible, once the airway is secure, the child should be reintubated nasally since this is better tolerated. Profuse secretions are always a problem, and frequent suction is necessary. Intubation is usually required for at least 2–3d, and bronchoscopy is indicated if an air leak around the tube fails to develop.
- With epiglottitis, intubation may be exceedingly difficult. Laryngoscopy often reveals an abnormal anatomy with no obvious glottic opening. Careful inspection may reveal movement of small amounts of mucus, indicating tidal flow. The child should be intubated, using a stylet, so that the ETT can be immediately railroaded, if necessary. The tube size will be smaller than predicted.
- Once intubation has been achieved, oedema rapidly settles. Following demonstration of a leak around the tube, extubation is normally possible within 36hr. Dexamethasone is often given prior to extubation to reduce laryngeal oedema.

Stabilization of the sick child (prior to PICU transfer)

- Anaesthetists may be required to assist with the stabilization of critically ill children, including difficult airway management, prior to surgery or transfer.
- Early contact and advice from the local paediatric intensive care retrieval team. Initial resuscitation remains the responsibility of the local medical teams.
- This will frequently involve the coordination of multidisciplinary teams, including paediatricians, intensivists, anaesthetists, and surgeons. Management of sick children should follow a systematic, evidence-based approach.
- These cases will often take place away from theatres and familiar surroundings. The availability of a trained assistant is essential.
- Checklists for drugs and equipment, as well as emergency 'grab bags', will improve readiness. 'Run-throughs' or simulation *in situ* will improve familiarity and identify potential problems with working in unfamiliar locations.

General principles

Airway and breathing

- Indications for intubation:
  - Control of ventilation (respiratory failure, head injury)
  - Protection of airway (low conscious level, facial trauma, burns).
- Cuffed tube, if possible (see ➔ p. 791). Avoid pre-cutting smaller tubes. End-tidal capnography recommended.
- If equipment, monitoring, or personnel are not optimal, consider risk/ benefits of moving location, e.g. theatres.
- Induction: ketamine (0.5–2mg/kg) with suxamethonium (1.5mg/kg) is becoming more popular. Must be fluid-resuscitated first. Use reduced doses, if unstable.
- Ventilation—pressure control ventilation usually appropriate. Aim for normocapnia and O_2 saturations of 94–98%. PEEP is helpful if volume-resuscitated.
- Sedation—various regimens. Morphine and midazolam infusions are popular (Table 34.14). Propofol is acceptable for short transfers (remember analgesia).

Circulation

- Isotonic fluid for boluses: 20mL/kg repeated. Be aware that intubation more likely after 40mL/kg (if blood loss is the cause, then consider giving blood early, e.g. after 40mL/kg of fluid).
- Inotropes after discussion (Table 34.14). Dopamine can be given peripherally.
- IV access. Consider intraosseous, if difficult. Central access may be needed.
- Arterial line may be useful, but rarely essential.

Table 34.14 Infusion regimes of selected PICU drugs

Medication	Dosing details
Morphine infusion (sedation)	20–80 micrograms/kg/hr
If <50kg, 1mg/kg in 50mL	1mL/hr = 20 micrograms/kg/hr
If >50kg, 50mg in 50mL	(approximate)
Midazolam infusion (sedation)	50–200 micrograms/kg/hr
If <10kg, 5mg/kg in 50mL	1mL/hr = 100 micrograms/kg/hr
If >10kg, 50mg in 50mL	(approximate)
Propofol	2–5mg/kg/hr; titrate to effect
Dopamine infusion	2–10 micrograms/kg/min
<15kg	15mg/kg in 50mL (central access)
	1mL/hr = 5 micrograms/kg/min of this mix
	Halve concentration if giving peripherally
Dopamine infusion	2–10 micrograms/kg/min
>15kg	200mg in 50mL (central access)
	80mg in 50mL (peripheral access)
Adrenaline infusion	0.1–0.5 micrograms/kg/min
<15kg	0.3mg/kg in 50mL
	1mL/hr = 0.1 micrograms/kg/min of this mix
Adrenaline infusion	0.1–0.5 micrograms/kg/min
>15kg	4mg in 50mL

Further reading

Guidelines and drug calculators. Many exist. Consider local retrieval service website.

Children's Acute Transport Service (CATS, North Thames). ℛ http://site.cats.nhs.uk/.

Managing Emergencies in Paediatric Anaesthesia (MEPA). [Simulation training.] ℛ https://mepa.org.uk.

Spotting the Sick Child. [Education and case studies.] ℛ http://www.spottingthesickchild.com/.

Sedation

- The expansion of imaging techniques, together with new diagnostic and therapeutic interventions, has led to a rise in demand for sedation services.
- Compared with GA, sedation is neither cheaper nor safer. Safety is paramount, and the requirements, in terms of personnel and resuscitation equipment, are the same.
- With current staff shortages, anaesthetists are not always available to administer sedation, and other medical or nursing personnel may be involved. Sedation guidelines are essential.[22]
- Facilities must include sufficient space for a trolley and monitoring and resuscitation equipment, together with all personnel necessary to sedate the child and carry out the specific procedure. All standard anaesthetic equipment should be available for resuscitation.
- Each sedated child must be supervised by an appropriate nurse or doctor trained in paediatric resuscitation. Experienced medical staff must be immediately available to assist with sedation problems or resuscitation. There must be a contingency for overnight admission if recovery is prolonged.
- The adult concept of sedation with verbal contact maintained is not practical in children. There may be little difference between deep sedation, as defined by the American Academy of Pediatrics, and uncontrolled anaesthesia. Ideal conditions achieve depression of the nervous system, allowing the relevant procedures to occur, with preservation of the airway reflexes. In practice, this is difficult to achieve.
- It is important not to confuse sedation with analgesia. Painful procedures may require a topical anaesthetic cream, infiltration with LAs, and occasionally systemic opioids.
- Contraindications include children with airway problems, apnoeic episodes, respiratory disease, raised ICP, risk of pulmonary aspiration, and epilepsy.
- The most frequently used oral sedative drugs are chloral hydrate (50–100mg/kg), triclofos (50–75mg/kg), and, to a lesser extent, benzodiazepines, alimemazine, and ketamine. Opioids are also used in combination with other sedatives.
- Midazolam (0.5mg/kg PO) or in incremental bolus doses of 0.05mg/kg IV, up to a maximum dose of 0.2mg/kg, can produce good conditions for sedation and has the additional property of amnesia. Ketamine (6mg/kg PO or 1–2mg/kg IV) is indicated for short, painful procedures and may be used in combination with midazolam. Emergence delirium is less of a problem with children, but a drying agent is often required.
- Propofol can be used alone or in combination with remifentanil for endoscopy sedation, but the use of both drugs should be reserved for anaesthetists.[23]
- Emergency physicians are increasingly using IV ketamine 'sedation' for short, painful procedures. This is a controversial practice in the UK. Anyone using anaesthetic agents must have the full range of skills required for their safe use.

- With appropriate planning, organization, and safety, nurse-led sedation services have been developed at several centres following strict protocols. The children are fasted conventionally but allowed unrestricted clear fluids. A pulse oximeter is mandatory. Surprisingly young children can tolerate scans awake with encouragement, careful explanation, and parental presence.

References

22 National Institute for Health and Care Excellence (2010). *Sedation in children and young people: sedation for diagnostic and therapeutic procedures in children and young people.* ℘ http://www.nice.org.uk/CG112.

23 Berkenbosch JW, Graft GR, Stort JM, Tobias J (2004). Use of a remifentanil-propofol mixture for paediatric flexible fiberoptic bronchoscopy sedation. *Paediatr Anaesth*, **14**, 941–6.

Further reading

Association of Paediatric Anaesthetists of Great Britain and Ireland. ℘ http://www.apagbi.org.uk.

Baum VC, O'Flaherty JE (1999). *Anaesthesia for genetic, metabolic and dysmorphic syndromes of childhood.* Philadelphia: Lippincott, Williams & Wilkins.

Bingham R, Lloyd Thomas A, Sury M, eds. (2007). *Hatch and Sumner's textbook of paediatric anaesthesia.* London: Hodder Arnold.

Black A, McEwan A (2004). *Paediatric & neonatal anaesthesia: anaesthesia in a nutshell.* Edinburgh: Butterworth-Heinemann.

Hammer G, Holzki J, Morton N (2009). The paediatric airway. *Paediatr Anaesth*, **19** (Suppl 1), 1–197.

National Confidential Enquiry into Patient Outcome and Death (NCEPOD) (2011). *Are we there yet? A review of organizational and clinical aspects of children's surgery.* ℘ http://www.ncepod.org.uk/2011sic.htm.

Online Mendelian Inheritance in Man. [Database of human genes and genetic disorders from Johns Hopkins University, with links to Medline and PubMed.] ℘ http://www.ncbi.nlm.nih.gov/omim.

Orphanet portal. [Summary of rare syndromes and diseases.] ℘ http://www.orpha.net.

Williams G (2012). Analgesic regimens for children. In: Johnston I, Harrop-Griffiths W, Gemmell L, eds. *AAGBI core topics in anaesthesia 2012.* Chichester: Wiley-Blackwell, pp. 72–87.

Table 34.15 Paediatric quick reference guide

Age	Approximate weight (kg)	Body surface area (m²)	Percentage of adult drug dose (approximate)	ETT size (mm)	ETT length (cm)	LMA size	Suxamethonium dose (mg) IV	Atropine dose (micrograms) IV
Term	3.5	0.23	12.5 (1/8th)	3.5	9	1	7	35
1 month	4.2	0.26	14.5	3.5	10	1	8	40
3 months	6	0.33	15	3.5	10	1.5	12	60
6 months	7.5	0.38	22	3.5/4.0	11	1.5	15	75
1yr	10	0.47	25 (1/4)	4.0	12	1.5/2	20	100
2yr	12	0.53	30	4.5	13	2	24	120
3yr	14	0.61	33	4.5/5	13/14	2	28	140
5yr	18	0.73	40	5.0/5.5	14.5	2.5	36	180
7yr	22	0.86	50 (1/2)	6.0	15.5	2.5	44	220
10yr	30	1.10	60	6.5 cuffed	17	3	60	300
12yr	38	1.30	75 (3/4)	7.0 cuffed	18	3 or 4	75	380

Note: weights are approximations only. Patients should be weighed accurately.

The critically ill patient

Jerry Nolan

Immediate trauma care

(See also ➜ p. 476.)

Trauma networks

Severely injured patients who are treated in specialized trauma centres have better outcomes than those treated in smaller hospitals that treat relatively few such patients. Severely injured patients are transferred directly to a major trauma centre (MTC), unless they have immediately life-threatening injuries that require initial stabilization at the nearest trauma unit (usually a district general hospital) before 2° transfer to the MTC.

Preparation

Advance warning before the arrival of a severely injured patient in the emergency department enables emergency department staff to alert the trauma team and prepare essential resuscitation drugs, fluid, and equipment before the patient's arrival.

The trauma team

Trauma patient resuscitation is most efficient if undertaken by a team of doctors and nurses; in this way, several tasks can be undertaken simultaneously.

Immediate care—Advanced Trauma Life Support®

The ATLS®[1] programme provides a framework on which the immediate management of the trauma patient is based. The initial management is considered in four phases:
- Primary survey
- Resuscitation
- Secondary survey
- Definitive care.

The first two phases are undertaken simultaneously. The secondary survey, or head-to-toe examination of the patient, is not started until the patient has been resuscitated adequately.

Reference

1 American College of Surgeons Committee on Trauma (2012). *Advanced Trauma Life Support®* for *doctors. Student course manual*, 9th edn. Chicago: American College of Surgeons.

Primary survey and resuscitation

The primary survey ('ABC principles') comprises a sequential search for immediately life-threatening injuries:
- Airway with cervical spine control.
- Breathing.
- Circulation and haemorrhage control.
- Disability—a rapid assessment of neurological function.
- Exposure—while considering the environment and preventing hypothermia.

Airway and the cervical spine

The priority during resuscitation of any severely injured patient is to ensure a clear airway and maintain oxygenation. Use basic airway manoeuvres, with or without adjuncts such as an oropharyngeal and nasopharyngeal airway. Give the patient high-concentration O_2; in the unintubated, spontaneously breathing patient, this is delivered with a mask and reservoir (non-rebreathing) bag—FiO_2 0.85.

Assume the presence of a spinal injury in any patient who has sustained significant blunt trauma, until clearance procedures have been completed. This implies that the patient has been examined by an experienced clinician and radiological procedures have been completed. A reliable clinical examination cannot be obtained if the patient:
- Has sustained a significant closed head injury.
- Is intoxicated.
- Has a reduced conscious level from any other cause.
- Has significant pain from an injury, which 'distracts' attention from the neck.

Tracheal intubation

Indications for immediate intubation of the severely injured patient include:
- Airway obstruction unrelieved by basic airway manoeuvres
- Impending airway obstruction, e.g. from facial burns and inhalation injury
- GCS <9 (to facilitate CT scanning, intubation is required in many patients with a GCS >9)
- Haemorrhage from maxillofacial injuries compromising the airway
- Respiratory failure 2° to chest or neurological injury
- The need for resuscitative surgery
- Uncooperative patients requiring further investigations.

The best technique for emergency intubation of a severely injured patient with a potential cervical spine injury is:
- Manual in-line stabilization of the cervical spine by an assistant whose hands grasp the mastoid processes and hold the head down firmly on to the trolley; this reduces neck movement during intubation. Do not apply traction to the neck
- Preoxygenation
- IV induction of anaesthesia. All induction drugs have the potential to produce or worsen hypotension, and the choice of drug is less important than the way it is used. Extreme caution is essential in patients who may be hypovolaemic; whenever possible, give fluid before anaesthetic induction. In the hypovolaemic patient, ketamine is less likely than other induction drugs to cause profound hypotension

- Paralysis with suxamethonium 1.5mg/kg (though, in experienced hands, rocuronium 1mg/kg is acceptable, especially if sugammadex is immediately available)
- Application of cricoid pressure—using one or two hands (there is no strong evidence supporting one technique over the other)
- Direct laryngoscopy and oral intubation.

Placing the patient's head and neck in neutral alignment will tend to make the view at laryngoscopy difficult—expect 20% of patients to have a grade 3 view of the larynx; use of a GEB and either a videolaryngoscope or a McCoy levering laryngoscope is recommended. If intubation is impossible, a supraglottic airway (e.g. ProSeal LMA or i-Gel) will provide a temporary airway but may not prevent aspiration. Surgical cricothyroidotomy, using a scalpel and a 6.0mm internal diameter ETT, is indicated if the patient cannot be intubated by conventional methods (see also ➔ p. 913 and p. 952).

Breathing—immediately life-threatening chest injuries

- **Tension pneumothorax.** Reduced chest movement, reduced breath sounds, and a resonant percussion note on the affected side, along with respiratory distress, hypotension, and tachycardia, indicate a tension pneumothorax. Deviation of the trachea to the opposite side is a late sign, and neck veins may not be distended in the presence of hypovolaemia. Treatment is immediate decompression with either a large cannula placed in the 2nd intercostal space in the mid-clavicular line on the affected side or a rapid thoracostomy (small incision into the pleural space) in the 5th intercostal space in the anterior axillary line. Once IV access has been obtained, insert a large chest drain (32FG) in the 5th intercostal space (anterior axillary line), and connect to an underwater seal drain.
- **Open pneumothorax.** Cover an open pneumothorax with an occlusive dressing, and seal on three sides; the unsealed side should act as a flutter valve. Insert a chest drain away from the wound in the same hemithorax.
- **Massive haemothorax** (defined as >1500mL of blood in a hemithorax) will cause reduced chest movement and a dull percussion note, in the presence of hypoxaemia and hypovolaemia. Start fluid resuscitation, and insert a chest drain. The patient is likely to require a thoracotomy if blood loss from the chest drain exceeds 200mL per hour, but this decision will depend also on the patient's general physiological state.

Cardiac tamponade

- Consider cardiac tamponade while examining the chest, particularly if the patient has sustained a penetrating injury to the chest or upper abdomen.
- Distended neck veins in the presence of hypotension are suggestive of cardiac tamponade, although, after rapid volume resuscitation, myocardial contusion may also present in this way. Tension pneumothorax may also mimic tamponade.
- Muffled heart sounds are meaningless in the midst of a busy resuscitation room.

- Ultrasound examination in the resuscitation room is the best way to make the diagnosis, and focused assessment sonogram in trauma (FAST) scanning is becoming routine in most emergency departments.
- If cardiac tamponade is diagnosed or suspected after a penetrating injury and the patient is deteriorating, despite all resuscitative efforts, an urgent thoracotomy and pericardiotomy will be required. This is best undertaken in an operating theatre; however, *in extremis*, resuscitative thoracotomy should be undertaken in the emergency room.
- In the absence of a suitably experienced surgeon, pericardiocentesis may provide temporary relief from the tamponade, while awaiting definitive treatment; however, needle pericardiocentesis is often unsuccessful, because the pericardial blood is often clotted or re-accumulates rapidly once aspirated.

Circulation—management of hypovolaemia

(See also ➲ p. 762, p. 1049, p. 1001.)

Control external haemorrhage with direct pressure. Hypovolaemic shock is divided into four classes, according to the percentage of total blood volume lost and the associated symptoms and signs. Table 35.1 provides a rough guidance only—several recent studies have challenged the reliability of this classification, which is derived from the ATLS® course.

Haemorrhage alone, in the absence of significant tissue injury, causes relatively less tachycardia and is easily overlooked, particularly in young, fit people who are able to compensate to a remarkable degree. A decrease in systolic pressure suggests a loss of >30% of total blood volume (~1500mL

Table 35.1 Classification of hypovolaemic shock, according to blood loss (adult)

	Class I	Class II	Class III	Class IV
Blood loss (%)	<15	15–30	30–40	>40
Blood loss (mL)	750	800–1500	1500–2000	>2000
Systolic BP	Unchanged	Normal	Reduced	Very low
Diastolic BP	Unchanged	Raised	Reduced	Unrecordable
Pulse (bpm)	Slight tachycardia	100–120	120 (thready)	>120 (very thready)
Capillary refill	Normal	Slow (>2s)	Slow (>2s)	Undetectable
Respiratory rate	Normal	Tachypnoea	Tachypnoea (>20/min)	Tachypnoea (>20/min)
Urine output (mL/hr)	>30	20–30	10–20	0–10
Extremities	Normal	Pale	Pale	Pale, cold, clammy
Complexion	Normal	Pale	Pale	Ashen
Mental state	Alert	Anxious or aggressive	Anxious, aggressive, or drowsy	Drowsy, confused, or unconscious

in a 70kg adult). Reduced consciousness caused by hypovolaemia implies at least 40–50% loss of blood volume.

- Insert two short, large-bore IV cannulae (14G); take blood samples for FBC and electrolytes, and cross-match from the 1st cannula.
- If peripheral access is difficult, use an external jugular vein or femoral vein (avoid in abdominal/pelvic/leg injury).
- The intraosseous route (usually via the proximal tibia or proximal humerus) is useful, and modern devices enable the infusion of fluids at up to 200mL/min, which makes this route useful for fluid resuscitation of adults as well as children.
- Insert an arterial cannula for continuous direct BP monitoring, and send a sample for ABG analysis—severely injured patients will have a marked base deficit, and its correction will help to confirm adequate resuscitation.

Fluids

(See also ➜ p. 1053.)

Aggressive fluid resuscitation before surgical control of the bleeding is harmful; in the presence of active bleeding, increasing the BP with fluid accelerates the loss of red blood cells and may hamper clotting mechanisms. However, untreated hypovolaemic shock is associated with microvascular hypoperfusion and hypoxia, leading to multiple organ failure. The balance is between the risk of inducing organ ischaemia and the risk of accelerating haemorrhage; until haemorrhage control is achieved, the current recommendation is to give 250mL boluses of crystalloid to maintain systolic BP of 80mmHg. Older patients and those with a significant head injury will require a higher BP. In an attempt to avoid high volumes of crystalloid in hypovolaemic trauma patients, blood and blood products are given much earlier. Observational data from both military and civilian settings have documented increased survival rates associated with earlier use of platelets and FFP, particularly when given with red cells in ratios approximating 1:1:1. More recently, it has been suggested that a red cells:FFP ratio of 2:1–1.5:1 may be optimal. Tranexamic acid (1g over 10min, given within 3hr of injury, and then an infusion of 1g over 8hr) reduces mortality from bleeding in trauma patients. The use of recombinant factor VII may be considered if coagulopathy persists, despite adequate treatment with other blood products, but the initial enthusiasm for this expensive product has waned following an RCT that showed no benefit.

A full cross-match will take 45min; group-specific red cells can be issued in 10min, and group O red cells can be obtained immediately. It is nearly always possible to wait for at least group-specific red cells; major incompatibility reactions when using group-specific red cells are extremely rare.

- Once haemorrhage control has been achieved, the goals of fluid resuscitation are to optimize O_2 delivery, improve microcirculatory perfusion, and reverse tissue acidosis. Fluid infusion should be targeted at a BP and cardiac output that result in an acceptable urine output and a falling lactate and base deficit (Table 35.2).

Warm all IV fluids; a high-capacity fluid warmer is necessary to cope with the rapid infusion rates used during resuscitation of trauma patients.

Table 35.2 Goals for resuscitation of the trauma patient
before haemorrhage has been controlled

Parameter	Goal
BP	Systolic 80mmHg. Mean 50–60mmHg
HR	<120bpm
Oxygenation	SaO_2 >95% (peripheral perfusion allowing oximeter to work)
Urine output	>0.5mL/kg/hr
Mental state	Following commands accurately
Lactate level	<1.6mmol/L
Base deficit	>-5
Hb	>8.0g/dL

Hypothermia (core temperature <35°C) is a serious complication and is
an independent predictor of mortality. Hypothermia has several adverse
effects:

- It causes a gradual decline in HR and cardiac output, while increasing
  the propensity for myocardial dysrhythmias and other morbid
  myocardial events
- The oxyhaemoglobin dissociation curve is shifted to the left by a
  decrease in temperature, thus impairing peripheral O_2 delivery in the
  hypovolaemic patient at a time when it is most needed
- Shivering may increase O_2 consumption and compound the lactic
  acidosis that typically accompanies hypovolaemia
- Even mild hypothermia inhibits coagulation significantly and increases the
  incidence of wound infection.

Disability—rapid neurological assessment

Check the pupils for size and reaction to light, and assess the GCS score
rapidly (see ⊃ p. 852).

If the patient requires urgent induction of anaesthesia and intubation,
remember to perform a quick neurological assessment first.

Exposure/environmental control

Undress the patient completely, and protect from hypothermia with warm
blankets.

Tubes

Insert a urinary catheter; urine output is an excellent indicator of the
adequacy of resuscitation. Place a gastric tube; this will enable stomach
contents to be drained and reduce the risk of aspiration. If there is any
suspicion of a basal skull fracture, use the orogastric route.

Imaging

Advances in the image quality and speed of CT, combined with increasing recognition of the limitations of plain radiographs, have led to a much

greater reliance on whole-body CT as the 1° radiological investigation in severely injured patients. Today's standard is to obtain a CT scan within 30min of patient arrival in the emergency department. Chest and pelvic X-rays are considered if the patient is going directly to the operating room or they are haemodynamically very unstable (e.g. systolic BP <90mmHg or HR >120bpm despite 2U of group O-negative blood). Any X-rays must be taken without interrupting the resuscitation process—this is achievable if members of the trauma team are wearing lead coats. There is no indication for a lateral X-ray of the cervical spine in the severely injured patient—it will not change the patient's management, and a cervical spine injury is assumed until ruled out with a CT scan, with or without clinical examination.

Further reading

Harris T, Thomas GOR, Brohi K (2012). Early fluid resuscitation in severe trauma. *BMJ*, **345**, e5752.

The secondary survey

A detailed head-to-toe survey of the trauma patient is not undertaken until the vital signs are relatively stable. Re-evaluate the patient repeatedly, so that ongoing bleeding is detected early. Patients with exsanguinating haemorrhage may need a laparotomy as part of the resuscitation phase.

Head injuries

Most potentially preventable head injury morbidity is caused by a delay in diagnosing and evacuating an intracranial haematoma or the failure to correct hypoxia and hypotension.

- Inspect and palpate the scalp for lacerations, haematomas, and depressed fractures.
- Check for signs of a basal skull fracture: 'panda' eyes (Battle's sign), bruising over the mastoid process, subhyaloid haemorrhage, scleral haemorrhage without a posterior margin, haemotympanum, CSF rhinorrhoea, and otorrhoea.
- Brain injury can be divided into 1° injury (concussion, contusion, and laceration) and 2° brain injury (hypoxia, hypercapnia, and hypotension). Resuscitation goals include:
  - MAP at least 90mmHg—allows for CPP of 70mmHg in the presence of slightly raised ICP (e.g. 20mmHg)
  - SpO_2 >95%
  - $PaCO_2$ 4.5–5.0kPa (34–38mmHg) (if mechanically ventilated)
  - Hb >10g/dL.
- The conscious level is assessed using the GCS. The trend of change in the conscious level is more important than one static reading. Record the pupillary response and the presence of any lateralizing signs (Tables 35.3 and 35.4).

Table 35.3 Glasgow Coma Scale

	Response	Score
Best motor response	Obeys commands	6
	Localizes pain	5
	Normal flexion withdrawal (stimulus to supraorbital notch)	4
	Abnormal flexion to pain	3
	Extension to pain	2
	Nothing	1
Best verbal response	Orientated	5
	Confused	4
	Inappropriate words	3
	Inarticulate sounds	2
	Nothing	1
Eye opening	Eyes open	4
	Eyes open to speech	3
	Eyes open to pain	2
	No eye opening	1

Reprinted from *The Lancet*, 304:7872, Teasdale G, Jennett B, Assessment of coma and impaired consciousness, pp. 81–84, Copyright (1974), with permission from Elsevier.

Table 35.4 Modification of GCS for children under 5

	Response	Score
Best motor response	Obeys commands (>2yr)	6
	Localizes to pain (<2yr)	5
	Normal flexion to pain (>6 months)	4
	Abnormal flexion to pain	3
	Extension to pain	2
	Nothing	1
Best verbal response	Orientated (>5yr)	5
	Words (>1yr)	4
	Vocal sounds (>6 months)	3
	Cries (<6 months)	2
	None	1
Eye opening	Eyes open	4
	Eyes open to speech	3
	Eyes open to pain	2
	No eye opening	1

Using this scoring system, the maximum GCS is 9 at 0–6 months, 11 at 6–12 months, 13 at 1–2yr, and 14 at 2–5yr.

Indications for intubation and ventilation after head injury

- GCS <9.
- Loss of protective laryngeal reflexes.
- Ventilatory insufficiency (PaO_2 <13kPa (100mmHg) on O_2, $PaCO_2$ >6kPa (45mmHg)).
- Spontaneous hyperventilation causing $PaCO_2$ <4kPa (30mmHg).
- Respiratory arrhythmia.
- To enable CT scanning.
- Before transfer to a regional neurosurgical unit:
  - Significantly deteriorating conscious level, even if not in coma
  - Unstable fractures of the facial skeleton
  - Copious bleeding into the mouth (e.g. skull base fracture)
  - Seizures.

Management of intubation in the head-injured patient

- An RSI is required with cricoid pressure and manual in-line stabilization of the head and neck.
- Give thiopental 3–5mg/kg or propofol 1–3mg/kg with suxamethonium 1–2mg/kg and fentanyl 2–5 micrograms/kg or alfentanil 15–30 micrograms/kg.
- Ventilate to a $PaCO_2$ of 4.5–5.0kPa (34–38mmHg).
- Maintain oxygenation (SpO_2 >95%).
- Maintain sedation with a propofol infusion (1–3mg/kg/hr).

- Insert an orogastric tube—NGTs are contraindicated until a fractured base of the skull has been excluded.
- Restore normovolaemia (0.9% NaCl), and give vasopressors to maintain a mean arterial BP of 90mmHg.

Criteria for immediate request for CT scan of the head (adults)
- GCS <13 on initial assessment in the emergency department.
- GCS <15 at 2hr after the injury on assessment in the emergency department.
- Suspected open or depressed skull fracture.
- Any sign of basal skull fracture (haemotympanum, 'panda' eyes, CSF leakage from the ear or nose, Battle's sign).
- Post-traumatic seizure.
- Focal neurological deficit.
- >1 episode of vomiting.
- Amnesia for events >30min before impact.

Criteria for immediate request for CT scan of the head, provided the patient has experienced some loss of consciousness or amnesia since the injury (adults)
- Age 65yr or older.
- Coagulopathy (history of bleeding, clotting disorder, current treatment with warfarin).
- Dangerous mechanism of injury (a pedestrian or cyclist struck by a motor vehicle, an occupant ejected from a motor vehicle, or a fall from a height of >1m or five stairs).

Indications for referral to a regional neurosurgical unit
- All patients with an intracranial mass.
- 1° brain injury requiring ventilation.
- Compound or depressed skull fracture.
- Persistent CSF leak.
- Penetrating skull injury.
- A seizure without full recovery.
- Patients deteriorating rapidly with signs of an intracranial mass lesion.

Management of seizures
- Lorazepam 25–30 micrograms/kg IV.
- Phenytoin 15mg/kg over 15min.
- Thiopental 3mg/kg, if required.
- Recheck ABC.

Management of increased intracranial pressure
- Give mannitol 0.5g/kg [Weight (kg) × 2.5 = mL of 20% mannitol] or 100mL of 5% hypertonic saline and furosemide 10–20mg.
- Manually hyperventilate the patient's lungs for 30s, and reassess the pupillary response.

Transfer to a regional neurosurgical unit

Critically ill patients with acute brain injuries must be accompanied by a doctor with suitable training, skills, competencies, and experience of brain injury transfer.[2,3] A dedicated trained assistant must be provided for the escorting doctor. This might be an appropriately trained operating department practitioner, nurse, or paramedic. The patient should receive the same standard of physiological monitoring during transfer as they would receive in an ICU. All notes (or photocopies), radiographs, blood results, and cross-matched blood should accompany the patient. The transfer team should carry a mobile phone. Head-injured patients must be resuscitated adequately before transfer. Cervical spine protection should be continued, and pupillary responses reassessed every 15min (see also ➜ p. 881).

Essential equipment for patient transfer

- Portable mechanical ventilator, with supply of O_2.
- Portable, battery-powered monitors—ECG, IABP, CVP, SpO_2, $ETCO_2$, temperature.
- Suction, defibrillator, battery-powered syringe pumps.
- Airway and intubation equipment.
- Venous access equipment.

Essential drugs for patient transfer

- Hypnotics—a propofol infusion is ideal for sedating intubated patients.
- Neuromuscular-blocking drugs and analgesics, e.g. fentanyl.
- Mannitol 20%: mannitol (0.5g/kg) may be given after discussion with the neurosurgeon. This may reduce ICP and will buy time before surgery.
- Vasoactive drugs, e.g. metaraminol, noradrenaline.
- Additional resuscitation drugs.

References

2 Association of Anaesthetists of Great Britain and Ireland (2006). *Recommendations for the safe transfer of patients with brain injury*. London: Association of Anaesthetists of Great Britain and Ireland.

3 Intensive Care Society (2002). *Guidelines for the transport of the critically ill adult*. London: Intensive Care Society.

Chest injuries

There are six potentially life-threatening injuries (two contusions and four 'ruptures'):
- Pulmonary contusion
- Cardiac contusion
- Aortic rupture—blunt aortic injury
- Ruptured diaphragm
- Oesophageal rupture
- Rupture of the tracheobronchial tree.

Pulmonary contusion
- Inspection of the chest may reveal signs indicating considerable decelerating forces such as seat belt bruising.
- Pulmonary contusion is the commonest potentially lethal chest injury.
- Young adults and children have particularly compliant ribs, and considerable energy can be transmitted to the lungs in the absence of rib fractures.
- The earliest indication of pulmonary contusion is hypoxaemia (reduced PaO_2/FiO_2 ratio).
- The chest radiograph shows patchy infiltrates over the affected area but may be normal initially.
- Increasing the FiO_2 may provide sufficient oxygenation; if not, the patient may require mask CPAP or tracheal intubation and positive pressure ventilation.
- Use small V_T (5–7mL/kg—based on IBW) to minimize volutrauma. Try to keep the peak inspiratory pressure $<35cmH_2O$.
- The patient with chest trauma requires appropriate fluid resuscitation, but fluid overload will compound the lung contusion.

Myocardial contusion
- Cardiac contusion must be considered in any patient with severe blunt chest trauma, particularly those with sternal fractures.
- Cardiac arrhythmias, ST changes on the ECG, and elevated serum concentrations of cardiac troponin suggest cardiac contusion.
- Elevated CVP in the presence of hypotension is the earliest indication of myocardial dysfunction 2° to severe cardiac contusion, but cardiac tamponade must be excluded.
- Echocardiography is the best method of confirming a cardiac contusion.
- Patients with severe cardiac contusion tend to have other serious injuries that will mandate their admission to an ICU—the decision to admit a patient to ICU rarely depends on the diagnosis of cardiac contusion alone.
- The severely contused myocardium will require inotropic support (e.g. dobutamine).

Blunt aortic injury
- The thoracic aorta is at risk in any patient sustaining a significant decelerating force (e.g. fall from a height or high-speed road traffic accident). Only 10–15% of these patients will reach hospital alive;

without surgery, two-thirds of these survivors will die of delayed rupture within 2wk.

- The commonest site for aortic injury is at the aortic isthmus, just distal to the origin of the left subclavian artery at the level of the ligamentum arteriosum. Deceleration produces large shear forces at this site, because the relatively mobile aortic arch travels forward relative to the fixed descending aorta.
- The tear in the intima and media may involve either part or the whole of the circumference of the aorta, and, in survivors, the haematoma is contained by an intact aortic adventitia and mediastinal pleura.
- Patients sustaining a blunt aortic injury usually have multiple injuries and may be hypotensive at presentation. However, upper extremity hypertension is present in 40% of cases, as the haematoma compresses the true lumen, causing a 'pseudocoarctation'.
- The supine chest radiograph will show a widened mediastinum in the vast majority of cases. Although this is a sensitive sign of a blunt aortic injury, it is not very specific—90% of cases of a widened mediastinum are due to venous bleeding.
- Signs on the chest radiograph suggesting a possible blunt aortic injury are: *a wide mediastinum, pleural capping, left haemothorax, deviation of the trachea to the right, depression of the left mainstem bronchus, loss of the aortic knob, deviation of the NGT to the right, fractures of the upper three ribs*, and *fracture of the thoracic spine*.
- If the chest radiograph is suspicious, further investigation will be required. **Contrast-enhanced CT** is the standard investigation for the diagnosis of a blunt aortic injury.
- If a blunt aortic injury is suspected, the patient's BP should be maintained at 80–100mmHg systolic (using a β-blocker such as esmolol), in an effort to reduce the risk of further dissection or rupture. The use of pure vasodilators increases the pulse pressure and will not reduce the shear forces on the aortic wall. Once stable, the patient must be transferred immediately to the nearest cardiothoracic unit (see ➲ p. 881).

Rupture of the diaphragm

- Rupture of the diaphragm occurs in about 5% of patients sustaining severe blunt trauma to the trunk.
- It can be difficult to diagnose initially—the diagnosis is often made late.
- ~75% of ruptures occur on the left side. The stomach or colon commonly herniates into the chest, and strangulation of these organs is a significant complication.
- Signs and symptoms may include diminished breath sounds, chest and abdominal pain, and respiratory distress.
- Diagnosis can be made on a plain radiograph (*elevated hemidiaphragm, gas bubbles above the diaphragm, shift of the mediastinum to the opposite side, NGT in the chest*). The definitive diagnosis may be made by instilling contrast media through the NGT and repeating the radiograph or, more usually nowadays, by CT scan.
- Once the patient has been stabilized, the diaphragm will require surgical repair (see ➲ p. 385).

Oesophageal rupture

- A severe blow to the upper abdomen may tear the lower oesophagus, as gastric contents are forcefully ejected.
- The conscious patient will complain of *severe chest and abdominal pain*, and *mediastinal air may be visible on the chest radiograph*.
- Gastric contents may appear in the chest drain.
- The diagnosis is confirmed by contrast study of the oesophagus or endoscopy.
- Urgent surgery is essential—mediastinitis carries a high mortality (see ➔ p. 385).

Tracheobronchial injury

- Laryngeal fractures are rare.
- Signs of laryngeal injury include *hoarseness, SC emphysema*, and *palpable fracture crepitus*.
- Total airway obstruction and severe respiratory distress are managed by intubation or a surgical airway—tracheostomy is indicated, rather than cricothyroidotomy.
- Less severe laryngeal injuries may be assessed by CT before any appropriate surgery.
- Transections of the trachea or bronchi proximal to the pleural reflection cause massive mediastinal and cervical emphysema.
- Injuries distal to the pleural sheath lead to pneumothoraces—these will not resolve after chest drainage, since the bronchopleural fistula allows a large air leak.
- Most bronchial injuries occur within 2.5cm of the carina, and the diagnosis is confirmed by bronchoscopy.
- Tracheobronchial injuries require urgent repair through a thoracotomy (see ➔ p. 386).

Abdominal injuries

- The priority is to determine quickly the need for laparotomy and not to spend considerable time trying to define precisely which viscus is injured.
- Inspect the abdomen for bruising, lacerations, and distension. Careful palpation may reveal tenderness.
- FAST scanning will detect significant free fluid in the regions defined by the four Ps: pericardial, perihepatic, perisplenic, and pelvic. While ultrasound is good for detecting blood, CT will provide information on specific organ injury; however, CT may miss some GI, diaphragmatic, and pancreatic injuries (Table 35.5).
- In patients with multiple injuries, 'damage control' surgery is often undertaken. This emphasizes a rapid, but definitive, haemostasis, closure of all hollow viscus injuries, or performing only essential bowel resections, and delaying the more standard reconstruction until after the patient has been stabilized and all physiological parameters have been corrected.

Table 35.5 Imaging the injured abdomen

	Ultrasound	CT scan
Indication	Screening for free fluid or solid organ injury in all blunt trauma patients	Diagnosis of organ injury in haemodynamically stable patients
Advantages	Fast, sensitivity 83–87%, can detect free fluid and solid organ injury	Most specific for injury (92–98%)
Disadvantages	Operator-dependent, misses diaphragm, bowel, and some pancreatic injuries	Takes time to transfer to scanner, misses diaphragm, bowel, and some pancreatic injuries

Pelvic fractures

- Pelvic fractures can cause life-threatening haemorrhage. *In the hypovolaemic, shocked patient, the blood is either on the floor, in the chest, in the abdomen, or in the pelvis.*
- Bleeding associated with pelvic fractures arises mainly from the shearing and tearing of large veins lining the posterior pelvis. Bleeding can also arise from the raw, cancellous bony surfaces. Arterial bleeding accounts for major bleeding in <10% of cases.
- The two main fracture types responsible for severe haemorrhage are the open book type (or AP compression) and the vertical shear pattern.
- Suspect pelvic fracture after motor vehicle accidents, especially where the victim has been ejected from the vehicle, pedestrian–vehicle contact, motorcycle accidents, and falls from >3m.
- Clinical signs are variable and unpredictable, and the diagnosis is made with an AP pelvic radiograph at the end of the primary survey. Widening of the symphysis of >2cm or vertical displacement of one side of the pelvis indicates severe disruption and a high likelihood of major haemorrhage.

Treatment

- A widening or diastasis of the symphysis of >2cm doubles the pelvic volume. Emergency treatment aims to reduce this volume and tamponade the bleeding vessels. In the emergency room, 'closing the book' using a folded sheet or purpose-made binder wrapped around the pelvis and tying the legs together can reduce bleeding significantly.
- After stabilization of the airway and breathing, the next step is rapid emergency surgical stabilization of the pelvis with an external fixator. Threaded self-drilling pins are inserted into the wings of the pelvis, enabling the 'book' to be closed by clamping both halves of the pelvis together, tamponading the underlying venous bleeding.
- Application of an external fixator takes precedence over laparotomy in the presence of an open book or vertical shear pelvic fracture, otherwise the loss of tamponade associated with the laparotomy incision can lead to catastrophic retroperitoneal bleeding. Once the external fixator is applied, diagnostic peritoneal lavage can be performed (above the umbilicus to avoid pelvic haematoma). Alternatively, emergency focused ultrasound may exclude associated intraperitoneal bleeding. Laparotomy can be undertaken easily with the external fixator in place.
- The external fixator can be applied in the resuscitation room or the operating theatre, depending on local policy.

Associated injuries

- Bladder injury 20%, urethral injury 14%, liver and splenic injury, spinal fracture, other limb injuries.

Pitfalls

- Open fractures of the pelvis involving perforation of the vagina or rectum may be difficult to diagnose and are associated with a mortality of 30–50%.
- Beware urethral injury; do not attempt to catheterize if there is marked pelvic disruption on the radiograph or marked perineal bruising and urethral bleeding. Call a surgeon to undertake an emergency urethrogram.
- If there is no improvement in the vital signs after external fixation, look for other causes of the bleeding, i.e. intraperitoneal (laparotomy) or arterial (angiography). Discuss with a radiologist the possibility of embolizing bleeding pelvic vessels.

Anaesthetic considerations

- These patients are usually in class III shock and need early blood transfusion. Fixators may be applied under LA or GA.
- Patients with a fractured pelvis need analgesia; opioids are the easiest early treatment, but an epidural is effective, if not contraindicated.

Spinal injuries

(See also ➋ p. 237.)

- If a spinal board has been used to transfer the patient to hospital, remove it as soon as possible; spinal boards are designed for extrication, not transport—they are very uncomfortable to lie on and will cause pressure sores quickly. Log roll the patient to enable a thorough inspection and palpation of the whole spine. A safe log roll requires five people: three to control and turn the patient's body, one to maintain the cervical spine in neutral alignment with the rest of the body, and one to palpate the spinous processes for tenderness/deformities.

The person controlling the cervical spine commands the team. Thorough clearance of the patient's spine can be complex.

- In the patient who is awake, alert, sober, neurologically normal, and without distracting injuries, the spine may be cleared if there is no pain at rest, and subsequently on flexion and extension.
- All other patients will require some form of radiological imaging—lateral, AP, and open-mouth radiographs can be used to clear the cervical spine; CT scans may be used to image C1–C2 and/ or C7–T1 if these areas are not seen clearly on the radiographs. In the unconscious patient and those with multiple injuries, it is now standard practice to image the entire cervical spine with CT and use 3D reconstruction to rule out significant injury. This is undertaken as part of the standard trauma CT scan. Most experts now accept the small possibility of missing a ligamentous injury on the CT scan in unconscious patients and 'clear' the cervical spine to enable optimal treatment and positioning on the ICU.
- In the obtunded patient and those with multiple injuries, the thoracolumbar spine is also cleared with CT.
- In the conscious patient, a detailed neurological examination should detect any motor or sensory deficits.
- Spinal cord injury can be categorized as:
  - Incomplete or complete paraplegia
  - Incomplete or complete quadriplegia.

Any motor or sensory function below the level of injury indicates an incomplete injury. A cervical or high thoracic injury may cause loss of vasomotor tone, with hypotension and bradycardia; this requires fluid and vasopressor therapy. The principles of resuscitation for the spinal-injured patient are much the same as for the head-injured patient; the cord perfusion pressure should be maintained, and hypoxia avoided. High-dose methylprednisolone therapy is used only rarely in the UK.

Limb injuries

(See also ⮊ p. 481.)

Limb injuries are rarely immediately life-threatening but should be examined to ensure an adequate circulation and the absence of a neurological deficit. The priority is to detect injuries that may be limb-threatening. Align fractures carefully, and splint appropriately, checking for pulses after each intervention. Tibial and forearm fractures are at particularly high risk of causing a **compartment syndrome**. The signs and symptoms of a compartment syndrome are:

- Pain greater than expected and increased by passive stretching of the muscles
- Paraesthesiae
- Decreased sensation or functional loss of the nerves traversing the compartment
- Tense swelling of the involved compartment
- Loss of pulses is a very late sign—a distal pulse is usually present in a compartment syndrome.

Definitive diagnosis of a compartment syndrome is made by measurement of compartment pressures using a cannula connected to a transducer. In patients with normal BP, compartment pressures in excess of 30–35mmHg are indicative of a compartment syndrome requiring urgent surgical decompression (see also ⮊ p. 483).

Burns: early management

(See also ➔ p. 507.)

General considerations

- Treat immediately life-threatening injuries first.
- Fire is the commonest cause of burns in adults; scalding is the commonest cause in children. Most injuries occur at home.
- Burns may be associated with alcohol intoxication, epilepsy, or a psychiatric illness. Consider the possibility of non-accidental injury in children.
- Mortality is related to age, total body surface area (TBSA) burnt, and burn depth.

Airway (with cervical spine control)

- Burns to the head and neck may rapidly cause airway obstruction from massive oedema. Inhalation of hot gases usually causes airway injury above the larynx. Signs of potential airway compromise include singed nasal hairs, hoarse voice, productive 'brassy' cough, and soot in the sputum.
- Clinical judgement will determine the need for immediate intubation, particularly if the patient is to be transferred. Maximum wound oedema occurs 12–36hr after injury, although the airway may be compromised much earlier. *If in doubt, intubate early using an uncut ETT; the subsequent oedema can be considerable.*

Breathing

- Give O_2 15L/min, using a face mask with a reservoir bag.
- Intubation and mechanical ventilation may be required in patients who are:
  - Unconscious from coexisting trauma or from the inhalation of toxic substances such as CO
  - Developing acute respiratory failure due to smoke inhalation or blast injury
  - In need of extensive resuscitation, sedation, and analgesia following a major burn.

Circulation (with haemorrhage control)

- Burns >25% TBSA produce a marked systemic inflammatory response, accompanied by an increase in capillary permeability and generalized oedema.
- Insert cannulae through intact skin, wherever possible. Start IV fluids for burns:
  - >15% TBSA in adults
  - >10% TBSA in children.
- Hartmann's solution is the preferred resuscitation fluid for burns.
  - The fluid requirement in the 1st 24hr in adults and children is 4mL/kg/% TBSA. *Give half the calculated fluid in the 1st 8hr from the time of injury, and give the remainder in the next 16hr.*
  - Maintenance fluids are required, in addition to the calculated resuscitation fluid.

- These calculated values are merely an estimate—the precise volumes required will be guided by the urine output (>0.5–1.0mL/kg) and CVS response.
- Test the urine for haemochromogens (myoglobin/Hb) arising from muscle damage and red cell breakdown. If positive:
  - Increase the urine output to 1–2mL/kg/hr
  - Alkalinize urine—infuse 1.25% sodium bicarbonate solution
  - Promote diuresis—add 12.5g of mannitol to each litre of Hartmann's solution.

Neurological deficit

- Head injury is common in burns associated with road traffic crashes, falls, blasts, and explosions.
- CO poisoning and alcohol intoxication are common causes of altered consciousness.

Exposure (with temperature control)

- Remove all clothing to assess the extent of burn injury. If clothing is stuck to the skin, cut around the area, leaving the adherent fabric in place. Keep the patient warm.
- Assess the percentage TBSA burnt by reference to an adult or paediatric burn chart. The '**rule of nines**' conveniently divides the adult body surface into multiples of 9%; this is inaccurate for small children. The palmar surface of a patient's hand and fingers is ~1% TBSA. Detailed assessment of the burn area is made by referring to a Lund and Browder chart (Fig. 35.1, Table 35.6).
- Assess the burn depth—burn wounds may be superficial or deep; in practice, most injuries are a mixture of both.
  - Superficial—consist of burns to the epidermis only (sunburn, flash burns) or involving the superficial part of the dermis (producing a blister); these burns are painful, and pinprick sensation is preserved. Healing will occur without the need for grafting.
  - Deep—consist of deep dermal burns (no capillary refill beneath the blister, since blood vessels are destroyed) or full-thickness (involving the entire epidermis and dermis, possibly including underlying structures). Burns may have a white, waxy appearance. Pinprick sensation is lost.

Immediate wound care

- Cool the burn wound with cold running water—this helps reduce the production of inflammatory mediators and reduces tissue damage. Continue cooling for at least 20min, taking care to prevent hypothermia, especially in the young child. Cooling the burn is an effective analgesic.
- Burn wounds are initially sterile. Cover with 'cling film' to limit evaporation and heat loss and reduce pain.

Monitoring

- Monitor SpO_2, ECG, urine output, core temperature, and NIBP. The pulse oximeter cannot detect COHb and will over-read the O_2

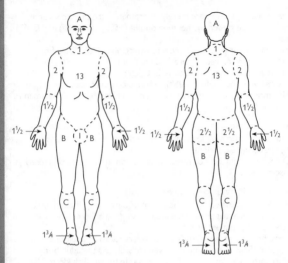

Fig. 35.1 Lund and Browder chart.

Table 35.6 Relative percentage of area affected by growth (age in years)

	0	1	5	10	15	Adult
A: half of head	91/2	81/2	61/2	51/2	41/2	31/2
B: half of thigh	23/4	31/4	4	41/2	41/2	43/4
C: half of leg	21/2	21/2	23/4	3	31/4	31/2

saturation of Hb; use a co-oximeter to obtain an accurate estimation of the percentage of oxyhaemoglobin.
- Insert an arterial line for unconscious patients and those with major burns and/or inhalational injury.
- Insert an NGT for large burns (>20% TBSA adult, >10% TBSA child); gastroparesis is common.
- Check the FBC (including Hct), urea/creatinine, electrolytes, glucose, and COHb, and cross-match some blood.

Analgesia
- All burns are painful; although skin sensation is lost over deep burns, the surrounding area is very painful.
- Give morphine IV, titrated to effect, and continue with a morphine infusion or PCA.

Escharotomy

- Eschar is the coagulated dead skin of a full-thickness burn; it cannot expand, as tissue oedema progresses. Circumferential burns to limbs may result in limb ischaemia; circumferential burns to the trunk may reduce chest wall compliance and impede ventilation.
- Escharotomy, the release of the burn wound by incision down to SC fat, is performed in the operating room. Incisions are made longitudinally along the medial and lateral sides of the limbs; on the trunk, incisions are made along the anterior axillary line down to the upper abdomen. Ensure blood is available; bleeding can be extreme.
- Patients are often already sedated and ventilated. Conscious patients will need additional sedation and analgesia. Full-thickness burns are painless, but incisions will extend onto normal skin for a short distance.

Special circumstances

Inhalation of toxic substances

CO poisoning is common; check COHb. The severity of symptoms may not correlate well with the COHb level. Poisoning may mimic alcohol intoxication.

- **CO** reduces the capacity of blood to carry O_2 and causes tissue hypoxia. The PaO_2 is normal. CO also binds avidly to other haem-containing compounds, especially the cytochrome system. The half-life of COHb is 250min when breathing room air; this is reduced to 40min when breathing 100% O_2. O_2 therapy should be continued, since a 2° peak of COHb occurs after 24hr and is attributed to washout of CO from cytochromes.
- Hyperbaric O_2 therapy reduces the half-life of COHb to just 15–30min; however, the precise role of hyperbaric O_2 is controversial and is highly subject to the availability of hyperbaric facilities. Indications for discussion with the nearest hyperbaric facility include:
  - Any neurological abnormality or cognitive impairment
  - Chest pain, abnormal ECG, and cardiac enzymes
  - Pregnancy
  - History of loss of consciousness
  - Inability to assess adequately.
- Symptoms of COHb poisoning are shown in Table 35.7.
- Other toxic products of combustion may include cyanide, ammonia, phosgene, hydrogen chloride, fluoride, bromide, and complex organic compounds. These toxic substances may produce:
  - A chemical burn to the respiratory tract
  - Interstitial lung oedema, impaired gas exchange, and ARDS
  - Systemic acid–base disturbances
  - Hydrofluoric acid binds serum Ca^{2+} and causes hypocalcaemia.

Chemical burns

- Hands and upper limbs are the most frequently affected areas.
- Staff must protect themselves with gloves, apron, and face mask.
- Remove contaminated clothing as early as possible—store in a secure container for disposal.

Table 35.7 Symptoms of carbon monoxide toxicity

COHb (%)	Symptoms
0–15	None (smokers)
15–20	Headache, mild confusion
20–40	Nausea and vomiting, disorientation, fatigue
40–60	Hallucinations, ataxia, fits, coma
>60	Death

- Industrial or household alkalis and acids are commonly used chemicals, e.g. bleach, washing powder, disinfectants, drain cleaner, paint stripper. Immersion in complex hydrocarbons (petrol, diesel) without ignition may cause systemic toxicity. Phosphorus burns may result from fireworks or military applications.
- Tissue damage continues, until the chemical is neutralized or diluted by washing with water. Early, continuous, and prolonged (1hr) irrigation with cold water is vital for all burns (except elemental Na, K, and lithium).
- Specific treatments include:
  - **Hydrofluoric acid**, used in the glass industry, is highly toxic. Burns of 2% TBSA can be fatal. Tissue penetration by fluoride ions causes deep chemical burns. Inactivate toxic fluoride ions by application of topical calcium gluconate burn gel and 10% gluconate local injections into the burn wound (0.5mL of a 10% solution/cm^2 of surface burn, extending 0.5cm beyond the margin of involved tissue; do not use the chloride salt, because it is an irritant and may cause tissue damage), and consider intra-arterial (infuse a solution of 10mL of 10% calcium gluconate in 40mL of 5% glucose over 4hr) or IV (Bier's block—10–15mL of 10% calcium gluconate plus 5000U heparin, diluted up to 40mL in 5% glucose)
  - **Phosphorus**: white phosphorus ignites spontaneously when exposed to air; it can be extinguished by water. Apply copper sulphate solution which converts phosphorus to black cupric phosphide
  - **Bitumen**: common injury in the UK from road maintenance. It is liquid at 150°C and causes thermal burns. Cool with water; remove the bitumen with vegetable or paraffin oil.

Electrical burns

- Low voltage (<1000V) causes a local contact burn. The 50Hz alternating current (AC) domestic supply is particularly likely to cause cardiac arrest. Muscle spasm may prevent release of the electrical source. There is no associated deep tissue damage.
- High voltage (>1000V) causes flash burn or deep tissue damage due to current transmission. High-voltage cables carry 11 000 or 33 000V; electrocution produces an entrance and exit wound, which may require fasciotomy under GA. Haemochromogens released from muscle and damaged red cells may cause renal failure.

- A direct strike by lightning (ultra-high voltage, high current) has a very high mortality. Side flash is commoner; a nearby lightning strike produces a current that flows over the surface of the victim, causing superficial burns. Current may flow up one leg and down the other, producing an entry and exit wound. Respiratory arrest is common.

British Burn Association criteria for transfer to a burns centre

- Burn >10% TBSA (adult) or >5% TBSA (child), and any patient with full-thickness burn >5% TBSA.
- Burn to the face, hands, feet, genitalia, perineum, or major joints.
- Electrical and chemical burns.
- Inhalational injury.
- Circumferential burn to the limbs or chest.
- Patients at extremes of age.
- Patients with poor medical conditions, which may complicate treatment.

Analgesia for the injured patient

- Give effective analgesia to the injured patient as soon as practically possible.
- If the patient needs surgery imminently, then immediate induction of GA is a logical and very effective solution to the patient's pain; if not, titrate IV opioid (e.g. fentanyl or morphine) to the desired effect.
- Head-injured patients require adequate pain relief for any other injuries; careful titration of IV morphine or fentanyl will provide effective pain relief, without significant respiratory depression.
- Regular IV paracetamol will reduce the dose of opioid required.
- NSAIDs provide moderate analgesia but are relatively contraindicated in patients with hypovolaemia; these patients depend on renal prostaglandins to maintain renal blood flow.
- Entonox® is useful for short procedures such as fracture splintage.
- LA blocks are ideal for the acute trauma patient; unfortunately, relatively few blocks are both simple and effective. Femoral nerve blockade will provide analgesia for a fracture of the femoral shaft. Intercostal nerve blocks will provide analgesia for rib fractures, but the duration is relatively short. Continuous thoracic epidural analgesia will provide excellent pain relief for patients with multiple rib fractures.

Anaesthesia for major trauma

(See also ➡ p. 476.)

General considerations

The following considerations are of relevance to the anaesthetist during surgery for the severely injured patient:

- Prolonged surgery—the patient will be at risk from pressure areas and from heat loss. Anaesthetists (and surgeons) should rotate to avoid exhaustion. Avoid N_2O in those cases expected to last >6hr.
- Fluid loss—be prepared for heavy blood and '3rd space' losses. The combination of hypothermia and massive transfusion will result in profound coagulopathy. Expect to see significant metabolic acidosis in patients with major injuries. This needs frequent monitoring (ABGs) and correction with fluids and inotropes, as appropriate.
- Massive haemorrhage is treated with red cells, FFP, and platelets in a ratio of 1:1:1 or 1.5:1:1. Cryoprecipitate is given if the fibrinogen concentration is <1.5g/L. Give 10mL of calcium chloride if ionized Ca^{2+} <0.9mmol/L. Give tranexamic acid 1g over 10min, followed by an infusion of 1g over 8hr. Consider giving rFVIIa if coagulopathy persists, despite adequate treatment with other blood products (usually 10U of red blood cells, 8U of FFP, two adult therapeutic doses of platelets, and two packs of cryoprecipitate will have been given). Give rFVIIa 100 micrograms/kg. To avoid any wastage, round the dose up or down to the nearest 1.2mg vial. Clinical response is usually obvious within 20min. If no response within 20min, consider a 2nd dose of rFVIIa 100 micrograms/kg.
- Multiple surgical teams—it is more efficient if surgical teams from different specialties are able to work simultaneously. However, this may severely restrict the amount of space available to the anaesthetist.
- ALI—trauma patients are at significant risk of hypoxia resulting from ALI. This may be 2° to direct pulmonary contusion or due to fat embolism from orthopaedic injuries. Advanced ventilatory modes may be required to maintain appropriate oxygenation.

Regional anaesthesia

Regional anaesthesia may be considered as an adjunct, although preoperative urgency, haemodynamic instability, coagulopathy, and the possibility of a compartment syndrome often make it impractical.

Problems

- **Unexplained hypotension** and tachycardia: consider hypovolaemia, pneumothorax, or pericardial tamponade.
- **Unexplained hypoxia** is often associated with a rise in inflation pressure; consider tension pneumothorax.
- **Unexplained hypertension**: consider pain, raised ICP (search for associated neurological signs; obtain a brain CT scan), or rarely traumatic disruption of the thoracic aorta (causing a pseudocoarctation effect).

The multiply injured patient: common dilemmas

- The head-injured patient with an abdominal injury—which of a laparotomy and brain CT should be undertaken first? If the patient is haemodynamically unstable, the laparotomy has priority. Hypotension will compound any brain injury, and bleeding must be controlled rapidly. If the patient is haemodynamically stable, a CT scan of both the brain and the abdomen may be appropriate.
- The head-injured patient with lower limb fractures—in general, in the haemodynamically stable patient, limb fractures should be stabilized as soon as possible. In the presence of a significant brain injury, the ICP should be monitored before intramedullary nailing of limb fractures.
- The patient with pulmonary contusion and lower limb fractures—intramedullary reaming will cause some degree of fat embolism. Whether this results in significant risk to the patient is contentious. In the presence of severe pulmonary contusion, it may be wise to stabilize lower limb fractures temporarily with an external fixator (damage control orthopaedic surgery) before undertaking definitive nailing later.

Post-cardiac arrest resuscitation care

Following cardiac arrest, restoration of a spontaneous circulation (ROSC) is just the 1st step in what may be a prolonged period of treatment. Unless the duration of cardiac arrest is very short, the patient is likely to develop the post-cardiac arrest syndrome, which is associated with a marked systemic inflammatory response. The anaesthetist may be expected to initiate treatment in the emergency department, the operating room, the critical care unit, or on the general ward. The aims of post-resuscitation care are to:

- Prevent a further cardiac arrest
- Define the underlying pathology
- Limit organ damage
- Predict non-survivors.

Prevention of further cardiac arrest

- Optimize oxygenation—after an immediate return to full consciousness following a short-duration cardiac arrest, give O_2 via a face mask.
- Other patients may require assisted ventilation via an ETT. Aim to achieve normoxia—hyperoxia may exacerbate neurological injury. Maintain adequate sedation with a propofol infusion, combined with an opioid, as required.
- Provide ventilation to maintain normocapnia—excessive ventilation will cause hypocarbia and cerebral ischaemia from cerebral vasoconstriction.
- Correct electrolyte disturbances, particularly K^+, Mg^{2+}, and Ca^{2+}.
- Control the blood glucose; treat the blood glucose with insulin if it exceeds 10mmol/L; maintain in the range of 4–10mmol/L.

Defining the underlying pathology

- Establish the patient's pre-arrest medical condition.
- Confirm correct placement of the ETT, and exclude a pneumothorax.
- Listen to the heart for evidence of murmurs, and seek evidence of ventricular failure.
- Record the GCS (see ➔ p. 852).

Limiting organ damage

- If there is evidence of ST-elevation myocardial infarction (STEMI), coronary artery reperfusion therapy must be started rapidly. This is best achieved by immediate PCI.
- Patients remaining comatose after ROSC, particularly after an out-of-hospital cardiac arrest, should have their temperature controlled, so that hyperthermia is prevented. The target temperature has been 32–34°C for 12–24hr, but a recent study has shown no difference in neurological outcome when using a temperature of 36°C. After 24hr, the patient is rewarmed slowly. Cooling is started with ice-cold IV saline 20–30mL/kg, and the application of wet towels to the torso and ice to the groins, axillae, and neck. Cooling is continued either externally or internally (intravascular).

Prediction of non-survivors

- ~8% of those sustaining an out-of-hospital cardiac arrest will survive to hospital discharge; the figure for in-hospital cardiac arrest is about 18%.
- Short duration of cardiac arrest/CPR correlates with a more rapid ROSC and better neurological outcomes.
- Prognostication in unconscious patients after more protracted CPR remains unreliable for at least 72hr after ROSC. If therapeutic hypothermia is used, this time may need to be extended to 72hr after normothermia has been restored. Regardless of when prognostic tests are undertaken, it is essential to ensure that sedative drugs have been cleared.
- Myocardial, neurological, and other organ function may all improve slowly, given the appropriate support over a period of time; at least 3–5 days of intensive care should be considered in the comatose patient with ROSC following a cardiac arrest.[4]

Reference

4 Nolan JP, Neumar RW, Adrie C, et al. (2008). Post-cardiac arrest syndrome: epidemiology, pathophysiology, treatment, and prognostication. A Scientific Statement from the International Liaison Committee on Resuscitation; the American Heart Association Emergency Cardiovascular Care Committee; the Council on Cardiovascular Surgery and Anesthesia; the Council on Cardiopulmonary, Perioperative, and Critical Care; the Council on Clinical Cardiology; the Council on Stroke. *Resuscitation*, **79**, 350–79.

Further reading

Deakin CD, Nolan JP, Soar J, et al. (2010). European Resuscitation Council Guidelines for Resuscitation 2010 Section 4. Adult advanced life support. *Resuscitation*, **81**, 1305–52.

Septic shock

Definitions

- **Infection**: the inflammatory response to the presence of microorganisms or the invasion of normally sterile host tissue by those organisms.
- **Bacteraemia**: the presence of viable bacteria in the blood.
- **SIRS**: the patient exhibits two of the following four abnormalities:
  - Temperature >38°C or <36°C
  - HR >90bpm
  - Respiratory rate >20 breaths/min or $PaCO_2$ <4.3kPa (32mmHg)
  - WCC >12 000 cells/mm^3 or <4000 cells/mm^3 or >10% immature cells (band forms).
- **Sepsis**: SIRS resulting from infection.
- **Severe sepsis**: sepsis associated with organ dysfunction, hypoperfusion, or hypotension. Hypoperfusion and perfusion abnormalities include lactic acidosis, oliguria, and an acute alteration in the mental status.
- **Septic shock**: sepsis with hypotension (systolic BP <90mmHg or a reduction of >40mmHg from baseline) and perfusion abnormalities or the requirement for vasoactive drugs despite adequate fluid resuscitation in the absence of other causes for hypotension.

Pathology

- The response to sepsis is complex and involves many pro- and anti-inflammatory mediators; the severity of illness is determined more by the nature of the inflammatory response than by the infection.
- Most abdominal sepsis is caused by Gram-negative bacteria, which contain endotoxin in their outer membrane. **Endotoxin** is a lipopolysaccharide implicated in macrophage and monocyte activation and the release of numerous mediators, including TNF, IL-1, and other cytokines, plus prostaglandins, leukotrienes, the complement and fibrinolytic systems, platelet-activating factor, and NO.
- Pathological effects caused by these mediators include vasodilatation, increased capillary permeability, impaired tissue O_2 utilization, and myocardial depression.
- Tissues may become hypoxic for several reasons, including hypotension (vasodilatation, hypovolaemia, myocardial depression); microvascular thrombosis (activation of coagulation); tissue oedema acting as a barrier to O_2 diffusion; and shunting past some capillary beds. This results in anaerobic metabolism and lactic acidosis. In sepsis, despite adequate O_2 delivery, lactic acidosis may also be caused by mitochondrial dysfunction. Reperfusion of previously hypoxic tissues can cause further release of damaging reactive O_2 species.

Resuscitation

The resuscitation of a septic patient is started as soon as the condition is recognized and must not be delayed, pending admission to the ICU or transfer to the operating room. Induction of anaesthesia in the septic patient is hazardous, and every effort should be made to resuscitate the patient adequately preoperatively; whether or not this is achievable will depend on the urgency of the surgery. International guidelines for the treatment of severe sepsis and septic shock have been updated recently.[5]

- Anaesthetic induction drugs and volatile agents will compound the vasodilatory and negative inotropic effects of sepsis. Surgery may initially worsen the septic state by further releasing bacteria, endotoxins, and cytokines, and causing haemorrhage and fluid loss.
- Establish vascular access and monitoring as soon as possible and before induction of anaesthesia:
  - Two functioning, large-bore IV cannulae
  - CVP line
  - Arterial line
  - Urinary catheter
  - In the presence of advanced sepsis, consider non-invasive cardiac output monitoring using the method preferred locally. Measurement of $ScvO_2$ may be valuable.
- While establishing monitoring, give O_2 and fluid. Use crystalloids; consider adding albumin solution if large volumes of crystalloid are required.
- **Resuscitation goals** during the 1st 6hr of resuscitation include:
  - CVP 8–12mmHg (use a higher target CVP of 12–15mmHg in the presence of mechanical ventilation)
  - MAP ≥65mmHg
  - Urine output ≥0.5mL/kg/hr
  - (SVC) $ScvO_2$ ≥70%.
- Once adequate fluid has been given, start a **noradrenaline** infusion to maintain MAP ≥65mmHg.
- Give IV hydrocortisone (50mg 6-hourly) if hypotension remains poorly responsive to adequate fluid resuscitation and vasopressors.
- Ensure blood is available—Hb concentration will decrease due to haemodilution, and coagulopathy may cause excessive blood loss. Maintain Hb >7.0g/dL—a higher target value will be appropriate in the presence of CAD, acute haemorrhage, and persistent lactic acidosis.
- Begin IV antibiotics as early as possible, and always within the 1st hour of recognizing severe sepsis and septic shock.
- Obtain appropriate cultures before starting antibiotics, provided this does not significantly delay the antibiotics. The choice of antibiotics is guided by local microbiology policies.
- If the patient requires surgery, discuss with critical care staff, so plans can be made for admission to an appropriate unit for level 2 or 3 care.

Interpretation of investigations in the septic patient

- FBC: expect a high WCC with neutrophilia (a low WBC is evidence of overwhelming sepsis); a low platelet count is common.
- U&Es: urea and Na^+ raised proportionately more than creatinine indicates dehydration; high creatinine indicates renal impairment.
- Coagulation screen: increased INR indicates septic coagulopathy (unless on warfarin).
- Blood glucose: usually raised; low glucose indicates advanced sepsis or hepatic dysfunction.

- ABGs: metabolic acidosis is common; there may be compensatory hyperventilation, unless the patient is obtunded. Hypoxia is common in severe sepsis.
- Blood lactate: a high blood lactate indicates tissue hypoxia. If there is acidaemia with a normal lactate, check the creatinine and urine output (renal failure is the most likely cause of non-lactic acidosis in the septic patient; another cause is diabetic ketoacidosis).
- The chest radiograph may show evidence of non-cardiogenic pulmonary oedema, indicating the development of ARDS.

Induction and maintenance of anaesthesia

- RSI is normally used in any patient with severe sepsis; however, many experienced intensive care clinicians prefer to titrate the induction drugs slowly in an attempt to avoid causing CVS collapse.
- All induction drugs will cause hypotension—use reduced doses. Use of a short-acting opioid, such as alfentanil, will enable a significant reduction in the dose of the induction drug. Avoid etomidate in critically ill patients—a single dose suppresses the adrenocortical axis for at least 24hr and is associated with increased mortality in septic patients. The use of ketamine 1–2mg/kg is increasingly popular as an induction drug in the critically ill.
- Ensure vasopressor drugs are available before inducing anaesthesia; **adrenaline** drawn up in two concentrations (10mL of 1:10 000 and 1:100 000) provides the flexibility to reverse the CVS effects of induction drugs.
- Insert an NGT, if not already in place.
- The use of epidural blockade for analgesia is controversial in sepsis, although, depending on the precise circumstances, some experienced clinicians still consider the benefits outweigh the risks.
  - A potential bacteraemia may be considered to be a contraindication.
  - Coagulopathy will preclude insertion.
  - Hypotensive effects are likely to be exaggerated.
  - If insertion of an epidural is not contraindicated by other factors, consider inserting a catheter, but waiting until the patient is stable before establishing the block.
- Maintain anaesthesia with a volatile anaesthetic or propofol. **Noradrenaline** infusion counteracts hypotension and maintains MAP ≥65mmHg.
- The effects and duration of action of opioids, other than remifentanil, will be increased by impaired hepatic and renal perfusion.
- Avoid NSAIDs in patients who are persistently hypotensive or septic.

Maintaining tissue oxygenation in the operating room

Fluids

- Continue to give crystalloid, aiming for CVP 12–15mmHg (assuming mechanical ventilation).
- Monitor ABGs regularly, and give blood to maintain an Hb concentration of 7–9g/dL.

Inotropes/vasoconstrictors

Having ensured adequate fluid resuscitation, use noradrenaline to maintain the MAP ≥65mmHg—this will counteract the vasodilatation associated with sepsis and also provides some inotropic effect. If the cardiac output is thought to be inadequate, despite fluid and noradrenaline, consider adding dobutamine or adrenaline.

Oxygen and positive end-expiratory pressure

- Critically ill patients should be anaesthetized with equipment that can provide PEEP and variable I:E ratios.
- Oxygenation may be impaired by non-cardiogenic pulmonary oedema, which is caused by the increased capillary permeability in sepsis.
- Increase the FiO_2 until SaO_2 is at least 90%, and use 5cmH$_2$O PEEP.
- Increase the PEEP to 10cmH$_2$O if the patient is still hypoxic, despite FiO_2 of 0.5. Consider an alveolar recruitment manoeuvre (hold the lungs in inspiration at 40cmH$_2$O for up to 40s).

Ventilation

- Increased capillary permeability in sepsis may reduce lung compliance and produce high airway pressures.
- Shear forces caused by ventilation with high V_T or high inspiratory pressures will exacerbate lung injury. In patients with early ARDS, every effort should be made to limit the peak airway pressure to 30cmH$_2$O and V_T to 6–8mL/kg of the IBW. These target values can be reconsidered if the resultant minute ventilation fails to achieve a pH >7.15.
- Monitor ABGs regularly; a base deficit or raised lactate indicates inadequate resuscitation, although both of these abnormalities can be associated with an adrenaline infusion.
- An ScvO$_2$ <70% implies inadequate O$_2$ delivery. Fluids and inotropic treatment may be indicated. Non-invasive measurement of the cardiac output will assist treatment.
- The trends indicated by these monitors are valuable; single readings taken in isolation are difficult to interpret.

Reference

5 Dellinger RP, Levy MM, Rhodes A, et al. (2013). Surviving Sepsis Campaign: international guidelines for management of severe sepsis and septic shock: 2012. *Crit Care Med*, 41, 580–637.

The ICU patient going to theatre

The planning, transfer, and monitoring of a critically ill patient on the ICU needing surgery can be challenging. Physiological instability should be anticipated, detected, and acted upon promptly and effectively. Senior anaesthetists and surgeons must be involved.

Consent

Informed consent is often impossible, as the patient may be sedated or comatose. While the family is not able to give consent in law, the reasons for surgery and risks should be discussed with them, whenever possible.

Preoperative assessment

- Routine aspects of the preoperative assessment (e.g. history of previous anaesthetics, chronic medical conditions, allergies) are just as relevant to the critically ill patient as they are to the elective case.
- Assess the patient's current condition from discussion with the critical care team and from information on the observation and drug charts.
- Note the current fluid requirements and rate/concentration of inotrope infusions; ensure that there is an adequate supply of inotrope prepared for theatre; consider which vasopressors may be required.
- Note the patient's O_2 requirement, lung compliance, minute volume, PEEP, etc. to enable prediction of the ventilator settings that will be necessary in theatre. In the absence of a suitable ventilator in the operating room, it will be necessary to use a ventilator from the ICU.
- Check IV access, and consider if any additional cannulae may be required. Many ICU patients have had all peripheral access removed.
- Check which antibiotics the patient is receiving and whether any doses will be due in theatre.
- Check the most recent FBC, U&Es, and ABG, and ensure that blood is available.
- If the patient is being transferred to a more remote facility, such as the X-ray department, ensure adequate anaesthetic assistance. If the patient's lungs have poor compliance and are requiring high PEEP, it may be necessary to use an ICU ventilator.
- On occasions, it may be necessary to undertake an MRI scan on a critically ill patient—the inability to take ferrometallic objects into the scan room is problematic (see ➜ p. 699).

Transfer to the operating room

- Familiarize yourself with the transport equipment, and ensure it is functioning before leaving the ICU.
- If the patient is already ventilated, establish on the transfer ventilator before leaving the ICU to ensure adequate ventilation can be maintained. Modern transfer ventilators provide many of the functions of an ICU ventilator.
- Consider increasing the patient's sedation for the transfer.
- If the patient is not already sedated and ventilated, decide whether to induce in the ICU, the anaesthetic room, or theatre; factors influencing

the decision will be safety, available assistance, haemodynamic instability, and patient comfort.
- Monitor the patient fully en route.
- Disentangle all lines; re-establish full monitoring, and check IV access before the start of surgery.

Transfer back to the intensive care unit
- Inform the ICU staff when surgery is about to finish; this enables them to prepare to receive the patient, and possibly to assist in the transfer.
- Ensure that a full verbal and written handover is given to the ICU medical and nursing staff, and communicate the post-operative requirements.

Further reading
Dellinger RP, Levy MM, Rhodes A, et al. (2013). Surviving Sepsis Campaign: international guidelines for management of severe sepsis and septic shock: 2012. *Crit Care Med*, **41**, 580–637. Also available at: ℘ http://www.survivingsepsis.org.

Transferring the critically ill

Safe transfer demands experienced staff and careful preparation. Several studies have demonstrated that patients are often inadequately resuscitated and monitored during transfer. Specialized transport teams improve outcome but are not always available or appropriate. Before transferring any critically ill patient, the risks of transfer should be weighed against the potential benefits of treatment at the receiving unit.

Dangers of transfer

- Deranged physiology, worsened by movement (acceleration/deceleration leads to CVS instability)—15% of patients develop avoidable hypoxia and hypotension.
- Cramped conditions, isolation, and temperature and pressure changes.
- Vehicular crashes.

Principles of safe transfer

- Staff experienced in intensive care and transfer—specialist transport teams may improve outcome but may cause delay.
- Use of appropriate equipment and vehicle, extensive monitoring, careful stabilization, continuing reassessment, direct handover, documentation, and audit.

The transfer vehicle

- Adequate space, light, gases, electricity, and communications.
- Mode: consider urgency, mobilization time, geography, weather, traffic, and costs.
- Consider air if over 150 miles (remember decreasing PaO_2 at altitude, expanding air spaces requiring NGT/orogastric tube, temperature, noise, and vibration).

Aeromedical transfer

- Hazards depend on whether the craft is rotary (helicopter) or fixed-wing (aeroplane).
- Helicopters fly at relatively low altitude and therefore avoid some of the problems of aeroplanes.
- High altitude decreases the partial pressure of O_2—at 1500m, the arterial PaO_2 is about 10kPa (75mmHg). Most aircraft are pressurized to 1500–2000m.
- Decreased barometric pressure leads to expansion of gas-filled cavities (patients should have NGTs and may need chest drains).
- Pressurizing the cabin pressure to sea level can decrease these problems but increases fuel costs!
- Air in the ETT cuff should be replaced by saline.

Problems during transfer

- Vibration leads to failure and inaccuracy of NIBP monitoring. Invasive monitoring should be used, if at all possible.
- Access to the patient may be limited.
- Acceleration/deceleration may lead to CVS instability.
- Hypothermia, particularly during transfer between vehicles.

Specific considerations for children

- Hypothermia is a greater risk, particularly in the infant. Monitor the central temperature, and use warming mats, 'bubble wrap', hats, etc. to maintain temperature.
- A secure IV access is paramount before departure.

Calculating oxygen reserves

Anticipate your length of journey, and ensure you have plenty of spare O_2 available for unanticipated delays. Table 35.8 gives the approximate operating times for different O_2 cylinders venting at different rates. See also Table 43.3.

Table 35.8 Operation time (in min) for different minute volumes at FiO_2 1.0

Size of O_2 cylinder (volume, L)	Minute volume 5L/min	Minute volume 7L/min	Minute volume 10L/min
D (340)	56	42	30
E (680)	113	85	61
F (1360)	226	170	123

Battery life

- This can vary greatly, depending on the manufacturer, but must be known (Table 35.9).
- The charge time is usually considerable.
- Battery life will vary, depending on the rate of infusion.

Table 35.9 Examples of battery lives for pumps running at 5–10mL/hr

Type	Battery life (estimated) (hr)	Charge time (estimated) (hr)
Graseby 3100	3	14
Alaris IVAC	6	24
Graseby Omnifuse	8	18

Preparation

- Ensure meticulous stabilization prior to transfer.
- Take a full history, and make a thorough examination.
- Full monitoring, including invasive BP and CVP where indicated.
- Blood tests, radiographs, and CT prior to transfer.
- Explain the procedure to the patient and family.
- Use the checklist in Table 35.10.
- It is sensible to have a transfer pack already prepared with the things you are most likely to need. Table 35.11 gives a list of recommended items to consider.

Table 35.10 Checklist for preparation to transfer a patient

A: airway	• •	Is the airway safe? If in doubt, intubate.
	• •	Cervical spine control.
B: breathing	• •	Portable ventilator settings. Check ABG before departure after 15min on the portable ventilator.
	• •	Self-inflating bag–valve device in the event of a ventilator/O_2 failure.
	• •	Suction.
	• •	Adequate sedation, analgesia, and relaxation.
	• •	Adequate O_2 reserves.
	• •	Insert a chest drain if there is a possibility of a pneumothorax (e.g. fractured ribs).
C: circulation	• •	Stable circulation with good access.
	• •	Controlled external bleeding.
	• •	Invasive BP and CVP, when indicated.
	• •	Inotropes—if in doubt, have them prepared and ready to run.
	• •	Pumps and batteries.
	• •	Insert a urinary catheter, and monitor output.
D: disability	• •	GCS (mannitol, IPPV), pupillary signs.
	• •	NGT/orogastric tube.
E: exposure	• •	Temperature loss.
	• •	Splint long bones.
F: forgotten?	• •	All notes, referral letter, results, radiographs (including CT scans), and blood products.
	• •	Inform the receiving unit that you are leaving the base hospital.
	• •	Inform relatives.
	• •	Take contact numbers.
	• •	Take warm clothing, mobile phone, food, and credit card/money for the team!
	• •	Plan for the return journey.
	• •	Medical indemnity and insurance for death or disability of transfer staff.

Table 35.11 Equipment and drug box guidelines

Airway and breathing	
Suction equipment	Tracheal tubes, connectors, ties
Stethoscope	Tracheostomy tubes (if appropriate)
Face masks, airways, self-inflating bag with reservoir	Laryngoscopes, spare batteries
Gum elastic bougie	

Circulation	
Cannulae plus IV dressings and tape	IV fluids and giving set
Syringes and needles	Mini-sharps receptacle

Resuscitation drugs	
Adenosine	Noradrenaline
Hydrocortisone	Lorazepam
Adrenaline	Salbutamol nebulizers
Lidocaine	Glucose
Amiodarone	Sodium bicarbonate
Metoprolol	Furosemide
Atropine	Saline ampoules
Naloxone	GTN spray
Calcium chloride	Plain drug labels

Sedation/muscle relaxants	
Propofol	Midazolam
Atracurium or rocuronium	Suxamethonium

Paediatric equipment—extras	
Paediatric O$_2$ mask with reservoir bag	Tracheal tubes
Small cannulae	Paediatric drug doses
Appropriate self-inflating bag with reservoir	Laryngoscope and stylets
Intraosseous needle	Magill forceps and suction catheters
Masks and airways	10% glucose for infusion

Anaesthetic emergencies

Andrew McIndoe

See also:

Introduction

Anaesthetic emergencies may develop rapidly into life-threatening conditions that cannot be managed effectively by an individual and require a team response. Although critical incidents frequently occur in the presence of a theatre team, the anaesthetist is likely to be the person present with the specialist knowledge and skills to deal with the problem. This can give rise to intense pressure. Always send for help early. An extra pair of hands and an independent pair of eyes and ears are invaluable assistance, even if only to reassure you that you are already dealing with the situation appropriately. Critical incident protocols and drills have been designed to aid in the management of the more complex or common emergencies, and some are detailed below. However, a protocol-driven approach is heavily reliant upon recognition that a serious problem exists.

General considerations to help deal with any unanticipated anaesthetic crisis

Communication

- Declare problems early to the rest of the theatre team, before you lose control of the situation. Basic resuscitation measures should be ongoing, while you figure out the diagnosis.
- No matter whatever or whoever 'caused' the crisis, use objective and non-judgemental comments. Insults tend to provoke an aggressive or withdrawal response from the recipient and inhibit team function.
- To communicate effectively, your messages or commands must be: ADDRESSED—ask specifically named individuals to perform tasks; HEARD—reduce background noise and distractions by turning off the radio, etc.; UNDERSTOOD—if you make a complex request, ask the recipient to repeat it back to you.
- If the cause of the problem is unknown, say so. Say what you do not know as well as what you do know. Encourage others to contribute.
- Reappraise the situation regularly. Update the rest of the team with new information. If you are still unsure about what to do, send for help—a 2nd person with a fresh approach may pick up on missed clues.

Invoke a team approach

- A team should have one clearly identified leader, who should make effective use of the mixture of skills and resources available.
- A good team leader is able to step back from the situation to consider the whole picture. This can only be achieved by delegation of responsibility for tasks to other members of the team.
- A repeated and systematic ABC approach helps render the patient 'safe', buys thinking time, and increases the likelihood of detecting signs that may lead to a definitive diagnosis.
- Most members of an impromptu emergency team will need to adopt the role of 'team players'. A good team player is adaptable, assumes complete responsibility for delegated problems, and feels comfortable enough to advocate an opinion or feed back information to the rest of the team.

Adult basic life support

Aims when managing a 'collapsed' patient in a hospital
- Algorithm given in Fig. 36.1.
- Immediate recognition of cardiorespiratory arrest.
- Help summoned quickly by telephone.
- CPR to be started immediately using airway adjuncts.
- If indicated, defibrillation attempted rapidly (within 3min at most).

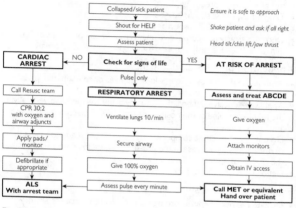

Fig. 36.1 Adult basic life support algorithm.

Patient assessment
- Turn the patient onto their back.
- Optimize the airway, and remove any visible obstruction.
- Look, listen, and feel for signs of life. Put your ear by the patient's mouth, while observing for chest/abdominal movements and feeling for a carotid pulse. Take no more than 10s.
- Occasional gasps or slow laboured breathing are indicative of an actual or impending cardiac arrest.

Chest compressions
- Give cycles of 30 compressions followed by two ventilations.
- Rate of delivery at 100–120/min.
- Finding the right place—do not waste time. Ideally, locate the middle of the lower half of the sternum. Place the heel of one hand there, with the other hand on top of the first. Interlock the fingers of both hands, and lift them to ensure that pressure is not applied over the patient's ribs. Do not apply any pressure over the upper abdomen or bottom tip of the sternum.

- Aim to depress the sternum ~5–6cm (or one-third of the chest depth), and apply only enough pressure to achieve this.
- The pressure should be firm, controlled, and applied vertically. Erratic or violent action is dangerous.
- About the same time should be spent in the compression phase as in the released phase (allow the chest wall to recoil fully).

Breathing
- Give 30 chest compressions, before giving TWO ventilations.
- Use an inspiratory time of 1s and sufficient volume to make the chest rise as in normal breathing.
- Time off the chest should be <5s.
- Add supplemental O_2 as soon as it is available.
- Once the airway is secured, give uninterrupted compressions at 100/min, and simultaneously ventilate the lungs at a rate of 10 breaths/min.

Application of defibrillation pads
- Analyse the rhythm using 'quick-look' paddles or self-adhesive pads as soon as is possible.
- Apply self-adhesive defibrillation pads over the sternum and vertically in the mid-axillary line at the position of the V_6 ECG electrode (lateral to any breast tissue).
- Do not interrupt chest compressions, until you are ready to assess the rhythm. Every 5s increase in the pre-shock pause in compressions halves the chance of a successful defibrillation.
- Defibrillation is indicated for VF/VT.

Suspected cervical spine injury
- Despite the risk of spinal cord damage, untreated cardiorespiratory arrest will kill the patient.
- Potential 2° damage will be minimized by in-line immobilization of the C-spine.
- Try to use a jaw thrust and/or a Guedel airway to open the airway, rather than tilting the neck.
- Avoid placing the patient in the recovery position.

At-risk patients
- Collapsed patients with signs of life (breathing and a pulse) often require urgent medical assessment and intervention to prevent a cardiorespiratory arrest.
- Give 100% O_2; obtain IV access, and establish ECG, SpO_2, BP, respiratory rate, and temperature monitoring.
- Look for correctable pathophysiology/biochemistry, and establish higher dependency care.

Further reading
Resuscitation Council (UK). *Resuscitation guidelines 2010.* ℘ http://www.resus.org.uk/pages/GL2010.pdf.

Adult advanced life support

The ALS algorithm is given in Fig. 36.2.

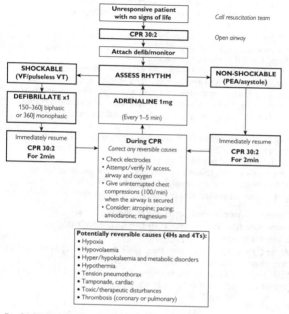

Fig. 36.2 Adult advanced life support algorithm.

Defibrillation

- For monophasic defibrillators, all shocks should be delivered at 360J.
- For biphasic defibrillators, use 150–200J for the 1st shock, and 150–360J for subsequent shocks.
- Electrode polarity is unimportant. Use defibrillation pads to improve electrical contact. One pad is placed to the right of the sternum below the clavicle, the other over the lower left ribs in the mid-axillary line (level with the V_6 ECG electrode), avoiding placement over breast tissue. Put the long axis of this pad vertical, and make sure it is lateral to the cardiac apex.
- Do not attempt to reposition pads that have already been stuck on the chest—it is more important to deliver the shock quickly.
- Remove transdermal patches to prevent arcing, and place defibrillator pads/paddles 12–15cm away from implanted pacemakers.

- For safety reasons, charge the defibrillator only when the pads/paddles are in contact with the patient, but continue chest compressions while charging. Hold the O_2 mask away from the patient during the actual defibrillation, but leave the bag connected to the ETT.
- Recheck the rhythm trace on the monitor immediately prior to shock delivery.
- It is the responsibility of the defibrillator operator to visually check that everyone is clear and to state STAND CLEAR prior to delivery of each shock, but aim to stop compressions for <5s.
- VT and pulseless VT are the commonest causes of reversible cardiac arrest in adults. These are the most 'recoverable' rhythms, and it is therefore always worthwhile persisting with CPR while they are present. However, successful resuscitation does depend on early defibrillation. BLS, IV access, and airway control should not delay the delivery of shocks.
- Resume CPR IMMEDIATELY after delivering a shock. Delay the next rhythm check for 2min. Then shock again if still in VF/VT, before resuming CPR for another 2min.
- After three shocks, follow with adrenaline 1mg IV and amiodarone 300mg IV, while simultaneously resuming 2min of CPR.
- Give further adrenaline 1mg IV after alternate shocks

Witnessed monitored ventricular tachycardia/ ventricular fibrillation arrest in the catheterization lab/after cardiac surgery

- As on p. 889, but give up to three quick successive (stacked) shocks immediately (instead of just one) if the initial rhythm is VF/VT.
- Start 2min of CPR immediately after delivery of the 3rd shock, without pausing to assess the pulse or heart rhythm.

Ventilations

- Once the trachea is intubated, chest compressions should continue uninterrupted (except for pulse checks and defibrillation) at a rate of 100–120/min, while ventilations are administered simultaneously at a rate of 10/min.
- A pause in chest compressions allows the coronary perfusion pressure to fall substantially and is followed with a delay before the original perfusion pressure is restored after external cardiac massage is recommenced.

Circulatory access

- Follow all peripherally injected drugs with at least 20mL of flush.
- Use an intraosseous access (e.g. tibia, humerus) if IV access cannot be established in <2min. Avoid sites with proximal fractures.

Adrenaline

- Give adrenaline as soon as IV access is secured for PEA/asystole or after a 3rd shock for VF/VT.
- Then give 1mg every 3–5min (or alternate shock cycles in VF/pulseless VT), without interrupting CPR.

Calcium

- Consider 10mL of calcium chloride 10% slow IV if PEA is thought to be caused by hyperkalaemia, hypocalcaemia, overdose of calcium channel blockers, or magnesium.

Antiarrhythmics

- Give amiodarone 300mg IV bolus injection after a 3rd shock for VF/VT. A further dose of 150mg may be given for recurrent or refractory VF/pulseless VT, followed by an infusion of 900mg over 24hr.
- Consider lidocaine 1mg/kg as an ALTERNATIVE treatment.
- Give magnesium sulphate 8mmol (4mL of 50% solution) for refractory VF if the patient has hypomagnesaemia (e.g. diuretic-induced), torsade de pointes, or digoxin toxicity.
- Is no longer recommended for asystole or PEA.

Bicarbonate

- Consider bicarbonate 50mmol in the presence of hyperkalaemia or tricyclic antidepressant overdose.
- Remember that $HCO_3^- + H^+ = H_2O + CO_2$, therefore bicarbonate administration requires an increase in minute ventilation. Check ABGs before repeating the dose.

Subsequent management

(See also ➲ p. 873.)
- CXR, 12-lead ECG, ABG, U&Es.
- Reverse any biochemical abnormalities.
- Unless the period of arrest has been very brief (<3min), the patient should remain intubated and be transferred to the ICU.
- Target IV fluids and MAP to achieve 1mL/kg/hr of urine output and decreasing plasma lactate values.
- Consider the use of an IABP and/or inotropes for low cardiac output.
- Maintain blood glucose ≤10mmol/L.
- Consider inducing mild hypothermia (32–34°C).
- Control seizures with benzodiazepines/phenytoin/sodium valproate/propofol.

Further reading

Resuscitation Council (UK). *Resuscitation guidelines 2010.* ℘ http://www.resus.org.uk/pages/GL2010.pdf.

Severe bradycardia

(See also ➔ p. 79.)

The algorithm for managing severe bradycardia is given in Fig. 36.3.

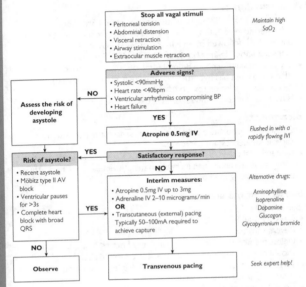

Fig. **36.3** Severe bradycardia.

Notes

- If adverse signs are present, give atropine 500 micrograms IV, and, if necessary, repeat every 3–5min up to 3mg.
- Atropine will not work if the patient has a heart transplant.
- A transvenous pacing wire can be passed via a PAFC introducer.
- A 3rd-degree AV block and 2nd-degree Möbitz type II AV block will result in significant bradycardia, haemodynamic instability, and the possibility of asystole. Other significant risk factors for asystole include a recent episode of asystole and ventricular pauses of >3s.
- Indications for referral for preoperative pacing:
  - 2nd-degree AV block—Möbitz type II or 2:1 block
  - Complete heart block
  - Symptomatic sinus node disease
  - Asymptomatic bundle branch block, bifascicular, trifascicular, and 1st-degree heart block are not indications for preoperative pacing. Pacing is not usually required for Möbitz type I 2nd-degree AV block (Wenckebach), unless the patient is symptomatic.

Narrow complex tachycardia

(See also ➲ p. 73.)

The algorithm for managing narrow complex tachycardia is given in Fig. 36.4.

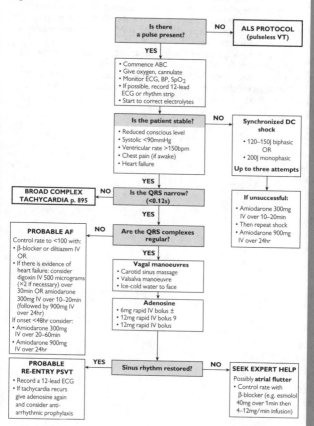

Fig. 36.4 Narrow complex tachycardia.

PSVT, paroxysmal supraventricular tachycardia.

Notes

- Exclude light anaesthesia/inadequate analgesia.
- Narrow complex tachycardia in an unstable patient (reduced conscious level, and/or chest pain (if awake), LV failure, systolic BP <90mmHg;

ventricular rate >150bpm; ischaemia) requires urgent synchronized DC shock.
- Differentiating narrow from broad complex tachycardia can be difficult, especially at high ventricular rates. Vagal manoeuvres or adenosine should slow AV conduction of an SVT, but not a VT.
- Theophylline interacts with adenosine and tends to block its effect.
- Dipyridamole and carbimazole potentiate the effects of adenosine.
- **Adenosine** should be used with caution in WPW syndrome and should be avoided in asthmatics.
- AF may require anticoagulation of the patient prior to cardioversion (patients with AF >48hr should be anticoagulated for 3wk prior to cardioversion, unless checked for absence of atrial thrombus with TOE).
- Verapamil should not be administered in the presence of β-blockade.
- Serum therapeutic range for digoxin is 0.8–2.0 micrograms/L.

Broad complex tachycardia

(See also ➋ p. 77.)

The algorithm for the management of broad complex tachycardia is given in Fig. 36.5.

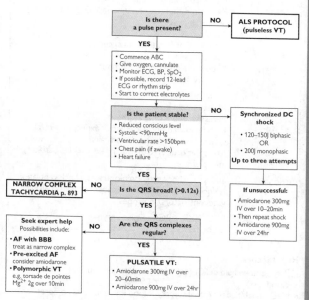

Fig. 36.5 Broad complex tachycardia.

Notes

- Broad complex tachycardia in an unstable patient (reduced conscious level, and/or chest pain (if awake), LV failure, systolic BP <90mmHg; ventricular rate >150bpm; ischaemia) requires urgent synchronized DC shock.
- 2° treatment is aimed at stabilizing the sinus rhythm and preventing recurrence (antiarrhythmics and electrolyte correction).
- Torsade de pointes is a polymorphic form of VT characterized by beat-to-beat variation, a constantly changing axis, and a prolonged QT interval. Stop all drugs that prolong the QT interval. Treat with magnesium 2g IV, and correct any electrolyte abnormalities such as hypokalaemia. The patient may need overdrive pacing.
- If the patient is not adversely affected by the tachyarrhythmia, correct electrolytes while giving antiarrhythmics.

Severe hypotension in theatre

Consider	**Patient:**
	Hypovolaemia
	Obstructed venous return
	Raised intrathoracic pressure, including tension pneumothorax
	Anaphylaxis
	Embolus (gas/air/thrombus/cement/fat/amniotic fluid)
	1° pump failure/tachyarrhythmia
	Systemic sepsis
	Technique:
	Measurement error
	Excessive depth of anaesthesia
	High regional block (including unexpected central spread from peribulbar/interscalene, etc.)
	Iatrogenic drug error, including LA toxicity, barbiturates plus porphyria
Action	100% O_2; check surgery/blood loss; check ventilation; reduce volatile; lift legs (if feasible); IV fluid challenge; vasoconstrictors/inotropes
Investigations	ECG, CXR, ABGs, cardiac enzymes

Risk factors

- Preoperative fluid deficit (dehydration, diarrhoea and vomiting, blood loss).
- Mediastinal/hepatic/renal surgery (blood loss and caval compression).
- Pre-existing myocardial disease/dysrhythmia.
- Multiple trauma.
- Sepsis.
- Carcinoid syndrome with liver or lung tumour/metastases (bradykinin).

Differential diagnosis

- Measurement error: palpate the distal pulse manually, while repeating NIBP; check when pulsation returns against the monitor deflation figure. Invasive BP—check the transducer height.
- Check peripheral perfusion; warm peripheries suggest excessive anaesthesia (GA/regional) or sepsis.
- Suspect tension pneumothorax (particularly following central line insertion) if IPPV and the trachea shifted away from a hyperresonant lung field, with diminished breath sounds. Neck veins may be engorged. Treat immediately by decompressing the pleural cavity with an open cannula placed in the 2nd intercostal space in the mid-clavicular line.
- Suspect hypovolaemia if the patient has HR >100bpm, respiratory rate >20bpm, capillary return >2s, cool peripheries, collapsed veins, a

narrow and peaked arterial line trace, or marked respiratory swing to either CVP or arterial line trace. Dehydration if the patient is thirsty, has a dry tongue, is producing dark concentrated urine, and has globally elevated blood cell, urea, creatinine, and electrolyte values.

- Suspect cardiac failure if the patient has HR >100bpm, respiratory rate >20bpm, engorged central veins, capillary return >2s, cool peripheries, pulmonary oedema, or worsening SpO_2 with fluid challenge.
- Suspect air or gas embolus if the patient had a pre-existing low CVP and open venous bed. Signs are variable but may include sudden ↓ $ETCO_2$, ↓ SpO_2, loss of palpable pulse, PEA, and rise in CVP.
- Suspect fat embolus or cement reaction in the presence of multiple bony injuries or long bone intramedullary surgery.
- Iatrogenic drug response: histamine release or wrong dilution.
- High central neural blockade may be heralded by Horner's syndrome (small pupil, ptosis, stuffy nose, anhidrosis).
- Anaphylaxis—CVS collapse 88%, erythema 45%, bronchospasm 36%, angio-oedema 24%, rash 13%, and urticaria 8.5%.

Immediate management

- **ABC**—check what the surgeons are doing (caval compression/blood loss/high pneumoperitoneal pressure); prevent further losses by clamp or direct pressure. Administer high FiO_2. Maintenance of organ perfusion and oxygenation is more important than achieving BP alone. BP = SVR × CO (cardiac output), therefore improvement in cardiac output may help ameliorate low perfusion pressure.
- **Optimize preload** (check initial CVP if already sited; change in CVP is more informative than actual CVP). Lifting the legs returns blood into the central venous compartment and also increases afterload. Fluid challenge of 10mL/kg of crystalloid/colloid using a pressure infusor. Assess response (BP/HR/CVP), and repeat if appropriate.
- **Increase contractility**: ephedrine 6mg IV (mixed direct and indirect action); adrenaline 10 micrograms IV ($\beta_{1,2}$ and α activity); consider calcium slow IV (up to 10mL of 10% calcium chloride).
- **Systemic vasoconstriction** (note: α-agonists increase perfusion pressure but may reduce cardiac output). Metaraminol 1–2mg IV; phenylephrine 0.25–0.5mg IV; adrenaline 10 micrograms IV.

Subsequent management

- Correct acidosis to improve myocardial response to inotropes. Check ABGs, and correct respiratory acidosis first. If a severe metabolic acidosis exists (art pH <7.1, base excess <−10), consider using bicarbonate 50mmol (50mL of 8.4% sodium bicarbonate).
- Maintenance infusion of vasoconstrictor (e.g. adrenaline or noradrenaline) or inotrope (e.g. dobutamine), if required.

Other considerations

- **Adrenaline** 1:10 000 = 100 micrograms/mL; 1 in 10 dilution results in a 1:100 000 solution (10 micrograms/mL).
- Patients taking β-blockers may not demonstrate tachycardia, despite significant hypovolaemia.

Severe hypertension in theatre

Consider	Inadequate depth of anaesthesia/analgesia Measurement error Hypoxia/hypercapnia Iatrogenic drug error Pre-eclampsia Raised ICP Thyroid storm Phaeochromocytoma
Action	Stop surgery until controlled; confirm readings; increase depth of anaesthesia; analgesia; vasodilators; β-blockade; α-blockade
Investigations	ECG, cardiac enzymes, thyroid function tests, 24hr urinary catecholamine excretion

Risk factors

- Untreated or 'white coat' hypertension preoperatively (increased lability).
- Aortic surgery (cross-clamp may ↑↑ SVR).
- Drugs: MAOIs (plus pethidine); ketamine; ergometrine.
- Family history of MEN (type 2) syndrome, medullary thyroid carcinoma, Conn's syndrome.
- Acute head injury.

Differential diagnosis

- Hypoxia/hypercapnia: go through ABC, and check for patient colour and SpO_2.
- Inadequate depth of anaesthesia: check volatile agent concentration; sniff test (smell gases); check TIVA pump, line, and IV cannula.
- Inadequate analgesia: if in doubt, administer alfentanil 10–20 micrograms/kg, and observe effect.
- Measurement error: palpate the distal pulse manually, while repeating NIBP; check when pulsation returns against the monitor deflation figure. Invasive BP—check the transducer height.
- Iatrogenic drug response: cocaine, wrong drug such as ephedrine, adrenaline, or wrong dilution (remember surgical drugs, e.g. adrenaline with LA, Moffett's solution, phenylephrine).
- Pre-eclampsia: if over 20wk pregnant, check for proteinuria, platelet count ± clotting studies, and LFTs.
- Thyroid storm causing elevated T_4 and T_3 levels.
- Phaeochromocytoma causing elevated plasma noradrenaline levels. Adrenaline will also cause tachydysrhythmias.
- Cushing response—hypertension and reflex bradycardia (baroreceptor-mediated). This intracranially mediated response maintains cerebral perfusion in the presence of ↑ ICP (see ➲ p. 899).

Immediate management

- ABC—assuming this is not a physiological response to a correctable cause, the overall aim of symptomatic management is to prevent hypertensive stroke or subendocardial ischaemia/infarct. Apart from increasing the depth of anaesthesia and analgesia (systemic or regional), treatment options at CVS effector/receptor level include:
  - **Vasodilators** (may cause tachycardia): ↑ volatile concentration—this is most rapidly achieved by simultaneously increasing FGF, but beware of increasing desflurane which may cause sympathetic activation at >1.5 MAC. Hydralazine 5mg slow IV every 15min. GTN (50mg/50mL; start at 3mL/hr, and titrate to BP) or sodium nitroprusside. Magnesium sulfate 2–4g slow IV (8–16mmol) over 10min, followed by infusion of 1g/hr
  - **β-blockade** (particularly in the presence of ↑ HR or dysrhythmias): esmolol 25–100mg, then 50–200 micrograms/kg/min. (Note that esmolol is supplied as 10mg/mL and 250mg/mL solutions.) Labetalol 5–10mg IV PRN (1–2mL increments from a 100mg/20mL ampoule). β:α block ratio = 7:1
  - **α-blockade** (particularly in the presence of normal or ↓ HR): phentolamine 1mg IV PRN (10mg ampoule made up to 10mL, in 1mL increments).

Subsequent management

- For intense analgesia, try remifentanil 0.25–0.5 micrograms/kg/min, titrated to BP.
- Check for myocardial damage with an ECG, serial cardiac enzymes, including CK-MB, and/or troponins.
- Thyroid function tests, 24hr urine collection for noradrenaline, adrenaline, and dopamine excretion.

Other considerations

- Hypertension in the presence of raised ICP requires CT head and urgent neurosurgical intervention. Maintain MAP >80mmHg, normocapnia, head-up tilt, unobstructed SVC drainage, low airway pressures, and good oxygenation. Consider mannitol 0.5g/kg. Bradycardia can be treated with anticholinergics.

Severe hypoxia in theatre

Consider	**Hypoxic gas mixture:** • Incorrect flow meter settings • Second gas effect (especially on extubation) • O_2 failure • Anaesthetic machine error **Failure to ventilate:** • Ventilatory depression or narcosis (note: regional block after opioids) • Inadequate IPPV • Disconnection • Misplaced ETT (oesophagus/endobronchial) • Obstruction to airway, ETT, filter, mount, circuit, etc. • ↑ airway resistance (laryngospasm, bronchospasm, anaphylaxis) • ↓ FRC (pneumothorax, ↑ intra-abdominal pressure, morbid obesity) **Shunt:** • Atelectasis • Airway secretions • ↓ hypoxic pulmonary vasoconstriction (vasodilators or β_2-agonists) • CCF with pulmonary oedema • Aspiration of gastric contents • Pre-existing pathology (e.g. VSD, ASD plus ↓ SVR with reversal of flow) **Poor O_2 delivery:** • Systemic hypoperfusion (hypovolaemia, sepsis) • Embolus (gas/air/thrombus/cement/fat/amniotic fluid) • Local problems (cold limb, Raynaud's, sickle) **Increased O_2 demand:** • Sepsis • MH
Action	100% O_2; check FiO_2; expose patient, and check for central cyanosis; check ventilation bilaterally; hand-ventilate on a simple system giving 3–4 large breaths initially to recruit alveoli; secure airway; endotracheal suction; initially remove any PEEP; give adrenaline if accompanied by poorly palpable pulses
Investigations	SpO_2; capnography; CXR; ABGs; CVP ± PAOP; echocardiography

Risk factors

- Reduced FRC (obesity, intestinal obstruction, pregnancy) reduces O_2 reserves.
- Failure to preoxygenate exacerbates any airway difficulties at induction.
- Laryngospasm can result in negative-pressure pulmonary oedema.
- Head and neck surgery (shared access to the airway) increases the risk of undetected disconnection.
- History of CHD or detection of a heart murmur (left-to-right communication).
- Chronic lung disease.
- SCD.
- Methaemoglobinaemia (interpreted as deoxyhaemoglobin by pulse oximeters).

Differential diagnosis

- FiO_2: use an O_2 analyser at all times.
- Ventilation: cross-check rise and fall of the chest with auscultation over the stomach and in both axillae, capnograph trace, measured expired V_T, and airway pressure.
- Measurement error: does the patient appear cyanotic? Beware in anaemia when 5g/dL of deoxyhaemoglobin may not be visible.
- Aspiration/airway secretions: auscultate, and aspirate using a tracheal suction catheter ± litmus paper.
- Suspect tension pneumothorax (particularly following central line insertion) if IPPV and the trachea shifted away from a hyperresonant lung field, with diminished breath sounds. Neck veins may be engorged. Treat immediately by decompressing the pleural cavity with an open cannula placed in the 2nd intercostal space in the mid-clavicular line.
- Suspect hypovolaemia if the patient has HR >100bpm, respiratory rate >20 breaths/min, capillary return >2s, cool peripheries, collapsed veins, a narrow and peaked arterial line trace, or marked respiratory swing to either CVP or arterial line trace.
- Suspect cardiac failure if the patient has HR >100bpm, RR >20 breaths/min, engorged central veins, capillary return >2s, cool peripheries, pulmonary oedema, or worsening SpO_2 with fluid challenge.
- Suspect air or gas embolus if the patient had a pre-existing low CVP and open venous bed. Signs are variable but may include sudden ↓ $ETCO_2$, ↓ SpO_2, loss of palpable pulse, PEA, and subsequent rise in CVP.
- Suspect fat embolus or cement reaction in the presence of multiple bony injuries or long bone intramedullary surgery.
- Malignant hyperthermia: especially if accompanied by ↑ $ETCO_2$, ↑ respiratory rate, ↑ HR, ↑ ectopics.
- Anaphylaxis—CVS collapse 88%, erythema 45%, bronchospasm 36%, angio-oedema 24%, rash 13%, and urticaria 8.5%.

Immediate management

- ABC—expose the chest, all the breathing circuit, and all airway connections. Administer 100% O_2 by manual ventilation—at least 3–4 large breaths initially will help to recruit collapsed alveoli (and gives continuous tactile feedback about the state of the airway). If no improvement:

- **Confirm FiO$_2$**: if there is any doubt about the inspired O$_2$ concentration from the anaesthetic machine, use a separate cylinder supply (as a last resort, use room air via a self-inflating bag = 21% O$_2$)
- **Misplaced ETT**—cross-check rise and fall of the chest with auscultation over the stomach and in both axillae and the capnograph trace
- **Ventilation problem**: simplify the breathing system until the problem is removed, i.e. switch to bag, rather than the ventilator; use a Bain circuit, instead of the circle system; try a self-inflating bag plus mask, rather than an ETT, etc.
- **Diagnosis** of the source of a leak or obstruction: is not as important initially as oxygenation of the patient. Make the patient safe first, then use a systematic approach. The fastest way to isolate the problem is probably by division. For instance, does breaking the circuit at the ETT connector leave the problem on the patient side or the anaesthetic machine side?
- **Severe right-to-left shunt**: severe hypoxia occurs when blood starts flowing through a congenital heart defect in the presence of low SVR, thus bypassing the pulmonary circulation. The resultant hypoxaemia then exacerbates the problem by causing hypoxic pulmonary vasoconstriction which increases PVR and increases the tendency for blood to shunt across the cardiac defect. Treatment is therefore 2-fold: (1) increase SVR—by lifting the legs and giving adrenaline and IV fluid, especially in sepsis; (2) minimize PVR—by removing PEEP, avoiding high intrathoracic pressure, and maximizing FiO$_2$.
- **Bronchospasm**: eliminate ETT obstruction by sounding ETT with a GEB. Treat by increasing the volatile agent concentration, IV salbutamol (250 micrograms)—see Status asthmaticus, ➔ p. 909).

Other considerations

- In chronic bronchitis, the bronchial circulation can shunt up to 10% of the cardiac output.
- The foramen ovale remains patent in 20–30% of patients but is normally kept closed, because the left atrial pressure is usually higher than the right atrial pressure. IPPV, PEEP, breath-holding, CCF, thoracic surgery, and PE can reverse the pressure gradient and result in shunt.
- Always check the SpO$_2$ probe is well positioned and has a good trace.

Severe laryngospasm

Condition	Acute glottic closure by the vocal cords
Presentation	Crowing or absent inspiratory sounds and marked tracheal tug
Immediate action	Avoid painful stimuli; 100% O_2; CPAP; jaw thrust; remove irritants from the airway; deepen anaesthesia; Larson's manoeuvre
Follow-up action	Muscle relaxation, if intractable
Also consider	Bronchospasm Laryngeal trauma/airway oedema (especially if no leak with paediatric ETT) Recurrent laryngeal nerve damage Tracheomalacia Inhaled foreign body Epiglottitis; croup

Risk factors

- Barbiturate induction or light anaesthesia, especially in anxious patients.
- Intense surgical stimulation: anal stretch; cervical dilatation; incision and drainage of abscesses.
- Extubation of a soiled airway.
- Thyroid surgery.
- Hypocalcaemia (neuromuscular irritability).
- Multiple crowns (inhaled foreign body).

Immediate management

- Remove the stimulus that precipitated the laryngospasm.
- Check that the airway is clear of obstruction or potential irritants.
- Give high-concentration O_2, with the expiratory valve of the circuit closed, and maintain a close seal by mask with two hands, if necessary, to maintain CPAP. The degree of CPAP can be controlled by intermittently relaxing the airway seal at the level of the mask.
- If the laryngospasm has occurred at induction, it may be relieved by deepening anaesthesia using further increments of propofol (disadvantage: potential ventilatory depression) or by increasing the volatile agent concentration (disadvantage: irritation of the airway, less so with sevoflurane, more with isoflurane). Do not use N_2O, as it will decrease O_2 reserves.
- If the laryngospasm fails to improve, remove any airways that may be stimulating the pharynx.
- Suxamethonium 0.25–0.5mg/kg will relieve laryngospasm. If IV access is impossible, consider giving 2–4mg/kg IM or sublingually.

Subsequent management
- Monitor for evidence of pulmonary oedema.
- CPAP may have inflated the stomach with gas, so decompress it with an orogastric tube, and recover the patient in the lateral position.

Other considerations
- Risk of laryngospasm may be reduced by co-induction with IV opioids, IV lidocaine, or by topical lidocaine spray prior to laryngoscopy (do not use >4mg/kg).
- Unilateral recurrent laryngeal nerve trauma results in paralysis of one vocal cord and causes hoarseness, ineffective cough, and the potential to aspirate. Bilateral vocal cord paralysis is more serious, leading to stridor on extubation—this may mimic laryngospasm but does not get better with standard airway manoeuvres. The patient will require reintubation, and possibly tracheostomy.
- Tracheomalacia is likely to cause more stridor with marked negative inspiratory pressure, so treat initially with CPAP. Reconstructive surgery may be necessary.

Air/gas embolism

(See also ⊃ p. 413.)

Condition	Venous gas produces airlock in RV and obstructs pulmonary capillaries
Presentation	↓ ETCO$_2$, ↓ SpO$_2$, loss of palpable pulse, PEA, ↑ CVP then ↓ CVP
Immediate action	Remove source of embolus; flood wound; compress drainage veins
Follow-up action	↑ venous pressure; turn off N$_2$O; left lateral head-down tilt; CVS support
Investigations	Auscultation; Doppler; ECG; CXR
Also consider	Breathing circuit disconnection (loss of ETCO$_2$ trace and ↓ SpO$_2$) Pulseless cardiac arrest—other causes of PEA (4Ts and 4Hs) Cement reaction Pulmonary thromboembolism AFE

Risk factors

- Patient: SV (negative CVP); patent foramen ovale (risk of paradoxical emboli).
- Anaesthesia: hypovolaemia; any open vascular access point; operation site higher than the heart; pressurized infusions.
- Orthopaedic surgery: multiple trauma; long bone surgery—especially intramedullary nailing; hip surgery.
- General surgery: laparoscopic procedures; hysterectomy; neck surgery; vascular surgery.
- ENT surgery: middle ear procedures.
- Neurosurgery: posterior fossa operations in the sitting position (almost historical).

Diagnosis

- 'At-risk' patient, dramatic fall/loss of the ETCO$_2$ trace, and fall in SpO$_2$.
- Awake patients complain of severe chest pain.
- HR may rise.
- Sudden rise in CVP due to a fall in cardiac output and rise in PVR.
- Classically, a 'millwheel' murmur can supposedly be heard.
- Doppler ultrasound is an extremely sensitive (0.25mL of air!) diagnostic tool.
- PEA arrest may occur. ECG may show signs of acute ischaemia, e.g. ST-segment depression of >1mm.
- It is claimed that symptoms/signs of an air embolus appear following 0.5mL/kg/min of intravascular gas.

Immediate management

- **ABC**—eliminate breathing circuit disconnection; give 100% O_2; check the ECG trace and pulse.
- **Prevent further gas/air** from entering the circulation. Get the surgeon to apply compression to major drainage vessels, and flood the wound with irrigation fluid, or cover with damp pack, stop reaming, etc.
- **Decompress** any gas-pressurized system/cavity, e.g. the abdomen during laparoscopy.
- **Lower** the operation site to below the heart level.
- **Turn off** N_2O (because it will expand any intravascular gas volume).
- Increase VP with rapid IV infusion of fluids ± vasopressors.
- If **PEA** arrest occurs, start chest compressions, and adopt the ALS protocol for non-VF/VT cardiac arrest.
- **Aspirate the central venous line.** Classic teaching is to tip the patient head-down in the left lateral position to keep the bubble in the right atrium or apex of the RV, until it dissolves or can be aspirated via a central line advanced into the right atrium. In practice, if there is not already a CVP line *in situ*, aspiration is likely to be difficult.
- **Moderate CPAP** has been advocated as a means of rapidly increasing the intrathoracic pressure, and therefore CVP, in the event of a gas embolus. While this manoeuvre may limit the extent and progress of an air embolus, it must be borne in mind that 10% of patients may have a patent foramen ovale. Sustained rise in right atrial pressure may then lead to a right-to-left shunt and paradoxical air embolism to the cerebral circulation.

Subsequent management

- Ask the surgeon to apply bone wax to exposed bone edges.
- Correct any pre-existing hypovolaemia.
- Avoid N_2O for the remainder of the anaesthetic, and maintain a high FiO_2.
- Perform a 12-lead ECG to look for ischaemia. Air in coronary arteries is suggestive of paradoxical air embolism.
- Consider hyperbaric therapy, if available. Increased ambient pressure (3–6 bar) will decrease the volume of gas emboli.

Other considerations

CO_2 is the safest gas to use for laparoscopic insufflation. It is non-flammable and more soluble than other agents. Should a gas embolus occur, it will dissolve over time. The priority of management should therefore be to limit the extent and central progress of the gas 'bubble', thereby minimizing its systemic CVS effect.

Aspiration

Condition	Chemical pneumonitis; foreign body obstruction and atelectasis
Presentation	Tachypnoea; tachycardia; ↓ lung compliance; ↓ SpO₂
Immediate action	Minimize further aspiration; secure the airway; suction
Follow-up action	100% O₂; consider CPAP; empty the stomach
Investigations	CXR; bronchoscopy
Also consider	Pulmonary oedema Embolus ARDS

Risk factors
- Full stomach/delayed emptying (many causes).
- Known reflux.
- Raised intragastric pressure (intestinal obstruction, pregnancy, laparoscopic surgery).
- Recent trauma.
- Perioperative opioids.
- Diabetes mellitus.
- Topically anaesthetized airway.

Diagnosis
- Clinical: auscultation may reveal wheeze and crepitations; tracheal aspirate may be acidic (but a negative finding does not exclude aspiration).
- CXR: diffuse infiltrative pattern, especially in the right lower lobe distribution (but often not acutely).

Immediate management
- Avoidance of GA in high-risk situations. Use of a rapid sequence technique when appropriate.
- Administer 100% O₂, and minimize the risk of further aspirate contaminating the airway.
- If the patient is awake or nearly awake, suction the oro-/nasopharynx, and place in the recovery position.
- If the patient is unconscious but breathing spontaneously, apply cricoid pressure. Avoid cricoid pressure if the patient is actively vomiting (risk of oesophageal rupture), and place the patient in a left lateral head-down position. Intubate if tracheal suction and ventilation indicated.

- If the patient is unconscious and apnoeic, intubate immediately, and commence ventilation.
- Treat as an inhaled foreign body; minimize positive pressure ventilation, until the ETT and airway have been suctioned and all aspirates are clear.

Subsequent management

- Empty the stomach with a large-bore NGT prior to attempting extubation.
- Monitor respiratory function, and arrange a CXR. Look for evidence of oedema, collapse, or consolidation.
- If SpO_2 remains 90–95%, atelectasis can be improved with CPAP ($10cmH_2O$) and chest physiotherapy.
- If SpO_2 remains <90%, despite 100% O_2, there may be solid food material obstructing part of the bronchial tree. If the patient is intubated, consider using fibreoptic/rigid bronchoscopy or bronchial lavage using saline to remove any large foreign bodies or semi-solid material from the airway. Refer to ICU post-operatively.

Other considerations

- Corticosteroids may modify the inflammatory response early after aspiration, but do not alter the outcome, except by potentially interfering with the normal immune response.
- Prophylactic antibiotics are not generally given routinely (unless infected material aspirated) but may be required to treat subsequent 2° infections.
- If the gastric aspirate has been buffered to pH 7, the resulting aspiration pneumonitis is less severe, volume for volume, than if it is highly acidic. However, solid food material can produce prolonged inflammation, even if the overall pH is neutral.
- Blood, although undesirable, is generally well tolerated in the airway.

Status asthmaticus

Condition	Intractable bronchospasm[1]
Presentation	↑ airway pressure; sloping expiratory capnograph trace
Immediate action	100% O_2; salbutamol 250 micrograms IV/2.5mg neb; aminophylline 250mg slow IV; magnesium sulphate 2g IV has been shown to be effective
Follow-up action	Hydrocortisone 200mg
Investigations	CXR; ABGs
Also consider	Breathing circuit obstruction Kinked ETT/cuff herniation Endobronchial intubation/tube migration Foreign body in airway Anaphylaxis Pneumothorax

Risk factors

- Asthma, particularly with previous acute admissions, especially to ICU, and/or systemic steroid dependence.
- Intercurrent respiratory tract infection.
- Carinal irritation by ETT.

Diagnosis

- Increased airway pressure, prolonged expiratory phase to capnograph trace.
- Central trachea, with bilaterally hyperexpanded and resonant lung fields ± expiratory wheeze (absent if severe).
- Severe bronchospasm is a diagnosis of exclusion. The quickest method of ascertaining the source of increased airway resistance is to break the breathing circuit distal to all connectors/filters and to try ventilating directly with a self-inflating bag. If the inflation pressure still feels too high, the problem is due to airway/ETT obstruction or reduced compliance.
- Eliminate ETT obstruction by 'sounding' the ETT with a graduated GEB (note the distance it can be inserted down the ETT, and compare it with the external tube markings).

Immediate management

- ABC—100% O_2.
- Increase the volatile agent concentration—sevoflurane is the least irritant and is less likely to precipitate dysrhythmias in the presence of hypercapnia.
- Salbutamol 250 micrograms IV or 2.5mg by nebulizer up to 5mg every 15min. Alternatively (as an immediate measure), administer 2–6 puffs

of a β-agonist inhaler into the airway by placing the device in the barrel of a 50mL syringe. Attach the syringe by a Luer lock to a 15cm length of fine-bore infusion/capnograph tubing, which can then be fed directly down the ETT. The inhaler can be discharged by pressure applied via the syringe plunger. Use of the fine-bore tubing decreases deposition of the drug on the ETT.
- Aminophylline 250mg by slow IV injection (up to 5mg/kg).

Subsequent management
- If immediate treatment fails or is unavailable, consider ipratropium bromide (0.25mg nebulizer, up to 0.5mg 4- to 6-hourly), adrenaline IV boluses (10 micrograms = 0.1mL of 1:10 000), ketamine (2mg/kg IV), magnesium (2g slow IV).
- Hydrocortisone 200mg IV.
- Check the drug chart and notes for possible drug allergies to agents already administered.
- Arrange CXR—check for pneumothorax and ETT tip position (withdraw if carinal).
- Check ABGs and electrolytes (prolonged use of $β_2$-agonists causes hypokalaemia).
- Refer to ICU.

Other considerations
- **Gas trapping**: raised mean intrathoracic pressure may result from IPPV in the presence of severe bronchospasm. If pulse pressure falls and neck veins appear distended, consider obstructed venous return and a dependent fall in cardiac output. Intermittently disconnect the ETT from the circuit, and observe the (connected) capnograph trace for evidence of prolonged expiration and return of pulse pressure.
- Ventilator setting advice during this phase: 100% O_2, initially by hand, may need high pressures, slow rate, and prolonged expiration; do not worry about CO_2 levels, provided SpO_2 is adequate. May be necessary to accept a reduced ventilatory rate to allow adequate expiration to occur (**permissive hypercapnia**).[1]

Reference
1 British Thoracic Society, Scottish Intercollegiate Guidelines Network (2008). *British guideline on the management of asthma. A national clinical guideline.* Revised January 2012. ℘ https://www.brit-thoracic.org.uk/document-library/clinical-information/asthma/btssign-guideline-on-the-management-of-asthma/.

Pulmonary oedema

Condition	↑ Hydrostatic pressure; ↑ vascular permeability; ↓ plasma colloid osmotic pressure; negative inter-stitial pressure; obstructed lymphatic drainage
Presentation	Pink frothy sputum; ↑ HR; ↑ respiratory rate; ↓ SpO_2; ↑ CVP; ↑ PAOP
Immediate action	100% O_2; ↓ PAOP by posture
Follow-up action	Opioids; diuretics; vasodilators
Investigations	CXR; ECG; ABG; consider PA catheter studies
Also consider	Asthma
	MI
	ARDS
	Drug reaction
	Aspiration

Risk factors

- MI or pre-existing myocardial disease (pump failure).
- Drugs/toxins (drug reaction, myocardial depression).
- Fluid overload (especially in renal failure and the elderly).
- Aspiration (chemical pneumonitis).
- Pre-existing lung disease or infection (increased capillary permeability).
- Malnutrition (low oncotic pressure)—rare.
- Acute head injury or intracranial pathology (neurogenic).
- Severe laryngospasm or airway obstruction (negative intrathoracic pressure).
- Severe hypertension; LV failure; mitral stenosis (high pulmonary vascular hydrostatic pressure).
- Lateral decubitus position (unilateral).
- Impairment of lymphatic drainage (e.g. malignancy).
- Rapid lung expansion (e.g. re-expansion of a pneumothorax).
- Following pneumonectomy.

Diagnosis

- Clinical: wheeze; pink, frothy sputum; fine crackles; quiet bases; gallop rhythm; ↑ JVP; liver engorgement.
- Monitors: ↑ HR; ↑ RR; ↓ SpO_2; ↑ airway pressure; ↑ CVP; ↓ PAOP (>25–30mmHg).
- CXR: basal shadowing; upper lobe diversion; 'bat's wing' or 'staghorn' appearance; hilar haze; bronchial cuffing; Kerley B lines; pleural effusions; septal/interlobar fluid lines.
- ECG: evidence of right heart strain; evidence of MI.

Immediate management

- ABC—then management depends upon the current state of the patient.
- If awake and breathing spontaneously: sit up to offload the pulmonary vasculature and improve FRC; high-flow 100% O_2 via mask with reservoir bag; furosemide 50mg IV; diamorphine 5mg IV; consider using CPAP 5–10mmHg, and a vasodilator if hypertensive (e.g. GTN 0.5–1.5mg sublingually, or 10mg transcutaneous patch. Beware of IV GTN administration in the absence of invasive BP monitoring).
- If anaesthetized and intubated: commence IPPV with PEEP (5–10cmH$_2$O) in a 15 head-up position to reduce atelectasis and improve FRC; aspirate free fluid from the trachea intermittently; drug therapy as above.

Subsequent management

- Optimize fluid therapy, and maintain plasma colloid oncotic pressure on the basis of serial CVP measurements. If in doubt, measure PAOP via a PA catheter.
- Consider inotropic support with a β-agonist (e.g. dobutamine) or venesection (500mL) if filling pressures remain high or signs of inadequate circulation persist.

Failed intubation

(See also ➲ p. 952 and p. 749.)

Condition	Patients die from failure to oxygenate, NOT failure to intubate
Presentation	One in 65 patients is likely to present difficulties with intubation
Immediate action	Establish a patent airway with 100% O_2
Follow-up action	Do you need to intubate? Should you continue or wake the patient up?
Investigations	ETT confirmation—capnograph; negative-pressure ETT aspiration (bladder syringe); fibreoptic scope
Also consider	Regional anaesthesia or AFOI

Diagnosis of misplacement

- Retain a high index of suspicion after difficult intubation.
- Suspect oesophageal placement if you cannot confirm; normal breath sounds in both axillae and absent sounds over the stomach; rise AND fall of the chest; normal $ETCO_2$ trace; normal airway pressure cycle.
- The trachea is a rigid structure; the oesophagus is not. If negative pressure is applied to the ETT, failure to aspirate air (e.g. with a bladder syringe directly attached to the ETT) suggests an oesophageal placement.
- Confirm ETT placement with a fibrescope.
- Remember—if in doubt, pull it out, and apply bag-and-mask ventilation.

Other considerations

- Head-down left lateral position used to be advocated as a part of the failed intubation drill. However, for the majority of anaesthetists, the ability to manipulate an obstructed airway will be greater with the patient left in the more familiar supine position. In a spontaneously breathing patient who is waking up, the airway is often better in the lateral position. Use whichever is most effective, but keep help available to turn the patient, if needed.
- If the patient remains well oxygenated, while asleep, with an LMA *in situ*, consider attempting intubation via the LMA using an Aintree catheter loaded onto a 4.2mm fibreoptic laryngoscope, then, after withdrawal of the LMA and with the aid of a laryngoscope, railroad a 7.0mm ETT (with the tip anterior) over the Aintree catheter.

Immediate management

The Difficult Airway Society (DAS) algorithm for failed intubation is given in Fig. 36.6.

Further reading

Difficult Airway Society. [UK guidelines] ✍ http://www.das.uk.com.

Failed intubation, increasing hypoxaemia, and difficult ventilation in the paralysed anaesthetized patient: rescue techniques for the 'Cannot intubate, cannot ventilate' situation

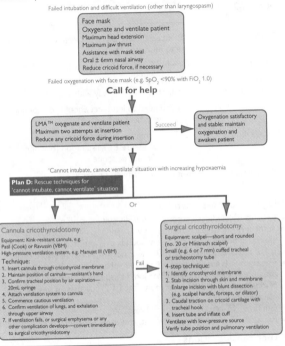

Failed intubation and difficult ventilation (other than laryngospasm)

> **Face mask**
> Oxygenate and ventilate patient
> Maximum head extension
> Maximum jaw thrust
> Assistance with mask seal
> Oral ± 6mm nasal airway
> Reduce cricoid force, if necessary

Failed oxygenation with face mask (e.g. SpO₂ <90% with FiO₂ 1.0)

Call for help

> LMA™ oxygenate and ventilate patient
> Maximum two attempts at insertion
> Reduce any cricoid force during insertion

Succeed →

> Oxygenation satisfactory and stable: maintain oxygenation and awaken patient

'Cannot intubate, cannot ventilate' situation with increasing hypoxaemia

Plan D: Rescue techniques for 'cannot intubate, cannot ventilate' situation

Or

Cannula cricothyroidotomy
Equipment: Kink-resistant cannula, e.g. Patil (Cook) or Ravussin (VBM)
High-pressure ventilation system, e.g. Manujet III (VBM)
Technique:
1. Insert cannula through cricothyroid membrane
2. Maintain position of cannula—assistant's hand
3. Confirm tracheal position by air aspiration—20mL syringe
4. Attach ventilation system to cannula
5. Commence cautious ventilation
6. Confirm ventilation of lungs, and exhalation through upper airway
7. If ventilation fails, or surgical emphysema or any other complication develops—convert immediately to surgical cricothyroidotomy

Fail →

Surgical cricothyroidotomy
Equipment: scalpel—short and rounded (no. 20 or Minitrach scalpel)
Small (e.g. 6 or 7 mm) cuffed tracheal or tracheostomy tube
4-step technique:
1. Identify cricothyroid membrane
2. Stab incision through skin and membrane Enlarge incision with blunt dissection (e.g. scalpel handle, forceps, or dilator)
3. Caudal traction on cricoid cartilage with tracheal hook
4. Insert tube and inflate cuff
Ventilate with low-pressure source
Verify tube position and pulmonary ventilation

Notes:
1. These techniques can have serious complications—use only in life-threatening situations
2. Convert to definitive airway as soon as possible
3. Post-operative management—see other difficult airway guidelines and flow charts
4. 4mm cannula with low-pressure ventilation may be successful in patient breathing spontaneously

Difficult Airway Society guidelines flow charts 2004 (use with DAS guidelines paper)

Fig. 36.6 Failed intubation.
Reproduced with permission of J. J. Henderson, M. T. Popat, I. P. Latto, A. C. Pearce, *Difficult Airway Society guidelines for management of the unanticipated difficult intubation*, John Wiley & Sons, Inc.

Cannot intubate, cannot ventilate

(See also ➐ p. 957.)

Condition	Failure to oxygenate by ETT/face mask/LMA/ ProSeal LMA/ILMA
Presentation	One in 10 000 anaesthetics
Immediate action	Summon help; 100% O_2; CPAP; wake patient up, if possible
Follow-up action	Needle or surgical cricothyroidotomy
Also consider	Emergency tracheostomy; fibreoptic intubation; blind nasal approach

Immediate management

- Call for help, but retain your trained assistant.
- Attempt oxygenation, even if it appears futile. Insert both an oral AND a nasopharyngeal airway. Emergency O_2 flush. Apply a close-fitting face mask with two hands, and lift/dislocate the mandible firmly forwards (jaw thrust). Although an assistant may help by bag-squeezing, it may be easiest to attempt ventilation by allowing an intermittent leak around the mask.
- Consider using a conventional LMA, ILMA, ProSeal LMA, or i-Gel. No single airway adjunct has clear advantages over another. This is not a time to experiment with unfamiliar devices, so stick to whatever you feel comfortable with, and abandon them early if they prove to be of no benefit.
- If the patient is making spontaneous effort and respiratory noise, maintain CPAP and 100% O_2 until they awaken.

Subsequent management

- **Cricothyroidotomy**: the decision to attempt transtracheal oxygenation is not an easy one to make. However, remember that it is likely to take over a minute to achieve access, and, even then, the ability to oxygenate will be severely limited. Speed is essential in order to prevent hypoxic cardiac arrest and brain damage.
- Options are surgical cricothyroidotomy and needle cricothyroidotomy.
- **Needle cricothyroidotomy**: extend the neck. You may find access easier if someone else does this for you and simultaneously fixes the skin by applying slight traction bilaterally to the soft tissues of the neck.
- Find the cricothyroid membrane (lies between the superiorly notched thyroid cartilage and the cricoid cartilage) (Fig. 36.7).
- Attach a 20mL syringe containing 10mL of saline to a large-bore needle or cannula (14–16G). Advance through the cricothyroid membrane in a slightly caudally inclined direction, aspirating until air bubbles freely into the syringe.

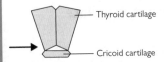

Fig. 36.7 Location of the cricothyroid membrane.

- If you have used a needle, hold it firmly in place. If you have used a cannula, guard against kinking.
- There are several ways of connecting a needle/cannula to a standard breathing circuit:
  - Connect a 10mL syringe; remove the plunger, and intubate the barrel with a cuffed ETT
  - Insert an ETT connector from a neonatal 3.5mm ETT to the hub of the needle/cannula
  - Unscrew the capnograph tubing from the monitor; attach the Luer lock end to the hub of the needle/cannula. Take the other end, and attach the sampling end (T-piece) to the common gas outlet. Use your thumb to intermittently occlude the other end of the T-piece
  - Use a Sanders injector or similar jetting device attached by a Luer lock. Beware—high-pressure O_2 can cause catastrophic surgical emphysema via a misplaced cannula. Check for rise and fall of the chest wall.
- Transtracheal oxygenation by needle/cannula is a temporary emergency measure. Fully effective ventilation will not be possible, but there should be a flow of O_2 down the bronchial tree to the alveoli.
- If there is significant O_2 leakage upwards, occlude the mouth and nose during the inspiratory phase of ventilation.
- Call urgently for an ENT surgeon to perform an emergency tracheostomy. If possible, improve transtracheal access with a 'Minitrach' or similar device. There are several easy-to-use commercial kits that exist, based around a Seldinger method of insertion. If the patient remains paralysed, attempt fibreoptic/blind nasal intubation.
- Consider transtracheal jet ventilation, but stop ventilating immediately if surgical emphysema forms in the neck.
- **Surgical cricothyroidotomy** requires a scalpel, tracheal hook/forceps/clamp, and a small tube (6–7mm).
  - Make a stab incision through the cricothyroid membrane.
  - Enlarge the incision with blunt dissection using forceps/clamp.
  - Keep the hook/clamp/forceps in the wound to avoid losing access.
  - Apply caudal traction on the cricoid cartilage, while inserting the tube.

Other considerations
- The best treatment is prevention, or at least anticipation of potential airway difficulties. Avoidance of muscle relaxants is prudent, until one has determined that ventilation can be achieved manually. Thorough preoxygenation will ensure that the FRC contains ~1L of O_2, rather than

0.5L at induction. Have the kit and personnel required for the creation of a surgical airway close at hand if you anticipate difficulties intubating.
- Reversal of recent rocuronium-induced paralysis (and, to some extent, vecuronium-induced paralysis) can be achieved in 1.5min with sugammadex 16mg/kg IV.
- If the problem is an inability to achieve a seal due to the presence of a beard, quickly apply a large transparent self-adhesive dressing over the whole of the lower face. Make a large hole in it for the mouth and nostrils, and reapply the mask ± an airway.
- If the problem is an inability to pass a small enough ETT tube down a narrowed trachea (either ETT too short or size unavailable), consider passing an airway exchange catheter. This is a robust guide that resembles a yellow, but hollow, GEB. It comes with either a Luer lock or 15mm connector, allowing O_2 to be passed through it into the distal airway, while a more definitive airway is established either by railroading a larger tube over it or by surgical tracheostomy.
- Commercially available transtracheal needles and injectors are now widely available.
- Check that your theatres have a well-stocked difficult/failed intubation trolley available at all times.
- YouTube (⌨ http://www.youtube.com) has some good examples of different techniques of cricothyroidotomy.

Further reading

Difficult Airway Society. [UK guidelines] ⌨ http://www.das.uk.com.

Malignant hyperthermia

(See also ➋ p. 255.)

Condition	Hypermetabolism due to increased skeletal muscle intracellular Ca^{2+}
Presentation	↑ $ETCO_2$; ↓ SpO_2; ↑ HR; CVS instability; dys-rhythmias; ↑ core temperature
Immediate action	Stop triggers (volatile agents plus suxametho-nium); hyperventilate with high-flow 100% O_2; dantrolene 1–10mg/kg
Follow-up action	Cool; correct DIC, acidosis/↑ K^+; promote diuresis (ARF risk)
Investigations	Clotting studies, ABGs, K^+; urine myoglobin; CK
Also consider	Rebreathing Sepsis Awareness Neuroleptic malignant syndrome Ecstasy Thyroid storm

Risk factors

- Family history.
- Exposure to suxamethonium or volatile agents (even if previous exposures were uneventful).
- Exertional heat stroke. Exercise-induced rhabdomyolysis, central core disease, scoliosis, hernias, strabismus surgery.

Diagnosis

- Sustained jaw rigidity after suxamethonium (masseter spasm).
- Unexplained tachycardia, together with an unexpected rise in $ETCO_2$ (IPPV) or minute volume (SV).
- Falling SpO_2, despite increased FiO_2.
- CVS instability, dysrhythmias, especially multiple ventricular ectopics, peaked T waves on ECG.
- Generalized rigidity.
- Core temperature rise of 2°C/hr.

Immediate management

- **Check ABC**—turn off all volatile agents; do not administer any further doses of suxamethonium.
- **Hyperventilate** with 100% O_2 using a high FGF to flush out the volatile agent and expired CO_2.
- Tell the rest of the theatre team what the problem is. Ask for more help, and obtain dantrolene immediately.

- Use a fresh breathing circuit ± a 'vapour-free' machine if it is easy to do so, but not if it results in rebreathing of expired CO_2 or a low FiO_2, or delays administration of dantrolene.
- When available, give **dantrolene** 2–3mg/kg IV (it comes in 20mg ampoules, so about four are required). Usually about 2.5mg/kg is required in total, but up to 10mg/kg may be given.
- **Stop surgery**, if feasible; otherwise maintain anaesthesia with TIVA (propofol).
- **Reduce core temperature** by: evaporation; ice to the groin and axillae; cold fluids into IV lines, the bladder via a urinary catheter, the stomach via an NGT, or the peritoneal cavity if open.
- **Check ABGs and K^+**, especially if dysrhythmias occur, and correct acidosis/hyperkalaemia where appropriate.
- **Surgical team**—call for senior help to conclude the operation as quickly as is safely possible.

Subsequent management
- Place invasive BP and CVP monitoring lines.
- Send a clotting screen for DIC, and serum CK assay (up to 1000 times normal).
- Send a urine sample for myoglobin estimation 2° to muscle breakdown.
- Monitor for ARF, and promote diuresis with fluids and mannitol.
- Refer to the MH Investigation Unit for IVCTs.

Other considerations
- Dantrolene is formulated with 3g of mannitol per ampoule.
- Emptying several ampoules into a sterile dish and adding a large volume of sterile water may help mix dantrolene more rapidly.
- Follow-up involves muscle biopsy under LA and *in vitro* halothane, caffeine, ryanodine, and chlorocresol contracture tests.
- Beware of using bicarbonate to correct acidosis, since the reaction with H^+ produces an increased CO_2 load.
- AVOID calcium channel blockers; treat arrhythmias with magnesium or amiodarone or metoprolol, and correct electrolytes.

Further reading
Association of Anaesthetists of Great Britain & Ireland (2011). *Malignant hyperthermia crisis. AAGBI safety guideline.* ℘ http://www.aagbi.org/sites/default/files/MH%20guideline%20for%20web%20v2.pdf.
British Malignant Hyperthermia Association. ℘ http://www.bmha.co.uk.

Useful contact
(See also ➲ p. 260.)
UK MH Investigation Unit, Academic Unit of Anaesthesia, Clinical Sciences Building, St James' University Hospital Trust, Leeds LS9 7TF. Emergency telephone number 07947 609601.

Anaphylaxis

(See also ➲ p. 993.)

Condition	IgE-mediated type 1 hypersensitivity reaction to an antigen, resulting in histamine and serotonin release from mast cells and basophils
Presentation	CVS collapse; erythema; bronchospasm; oedema; rash
Immediate action	Remove trigger; 100% O_2; elevate legs; adrenaline 50 micrograms; fluids
Follow-up action	Chlorphenamine 10–20mg; hydrocortisone 100–300mg; ABGs
Investigations	Plasma tryptase; urinary methylhistamine
Also consider	1° myocardial/CVS problem Latex sensitivity Airway obstruction Asthma Tension pneumothorax

Risk factors

- IV administration of the antigen.
- Note that cross-sensitivities with NSAIDs and muscle relaxants mean that previous exposure is not always necessary.
- True penicillin allergy is a reaction to the basic common structure present in most penicillins (the β-lactam ring).
- Muscle relaxants, antibiotics, and NSAIDs are the most frequent triggers.
- Reactions to dyes (e.g. patent blue) and chlorhexidine are becoming more commonplace.

Diagnosis

- CVS collapse (88%).
- Erythema (45%).
- Bronchospasm (36%.)
- Angio-oedema (24%).
- Rash (13%).
- Urticaria (8.5%).

Immediate management

- Check ABC—stop the administration of any potential triggers, particularly IV agents.
- Call for help.
- Maintain the airway, and give 100% O_2.
- Lay the patient flat, with the legs elevated.

- Give adrenaline in 50 micrograms IV increments (0.5mL of 1:10 000 solution) at a rate of 100 micrograms/min, until pulse pressure or bronchospasm improves. Alternatively, give adrenaline 0.5–1mg IM (repeated after 10min, if necessary).
- Give IV fluid (colloid or suitable crystalloid).

Subsequent management

- Antihistamines: give chlorphenamine 10–20mg slow IV.
- Corticosteroids: give hydrocortisone 100–300mg IV.
- Catecholamine infusion, as CVS instability may last several hours: adrenaline 0.05–0.1 micrograms/kg/min (= 4mL/hr of 1:10 000 or 5mg/50mL of saline—70kg adult). Noradrenaline 0.05–0.1 micrograms/kg/min (= 4mL/hr of 4mg/40mL of 5% glucose—70kg adult).
- Check ABGs for acidosis, and consider bicarbonate 0.5–1.0mmol/kg (8.4% solution = 1mmol/mL).
- Check for the presence of airway oedema by letting down the ETT cuff and confirming a leak prior to extubating.
- Consider bronchodilators (see Status asthmaticus, ➲ p. 909) for persistent bronchospasm.

Other considerations

- Investigations can wait until the patient has been stabilized. Take a 10mL clotted blood sample 1hr after the start of the reaction, to perform a tryptase assay. The specimen needs to be spun down, and the serum stored at −20°C.
- The anaesthetist should follow up the investigation, report reactions to the Committee on Safety of Medicines (CSM), and arrange testing with an immunologist (see ➲ p. 993).

Further reading

Harper NJ, Dixon T, Dugué P, et al.; Working Party of the Association of Anaesthetists of Great Britain and Ireland (2009). Suspected anaphylactic reactions associated with anaesthesia. *Anaesthesia*, **64**, 199–211. Also available at: ⌨ http://www.aagbi.org.

Resuscitation Council (UK). [UK Resuscitation Council guidelines.] ⌨ http://www.resus.org.uk.

Intra-arterial injection

Condition	Chemical endarteritis characterized by: arterial vasospasm and local release of noradrenaline; crystal deposition within the distal arteries (thiopental); subsequent thrombosis and distal ischaemic necrosis
Presentation	Intense burning pain on injection; distal blanching; blistering
Immediate action	Stop injection, but leave the cannula *in situ*, and administer 1% lidocaine 5mL and papaverine 40mg, and flush with heparinized saline
Follow-up action	Regional sympathetic blockade; anticoagulation
Investigations	Monitor anticoagulation
Also consider	Extravasation Dilution error of drug administered

Risk factors
- Antecubital lines: inadvertent cannulation of the brachial artery or aberrant ulnar artery.
- Radial aspect of the wrist: inadvertent cannulation of the superficial branch of the radial artery.
- Arterial injection is more likely to cause damage with a stronger drug concentration (e.g. 5% thiopental).
- A cannula that has been inserted previously and only been flushed with saline (not painful) may present later.

Diagnosis
- Awake patients complain of intense burning pain on injection that may last for several hours.
- Blanching of the skin.
- Blistering.
- Within 2hr: oedema; hyperaesthesia; motor weakness.
- Later: signs of arterial thrombosis ± gangrene.

Immediate management
- Stop injecting!
- Principles of treatment are to dilute the irritant, reverse vasospasm, and prevent thrombosis.
- Keep the cannula *in situ*—you will need access to reverse local vasoconstriction within the distal arteriolar tree.
- If the drug administered was highly irritant, flush the vessel with isotonic saline or Hepsal®.

- Administer LA via the cannula to reduce vasospasm and reduce pain (e.g. 5mL of 1% lidocaine).
- Administer a vasodilator (e.g. papaverine 40mg).
- Once the immediate reaction has subsided, if the hand is well perfused and pink, remove the cannula, and apply sufficient pressure to the puncture site to minimize local haematoma formation.

Subsequent management

- Sympathetic blockade and anticoagulation to reduce the risk of thrombosis:
  - **Sympathectomy** via stellate ganglion or brachial plexus block—probably most easily achieved via the axillary approach, or
  - **Guanethidine** block: performed like a Bier's block (guanethidine 10–20mg IV plus heparin 500U in 25–40mL of saline, cuff left inflated for 20min). Guanethidine blocks α-adrenergic neurones and depletes noradrenaline stores. The effects can last for several weeks. Ask for assistance from a consultant with a special interest in chronic pain, since this block is also used to treat complex regional pain syndrome (CRPS)
  - **Heparinize** after achieving sympathetic blockade to minimize the risk of late arterial thrombosis.

Other considerations

Nerve supply to the arm = C5–T1. The sympathetic nerve supply to the arm comes from T1 via the sympathetic chain and the stellate ganglion (fusion of the inferior cervical ganglion and the 1st thoracic ganglion).

Unsuccessful reversal of neuromuscular blockade

(See also ➋ p. 1024 and p. 1028.)

Condition	Competitive antagonism at nicotinic acetylcholine receptor of neuromuscular junction
Presentation	Uncoordinated, jerky movements during the recovery phase. Inability to maintain an airway OR inadequate minute ventilation
Immediate action	Maintain and protect airway, and provide adequate ventilation
Follow-up action	Maintain anaesthesia, if appropriate; correct the cause Consider reversal of aminosteroids (rocuronium, vecuronium, pancuronium) with sugammadex
Investigations	Nerve stimulator train-of-four, post-tetanic count; double-burst stimulation
Also consider	Non-functional peripheral nerve stimulator (check the battery charge) Volatile agent concentration (maintained by hypoventilation) Hyperventilation ($ETCO_2$ <4kPa (30mmHg)) or CO_2 narcosis (over about 9kPa (68mmHg)) Undiagnosed head injury (examine pupils) CVA Hypoglycaemia

Risk factors

- Recent dose of relaxant/backflow in IVI/drug error.
- Renal and hepatic impairment, causing delayed elimination of the relaxant in long cases (except atracurium).
- Perioperative administration of magnesium (especially above the therapeutic range 1.25–2.5mmol/L).
- Hypothermia.
- Acidosis and electrolyte imbalance.
- Co-administration of aminoglycoside antibiotics.
- Myasthenia gravis (reduced number of receptors).
- Low levels of plasma cholinesterase (pregnancy, renal and liver disorders, hypothyroidism) or competition with drugs also metabolized by plasma cholinesterase (etomidate, ester LAs, and methotrexate).
- Abnormal plasma cholinesterase (suxamethonium apnoea).

Diagnosis

- Uncoordinated, jerky patient movements are suggestive of an inadequate reversal of NMB. Sustained head lift off the pillow for 5s is a good clinical indicator of adequate reversal.
- Train-of-four is classically measured as adductor pollicis twitches in response to supramaximal stimulation via two electrodes placed over the ulnar nerve (see ⟶ p. 1027).
- Double-burst stimulation is said to be more accurate as a means of quantifying the train-of four-ratio (see ⟶ p. 1027).
- Post-tetanic count is used to monitor deep relaxation when the train-of-four will not show any twitches. First, establish that the PNS is actually working and has an adequate battery charge. A 50Hz tetanic stimulus is applied for 5s, followed by single stimuli at 1Hz. Post-tetanic facilitation in the presence of non-depolarizing blockade allows a number of twitches to be seen. Reversal with an anticholinesterase should be possible with a count of >10.

Immediate management

- ABC—then check for signs of awareness; assess the anaesthetic depth, and check ETCO₂.
- If you have already given a dose of neostigmine, ensure it was adequate (0.05mg/kg) and that it did actually enter the circulation (check the IV line for backflow and the site of cannulation for swelling).
- If you have used an aminosteroid muscle relaxant (rocuronium, vecuronium, or pancuronium), consider administering sugammadex at a dose of 2–4mg/kg.
- Hypothermia, electrolyte imbalance, and acidosis will impair reversal and should be corrected.
- Aminoglycoside or Mg^{2+}-induced poor reversal may improve with calcium gluconate (10mL of 10%) titrated IV.

Subsequent management

- Wait patiently—this is not an emergency!
- Suspected myasthenia gravis should be confirmed post-operatively with an edrophonium test.
- If the patient has suffered a period of awareness while paralysed, admit it, explain it, apologize, and ensure that the patient has access to professional counselling, if required.

Other considerations

- A dual (phase II) blockade occurs when large amounts of suxamethonium are used and the depolarizing block is gradually replaced by one with non-depolarizing characteristics (fade, etc.).

Further reading

Lenz A, Hill G, White PF (2007). Emergency use of sugammadex after failure of standard reversal drugs. *Anesth Analg*, **104**, 585–6.

Naguib M (2007). Sugammadex: another milestone in clinical neuromuscular pharmacology. *Anesth Analg*, **104**, 575–81.

Paediatric emergencies: advanced life support

(See also ➲ p. 838.)

Adopt a SAFE approach

- Shout for help.
- Approach with care.
- Free the patient from immediate danger.
- Evaluate the patient's ABC.

Assess the airway and breathing first. Give FIVE RESCUE BREATHS (chest seen to rise and fall) before assessing the circulation. Each breath should take about 1–1.5s. Check the carotid pulse in a child, but use the brachial pulse in an infant. Feel for no more than 10s.

The commonest arrest scenario in children is bradycardia proceeding to asystole—a response to severe hypoxia and acidosis. BLS aimed at restoring early oxygenation should therefore be a priority of management (Fig. 36.8). VF is relatively uncommon but may complicate hypothermia, tricyclic poisoning, and children with pre-existing cardiac disease (Fig. 36.9).

- All children over 1yr should be given BLS at a ratio of 15:2 (compressions:ventilations), aiming for 100–120 compressions/min (five cycles).
- Chest compressions should be started if a central pulse cannot be palpated or the child has a pulse rate <60bpm with poor perfusion.
- Where no vascular access is present, immediate intraosseous access is recommended.
- Once the airway has been secured, chest compressions should be continued at 100–120/min uninterrupted, with breaths administered at a rate of 10–12/min.
- When circulation has been restored, ventilate the child at 12–20 breaths/min to normalize PCO_2.

Asystole or pulseless electrical activity

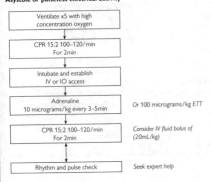

Fig. 36.8 Asystole or pulseless electrical activity.

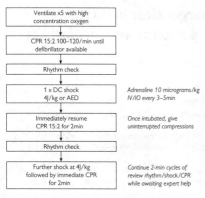

Fig. 36.9 Ventricular fibrillation or pulseless ventricular tachycardia.

Notes

Consider the following:

- Hypoxia
- Hypovolaemia
- Hyper-/hypokalaemia
- Hypothermia
- Tension pneumothorax

- Cardiac tamponade
- Toxin/drug overdose
- Thromboemboli
- Metabolic disturbances.

Further reading

Resuscitation Council (UK) (2010). *Paediatric advanced life support.* ℘ https://www.resus.org.uk/
pages/pals.pdf.

Paediatric emergencies: ventricular fibrillation or pulseless ventricular tachycardia

(See also ➜ p. 889.)

Notes

- Continue shocks every 2min.
- Standard automated external defibrillators (AEDs) may be used in children over 8yr.
- Purpose-made paediatric pads are recommended for children aged between 1yr and 8yr, but an unmodified adult AED may be used for children older than 1yr.
- Adrenaline 10 micrograms/kg (= 0.1mL/kg of 1:10 000 solution) and amiodarone 5mg/kg after a 3rd shock, once compressions have been resumed.
- Repeat adrenaline every alternate cycle (3–5min).
- Consider hypokalaemia, hypothermia, and poisoning.
- Further antiarrhythmic agents:
  - 1st line: repeat amiodarone 5mg/kg IV after 5th shock
  - 2nd line: lidocaine 1mg/kg IV if amiodarone is not available
  - Torsade de pointes: magnesium sulfate 25–50mg/kg
  - There is no evidence that atropine confers any benefit in asphyxial bradycardia or asystole.

Further reading

Resuscitation Council (UK) (2010). *Paediatric advanced life support.* ℛ https://www.resus.org.uk/pages/pals.pdf.

Paediatric emergencies: neonatal resuscitation

Condition	Acute neonatal asphyxia during the birth process
Presentation	Floppy, blue, or pale, HR <60bpm, diminished respiratory effort
Immediate action	Delay cord clamping for at least 1min. Dry, wrap, and warm the baby. Open and clear airway, five inflation breaths with air (2–3s at 30cmH$_2$O)
Follow-up action	Cardiac compressions (3:1) at 120/min if <60bpm, review ventilation
Investigations	Record Apgar scores (Table 36.1)
Also consider	Hypovolaemia, diaphragmatic hernia, pneumothorax, therapeutic hypothermia

Risk factors

- Known fetal distress; category 1 emergency Caesarean section; meconium-stained liquor.
- Prolonged delivery; instrumental delivery; shoulder dystocia; multiple births.
- Maternal drugs: opioids, GA for Caesarean section.
- Preterm delivery (survival is very poor if gestation <23wk, and resuscitation is not recommended).

Diagnosis

- A normal newly delivered baby is pink, breathes spontaneously within 15s, has an HR >100bpm, has good muscle tone, and is vocal.
- A baby requiring resuscitation is floppy, silent, blue, or pale, has an HR <100bpm, and with gasping, diminished, or absent respiratory effort. See Apgar scores in Table 36.1.

Table 36.1 Apgar scores

	0	1	2
Colour	Pale/blue	Blue extremities	Pink
HR (bpm)	Absent	<100	>100
Response to stimulation	Nil	Movement	Cry
Muscle tone	Limp	Some flexion	Well flexed
Respiratory effort	Absent	Poor effort/weak cry	Good

Immediate management

- Keep the theatre warm. Dry and wrap the baby. Keep warm under a radiant heater. Use food-grade plastic wrapping for preterm babies (30wk and below).
- Open and clear the airway, but keep the neck in a neutral position.
- Give FIVE effective inflation breaths (2–3s at 30cmH$_2$O) of air or O$_2$.
- HR should increase; continue ventilating at 30–40/min, until spontaneous effort is adequate.
- If HR remains <60bpm, commence chest compressions with thumbs around the chest, at a compression rate of 120/min and a ratio of 3:1 breaths. Compress the chest diameter by one-third.
- Reassess HR every 30s.

Subsequent management

- In the neonate that remains unresponsive despite oxygenation, consider intubation and drugs (Table 36.2).

Table 36.2 Resuscitating the neonate

	40/40 gestation	35/40 gestation	30/40 gestation
Weight (kg)	3.5	2.5	1.5
ETT internal diameter (mm)	3.5	3.0	2.5
ETT length (cm)	9.5	8.5	7.5
Adrenaline 1/10 000 (intraosseous/IV) (mL)	0.35–1.0	0.25–0.75	0.15–0.45
Sodium bicarbonate 4.2% IV(mL)	3.5–7	2.5–5	1.5–3
Glucose 10% IV (mL)	17–35	12–25	7–15
Volume IV (O-negative/0.9% NaCl) (mL)	35–70	25–50	15–30

Other considerations

- If response to resuscitation is prompt (requiring only support breaths), return the baby to the parents.
- For ventilatory depression thought to be due to maternal opioids, give naloxone 200 micrograms IM.
- Reasons to transfer to special care baby unit: ongoing ventilation, major congenital abnormality, prematurity.

Further reading

Resuscitation Council (UK) (2010). *Newborn life support.* ℬ https://www.resus.org.uk/pages/nls.pdf.

Paediatric emergencies: collapsed septic child

Condition	Sepsis with multiorgan failure, capillary leak, and hypoperfusion
Presentation	Fever >38°C, ↓ BP, ↑ HR, ↑ respiratory rate, oliguria, altered conscious level
Immediate action	100% O$_2$, fluid resuscitation, inotropes, antibiotics
Follow-up action	Referral to a specialist paediatric critical care unit
Investigations	FBC, clotting, U&Es, glucose, blood cultures
Also consider	Hypovolaemia/blood loss, anaphylaxis, poisoning, cardiac abnormality

Risk factors
- Immune deficiency, chronic illness.
- Exposure to Gram-positive/negative bacteria, *Listeria*, *Rickettsia*, herpesvirus.

Diagnosis
- 'Warm shock' presents early as vasodilatation and often responds to volume resuscitation.
- 'Cold shock' is more serious with lower BP, particularly diastolic hypotension, cold peripheries, capillary refill >2s, and oliguria, requiring significant circulatory support.
- Fever >38°C, altered level of consciousness, high WCC.

Immediate management
- **ABC**—100% O$_2$ via a non-rebreathing mask ± ventilatory support/intubation.
- **Fluid boluses** of 20mL/kg of crystalloid/colloid, up to 100mL/kg, to restore normovolaemia.
- **Inotropic support** with dobutamine (up to 20 micrograms/kg/min) if fluids ineffective.
- **Correct hypoglycaemia** with 10–20% glucose.
- If IV fluid and dobutamine are ineffective at maintaining BP, consider:
  - Dopamine (up to 20 micrograms/kg/min)
  - Adrenaline (0.1–1.0 micrograms/kg/min)
  - Noradrenaline (0.1 micrograms/kg/min).
- If pH <7.1 on ABGs and ventilation is adequate, correct acidosis with 8.4% sodium bicarbonate (4.2% in neonates), according to the following formula: *sodium bicarbonate required for full correction (mmol) = (weight in kg × 0.3 × base deficit)*. Give 50% correction first, then repeat ABGs and reassess.

- Antibiotics: cefotaxime 50mg/kg IV 6-hourly for older children or ampicillin plus gentamicin for neonates (seek the microbiologist's or PICU advice for up-to-date guidelines about doses for different ages).

Subsequent management

- Obtain specialist help early. Contact the nearest regional centre/PICU department for advice.
- Consider the possibility of raised ICP (bulging fontanelle, papilloedema, altered pupils). If suspected, catheterize the patient; ventilate to normocapnia, and give mannitol 0.5–1.0g/kg or furosemide 1mg/kg. Avoid LP. CT head.
- Consider the possibility of meningitis/encephalitis. Look for fever, lethargy, irritability, vomiting, headache, photophobia, convulsions, neck stiffness, and raised ICP. Look carefully for purpuric non-blanching spots.
- Consider DIC if mucosal surfaces are bleeding.
- Stabilize for transfer. A retrieval service may be provided by the receiving unit—prepare a handover.

Other considerations

- Significant capillary leakage in severe sepsis may result in pulmonary oedema 2° to fluid resuscitation. This may be reduced by using 4.5% HAS.
- If drugs are required to intubate the child, anticipate an exaggerated fall in BP, and adjust the dose accordingly. It is wise to start inotropes and fluid resuscitation before induction.

Paediatric emergencies: major trauma

(See also ➲ p. 844.)

Condition	Serious injury to chest/abdomen/pelvis/spine/head
Presentation	↑ HR, ↓ capillary refill, ↑ respiratory rate, ↓ conscious level, bony/visceral injuries
Immediate action	ABCDE, 100% O$_2$, 2 × IVs or intraosseous access, 20mL/kg of IV fluids
Follow-up action	2° survey, stabilize for transfer to theatre or critical care
Investigations	CXR, C-spine, ABG, ECG, G&S, blood glucose, CT head, ultrasound abdomen
Also consider	Non-accidental injury, poisoning, fitting

Risk factors

- Pedestrian/cyclist struck by vehicle, unrestrained passenger in road traffic accident.
- Head injuries account for 40% of trauma deaths in children.
- At-risk register.

Diagnosis

- Dependent upon the cause and 1° mode of injury. Usually involves blood loss, with resultant tachycardia and peripheral vasoconstriction. Respiratory rate increased.
- Diminished level of consciousness, respiratory/ventilatory compromise if chest injured.
- Immediately life-threatening conditions include airway obstruction, tension pneumothorax, cardiac tamponade, PEA cardiac arrest.

Immediate management

- *Airway*—100% O$_2$ (15L/min via non-rebreathing mask). In-line C-spine stabilization and RSI.
- *Breathing*—assess for bilateral expansion, breath sounds, and evidence of pneumothorax.
- *Circulation*—assess for tachycardia, capillary refill >2s, two IV cannulae, 20mL/kg of crystalloid.
- *Disability*—pupils and AVPU (Alert/responds to Voice/responds to Pain/Unresponsive).
- *Exposure*—remove clothes to assess, but keep warm. Look for evidence of visceral injuries (CSF leak, bloodstained sputum, bloodstained urine).

Subsequent management

- If repeated fluid boluses of 20mL/kg are required, blood should be given for the 3rd and subsequent boluses. Surgical intervention is likely if an external bleeding point has not been identified and controlled. Likely sites for internal bleeding are the abdomen, thorax, and pelvis. There may be large blood loss from scalp wounds or into the subdural space in children with head injuries, particularly infants.
- Place a urinary catheter and an orogastric tube/NGT.
- Unconscious patients should be ventilated to normocapnia with muscle relaxants, but beware of masking seizures.
- Perform a more detailed 2° survey after initial stabilization.
- Assess the need for surgical intervention.
- Stabilize before transferring out of the department.

Other considerations

- If IV cannulation proves difficult at conventional sites, attempt femoral venous access.
- **Intraosseous cannulation**: useful in all children if IV access is difficult. The most suitable site is the proximal tibia, 1–3cm (children) or 0.5–1cm (babies) below and just medial to the tibial tuberosity on the flat, medial aspect of the tibia where the bone lies SC. The anterior distal femur or humerus is an alternative if the tibia is fractured. Insert an 18–12G smooth or threaded needle at right angle, with the needle directed slightly caudally (away from the growth plate), until loss of resistance is felt and fluid can be injected easily without evidence of extravasation.

Paediatric emergencies: acute severe asthma

(See also ➲ p. 909.)

Condition	Severe bronchospasm
Presentation	Respiratory exhaustion; wheezy/silent chest; ↑ respiratory rate, ↑ HR
Immediate action	100% O₂, nebulized salbutamol 2.5mg, and ipratropium 250 micrograms
Follow-up action	Hydrocortisone 4mg/kg, consider adrenaline/ aminophylline/magnesium sulfate
Investigations	ABG, CXR, serum theophylline (if already taking this)
Also consider	Anaphylaxis, inhaled foreign body, pneumonia, epiglottitis, pneumothorax

Risk factors
- History of asthma, especially with acute respiratory tract infection.
- Exposure to known triggers (e.g. cold, smoke, allergen, exercise).
- Prematurity and low birthweight.

Diagnosis
- Confused or drowsy from exhaustion, maximal use of accessory muscles, unable to talk.
- Respiratory rate >30 breaths/min (>5yr) or >50 breaths/min (2–5yr), especially with a silent chest.
- PEFR <33% predicted [predicted PEFR in L/min = 5 × (height in cm − 80)].
- SpO_2 <92% or PaO_2 <8kPa (60mmHg) in air.
- $PaCO_2$ often normal initially but rises peri-arrest.
- HR >140bpm.

Immediate management
- Check ABC—100% O_2.
- Nebulized salbutamol 2.5–5mg (ten puffs via inhaler and spacer).
- Nebulized ipratropium bromide 250 micrograms.
- IV hydrocortisone 4mg/kg.
- Review ABC—consider intubation and ventilation (note gas trapping, so slow respiratory rate preferable).
- If still unresponsive:
  - IM adrenaline 10 micrograms/kg ± IV adrenaline infused at 0.02–0.1 micrograms/kg/min (or consider nebulized adrenaline 2.5–5mg or IV adrenaline 1 micrograms/kg, with ECG monitoring)
  - IV salbutamol titrated to effect, up to 15 micrograms/kg IV, over 10min, then infused at 1–5 micrograms/kg/min
  - IV aminophylline 5mg/kg loading dose, then infused at 1mg/kg/hr
  - IV magnesium sulfate 40mg/kg (max 2g).

Subsequent management
- Rehydrate with 10–20mL/kg of crystalloid.
- Oral prednisolone 20mg (2–5yr), 30–40mg (>5yr) for 3d.
- Repeat nebulizers every 20–30min, if necessary, otherwise 3- to 4-hourly.
- CXR to exclude pneumothorax.

Other considerations
- IPPV in severe bronchospasm is difficult and may result in gas trapping and CVS compromise 2° to raised intrathoracic pressure. Consider extending the expiratory phase and allowing hypercapnia to occur.
- Volatile agents and ketamine have been used to relieve intractable bronchospasm.
- Avoid the use of known histamine-releasing drugs (e.g. thiopental) and NSAIDs.

Further reading
British Thoracic Society, Scottish Intercollegiate Guidelines Network (2014). *British guideline on the management of asthma. A national clinical guideline, October 2014.* ℜ http://www.sign.ac.uk/pdf/SIGN141.pdf.

Paediatric emergencies: anaphylaxis

(See also ➲ p. 920 and p. 993.)

Condition	IgE-mediated type B hypersensitivity reaction
Presentation	Stridor, wheeze, cough, ↑ SpO_2, CVS collapse, respiratory distress
Immediate action	100% O_2, remove trigger, adrenaline IM, 20mL/kg of IV fluid
Follow-up action	Chlorphenamine IM/slow IV; hydrocortisone IM/slow IV
Investigations	ABGs, CXR, plasma tryptase, urinary methylhistamine
Also consider	Tension pneumothorax, latex allergy, sepsis, acute severe asthma

Risk factors

- Previous allergic reaction.
- History of asthma or atopy.
- Absence of an airway/circuit filter (latex allergy via aerosolized particles).
- Cross-sensitivities (e.g. latex and kiwi fruit/bananas; NSAIDs).
- Use of known allergens (nut extracts in ENT, radiographic contrast media, penicillins).

Diagnosis

- Common signs: stridor, wheeze, cough, arterial desaturation, respiratory distress, CVS collapse.
- Less commonly: rash, urticaria, oedema.

Immediate management

- ABC—100% O_2. (NB beware of sudden loss of airway control due to oedema.)
- Remove direct contact with all potential triggers (most commonly muscle relaxants/NSAIDs).
- Give IM adrenaline 1:1000 solution (10 micrograms/kg = 0.01mL/kg of 1:1000): <6 months, 50 micrograms (0.05mL); 6 months to 6yr, 120 micrograms (0.12mL); 6–12yr, 250 micrograms (0.25mL); >12yr, 500 micrograms (0.5mL) (Table 36.3).
- Give IV fluid volume resuscitation with 20mL/kg of crystalloid or colloid, and secure more IV access sites.

Subsequent management

- Antihistamine: chlorphenamine IM/slow IV (1–6yr, 2.5–5mg; 6–12yr, 5–10mg; >12yr, 10–20mg) (Table 36.3).
- Steroids: hydrocortisone IM/slow IV (1–6yr, 50mg; 6–12yr, 100mg; >12yr, 100–500mg).
- Frequent and careful review of the unsecured airway.

Table 36.3 Treatment of anaphylaxis in children

Age range	Adrenaline (IM) 1:1000	Chlorphenamine (IV)	Hydrocortisone (IV)
<6 months	50 micrograms (0.05mL)	–	–
6 months to 6yr	120 micrograms (0.12mL)	2.5–5mg (>12 months)	50mg (>12 months)
6–12yr	250 micrograms (0.25mL)	5–10mg	100mg
>12yr	500 micrograms (0.5mL)	10–20mg	100–500mg

Other considerations
- Chlorphenamine should not be given to neonates.
- IV adrenaline 1 microgram/kg (0.01mL/kg of 1:10 000) can be given incrementally, titrated to response, as an alternative to the IM route, but it must be done with ECG monitoring due to the risk of provoking dysrhythmias.
- Complete a yellow CSM notification, and refer to a clinical immunologist for skin-prick testing.

Further reading
Harper NJ, Dixon T, Dugué P, *et al.*; Working Party of the Association of Anaesthetists of Great Britain and Ireland (2009). Suspected anaphylactic reactions associated with anaesthesia. *Anaesthesia*, **64**, 199–211. Also available at: ℘ http://www.aagbi.org.
Resuscitation Council (UK). [Guidelines.] ℘ http://www.resus.org.uk.

Paediatric doses and equipment

Weight/blood pressure estimation (1–10yr)

- Child's weight in kg = 2 × (age in yr + 4)
- Normal systolic BP in mmHg = (age in yr × 2) + 80

Airway

- ETT internal diameter in mm = (age in yr / 4) + 4
- ETT length (oral) to lips in cm = (age in yr / 2) + 12
- ETT length (nose) to lips in cm = (age in yr / 2) + 15
- LMA#1 (cuff volume 4mL): <6.5kg
- LMA#2 (cuff volume 10mL): 6.5–20kg
- LMA#2.5 (cuff volume 14mL): 20–30kg
- LMA#3 (cuff volume 20mL): >30kg

Estimated drug doses

(See also p. 842.)

- Adrenaline   10 micrograms/kg
- Aminophylline   5mg/kg
- Amiodarone   5mg/kg
- Atropine   10–20 micrograms/kg
- Bicarbonate   1mmol/kg
- Calcium chloride   0.2mL/kg of 10% solution slowly
- Calcium gluconate   0.6mL/kg of 10% solution
- Cefotaxime   50mg/kg
- Diazepam   0.1mg/kg IV 0.5mg/kg PR
- Glucose (10%)   5mL/kg
- Ketamine   2mg/kg
- Lidocaine   1mg/kg
- Lorazepam   0.1mg/kg recommended for status epilepticus
                         (repeatable after 10min)
- Magnesium   25–50mg/kg
- Naloxone   0.1mg/kg
- Neostigmine   50 micrograms/kg
- Paraldehyde   0.1mg/kg
- Phenytoin   20mg/kg
- Salbutamol   2.5mg nebulizer

Circulation

- Blood volume 75mL/kg (1–10yr) 70mL/kg (>10yr)
- Fluid bolus 20mL/kg

These estimations are not valid for premature infants and are intended as rough guides only.[2,3]

References

2 Resuscitation Council (UK) (2010). *Resuscitation guidelines 2010.* ⌖ http://www.resus.org.uk/pages/GL2010.pdf.
3 European Resuscitation Council (2010). *ERC guidelines 2010.* ⌖ http://www.cprguidelines.eu/2010/.

Airway assessment and management

Jules Cranshaw and Tim Cook

Airway assessment

The difficult airway is *the* most important cause of anaesthesia-related morbidity and mortality. ~30% of deaths attributable to anaesthesia are associated with inadequate airway management.

- Most catastrophes are due to unexpected difficulty or poor planning in patients with known difficulty.
- Airway assessment has traditionally focused on predicting difficult direct laryngoscopy.
- Equally important is predicting difficult mask ventilation, SAD placement, and other rescue techniques.
- Mask ventilation is difficult in ~1:20 cases, and impossible in ~1:1500.
- Intubation is difficult in ~1:50 cases, and impossible in ~1:2000 (**~1:300 for emergencies**).
- Rescue techniques fail in ~1:20 cases.
- Patients with multiple predictors of difficulty or risk factors for rapid hypoxaemia (e.g. pregnancy, obesity, children) need great care.
- History, examination, and investigations must assess the risks of difficult airway maintenance, ventilation, and oxygenation, and not just difficult direct laryngoscopy. They must lead to plans that anticipate and avoid predicted difficulties or mitigate their effects.

History

- Congenital airway difficulties (e.g. Down's, Klippel–Feil, craniofacial syndromes).
- Acquired airway difficulties (e.g. pregnancy, obesity, diabetes, RA, ankylosing spondylitis, acromegaly, Still's disease, snoring, OSA).
- Iatrogenic problems (e.g. C-spine fusion, oral/pharyngeal radiotherapy, laryngeal/tracheal surgery, temporomandibular joint (TMJ) surgery).
- Reported previous anaesthetic problems, e.g. dental damage or severe sore throat. Check anaesthetic notes, med-alerts, and databases, if present.

Examination

- Adverse anatomical features (e.g. small mouth, receding chin, high arched palate, large tongue, bull neck, obesity, large breasts).
- Acquired problems (e.g. head/neck burns, goitre, tumour, haematoma, abscess, radiotherapy injury, restrictive scars).
- Mechanical limitation—reduced mouth opening and anterior temporomandibular movement (e.g. TMJ damage, quinsy, post-radiotherapy); poor C-spine movement, especially upper extension).
- Poor dentition (e.g. anterior gaps, sharp/loose/protruding awkward teeth).
- Orthopaedic/neurosurgical/orthodontic equipment (e.g. neck collar, halo traction, external fixator, stereotactic locator, dental wiring).
- If using the nasal route, check the patency of the nasal passages.
- Note: facial hair may hide adverse anatomical features.

Radiology

- A *recent* CT or MRI may define a potentially difficult anatomy.
- On plain C-spine X-rays, occipito-atlanto-axial disease is more predictive of difficult direct laryngoscopy than disease below C2.
- Loss of disc space (e.g. rheumatoid) predicts difficult intubation and instability, but plain X-rays are poor predictors of cervical stability.
- If indicated, flexion/extension or dynamic studies of the C-spine can confirm instability.

Predictive tests of difficult direct laryngoscopy

Direct laryngoscopy requires a clear line of sight from the upper teeth to the glottis. It entails mouth opening, extension of the upper C-spine, and moving the tissue within the arch of the mandible out of the way. Most tests check one or more of these capabilities, but, by comparison to predicting difficult airway maintenance, ventilation, and oxygenation, predicting difficult direct laryngoscopy should be de-emphasized.

Problems with predictive tests of difficult direct laryngoscopy include:

- Low sensitivity, specificity, and positive predictive value, and frequent false positives (i.e. >50% are not predicted, and <5% are difficult) (studies developing the tests find higher sensitivities and specificities than routine practice)
- Combining tests increases the specificity (i.e. reduces false positives) but decreases the sensitivity (i.e. misses more of the difficult cases)
- Definitions of 'difficult' vary. Cormack and Lehane's graded laryngeal views (Fig. 37.1) correlate modestly with difficulty in placing a tube in the trachea. Modifications have therefore been proposed (Fig. 37.2).

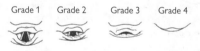

Fig. 37.1 Cormack and Lehane classification of glottic visualization.

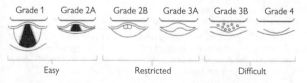

Fig. 37.2 Cook's modified classification of the laryngeal view.

Grades 1–4 refer to Cormack and Lehane classification. In Cook's classification, 'easy' views require no adjuncts; 'restricted' views require a bougie; 'difficult' views require advanced techniques to intubate

Interincisor gap (II gap)
- The distance between the incisors (or alveolar margins), with the mouth open maximally.
- Affected by the TMJ and upper C-spine mobility.
- <3cm makes intubation difficulty more likely.
- <2.5cm—LMA insertion will also be difficult.

Protrusion of the mandible
- Class A: can protrude the lower incisors anterior to the upper incisors.
- Class B: can protrude the lower incisors to, but not beyond, the upper incisors.
- Class C: cannot protrude the lower incisors to the upper incisors.

Classes B and C are associated with an increased risk of difficult laryngoscopy.

Mallampati test (with Samsoon and Young's modification)
(See Fig. 37.3.)
   Examine the patient's oropharynx from opposite the patient's face, while the patient opens their mouth maximally and protrudes their tongue without phonating.

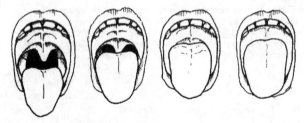

Fig. 37.3 Modified Mallampati classes 1, 2, 3, and 4.

- Class 1: faucial pillars, soft palate, and uvula visible.
- Class 2: faucial pillars and soft palate visible—uvula tip masked by base of tongue.
- Class 3: only soft palate visible.
- Class 4: soft palate not visible (class added by Samsoon/Young).

Class 3 and 4 views (i.e. when there is no view of the posterior pharyngeal wall) are associated with an increased risk of difficult laryngoscopy. This test is prone to interobserver variation. Used alone, it correctly predicts about 50% of difficult laryngoscopies and has a false positive rate of >95%.

Extension of the upper cervical spine
- When limited (<90°), the risk of difficult laryngoscopy is increased.
- Movement may be assessed by:
   - Flexing the head on the neck, immobilizing the lower C-spine with one hand on the neck, then fully extending the head. Placing a

pointer on the vertex or forehead allows the angle of movement to be estimated
- Placing one finger on the patient's chin and one finger on the occipital protuberance, and extending the head maximally
  - With normal C-spine mobility, the finger on the chin is higher than the one on the occiput. Level fingers indicate moderate limitation. If the finger on the chin remains lower than the one on the occiput, there is severe limitation.

Thyromental distance (Patil test)

The distance from the tip of the thyroid cartilage to the tip of the mandible, with the neck fully extended.
- Normal >7cm; <6cm predicts ~75% of difficult laryngoscopies.
- Combined Patil and Mallampati tests (<7cm and classes 3–4) increases the specificity (97%) but reduces the sensitivity (81%).

Sternomental distance (Savva test)

The distance from the sternal notch to the tip of the mandible, with the neck fully extended and mouth closed.
- <12.5cm associated with difficulty (positive predictive value 82%).

Wilson score

Five factors—weight; upper C-spine mobility; jaw movement; receding mandible; protruding upper teeth. Each scored from 0 to 2 (subjectively normal to abnormal).
- A total score of ≥2 predicts 75% of difficult intubations; 12% false positives.

Predictors of difficult mask ventilation

Mask ventilation requires a face mask producing an effective seal around the mouth and nose and an open airway.
Predictors of difficulty include:
- Age >55yr
- BMI >26kg/m^2
- History of snoring
- Beard
- Absence of teeth (the presence of two of the above factors has a >70% sensitivity and specificity)
- Facial abnormalities
- Receding or markedly prognathic jaw
- OSA
- Mallampati classes 3–4.

Predictors of problems with airway rescue techniques

Supraglottic airway device insertion

SAD (often laryngeal mask) insertion is likely to be part of a rescue plan. Laryngeal mask insertions fail in ~1% and are higher with some other SADs. Factors associated with difficult laryngeal mask placement are mouth opening <2.5cm (impossible if <2.0cm), intraoral/pharyngeal masses (e.g. lingual tonsils), obesity, and poor dentition. 'Classic' laryngeal masks lose their seal at ~15–20cmH$_2$O. Higher pressures may be obtained with other SADs (e.g.

ProSeal or ILMA). This may be important in restoring oxygenation by ventilation in patients with low chest compliance.

Direct tracheal access

If emergency tracheal access is contemplated, in the neck position in which it will be attempted (usually fully extended), check and mark:
- The position of the larynx and trachea; ultrasound may be useful
- The accessibility of the cricothyroid membrane and trachea.

Beware obesity, goitre, other anterior neck masses, infection or scarring, deviated trachea, fixed neck flexion, previous radiotherapy, surgical collar, or an external fixator preventing access. Inspect a recent CT or MRI. Be familiar with your access device (e.g. with obesity, will it reach the trachea?).

Awake techniques, including fibreoptic intubation

The most important predictors of difficult AFOI are lack of patient cooperation and operator inexperience. Blood or unmanageable secretions in the airway also predict failure. Use of AFOI in cases of airway obstruction is controversial.

Aggregation of difficulties

Patients in whom one airway management technique is difficult or fails are at greatly increased risk of difficulty and failure of other techniques. Beware, and be prepared!

Further reading

Cook TM (2000). A new practical classification of laryngeal view. *Anaesthesia*, **55**, 274–9.

Cook TM, MacDougall-Davis SR (2012). Complications and failure of airway management. *Br J Anaesth*, **109** Suppl 1, i68–85.

Cormack RS, Lehane J (1984). Difficult tracheal intubation in obstetrics. *Anaesthesia*, **39**, 1105–11.

Kheterpal S, Han R, Tremper KK, et al. (2006). Incidence and predictors of difficult and impossible mask ventilation. *Anesthesiology*, **105**, 885–91.

Kheterpal S, Healy D, Aziz MF, et al.; Multicenter Perioperative Outcomes Group (MPOG) Perioperative Clinical Research Committee (2013). Incidence, predictors, and outcome of difficult mask ventilation combined with difficult laryngoscopy: a report from the multicenter perioperative outcomes group. *Anesthesiology*, **119**, 1360–9.

Langeron O, Masso E, Huraux C, et al. (2000). Prediction of difficult mask ventilation. *Anesthesiology*, **92**, 1229–36.

Mallampati SR, Gugino LD, Desai S, Waraksa B, Freiberger D, Lui PL (1983). Clinical sign to predict difficult tracheal intubation. *Can Anaesth Soc J*, **30**, 316–17.

Patil VU, Stehling LC, Zauder HL (1983). Predicting the difficulty of intubation using an intubation gauge. *Anesthesiol Rev*, **10**, 32–3.

Ramachandran SK, Mathis MR, Tremper KK, Shanks AM, Kheterpal S (2012). Predictors and clinical outcomes from failed Laryngeal Mask Airway Unique™: a study of 15,795 patients. *Anesthesiology*, **116**, 1217–26.

Samsoon G, Young JR (1987). Difficult tracheal intubation: a retrospective study. *Anaesthesia*, **42**, 487–90.

Savva D (1994). Prediction of difficult intubation. *Br J Anaesth*, **73**, 149–53.

Shiga T, Wajima Z, Inoue T, Sakamoto A (2005). Predicting difficult intubation in apparently normal patients: a meta-analysis of bedside screening test performance. *Anesthesiology*, **103**, 429–37.

Wilson ME (1993). Predicting difficult intubation. *Br J Anaesth*, **71**, 333–4.

Yentis S (2002). Predicting difficult intubation—worthwhile exercise or pointless ritual? *Anaesthesia*, **57**, 105–9.

Unanticipated difficult airway

- Despite careful assessment, ~50% of airway difficulties arise unexpectedly from:
  - Difficult/failed intubation
  - Difficult/failed mask ventilation
  - Both.
- Unexpected difficulty is more likely in emergencies, obstetric cases, and with inexperience. *When difficulties occur, patients do not die from failure to intubate, but from failure to oxygenate.* Preoxygenation of all cases prolongs the period before desaturation and 'buys time'. Switch to 100% O_2 whenever an airway problem develops. Ensure anaesthesia and muscle relaxation are effective. *Difficult ventilation makes oxygenation harder to restore.*
- The 4th National Audit Project (NAP 4) report highlighted that, compared to anaesthesia, complications from difficult airway management occur more frequently in the emergency department, and especially in intensive care. Complications in these environments are also more likely to be managed suboptimally and cause harm. These places should be considered 'high-risk areas' for airway management.

Difficult intubation

Management of unpredicted difficult intubation can be considered a four-step process:

A. 1° intubation attempt with optimal muscle relaxation, patient position, blade or laryngoscope*, external laryngeal manipulation, and careful use of a GEB or stylet.

B. **2° intubation attempt** through an SAD, preferably with fibreoptic-guided assistance. An Aintree intubation catheter (AIC) over the fibrescope and a small ETT increase ease (omit in RSI).

C. **Abandoning intubation attempt.** Maintain/restore oxygenation by face mask ventilation, or with an SAD if this fails. If it is feasible and will provide a better airway and oxygenation, re-establish SV and the previous airway tone as quickly as possible. Wake the patient, if indicated and feasible.

D. **Rescue.** Invasive tracheal techniques (needle or cannula cricothyroidotomy, surgical airway).

The decision to proceed from A to B to C to D depends on failure of each technique. In most cases, senior help should be called when plan A fails. Plan D should be reserved for situations of CICV and failed SAD with progressive desaturation despite optimal attempts to oxygenate.

Difficult intubation with easy ventilation (no aspiration risk)
- A calm stepwise approach can be used. If plan A fails, plan B will usually succeed. When plans A and B fail, plan C is usually successful (see Failed intubation, ➜ p. 913 and p. 952).

---

* In experienced hands, the 1° attempt might include a videolaryngoscope (e.g. Airtraq, C-Mac, Glidescope, etc.).

Difficult intubation with difficult/impossible ventilation
(cannot intubate, cannot ventilate)
- This situation is an emergency and becomes life-threatening if managed incorrectly. If mask ventilation is difficult, an SAD—that inserts reliably and achieves a high pressure airway seal, e.g. ILMA, i-Gel, LMA Supreme™, or ProSeal LMA—will rescue the airway and oxygenation in >90% of cases. Where ventilation remains impossible and oxygenation cannot be maintained, invasive techniques (plan D) can be lifesaving. If the patient is not already paralysed, a muscle relaxant should be administered before attempting invasive tracheal access. Anaesthetists must be equipped and prepared to use such techniques when the need arises and should be able to perform >1 technique (see ➲ p. 915 and p. 957).

Difficult intubation during rapid sequence intubation
- After two attempts at intubation, proceed directly to plan C (omit plan B), and, if feasible, wake the patient (see Rapid sequence induction, ➲ p. 963).

Unanticipated difficult tracheal intubation
See Fig. 37.4.

Failed mask ventilation
This may arise as a result of:
- Anaesthetic circuit problems (e.g. blockage, disconnection, leak)
- Failure to achieve an adequate seal between the mask and face (consider leaving well-fitting dentures)
- Failure to maintain upper airway patency (commonest problem)
- Laryngospasm (see ➲ p. 903.)
- Laryngeal pathology (rare; cricothyroidotomy may be lifesaving)
- Bronchospasm (may occur in smokers and asthmatics (see ➲ p. 909, p. 98 and p. 97) and may be part of anaphylaxis (see ➲ p. 920))
- Lower airway pathology.

This is always an emergency—an extra pair of hands is helpful. Call for help early, but do not let your assistant leave.

Circuit problems and mask seal problems
- Prior checking of the entire circuit (including mask and catheter mount) should avoid problems. If suspected, change to a self-inflating bag and new mask. Mask seal problems require good technique, experience, and often assistance.

Failure to maintain airway patency
(This is plan C as mentioned on ➲ p. 949.)
- Place the head and neck in the optimal position (lower neck flexed on shoulders, and upper neck extended—'sniffing the morning air'). Obese patients will be better in the 'ramped-up' position.
- Use two-person mask ventilation (one to provide jaw thrust and face mask seal, and one to squeeze the reservoir bag). An additional helper may take over the jaw thrust (three-person mask ventilation).

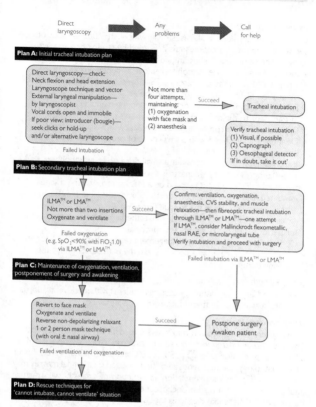

Fig. 37.4 Unanticipated difficult tracheal intubation.

Reproduced with permission of J. J. Henderson, M. T. Popat, I. P. Latto, A. C. Pearce, Difficult Airway Society guidelines for management of the unanticipated difficult intubation, John Wiley & Sons, Inc.

- Insert an oral and, if this is inadequate, a soft lubricated nasal airway carefully to avoid bleeding.
- If still unable to ventilate by face mask, insert an SAD. If cricoid force has been applied, reduce or release it, but be ready with suction.
- If not already done and rapid waking is not feasible, the patient should be paralysed at this stage.
- If unable to intubate, with progressive severe desaturation, proceed to plan D before cardiac arrest.

Laryngospasm

Can be fatal. Consider in all cases of airway obstruction without obvious supraglottic causes. Sometimes it is preceded by stridor or a characteristic 'crowing' noise but may be instant, complete, and silent.

- Inspect the airway. Use suction to remove all contaminants.
- Apply CPAP, with the expiratory valve closed, and 100% O_2. Attempt manual ventilation. This needs two people.
- Forcible jaw thrust or anterior pressure on the mandibular rami just anterior to the mastoid process (Larson's point) may 'break' laryngospasm by a combination of stimulation and airway opening.
- Deepening anaesthesia with a small dose of propofol (20–50mg) may relax spasm.
- If oxygenation is falling, consider a small dose of suxamethonium (0.1–0.5mg/kg). If laryngospasm is severe, a full dose of suxamethonium (1mg/kg) should be administered, and the trachea intubated. If there is no venous access, suxamethonium may be administered IM or into the tongue (3mg/kg).
- As laryngospasm starts to 'break', anaesthesia may be deepened with further doses of the IV agent, as appropriate.
- Consider a change in airway management (e.g. exchange a ETT for an SAD), prior to further attempts to wake the patient, to reduce the risk of recurrence.

Laryngeal pathology

Unexpected laryngeal pathology causing problems with mask ventilation is a very rare scenario. Cricothyroidotomy may be lifesaving.

Lower airway pathology

Acute severe bronchospasm may present as difficulty in mask ventilation. This may occur in smokers and severe asthmatics or may be part of an adverse drug reaction (see p. 98, p. 909, and p. 920). Very rarely, lower airway pathology due to diagnosed or undiagnosed mediastinal masses may present as difficulty with ventilation at induction of anaesthesia. Tracheal intubation or use of a rigid bronchoscope to maintain airway patency may be lifesaving. Differential diagnosis includes a foreign body (inhaled object from the anaesthetic circuit, inhaled teeth, blood clot, mucus plug, etc.) which may mimic severe bronchospasm. This should be considered and, if necessary, excluded by fibreoptic inspection.

Paediatric implications

- Difficulty with tracheal intubation in the absence of structural abnormalities is uncommon, but invasive tracheal access is more difficult.
- Laryngospasm is commoner. Beware inflating the stomach during ventilation attempts. This can trigger vagal reflexes and regurgitation, and compromise the diaphragm.
- Foreign bodies are commoner.
- Hypoxia occurs rapidly in children if ventilation is inadequate.
- Airway manipulation or use of suxamethonium in the presence of hypoxia may lead to bradycardia and cardiac arrest.
- Specific paediatric difficult intubation guidelines exist for children.

Special considerations

All patients who have airway difficulties should be informed after they have recovered. Inform the patient and GP, and document fully in the notes and databases, as appropriate. Complete an 'airway alert', if in use. The Read code for difficult intubation is SP2y3 and should be included where relevant.

Failed intubation

(See also ➲ p. 913.)

The commonest cause is difficult laryngoscopy. Patients do not die from failure to intubate, but from failure to oxygenate.

Optimizing primary intubation attempts

Following a few simple rules will eliminate the majority of difficulties.

- Optimize the position of the head and neck (flexion of the lower C-spine with extension at the upper C-spine—'sniffing the morning air'). One pillow. 'Ramping' for obese patients.
- Optimal anaesthesia: an unconscious patient with a fully working relaxant.
- Optimal laryngeal position. If difficulty is encountered, use optimal external laryngeal manipulation (OELM) or backwards, upwards, and rightwards pressure (BURP) during cricoid pressure.
- Use of an effective laryngoscope *that the user is trained to use*. There are increasing choices: a long blade, a McCoy blade, and a straight blade.
- Increasingly, videolaryngoscopes are accepted as having a role here. The technique often differs from direct laryngoscopy, and users must be trained before using in a clinical crisis.
- Use a GEB (or stylet in paediatrics).

Diagnosis of misplacement of the tracheal tube (oesophageal intubation)

- Patients continue to die of this (avoidable and unacceptable) complication. Avoiding it should be a constant priority.
- Retain a high index of suspicion after a difficult intubation.
- Capnography is the gold standard for confirmation of tracheal intubation. Do not proceed with elective anaesthesia without a working capnograph.
- In the absence of capnography (which should be vanishingly rare), suspect oesophageal placement if you cannot confirm the following: normal breath sounds in both axillae, with absent sounds over the stomach; rise and fall of the chest; normal airway pressure cycle; and patient stability. However, none are foolproof. Beware 'confirmation bias'. You see and hear what you expect and want.
- Use an 'oesophageal detector'. If negative pressure is applied to the ETT, the trachea (a rigid structure) does not collapse, while the oesophagus (not rigid) does. Failure to aspirate air with a bladder syringe directly attached to the ETT suggests oesophageal placement.
- Confirm ETT placement with a fibreoptic scope.
- Where there is doubt, take it out, and apply bag-and-mask ventilation.
- Note: delay in diagnosis of oesophageal intubation leads to CVS collapse, and the diagnosis is then easy to overlook.

Failed elective intubation with easy ventilation

(See ➲ p. 954.)

In these cases, when the patient has received a full dose of an NDMR, and mask ventilation is easy, it may be appropriate to try a full range of 2° intubation techniques (plan B on ➲ p. 949).

Failed intubation during rapid sequence induction

(See Rapid sequence induction, **→** p. 963.)

Proceed directly to plan C.

Failed elective intubation with difficult ventilation

(See Cannot intubate, cannot ventilate, **→** p. 915 and p. 957.)

The options here are only to wake the patient (i.e. continue with plan C) or to move rapidly to plan D.

Further reading

Cook TM, MacDougall-Davis SR (2012). Complications and failure of airway management. *Br J Anaesth*, **109** Suppl 1, i68–85.

Cook TM, Woodall N, Harper J, Benger J; Fourth National Audit project (2011). Major complications of airway management in the UK: results of the Fourth National Audit Project of the Royal College of Anaesthetists and the Difficult Airway Society. Part 2: intensive care and emergency departments. *Br J Anaesth*, **106**, 632–42.

Difficult Airway Society (2012). *Paediatric difficult airway management guidelines*. ℘ http://www.das.uk.com/guidelines/paediatric-difficult-airway-guidelines.

Henderson JJ, Popat MT, Latto IP, Pearce AC; Difficult Airway Society (2004). Difficult Airway Society guidelines for management of the unanticipated difficult intubation. *Anaesthesia*, **59**, 675–94.

Techniques for management of elective difficult intubation

Gum elastic bougie

The GEB (e.g. Eschmann TT introducer (reusable), Smiths Portex Ltd) should enable intubation where the laryngeal inlet is partially visible and some where it is not (laryngoscopy grades 2a–3a; see ➲ p. 943), and is probably the single most useful piece of difficult intubation equipment. Keep the bougie anterior and in the midline to ensure it does not enter the oesophagus or either piriform fossa. The signs of correct placement are 'bumping' as it rubs along tracheal rings, and the anaesthetic assistant may 'feel' it as it passes the larynx. Use of signs, such as rotation as the GEB enters the main bronchi and 'hold-up' at ~40cm, are no longer recommended, as they rely on excessive insertion. There is no need to insert the GEB beyond the carina (~24–26cm). When railroading the ETT, keep the laryngoscope in the mouth, and rotate the tube 90° counterclockwise to ensure the bevel is correctly orientated to avoid catching on the larynx during passage. A small ETT will 'railroad' better than a large one.

There are numerous newer designs of bougies, but performance varies considerably, as does their rigidity and potential to cause airway trauma. A recent development is a 'traffic light bougie' which is colour-coded to indicate 'safe' (green), 'at-risk' (orange), or 'excessive' (red) depth of insertion.

Intubation via a supraglottic airway device

These techniques use an SAD as a 'dedicated airway'. This allows oxygenation and ventilation during intubation and provides a guiding channel through which to attempt intubation (Table 37.1). 'Blind' intubation via the classic LMA (cLMA) is rarely (<20%) successful. A fibrescope increases success to near 100%. A recommended technique involves placement of an AIC (ID 4.7mm, ED 7.0mm, Cook Critical Care) to the carina over a fibrescope, then removal of the LMA and the fibrescope. The AIC remains in place and has connectors that enable ventilation and oxygenation at this point. A ETT (ID 7.0mm) is then railroaded over the catheter. The same technique is suitable for a number of SADs—in particular the i-Gel and ProSeal LMA. It is less well suited to the LMA Supreme™ or laryngeal tubes, because narrow parts of the airway device interfere with railroading.

The ILMA (Teleflex) is a modification of the cLMA, designed to facilitate blind or fibreoptic oral intubation, in asleep or very cooperative awake patients. It comprises a rigid anatomically curved airway tube, terminating in a standard 15mm connector, integral with a rigid metal handle. The mask has an epiglottic elevating bar, replacing the two bars of a cLMA. As the ETT exits the airway, it is centralized by a funnel and then lifts the epiglottis from the route of passage of the ETT. Sizes 3–5 enable intubation in large children and adults. Specific ILMA ETTs (silicone-tipped, wire-reinforced, size 6–8mm) are designed for use with all ILMAs and decrease intubation failure/trauma. Standard PVC ETTs should not be used because of the risk of trauma. Fibreoptic guidance improves success and is advocated for all, but considerable, emergencies.

Table 37.1 Tracheal tube size fitting through Teleflex LMAs (if cuffed tracheal tube, take off 0.5mm)

	Size	ID (mm)	Distance to bars (mm)
cLMA	1	3.5[1]	108
	1.5	4.5	135
	2	5.0	140
	2½	6.0	170
	3	6.5	200
	4	6.5	205
	5	7.0	230
fLMA (flexible LMA)	2	3.5[1]	140[2]
	2½	3.5[1]	205[2]
	3	5.5	237
	4	5.5	237
	5	6.0	284
ProSeal LMA	3	6.0	190
	4	6.5	190
	5	6.5	195
ILMA	6.0–8.0mm ILMA tubes, distance to epiglottic elevator 160mm		

[1] A tube larger than this cannot pass the proximal end of the LMA, at the site of the 15mm connector.

[2] This is longer than an uncut ETT of this size, so not suitable for this technique; fLMA cannot be recommended for this technique!

Videolaryngoscopes

This term describes rigid fibreoptic intubation aids—though not all have video screens, and not all use fibreoptics! Numerous new and older devices are available, too many to describe. Many are poorly evaluated, and their clinical value for difficult intubation is promoted but largely unproven. They will all become useless if their 'eye' is covered by airway secretions, blood, or other matter. They are therefore likely to be more effective as the 1st or 2nd choice of laryngoscope. Most use fibreoptics to 'see round corners', obviating the need for a direct 'line of sight' and enabling the use of lower forces, or even awake use. There are three main groups.

Bladed videolaryngoscopes

Generally curved bladed devices: curvature varies, and the blade may be metal/plastic and reusable/single-use. A fibreoptic bundle takes light to a lens and transmits a picture to an integral or remote viewer. The blade enables manipulation of tissues. May be inserted in standard, midline, or paramedian approaches, and some can be simultaneously used as direct laryngoscopes. May require stylets and specialized techniques to convert easy laryngoscopy to easy intubation. Include Bullard, WuScope, McGrath5, McGrath Mac, Glidescope, and C-Mac.

Conduited videolaryngoscopes

These devices (including the non-fibreoptic Airtraq; single-use and prism and mirror image delivery) have a channel parallel with the camera to guide a ETT to where the camera is pointing and thus improve intubation success. Choice of tube size and type relative to the conduit may affect intubation success. Include Upsherscope, Pentax AWS, Airtraq, and Venner AP Advance.

Optical stylets

Preformed rigid or malleable metal guides, containing an optical bundle or distal camera, project the image to an eyepiece or screen. A ETT is preloaded, manipulated to the glottis, and then advanced into the trachea. Stylets require minimal mouth opening but have limited ability to manipulate tissues. May be used awake and as lightwand. O_2 can be administered during use (via the ETT) in most, including the Bonfils, Shikani, Levitan, and Trachway devices.

Note: all these devices have learning curves and have 'tricks of the trade'. Use of these without adequate training in the circumstances of intubation difficulty is poor practice.

Further reading

Behringer EC, Kristensen MS (2011). Evidence for benefit vs novelty in new intubation equipment. *Anaesthesia*, 66 Suppl 2, 57–64.

Dhara SS (2009). Retrograde tracheal intubation. *Anaesthesia*, 64, 1094–104.

Henderson JJ, Popat MT, Latto IP, Pearce AC; Difficult Airway Society (2004). Difficult Airway Society guidelines for management of the unanticipated difficult intubation. *Anaesthesia*, 59, 675–94.

Mihai R, Blair E, Kay H, Cook TM (2008). A quantitative review and meta-analysis of performance of non standard laryngoscopes and rigid fibreoptic intubation aids. *Anaesthesia*, 63, 745–60.

Waters DJ (1963). Guided blind endotracheal intubation. *Anaesthesia*, 18, 158–62.

Cannot intubate, cannot ventilate

(See Fig. 37.5 and also ➔ p. 915.)

Inability to intubate the trachea and ventilate the lungs *is always a life-threatening situation*. Managed badly, it will lead to morbidity or death. It occurs in <1:5000 routine anaesthetics. It is commoner during emergency anaesthesia, intubation in the emergency department, after multiple attempts at intubation, and with inexperienced anaesthetists. This is plan D

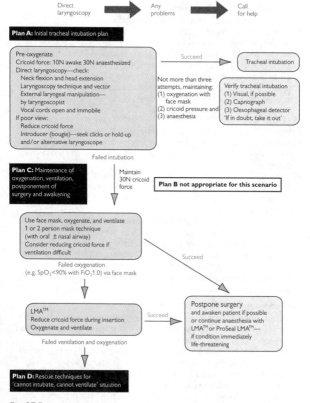

Fig. 37.5 Cannot intubate, cannot ventilate.

Reproduced with permission of J. J. Henderson, M. T. Popat, I. P. Latto, A. C. Pearce, Difficult Airway Society guidelines for management of the unanticipated difficult intubation, John Wiley & Sons, Inc

of the DAS guidelines (see ➲ p. 949). NAP 4 reported high failure rates when cricothyroidotomy was performed by anaesthetists. NAP 4 recommended improved training in both needle and surgical techniques for all anaesthetists.

Rescue techniques for the 'cannot intubate, cannot ventilate' situation

- These techniques may cause complications of placement (pneumothorax, adjacent tissue damage, bleeding) and of ventilation (barotrauma if using high-pressure source ventilation (SC emphysema, pneumothorax, pneumomediastinum, and hypoventilation with larger uncuffed devices)). The complications of NOT performing them when indicated are hypoxic brain damage and death.
- Remember insertion of an appropriate SAD will rescue the airway in >90% of cases. It would be rare to attempt an invasive procedure without first trying to rescue the airway with an SAD. Once inserted, the SAD should be left in place during and after invasive tracheal access; it may provide some oxygenation and a route of exhalation, which is needed if high-pressure source (jet) ventilation is used. This takes time to set up and should be done simultaneously by an assistant.

Needle and cannula cricothyroidotomy

- Invasive techniques rely on palpable external tracheal landmarks. In obesity, ultrasound may help. Identification takes practice. The cricothyroid membrane appears as a bright white line, and the larynx moves with phonation.[1]
- In the 'CICV' situation with progressive desaturation, emergency tracheal access is required. Needle cricothyroidotomy is quicker than formal tracheostomy. It is performed at the level of the cricothyroid membrane.
- Appropriate techniques include a cannula-over-needle technique (e.g. <2mm ID, non-kinking cannula, such as the Ravussin cannula) or larger catheters placed with a Seldinger technique (e.g. Cook Melker cricothyroidotomy catheter, 5.0mm ID, cuffed).
- Length is important. Some cannulae are <5cm long and may not reach the trachea in oedematous or obese patients—perhaps typical of those needing these techniques.

Small cannulae (2–4mm internal diameter)

- Cannulae of <4.0mm ID require a high-pressure source for adequate ventilation and rely on exhalation via the native upper airway. Maximize its patency (e.g. SAD), or barotrauma may result.
- Position must be confirmed by aspiration of air or capnography before ventilating. Ventilation requires a high-pressure source (e.g. piped O_2 and an injector or 'wall' O_2). A breathing system, anaesthetic machine O_2 flush, or self-inflating bag are ineffective. If using 'wall' O_2, insert a control mechanism (e.g. a three-way tap or hole) in the tubing connecting the flowmeter to the cannula.
- If exhalation is impossible by the native upper airway, O_2 flow *must be reduced* to the basal rate (<0.5L/min). This may provide some O_2

and will avoid barotrauma but will not rapidly re-establish FRC and oxygenation.
- The Ventrain device attached to a narrow cannula enables active exhalation by entrainment of expired gas. This may lessen the risk of both failed ventilation and barotrauma.

Wide-bore cannulae (>4mm internal diameter)
- Catheters of >4.0mm ID are suitable for conventional ventilation but will only provide adequate ventilation if they are cuffed or the upper airway is obstructed.

Surgical airway (surgical cricothyroidotomy)
- This technique allows the introduction of an ETT; a size of 6.0mm ID ETT is recommended.
- As with needle and cannula techniques, it is performed through the cricothyroid membrane.
- A scalpel (ideally size 20) is used to make an incision through the skin and cricothyroid membrane. A hole (~8mm in diameter for easier ETT passage) should be created 'bluntly' and maintained by forceps, tracheal dilators, or cricoid hook(s) to avoid loss of definition of tissue planes and creation of a false track.
- It is important that the incision is kept patent to avoid closure of the hole, loss of definition of tissue planes, and creation of a false track. A bougie may be inserted before the ETT to ease passage—a 5.0–5.5mm ID ETT is best to railroad over this.
- In expert hands, this technique establishes a secure airway in 30s after arrival of the equipment. An advantage, over cricothyroidotomy, is the absence of problems with ventilation once a cuffed ETT is inserted.

Special considerations
- Multiple intubation attempts lead to airway trauma and increase the likelihood of a CICV situation. If one technique has failed twice, it is unlikely to work on further attempts. Try something new!
- Anaesthetists should be willing (and able) to switch to a different method of cricothyroidotomy if their 1st choice is not working.
- Difficult and failed intubation is associated with an increased incidence of aspiration.
- After rescuing the airway, it is necessary to establish a definitive airway as a matter of urgency. ENT assistance is recommended.
- After prolonged obstruction, pulmonary oedema may develop.

Further reading
Cook TM, Nolan JP, Cranshaw J, Magee P (2007). Needle cricothyroidotomy. *Anaesthesia*, **62**, 289–90.

Cook TM, Woodall N, Frerk C; Fourth National Audit Project (2011). Major complications of airway management in the UK. Results of the Fourth National Audit Project of the Royal College of Anaesthetists and Difficult Airway Society. Part 1: anaesthesia. *Br J Anaesth*, **106**, 617–31.

Henderson JJ, Hamaekers AE (2011). Equipment and strategies for emergency tracheal access in the adult patient. *Anaesthesia*, **66** Suppl 2, 65–80.

Henderson JJ, Popat MT, Latto IP, Pearce AC; Difficult Airway Society (2004). Difficult Airway Society guidelines for management of the unanticipated difficult intubation. *Anaesthesia*, **59**, 675–94.

Management of the obstructed airway

(See also ➲ p. 628.)

The approach to the patient with an obstructed airway differs, according to:

- Urgency of intervention
- Level of obstruction
- General condition of the patient.

These cases are always difficult. If planned or managed poorly, life-threatening problems will develop. Management is controversial—airway obstruction is likely to get worse during anaesthesia due to loss of airway tone and reflexes. All approaches have potentially life-threatening complications (complete obstruction on induction, airway haemorrhage, swelling). Experienced anaesthetic and surgical involvement are essential. Planning a strategy is critical: *have a backup plan, and ensure that all those involved understand it.*

- If time, obtain appropriate investigations to define the site, extent, and severity of the obstruction and involvement of related structures.
- Where previous investigations and records are available, interpret them intelligently, as lesions may progress over a short period of time, leading previously successful techniques to fail. Useful investigations may include:
  - Nasendoscopy
  - CT/MRI
  - Lung function tests with flow–volume loops
  - Echocardiography if pulmonary vessel involvement suspected.
- Assess the:
  - Level—oral; supraglottic; laryngeal; mid-tracheal; lower tracheal. Several levels may be affected. Inspiratory stridor and voice changes indicate laryngeal obstruction; intrathoracic obstruction may cause expiratory stridor (monophonic wheeze)
  - Severity—respiratory distress; accessory muscle use; stridor; hypoxaemia; silent chest; dysphagia; nocturnal panic
  - Lesion—mobility and friability
  - Neck—examine ease of invasive tracheal access
  - Effect of patient position—find the patient's 'best breathing position'. Ask about any tendency to obstruction when lying flat.

Oral, supraglottic, and laryngeal obstruction

Most commonly due to trauma, burns, tumour, and infection.

- In semi-elective cases, nasendoscopy may help in predicting difficulties but must be performed with great care.
- If emergency access to the trachea is needed (e.g. cricothyroidotomy), this should be unimpeded by any lesion.
- An experienced surgeon who is an engaged participant in the 'airway strategy' and is scrubbed, equipped, assisted, and ready to perform an emergency cricothyroidotomy (preferably) or a *very* rapid tracheostomy must be available, in case an irreversible, life-threatening obstruction occurs. Remember, elective awake (with LA) cricothyroidotomy or

tracheostomy are also choices (though these are not easy in these situations either).
- Consider:
  - AFOI
  - SV induction (inhalational or by slow incremental TCI of propofol), then fibreoptic laryngoscopy or, if unavailable, careful direct laryngoscopy
  - Inserting a prophylactic cricothyroid cannula (even if planning an alternative technique) for use if the situation deteriorates.
- If available, a rigid bronchoscope (requires maximal neck extension) may provide an emergency airway in some cases.
- If an unexpected airway obstruction occurs, an SAD may assist ventilation during emergency tracheal access.
- *IV induction and attempted laryngoscopy (with or without paralysis) without a clear backup plan cannot be recommended for upper airway obstruction.* IV induction has been recommended for laryngeal lesions but requires skill, specific experience, and very clear backup plans.

Mid-tracheal

Commonly tumour or retrosternal goitre—often present semi-electively but may expand suddenly with haemorrhage. Knowing the site of obstruction is vital. Laryngoscopy is usually not impeded (though the trachea may be displaced), but difficulties may develop when the tube is inserted into the trachea.
- The site of the lesion may preclude cricothyroidotomy or tracheostomy—attempts risk bleeding and complete obstruction.
- Inhalational induction may be very slow, difficult, and complicated by worsening airway obstruction. It is rarely 1st choice.
- AFOI may be indicated if inability to ventilate is a significant possibility. However, coughing and distress may lead to increased obstruction. Passage of the fibrescope and/or the ETT through the narrowing may hinder SV and be unpleasant for the patient ('cork-in-a-bottle' phenomenon). An AIC is narrow (6.3mm outside diameter) and can be useful.
- An ETT, endobronchial tube, or hollow intubation bougie that also enables high-pressure source ventilation (e.g. Cook airway exchange catheter) may pass the narrowing. A route of exhalation must be ensured.
- The obstruction must be high enough in the trachea to allow the bevel of the device to sit safely below it and above the carina.
- IV induction, rapid NMB, and early passage of a rigid bronchoscope are used for marked tracheal obstruction requiring thoracic surgery (e.g. resection, laser, or stent insertion).
- The rigid bronchoscope establishes airway patency and is then used as a dedicated airway for further assessment, oxygenation, ventilation, and surgery.
- To avoid awareness, anaesthesia will need to be maintained with an IV technique.

Lower tracheal lesions and bronchial obstruction

Commonly due to tumours, trauma, and large mediastinal masses.

- Best managed by experienced specialists in thoracic centres.
- CPB is sometimes necessary (e.g. in the case of PA compression). This requires planning and preparation before the case is started!
- IV induction, rapid NMB, and passage of a rigid bronchoscope may be lifesaving.
- Use of laser resection and/or stents may then be deployed to maintain a patent airway.

Further considerations

- A specific tissue diagnosis may allow shrinking of a lesion with antibiotics, steroids, chemotherapy, or radiotherapy where time allows.
- Have a management plan for extubation, which may need to be delayed. Prolonged instrumentation may cause upper airway oedema.
- Heliox (premixed helium/O_2 containing 21–30% O_2) may improve flow through narrowed airways but reduces the FiO_2. Use of a 'Y' connector and an O_2 cylinder may increase the FiO_2 but reduce the effect of the helium. New delivery systems for helium (including ventilators) are marketed. Heliox may be useful for obstruction at any level but is usually only effective as a temporary measure while organizing definitive management.

Further reading

Cook TM, Morgan PJ, Hersch PE (2011). Equal and opposite expert opinion. Airway obstruction caused by a retrosternal thyroid mass: management and prospective international opinion. *Anaesthesia*, **66**, 828–36.

Gerig HJ, Schnider T, Heidegger T (2005). Prophylactic percutaneous transtracheal catheterisation in the management of patients with anticipated difficult airways: a case series. *Anaesthesia*, **60**, 801–5.

Nouraei SA, Giussani DA, Howard DJ, Sandhu GS, Ferguson C, Patel A (2008). Physiological comparison of spontaneous and positive-pressure ventilation in laryngotracheal stenosis. *Br J Anaesth*, **101**, 419–23.

Ovassapian A, Yelich SJ, Dykes MHM, Brunner EE (1983). Fibre-optic nasotracheal intubation—incidence and causes of failure. *Anesth Analg*, **63**, 692–5.

Patel A, Pearce A, Pracy P (2011). Head and neck pathology. In: Cook TM, Woodall N, Frerk C, eds. *4th National Audit Project of the Royal College of Anaesthetists and the Difficult Airway Society. Major complications of airway management in the United Kingdom. Report and findings, March 2011.* London: The Royal College of Anaesthetists, pp. 143–54. http://www.rcoa.ac.uk/nap4.

Rapid sequence induction

RSI (Fig. 37.6) involves IV induction, immediately followed by muscle relaxation to aid tracheal intubation, combined with cricoid pressure to reduce the risk of pulmonary aspiration in those considered to be at increased risk.

If airway assessment indicates intubation may be difficult, consider a local/regional technique or AFOI.

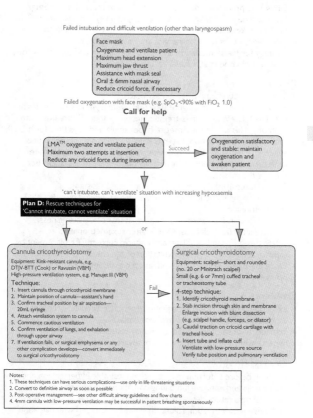

Fig. 37.6 Unanticipated difficult tracheal intubation (rapid sequence induction).

Reproduced with permission of J. J. Henderson, M. T. Popat, I. P. Latto, A. C. Pearce, Difficult Airway Society guidelines for management of the unanticipated difficult intubation, John Wiley & Sons, Inc.

Checks

- Anaesthetic machine, vaporizers, breathing system, ventilator, suction, intubation aids, and rescue equipment.
- Two functioning laryngoscopes and ETT cuff.
- Patient on a tipping trolley or bed.
- Routine monitoring applied, including capnography.
- Head in the 'sniffing' position—extended on neck, cervical spine flexed on the thorax—with a pillow. 'Ramped' position for obese patients.
- Reliable wide-bore IV cannula with fluid running.
- Drawn-up predefined dose of induction agent (propofol 1–2.5mg/ kg; ketamine 1–2mg/kg; thiopentone 2–5mg/kg) and suxamethonium (1–1.5mg/kg). Ketamine is increasingly favoured in unstable patients.
- Emergency drugs (anticholinergics and vasopressors).
- Strategy for failed intubation and failed ventilation. Difficult intubation may occur in one in 20 cases—failure in one in 200.

Procedure

- Switch on suction, and place in easy reach.
- Preoxygenate through a tight-fitting mask with high-flow O_2 for 3min, until ETO_2 is >90% or, in extreme emergency, four VC breaths (with O_2 flush on). This delays the onset of hypoxaemia and buys time for muscle relaxation and intubation. Patients who are pregnant, obese, septic, anaemic, paediatric, and those with respiratory disease desaturate faster. Any entrainment of air partially undoes the process. Do not remove the mask until laryngoscopy.
- Cricoid force 10N (1kg) is applied by a trained assistant.
- Administer the induction agent, immediately followed by suxamethonium.
- Cricoid force is increased to 30N (3kg) at loss of consciousness.
- Intubate after fasciculations, 45–60s after suxamethonium.
- Inflate the cuff, hand-ventilate, and confirm correct ETT placement by capnography and bilateral auscultation of the chest and stomach.
- Once the ETT is correctly placed, ask the assistant to remove cricoid pressure.

Problems

- Excessive dose of induction agent may produce circulatory collapse, especially in the presence of hypovolaemia.
- Inadequate dose of induction agent may cause tachycardia and hypertension and increase the risk of awareness (perhaps particularly with thiopental).
- Alfentanil (10–30 micrograms/kg) or remifentanil (1–2 micrograms/ kg) 1min before induction may reduce undesirable hypertension and tachycardia and improve intubating conditions. (In obstetrics, beware neonatal respiratory depression if given to the mother on induction). In the event of intubation failure, this may be reversed with naloxone (400–800 micrograms).
- Increased risk of airway difficulty due to lack of time and cricoid pressure.

Cricoid force (pressure)

- This is a trained, practised skill.
- The cricoid cartilage is held between the thumb and middle finger, and pressure is exerted mainly with the index finger posteriorly.
- Bimanual force (other hand behind the neck) has not been shown to be of any benefit in supine patients and uses up one of the assistant's hands. It is not recommended.
- Some patients may only tolerate cricoid force after induction, e.g. distressed children.
- Correct application of cricoid force improves the view at laryngoscopy and does not occlude the airway.
- BURP may improve the laryngeal view but increases the likelihood of airway obstruction. Therefore, if intubation fails and ventilation is required, remove BURP.
- Excessive force (>50N, >5kg) produces airway obstruction and makes intubation more difficult.
- Cricoid force is often poorly applied; this is an issue of training, not of the technique.
- If intubation is difficult, cricoid force is often the cause; it should be reduced and then removed to see if it leads to an improved view that enables intubation. Suction should be immediately available.
- If a patient vomits after application of cricoid force, but before induction, it should be released. Vomiting does not occur after loss of consciousness.
- A tiring assistant may not be able to maintain cricoid force for >5min.
- The correct force to apply is easily practised on an air-filled sealed syringe positioned vertically on the plunger; compressing 20mL of air to 12mL or 50mL to 32mL requires ~3kg of force.

Controversies

- RSI with cricoid force is not proven to reduce aspiration and is known to increase the risk of failed intubation.
- Many add rapid, but short-acting, opioids to 'smooth' induction and intubation; there is no evidence of harm from this technique, but avoiding muscle relaxants altogether is rarely practised.
- Classic RSI prohibits mask ventilation before intubation. However, effective cricoid force significantly reduces the risk of gastric inflation. Ventilation may be safer, particularly if the patient is becoming hypoxaemic.
- If suxamethonium is to be avoided, rocuronium is an alternative. A dose of 0.9–1.0mg/kg and co-administration of propofol (2mg/kg) and a rapid-onset opioid are usually required to achieve optimal laryngoscopy conditions in <1min. Duration of muscular blockade will exceed 30min with this technique, though sugammadex may now be used to reverse this in <3min.
- Sugammadex reverses the NMB of rocuronium very rapidly. However, it can only be used once prepared, and *it does not reverse airway obstruction due to mechanical factors*. A strategy of RSI using rocuronium with sugammadex to manage airway difficulty requires careful consideration of the likely cause of difficulty and for the drug to be immediately available and drawn up.

Failed intubation (plan C in Difficult Airway Society guidelines)

- It is a fallacy that 'RSI is safe, because the patient will wake if there are airway complications'. In the event of failed intubation, whatever drug combination is used, induction agents/NMB are very unlikely to wear off before the onset of life-threatening hypoxia (and awareness).
- Oxygenation is essential. Gentle manual ventilation should be part of any failed intubation protocol.
- If ventilation is difficult, cricoid force should be reduced or released.
- Airway rescue is likely to be required—an SAD with an oesophageal drain tube is the logical choice, e.g. ProSeal LMA, LMA Supreme™, or i-Gel, and a 'CICV' protocol adopted (see ➔ p. 915 and p. 957).

Paediatric considerations

- Effective cricoid force has not been established.
- Young children are unlikely to cooperate with preoxygenation and cricoid force. Children desaturate more quickly than adults. RSI may therefore need to be modified with gentle mask ventilation after induction to prevent hypoxaemia before or during laryngoscopy. Beware effects of stomach inflation, vagal reflexes, regurgitation, and diaphragm splinting.
- Difficult laryngoscopy and tracheal intubation are fortunately much less common in children.

Further reading

Heier T, Feiner JR, Lin J, Brown R, Caldwell JE (2001). Hemoglobin desaturation after succinylcholine-induced apnea: a study of the recovery of spontaneous ventilation in healthy volunteers. *Anesthesiology*, **94**, 754–9.

Li CW, Xue FS, Xu YC, *et al.* (2007). Cricoid pressure impedes insertion of, and ventilation through, the ProSeal laryngeal mask airway in anesthetized, paralyzed patients. *Anesth Analg*, **104**, 1195–8.

McLelland CH, Bogod DG, Hardman JG (2009). Pre-oxygenation and apnoea in pregnancy: changes during labour and with obstetric morbidity in a computational simulation. *Anaesthesia*, **64**, 371–7.

Neilipovitz DT, Crosby ET (2007). No evidence for decreased incidence of aspiration after rapid sequence induction. *Can J Anaesth*, **54**, 748–64.

Sellick BA (1961). Cricoid pressure to control regurgitation of stomach contents during induction of anaesthesia. *Lancet*, **2**, 404–6.

Vanner R, Asai T (1999). Safe use of cricoid pressure. *Anaesthesia*, **54**, 1–3.

Inhalational induction

Indications
- To avoid IV induction—children, needle phobia, difficult IV access.
- To maintain airway patency and SV during induction:
  - Anticipated difficult intubation and/or difficult manual ventilation, e.g. acute epiglottitis, perilaryngeal tumours
  - Inhaled foreign body
  - Bronchopleural fistula.

Preparation and practice
Explain the process to the patient/parents on the ward. Warn parents about the excitation phase. Some anaesthetists prescribe an antisialogogue. Apply routine monitoring whenever possible. A close-fitting face mask speeds induction, but, in young children, a cupped hand to deliver the fresh gas supply is preferred by some. When inhalational induction is used, for reasons of anticipated airway difficulty, have a backup plan.

- Inhalational induction is frequently used prior to IV access. In complicated cases, have a skilled assistant/2nd anaesthetist present to secure cannulation.
- Sevoflurane and halothane are the best tolerated agents. Sevoflurane is faster in onset and less arrhythmogenic. Use of a 50:50 $N_2O:O_2$ mix improves tolerance and speeds the onset of anaesthesia. However, with an actual or anticipated airway obstruction, 100% O_2 is sensible.
- Sevoflurane can be introduced at 8%. Halothane may be introduced at 0.5–1% and increased every four breaths or as tolerated.
- Single VC breath induction from a 4L reservoir bag containing 4–5% halothane or 8% sevoflurane in O_2 is a recognized, but rarely used, technique. The patient typically loses consciousness in under a minute.

Difficulties with inhalational induction
- A leak around the mask, low alveolar ventilation (partial/intermittent obstruction, stridor, breath-holding), and high cardiac output slow induction.
- The correct stage of anaesthesia to cannulate veins, instrument the airway, apply cricoid pressure, or intubate is a matter of experience and may be misjudged.
- Rapid offset with sevoflurane may cause lightening of anaesthesia during airway intervention.
- The excitement stage may be long and associated with complications. Induction will only progress past this phase if the airway is patent.
- Application of CPAP may be useful, as may gentle assisted ventilation.
- The traditional view that inhalation induction is safe because, if the patient obstructs, they will automatically lighten, unobstruct, and start ventilating again is *not true*; persistent obstruction, laryngospasm, hypoxia, and arrhythmias may all lead to morbidity, and even mortality. This was noted as a significant cause of morbidity in NAP 4.
- In safe circumstances, additional judicious IV induction, while maintaining spontaneous breathing, may sometimes be appropriate.

- Although inhalational induction may permit indirect and direct laryngoscopy and assessment of ease of intubation past an upper airway obstruction, have a backup plan prepared (e.g. equipment for cricothyroidotomy or experienced surgical assistance ready and waiting if an emergency surgical airway may be necessary).

Slow spontaneous breathing induction of anaesthesia with incremental target-controlled infusion of propofol

Advantages over gaseous induction:
- Low-dose propofol provides excellent anxiolysis, assisting the progress of anaesthesia.
- Increasing the depth of anaesthesia is independent of the patient's ventilation.
- Allows the rate of increase of the depth of anaesthesia to be titrated carefully by the anaesthetist (not dictated by the patient).
- If difficulty is encountered, stopping the infusion rapidly enables anaesthesia to lighten, without requiring a patent airway.
- Airway reflexes are rapidly obtunded.
- Secretions are not increased.
- Coughing is very rare as is bucking, laryngospasm, or worsening obstruction.
- Assisted ventilation may be attempted at a much earlier stage; in many cases, patients will tolerate gentle manual ventilation, even when still responsive to verbal stimulus.
- Airway adjuncts (e.g. Guedel airway) are tolerated considerably earlier.
- The technique does demand scrupulous attention to detail to detect problems with the airway early and an understanding of the potential effects of pre-programmed pharmacokinetic models as they relate to weight, especially in the obese.

Paediatric considerations

- Parental explanation and support are essential, as their assistance is often useful during induction.
- Optimal positioning will depend on child size. Between the ages of 2 and 5yr, sitting the child on the parent's lap and encouraging them to cuddle/gently restrain them during induction is a useful technique. For older and younger children, the trolley may be more appropriate.

Further reading

Patel A, Pearce A, Pracy P (2011). Head and neck pathology. In: Cook TM, Woodall N, Frerk C, eds. *4th National Audit Project of the Royal College of Anaesthetists and the Difficult Airway Society. Major complications of airway management in the United Kingdom. Report and findings, March 2011.* London: The Royal College of Anaesthetists, pp. 143–54. ॐ http://www.rcoa.ac.uk/nap4.

Awake fibreoptic intubation

Indications

- Known or anticipated difficult airway: particularly where there is a high risk that backup techniques will not be successful.
- Known or suspected cervical cord trauma or unstable neck (e.g. RA).
- After failed intubation.
- Consider in cases of obesity, OSA, and risk of aspiration.

Contraindications

- Patient refusal or patient so uncooperative as to render the procedure unsafe.
- Severe coagulopathy: bleeding danger, particularly via the nasal route.
- Periglottic masses causing partial airway obstruction: risk of complete airway obstruction or laryngospasm.

Patient

- Give explanation, and obtain consent.
- Consider premedication and anticholinergic.
- Equipment: as per checklist (Table 37.2).

Table 37.2 Awake fibreoptic intubation checklist

Decongestant	Xylometazoline 0.1% or phenylephrine 1% nasal spray—administered in advance, if possible
Anticholinergic	Glycopyrronium 400 micrograms IM 30min before or 100–200 micrograms IV in theatre
LA	Lidocaine 10% throat spray; 2–4% for nose, larynx, trachea
O_2	Continuously by mask, nasal cannula, or via fibrescope
Monitoring	Minimum SpO_2, BP, ECG, capnography, conscious level
Conscious sedation	Choose from short-acting opioid (remifentanil, alfentanil, fentanyl), propofol, or midazolam
Airway adjuncts	Bite blocks (Berman, BreatheSafe) for oral route
Assistance	Trained assistant, familiar with technique, able to assist with monitoring, and briefed
ETT	Small: nasal 6–6.5mm ID, oral 6–7mm ID.
	ILMA ETT optimal
Fibrescope	Appropriate size, sterilized, leak-tested
Suction	Attached to fibrescope
Light source	Light box recommended if using remote screen
Monitor	Remote screen with image capture/download facility. White-balanced

Tracheal tube

- Unless there is a specific indication, a small tube that fits snugly over the fibrescope will reduce 'hold-up' during passage and minimize airway trauma. Small tubes are particularly indicated in airway difficulty.
- Recommended: ILMA size 6mm ID. Lubricated.
- Alternatives: reinforced ETT softened with warm water, or Blue Ivory (Portex).
- AIC (ED <7mm) may be useful for severely narrowed lesions.

Topical anaesthesia

Specific nerve blocks (sphenopalatine, ethmoid, glossopharyngeal, superior laryngeal nerve, recurrent laryngeal nerve) are described in other texts. Here we describe topical anaesthesia.

Nose

- Assess nasal passages for patency (history and examination) and history of epistaxis. Vasoconstriction: co-phenylcaine. Topical 4% lidocaine with gauze or cotton buds.
- Alternative is serial dilation: Hegar cervical dilators coated in lidocaine gel (or nasopharyngeal airways). Risks bleeding.

Oropharynx

- Lidocaine 10% spray (ten sprays) or gargle lidocaine gel.

Larynx

- Spray lidocaine under direct vision (e.g. dropwise via an epidural catheter). Nebulized lidocaine may reach the larynx.

Trachea

- Lidocaine 2% via cricothyroid injection (2mL via a 20G cannula) very effectively anaesthetizes the trachea and larynx. Although invasive, it is well tolerated and ensures the anaesthetist has carefully examined the front of the neck.

Note: the total dose of lidocaine should not exceed 7mg/kg.

Sedation

- Critical airway: may need to avoid sedation.
- Non-critical airway: target is a relaxed, awake patient, comfortable, but able to communicate and cooperate. Include hypnosis and analgesia. TCI technique suitable, if familiar.

Position

- Patient sitting up at 45°. Operator facing the patient.

Oxygen

- Always give, and always monitor. O_2 via a nasal catheter or Hudson mask with a 'window' cut out to allow access for intubation. O_2 2L/min via a fibrescope suction channel will oxygenate, clear secretions from the tip, and aid atomization of injected LA.

Technique

- The nasal technique is most frequently used; it allows easy access to the glottis, and topical anaesthesia is easier. General aspects of the technique are described below.
- Check the ETT is mounted on the fibrescope, lubricated, and fixed. Pass the fibrescope under direct vision via the nasal route, identifying all structures en route to the pharynx. With the fibrescope above the cords, dribble lidocaine onto the cords, prior to entering with the fibrescope. Advance the fibrescope to sit just above the carina, then railroad the ETT gently. Use gentle rotation if 'hold-up' (ILMA ETT avoids this). Visually confirm the position of the ETT during withdrawal of the fibrescope. Connect the circuit, and reconfirm the position with capnography. Cuff inflation may be uncomfortable; warn patients.

Post-technique care

- If the airway remains at risk post-operatively, plan extubation (and potential reintubation) carefully. Extubation may need to be delayed.
- Patient to remain starved until airway anaesthesia has worn off. If to remain intubated, change the ILMA ETT to conventional (with exchange catheter).
- Fibrescope to be cleaned and sucked through with 1L of sterile water before transfer for formal decontamination.

Hints for difficulty

- Black is a cavity—aim for black! 'Red out' indicates the fibrescope is not in an airspace—withdraw until recognizable structures are seen, then advance more slowly, staying away from the mucosa. Ask the patient to take deep breaths as the tube approaches the glottis. Ask the patient to protrude the tongue if negotiating the oropharynx is difficult. Alternatively, the assistant may use jaw thrust, pull the tongue with gauze, or insert a laryngoscope. A small ILMA ETT will avoid most railroading problems. Lubrication really helps! Other railroading problems may be overcome by increasing the degrees of gentle tube rotation.

Complications

- Poor compliance/coughing, bleeding in airway (from nasal dilatation), excess secretions, laryngospasm, vomiting, aspiration, airway obstruction. All should be rare in a well-prepared patient.

Oral route

- This route is less frequently used; it is less easy to topically anaesthetize, and entering the glottis requires more advanced control of the fibrescope. Topicalization may include lidocaine nebulizer (5–10mL of 2%), tetracaine (amethocaine) lozenges, or gargle of lidocaine.
- Use of a conduit (e.g. Berman Airway: holds the tongue forward and keeps the scope in midline) will protect the fibrescope and facilitate intubation.

Further reading

Ovassapian A, Krejcie TC, Yelich SJ, Dykes MHM (1989). Awake fibreoptic intubation in the presence of a full stomach. *Br J Anaesth*, **62**, 13–16.

Ovassapian A, Yelich SJ, Dykes MHM, Brunner EE (1983). Fibre-optic nasotracheal intubation—incidence and causes of failure. *Anesth Analg*, **63**, 692–5.

Popat M (2001). *Practical fibreoptic intubation*. Oxford: Butterworth-Heinemann.

Walker A, Smith A (2007). Promoting awake fibreoptic intubation. *RCoA Bulletin*, **46**, 2329–33.

Woodall NM, Harwood RJ, Barker GL (2008). Complications of awake fibreoptic intubation without sedation in 200 healthy anaesthetists attending a training course. *Br J Anaesth*, **100**, 850–5.

Extubation after difficult intubation

After difficult intubation, the airway may occlude when the ETT is removed. Reintubation may then be much more difficult than before due to:
- Airway bruising and swelling
- Airway contamination with clot, pus, or regurgitated material
- New impairments to airway access (e.g. cervical fusion, external fixators, dental wiring)
- Laryngospasm and laryngeal dysfunction (e.g. recurrent laryngeal nerve injury). Paralysis will overcome these.

In NAP 4, one in three of all complications occurred during emergence or recovery; all of these involved airway obstruction, and one in three involved blood in the airway.

Extubation must be planned

Assessing extubation risk must include the risk of requiring reintubation and of its potential difficulty. If indicated, prepare and check the same equipment, and assemble and brief the same skilled personnel as for a difficult intubation. Have a plan and a backup plan. If an emergency surgical airway could still be required, consider:
- Delaying extubation, ventilating on ICU, and reassessing later
- Corticosteroid therapy (dexamethasone 0.5mg/kg to a maximum of 10mg 6-hourly for 24–48hr) before extubation to reduce oedema
- An elective tracheostomy.

Before extubating

- Clear the entire upper airway carefully, and suction the trachea.
- Ensure good haemostasis. Can the airway be improved surgically—evacuation of haematoma, relocation of the arytenoids, stitches to bring the tongue forward?
- Empty the stomach, if necessary.
- Perform a leak test. Deflate the cuff (if present), and ventilate to check there is a low pressure leak around the tube. If no leak is present, re-evaluate. This test is unreliable, but no leak at all should lead to consideration of delaying extubation.
- Place the patient in their most advantageous position for SV and airway maintenance. This is often sitting up.
- Preoxygenate; fully reverse any muscle relaxant; wake the patient, and extubate when obeying commands. Use of drugs with rapid offset is advantageous.
- Provide high-flow O_2 after extubation. CPAP may be indicated.
- Monitor closely in the recovery period for as long as necessary.

Difficult Airway Society extubation guidelines (2012)

(See Figs. 37.7 and 37.8.)
- The principles are plan, prepare, and perform, and post-extubation care.
- Planning is divided into 'low-risk' and 'at-risk' extubation.
- The guidelines emphasize awake extubation as a default.

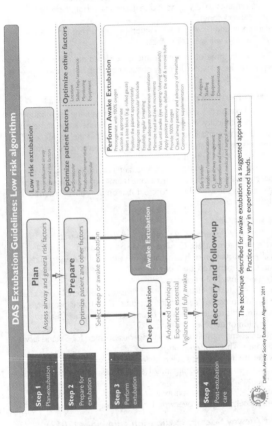

Fig. 37.7 Difficult Airway Society Extubation Guidelines: low-risk algorithm.
Reproduced with permission of J. J. Henderson, M. T. Popat, I. P. Latto, A. C. Pearce, Difficult Airway Society guidelines for management of the unanticipated difficult intubation, John Wiley & Sons, Inc.

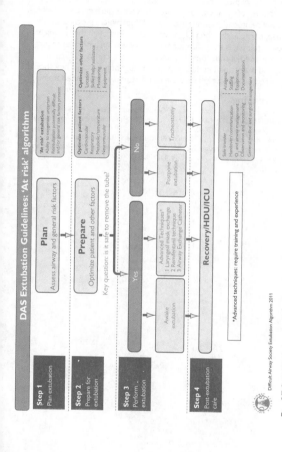

Fig. 37.8 Difficult Airway Society Extubation Guidelines: at-risk algorithm.

Reproduced with permission of J. J. Henderson, M. T. Popat, I. P. Latto, A. C. Pearce, Difficult Airway Society guidelines for management of the unanticipated difficult intubation, John Wiley & Sons, Inc.

- For at-risk extubation, three advanced techniques are recommended:
  - Use of remifentanil to enable a smooth unstimulated extubation
  - Insertion of an airway exchange catheter as a conduit for reintubation
  - Exchange for an SAD.
- All these techniques require practice and attention to detail. In particular, use of an airway exchange catheter is perhaps controversial. Successful reintubation is not guaranteed. Morbidity associated with their use, particularly when O_2 is administered through them, which risks barotrauma, is a significant concern. Where an airway exchange catheter is used, it must be positioned above the carina ($\leq25cm$ in adults) and maintained in that position throughout its use. They should not be used outside a high care area, and attending staff need training.

Further reading

Difficult Airway Society Extubation Guidelines Group, Popat M, Mitchell V, Dravid R, Patel A, Swampillai C, Higgs A (2012). Difficult Airway Society Guidelines for the management of tracheal extubation. *Anaesthesia*, **67**, 318–40.

Maclean S, Lanam C, Benedict W, Kirkpatrick N, Kheterpal S, Ramachandran S (2013). Airway exchange failure and complications with the use of the Cook airway exchange catheter: a single centre cohort of 1177 patients. *Anesth Analg*, **117**, 1325–7.

Practical anaesthesia

Herbal medicines and anaesthesia

- ~5–14% of patients take perioperative herbal medication.
- Of these, 70% do not disclose this fact to their doctor.
- Content and concentrations of herbal remedies may vary dramatically.
- Most herbal remedies are harmless, but some may have important consequences for anaesthesia (Table 38.1).
- The ASA recommends that patients stop herbal medications 2 weeks before surgery.

Table 38.1 Herbal medicines which may affect anaesthesia

Drug (*common name*)	Potential uses	Perioperative concerns
Echinacea (*purple coneflower root*)	Boosts immune system (stimulates cell-mediated immunity)	Immunosuppression in long-term use. Avoid in transplant surgery. May cause hepatotoxicity[1]
Ephedra (*Ma huang*)	Promotes weight loss. Used for asthma and bronchitis (direct and indirect sympathomimetic)	Increased risk of cardiac arrhythmias, hypertension, strokes, and MIs.[2] May cause ventricular arrhythmias with halothane. Life-threatening interaction with MAOIs[1]
Garlic	Treatment of hypertension, hyperlipidaemia, atherosclerosis	Increased risk of bleeding due to antiplatelet effects[3]
Ginkgo (*duck foot tree, maidenhair tree, silver apricot*)	Used to improve mental alertness (antiplatelet activity)	Increased risk of bleeding when combined with anticoagulant and antithrombotic medication[4]
Ginseng (*American, Asian, Chinese, Korean ginseng*)	Aimed at increasing physical and mental stamina	May lower blood concentration of warfarin. May cause hypoglycaemia.[1] May see tachycardia and hypertension
Kava-kava (*intoxicating pepper, kawa*)	Anxiolytic and muscle relaxant	Can increase sedative effect of anaesthetic[1]
St John's wort (*amber, goat weed, hardhay, Hypericum, klamatheweed*)	Antidepression, anxiolytic, and used in sleep disorders (inhibits neurotransmitter reuptake)	Induction of cytochrome P450 liver enzymes. Deceases serum digoxin levels.[1] Avoid in transplant surgery.[5] Associated with hypertensive crisis[6]
Valerian (*All heal, garden heliotrope, vandal root*)	Sleeping aid	Potentiates anaesthetic agents[1]

References

1 Ang-Lee MK, Moss J, Yuan CS (2001). Herbal medicines and perioperative care. *JAMA*, **286**, 208–16.
2 Haller CA, Benowitz NL (2000). Adverse cardiovascular and central nervous system events associated with dietary supplements containing ephedra alkaloids. *N Engl J Med*, **343**, 1833–8.
3 Wong A, Townley S (2011). Herbal medicines and anaesthesia. *Contin Educ Anaesth Crit Care Pain*, **11**, 14–17.
4 Bebbington A, Kulkarni R, Roberts P (2005). Ginkgo biloba: persistent bleeding after total hip arthroplasty caused by herbal self-medication. *J Arthroplasty*, **20**, 125–6.
5 Ernst E (2002). St John's wort supplements endanger the success of organ transplantation. *Arch Surg*, **137**, 316–19.
6 Patel S, Robinson R, Burk M (2002). Hypertensive crisis associated with St John's wort. *Am J Med*, **112**, 507–8.

Further reading

Skinner CM, Rangasami J (2002). Preoperative use of herbal medicines: a patient survey. *Br J Anaesth*, **89**, 792–5.

Blood exposure incidents

Blood exposure incidents, sometimes referred to as inoculation or needle-stick injuries, are common in health-care settings (1–5 per 100 person-years).[7] These incidents can lead to exposure to blood-borne viruses (BBVs), such as HBV and human immunodeficiency virus (HIV), but the commonest encountered in the UK is HCV. Other microorganisms can also be transmitted, leading to local or systemic infection.

A significant number of these exposures are avoidable by ensuring you are immunized against HBV, adherence to universal precautions, and safe disposal of clinical waste.

Routes of exposure

- Percutaneous injury, usually involving a needle (the commonest) or sharp instrument.
- Contact with broken skin, e.g. cuts, abrasions, and eczema.
- Splashes to mucous membranes such as the mouth or eye.

Risk of infection following exposure

The risk of infection will depend upon several factors associated with the injury and the volume of inoculum. An increased risk is associated with:

- Deep penetrating injury
- Large-bore hollow needles
- High viral load of the source patient (donor)
- Injury from a needle that has been in an artery or vein.

Risk of seroconversion following needle-stick injury

- HBV 30%.
- HCV 1.5–3%.
- HIV 0.3%.

Immediate management after exposure

- Immediately wash the area with soap and water, without scrubbing.
- Encourage bleeding of the puncture wound.
- If splash to the eye or mouth, irrigate with water/saline.

Post-exposure management

- Follow your hospital's policy and procedure for blood exposure incidents. The injury requires rapid assessment. In most hospital settings, the occupational health service (OHS) is responsible for this in working hours, and, out of hours, the emergency department is often responsible, but different arrangements may be in place.
- The assessment will consider:
  - The nature of the exposure
  - The likelihood of the source patient being infected with a BBV (see ➲ p. 982)
  - The likelihood that the source patient or a 3rd party has been exposed to your blood.

- The OHS will liaise with the source patient's clinical team to obtain consent for testing for BBVs. Most units test routinely for all three BBVs, provided consent is given to do so.
- Assessment and consent should be carried out as quickly as possible, as post-exposure prophylaxis (PEP) for HIV should be given within 1hr if deemed appropriate.
- If consent cannot be obtained or is refused, a risk assessment of the source patient's status will be required to determine the need for PEP.
- The source patient cannot be tested without their informed consent, even if they are incapacitated (anaesthetized or sedated on intensive care).
- It is important to consider whether your injury has led to the source patient or anyone else being exposed to your blood.
- Complete an incident form. Important to record the event in case of health problems developing later.

If occupational health help is not available

Assess the significance of the injury.[8] If exposure has been significant:
- A colleague must assess the source patient
- Check to see if results of previous testing are available
- Obtain informed consent for testing for BBVs
- If consent unavailable, obtain clinical/social history to assess risk factors for possible infection (see ➔ p. 982)
- If exposure to BBV is likely, contact the on-call microbiologist, consultant in communicable disease control, or genitourinary medicine specialist.

Post-exposure prophylaxis

- PEP is used following exposure to HBV and HIV. (Antibiotics or antiviral therapy may also be considered after exposures to blood or body fluids of patients suffering from other infectious illnesses.)
- PEP may be started as a result of a risk assessment of the injury, while awaiting consent of the source patient or test results.
- Follow-up serology at 6, 12, and 24wk identifies early disease and allows active management. No practice restrictions are required during this period, unless seroconversion occurs.
- HBV—depending on the immunization status, victims will receive HBV vaccine alone or in combination with HBV immunoglobulin.
- Treatment should begin within 48hr of injury.
- HIV—ideally PEP should commence within 1hr but may be given up to 1wk following injury. Currently, a combination of antiretroviral agents is recommended for 4wk. The protocol may require alteration if the source patient is not treatment-naïve. PEP can produce unpleasant side effects, as it is toxic to the liver, kidneys, and bone marrow, and their function is monitored during treatment. A significant proportion of injured health-care workers discontinue treatment because of side effects.
- HCV—no PEP is recommended. Early treatment of acute disease with α-interferon ± ribavirin has been shown to be successful in reducing the risk of long-term chronic liver disease.

The rights of the source patient

- Be aware that the injured health-care worker's blood may have contaminated the source patient as well. Alert senior colleagues if this may have occurred.
- Informed consent must be obtained prior to testing for BBV; the only exception to this is if the test is likely to be in the immediate clinical interests of the patient.
- Informed consent cannot be gained while the patient is recovering from anaesthesia or under the influence of sedatives.
- If consent is not obtained or refused, then a risk assessment should be made to assess the requirement of PEP for the health-care worker.
- Consent discussion should cover:
  - Reason for test—injured health-care worker, possible need for prophylaxis
  - Routine to test for all three BBVs
  - Advantages for the source patient—early diagnosis, with early treatment and protection for sexual partners
  - Potential disadvantages—distress at serious diagnosis, impact on relationships, and difficulty obtaining insurance (but not if negative result)
  - Confidentiality and who will need to know result if positive.

Risk assessment

- In order to assess the need for PEP, a risk assessment of the source patient status must be made.
- History consistent with an increased risk of infection with BBVs includes:
  - Domicile in a country of high prevalence
  - IV drug abuse
  - Blood/blood product transfusion, especially abroad
  - ♂/♂ sex, sex with prostitutes, casual sex, especially abroad (HBV, HIV)
  - History of jaundice.

The infected doctor

- Doctors infected with BBVs may represent a risk of infection to patients, particularly if they participate in exposure-prone procedures (EPPs).
- Occupational health advice must be sought on the range of activities that can be undertaken by infected doctors.
- Currently, participation in EPPs is barred for doctors in the UK who are:
  - HBV-infected (e-antigen positive or s-antigen positive with a viral load of ≥1000 genome copies/mL)
  - HCV-infected and HCV polymerase chain reaction (PCR) positive
  - HIV-infected.
- Most clinical procedures carried out by anaesthetists do not fall within the definition of EPP. Procedures that may be exposure-prone, depending on the technique used, include the placement of portacaths and insertion of chest drains in trauma cases where there may be multiple rib fractures.
- Mouth-to-mouth resuscitation can be undertaken by an EPP-restricted worker if no competent non-restricted colleague is available, as the benefit to the patient greatly outweighs the small risk of BBV transmission in these circumstances.

References

7 White SM (2007). Needlestuck. *Anaesthesia*, **62**, 1199–201.

8 Department of Health (2008). *HIV post-exposure prophylaxis: guidance from the UK Chief Medical Officers' Expert Advisory Group on AIDS*. ℘ http://webarchive.nationalarchives.gov. uk/20130107105354/http://www.dh.gov.uk/prod_consum_dh/groups/dh_digitalassets/@ dh/@en/documents/digitalasset/dh_089997.pdf.

Further reading

Benn P, Fisher M, Kulasegaram R; BASHH; PEPSE Guidelines Writing Group Clinical Effectiveness Group (2011). UK guideline for the use of post-exposure prophylaxis for HIV following sexual exposure. *Int J STD AIDS*, **22**, 695–708. ℘ http://www.bhiva.org/documents/Guidelines/PEPSE/PEPSE2011.pdf.

Department of Health (2007). *Health clearance for tuberculosis, hepatitis B, hepatitis C and HIV: new healthcare workers*. ℘ http://webarchive.nationalarchives.gov.uk/20130107105354/http://www.dh.gov.uk/prod_consum_dh/groups/dh_digitalassets/@dh/@en/documents/digitalasset/dh_074981.pdf.

Department of Health (2007). *Annex A: examples of UKAP advice on exposure prone procedures*. In: Department of Health. *HIV infected health care workers: guidance on management and patient notification*. ℘ http://webarchive.nationalarchives.gov.uk/+/www.dh.gov.uk/en/Publicationsandstatistics/Publications/PublicationsPolicyAndGuidance/Browsable/DH_5368137.

Target-controlled infusions

(See also ➲ p. 1007.)

TCI allows the anaesthetist to achieve a target plasma concentration of a drug for a given patient. The system maintains a target concentration by continually delivering and adjusting the required amount of drug, optimized by weight, age, ± gender, ± height. Propofol has been studied extensively, and population pharmacokinetics were incorporated into the *Diprifusor* TCI system. 'Open' TCI systems are now available, offering the advantage of using generic propofol, as well as other drugs such as remifentanil.

Basic pharmacokinetics

A three-compartment model is often used to describe the redistribution and elimination of drugs such as propofol:

- Drug is delivered to the central compartment V_1 and then distributed throughout the body. The initial bolus is calculated according to the estimated volume of V_1.
- Drug is then distributed to compartments V_2 and V_3. The movement of the drug between the compartments is governed by intercompartmental rate constants (e.g. K_{eo} for brain/effect site concentration).
- The number and size of each compartment and the intercompartmental movement in any algorithm is dependent on many factors, including the pharmacodynamics and pharmacokinetics of the drug in question.

Accuracy

- During infusion, measured plasma concentrations tend to be higher than predicted.
- Once infusion is stopped, this bias is close to zero.
- Because pharmacodynamic variation is much greater than pharmacokinetic variation, the target concentration must be titrated to achieve the required effect in any individual patient.

Which numbers to use

With inhalational agents, the vaporizer is adjusted to the clinical situation, guided by MAC. For propofol, the EC_{50} (effective concentration required to prevent 50% of patients from moving in response to a painful stimulus) is 6–7 micrograms/mL with O_2-enriched air, and 4–5 micrograms/mL with 67% N_2O, in ASA 1–2 patients.

- Interindividual variations in pharmacokinetics and pharmacodynamics, as well as the interaction between drugs, account for the different responses between patients. The target should be titrated according to the clinical situation. Patients with liver and renal dysfunction show greater pharmacokinetic variability, as the drug has altered the distribution/elimination.
- Elderly patients have a smaller volume of distribution, with an increased sensitivity to drugs. Doses therefore should be titrated in small steps.
- Children require a different set of pharmacokinetic variables for propofol, which have been incorporated into the *Paedfusor* and Alaris Asena PK system.
- Benzodiazepine premedication, N_2O, and opioids all reduce propofol requirements.

Induction of anaesthesia
- Select a target concentration less than anticipated (4–6 micrograms/mL is the requirement in the majority of patients).
- Allow time for the effect site concentration to increase towards the target blood concentration. O_2 should be administered during the induction phase to ensure an adequate SpO_2.
- Increase the target concentration to achieve the desired level of anaesthesia for the procedure, the individual patient, and the balance of other agents such as analgesics.

Rapid induction of anaesthesia using target-controlled infusion
- Choose a high target, such as 6–8 micrograms/mL, but only in young, fit patients.
- Wait to allow for the effect site concentration to rise towards the target concentration.
- Reduce the target value, as propofol continues to be redistributed.

Target-controlled infusion for high-risk patients
- Select a low target such as 1 microgram/mL.
- Wait to allow for the effect site concentration to rise.
- Increase the target in small steps (0.5–1 micrograms/mL), until the desired effect is achieved.

Maintenance of anaesthesia
- Three to 6 micrograms/mL is required in the majority of patients, but the exact value will depend on the patient, premedication, analgesia, and degree of surgical stimulation.
- Titrate to effect.
- The majority of patients will wake at 1–2 micrograms/mL.
- When patients are breathing spontaneously, respiratory rate and $ETCO_2$ are good indicators as to the adequacy of anaesthesia.
- The use of N_2O or moderate doses of opioid analgesics, e.g. remifentanil, will allow a lower target concentration of propofol to be used—up to one-third.

Sedation only
Target concentrations of 0.5–2.5 micrograms/mL are usually required to produce good-quality sedation during surgery performed under LA/regional anaesthesia. One to 2mL of 1% lidocaine can be injected through the cannula prior to starting the infusion, to avoid the discomfort from propofol in the lightly sedated patient.

Open target-controlled infusion systems
Open TCI systems offer the possibility of targeting the estimated effect site concentration, rather than the plasma concentration.
- The different pharmacokinetic models available, in the different systems, result in different drug doses delivered for any given effect concentration. Therefore, one should always titrate to the clinical response.

- As open TCI systems allow the use of different drugs and drug concentrations, vigilance is needed to ensure that the correct drug and concentration are used.
- The models used in the available TCI systems calculate dose requirements in obese patients differently. This may result in over-/underestimating the amount of drug required. There is little available evidence regarding the use of TCI in morbidly obese patients, and many anaesthetists input values between the IBW and the total body weight, and then titrate to response.[9]

Intravenous access

- TCI requires secure IV access of adequate size to allow the infusion pump to run at its maximum rate of 1200mL/hr (20G or larger). Ideally, this access should be visible at all times to ensure the infusion is not disrupted. Minimize the use of extensions to reduce the dead space.
- If TCI and IV fluids are connected to the same cannula by means of a T-piece or three-way tap:
  - Ensure that the fluids are running
  - Prevent reflux by using a one-way valve.
- Co-administration of drugs by the same giving set is not ideal, as a change in the rate of one infusion can affect the other, especially if there is a significant dead space after the common connection.
- The most reliable method is to use a separate, dedicated access site.

Benefits of total intravenous anaesthesia

- Decreases the incidence of PONV (unless using N_2O).
- Beneficial in laryngoscopy/bronchoscopy, where delivery of an inhaled agent may be difficult, and in thoracic surgery where it does not appear to inhibit the hypoxic vasoconstrictor reflex.
- Safe to use in patients with a history of MH.
- Recovery with minimal 'hangover'.

Disadvantages

- Increased cost, compared with some volatile agents.
- Inability to monitor the drug concentration.
- Slow recovery following long operations, unless the dose of propofol is decreased by combination with remifentanil.
- Interruption to the delivery of propofol may take longer to recognize.

Target-controlled infusion of remifentanil

Remifentanil has a rapid onset of action, a short elimination half-life, and a context-sensitive half-time of ~3min, which does not change as the infusion time increases. The pharmacokinetics of remifentanil allow the drug to be easily titrated against patient response, using the TCI system. It is often used in combination with propofol TCI, and target values of 3–8ng/mL can provide adequate analgesia. Higher values may be required, depending on the type of surgery and should be titrated to patient response and the dose of hypnotic agent used. Adequate post-operative analgesia needs to be instituted prior to the end of surgery. Low-dose remifentanil TCI can also be used to provide analgesia for labour and AFOI.

Reference

9 Absalom AR, Mani V, De Smet T, Struys MMRF (2009). Pharmacokinetic models for propofol—defining and illuminating the devil in the detail. *Br J Anaesth*, **103**, 26–37.

Further reading

Hill SA (2004). Pharmacokinetics of drug infusions. *Contin Educ Anaesth Crit Care Pain*, **4**, 76–80.

Death on the table

All anaesthetists experience a patient dying on the operating table at some time. In some cases, death is anticipated, and the cause is understood—the patient's relatives and theatre staff will have been informed about the high risk of mortality and are prepared for the event. When death is unexpected, however, the experience can be shattering for all concerned. Added to this is the stress of potential litigation.

Guidelines help to ensure that the legal requirements following a death on the table are fulfilled and may reduce the trauma of the situation. The coroner or equivalent (Procurator Fiscal in Scotland) must be notified of all deaths that occur during anaesthesia or within 30d of an operation.

- **The patient**—all lines and tubes must be left in place, and the patient should be transferred to a quiet area where the relatives can attend.
- **The relatives**—break the news to the relatives in a sympathetic and considerate way. This should be done by a team of senior staff (surgeon, anaesthetist, and nurse). Interpreters, a chaplain, or social workers may be indicated in specific circumstances. It is highly inadvisable to let any single clinician see the relatives alone, as misunderstandings can occur. The initial interview should convey brief facts about the case to allow the relatives to take in the bad news. A nurse or carer should stay with the family to comfort them and offer practical help, as required. After a suitable interval, the team should return and provide further details, as appropriate, and answer the family's questions. Any queries should be answered as fully and accurately as possible.
- **Notifications**—the supervising consultant must be contacted, if not already present. The patient's family doctor and the coroner should be informed by telephone at the earliest opportunity.

Unexpected death

When death is unexpected, the cause of death may not be known at the time. The event needs to be accurately documented, and, in addition to the procedures outlined above, the following must be addressed:

- **Equipment**—the anaesthetic machine and drug ampoules used should be isolated and checked by a senior colleague, preferably someone unconnected with the original incident. An accurate record of these checks must be kept for future reference. Drug checks should include the identity, doses used, expiry dates, and batch numbers. The drug ampoules and syringes should be kept in case further analysis is required.
- **The theatre team**—the rest of the operating list should be delayed, until another team can take over, or cancelled.
- **Documentation**—ensure that the medical record is complete and accurate. If possible, a digital record of the recorded values should be downloaded from the monitors in the anaesthetic room and theatre. The medical physics department may be able to help with this. All entries in the patient's notes should be dated and signed. Details of the case should be clearly documented on an incident form (or equivalent), and copies delivered to the Medical Director and Clinical Director.

A copy should also be retained by the anaesthetist for the medical defence organization. These should not be filed in the case notes.

- **The mentor**—a senior colleague should be allocated to act as mentor for the anaesthetist, to provide guidance and support. The mentor should help with the notifications, assist in the compilation of reports, liaise with the anaesthetist's family, and offer support, as necessary.
- **The theatre team**—a debriefing session should be arranged to help the staff understand the event and come to terms with it. Group counselling may help to reduce post-event psychological trauma.

Preparing for legal proceedings

If legal proceedings do ensue, it may be a long time after the event. The medical records will assume utmost importance and form the basis of the case. Anything not recorded in the notes may be assumed not to have been done. The records should be completed within a few hours of the event and must not be altered in any way. An electronically recorded printout alone is insufficient. The record needs to show the reasoning behind the action taken and some indication of the working diagnosis.

The anaesthetist may find it helpful to record a detailed account of the case within a few days of the death, including all the preoperative discussions with the patient and the perioperative events, noting the personnel and times involved. This can be kept in a confidential and secure personal file and used as an aide-memoire. The anaesthetist's medical defence organization should be consulted for help and further advice. Other health-care staff should also make statements about the case—normally this is coordinated by the Trust.

Further reading

Association of Anaesthetists of Great Britain and Ireland (2005). *Catastrophes in anaesthetic practice: dealing with the aftermath.* ℛ http://www.aagbi.org/sites/default/files/catastrophes05.pdf.

Bacon AK (1989). Death on the table. *Anaesthesia*, **44**, 245–8.

Bacon AK, Morris RW, Runciman WB, Currie M (2005). Crisis management during anaesthesia: recovering from a crisis. *Qual Saf Health Care*, **14**, e25.

Dealing with a complaint

Most doctors receive complaints, the majority of which can be resolved without legal proceedings. Seventy-five per cent of complaints are due to a failure in communication, and only 25% due to a failure to investigate or treat. Patients are more likely to proceed to a legal claim if there is inadequate information or concern initially. The average acute hospital will investigate 120–160 formal complaints per 1000 doctors annually, but very few are followed by a legal claim, and fewer still by a trial. In any service, it is recognized that mishaps will occur, and mechanisms need to be in place to identify and rectify the causes. There is increasing awareness of the role of 'systems failure' in these cases. Usually a series of mistakes is involved, resulting in the adverse incident. The adoption of a 'no blame' culture enables open, honest reporting of failures, which allows appropriate changes to be made, thereby improving patient safety.

Background

In the UK, Crown Indemnity was introduced in 1990, and it is the Trust (hospital) or Health Authority that is sued and is liable, not the individual doctor. The actions of the doctor are considered separately, if required, by the Clinical Director or Medical Director. Crown Indemnity does not cover work performed outside the National Health Service (NHS) contract (e.g. private practice, 'Good Samaritan' deeds), and separate medical defence organization insurance should be arranged to cover this work. The defence organization will also provide support for doctors who become the subject of disciplinary proceedings.

Local resolution

Complaints can often be resolved quickly and to the satisfaction of all involved. The aim is to answer the complaint, offer an apology if that is appropriate, amend faulty procedures or practices (for the benefit of others), and clarify if the complaint is groundless.

Verbal complaints

- **Speak to the patient** as soon as you hear of any problem. Give the patient a full, clear explanation of the facts, and try to resolve any difficulty.
- **Speak to a senior colleague** for guidance and support. Consider asking a senior consultant or the Clinical Director to see the patient with you, as the patient may value their advice and you may value their reassurance.
- **Apologize**—saying sorry is not an admission of liability. Patients will appreciate your concern. However, do not apologize for the actions of others or blame anyone without allowing them to comment.
- **Documentation**—always make a detailed entry in the patient's notes of any dissatisfaction expressed and the action taken in response. Discuss with the Trust complaints manager.

Formal written complaints

Trusts must comply with national guidelines and, in England, acknowledge formal complaints within 3 working days. The complainant must be informed of the procedure to be followed and contacted to discuss the matter with the Trust's complaints manager, so that a time frame for investigating the problem can be agreed. This will involve copying the correspondence to all the relevant clinical staff and clinical directors for their explanation. The information provided is used to produce a report explaining the course of events and any necessary action taken. When replying:

- Speak to a senior consultant/clinical director. They may have experience of similar events and can help to clarify the issues with you.
- The hospital will have an experienced manager who has responsibility for complaints who should be contacted.
- Inform your medical defence organization who will provide advice and support.
- Record-keeping—keep a full account of the details of the incident.
- Leave a forwarding address if you move. A legal claim may be made many months after the event.

Independent review

Any patient not satisfied with the hospital's response should be reminded that they can refer the case to the Health Service Ombudsman (Public Services Ombudsman in Wales; Northern Ireland Commissioner of Complaints; Scottish Public Services Ombudsman).

Legal proceedings

A legal claim may be made several months after the incident or whenever the post-event problem becomes manifest. Initially, you will be asked for a statement of your involvement in the patient's care. The hospital's legal team will need to work with you and your Clinical Director to produce this.

Preparing a statement

This should include the following:
- Full name and qualifications.
- Grade and position held (including duration).
- Full names and positions of others involved (patients, relatives, staff).
- Date(s) and time(s) of all the relevant matters.
- Brief summary of the background details (e.g. patient's medical history).
- Full and detailed description of the matters involved.
- Date and time that your statement was made, and your signature on every page.
- Copies of any supporting documents referred to in the statement (initialled by you).

The statement should accord with the following points:
- **Accuracy.** There should be no exaggeration, understatement, or inconsistencies. Check the details with the patient's notes.
- **Facts.** Keep to the facts, particularly those that determined your decision-making, and avoid value judgements.
- Avoid hearsay. Try to avoid including details that you have not witnessed yourself. If reference has to be made to such information, record the name and position of the person providing it to you, when it was provided, and how.
- **Be concise.** State the essential details in a logical sequence, and avoid generalizations.

- **Relevance**. Include only the details required to understand the situation fully.
- **Avoid jargon**. Give layman's explanations of any clinical terms used, and avoid abbreviations.

Discuss the statement with your Clinical Director and hospital legal department to ensure a clear factual account. Only sign the statement when you are completely happy with the text, and keep a copy for your own reference. The hospital's legal team should provide advice on the subsequent legal process and discuss the management of the claim with you. Remember good record-keeping will help to support your case. Poor records give the impression of poor care. The medical records are the only proof of what occurred, and anything not written down may be assumed to have not happened. Any later additions to the notes should be signed and dated, with an explanation of the reasons why the entry was not made earlier.

Awareness

Complaints of awareness must be pursued promptly. It is important to confirm what the patient may have heard or felt and document this accurately. An explanation of the events and causes, if any, should be given to the patient and documented. The patient needs reassurance that steps can be taken to reduce the risk of awareness during subsequent anaesthetics. Post-traumatic stress disorder can develop, and it is important that these patients are offered counselling and given details of support groups that may be helpful.

Further reading

Department of Health (2009). *Listening, responding, improving—a guide to better customer care.* ℘ http://webarchive.nationalarchives.gov.uk/+/www.dh.gov.uk/en/publicationsandstatistics/publications/publicationspolicyandguidance/dh_095408.

Health Rights Information Scotland (2006). *Making a complaint about the NHS.* Glasgow: Health Rights Information Scotland.

NHS Choices. *Making a complaint.* ℘ http://www.nhs.uk/choiceintheNHS/Rightsandpledges/complaints/Pages/NHScomplaints.aspx.

NHS Wales (2006). *Complaints about NHS treatment and care. A guide to making a complaint about the NHS in Wales.* ℘ http://www.wales.nhs.uk/sitesplus/documents/903/Complaints_about_NHS_leafle2.pdf.

Northern Ireland Department of Health, Social Services and Public Safety (2009). *Complaints in health and social care: standards and guidelines for resolution and learning.* ℘ http://www.dhsspsni.gov.uk/hsc_complaints_revised_standards_and_guidelines_for_resolution_and_learning_updated_february_2015_-2.pdf

Anaphylaxis follow-up

- For immediate management of acute anaphylaxis, see ➋ p. 920.
- Information about reporting UK suspected anaphylactic reactions is at ℘ http://www.aagbi.org/safety/allergies-and-anaphylaxis.

Drugs given IV bypass the body's 1° defence systems. Potentially noxious chemicals are presented rapidly to sensitive cells such as polymorphs, platelets, and mast cells. Degranulation, whether immune or non-immune, releases inflammatory mediators—histamine, prostaglandins, and leukotrienes.

Apparent 'anaesthetic adverse drug reactions' (AADRs) may be due to non-drug mechanisms:
- Underlying pathology, e.g. asthma, systemic mastocytosis, MH
- Medical cause, e.g. septicaemia, severe asthma, cardiac pathology, pneumothorax, PE, air embolism
- Blood loss
- Adverse pharmacological effect related to genetic status, e.g. angio-oedema
- Machine or operator error
- Vasovagal episode
- Allergy to other exposed substances, e.g. latex, chlorhexidine, contrast dyes, and IV infusions (colloids, blood, plasma).

Drug-involved reactions may be:
- Exaggerated pharmacological response—hypotension with propofol, bradycardia and hypotension with opioids
- True allergic reactions—type 1 anaphylaxis (IgE-mediated) or type 3 immune complex (IgG-mediated)
- Pseudoallergic or anaphylactoid reactions—direct histamine release by active agent or indirect release by complement activation.

Clinically, anaphylactic reactions may be indistinguishable from anaphylactoid responses—the endpoint in both is mast cell degranulation. Life-threatening reactions are more likely to be immune-mediated, implying past exposure.
- Neuromuscular-blocking drugs are responsible for 60–70% of serious AADRs, frequently on 1st contact.
- The quaternary ammonium group found in neuromuscular-blocking drugs is widely present in other drugs, foods, cosmetics, and hair care products. Previous sensitization is possible, predominantly in ♀.

Antibiotic sensitivity

- Penicillin reactions may be IgE-mediated but are seldom as severe as AADRs.
- If previous penicillin anaphylaxis, 1st-generation cephalosporins should be avoided.
- The risk of reactivity to carbepenems is very low, particularly if a skin-prick test (SPT) is negative.
- Cross-reactivity to 3rd- or 4th-generation cephalosporins and aztreonam in patients with penicillin allergy is uncertain, and these can be given to most patients who declare themselves as 'penicillin-allergic'—give slowly and incrementally in case of an anaphylactoid (dose-related) response.

Incidence

The incidence of AADRs appears to be between 1 in 10 000 and 20 000 anaesthetics, with a preponderance for ♀.[10]

Presentation of anaphylactoid or anaphylactic reactions

- Isolated cutaneous erythema is commonly seen following IV thiopental or atracurium. If there are no further histaminoid manifestations, investigation is unwarranted. However, this may be the 1st clinical feature in severe reactions.
- Timing is important. Onset is usually rapid following an IV drug bolus. Slower onset is expected if, for example, gelatin infusion, latex sensitivity, or diclofenac suppository responsible.
- CVS collapse has been reported in 88% of cases, bronchospasm in 36%, and angio-oedema in 24% of AADRs, with cutaneous signs in ~50%.

Investigation of reactions

Referral to anaesthetic allergy clinic

The referral to an allergy clinic is the responsibility of the anaesthetist and should include:

- Anaesthetic chart
- Drug chart
- Timings of all administered substances
- Anaesthetic charts
- Tryptase results and timings.

Serum tryptase evaluation

Tryptase is a neutral protease released from secretory granules of mast cells during degranulation. *In vivo* half-life is 3hr (compared with 3min for histamine), and it is stable in isolated plasma or serum. Level is unaffected by haemolysis, as it is not present in red and white cells.

- Three venous blood samples preferable—immediately after resuscitation, at 1–2hr (not later than 6hr), and baseline levels at 24hr or later. Serum should be separated and stored at −20°C for onward transmission to an appropriate laboratory.
- Basal plasma tryptase concentration is usually <11ng/mL. Levels up to 15ng/mL are seen in pseudoallergy, i.e. non-specific, anaphylactoid reactions, and non-life-threatening anaphylaxis. Higher values are more likely to indicate IgE mediation.

Radioallergosorbent/CAP tests

- Radioallergosorbent tests (RASTs) for antigen-specific IgE antibodies have now been largely superseded by the CAP system (Phadia).
- An antigen-coated CAPsule is exposed to the patient's serum under laboratory conditions. If the serum contains antigen-specific IgE, a measurable colour change is produced.
- Currently, only helpful in confirming penicillin, suxamethonium, chlorhexidine, and latex allergy. Sensitivity is low, and a negative result still requires skin testing.

Skin testing

- Diagnosing an AADR depends on SPT or intradermal testing (IDT). In proven neuromuscular-blocking drug anaphylaxis, no *in vitro* test has been shown to have comparable specificity and sensitivity. Skin testing is probably diagnostic in anaphylaxis, but not in anaphylactoid reactions. Refer the patient to a centre experienced in investigating AADRs.
- Tests should take place at 4–6wk post-event to allow the regeneration of IgE.
- Antihistamines should not have been given within the last 5d.
- SPT is used initially. Some drugs, e.g. atracurium and suxamethonium, can produce a false positive result with IDT.
- Testing is required to all drugs given before the event. Remember antibiotics, latex, chlorhexidine, and lidocaine, if mixed with propofol. Suspected LA allergy is best tested by challenge.[11]
- Negative control is with saline (to exclude dermographia). Positive control is with a commercially available histamine solution. The latter demonstrates a normal skin response. Wheal and flare gives a reference for reactions to test drugs.
- Wheal >2mm wider than the saline control is interpreted as positive. Positive test with undiluted drug is repeated with 1:10 dilution to reduce the chance of a false positive.
- Following a positive result, other drugs in the same pharmacological group are tested. In neuromuscular-blocking drug allergy, up to 60% of people may be sensitive to other relaxants.
- If there is a strong history, but negative SPT, diluted drugs can be tested by IDT.

After testing

- The patient must know the importance and implications of the diagnosis. MedicAlert (𝓜 www.medicalert.org) can provide a warning bracelet at the patient's own expense.
- In the absence of positive skin testing, best advice is given based on the clinical history.
- Ensure hospital notes are marked. Inform the GP.
- Report the reaction to MHRA ('yellow card system'). AADRs are currently under-reported.

Future anaesthesia

- Avoid all untested drugs related to the original culprit.
- Do not use IV 'test' doses—unsafe if a true allergy exists.
- If any doubt about induction agents, use inhalational induction. There are no reports of anaphylaxis to inhalational anaesthetics.
- If neuromuscular-blocking drug reaction, give relaxant-free anaesthetic, if possible.
- If a neuromuscular-blocking drug must be used, ideally test your chosen drug by SPT preoperatively.
- In proven neuromuscular-blocking drug allergy, give chlorphenamine (10mg IV) and hydrocortisone (100mg IV) 1hr prior to induction.

References

10 Laxenaire MC, Mertes PM (2001). Anaphylaxis during anaesthesia. Results of a two year study in France. *Br J Anaesth*, **87**, 549–58.

11 Fisher MM, Bowey CJ (1997). Alleged allergy to local anaesthetics. *Anaesth Intensive Care*, **25**, 611–14.

Further reading

Association of Anaesthetists of Great Britain and Ireland (2009). Suspected anaphylactic reactions associated with analgesia. *Anaesthesia*, **64**, 199–211. ✍ http://www.aagbi.org/sites/default/files/anaphylaxis_2009.pdf.

Dewatcher P, Mouton-Faivre C, Emala C (2009). Anaphylaxis and anesthesia: controversies and new insights. *Anesthesiology*, **111**, 1141–50.

Ewan PW, Dugué P, Mirakian R, Dixon TA, Harper JN, Nasser SM; BSACI (2009). BSACI guidelines for the investigation of suspected anaphylaxis during general anaesthesia. *Clin Exp Allergy*, **40**, 15–31.

Fisher MM, Bowey CJ (1997). Intradermal compared with prick testing in the diagnosis of anaesthetic allergy. *Br J Anaesth*, **79**, 59–63.

Solensky R, Khan DA (2010). Drug allergy: an updated practice parameter. *Ann Allergy Asthma Immunol*, **105**, 259–73.

Latex allergy

Latex is derived from the sap of *Hevea brasiliensis* (rubber tree). Hev b proteins within latex act as the major allergens (there are 14 types—Hev b1–14).[12] Studies have suggested that latex hypersensitivity is the second commonest cause for anaesthetic-related anaphylaxis.[13]

Latex may be found in the following anaesthetic equipment: urinary catheters, gloves, syringes, drug vial stoppers, IV giving sets, IV cannulae, injection ports, masks, airways, ETTs, rebreathing bags, BP cuffs, bellows, and circuits. Many surgical pieces of equipment may also contain latex: drains, bulb irrigation syringes, vascular tags, rubber-covered clamps, and certain elastic that may be found in hats/compression stockings/underpants.

Classification of reaction

- **Irritant contact dermatitis**: non-allergic irritant contact dermatitis, presenting over minutes to hours with damage of the skin due to the exogenous substance causing irritation.
- **Contact dermatitis**: a type IV (delayed) hypersensitivity reaction, based on allergic sensitization mediated by T lymphocytes. Presents over 48–72hr with an eczematous eruption. This can progress to lichenification and scaling on chronic exposure.
- **Type I hypersensitivity**: development of latex sensitivity is dependent on previous exposure. IgE-mediated type I hypersensitivity has been attributed to Hev b proteins in latex. The three main presentations are:
  - Contact urticaria: particularly of health-care workers, typically 10–15min following, and usually at the site of, exposure. This may develop into a more severe reaction
  - Asthma and rhinitis: characterized with bronchospasm and secretions. Inhalations of airborne latex particles from powdered gloves have been implicated
  - Anaphylaxis: this is more commonly encountered intraoperatively. IV and membrane inoculation are the commonest triggers; however, donning of gloves and indirect contact have also been described.

High-risk individuals

Eight per cent of the population is sensitized to latex; however, 1.4% of the population exhibit a latex allergy. Latex anaphylaxis appears to be commoner in ♀.[13] There are certain groups at particular risk of developing latex sensitivity:

- **Multiple surgical procedures**: patients with repeated exposure to latex have an increased risk. This is more pronounced in children, especially at a very young age. Therefore, latex-free precautions need to be taken to avoid sensitization
- **Neural tube defects** (including spina bifida): incidence of latex sensitivity due to recurrent bladder catheterization is 20–65%
- **Associated medical conditions**: patients with atopy, asthma, rhinitis, and severe dermatitis have an increased incidence of sensitivity[14]
- **Health-care workers**: prevalence of sensitivity can be between 3 and 12%[12]

- **Occupation**: rubber industry workers, occupations involving the use of protective equipment (policemen, hairdressers, service food workers)
- **Fruit allergens**: patients allergic to fruit have an 11% risk of a latex reaction. Cross-reactivity has been demonstrated with certain fruit allergens (banana, chestnut, avocado, passion fruit, tomato, grape, celery, peach, watermelon, cherry, and kiwi fruit).[12]

Prevention of latex anaphylaxis

Preoperative assessment

- A quarter of patients who developed intraoperative latex anaphylaxis had a history suggestive of a latex allergy.[13] It is important to determine whether contact with balloons, condoms, or latex gloves causes itching, rash, or swelling. Ask about the occupational history.
- Patients with a positive clinical history may be referred for testing before surgery. This may not be possible in an emergency. Current tests have a sensitivity of 75–90%. This includes a blood test specifically for latex-specific IgE or an SPT (performed by trained staff).[15] If these tests are unclear or negative despite a clear history, consider other tests, such as provocation testing, to be performed by a specialist.

Perioperative precautions

- All team members need to be alerted when a patient has a latex allergy.
- The operating theatre should be prepared the night before, and the patient should be scheduled 1st on the list. This reduces the number of latex particles in the air.
- 'Latex allergy' notices should be placed on the anaesthetic and theatre doors.
- Only use latex-free equipment within the anaesthetic and surgical areas. Each theatre suit should have a list detailing which equipment is guaranteed latex-free. LMAs (Intavent), most ETTs, and airways are latex-free.
- Remove non-essential equipment from the vicinity of the patient.
- Limit staff traffic during surgery.
- Resuscitation equipment must be latex-free.
- There is no evidence to support prophylactic use of antihistamines and corticosteroids.

Clinical features of latex anaphylaxis

Onset is normally 20–60min following exposure and progressively worsens over 5–10min. Patients present with hypotension, bronchospasm, and commonly a rash. It may be difficult to exclude an anaphylaxis from anaesthetic drugs, as this presents in a similar manner. It is important to recognize anaphylaxis and remove any latex-containing objects from the patient. Treat as for anaphylaxis (see p. 920). Subsequent analysis of serum mast cell tryptase confirms anaphylaxis.

Hospital latex allergy policy

- There should be a lead clinician for latex allergy, and available instructions for access to latex allergy testing.
- Follow latex allergy precautions on the ward and in theatre.
- This should include a latex-free trolley containing the following latex-free equipment: gloves (synthetic rubber), masks and airways (plastics), ETTs (PVC), reservoir bags (neoprene), valves (silicone), IV tubing, IV cannulae (Teflon™), syringes, bellows, and circuits. There should also be barrier protectors for placement between latex-containing items and the patient's skin (e.g. Webril).
- Measures should be in place to avoid latex sensitization with hospital staff.

References

12 Hepner DL, Castells MC (2003). Latex allergy: an update. *Anesth Analg*, **96**, 1219–29.

13 Harper NJ, Dixon T, Dugué P, *et al.* (2009). Suspected anaphylactic reactions associated with anaesthesia. *Anaesthesia*, **64**, 199–211.

14 Bousquet J, Flahault A, Vandenplas O, *et al.* (2006). Natural rubber latex allergy among health care workers: a systematic review of the evidence. *J Allergy Clin Immunol*, **118**, 447–54.

15 Suli C, Lorini M, Mistrello G, Tedeschi A (2006). Diagnosis of latex hypersensitivity: comparison of different methods. *Eur Ann Allergy Clin Immunol*, **38**, 24–30.

Further reading

Cullinan P, Brown R, Field A, *et al.*; British Society of Allergy and Clinical Immunology (2003). Latex allergy. A position paper of the British Society of Allergy and Clinical Immunology. *Clin Exp Allergy*, **33**, 1484–99.

Lieberman P, Nicklas RA, *et al.* (2010). The diagnosis and management of anaphylaxis practice parameter: 2010 update. *J Allergy Clin Immunol*, **126**, 477–80.

Military anaesthesia

- Techniques of resuscitation, anaesthesia, and transportation of critically injured soldiers and civilians are continuously being developed and improved during conflict.
- Injuries may be the result of ballistic injuries from improvised explosive devices (IEDs), penetrating injuries from gunshot wounds, or non-battlefield injuries such as road traffic accidents.
- Military medical care starts immediately with soldiers trained to stop bleeding, apply tourniquets, and administer analgesia. More advanced first aid is given by combat medical technicians (CMTs). Uncontrolled haemorrhage is the commonest cause of death in conflict.
- Early intervention in the battlefield area and moving the patient rapidly to an appropriate emergency medical facility is making a major impact on survival.
- Simultaneous haemostatic resuscitation, major haemorrhage protocols, and damage control surgery (DCS), followed by a short period of stabilization in intensive care, is the norm prior to onward transportation to definitive care in Birmingham (UK). The aim is to do this within 24hr of injury.
- Anaesthetists are expected to work in a wide range of roles, including being deployed via land, sea, or air, via parachute or helicopter insertion, which often includes life-threatening exposure to conflict in our prehospital care role and extremes of cold/heat.
- Facilities for military anaesthesia are designed to be highly capable but mobile, allowing the setting up of full trauma resuscitation/surgery facilities within 45min of insertion.
- Anaesthesia includes IV, drawover, and regional/local anaesthesia techniques.

Damage control resuscitation

(See also ➔ p. 476, p. 871, p. 847 and p. 1049.)

- Damage control resuscitation (DCR) comprises haemostatic resuscitation, a massive haemorrhage protocol (MHP), and DCS.
- Haemorrhage remains the leading cause of combat casualty death. Haemostatic resuscitation is defined as the rapid proactive treatment of coagulopathy associated with major trauma. Hypoperfusion, hyperfibrinolysis, activation of protein C, and upregulation of thrombomodulin pathways all contribute to **acute coagulopathy of trauma shock (ACoTS)**. Aggressive treatment of the lethal triad of *hypothermia, acidosis, and coagulopathy* is essential to countering ACoTS.
- DCR relies on excellent effective and current communication between personnel from the medical emergency response team (MERT), emergency department, anaesthesia, surgery, nursing, and laboratory teams.
- Ensure everyone in the resuscitation area or theatre is aware of their role beforehand. Among the most important are those managing blood products, the rapid infusor, and the scribe. Be clear who the team leader is.

Rapid sequence induction of anaesthesia

- Excellent teamwork is key.
- Preoxygenation using a 'Waters circuit' ensures high FiO_2 and a degree of PEEP, which can be useful in chest trauma. Consider using nasal O_2 cannulae at 15L/min placed pre-intubation if SpO_2 <90%.
- Connect face mask–catheter mount–HME–CO_2–Waters, in that order.
- Ketamine at a dose of 0.7–1.5mg/kg (80mg/150mg) or thiopental 10–50% of the normal dose for normotensive head injuries.
- Rocuronium 1.2mg/kg (suxamethonium 1.5mg/kg as 2nd choice).

Intubation

- Aim for 'first time, every time'.
- An 8mm cuffed oral ETT for adults. Use Parker Flex-Tip, if available.
- Introducer pre-primed in ETT at 20cm, with a 10mL syringe attached.
- Size 4 Macintosh blade with a stubby handle or Glidescope/Airtraq.

Intravenous access

- Large-bore central access 8.5Fr (PAFC introducer/Arrow MAC) into the right/left subclavian vein (avoid going below the diaphragm).

Haemostatic resuscitation

- Initial resuscitation is empiric and fast.
- 'Shock packs' of 4U each of thawed FFP and blood (packed red blood cells, PRBCs) are made available for each severely injured patient.
- Give 1:1 ratio of **warmed** FFP:PRBCs.
- Ensure a platelet pool is made available, and give early if the anticipated blood product demand is high. Giving one platelet pool every 4–5 FFP:PRBCs maintains a 1:1:1 optimum ratio.

- Give 15mg/kg of **tranexamic acid** (1g) ASAP, if not already given.
- Give 10mL of 10% calcium chloride every 5U or if ionized calcium <1.0mmol/L, to avoid hypocalcaemia due to citrate in FFP.
- Avoid vasoconstrictors in the early period, and administer blood products until a palpable radial pulse or systolic BP of 90mmHg is achieved. Conscious level is also a good indicator pre-intubation of cerebral perfusion.
- Change from 'shock packs' to type-specific blood ASAP.
- Further haemostatic resuscitation should be guided by the base deficit/ lactate clearance and ROTEM/TEG (initial sample taken on admission). Repeating blood samples intelligently guides an evolving resuscitation.
- If hyperkalaemic, consider 50mL of 50% glucose and 15U of insulin infusion over 20 min to maintain K^+ 3.5–4.5mmol/L (especially important in blast injury and during MHP).
- Administer cryoprecipitate or fibrinogen concentrate, guided by ROTEM/TEG results (maintain **at least** a fibrinogen level of >1.0g/L, and preferably >2.5g/L).

Hypothermia management
- ESSENTIAL to try to achieve a core temperature >36°C.
- Use an oral oesophageal temperature probe.
- Fluid warming is the priority.
- Undermattress heater and forced warm air blankets.
- Head warmer or Gamgee around the head.
- Warm humidified breathing circuit.

Clinical tips
- Avoid crystalloid. If absent radial pulse or systolic BP <90mmHg, give blood products, if available.
- Do not attempt arterial line insertion until systolic BP >90mmHg.
- Use venous blood gas for pH, lactate/base deficit.
- Give recently donated blood (<14d old), if requiring >5U.
- For anaesthesia maintenance, using isoflurane at 0.4–0.6 MAC, with increasing boluses of fentanyl (2–3mg total dose for case), provides simple, CVS-stable anaesthesia, with a degree of vasodilatation to aid the replacement of lost circulating fluid and lactate clearance.
- If pH <7.1, consider tris-hydroxymethyl aminomethane (THAM; avoids intracellular acidosis). Dose in mL of a 0.3M solution (= base deficit × lean mass in kg), or consider sodium bicarbonate.
- For very resistant coagulopathy, consider 100 micrograms/kg of rFVIIa, combined with 1U of cryoprecipitate, 1U of FFP, and 1U of platelets—also known as 'Bastion Glue'.
- Additional platelets may be required in heavy platelet consumers—warn the laboratory early.
- Consider fresh warm whole blood for resistant coagulopathy.
- Although patients initially may be hypocoagulable, they often become progressively hypercoagulable. Veno-thromboprophylaxis should be instigated early when warranted.

- Resuscitation should not be delayed for tests or line insertion.
- Constantly re-evaluate. When bleeding is controlled, slow down the rate of blood and product infusion to avoid fluid-overloading the patient—an important consideration in the presence of blast lung.
- The use of transthoracic echocardiography may be useful in trending the fluid status of the heart chambers during MHP for those trained in its use.

Medical emergency response team

Critical care is a process, not a place. The MERT aims to provide physician-led prehospital care[16] close to the site of injury. This model has been shown to improve outcome.[17]

Team composition

- Senior anaesthetist or emergency physician—clinical lead.
- Emergency nurse.
- Two paramedics.

Role of the medical emergency response team

The MERT aims to improve outcome by making appropriate life-/limb-saving interventions following injury, using the battlefield advanced trauma life support (BATLS) principles. Delivery of the team is usually (but not always) by helicopter. The team delivers advanced airway care (RSI/surgical airway), thoracostomy, thoracotomy, large-bore IV access[18] (e.g. subclavian PAFC introducer/Arrow MAC introducer), administration of warmed blood products[19] (plasma and red blood cells), and other agents in line with a prehospital transfusion algorithm aiming to avoid ACoTS. Triage of soldiers to the most appropriate facility is undertaken, depending on the injuries sustained. While resuscitation follows the paradigm of <C> ABC, the key points for the MERT are:

- Appropriate triage and positioning of patients onto an airframe.
- <C>: control of life-threatening haemorrhage. Pneumatic/manual tourniquets. Pressure into wounds/haemostatic ribbon gauze.
- A: airway—RSI, if indicated.
- B: breathing—thoracostomy post-RSI with IPPV/PEEP.
- C: circulation—large-bore IV/intraosseous/central access. Used for PRBC/FFP administration. All fluids warmed with in-line prehospital fluid warmers. Clam-shell thoracotomy, if required (non-blast, single penetrating chest trauma).
- Hypothermia mitigation: this is achieved with the use of proprietary warming systems, such as Blizzard Heat, and prehospital blood warmers such as Belmont buddy lite.

References

16 Bøtker MT, Bakke SA, Christensen EF (2009). A systematic review of controlled studies: do physicians increase survival with prehospital treatment? *Scand J Trauma Resusc Emerg Med*, **17**, 12.
17 Morrison JJ, Oh J, DuBose JJ, et al. (2013). En-route care capability from point of injury impacts mortality after severe wartime injury. *Ann Surg*, **257**, 330–4.
18 Fyntanidou B, Fortounis K, Amaniti K, et al. (2009). The use of central venous catheters during emergency prehospital care: a 2-year experience. *Eur J Emerg Med*, **16**, 194–8.
19 Dawes RJ, Thomas GOR (2009). Battlefield resuscitation. *Curr Opin Crit Care*, **5**, 527–35.

Drawover anaesthesia: the Triservice anaesthetic apparatus

Drawover anaesthesia uses atmospheric air as the carrier gas for volatile anaesthetic agents supplemented by O_2 (cylinder or concentrator). The UK military version of drawover is the Triservice anaesthetic apparatus (TSAA) (Fig. 38.1). It consists of two 50mL Oxford miniature vaporizers (OMVs) in series connected to the patient via a self-inflating bag. A valve at the patient end ensures no rebreathing. O_2 is added before the vaporizer into

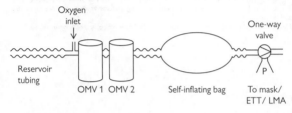

Fig. 38.1 The Triservice anaesthetic apparatus.

an open-ended reservoir tube of at least 500mL. When a ventilator is used, it replaces the inflating bag in the circuit.

Advantages of the Triservice anaesthetic apparatus
- Robust, modular, easy to transport, and simple to use.[20]
- Does not require electricity.
- Low O_2 requirement—typically 1L/min during maintenance, reducing the need to transport O_2 cylinders.
- Hypoxic gas mixture risk eliminated.
- OMV can use different volatile agents.
- Use of end-tidal gas monitoring overcomes the lack of temperature compensation.
- Can be used for SV or manual ventilation.
- Suitable for patients >10kg.[21]

Disadvantages
- Valve at patient end is bulky, especially when connected to attachments allowing scavenging, spirometry, and end-tidal monitoring.
- Not suitable for gaseous induction with sevoflurane.[22]
- Relatively inefficient.
- Vaporizers can be knocked over and spill contents.

Developing countries
- Drawover anaesthesia is commonly practised in resource-poor parts of the world where difficulties with compressed gas supplies and

maintenance occur. In general, the apparatus used in drawover is relatively simple to maintain, offering advantages in rural settings.
- Drawover anaesthesia equipment may be combined with an O_2 concentrator, allowing low-cost O_2 to be reliably produced (assuming electricity is available).
- Conditions of anaesthesia in developing countries differ from military circumstances (well-equipped and highly trained specialists treating severe trauma in well-run units).

References

20 Thompson MC, Restall J (1982). The Triservice anaesthetic apparatus. *Anaesthesia*, **37**, 778–9.
21 Bell GT, McEwen JPJ, Beaton SJ, Young D (2007). Comparison of work of breathing using drawover and continuous flow anaesthetic breathing systems in children. *Anaesthesia*, **62**, 359–63.
22 Mellor A, Hicks I (2005). Sevoflurane delivery via the Triservice apparatus. *Anaesthesia*, **60**, 1151.

Total intravenous anaesthesia: military uses

(See also ➲ p. 984.)

TIVA techniques depend on the overall clinical context of the patient and the type of infusion device available (e.g. TCI pumps or conventional syringe drivers). Secure, dedicated, visible IV access with suitable anti-reflux valves is recommended at all times.

Ketamine

Ketamine-based techniques in trauma, especially in hypovolaemia, are well proven. Concomitant use with propofol may reduce side effects, though emergence phenomena may still occur. Suggested regimes are shown in Fig. 38.2.

Propofol

Propofol–opioid techniques have been reported both in manual and TCI modes. However, haemodynamic compromise will determine the choice of such techniques, and their usefulness in the context of major battle-field trauma is yet to be determined. Manual infusion strategies employing propofol are shown in Figs. 38.3 and 38.4.

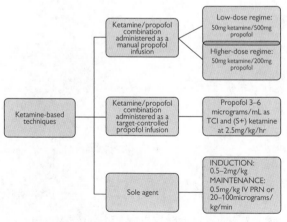

Fig. 38.2 Suggested ketamine regimes.

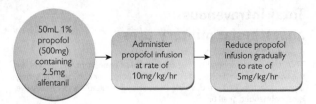

Fig. 38.3 A manual infusion strategy employing propofol and alfentanil.

Further reading

Absalom AR, Struys MMRF (2007). *An overview of TCI & TIVA*, 2nd edn. Ghent: Academia Press.
Cantelo R, Mahoney P (2003). An introduction to field anaesthesia. *Curr Anaesth Crit Care*, **14**, 126–30.

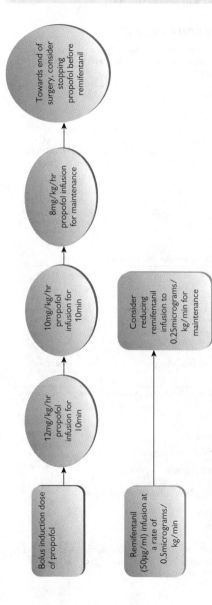

Fig. 38.4 A manual infusion strategy employing propofol and remifentanil concurrently.

Long-term venous access

Cannulae in peripheral veins last for only a few days. For longer-term access, several alternatives exist. Before deciding which to choose, the following should be considered:

• Indication and duration of proposed therapy requiring venous access.
• Proposed location for administration of therapy (hospital, GP/clinic, home).
• Risk of contamination of the catheter.
• Patient's clinical status (coagulation status, sepsis, CVS stability).
• Risk from sclerosant drugs.
• If long-term access is predicted, then it should be performed as soon as possible to reduce patient risks and discomfort from repeated short-term procedures.

The definition of long-term central venous access is not standardized, e.g. predicted use >6wk or presence of internal anchoring devices (Table 38.2). Anaesthetists are well placed to provide a service of inserting and removing such devices.

Table 38.2 Service life of various intravenous access device

Device	Normal duration
Peripheral cannulae	48–72hr
Midlines	14–21d
Non-cuffed, non-tunnelled CVCs	5–14d
Tunnelled, non-cuffed CVCs	5–21d
PICCs	Several months
Tunnelled, cuffed CVCs (Hickman line)	Months/years
SC ports	Months/years

CVC, central venous catheter; PICC, peripherally inserted central catheter; SC, subcutaneous.

Common indications
• Cancer chemotherapy.
• Long-term antibiotics.
• Home total parenteral nutrition.
• Haemodialysis.
• Repeated blood transfusions or repeated venesection.

Venous access devices

Short term
• Peripheral cannulae.
• Midlines (10–20cm soft catheter) are inserted via the antecubital fossa, with the tip of the device situated in the upper 3rd of the basilic or cephalic vein and short of the great vessels.

- Non-cuffed, non-tunnelled CVCs are used for resuscitation/central venous monitoring. Non-tunnelled CVCs are rarely used for >10–14d due to the risk of sepsis. Antimicrobial-coated catheters are available. Use a single-lumen catheter when possible.
- Tunnelled, non-cuffed catheters are used less frequently, as similar cuffed devices offer more secure fixation and a potential antimicrobial barrier.

Long term

- Peripherally inserted central catheters (PICCs) are advanced centrally from the antecubital fossa/upper arm veins. A PICC can last for several months, if managed correctly.
- Tunnelled, cuffed CVCs (Hickman-type lines) are tunnelled from the insertion site on either the chest or abdominal wall. They can be open-ended or contain a two-way valve (Groshong catheter). These are used for prolonged therapies and have a Dacron cuff which allows fibrotic tissue ingrowth to provide anchorage and a possible barrier to infection. It takes 3–4wk for fibrous adhesions to develop, and hence they should not be inserted for shorter-term use. Similar devices exist for dialysis (e.g. Tesio).
- SC ports made from either titanium or plastic offer a single or double injection port attached to a central catheter.
- A SC pocket is formed on the chest or abdominal wall to house the port. They are surgically placed and used for prolonged periods of intermittent therapy, e.g. antibiotics for CF. They are popular for children and enable bathing and immersion.

Site of access

- Anecdotal evidence suggests that catheters placed from the right side of the body have lesser risk of thrombosis due to a shorter, straighter route to the SVC. Easiest tip positioning is via the right internal jugular vein.
- Choose site dependent on patient factors, previous access, and clinician experience (Table 38.3).
- Look for evidence of thrombosis or stenosis, previous scars from long-term access, and venous collaterals (suggest great vein stenosis).
- Use ultrasound to assess the access site and guide needle puncture at all sites. Formal venography is helpful in difficult cases.

Ultrasound guidance

- Earlier UK NICE guidance was restricted to adult jugular veins; it is now recommended routinely for all sites and ages.
- Appropriate training required.
- Very useful in context of difficult/repeated long-term venous access.
- For subclavian access, move just lateral to the clavicle to allow visualization of the axillary vein with ultrasound.
- Note a patent vein at the access site does not guarantee central vein patency.
- Respiratory variation in the vein size suggests a patent central vein.

Table 38.3 Sites of central venous access

Site	Advantages	Disadvantages
Arm (cephalic/ basilic veins)	Simple to access—veins usually visible and palpable at elbow Fewer vital structures nearby. For patient comfort, use upper arm veins (if ultrasound-visible)	Failure to achieve central position. Higher incidence of thrombosis. Low infusion rates. Avoid elbow flexure, if possible
Right internal jugular	Simple to insert. Direct route to central veins. High flow rate—low risk of thrombosis. Lower risk of pneumothorax. Ideal for larger stiff catheters, e.g. dialysis	Patient discomfort. Possible higher risk of infection. Tunnelling more difficult to chest wall. Cosmetic considerations
Subclavian/ axillary	Less patient discomfort. Possibly lower risk of infection. Easy tunnelling	Curved insertion route. Thrombosis risk (swollen arm). Acute complications—pneumothorax, haemothorax, nerve damage. Catheter may be damaged between clavicle and 1st rib
Femoral	Tunnel to mid abdomen	High rate of infection/risk of thrombosis. More discomfort

Practical tips for insertion

Relevant to all devices

- Consider cosmetic and patient preferences for vein entry and exit sites.
- Ask patient to take a deep breath to facilitate central passage of guide-wire/catheter.
- Use a Terumo-type nitinol guide-wire and/or an angled catheter to access central veins around tight angles.
- Measure the catheter length required with a correctly positioned guide-wire (using fluoroscopy), or lay on the chest wall with the tip over the right side of the sternal angle.
- Approximate lengths for adults: right internal jugular vein 15cm, right axillary/subclavian 20cm, left internal jugular vein 20cm, left axillary/ subclavian 24cm.
- Take care with rigid sheaths and dilators to avoid central vessel damage. Do not insert too deeply (they are generally longer than required).
- Pinch the sheath on removal of the obturator to avoid bleeding and air embolism (some are valved).
- Sheaths readily kink—draw back until the catheter passes.
- Pass a long, thin guide-wire (70cm+, Terumo-coated type) through soft catheters to increase the torque if difficulties passing centrally.
- Screen the guide-wire, obturator sheath, and catheter insertion if any difficulty encountered. Use venography through needle, 4Fr sheath, or

catheter if uncertain as to position, e.g. 10mL of diluted contrast (check allergy), e.g. Ultravist 240® diluted 50:50 with 0.9% sodium chloride.
- Flush with saline/heparinized saline before and after use.
- Image the tunnelled section of the line to look for kinks.
- Do not accept poor central tip positions.

Peripherally inserted central catheters
- Use ultrasound guidance to allow puncture of the basilic or brachial veins in the upper arm above the elbow flexure. Cephalic vein less used due to smaller size and tortuous course on entry to the axillary vein.
- Use higher-resolution ultrasound to visualize and avoid the brachial artery, median nerve, and cutaneous nerves of forearm (around the basilic vein).
- Measure the projected length of the catheter from the puncture site to the right 3rd intercostal place, or, if using screening, insert the device to the optimal position, measure the external length, then remove and cut to length. Stop bleeding through the sheath by reinsertion of the dilator with a bung.

Tunnelled catheters
- Dissect the tunnel pockets further to straighten any kinks in the catheter.
- For fixed-length catheters (e.g. Groshong, dialysis), take care to choose the correct length for the site of access and an adequate length of tunnel tract to ensure correct tip position in the SVC.
- Move the catheter and cuff along the tunnel tract to adjust the catheter tip position.
- Choose puncture sites and tunnel tract to avoid tight bends; if necessary, use multiple puncture sites to avoid >90° bends and catheter kinks.
- Buried sutures can be inserted around the tunnelling rod, and hence the catheter, to trap the cuff.

Ports
- Ports can be inserted percutaneously under LA ± sedation or under GA. Smaller low-profile versions can be sited in the arm.
- Minimize the incision and pocket size by placing port anchor sutures within the pocket first, and then slide the port in over them and tie off.
- Access is gained by a specific 'non-coring' needle pushed through the silicone membrane to the reservoir below. Initial access to a port causes discomfort, and EMLA® cream can be applied 30min before. There is a distinct clunk as the needle hits the back wall of the port after penetrating the membrane.
- Leave the access needle *in situ*, if access required soon after insertion, to avoid a painful wound site (settles after a few days).
- Use buried subcuticular suture, Langer's lines (squeeze the skin), and lateral wounds for optimal cosmetic result.

Catheter tip position
This is important to reduce risks of thrombosis (with link to infection), catheter perforation into the pericardium, pleura, or mediastinum, and

migration with risk of extravasation injury. Optimal positioning is most consistently achieved with real-time fluoroscopy or serial X-rays.

- Tip should ideally lie in the SVC, in the long axis of the vein, i.e. not abutting the vein at an acute angle.
- It is traditionally recommended that the tip should lie above the pericardial reflection (to avoid perforation and tamponade). The carina can be used as a radiological landmark to define the approximate upper border of the pericardium.
- It may not be possible to get an adequate catheter tip position above the carina in catheters from the left side (left internal jugular or subclavian) or the right subclavian due to the angulation of the distal catheter segment. Aim to have the last 3–6cm of the catheter tip in the long axis of the SVC (this will approximate to the junction of SVC/right atrium or upper right atrium in such cases).
- ECG guidance may be used to confirm the central position but does not ensure a good tip position in the SVC (may be angled against the vein wall), particularly with left-sided catheters.
- Catheter tip may move between lying and sitting/standing. Assess on inspiration and expiration, with the patient table flat. It will generally appear much further centrally on supine/head-down imaging than on an erect PA film with deep inspiration.

Aftercare

It is essential that staff using such catheters have adequate training in use and use maximum sterile precautions at all times.

- Do not remove anchoring sutures for at least 3wk to allow the Dacron cuff to become adherent. Many centres use statlock-type adhesive anchors.
- When used in patients at high risk of thromboembolism, therapeutic doses of warfarin or LMWH may reduce the frequency of catheter-related thrombosis.
- Beware: some units still lock catheters with strong heparin (e.g. dialysis catheters)—always aspirate the catheter, and discard before use.
- Fibrin sleeves or thrombosed catheters can be unblocked with urokinase (5000U) or other thrombolytics. If totally blocked: suction all air through a three-way tap to collapse the catheter and create a vacuum. Then inject urokinase diluted in 2mL of saline, and repeat the sequence to get fluid into the catheter. Leave the drug *in situ* for some hours. Avoid excess syringe pressure that can rupture the catheter.

Removing a Hickman line

- Cuffed catheters usually pull out if *in situ* <3wk—before fibrous adhesions have anchored the cuff. Note: some operators insert internal cuff anchoring sutures.
- Heavily infected catheters usually pull out, as the infection breaks down adhesions.
- Push and pull the catheter to palpate the cuff shape and tethering. It is difficult to feel the cuff if it is just inside the exit site.
- Inject generous LA around the cuff site and tunnel tract.

- Cut down (1–1.5cm incision sufficient) just to the vein side of the cuff. Use forceps to feel the catheter as a solid structure that rolls under the forceps (incision too small for finger). Free up and remove the venous section first; a thin fibrin sheath/capsule will need to be incised to free the catheter. Pull the catheter out of the vein.
- Then dissect around the cuff to free adhesions.
- Try to avoid sharp dissection, until the venous section of catheter is removed, to reduce the risk of embolization from the cut catheter (catheters can pass to the RV/PA).
- Similar considerations apply to port removals where the port and catheter are encased in a tough fibrous sheath. Incise through the old scar.

Particular complications of long-term access

- **Catheter-related infection**. This is common and may be at the exit site, tunnel tract, or hidden internally. Some external infections can be managed with antibiotics—seek advice. Many such catheters are managed without dressings in the longer term. There is little evidence for the use of antiseptic dressing or devices for long-term catheters.
- **Catheter blockage**. Catheters can rupture between the clavicle and 1st rib (pinch off) or become thrombosed. External damage is common.
- **Fibrin sleeve** formation commonly obstructs the aspiration of blood but still allows injection of fluids.
- **Venous thrombosis** may require catheter removal and typically full anticoagulation.
- **Vein stenosis** and venous collateral formation are often asymptomatic due to gradual obstruction. Can be reopened by radiological stenting.

Use of devices in anaesthesia and critical care

- Long-term venous access devices can be used in the critical care setting if appropriate asepsis is maintained. Balance the risk/benefits of siting a new short-term CVC (e.g. coagulopathy).
- Valved catheters (Groschong) or those with a fibrin sleeve covering the tip may not give a CVP waveform and may cause intermittent drug bolusing during infusion (avoid for vasoactive drugs).
- Ports and other catheters are good options for a child requiring repeated IV anaesthetic induction.
- PICCs are increasingly used in the convalescent phases of critical care.
- Look out for these devices to give rapid access in the resuscitation situation.

Further reading

Galloway S, Bodenham AR (2003). Safe removal of long term cuffed Hickman type catheters. *Hosp Med*, **64**, 20–3.
Hudman L, Bodenham AR (2013). Practical aspects of long-term venous access. *Contin Educ Anaesth Crit Care Pain*, **13**, 6–11.
Lamperti M, Bodenham AR, Pittiruti M, *et al.* (2012). International evidence-based recommendations on ultrasound-guided vascular access. *Intensive Care Med*, **38**, 1105–17.
O'Leary R, Ahmed SM, McLure H, *et al.* (2012) Ultrasound-guided infraclavicular axillary vein cannulation: a useful alternative to the internal jugular vein. *Br J Anaesth*, **109**, 762–8.
Stonelake PA, Bodenham AR (2006). The carina as a radiological landmark for central venous catheter tip position. *Br J Anaesth*, **96**, 335–40.

Cardiac output monitoring

Enhanced recovery and fluid optimization

- Enhanced recovery is an evidence-based approach with the intention of helping patients recover faster from surgery. It involves a selected number of individual interventions, which, when implemented as a group, demonstrate a greater impact on outcome than when implemented as individual interventions.[23]
- Optimizing the stroke volume using goal-directed fluid therapy is only one of the 14 parts of the enhanced recovery framework, but it has been shown to be of benefit in several different patient groups.
- Delivering the right type of fluid at the right time in the right quantities is paramount to these principles.[24]
- Optimizing the stroke volume allows an adequate tissue O_2 delivery. This is achieved through a mixture of fluid administration and occasionally inotropic support.

Preoperative
- Good preoperative hydration.
- Carbohydrate drinks up to 2hr prior to surgery.
- Avoidance of bowel preparations.

Intra-operative
- Fluid management technologies to deliver individualized goal-directed fluid therapy, targeting the optimum stroke volume.

Post-operative
- Avoid the use of IV fluids where oral hydration can be administered.
- Use of isotonic IV electrolyte solutions where necessary.
- Early eating and drinking.

Use of fluid management technology is recommended for

- Major surgery, with a 30d mortality rate of >1%.
- Major surgery with anticipated blood loss of >500mL.
- Major intra-abdominal surgery.
- Intermediate surgery in high-risk patients.
- Unexpected blood loss requiring >2000mL of fluid replacement.
- Patients with evidence of ongoing hypovolaemia or tissue hypoperfusion (e.g. persistent lactic acidosis).

Cardiac output monitors

Invasive, minimally invasive, and non-invasive technologies are available to measure the cardiac output. Algorithms within these 'black boxes' can be calibrated or non-calibrated, and the parameters displayed can be directly measured or derived. All of these systems have their flaws, and none has been shown to be superior to the others.

Invasive cardiac output device—pulmonary artery catheters

- Regarded as the gold standard for measuring the cardiac output against which new devices are often measured.
- Cardiac output calculated by intermittent PA thermodilution technique.
- Reliability influenced by: mitral and tricuspid incompetence, shunt, and misplacement of the catheter tip.
- Additional measured parameters include: CVP, PAP, and mixed venous saturations.
- Use has declined due to the availability of new technologies, potential for rare, but life-threatening, complications, and lack of evidence.[25]

Minimally invasive cardiac output monitors

These devices fall into the following subtypes: pulse contour analysis, Doppler technology, applied Fick principle, and bioimpedance/reactance technologies.

Pulse contour analysis

Stroke volume is continuously estimated from the arterial pressure waveform obtained from an arterial line. The arterial waveform is not only affected by the stroke volume, but also vascular compliance, aortic impedance, and peripheral arterial resistance. Accuracy is dependent on the consistency of the waveform, arrhythmias, rapid changes in haemodynamic stability, and changes in intrathoracic pressure. Calibrated systems are more accurate and resistant to changes in haemodynamic stability but require recalibration regularly for accurate cardiac output measurements.

- PICCO*plus*™ (Pulsion Medical Systems):
  - Thermistor-tipped arterial catheter in the brachial or femoral artery to measure the arterial waveform. CVC for transpulmonary thermodilution calibration. Uses integration of the area under arterial pressure against the time curve to determine the cardiac output.
- LiDCO*plus*™ (LiDCO™):
  - Requires an arterial line and peripheral venous cannula, and utilizes the concept of the conservation of power within a system to derive cardiac output measurements. Measures pulse power, rather than pulse contour, and requires calibration using transpulmonary lithium indicator dilution. Reliability may be affected by interaction between lithium and high peak doses of muscle relaxants. LiDCO*rapid*™ is the uncalibrated LiDCO™ device.
- FloTrac™/EV1000™ (Edwards Lifesciences):
  - A FloTrac transducer is attached to an arterial catheter, which connects to the calibrated EV1000 monitor. Uses transpulmonary thermodilution to calibrate the sensor. The Vigileo™ monitor is the uncalibrated alternative for use with the FloTrac™.
- PulsioFlex™ (PULSION Medical Systems):
  - Uncalibrated pulse contour analysis device.
- Nexfin™ (Finapress Medical Systems):
  - Uncalibrated, non-invasive technology utilizing photoelectric plethysmography and a finger volume clamp to calculate pulse pressure.

Doppler technology

Oesophageal, transthoracic, and suprasternal Doppler probes are available as minimally invasive cardiac output monitoring devices. The oesophageal Doppler measures the flow in the descending aorta and multiplies the velocity by the estimated cross-sectional aortic area to calculate the cardiac output. Aortic diameter is estimated from a normogram. The most commonly used monitor is the Cardio-Q (Datex Medical). Limitations include: assumption that a fixed proportion of the cardiac output flows cephalad, probe positioning can be difficult, and the aortic diameter is dynamic.

Applied Fick principle

The Fick principle can be used in the intubated, sedated, and mechanically ventilated patient (NICO™, Philips Respironics). A rebreathing loop attached to the ventilator circuit allows rebreathing of CO_2, which is measured by an infrared sensor, along with airflow. $ETCO_2$ is used as a surrogate for arterial CO_2. CO_2 production is measured alone, and volume is calculated. At steady state, the amount of CO_2 entering the lungs via the PA is proportional to the cardiac output and equals the amount of CO_2 exiting via the pulmonary veins and the lungs. During 30s of rebreathing, the amount of CO_2 eliminated by expiration decreases, and $ETCO_2$ increases in proportion to the cardiac output, assuming the cardiac output does not change during rebreathing.

Bioimpedance/bioreactance

Cyclical changes in blood flow within the body induce changes in impedance and reactance to electrical current. Skin electrodes measure the electrical resistance of the thorax to a high-frequency, very low-magnitude current. Impedance to the current is proportional to the cardiac output. Newer technologies utilize reactance, rather than impedance.

Derived haemodynamic variables

These cardiac output monitoring technologies can be used to generate static measurements in the calibrated systems, treating the numbers accordingly. Alternatively, the uncalibrated systems can be used to show the trends of dynamic variables and the absolute values before and after fluid bolus administration. In this way, they are used to assess fluid responsiveness.

Commonly used dynamic variables

- Stroke volume variation (SVV) and pulse pressure variation (PPV) are functional haemodynamic variables available on many systems. Changes in intrathoracic pressure due to positive pressure ventilation induce changes in the stroke volume and pulse pressure as a result of a reduction in the preload. The greater the change in stroke volume or pressure, the greater the likelihood that the patient is intravascularly deplete. The reliability of these variables is adversely affected by arrhythmias, right heart failure, spontaneous breathing, and V_T <8mL/kg. Normal range for SVV and PPV is <10%.
- Corrected flow time (FTc) is the time blood is flowing in the aorta, corrected to an HR of 60bpm. Values are proposed to be in proportion to the LV end-diastolic volume or preload. Low values are indicative of hypovolaemia if inotropy is constant. Normal range is 330–360ms.

Targeting stroke volume—goal-directed fluid therapy

- When trying to optimize stroke volume, fluid is usually administered in boluses against a formalized protocol.
- Fluid is administered quickly, over 5min, in volumes of around 3mL/kg (200–250mL)
- Stroke volume is measured before and after fluid boluses.
- An improvement of >10% in stroke volume would suggest that the patient has moved up the Starling curve, and contractility has improved with an increase in end-diastolic volume. A further fluid bolus may improve the stroke volume further. Whether moving the patient further up the Starling curve is desirable or not is debatable, and there are some operations (thoracic/pancreatic/hepatic) where this algorithm may not be appropriate.
- No change or a reduction in stroke volume implies that the patient is at the top, or over the top, of the Starling curve, and further fluid administration would be disadvantageous.

References

23 Enhanced Recovery Partnership Programme (2010). *Delivering enhanced recovery: helping patients to get better sooner after surgery.* ℵ http://webarchive.nationalarchives.gov.uk/20130107105354/http://www.dh.gov.uk/prod_consum_dh/groups/dh_digitalassets/@dh/@en/@ps/documents/digitalasset/dh_115156.pdf.

24 Pearse RM, Ackland GL (2012). Perioperative fluid therapy. *BMJ*, **344**, e2865.

25 Harvey S, Harrison DA, Singer M, et al. (2005). Assessment of the clinical effectiveness of pulmonary artery catheters in management of patients in intensive care (PAC-Man): a randomised controlled trial. *Lancet*, **366**, 472–7.

Further reading

BAPEN (2011). *British consensus guidelines on intravenous fluid therapy for adult surgical patients (GIFTASUP)*. ℵ http://www.bapen.org.uk/pdfs/bapen_pubs/giftasup.pdf.

National Confidential Enquiry into Patient Outcome and Death (2011). *Knowing the risk. A review of the peri-operative care of surgical patients.* ℵ http://www.ncepod.org.uk/2011report2/downloads/POC_fullreport.pdf.

National Institute for Health and Care Excellence (2011). *CardioQ-ODM oesophageal Doppler monitor. NICE medical technology guidance (MTG3)*. ℵ http://www.nice.org.uk/guidance/MTG3.

Depth of anaesthesia monitoring

Patients expect that, while under GA, they will have no awareness of the surgery itself. The failure of this state of drug-induced loss of consciousness is termed awareness.

Awareness

Initial reports from the National Audit Project 5 (NAP 5) suggest that the incidence of awareness, with explicit recall, in the UK is around 1:15 000;[26] this is much lower than the previously reported 1:3000.[27] The incidence of implicit recall is higher and has been reported as 1:1421:1000.[27,28] Both types may lead to post-traumatic stress disorder. Types of awareness include:

• Explicit recall—spontaneously or provoked memory
• Implicit recall—not consciously recalled but may affect behaviour.

Awareness results from the failure to deliver enough anaesthetic agent to maintain loss of consciousness. Failure of anaesthetic delivery may be due to equipment failure or administration of less anaesthetic agent than required, either intentionally or unintentionally.[29] Many incidents of awareness can be prevented by careful technique and checking of equipment. In an ideal situation, anaesthetists could monitor the conscious level. Technology to do this reliably has proved difficult to develop, and, at present, the depth of anaesthesia is determined in the following ways.

Clinical parameters

Notoriously unreliable, HR, BP, pupil size, sweating, etc. rely on the sympathetic nervous system and can be profoundly affected by factors such as hypovolaemia, arrhythmias, preoperative drug therapy (β-blockers, antihypertensive agents), and epidural/subarachnoid block.

Monitoring anaesthetic gas concentrations

End-tidal anaesthetic agent monitoring provides the most precise estimate of brain anaesthetic agent concentration currently available, provided time is allowed for alveolar/blood/brain equilibration. MAC is normally distributed and has low biological variability (Table 38.4).

Variants of MAC

• MAC: the minimum alveolar concentration of anaesthetic at 1 atmosphere pressure producing immobility in 50% of subjects exposed to a standard noxious stimulus.
• MAC_{awake}: the minimum alveolar concentration of anaesthetic producing unconsciousness in 50% of subjects.
• MAC_{bar}: the minimum alveolar concentration of anaesthetic blocking the sympathetic nervous system response to a painful stimulus in 50% of subjects.

Table 38.4 Factors affecting MAC

Factors increasing MAC	Factors decreasing MAC
Hyperthermia	Increasing age
Hyperthyroidism	Hypothermia
Alcoholism	Hypoxia
	CNS depressants
	N_2O and other volatile agents
	α_2-agonists

MAC is decreased by hypothermia, hypoxia, acidosis, and CNS depressant drugs, and declines by 6% per decade after 1yr of age. Age-related MAC can be represented by iso-MAC charts, which calculate age-appropriate end-tidal volatile concentrations in various N_2O concentrations (see ➔ p. 1209). They may be useful in preventing awareness and also excessive administration of volatile agent in the elderly. Opioids reduce MAC, particularly MAC_{bar}; however, they are not anaesthetic themselves. It is therefore essential to administer enough volatile agent to prevent awareness (> MAC_{awake}), even when painful surgical stimuli are blocked by high doses of opioids or regional anaesthesia. Using an alarm and aiming to maintain 0.7 MAC of an inhaled anaesthetic prevents awareness as effectively as the use of a BIS monitor.[30]

Isolated forearm technique

A tourniquet is applied to the upper arm and inflated above systolic BP before muscle relaxation. Spontaneous movements or hand squeezing on command indicate impending or actual awareness. Not all patients who respond have explicit recall post-operatively, i.e. it is possible to have intra-operative awareness without recall. This technique is mainly used as a research tool.

Predicting anaesthetic drug concentrations

TIVA/TCI systems using pharmacokinetic models to estimate the arterial propofol concentration are widely used (see also ➔ p. 1007 and p. 984). There is moderate correlation between estimated and measured propofol concentrations for individual patients, and some interpatient variability in pharmacodynamic response. There is no equivalent of continuous end-tidal anaesthetic concentration measurement. Secure IV infusion is essential when IV agents are used to maintain hypnosis.

Electronic brain monitoring

Measurement of brain activity by standard EEG is impractical and time-consuming. There are two main types of modern depth of anaesthesia monitor using frontal electrodes now widely available: EEG-based and evoked potential-based. A change in either spontaneous cortical electrical activity or stimulus-evoked electrical activity is converted to an index of

Table 38.5 Bispectral index values and level of consciousness

Bispectral index values	Level of consciousness
100	Awake
65–85	Sedation
45–65	General anaesthesia
<40	Burst suppression
0	No electrical activity

depth of anaesthesia. The monitors then represent the depth of anaesthesia as a number between 100 (fully awake) and 0 (no electrical activity).

- *BIS* (Covidien, MA). Uses bifrontal electrodes; combined frequency information and phase relationships of the EEG's component sine waves, with pattern recognition of profound drug effect (burst suppression). BIS corresponds linearly to the hypnotic state (Table 38.5) and is agent-independent; however, the effects of N_2O, ketamine, and xenon are not well characterized by BIS. When using BIS to titrate IV and volatile anaesthesia, there is a modest reduction in anaesthetic usage and slightly faster emergence; however, this may encourage 'lighter' anaesthesia. Evidence that BIS monitoring reduces awareness is limited. The B-Aware study of 'high-risk' patients[29] had two reports of awareness in the BIS-guided group, and 11 reports in the routine care group (p = 0.022) of 2463 high-risk patients.
- *Narcotrend* (MT MonitorTechnik GmbH, Germany). Uses power spectral analysis and pattern recognition algorithms to classify the EEG into stages A to F.
- *M-Entropy* (GE Healthcare, UK). Entropy is a state of disorder. As anaesthesia deepens, there is an increase in regularity to the EEG, and disorder decreases. This change on EEG 'entropy' is displayed as an index on the monitor. Also displayed is an index of the frontalis EMG which also reduces as depth of anaesthesia increases. The EEG is referred to as 'state entropy', and the EMG as 'response entropy'.
- *Auditory evoked responses (AEPs)—aepEX* (Medical Device Management, UK). Early cortical EEG responses to auditory stimuli administered at 6–10Hz via headphones. As anaesthesia deepens, latency of the characteristic AEP waveform increases, and the amplitude of the wave decreases. Correlates with awake to asleep transition but predicts movement poorly. An index of 0–100 is displayed on the monitor.

Depth of anaesthesia monitors are credible adjuncts to patient care and are recommended as options by NICE[31] for patients receiving TIVA and patients at higher risk of adverse outcomes under GA.

Avoiding awareness

- Premedication with benzodiazepines or at induction reduces the incidence of awareness.
- Adequate doses of anaesthetic agents with a MAC of inhaled anaesthetic agents of 0.8–1.0

- Neuromuscular-blocking agents increase the risk of awareness so should be used only when necessary.
- Depth of anaesthesia monitoring may be useful in high-risk situations (Caesarean section, emergency surgery, surgery associated with large blood loss, and patients with previous history of awareness).[30]

What to do if a patient reports an episode of awareness

Complaints of awareness must be pursued promptly. It is important to confirm what the patient may have heard or felt and document this accurately. An explanation of the events and causes, if any, should be given to the patient and documented. The patient needs reassurance that steps can be taken to reduce the risk of awareness during subsequent anaesthetics. Post-traumatic stress disorder can develop, and it is important that these patients are offered counselling and given details of support groups that may be helpful.

Litigation following episodes of awareness is often successful, and poor anaesthetic technique is often blamed. Defence against these claims requires that the anaesthetist has made thorough records. It is advisable that routine documentation includes start and end time of surgery, timing and dosages of anaesthetic agents, and exhaled concentrations or plasma/effect site concentrations.[32]

References

26 Avidan MS, Mashour GA (2013). The incidence of intraoperative awareness in the UK: under the rate or under the radar? *Br J Anaesth*, **110**, 494–7.
27 Schwender D, Klasing S, Daunderer M, Madler C, Poppel E, Peter K (1995). Awareness during general anesthesia. Definition, incidence, clinical relevance, causes, avoidance and medicolegal aspects. *Anaesthesist*, **44**, 743–54.
28 Sandin RH, Enlund G, Samuelsson P, Lennmarken C (2000). Awareness during anaesthesia: a prospective case study. *Lancet*, **355**, 707–11.
29 Goddard N, Smith D (2013). Unintended awareness and monitoring of depth of anaesthesia. *Contin Educ Anaesth Crit Care Pain*, **13**, 213–17.
30 Avidan MS, Zhang L, Burnside BA, *et al*. (2008). Anaesthesia awareness and the bispectral index. *N Engl J Med*, **358**, 1097–108.
31 National Institute for Health and Care Excellence (2015). *Ensuring people with autism get the best treatment and care*. ℘ http://www.nice.org.uk/newsroom/pressreleases/DepthOfAnaesthesia MonitorsGuidance.jsp.
32 Hardman JG, Aitkenhead AR (2005). Awareness during anaesthesia. *Contin Educ Anaesth Crit Care Pain*, **5**, 183–6.

Neuromuscular blockers: reversal and monitoring

Suxamethonium

- The only depolarizing relaxant in clinical use.
- Has the most rapid onset of action of all relaxants.
- Used when a fast onset and brief duration of paralysis are required.
- A dose of 1–1.5mg/kg is recommended.
- Metabolized by plasma cholinesterase (see below).

Unwanted effects of suxamethonium

- Post-operative muscle pains: commoner in young muscular adults, and most effectively reduced by precurarization—the prior use of a small dose of a non-depolarizing relaxant, e.g. atracurium (5mg). A larger dose of suxamethonium (1.5mg/kg) is then required.
- Raised intraocular pressure: this is of no clinical significance in most patients but may be important in poorly controlled glaucoma or penetrating eye injuries (see ➲ p. 681).
- Hyperkalaemia: serum K$^+$ increases by 0.5mmol/L in normal individuals. This may be significant with pre-existing elevated serum K$^+$. Patients with burns or certain neurological conditions, e.g. paraplegia, muscular dystrophy, and dystrophia myotonica, may develop severe hyperkalaemia following administration. Patients who have sustained significant burns or spinal cord injuries can be given suxamethonium, if necessary, within the first 48hr following injury. Thereafter, there is an increasing risk of life-threatening hyperkalaemia, which reduces over the ensuing months. Avoid suxamethonium until 12 months have elapsed following a burns injury. There may be a permanent risk of hyperkalaemia with upper motor neuron lesions.
- Bradycardias, particularly in children or if repeated doses of the drug are given. Can be prevented or treated with antimuscarinic agents, e.g. atropine and glycopyrronium.
- MH (see ➲ p. 255 and p. 918): suxamethonium is a potent trigger for this condition in predisposed individuals.
- High or repeated doses (probably >8mg/kg) may create dual block which will prolong paralysis.

Cholinesterase

This enzyme occurs in two forms:

- Acetylcholinesterase (true cholinesterase): highly specific for acetylcholine
- Plasma cholinesterase (pseudocholinesterase or butyrylcholinesterase): capable of hydrolysing a variety of esters. A physiological function for this enzyme has yet to be discovered, but many drugs either interfere with its action or are metabolized by it. Plasma cholinesterase is synthesized in the liver, has a half-life of 5–12d, and metabolizes 70% of a 100mg bolus of suxamethonium within 1min. Genetically, it is encoded on the long arm of chromosome 3. Several variant genes can occur which result in reduced enzyme activity:
  - *The atypical gene.* Heterozygotes will not be sensitive to suxamethonium, unless other contributing factors (e.g. concurrent

illness, anticholinesterase administration) are present. Homozygotes have a prevalence of ~1:3000 and may remain paralysed for 2–3hr

- *The fluoride-resistant gene.* Homozygotes are much rarer (1:150 000) and are moderately sensitive to suxamethonium
- *The silent gene.* Heterozygotes would exhibit a prolongation of the action of suxamethonium, but homozygotes (1:10 000) are very sensitive and develop prolonged apnoea—usually 3–4hr but may last as long as 24hr
- Other variants (e.g. H-, J-, and K-type) also exist. Variant genes thus produce a spectrum of reduced activity of the enzyme, causing mild prolongation of the action of suxamethonium through to several hours of paralysis
- The activity of plasma cholinesterase can be measured by adding plasma to benzoylcholine and following the reaction spectrophotometrically. Abnormally low values can be further investigated for phenotype by carrying out the reaction in the presence of certain inhibitors such as cinchocaine (dibucaine), sodium fluoride, and a specific inhibitor known as Ro2–0683.

Reduced plasma cholinesterase activity can also occur for acquired reasons. This can occur in the following situations:

- Hepatic disease, renal disease, burns, malignancy, and malnutrition.
- Administration of drugs that share the same metabolic pathway, and therefore compete with suxamethonium for the enzyme, e.g. esmolol, MAOIs, methotrexate.
- Presence of anticholinesterases (e.g. edrophonium, neostigmine, ecothiopate eye drops), which inhibit plasma cholinesterase as well as acetylcholinesterase.
- Pregnancy where the enzyme activity is reduced by 25%.
- Plasmapheresis and CPB.

Many other drugs are metabolized by plasma cholinesterase. Individuals deficient in the enzyme may develop complications with:

- **Mivacurium**: muscle paralysis will be prolonged.
- **Cocaine**: toxicity is more likely.

Plasma cholinesterase also partially metabolizes diamorphine, esmolol, and remifentanil. Low enzyme activity does not currently appear to complicate their use.

Non-depolarizing agents

NDMRs are highly ionized, with a relatively small volume of distribution. Structurally, they are either benzylisoquinoliniums (e.g. atracurium and mivacurium) or aminosteroids (e.g. vecuronium and rocuronium). They can also be classified according to their duration of action:

- Short-acting compounds with a duration of action of up to 15min (mivacurium).
- Medium-acting compounds which are effective for ~40min (atracurium, vecuronium, rocuronium, cisatracurium).
- Long-acting compounds which have a clinical effect for 60min (pancuronium, d-tubocurarine).

Volatile agents prolong the duration of action of NDMRs. Other drugs may do the same, including aminoglycoside antibiotics, calcium channel blockers, lithium, and magnesium. NMB may also be prolonged by acidosis, hypokalaemia, hypocalcaemia, and hypothermia.

Choice of relaxant

Choice is based on individual preference, the length of procedure, and certain patient characteristics.

- **Suxamethonium** is the drug of choice for RSI.
- Many of the benzylisoquinoliniums release histamine, the amount of histamine released being related to the speed of injection. Avoid these drugs in severely atopic or asthmatic individuals. **Cisatracurium**, however, does not cause histamine release.
- Like suxamethonium, **mivacurium** is metabolized by plasma cholinesterase. Patients with reduced levels of this enzyme will exhibit prolonged paralysis.
- **Cisatracurium and atracurium** are mainly broken down by Hoffman degradation, a process that is pH- and temperature-dependent. This metabolism is not affected by the presence of renal failure, so these relaxants are ideal in those with renal impairment.
- **Rocuronium**, at doses of 0.6mg/kg or greater, gives satisfactory intubating conditions within 60s. Its speed of onset is significantly faster than all other non-depolarizing relaxants.
- **Mivacurium** is useful for short procedures. It does not need to be reversed routinely, provided sufficient time has elapsed (>20min) after a bolus and neuromuscular monitoring is used.

Practical tips when using relaxants

- Calculate dose requirements on lean body mass. NDMRs are highly ionized and do not penetrate well into vessel-poor fat areas.
- Monitor relaxants routinely. This will help you decide when to top up, when to reverse, and when muscle function has returned.
- Maintenance doses of NDMRs should be about a fifth to a quarter of the initial dose.
- Anticipate relaxant drugs wearing off, rather than waiting for the patient to cough or move.
- Do not attempt to reverse intermediate-duration NDMRs within 15min of administration.
- Do not wait for suxamethonium to wear off before giving an NDMR. On the very rare occasion that a patient has reduced cholinesterase levels, administering an NDMR will make little difference to the outcome.

Neuromuscular monitoring

PNSs allow the degree of NMB to be assessed. They should apply a supramaximal stimulus (strong enough to depolarize all axons) to a peripheral nerve, using a current of 30–80mA. Several peripheral nerves are suitable:

- Ulnar nerve. Electrodes are placed on the medial aspect of the wrist, proximal to the hypothenar eminence. Adductor pollicis muscle contraction is assessed.

- Common peroneal nerve. Stimulated immediately below the head of the fibula. Foot dorsiflexion is assessed.
- Facial nerve. Stimulated with electrodes placed in front of the hairline on the temple.

Modes of stimulation

(See Fig. 38.5.)

- **Train-of-four (TOF).** Four supramaximal stimuli are applied over 2s. If NDMR block is profound, no response will be elicited. As neuromuscular function starts to return, the 1st twitch reappears, followed by the 2nd, 3rd, and finally 4th. The number of twitches elicited is known as the *TOF count*. Fade (successive twitches reducing in amplitude) is a characteristic of partial non-depolarizing block. The train-of-four ratio (TOFR) is the ratio of amplitude of the 4th to the 1st response. Fully reversed patients have no fade and TOFRs of 1. Fade is difficult to assess clinically (visually or by tactile means), once the TOFR has reached 0.4.
- **Double-burst stimulation (DBS)** is a stronger stimulus where two short bursts of 50Hz tetanus are separated by 750ms. DBS and TOFRs correlate well, but fade is more accurately assessed with DBS, and an absence of fade is usually good evidence of reversal.
- **Post-tetanic count** can be used to assess deep relaxation when the TOF is zero. A 50Hz tetanic stimulation is applied for 5s, followed by 1Hz single twitches. Reversal should be possible at a post-tetanic count of 10 or greater.

These patterns of stimulation are usually assessed by visual or tactile means but can be assessed more objectively using mechanomyography, EMG, or accelerometry.

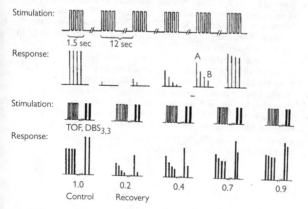

Fig. 38.5 Responses to TOF and DBS in non-depolarizing blockade.

It is preferable to assess the effect of stimulation before muscle relaxants are administered, preferably after the patient is unconscious. This enables the anaesthetist to place the electrodes in an optimal position, apply the minimum supramaximal stimulus required, and assess the onset of NMB once a relaxant has been given.

Muscle groups have differing sensitivities to NDMRs. In general, muscles that are bulkier and closer to the central circulation, e.g. respiratory and anterior abdominal wall muscles, exhibit a block that is less profound and wears off more rapidly. Smaller muscles at a greater distance from the heart, e.g. the muscles of the hand, are more sensitive and remain blocked for longer. Thus, if no residual block is apparent at peripheral muscles, more central muscle will be fully functional. The corollary of this is that patients may start to breathe or cough when there is minimal or no response to peripheral nerve stimulation.

The depth of NMB required depends on the type of surgery. Certain operations may need profound paralysis, e.g. laparotomies and retinal surgery. Otherwise an adequate non-depolarizing block can be maintained at two TOF twitches or one DBS twitch. At this degree of relaxation, patients will be adequately relaxed but also reversible.

Neuromuscular reversal

- Clinical signs of reversal: the ability to breathe is not a good indicator of adequate reversal, as a substantial degree of paralysis may be present with virtually normal V_T. Assessment of sustained muscle contraction is better, e.g. hand grip or head lift for 5s.
- Nerve stimulator: an acceptable recovery from block occurs when the TOFR has reached 0.9 or greater. The absence of any detectable fade with DBS indicates that the patient has reasonable recovery.
- At the completion of surgery, normal neuromuscular transmission can be facilitated by the use of anticholinesterase drugs.
- Reversal agents should not be given until there is evidence of return of neuromuscular transmission, e.g. at least two TOF twitches, one DBS twitch, or a post-tetanic count >10. Clinically, this might include evidence of breathing or spontaneous muscle movement. Intense NMB may not be reversible.
- Patients who are inadequately reversed exhibit jerky and uncoordinated muscle movements. If awake, they may appear dyspnoeic and anxious. If residual block is confirmed by TOF or DBS, one further dose of reversal agent may be administered. Agitated patients with reasonable respiratory function and otherwise normal vital signs may be given a small dose of a sedative (e.g. midazolam 1–5mg) while awaiting the return of full muscle function. If the block persists or if the patient is very distressed, anaesthesia, intubation, and artificial ventilation should be undertaken, and the cause sought.

Reversal drugs

- Conventional reversal drugs work by blocking acetylcholinesterase, thereby promoting the accumulation of acetylcholine. They include:
  - Neostigmine. A dose of 0.04mg/kg works within 2min and has a clinical effect for about 30min
  - Edrophonium. Onset time is faster, but it has a duration of action of only a few minutes. It is only used for the edrophonium test.
- Anticholinesterase drugs act at both nicotinic and muscarinic sites, thus producing unwanted side effects which include salivation, bradycardia, bronchospasm, and increased gut motility. They are therefore usually administered with antimuscarinic agents (atropine 10–20 micrograms/kg, glycopyrronium 10–15 micrograms/kg).
- Sugammadex is a novel reversal drug which rapidly immobilizes and inactivates certain aminosteroid NDMRs, particularly rocuronium (and vecuronium). Larger doses (4mg/kg) can reverse deep rocuronium blockade where there is no response to TOF or DBS. In doses of 16mg/kg, immediate reversal of an intubating bolus of rocuronium is possible. Conventional reversal drugs cannot do this. Its use is currently limited by expense.

Further reading

Caldwell JE, Miller RD (2009). Clinical implications of sugammadex. *Anaesthesia*, **64**, 66–72.

Davis L, Britten JJ, Morgan M (1997). Cholinesterase: its significance in anaesthetic practice. *Anaesthesia*, **52**, 244–60.

Kopman AF, Eikermann M (2009). Antagonism of non-depolarising block: current practice. *Anaesthesia*, **64**, 22–30.

Practising evidence-based anaesthesia

Evidence-based medicine (EBM)

Is defined as the conscientious, explicit, and judicious use of current best evidence in making decisions about the care of individual patients. It teaches how to ask a specific and relevant question arising from clinical practice, how to access and critically appraise up-to-date knowledge ('evidence') (Table 38.6), and then, using clinical experience and judgement, to determine whether the evidence is applicable to a clinical setting. Use of proven effective treatments should improve patient outcome.

- EBM depends on well-designed studies producing reliable results, with an emphasis on RCTs.
- Random assignment to treatment group and objective assessment of outcome are the best methods of avoiding bias. A consistent finding from several RCTs is very convincing, and so the pooled results of such trials constitute high level evidence.
- Small RCTs are prone to type II error—incorrectly accepting the null hypothesis—and so a beneficial (or harmful) effect of treatment might be missed.
- Large RCTs are needed to provide sufficient study power to identify effective treatments.
- Large multicentre RCTs, and meta-analyses of numerous RCTs, can include a broad range of patients and health-care settings to better reflect everyday clinical practice.
- Most studies in anaesthesia are too small to detect effective treatments that can prevent adverse outcomes; too often they focus only on surrogate endpoints.

Table 38.6 Levels of evidence

Level	Description
1	Meta-analysis of RCTs (with homogeneity) or individual RCT with narrow confidence interval
2	Low-quality RCT or cohort studies
3	Case-control study
4	Case series (and poor-quality cohort and case-control studies)
5	Expert opinion or based on basic science research

Finding the evidence

The anaesthetic literature is vast and difficult to access, without efficient search methods using electronic databases. Reliable web-based resources include:
- EBM:
  - ◈ http://www.cebm.net—the Oxford Centre for Evidence-Based Medicine; how to practise EBM

- • ℘ http://www.medicine.ox.ac.uk/bandolier—a premier EBM site with a focus on pain. Excellent examples of critical appraisal and assessment of effectiveness
- • ℘ http://www.nice.org.uk—the UK National Institute for Health and Care Excellence, which produces numerous evidence-based guidelines for clinical practice
- • ℘ http://www.tripdatabase.com—a useful search engine that links numerous databases of systematic reviews
- Search the literature:
  - • ℘ http://www.ncbi.nlm.nih.gov/pubmed—PubMed, an essential tool for literature searching
- Cochrane Collaboration:
  - • ℘ http://www.cochrane.org—a global network producing systematic reviews, with links to a teaching resource for meta-analysis
- Clinical trials and meta-analysis:
  - • ℘ http://www.jameslindlibrary.org—a collection of essays on the development and history of 'fair tests of treatments'.

How to interpret a meta-analysis

A systematic review is a process of examining all relevant studies. Meta-analysis is the statistical method used to pool the results.

- The effect on binary outcomes (complication/no complication) can be summarized by the risk ratio (RR) (Table 38.7) or odds ratio (OR). The RR is the probability of an event occurring in the exposed group versus a non-exposed group; the OR is the ratio of the odds of an event occurring in the exposed group versus a non-exposed group. The OR will approximate the RR for uncommon events but will otherwise overestimate the RR.
- An RR of 1.0 indicates no effect on risk, RR <1.0 reduced risk, and RR >1.0 increased risk.

Table 38.7 Interpreting risk ratio

Relative risk (RR)	Effect on risk
0.25	75% reduction in risk
0.5	50% reduction in risk
1.0	No effect
1.5	50% increase in risk
2.0	100% (or 2-fold) increase in risk

- The effects on numerical outcomes (e.g. cardiac index or opioid consumption) can be summarized as a weighted mean difference.
- Meta-analysis may be done using either a fixed effect model, which assumes that the individual study results are correlated with one another and probably represent similar study populations, or a random effects model, which does not require this assumption; the latter should be used if there is study heterogeneity.
- A forest plot can be used to graphically represent the individual studies contributing to a meta-analysis. Fig. 38.6 summarizes four trials comparing paravertebral block with epidural analgesia to reduce pulmonary complications:
  - The estimated effect (in this case, RR) of each trial is represented by the box and its 95% confidence interval (CI). The size of the box reflects the size of the study, and this is quantified by the study weight (%). The width of the 95% CI indicates the extent of uncertainty of this estimated RR—if the CI crosses the value 1.0 (the line of equality), then the individual study is not statistically significant
  - The pooled RR is 0.41, indicating a 59% reduction in risk of pulmonary complications
  - The CIs of this estimated RR range from 0.17 (83% risk reduction) to 0.95 (5% risk reduction); this is statistically significant, p = 0.04

- The width of the CI indicates the precision or reliability of the estimate. If either 95% confidence limit were the true effect, and if such a finding would change the conclusion of the study, then we are left with uncertainty
- In this case, the test for heterogeneity is not statistically significant, supporting the validity of pooling the studies. Similarly, the I^2 statistic indicates trivial inconsistency across the studies, with a value of >40% being of likely importance. These two statistics support the use of a fixed effect model for the meta-analysis.
- There are some weaknesses with a meta-analysis, e.g. publication bias (negative studies are less likely to be published), duplicate/repeated publication, heterogeneity, and inclusion of outdated studies; they probably inflate the risk of type I error. Meta-analyses that have minimal heterogeneity, narrow CIs, and a large number of study events and that include at least one large RCT tend to be more reliable.

Review: Paravertebral block
Comparison: 15 Pulmonary complications
Outcome: 01 Pulmonary complications

Study or sub-category	PVB n/N	Epidural n/N	RR (fixed) 95% CI	Weight %	RR (fixed) 95% CI
Leaver	2/14	3/15		17.30	0.71 [0.14, 3.66]
Kaiser	0/13	2/13		14.93	0.20 [0.01, 3.80]
Bimston	4/30	3/20		21.50	0.89 [0.22, 3.55]
Richardson 99	1/46	8/49		46.27	0.13 [0.02, 1.02]
Total (95% CI)	103	97		100.00	0.41 [0.17, 0.95]

Total events: 7 (PVB), 16 (Epidural)
Test for heterogeneity: Chi² = 3.06, df = 3 (P = 0.38); I² = 1.8%
Test for overall effect: Z = 2.08 (P = 0.04)

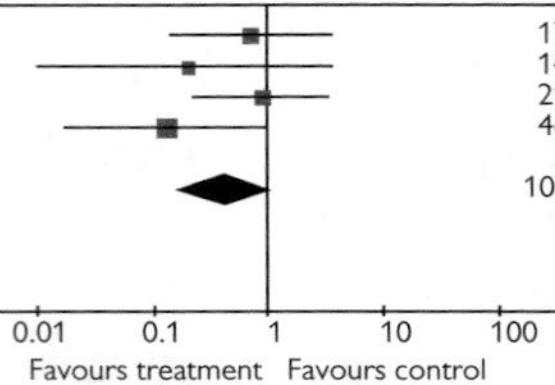

0.01 0.1 1 10 100
Favours treatment   Favours control

Fig. 38.6 Example forest plot showing four trials comparing paravertebral block with epidural analgesia to reduce pulmonary complications. See text for details.

Modified with permission from Davies RG, Myles PS, Graham JM (2006). A comparison of the analgesic efficacy and side-effects of paravertebral vs epidural blockade for thoracotomy—a systematic review and meta-analysis of randomized trials. *British Journal of Anaesthesia*, **96**, 418–426, by permission of Oxford University Press.

Evidence-based interventions in anaesthesia

There are some simple, effective techniques that should be used more widely, or, in some cases, abandoned because of lack of evidence or evidence of net harm to patients. These include the following.

- Chlorhexidine should be used for antisepsis when inserting intravascular (and probably major regional block) catheters.
- PONV prophylaxis should target at-risk patients only and include a multimodal regimen of dexamethasone, droperidol, and a 5-HT$_3$ antagonist.
- Epidural analgesia is superior to parenteral opioids in relieving post-operative pain after major surgery.
- Epidural analgesia reduces the risk of pneumonia after major surgery.
- The risk of stroke is comparable for both LA and GA in carotid surgery.
- Clonidine increases regional block duration (about 2hr) but has side effects of increased hypotension, bradycardia, and sedation.
- Intra-operative hypothermia reduces thermal comfort and increases bleeding/transfusion requirements and myocardial ischaemia. Avoiding intra-operative hypothermia reduces wound infection.
- Perioperative β-blockade can reduce MI but may increase the risk of stroke and death.
- Prophylactic antibiotics reduce sepsis complications after major abdominal surgery and should be given before skin incision.
- Volatile agents reduce the risk of MI and death after coronary artery surgery, when compared with IV anaesthetic techniques.
- Early enteral feeding reduces post-operative infection and hospital stay after abdominal surgery.
- There is no evidence that NG drainage speeds the return of bowel function or reduces the risk of wound infection or anastomotic leak after abdominal surgery.
- There is no evidence that intra-operative tight glucose control improves outcomes after major surgery, but the risk of hypoglycaemia is increased.
- Protective lung ventilation reduces the risk of respiratory failure in patients undergoing major abdominal surgery.
- HES 6% (130/0.4) increases the risk of renal failure in critically ill patients.
- α$_2$-agonists do not reduce perioperative cardiac events in non-cardiac surgery.
- It is unclear whether supplemental O$_2$ therapy improves outcomes after abdominal surgery.

Further reading

Collins R, MacMahon S (2001). Reliable assessment of the effects of treatment on mortality and major morbidity, 1: clinical trials. *Lancet*, **357**, 373–80.

Fisher DM (1994). Surrogate end points: are they meaningful? *Anesthesiology*, **81**, 795–6.

Higgins JP, Thompson SG, Deeks JJ, Altman DG (2003). Measuring inconsistency in meta-analyses. *BMJ*, **327**, 557–60.

Moher D, Cook DJ, Eastwood S, Olkin I, Rennie D, Stroup DF (1999). Improving the quality of reports of meta-analyses of randomised controlled trials: the QUOROM statement. Quality of Reporting of Meta-analyses. *Lancet*, **354**, 1896–900.

Møller A, Pederson T, eds. (2006). *Evidence-based anaesthesia and intensive care*. Cambridge: Cambridge University Press.

Myles PS (1999). Why we need large randomized studies in anaesthesia. *Br J Anaesth*, **83**, 833–4.

Pogue J, Yusuf S (1998). Overcoming the limitations of current meta-analysis of randomised controlled trials. *Lancet*, **351**, 47–52.

Tramer MR (2003). *An evidence based resource in anaesthesia and analgesia*, 2nd edn. London: BMJ Publishing Group.

Tunis SR, Stryer DB, Clancy CM (2003). Practical clinical trials: increasing the value of clinical research for decision making in clinical and health policy. *JAMA*, **290**, 1624–32.

National Institute for Health and Care Excellence and the Cochrane Collaboration

NICE and the Cochrane Collaboration are both independent bodies that systematically evaluate the evidence for both benefit and harm of medical interventions.

In 1979, the British epidemiologist Archie Cochrane stated, 'It is surely a great criticism of our profession that we have not organised a critical summary ... of all relevant randomised controlled trials'. By 1992, systematic reviews of interventions in perinatal care led to the foundation of the first Cochrane Centre in Oxford, followed by the launch of the international Collaboration the following year. About 30 000 people in 100 countries contribute to the preparation of systematic reviews and the maintenance and development of the Collaboration. Systematic reviews are divided thematically between review groups; anaesthesia, including prehospital care and critical care, was established in 2000 in Copenhagen (62 published reviews by April 2010; see website).[33]

NICE investigates three areas:
- Good health and prevention of illness: Centre for Public Health
- Technology and interventions: Centre for Health Technology Evaluation
- Specific disease management: Centre for Clinical Practice.

Guidance by NICE of interest to anaesthetists includes:[34]
- Ultrasound-guided central vein catheterization (09, 2002)
- Preoperative tests (06, 2003)
- Drotrecogin alfa for severe sepsis (09, 2004)
- Acutely ill hospitalized patients (07, 2007)
- Head injury (09, 2007)
- Epidural catheterization (01, 2008)
- Endocarditis prophylaxis (03, 2008)
- Perioperative hypothermia (04, 2008)
- Spinal cord stimulation for neuropathic pain (08, 2008)
- Surgical site infection (10, 2008)
- Ultrasound-guided nerve block (01, 2009)
- Critical illness rehabilitation (03, 2009)
- Child abuse (07, 2009)
- Percutaneous intradiscal electrothermal therapy for back pain (11, 2009)
- VTE prophylaxis (01, 2010)
- Drug treatment of neuropathic pain (03, 2010)
- Oesophageal Doppler in major surgery (03, 2011)
- BIS monitoring for awareness (11, 2012).

References

33 Cochrane Anaesthesia Group. ℘ http://www.carg.cochrane.org/our-reviews.
34 National Institute for Health and Care Excellence. ℘ http://www.nice.org.uk.

Blood products and fluid therapy

Richard Telford

Blood products

In 2012–2013, 1.9 million units of blood were issued by NHS Blood and Transplant.[1] There has been a steady fall in the number of units of packed red cells issued since 1999 which, in part, reflects the adoption of restrictive blood transfusion practices by clinicians. All donated blood is tested for HIV-1, HIV-2, HBV, HCV, human T cell lymphotrophic virus (anti-HTLV I and II), and syphilis. CMV antibody-negative blood components are available for immunosuppressed patients and neonates. In the UK, donated blood is routinely filtered to remove white cells, as a precaution against new vCJD, leaving a residual leucocyte count of $<1 \times 10^6$/U. This reduces the incidence of febrile transfusion reactions and alloimmunization to white cell (including HLA) antigens.

Whole blood

Blood is processed into blood components as follows (see also Table 39.1):
- **Packed red cells**: most of the plasma is removed, then packed red cells are resuspended in an optimal additive solution—saline, adenine, glucose, and mannitol (SAG-M). Total volume is 220–350mL, and Hct is 50–70%. Four mL per kg (280mL for a 70kg man) typically raises the Hb by 1g/dL. Irradiated cells (γ or X-ray) are used for patients at risk of transfusion-associated graft-versus-host disease (TA-GvHD)
- **Platelets**: one adult therapeutic dose (ATD) may be prepared from 4–6 donations of whole blood by centrifugation, or from a single donor by platelet apheresis. National Blood Services aim to produce 80% of platelets by apheresis (donors may give 2–3 ATDs in a single session). One ATD contains $250–500 \times 10^9$ platelets and typically increases the platelet count by $20–40 \times 10^9$/L. Platelets may be irradiated for use in TA-GvHD-susceptible patients
- **FFP and cryoprecipitate**: FFP is produced either by centrifugation of whole blood or by apheresis. Plasma is rapidly frozen to maintain the activity of labile clotting factors; this produces an average 'unit' of FFP of about 275mL. The Department of Health has recommended that, to minimize the risk of CJD transmission, children born, and patients likely to be, exposed to many doses of FFP should receive pathogen-reduced plasma (PRP). This is produced from non-UK-sourced plasma by two methods: methylthioninium chloride (methylene blue) treatment and solvent detergent treatment. Cryoprecipitate is obtained from controlled thawing of a single donation of FFP which precipitates high-molecular-weight proteins, including factor VIII, vWF, factor XIII, and fibrinogen. It is supplied as pooled units—each pooled unit contains cryoprecipitate from five donors. Two pooled units will typically raise the fibrinogen level by 1g/dL
- **Plasma derivatives**: albumin, immunoglobulin, and clotting factor concentrates. These products are derived from fractionation of plasma (non-UK-sourced).

Other products
- **rFVIIa**: licensed to treat bleeding in patients with haemophilia A or B with inhibitors of factors VIII or IX. rFVIIa has also been used in patients experiencing life-threatening haemorrhage unresponsive to blood

Table 39.1 Comparison of blood products

	Red cells	Platelet concentrate	Fresh frozen plasma	Cryoprecipitate
Storage temperature	2–6°C	20–24°C on an agitator rack	−30°C	−30°C
Shelf life	35d	5d	3yr (frozen)	3yr (frozen)
Longest time from leaving controlled storage to completing infusion	Transfuse within 30min of removal from blood fridge. Transfuse unit over maximum of 4hr	Start transfusion as soon as received from blood bank. Transfuse unit within 30min	Once thawed, should be transfused within 4hr	4hr
Unit cost (UK) 2014/15	£122	£208	£28	£193
Compatibility testing requirement	Must be compatible with recipient ABO and Rh D (RhD) type	Preferably ABO identical with patient. Rh-negative ♀ under the age of 45yr should be given RhD-negative platelets	FFP and cryoprecipitate should be ABO-compatible to avoid risk of haemolysis caused by donor anti-A or anti-B	
Administration	Infuse through a blood administration set—platelet concentrates should not be infused through giving sets that have been used for blood. Record details of each blood component infusion in the patient's case record; 100% traceability of blood products is mandatory			

product therapy, e.g. trauma, post-partum haemorrhage. An initial dose of 200 micrograms/kg, followed by two doses of 100 micrograms/kg, administered at 1 and 3hr following the 1st dose, has been recommended. A high risk of arterial thrombotic complications has recently been reported—the routine use of rFVIIa for non-haemophilia-related bleeding cannot be recommended outside well-designed clinical trials.

Practical uses

Red cells

Transfusion of red cells raises the Hb concentration, and thus the O_2-carrying capacity of blood. For indications for transfusion, see ➡ p. 1044.

Platelets

- **Prophylaxis for surgery:** a platelet count >100 × 10⁹/L is recommended before operations in critical sites, e.g. brain/eyes. Consensus guidelines suggest a platelet count of 80 × 10⁹/L for epidural anaesthesia (see also

➔ p. 1141, p. 772, and p. 758). For other invasive surgery and spinal anaesthesia, a platelet count of $>50 \times 10^9/L$ is acceptable.

- **Massive transfusion**: maintain count $>50 \times 10^9/L$ (expected after transfusion of two blood volumes). A higher target of $100 \times 10^9/L$ is recommended in multiple trauma or CNS injury. Many hospitals do not store platelets on site—the time for transfer from the blood centre must be factored into local protocols.
- **DIC**: administration of platelets should be guided by frequent platelet counts and rotational thromboelastometry. In the absence of bleeding, transfusion should not be given to correct a low platelet count.
- **CPB**: causes thrombocytopenia and platelet dysfunction—platelets should be readily available, but transfusion reserved for patients experiencing excessive post-operative bleeding in whom a surgical cause has been excluded. The decision to transfuse platelets is clinical, based on evidence of microvascular bleeding and excessive blood loss. Near-patient testing (TEG) leads to more rational blood product support.
- **Liver transplantation** (see ➔ p. 566): abnormalities may include reduced coagulation, thrombocytopenia, hyperfibrinolysis, and massive transfusion. Platelet and blood component therapy is guided by rotational thromboelastometry.
- **Contraindications** to platelet transfusion: TTP and HIT.

Fresh frozen plasma and cryoprecipitate

- **Vitamin K deficiency in the ICU**: prolonged PT in ICU patients may be caused by inadequate vitamin K intake. Vitamin K (10mg, three times per week) is the treatment of choice.
- **Reversal of warfarin**: FFP should no longer be used. Human PCC (Beriplex®, Octaplex®) is the treatment of choice.
- **Surgical bleeding and massive transfusion**: the decision to use FFP should be guided by laboratory-based tests of coagulation and near-patient testing where available. Many centres have moved to a formulaic replacement of blood and FFP in massive transfusion, administering red cells and FFP in a 1:1 ratio (see section on massive transfusion, ➔ p. 1049.
- FFP should not be used as a simple volume replacement, in plasma exchange (except for TTP), or to reverse a prolonged PT in the absence of bleeding.

Risks of transfusion

The commonest serious adverse event associated with blood transfusion is incorrect blood component transfused (IBCT). The majority of these events are associated with clerical and administrative errors, e.g. administration of the wrong blood component, phlebotomy, and laboratory error. In 2012, this contributed to over 250 wrong transfusions. As a consequence, the National Patient Safety Agency in the UK has recommended that all staff involved in the administration of blood products must undergo a triennial competency-based training and assessment.

- **Acute haemolytic transfusion reaction**: ABO incompatibility usually due to clerical error. Recipient antibodies bind to the transfused red cells, causing haemolysis and complement pathway activation. Inflammation, increased vascular permeability, and hypotension occur, which may cause shock and ARF.

- **Bacterial contamination**: signs and symptoms very similar to acute haemolytic transfusion reaction or severe acute allergic reaction with a rapid onset of hypo- or hypertension, rigors, and collapse. Bacterial contamination is rare but most frequently reported with platelets that are stored at room temperature.

- **Transfusion-related acute lung injury (TRALI)**: caused by antibodies in plasma of a single donor unit reacting with leucocyte antigens in the recipient. Incidence is 1:5–10 000U of products containing plasma transfused—most commonly FFP or whole blood. The risk is greatest with plasma-rich components—more cases are being attributed to FFP and platelets, now that leucodepleted packed red cells are used instead of whole blood. TRALI is probably underdiagnosed and should be considered if a patient develops acute-onset pulmonary oedema within 6hr of transfusion that is not due to circulatory overload. Management is the same as for ARDS/ALI of any cause. Donors of blood products implicated in TRALI tend to be women immunized against fetal leucocyte antigens in pregnancy. The blood bank should be notified, so that the donor may be contacted and, if necessary, taken off the donor panel.

- **Acute transfusion reactions (ATRs)**: defined as occurring up to 24hr following transfusion of blood or components. May range from full-blown anaphylaxis, manifesting as hypotension, bronchospasm, and oedema, to febrile non-haemolytic transfusion reactions.

- **Delayed haemolytic transfusion reactions (DHTRs)**: occurring >24hr after transfusion. Usually a delayed haemolytic reaction related to the development of red cell alloantibodies.

- **TA-GvHD**: this condition, usually occurring in immunocompromised individuals, is caused by engraftment and proliferation of transfused lymphocytes. They damage cells that carry HLA antigens in the skin, liver, spleen, and bone marrow. Fever, skin rash, diarrhoea, and dermatitis are seen. It is usually fatal. There has been a negligible incidence of this complication since the introduction of universal leucodepletion in 1999.

- **Transfusion-associated circulatory overload (TACO)**: acute or worsening pulmonary oedema within 6hr of transfusion. This may now be the commonest cause of transfusion-related death in developed countries. Elderly patients are particularly at risk, especially those with heart failure and renal impairment. Small elderly patients and children are at increased risk of receiving inappropriately high volume and rapid blood transfusion.

- **Infections transmissible by transfusion**: every donation is tested for hepatitis B surface antigen, hepatitis C antibody and RNA, HIV antibody, HTLV antibody, and syphilis antibody. It has been estimated that one donation over 2yr could transmit HIV, seven donations per year could transmit hepatitis B, and one donation per 7yr could transmit hepatitis C. Four cases of transmission of vCJD by transfusion have been reported, all prior to 2006. All four recipients had received transfusions of non-leucodepleted red blood cells between 1996 and 1999.

Indications and triggers for transfusion

Clinical guidelines for red cell transfusion

- Patients should be given information about the risks and benefits, wherever possible, and also be informed about possible alternatives, e.g. autologous transfusion. Patients have the right to refuse blood transfusion.
- Establish the cause of any anaemia. Red cell transfusions should not be given where effective alternatives exist, e.g. treatment of iron deficiency, megaloblastic, and autoimmune haemolytic anaemia.
- There is no absolute level of Hb at which transfusion of red cells is appropriate for all patients (transfusion trigger). Clinical judgement plays a vital role in the decision whether to transfuse or not (see below).
- In acute blood loss, crystalloids should be used for rapid acute volume replacement. The effects of anaemia need to be considered separately from those of hypovolaemia.
- Local arrangements should provide compatible blood urgently for patients with major bleeding, including emergency O RhD-negative blood.
- The reason for blood transfusion should be documented in the patient's records.

Indications for blood transfusion

Acute blood loss

First, attempt to quantify the amount of circulating volume lost (see ⊙ p. 762, p. 847, and p. 1001).

- Class I: <15% of circulating blood volume. Do not transfuse, unless blood loss is superimposed on a pre-existing anaemia or if the patient is unable to compensate for this level of blood loss because of reduced cardiorespiratory reserve.
- Class II: <30% of circulating blood volume. Will need resuscitation with IV fluids. Requirement for blood transfusion unlikely, unless patient has pre-existing anaemia, reduced cardiorespiratory reserve, or if blood loss continues.
- Class III: <40% of circulating blood volume. Rapid volume replacement is required; blood transfusion will almost certainly be required.
- Class IV: >40% of circulating blood volume. Rapid volume replacement, including blood transfusion.

Next consider the Hb. Plan a target level at which to maintain the patient's Hb:

- Blood transfusion is not indicated when the Hb level is >10g/dL.
- Transfusion is almost always indicated if the Hb level is <7g/dL.
- In patients who may tolerate anaemia poorly, e.g. patients over 65yr and those with CVS or respiratory disease, transfusion is indicated if the Hb is <8g/dL.
- It is debatable whether patients whose Hb levels are between 8 and 10g/dL should be transfused. Some will require a transfusion if

symptomatic of acute anaemia (fatigue, dizziness, shortness of breath, new or worsening angina).
- Finally, consider the risk of further bleeding from disordered haemostasis. Check the platelet count, and perform a coagulation screen.

'Group and screen' or cross-match?

- 'G&S': patient's blood sample is tested to determine ABO and RhD type and to detect red cell antibodies (in addition to anti-A or anti-B) that could haemolyse transfused red cells. The sample is held in the laboratory for 7d. If there is no historical sample on file, two samples, taken at different times, will be required by the laboratory before ABO-matched blood components can be issued. If there is a historical sample on file, only one sample is required. Current guidelines suggest that pre-transfusion testing should be performed on samples collected no more than 3d in advance of the transfusion.
- Provided the G&S sample shows no atypical antibodies, fully compatible blood can be electronically issued in 5min. This relies on the fact that, if the patient's ABO and RhD groups have been established and the antibody screen is negative, the possibility of issuing incompatible blood is negligible.
- If atypical antibodies are present in the G&S sample, then the issue of fully compatible blood will be delayed (up to 2hr), while a fully tested cross-match is performed.
- Institutions should have a regularly reviewed maximum surgical blood ordering schedule (MSBOS) that stipulates which operations require blood to be cross-matched.

Process for red cell or blood product transfusion

Procedures to ensure safe transfusion should include:
- Confirmation of the patient's identity verbally (if possible) and by identification band (first name, surname, date of birth, and hospital number) by two separate individuals.
- Check expiry date, blood group, and unit number match those on the laboratory-generated label attached to the pack.
- Inspect the bag to ensure integrity of the plastic casing. Look for discoloration or evidence of red cell clumping.
- Blood left out of the blood fridge for >30min should be transfused within 4hr or discarded.
- Be meticulous with your documentation. Sign the transfusion documentation, and record the details of the blood unit transfused on the anaesthetic chart or clinical notes.
- Document the reasons for transfusion.
- A 100% traceability of all allogeneic blood transfused is a legal requirement.

Reference

1 Norfolk D, ed. (2013). *Handbook of transfusion medicine*, 5th edn. ℰ http://www.transfusion-guidelines.org.uk/transfusion-handbook.

Blood conservation techniques

Blood conservation techniques rely upon:
- Increasing the patient's red blood cell mass.
- Decreasing perioperative blood loss.
- Optimizing blood transfusion practices, including both **allogeneic** (from another human) and **autologous** (reinfusion of the patient's own blood) transfusion.

Preoperative management
- Optimize preoperative Hb. Preoperative anaemia is a predictor of an increased risk of perioperative complications.
- Investigate and treat anaemia. Restrict diagnostic phlebotomy. If possible, stop antiplatelet and anticoagulant medication—this must be balanced against the risk of thrombosis.
- EPO: human recombinant EPO (rEPO) stimulates erythropoiesis and permits more aggressive preoperative autologous donation. EPO therapy should be started 3–4wk before surgery for maximum effect. It is an expensive method of increasing preoperative donation.
- Preoperative autologous donation (PAD): patients donate a unit of blood per week in the month prior to their operation. Blood transfusion may be commoner in patients undergoing PAD, possibly due to more liberal use of autologous blood. Disadvantages of PAD include: transfusion of the wrong blood due to clerical and laboratory errors, wastage of collected blood, and circulatory overload due to transfusion of whole blood. PAD is not widely used in the UK, mainly due to organizational difficulties.

Intraoperative management
- **Surgical**: techniques to minimize blood loss include: meticulous surgical technique, minimally invasive surgery (e.g. endoluminal grafts for AAAs), local vasoconstriction with adrenaline, topical haemostatic agents (fibrin glues), tourniquets, and surgical devices, e.g. ultrasonic/laser scalpels.
- **Anaesthetic techniques**: measures to reduce venous oozing include: avoidance of venous congestion (patient positioning), high intrathoracic pressures, hypercapnia, and hypothermia. Epidural and spinal anaesthesia minimize blood loss by reducing both arterial and venous pressures. Hypotensive anaesthesia has been used in selected patients; however, there is a risk of ischaemic cerebral and cardiac complications, especially in the elderly.
- **Pharmacological**: antifibrinolytic agents—aprotinin, a serine protease inhibitor, reduces the need for blood transfusion in cardiac and hepatic surgery but has been implicated with an increased risk of stroke, MI, and renal failure. It was temporarily withdrawn from prescription in 2007 and is currently recommended for use only in those patients with a particularly high risk of bleeding, in whom the benefits outweigh the risks.
- Tranexamic acid inhibits plasminogen activation and, at high concentration, inhibits plasmin. The CRASH-2 study supports its use at a loading dose of 1g IV over 10min, followed by 1g infused over 8hr.[2]

Autologous transfusion

Acute normovolaemic haemodilution

This involves perioperative collection of whole blood from the patient, with simultaneous infusion of crystalloid to maintain normovolaemia.[3] Blood may be collected from a large-bore IV cannula or an arterial line into citrated blood bags (available from the blood transfusion department). Once collected, bags should be labelled and stored at room temperature for reinfusion once surgical blood loss has ceased. They must be reinfused to the patient within 6hr. Mathematical models have suggested that significant haemodilution (Hct <20%) is required before acute normovolaemic haemodilution (ANH) is efficacious in reducing allogeneic blood transfusion. Risks of significant haemodilution, especially myocardial ischaemia, must be carefully considered.

- *Indications:* current UK guidelines state that ANH should be considered when the potential surgical blood loss is likely to exceed 20% of the blood volume with a preoperative Hb of >10g/dL.
- *Advantages:* no testing required, and minimal risk of an ABO-incompatible blood transfusion, as the units are not removed from the operating theatre.
- *Contraindications:* severe myocardial disease, e.g. moderate to severe LV impairment, unstable angina, severe AS, and critical left main stem CAD.

Intra-operative cell salvage

This involves collection and reinfusion of autologous red cells lost during surgery.[4] Most machines depend on a centrifugal principle using a collection bowl that spins and separates the red cells from plasma, white cells, and platelets. Shed blood is aspirated into a collection reservoir via heparinized or citrated tubing. The salvaged red cells are separated by centrifugation and finally washed in 1–2L of saline. This removes circulating fibrin, debris, plasma, leucocytes, microaggregates, complement, platelets, free Hb, circulating procoagulants, and heparin. Cell salvage produces packed red cells suspended in saline, with an Hct of 50–60%.

- *Indications:* cell washing devices can provide the equivalent of 10U of bank blood per hour in cases of massive bleeding. The technique is applicable to open heart surgery, vascular surgery, total joint replacements, spinal surgery, liver transplantation, ruptured ectopic pregnancy, some neurosurgical procedures, and massive obstetric haemorrhage (provided a leucocyte depletion filter is used).
- *Contraindications:* bacterial contamination of the operative field, malignant disease, and presence of fat or amniotic fluid in salvaged blood (risk of embolism and DIC). Topical clotting agents, such as collagen, cellulose, and thrombin, and topical antibiotics or cleansing agents used in the operative field should not be aspirated into a cell salvage machine. Complications have been reported in patients with SCD. However, there are scarce data to support some of these contraindications, and most contraindications are relative, rather than absolute.[5,6] Cell salvage can be used in obstetric haemorrhage, despite contamination of blood with amniotic fluid. A leucocyte depletion filter must be used. In cancer surgery, allogeneic blood transfusion may worsen the outcome, possibly by immunomodulation. Therefore, some

centres *advocate* cell salvage techniques in cancer surgery. The high cost of the machinery and the need for trained operators are drawbacks. Once set up, the disposable kits can process limitless units of packed red cells. Current disposable costs are very similar to the cost of 1U of leucodepleted red cells (£122).

Post-operative recovery of blood

This involves collection of blood from surgical drains, followed by reinfusion, with or without processing. The blood recovered is dilute, partially haemolysed/defibrinated, and may contain high concentrations of cytokines. Most experience has been gained in cardiac and orthopaedic surgery, especially total knee replacements. The safety and benefit of the use of unwashed blood remains questionable. Some groups have reported considerable savings in the use of bank blood.

References

2 CRASH-2 trial collaborators, Shakur H, Roberts I, Bautista R, *et al.* (2010). Effects of tranexamic acid on death, vascular occlusive events, and blood transfusion in trauma patients with significant haemorrhage (CRASH-2): a randomised, placebo-controlled trial. *Lancet*, **376**, 23–32.
3 Kovesi T, Royston D (2003). Pharmacological approaches to reducing allogeneic blood exposure. *Vox Sang*, **84**, 2–10.
4 Napier JA, Bruce M, Chapman J, *et al.* (1997). Guidelines for autologous transfusion II. Perioperative haemodilution and cell salvage. *Br J Anaesth*, **78**, 768–71.
5 The Association of Anaesthetists of Great Britain and Ireland (2009). *AAGBI safety guideline: blood transfusion and the anaesthetist. Intra-operative cell salvage.* ℬ http://www.aagbi.org/sites/default/files/cell%20_salvage_2009_amended.pdf.
6 Waters JH (2004). Indications and contraindications of cell salvage. *Transfusion*, **44**, 40S–44S.

Massive transfusion

(See also ➲ p. 762, p. 847, and p. 1001.)

Defined as loss of one blood volume in <24hr, 50% blood loss within 3hr, or blood loss of >150mL/min.

Many centres advocate early transfusion of FFP in a fixed ratio to red cells in massive haemorrhage to reduce coagulopathy and reduce bleeding. This approach has been extrapolated from military to civilian practice, but the true value is uncertain. Retrospective studies are confounded by 'survivor bias' (the most severely injured do not survive long enough to be transfused), and the civilian population is older and frequently less fit. All hospitals must have massive transfusion protocols in place. The principles are summarized in Table 39.2.

Table 39.2 Resuscitation from major haemorrhage

Goal	Procedure
Restore circulating volume	Two 14G IV cannulae. Resuscitation with warmed crystalloid/colloid. Warm patient. Consider arterial line/central venous access
Contact key personnel	Senior anaesthetist/surgeon/obstetrician. Blood bank/haematologist. Activate massive haemorrhage protocol
Arrest bleeding	Early surgical/obstetric intervention. Interventional radiology
Request laboratory investigations	FBC, PT, APTT, fibrinogen, cross-match—*check patient identity,* biochemistry, ABG. *Repeat clotting, FBC, fibrinogen after products/every 4hr. May need to give blood products before results available*
Request suitable red cells	Uncross-matched group O Rh-negative in extreme emergency, no more than 2U (Rh-positive acceptable if ♂ patient or post-menopausal ♀). Uncross-matched ABO group-specific when blood group known (laboratory will complete cross-match after issue). Fully cross-match (if time permits or irregular antibodies)
	Use blood warmer/rapid infusion device
	Consider cell salvage
Request platelets	Allow for delivery time from blood centre. Anticipate platelet count <50 × 10^9/L after twice blood volume replacement
	Target platelet count: 100 × 10^9/L for multiple/CNS trauma, for other situations >50 × 10^9/L
Request FFP (12–15mL/kg body weight)	Aim for PT and APTT <1.5 × control. Allow for 30min thawing time
Request cryo-precipitate, two packs (one pack represents pooled donations from five donors)	Replaces fibrinogen and factor VIII
	Low fibrinogen associated with microvascular bleeding. Deficiency develops early when plasma-poor red blood cells used for replacement. Aim for fibrinogen >1.5g/L
	Allow for delivery time plus 30min thawing time
Suspect DIC	Treat underlying cause, if possible

Jehovah's Witnesses

The Jehovah's Witness religious movement is 120 years old, with an estimated 6 million members worldwide. Most Jehovah's Witnesses will not accept a transfusion of blood or its 1° components, although absolute rules regarding specific blood products do not exist (Box 39.1).[7]

Box 39.1 Acceptability of blood products and transfusion-related procedures in Jehovah's Witnesses (with permission)

Unacceptable	Whole blood, packed red cells, plasma, autologous pre-donation
Acceptable	CPB, renal dialysis, acute hypervolaemic haemodilution, human rEPO, rFVIIa
May be acceptable ('matters of conscience')	Platelets, clotting factors, albumin, immunoglobulins, epidural blood patch, cell salvage

---

Ethical and legal issues

- Administration of blood or blood products to a competent patient who has refused blood transfusion against their wishes is unlawful and may lead to criminal and/or civil proceedings for assault against the doctor.
- Many Jehovah's Witnesses carry 'advance directives', which outline treatments accepted by the individual; the family and GP may hold copies.
- Anaesthetists have the right to refuse to anaesthetize Jehovah's Witnesses for elective surgery. However, the anaesthetist is obliged to provide care in emergency cases and must respect the patient's wishes.[8]
- **Emergencies**: if the patient's Jehovah's Witness status is unknown (e.g. unconscious), the doctor is expected to act in the best interests of the patient—this may include blood transfusion. Opinions of relatives or associates that the patient would not accept a blood transfusion must be verified; evidence of an advance directive should be sought.
- **Children**: the care of children of Jehovah's Witnesses (aged <16yr) may present particular difficulty. For elective procedures, preoperative discussion involving the surgeon, anaesthetist, parents, and child should occur. If the parents refuse permission for blood transfusion, it may be necessary to apply for a legal 'Specific Issue Order' via the High Court in order to administer a blood transfusion. Two consultants should document that blood transfusion is essential before this serious step is taken.
- In an emergency situation, when a child of Jehovah's Witnesses is likely to die without blood transfusion, blood should be given. Courts are likely to uphold this medical decision.

Preoperative management

- Early communication with the anaesthetic department is essential. Apart from minor surgery, a consultant anaesthetist should be available who is prepared to manage the patient.
- Meet the patient as early as possible preoperatively, with the results of relevant investigations to ascertain the degree of limitation of normal routine management.
- Involve other specialists, e.g. haematology, intensive care.
- There is a specific NHS consent form for Jehovah's Witnesses. At the preoperative visit, establish which treatments are acceptable, including an advance directive if signed. Make the patient aware of the risks of non-acceptance of blood and blood products.
- Specifically discuss and document whether strategies, such as ANH and perioperative cell salvage, may be used.
- Involve the local Jehovah's Witness hospital liaison committee in the discussions. Representatives can help avoid confrontation and assist the understanding of both parties. The address of the local committee may be obtained by contacting hospital information services (Britain)— tel: 0208 906 2211; email: his.gb@jw.org.
- Investigate and treat preoperative anaemia. Oral iron supplements can be used to improve iron stores (ferrous sulphate 200mg bd). Consider IV iron infusion (see ➋ p. 196). Human rEPO may be used pre-surgery, although the clinical response takes up to a month. Iron supplementation is usually required with rEPO therapy. Discussion of an individual case with a haematologist may be useful.
- Review the indications for anticoagulant and antiplatelet drugs, and consider stopping.
- Major operations can sometimes be staged to limit acute blood loss.

Intraoperative management

Preoperative assessment must determine which of these techniques are acceptable to the individual patient.

- **Surgical**: consider staged or laparoscopic surgery. Meticulous surgical technique, use of ultrasonic/laser scalpels, biological haemostats, e.g. alginate dressings, and fibrin glues and sealants.
- **Anaesthetic**: reduce venous oozing—avoid venous congestion (patient positioning), high intrathoracic pressures, and hypercapnia. Prevent hypothermia—leads to coagulopathy. Consider the use of invasive monitoring, even when the medical condition of the patient or the nature of the operation would not usually warrant it. The potential benefits and risks of hypotensive anaesthesia and regional anaesthesia should be considered.
- **Drug therapy**: antifibrinolytics, e.g. tranexamic acid. Desmopressin increases platelet adherence. Use of these drugs during major surgery may be considered.
- **Acute normovolaemic haemodilution**: ANH may be acceptable to Jehovah's Witnesses, even though it involves removal and storage of blood from the circulation, as long as the blood 'does not break contact'.

- **Intraoperative cell salvage**: acceptable to most Jehovah's Witnesses.
- **Red cell substitutes**: perfluorocarbons and Hb solutions may be acceptable to some Jehovah's Witnesses as an alternative to transfusion. These products are not available in the UK, although there are case reports of off-licence use.
- **Alternatives to clotting factors**: there are case reports of the successful use of rFVIIa in Jehovah's Witnesses undergoing major surgery.

Post-operative management

- Intensive care: low threshold for admission. Treat post-operative oozing aggressively. Remember simple measures such as direct compression. Early re-exploration is mandatory.
- Hyperbaric O_2 therapy: in severe blood loss or anaemia, this may swiftly reverse hypoxaemia. However, hyperbaric facilities are not readily available, and the technique has practical difficulties.

References

7 Milligan LJ, Bellamy MC (2004). Anaesthesia and critical care of Jehovah's Witnesses. *Contin Educ Anaesth Crit Care Pain*, 4, 35–9.

8 The Association of Anaesthetists of Great Britain and Ireland (2005). *Management of anaesthesia for Jehovah's Witnesses*, 2nd edn. ℘ http://www.aagbi.org/sites/default/files/Jehovah%27s%20 Witnesses_0.pdf.

Further reading

Association of Anaesthetists of Great Britain and Ireland (2005). *Blood transfusion and the anaesthetist: blood component therapy*. ℘ http://www.aagbi.org/sites/default/files/bloodtransfusion06. pdf.

Hébert PC, Wells G, Blajchman MA, *et al.* (1999). A multicenter randomised controlled trial of transfusion requirements in critical care. Transfusion Requirements in Critical Care Investigators, Canadian Critical Care Trials Group. *N Engl J Med*, 340, 409–17.

Mahdy AM, Webster NR (2004). Perioperative systemic haemostatic agents. *Br J Anaesth*, 93, 842–58.

McGill N, O'Shaughnessy D, Pickering R, *et al.* (2002). Mechanical methods of reducing blood transfusion in cardiac surgery: randomised controlled trial. *BMJ*, 324, 1299.

Shander A (2003). Surgery without blood. *Crit Care Med*, 31, S708–14.

Wallis JP (2003). Transfusion-related acute lung injury (TRALI)—under-diagnosed and under-reported. *Br J Anaesth*, 90, 573–6.

Fluid and electrolyte therapy

Fluid equilibrium (Table 39.3) may be disrupted by illness, anaesthesia, and surgery. This may elicit a combined metabolic, neuroendocrine, immunological, and inflammatory 'stress' response. This response is proportional to the degree of insult and is intended to be protective. It normally subsides within several days of surgery but may be exaggerated/inappropriate.

A short period of fasting in patients undergoing elective minor surgery is well tolerated and does not require fluid replacement. Small volumes of fluid given at the time of minor surgery may be associated with faster recovery and less PONV. Very small children and the elderly tolerate dehydration less well, and replacement should be considered.

Table 39.3 Normal water balance

Intake (2500mL)	Output (2500mL)
1500mL oral	1500mL urine
750mL food	100mL faeces
250mL metabolism	900mL insensible loss

Fluid and electrolyte balance in a 70kg man
See Tables 39.3, 39.4, 39.5, and 39.6.

Table 39.4 Daily requirements of common electrolytes

	Plasma concentration (mmol/L)	Daily requirement (mmol/kg/d)
Na^+	135–145	1–1.5
K^+	3.5–5.0	1–1.5
Mg^{2+}	0.75–1.05	0.1–0.2
Ca^{2+}	2.12–2.65 (total), 1.0 (ionized)	0.1–0.2
Cl^-	95–105	0.07–0.22
Phosphate	0.8–1.45	20–40

Table 39.5 Fluid compartments (70kg adult ♂)

Total body water 55–60% (of weight) = 45L	Intracellular 30L	
	Extracellular 15L	Interstitial 12L
		Intravascular 3L

Table 39.6 Physiological changes during the stress response

↑ Antidiuretic hormone (ADH)	Thirst, water retention, K^+ loss
↑ Cortisol (mineralocorticoid effect)	Na^+/water retention, K^+ excretion
↑ Renin–angiotensin–aldosterone axis	Na^+ reabsorption
↑ Organ osmo-/chemoreceptor activity	Endocrine/sympathetic catabolic state
↑ Systemic inflammatory response	Cytokine-induced capillary leak

Assessment of dehydration

- This is notoriously inaccurate—most patients are more dehydrated than they look, in spite of 'adequate' fluid maintenance therapy.
- Every effort should be made to identify and correct perioperative dehydration and hypovolaemia, as it is associated with considerable morbidity.
- This should begin with detailed clinical examination to identify signs and symptoms of dehydration (Table 39.7).
- Classical signs and symptoms may be absent, especially in chronic dehydration. Careful examination of fluid balance charts and assessment of periods of fluid restriction, GI losses, blood loss, drugs, bowel preparation, or specific disease states that impact on hydration status is essential.
- In particular, '3rd space' losses may account for a significant fluid volume loss, of which the electrolyte content may be large.
- Charting of vital signs over time is useful. Scrutinize trends in BP, pulse, temperature, urine output, and respiratory rate.
- Laboratory indices may be useful. Elevated plasma creatinine/urea/ Hct/albumin and low urine acidity/Na^+ concentration indicate significant dehydration. Plasma lactate/acid–base status may highlight metabolic derangement associated with hypovolaemia and tissue hypoperfusion (Table 39.6).
- CXR may help identify cardiomegaly/pulmonary oedema due to fluid overload.
- Creatinine clearance is a robust measure of renal function and can be estimated at the bedside (see ➔ p. 1055).
- More invasive monitoring (e.g. CVP, oesophageal Doppler, LiDCO™ rapid, Cheetah NICOM), especially with dynamic fluid challenges, is

Table 39.7 Signs and symptoms of dehydration

Body weight loss (%)	Signs and symptoms
5	Thirst, dry mouth
5–10	↓ peripheral perfusion, ↓ skin turgor, postural dizziness, oliguria, ↓ CVP, lassitude, tachycardia
10–15	↑ respiratory rate, hypotension, anuria, delirium, coma
>15	Life-threatening

probably the most reliable method of measuring (and replacing) lost fluid (see ⮞ p. 1016).

Estimation of creatinine clearance (Cockcroft and Gault formula)

$$\text{Creatinine clearance (mL/min)} = \frac{(140 - \text{age}) \times \text{weight (kg)}}{0.814 \times \text{serum creatinine (micromoles/L)}} \quad (\times\, 0.85 \text{ for women})$$

Replacing fluid

- In the fluid-replete adult undergoing a significant period of nil by mouth, replace total daily water requirements of 30–40mL/kg/d, plus total daily electrolyte requirements for Na^+, Cl^-, and K^+ (Table 39.4). In pyrexial patients, increase fluid by 15% for every 1°C rise in body temperature above normal.
- The perioperative period often proves difficult for assessment of fluid losses. In theatre, increased evaporative and 3rd space losses from an open abdomen will not be apparent and may require 10–15mL/kg/hr of crystalloid, in addition to calculated basal requirements.
- Most fluids lost are salt-containing and should be replaced with fluids of similar content. Isotonic formulations of crystalloid equilibrate with ECF (Table 39.5) and are the replacement fluid of choice.
- In the perioperative period, Na^+, Cl^-, and K^+ are often replaced routinely. In illness, Na^+ stores may be well conserved, while obligatory K^+ losses occur, and occult total body K^+ deficiency is common. This will not be reflected by plasma concentration.
- The daily volume and composition of various GI secretions is given in Table 39.8.
- A list of common IV fluid preparations and their constituents is given in Table 39.9.

Table 39.8 Daily volume and composition of GI secretions

	Flow (mL/d)	H^+ (nmol/L)	Na^+ (mmol/L)	Cl^- (mmol/L)	HCO_3^- (mmol/L)	K^+ (mmol/L)
Saliva	500–1000	0	30	10–35	0–15	20
Gastric	1500–2000	0–120	60	100–120	0	10
Bile	500	0	140	100	40–70	5–10
Pancreas	750	0	140	70	40–70	5–10
Small/large intestine	2000–4000	0	110	100	25	5–10

Table 39.9 Composition of common intravenous fluids

	Na⁺ (mmol/L)	K⁺ (mmol/L)	Ca²⁺(mmol/L)	Cl⁻ (mmol/L)	Other	pH	mOsmol/L	Cost (£/L)
NaCl 0.9% (normal saline)	154			154		5	308	1
Glucose 4% NaCl 0.18%	30			30	Glucose 40g	4	263	1
Glucose 5%					Glucose 50g	4	278	1
Hartmann's solution	131	5	2	111	Lactate 29mmol/L	6.5	278	2
Gelofusine®	154	<0.4	<0.4	125	Gelatin 40g	7.4		10
Albumin 4.5%	<160	<2		136	Albumin 40–50g	7.4		95

Dynamic fluid challenge

- Use boluses of 100–200mL of crystalloid.
- Assess clinical and intravascular endpoints, e.g. urine output, HR, SV, BP, CVP, and SVV.
- A sustained rise in CVP of >3mmHg or SVV <10% suggests the patient is well filled.
- An inadequate response is a failure to sustain clinical/CVS endpoint improvement.
- Repeat boluses, with frequent reassessment.
- This should not be considered as treatment for acute blood loss from the vascular compartment.

Crystalloids

- Cheap and effective, with relatively few adverse effects.

Balanced salt solutions

(e.g. Hartmann's (Ringer's lactate) solution)
- Physiological solutions.
- Osmolality is similar to ECF, and thus balanced salt solutions (BSS) are useful for restoring extracellular volume.
- 1st-line replacement therapy in the perioperative period.
- May reduce iatrogenic hyperchloraemic metabolic acidosis, associated with use of higher chloride-containing solutions.
- The addition of K^+ and Ca^{2+} to BSS may limit usefulness in hyperkalaemic states or with citrated blood transfusions.

Normal saline (sodium chloride 0.9%)

- Commonly used for electrolyte replacement.
- Contains high Na^+ and Cl^- concentrations and may be responsible for hyperchloraemic metabolic acidosis, which is of unknown significance.
- Remains the preferred fluid for hypovolaemic resuscitation in many countries, but the intravascular half-life may be limited to 15min. Useful for replacing electrolyte-rich GI losses.

Glucose solutions

(e.g. glucose 5%, glucose 4%–NaCl 0.18%)
- (Dextrose is the preferred name in the United States.)
- Glucose 5% is a convenient way of giving free water, used to restore dehydration associated with water loss. Perioperatively, hyponatraemia may occur with excessive use.
- Glucose in 10%, 20%, and 50% solutions are available to promote normoglycaemia but have little role in routine daily fluid management in adults.
- Sugar-containing solutions provide 4kcal/g of glucose (glucose 5% contains 5g/100mL) and are a considerable energy source, but their potential deleterious osmotic effects limit use, and they have no role as plasma expanders.

Colloids

Colloids are homogeneous, non-crystalline substances, consisting of large molecules or ultramicroscopic particles, which persist in the vascular compartment to expand the functional plasma volume (lasting several hours to several days). Duration of action is determined by physiochemical properties, integrity of the capillary membrane, and metabolic and clearance pharmacokinetics.

Human albumin solution
- Molecular weight (MW) 69 000.
- Available as a 4.5% solution for the treatment of hypovolaemia, and as a salt-poor 20% solution for the treatment of hypoalbuminaemia.
- Like other blood products, HAS is manufactured from fractionation of whole blood. Concern of theoretical transmission of vCJD has resulted in this product currently being imported from the US, and it is thus expensive in the UK.

Gelatins
- Succinylated gelatins (MW 30 000), e.g. Gelofusine® 4%.
- Often presented in NaCl solution.
- Manufactured from bovine collagen from bovine spongiform encephalopathy (BSE)-free herds—there have been no reports of vCJD. Succinylated gelatins undergo thermal degradation during manufacture. Succinic anhydride then replaces free amino acid groups with carboxyl groups, resulting in a conformational change in the molecule size. They have an initially powerful osmotic effect. Administration may rarely lead to histamine release causing bronchospasm, urticarial rash, hypotension, and tachycardia (see below). There is no limit on the total volume that may be administered.

Hydroxyethyl starches
- MW 70 000–450 000.
- Manufactured from hydrolysed amylase-resistant maize or sorghum. HES products differ widely and may be characterized by the concentration, molar substitution, MW, and degree of substitution (DS), which confers solubility and the degree of degradation. Thus there are hetastarches (DS 0.6–0.7), pentastarches (DS 0.5), and tetrastarches (DS 0.4). The greater the DS, the greater is the resistance to degradation, which means that plasma-expanding activity is prolonged.
- 1st-generation starches were associated with considerable side effects, including renal impairment, accumulation, pruritus, and clotting derangements and bleeding. Manufacturers recommend a maximum dose which varies with the formulation—newly formulated 2nd-/3rd-generation HES solutions, with lower MW, may reduce the incidence of unwanted side effects and may be given in volumes of 30 and 50mL/kg/d, respectively.

Adverse effects of colloid solutions
There are clinically important differences in safety among colloids. A 2004 systematic review of 113 publications showed that ~1.3 cases per million transfusions of albumin result in anaphylactoid reactions. Twofold and

4-fold increases are seen with dextran and HES solutions, respectively, while 12 times the anaphylactoid rate was seen with gelatin products.

HES products were withdrawn in the UK in 2013 because of safety concerns over their use as resuscitation fluids in critically ill patients and patients with pre-existing renal dysfunction. In contrast, in the US, the Food and Drug Administration (FDA) has not removed HES solutions completely but recommends that they are not used in patients in critical care or with pre-existing renal dysfunction.

Safety of albumin as a plasma expander

- The use of albumin, when compared to saline, in sepsis does not impair renal function. A meta-analysis of clinical trials of fluid resuscitation with albumin-containing fluids, compared with other resuscitation strategies, in sepsis showed a lower mortality among those receiving albumin. Although the Surviving Sepsis Campaign recommends crystalloids as the initial fluid of choice, it also recommends HAS in patients requiring 'substantial amounts' (precise volumes undefined) of crystalloid. Albumin should not be used as a resuscitation fluid in patients with a severe head injury, as its use is associated with a higher mortality rate.

Hypertonic saline in patients undergoing surgery

- Small-volume hypertonic saline has theoretical advantages for emergency plasma expansion, but a recent Cochrane review suggests that there are insufficient data available to recommend its use in the perioperative setting.

Fluid and goal-directed therapy

- In emergency surgery, there is good evidence that optimal fluid filling, as judged by cardiac stroke volume and cardiac index, reduces perioperative renal failure and reduces the length of hospital stay (see ➲ p. 1016). Only after fluid optimization and the persistence of organ hypoperfusion (elevated lactate, reduced mixed venous O_2 saturation, persisting base deficit) should the delivery of O_2 be increased by inotropic support.

Further reading

BAPEN (2011). *British consensus guidelines on intravenous fluid therapy for adult surgical patients (GIFTASUP).* ⌖http://www.bapen.org.uk/pdfs/bapen_pubs/giftasup.pdf.

Davies SJ, Wilson RJT (2004). Preoptimisation of the high-risk surgical patient. *Br J Anaesth*, **93**, 121–8.

Delaney AP, Dan A, McCaffrey J, Finfer S (2011). The role of albumin as a resuscitation fluid for patients with sepsis: a systematic review and meta-analysis. *Crit Care Med*, **39**, 386–91.

Dellinger RP, Levy MM, Rhodes A, et al. (2013). Surviving Sepsis Campaign: international guidelines for management of severe sepsis and septic shock: 2012. *Crit Care Med*, **41**, 580–637.

Finfer S, Bellomo R, Boyce N, French J, Myburgh J, Norton R; SAFE Study Investigators (2004). A comparison of albumin and saline for fluid resuscitation in the intensive care unit. *N Engl J Med*, **350**, 2247–56.

Gan TJ, Soppitt A, Maroof M, et al. (2002). Goal-directed intraoperative fluid administration reduces length of hospital stay after major surgery. *Anesthesiology*, **97**, 820–6.

Sinclair S, James S, Singer M (1997). Intraoperative intravascular volume optimisation and length of hospital stay after repair of proximal femoral fracture: randomised control trial. *Br J Anaesth*, **315**, 909–12.

Acute pain

Adrian Dashfield

Introduction

Problems with inadequate acute pain management

Severe post-operative pain and the stress response to surgery cause increased morbidity and mortality.

- CVS—tachycardia, hypertension, and increased peripheral vascular resistance cause increased myocardial O_2 consumption/demand and myocardial ischaemia. Altered regional blood flow (sympathetic stimulation), reduced mobility, venous stasis, and increased clotting cause venous thrombosis.
- Respiratory system—abdominal/thoracic pain results in diaphragmatic splinting and weakened cough. Reduction in lung volumes, atelectasis, and sputum retention cause chest infections and hypoxaemia.
- GI—delayed gastric emptying and reduced intestinal motility. This can be a direct effect of pain or as a side effect of opioids and surgery.
- Genitourinary—urinary retention.
- Metabolic/endocrine—release of vasopressin, aldosterone, renin, angiotensin, cortisol, glucagon, growth hormone, and catecholamines, and reduction in insulin and testosterone lead to increased protein breakdown, impairment of wound healing/immune function, sodium and water retention, increased fibrinogen and platelet activation, and increased metabolic rate.
- Chronic pain—there is increasing evidence that patients who suffer from acute pain are more likely to develop chronic pain.
- Psychological—poor acute pain management can lead to patient anxiety, sleeplessness, fatigue, and distress well into the post-operative period.

Measurement of pain

- **Verbal rating scales**—stratify pain intensity according to commonly used adjectives such as 'mild', 'moderate', and 'severe'. They are widely applied and easy for patients to use. The semi-quantitative nature makes them less suitable for research purposes.
- **Numerical rating scales**—take the two extremes of the pain experience and have a numerical scale in between 'no pain' and 'worst imaginable', for example. These scales are robust and reproducible and easy for patients to understand. A disadvantage is that a digital scale reduces the capacity to detect subtle changes, as the digits act as anchoring points.
- **Visual analogue scales**—similar to numerical rating scales, with two extremes of the pain experience on either end of the scale. The patient is asked to mark across the line of standard length (usually 100mm). The distance along this line is used. The continuous data generated make analysis easier than with verbal or numerical rating scales.

World Health Organization analgesic ladder

- In 1986, WHO proposed the analgesic ladder (Fig. 40.1). It was intended to be logical, safe, applicable to many different types of pain, and consist of drugs which are easily available in most countries.

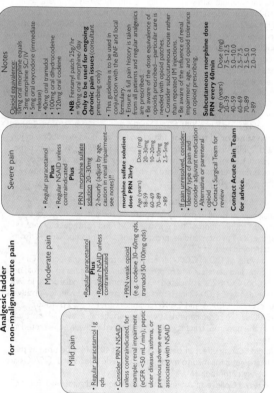

Analgesic ladder
for non-malignant acute pain

Mild pain

- Regular paracetamol 1 g qds
- Consider PRN NSAID unless contraindicated, for example: renal impairment (eGFR <50 mL/min), peptic ulcer disease, asthma, or previous adverse event associated with NSAID

Moderate pain

- Regular paracetamol
  Plus
- Regular NSAID unless contraindicated
- PRN weak opioid (e.g. codeine 30–60mg qds, tramadol 50–100mg qds)

Severe pain

- Regular paracetamol
  Plus
- Regular NSAID unless contraindicated
  Plus
- PRN morphine sulfate solution 20–30mg

2-hourly (adjust by age, caution in renal impairment see notes)‼

morphine sulfate solution dose PRN 2hrly

Age (years)	Dose (mg)
18–59	20–30mg
60–69	10–20mg
70–89	5–10mg
>89	2.5–5mg

- If pain unresolved, consider:
- Identify type of pain and consider adjuvant medication
- Alternative or parenteral opioid
- Contact Surgical Team for review

Contact Acute Pain Team for advice.

Notes

Opioid equivalence:
- 10mg oral morphine equals
- 3mg morphine SC/IV
- 5mg oral oxycodone (immediate release)
- 40mg oral tramadol
- 100mg oral dihydrocodeine
- 120mg oral codeine

- **NB.** Fentanyl patch 25μg/hr = 90mg oral morphine/day **Only to be used for ongoing chronic pain issues** (consultant prescribing only)

- This guideline is to be used in conjunction with the BNF and local formulary.
- Ensure a full pain history is taken from all patients and regular analgesics are prescribed.
- Be aware of the dose equivalence of opioids prescribed—particular care is needed with opioid patches.
- Consider subcutaneous route rather than repeated IM injections.
- Be aware of the influence of renal impairment, age, and opioid tolerance on opioid prescribing.

Subcutaneous morphine dose PRN every 60min

Age (years)	Dose (mg)
20–39	7.5–12.5
40–59	5.0–10.0
60–69	2.5–7.5
70–89	2.5–5.0
>89	2.0–3.0

Fig. 40.1 The WHO analgesic ladder.

Analgesic drugs

Paracetamol

- Action is via a number of central mechanisms, including effects on prostaglandin production, and serotonergic, opioid, NO, and cannabinoid pathways. Analgesic and antipyretic, without anti-inflammatory activity. Excreted renally after glucuronide and sulphate conjugation in the liver. A hepatotoxic metabolite N-acetyl-p-benzoquinoneimine is normally inactivated by conjugation with hepatic glutathione. In paracetamol overdose, this pathway is overwhelmed, leading to hepatic cell necrosis. Toxicity may occur, even within the recommended dose range, in certain patients because of altered metabolism.
- Usually given PO or PR, but available as an IV preparation. Particularly effective when administered IV.
- Recommended dose—4g/d in adults. Most effective when prescribed regularly, rather than PRN. The MHRA licensed dose of paracetamol is the same for all routes of administration in adults over 50kg. In July 2010, MHRA issued a Drug Safety Update for dosing IV paracetamol in neonates, infants, and children, following a number of cases of accidental overdose. The dose in children weighing ≤10kg is now 7.5mg/kg (>10kg: 15mg/kg).

Non-steroidal anti-inflammatory drugs

- Analgesic, anti-inflammatory, antiplatelet, and antipyretic actions are due to inhibition of the enzyme COX, and consequently the synthesis of prostaglandins, prostacyclins, and thromboxane A_2 from arachidonic acid.
- Two types of COX: **COX-1** is normally present in the kidney, GI mucosa, and platelets where prostaglandin contributes to normal organ function. **COX-2** is associated with inflammatory mediators following tissue damage. COX-2 inhibitors may be associated with fewer adverse effects than COX-1 and COX-2 inhibitors (but see ➔ p. 1066).
- NSAIDs have some central, as well as peripheral, activity. Absorption from the upper GI tract is rapid. Metabolized in the liver, excreted in the kidney.
- Opioid-sparing effect of between 20% and 40%. May be used as the sole analgesic for mild to moderate pain. Side effects with NSAIDs are relatively common.
- The Royal College of Anaesthetists has published guidelines[1] for the use of NSAIDs in the post-operative period, suggesting a number of precautions and contraindications (Table 40.1).
- The VIGOR study,[2] in which patients on low-dose aspirin were excluded, found an increased risk of MI for patients given rofecoxib, compared to naproxen. Rofecoxib and some other COX-2 inhibitors have been withdrawn from clinical practice because of further concerns about the risks of CVS events, including MI and stroke.[3] Celecoxib

and etericoxib remain available in the UK for the relief of pain in osteoarthritis, RA, and ankylosing spondylitis. IV parecoxib remains a useful analgesic drug in the perioperative period.

- In January 2010, MHRA assessed the increased thrombotic risk at three additional events per 1000 patient-years.[4] The increased risk relates mainly to MI and includes cerebrovascular and peripheral events in some studies. For the majority of patients, the potential increase in the thrombotic risk is small. In patients with pre-existing risk factors for, or a history of, cerebrovascular disease, the risk may be higher, and therefore coxibs are contraindicated in patients with IHD, cerebrovascular disease, peripheral arterial disease, and moderate or severe heart failure. Caution should be applied to patients with a history of LV dysfunction, hypertension, oedema for any reason, and those with other risk factors for heart disease (Table 40.2).
- The effect of conventional NSAIDS and coxibs on bone healing is unclear. After a fracture, COX-2 results in local release of prostaglandins as part of the acute inflammatory response, which plays a role in the induction of osteoblasts to promote bone healing. Ketorolac has been linked to higher non-union rates after spinal fusion surgery, but studies are often of poor quality and design. There is no robust scientific evidence to discard the use of NSAIDs or coxibs in patients suffering from a fracture, especially if prescribed for a short period of time, to treat acute pain.

Table 40.1 Contraindications to NSAIDs

Relative contraindications	Absolute contraindications
Impaired hepatic function, diabetes, bleeding or coagulation disorders, vascular disease	History of GI bleeding or ulceration
Operations with a high risk of intra-operative haemorrhage (e.g. cardiac, vascular, and hepatobiliary surgery)	Known hypersensitivity to NSAIDs
	Severe liver dysfunction
Operations where an absence of bleeding is important (eye surgery, neurosurgery)	Cardiac failure (NSAIDs cause sodium, potassium, and water retention)
Non-aspirin-induced asthma	
Concurrent use of ACE inhibitors, potassium-sparing diuretics, anticoagulants, methotrexate, ciclosporin, antibiotics such as gentamicin	Dehydration, hypovolaemia, hypotension
	Hyperkalaemia
Pregnant and lactating women	Pre-existing renal impairment
Age >65yr (risk of renal impairment)	Uncontrolled hypertension
	Aspirin-induced asthma

Table 40.2 Comparison of NSAIDs and COX-2

	NSAIDs	COX-2
Efficacy for moderate to severe acute pain (NNT)	Diclofenac 50mg (2.3) Ibuprofen 400mg (2.4) Ketorolac 10mg (2.6)	Celecoxib 200mg (4.5) Parecoxib 20mg (3.0) Valdecoxib 20mg (1.7)
Renal function	Can affect renal function post-operatively	Similar adverse effects on renal function
GI	Acute gastroduodenal damage and bleeding can occur. Risk increased with higher doses, history of GI ulceration, long-term use, and elderly	Less clinically significant peptic ulceration than NSAIDs (VIGOR and CLASS studies)
Platelet function	Inhibit platelet function but do not significantly increase surgical blood loss in normal patients. Associated with higher incidence of post-tonsillectomy haemorrhage	Do not impair platelet function
Aspirin-exacerbated respiratory disease	10–15% of asthmatics affected when given aspirin. Cross-sensitivity with NSAIDs	Do not produce bronchospasm
Bone healing	Impaired in animal models. No good evidence of clinical importance	Similar to NSAIDs

NNT, number needed to treat.

Inhalational analgesia
- **Entonox®** (50% N_2O, 50% O_2) is a quick-acting, potent analgesic of short duration which relies on self-administration.
- **Isonox®** (isoflurane 0.2–0.75% in Entonox®). Lower concentrations of isoflurane produce less drowsiness.[5]
- Ideal for procedures of short duration such as dressing changes, removal of drains, catheterization, labour pain, and application of traction.
- Side effects of Entonox® include drowsiness, nausea, excitability, and augmentation of respiratory depressant drugs.
- Entonox® diffuses rapidly into and increases gas-containing cavities. Contraindications thus include pneumothorax, decompression sickness, intoxication, bowel obstruction, bullous emphysema, and head injury.

Opioids

Opioid drugs act as agonists at opioid receptors, found mainly in the brain and spinal cord, but also peripherally. There are three principal classes of opioid receptor:

- μ—analgesia, nausea and vomiting, bradycardia, respiratory depression, miosis, inhibition of gut motility, pruritus. Endogenous agonists are β-endorphins
- κ—analgesia, sedation, dysphoria, diuresis. Endogenous agonists are dynorphins
- δ—analgesia. Endogenous agonists are enkephalins.

Morphine—remains the gold standard against which all new analgesics are compared. It is the least lipid-soluble opioid in common use. Metabolized in the liver, with only 10% excreted unchanged by the kidney. The metabolite morphine-6-glucuronide is more potent than morphine. The other main metabolite is morphine-3-glucuronide which has no analgesic activity. Both metabolites are excreted in the kidney. Accumulation can occur after prolonged use in patients with impaired renal function. Dose ranges and dose intervals vary according to the route of administration.

Diamorphine—a prodrug (diacetylmorphine) rapidly hydrolysed to 6-monoacetylmorphine and then morphine. Diamorphine is much more lipid-soluble than morphine and thus has a more rapid onset of action than morphine when given by epidural or IV route.

Fentanyl—highly lipid-soluble synthetic opioid with a short duration of action because of rapid tissue uptake. The high lipid solubility makes it suitable for transdermal administration. Metabolites of fentanyl are inactive. Fentanyl is commonly administered IV, epidurally, intrathecally, buccally, or via the nasal mucosa as a spray.

Pethidine—analgesic with anticholinergic and some LA activity. Primarily metabolized in the liver, with metabolites excreted in the urine. One of the main metabolites is norpethidine with a half-life of 15–20hr. Norpethidine is a potent analgesic. High blood concentrations can lead to CNS excitation. Patients with impaired renal function are at risk. Pethidine can be used to treat post-operative shivering associated with volatile anaesthetic agents, and epidural and spinal anaesthesia.

Codeine is a prodrug for morphine. Usually administered for the treatment of mild to moderate pain. About 10% of the dose is converted to morphine. Metabolism to morphine requires an enzyme (CYP2D6) which is part of the cytochrome P450 system; 8–10% of Caucasians lack this enzyme, obtaining little or no benefit.

Tramadol—synthetic, centrally acting opioid-like drug. Less than half of its analgesic activity is at the μ-opioid receptor. It inhibits noradrenaline and serotonin uptake at nerve terminals. Lower tolerance and abuse potential, less respiratory depression and constipation reported, compared to other opioids. Metabolized in the liver and excreted in the kidney. The main metabolite of tramadol is O-desmethyltramadol (M1) which is more potent. Formation of M1 also depends on the presence of CYP2D6 within the cytochrome P450 system (see Codeine earlier).

All opioids are equianalgesic if adjustments are made for the dose and route of administration. Allowance should be made for long-term opioid therapy, incomplete cross-tolerance between opioids, differing half-lives, and interpatient variability (Table 40.3).

Table 40.3 Equianalgesic dosages

Opioid	IM/IV (mg)	Oral (mg)
Morphine	10	25
Diamorphine	5	–
Fentanyl	0.15–0.2	–
Pethidine	100	250
Codeine	–	175
Tramadol	100	100

Opioids have a similar spectrum of side effects. There is considerable inter-patient variability, and some patients may suffer from more side effects with one particular drug compared to another.

Side effects include respiratory depression (decreased respiratory rate, V_T, and irregular respiratory rhythm), sedation, euphoria, dysphoria, nausea and vomiting, muscle rigidity, miosis, bradycardia, myocardial depression, vasodilatation, delayed gastric emptying, constipation, and pruritus.

Opioid antagonists act at all opioid receptors. *Naloxone* is the most commonly used. By titrating the dose of naloxone administered, it is possible to reverse side effects such as respiratory depression, nausea and vomiting, and sedation, without antagonizing the analgesic effects. It must be remembered that naloxone is effective for about 60min.

Opioids—routes of administration
• *Oral.* Oral bioavailability of most opioids is limited due to first-pass metabolism. The slower onset and longer duration of controlled-release formulations make rapid titration impossible. Immediate-release oral opioids (e.g. morphine syrup, oxycodone) are preferred for early management of acute pain. Oral fentanyl should be restricted to treating breakthrough pain in patients receiving opioid therapy for chronic cancer pain.
• *Intermittent SC or IM opioids.* Traditional route of administration ordered 4-hourly PRN. A reluctance to give opioids more frequently than 4-hourly often leads to failure of regimens. Blood levels of an opioid need to reach a minimum effective analgesic concentration (MEAC) before any relief of pain is perceived. This requires an adequate initial dose. The only way to achieve good pain relief is to titrate the dose of opioid for each patient.
• *Intermittent IV opioids.* To achieve sustained pain relief without excessive drowsiness and respiratory depression, small doses of opioids should be given often. This technique of opioid administration is suitable for recovery wards, but not for routine maintenance of analgesia by

untrained staff. Commonly used regimens are 1–3mg of morphine or 20–60 micrograms of fentanyl every 5min, until the patient is comfortable. Morphine can take up to 15min to exhibit its full effect.

- *Continuous IV infusion*. To avoid peaks and troughs in blood opioid concentrations associated with intermittent administration, continuous opioid infusions are sometimes used. Close observation and monitoring of the patient is essential. Patients are best made comfortable with IV boluses to 'load' the patient.
- *Intrathecal opioids*. Intrathecal opioids are administered at the same time as the intrathecal LA during spinal anaesthesia. Fentanyl 10–30 micrograms has a rapid onset (10–20min) and a short duration of action (4–6hr). After a single administration, it can be used in day-case arthroscopic surgery to enhance analgesia, without prolonging hospital stay. Diamorphine 0.3–0.4mg is used for analgesia after an elective Caesarean section. Doses up to 1mg of diamorphine have been used. Intrathecal morphine 0.1–0.2mg has been shown to give good post-operative pain relief following hip arthroplasty; 0.3–0.5mg of morphine similarly provides good post-operative relief following knee arthroplasty.
- *Intranasal diamorphine*. Very effective in children (>1yr) needing acute analgesia. A suitable dosing regime is 0.1mg/kg in 0.2mL of saline (0.1mL to each nostril). To prepare the solution, add 10mg of diamorphine to 20/weight (kg) of saline (mL), and draw up 0.2mL. Fentanyl nasal spray is available as a 50 microgram or 100 microgram metered spray. Use should be restricted to treating breakthrough pain in patients receiving opioid therapy for chronic cancer pain.
- *Transmucosal administration*. Fentanyl lollipops (oral transmucosal fentanyl citrate) allow absorption from the oral mucosa. More frequently used for anaesthetic premedication in children. Can be used for breakthrough analgesia in opioid-tolerant patients with cancer.
- *Transdermal administration*. Very lipid-soluble opioids are absorbed through the skin. Fentanyl patches are available in five sizes (12–100 micrograms/hr), and patches are replaced every 72hr. Buprenorphine patches are available as low-dose 7d-release patches or in higher-dose patches replaced every 72hr. Steady plasma concentrations occur, on average, 12hr after application of the transdermal patch. Dangerously high plasma concentrations can occur if patients are actively warmed while wearing a transdermal patch. Although not suitable for acute pain management, in chronic pain, the recommended dose, based on the daily parenteral morphine dose, is shown in Tables 40.4 and 40.5.
- The Oxford league table of analgesic efficacy is a helpful synthesis of all the available evidence about the relative efficacy of commonly used analgesics. An extract of the league table is provided in Table 40.6.

Table 40.4 Transdermal fentanyl versus morphine

Transdermal fentanyl dose (micrograms/hr)	Oral morphine dose in 24hr	Parenteral morphine dose in 24hr
12	30	4–11
25	60	8–22
50	120	23–37
75	180	38–52
100	240	53–67
125	450	68–82
150	540	83–97

Table 40.5 Transdermal buprenorphine versus morphine

Transdermal buprenorphine dose (micrograms/hr)	Oral morphine dose in 24hr	Parenteral morphine dose in 24hr
5	12	1–3
10	24	2–5
20	48	4–9
35	84	6–15
52.5	126	8–22
70	168	14–22

References

1 Royal College of Surgeons and College of Anaesthetists (1990). *Report of the Working Party on pain after surgery.* London: Royal College of Surgeons of England.

2 Bombardier C, Laine L, Reicin A, *et al.* (2000). Comparison of upper gastrointestinal toxicity of rofecoxib and naproxen in patients with rheumatoid arthritis. VIGOR Study Group. *N Engl J Med*, 343, 1520–8.

3 US Food and Drug Administration (2004). *FDA public health advisory: safety of Vioxx.* http://www.fda.gov/drugs/drugsafety/postmarketdrugsafetyinformationforpatientsandproviders/ucm106274.htm.

4 Medicines and Healthcare Products Regulatory Agency. *MHRA public assessment report. Non-steroidal anti-inflammatory drugs and cardiovascular risks in the general population, January 2010.* http://www.mhra.gov.uk/safety-public-assessment-reports/CON105663.

5 Ross JAS (2000). Isoflurane entonox mixtures for pain relief during labour. *Anaesthesia*, 55, 711–12.

Table 40.6 The Oxford league table of analgesic efficacy

Analgesic	Number of patients in comparison	At least 50% pain relief (%)	NNT	Lower CI	Higher CI
Diclofenac 100mg	411	67	1.9	1.6	2.2
Paracetamol 1000mg + codeine 60mg	197	57	2.2	1.7	2.9
Parecoxib 40mg (IV)	349	63	2.2	1.8	2.7
Diclofenac 50mg	738	63	2.3	2.0	2.7
Ibuprofen 600mg	203	79	2.4	2.0	4.2
Ibuprofen 400mg	4703	56	2.4	2.3	2.6
Ketorolac 10mg	790	50	2.6	2.3	3.1
Paracetamol 650mg + tramadol 75mg	679	43	2.6	2.3	3.0
Ibuprofen 200mg	1414	45	2.7	2.5	3.1
Diclofenac 25mg	204	54	2.8	2.1	4.3
Pethidine 100mg (IM)	364	54	2.9	2.3	.9
Morphine 10mg (IM)	946	50	2.9	2.6	3.6
Parecoxib 20mg (IV)	346	50	3.0	2.3	4.1
Ketorolac 30mg (IM)	359	53	3.4	2.5	4.9
Paracetamol 500mg	561	61	3.5	2.2	13.3
Paracetamol 1000mg	2759	46	3.8	3.4	4.4
Paracetamol 600/650mg + codeine 60mg	1123	42	4.2	3.4	5.3
Aspirin 600/650mg	5061	38	4.4	4.0	4.9
Tramadol 100mg	882	30	4.8	3.8	6.1
Tramadol 75mg	563	32	5.3	3.9	8.2
Paracetamol 300mg + codeine 30mg	379	26	5.7	4.0	9.8
Tramadol 50mg	770	19	8.3	6.0	13.0
Codeine 60mg	1305	15	16.7	11.0	48.0

Courtesy of Pain Research Unit, Oxford—http://www.ebandolier.com.

Patient-controlled analgesia

PCA refers to self-administration of IV opioids and helps overcome the marked variability in response to post-operative opioids. Patients titrate their plasma opioid concentration to remain in the analgesic window (above the MEAC and below the minimum toxic concentration (MTC)). The inherent safety of PCA lies in the fact that excessive doses of opioid will not be delivered, should the patient become sedated. No one but the patient is allowed to operate the PCA demand button.

Patient-controlled analgesia regimens

- The most commonly used opioid is morphine. Fentanyl, pethidine, tramadol, and other opioids have also been used. No opioid is noticeably superior to any other, although a greater incidence of pruritus may be seen with morphine; on an individual basis, one opioid may be better tolerated than another.
- The optimal bolus dose consistently results in analgesia without side effects. Initial values for PCA variables are given in Table 40.7.
- For paediatric use of PCA, see ➔ p. 808.

Table 40.7 PCA regimes

PCA variable	Drug and dose	Comments
Loading dose	0mg	Patients should be comfortable before starting PCA
Bolus dose	Morphine 1mg	Patients over the age of 70yr may require half this amount
	Pethidine 10mg	
	Fentanyl 20 micrograms	
	Diamorphine 0.5mg	
	Tramadol 10mg	
Concentration	Varies, depending on pumps used and hospital protocols	Should be standardized in hospital protocols for each drug
Lockout interval	5min is usual	
Background infusion	0mg/hr	If used, the background infusion rate (mg/hr) usually should not exceed the bolus dose (mg)
Dose limit	30mg morphine or equivalent in 4hr	No clear opinion on how this facility should be used. Often no dose limit is set

Complications

- Equipment malfunction is rare. Interference in pump operation has been reported following current surges and static electricity. Modern PCA pumps have a number of fail-safe design features where the program defaults to the lowest setting possible for a bolus dose. Most machines have a battery backup lasting up to 8hr. Failure of anti-reflux valves has led to cases of respiratory depression.
- Operator error is much commoner. Programming errors, the use of the wrong drug or incorrect drug concentrations, and incorrect background infusions have all been reported and have led to fatalities due to respiratory depression.
- Side effects related to opioid use include nausea and vomiting, pruritus, sedation, respiratory depression, urinary retention, confusion, constipation, and hypotension.

Troubleshooting

- Nausea and vomiting—consider:
  - Adding an antiemetic to the PCA (ondansetron 4mg, cyclizine 50–100mg, haloperidol 2mg)
  - Prescribe an antiemetic on a regular basis
  - Change the opioid.
- Breakthrough pain: add regular NSAID and paracetamol, if not contraindicated. Increase the bolus dose, or consider a background infusion, if severe.
- Respiratory depression: this is caused by the direct action of opioids on the respiratory centre. All opioids, given in equianalgesic doses, have the same potential for respiratory depression. This is a relatively uncommon side effect, and, if doses are properly titrated, the risk is small. The best early clinical indicator of respiratory depression is increasing sedation. Opioid doses are adjusted, so that the sedation score remains below 2 (Table 40.8). Respiratory depression (respiratory rate <8/min) is reversed with IV naloxone (100–400 micrograms).

Table 40.8 Sedation scores

Sedation score	
0	Patient wide awake
1	Mild drowsiness. Easy to rouse
2	Moderate drowsiness. Easy to rouse
3	Severe drowsiness. Difficult to rouse
4	Asleep but easy to rouse

Epidural analgesia

Epidural analgesia is considered by many to be the gold standard analgesic technique for major surgery. It can provide complete analgesia for up to 3d. Patients can mobilize and resume normal activities more quickly, compared to parenteral opioids. Beneficial effects of epidural analgesia result from attenuation of the stress response following surgery.

- The efficacy of epidural analgesia, regardless of the agent used, location of catheter, type of surgery, time or type of pain assessment, has recently been demonstrated.[6]
- The incidence of post-operative atelectasis and pulmonary infection is reduced, improving oxygenation.[7] Effective pain relief allows the patient to cough, breathe deeply, and cooperate with physiotherapy.
- The incidence of post-operative MI is reduced. The myocardial O_2 supply:demand ratio is improved by the reduction of sympathetic activity, improved pulmonary function, and reduced thrombotic tendency.
- The hypercoagulable response to surgery is attenuated, and fibrinolytic function is improved by attenuation of the stress response. This has been shown to be of benefit for graft survival in patients undergoing lower limb revascularization.
- Increased post-operative mobility reduces the incidence of DVT.
- Epidural analgesia improves intestinal motility by blocking nociceptive and sympathetic reflexes and limiting systemic opioid use. The duration of post-operative ileus is reduced, so permitting earlier feeding.
- Intra-operative neuraxial block reduces post-operative blood transfusion requirements.
- There is, however, no survival benefit in high-risk patients, despite being beneficial in terms of pain relief and respiratory function.[8]

Contraindications

- Patient refusal—a full explanation of the risks and benefits of the technique must be given to every patient.
- Untrained staff—staff must have a good understanding of the techniques used and be able to recognize and treat complications.
- Contraindications to catheter or needle placement include local or general sepsis, hypovolaemia, coagulation disorders, concurrent treatment with anticoagulant drugs, and some central neurological diseases (see ➲ p. 722, p. 759, p. 1141).

Troubleshooting

- Breakthrough pain—consider:
  - Adding regular PO/PR/IV NSAID and paracetamol, if not contraindicated
  - Bolus dose (3–5mL), followed by increased infusion rate
  - Check all connections and insertion site
  - Check the block level (with ice or touch). If block patchy or unilateral, withdraw the catheter to 2cm in space
  - Bolus dose of opioid only (fentanyl 50–100 micrograms, diamorphine 2–3mg)

- Pruritus—give naloxone (50–100 micrograms), and consider adding 300 micrograms to infusion fluids or removing the opioid from the epidural infusion. Antihistamines may give some relief [6–8]
- Hypotension—check fluid status of the patient, probably relatively hypovolaemic. Check block height. Consider reducing the infusion rate. If acute/severe, raise the legs; give fluid bolus and vasopressor
- Motor block—reduce the infusion rate. Consider reducing LA concentration
- Complications of epidural analgesia are summarized in Table 40.9 (see also ➲ p. 729).

Table 40.9 Complications of epidural analgesia[9]

Complication	Incidence (%)	Management
Dural puncture	0.16–1.3	Bed rest, analgesia, hydration, blood patch (see ➲ p. 732)
Headache	16–86	Bed rest, analgesia, hydration; suspect dural puncture
Nerve or spinal cord injury	0.016–0.56	Immediate neurological assessment (see ➲ p. 1142 and p. 24)
Catheter migration	0.15–0.18	Remove catheter, and resite if appropriate
Epidural haematoma	0.0004–0.03	MRI or CT scan. Immediate neurosurgical assessment. Antibiotics (see also ➲ p. 24 and p. 1142)
Epidural abscess	0.01–0.05	
Respiratory depression	0.13–0.4	Decrease in opioid concentration may be required
Hypotension	3–30	IV fluids ± vasopressors. Temporarily reduce or stop infusion
Pruritus	10	Naloxone IV (50–100 micrograms) ± antihistamine
Urinary retention	10–30 (in ♂)	Catheterization
Motor block	3	Check for catheter migration. Temporarily cease infusion. Consider epidural haematoma (see ➲ p. 1142)
Other		Possible increased risk of anastomotic leakage after bowel surgery. No evidence to support this

Drugs used for epidural analgesia

To minimize the side effects of each class of drug and provide optimal analgesia, a combination of an opioid and a low concentration of LA solution is given by continuous infusion. Commonly used mixtures are:
- Bupivacaine 0.125% with 5 micrograms/mL of fentanyl or 100–125 micrograms/mL of diamorphine

- Bupivacaine 0.1% with 5 micrograms/mL of fentanyl or 100 micrograms/mL of diamorphine
- Bupivacaine 0.0625% with 2 micrograms/mL of fentanyl or 50 micrograms/mL of diamorphine.

There is no universally accepted optimal combination of drugs. Infusion rates vary, according to the concentration, surgical site, and dermatomal level of the epidural catheter placement. Usual infusion rates for the above solutions are 8–15mL/hr for adult patients, and reduced rates of 4–8mL/hr in patients over 70yr of age. Some anaesthetists reduce or avoid epidural opioids in the very elderly and use LA solutions only.

Intrathecal opioids

Opioids can be administered intrathecally, in combination with LA, during spinal anaesthesia. The opioid is delivered directly into the CSF, so avoiding distribution into epidural fat and blood vessels. Consequently, the doses used are much smaller, compared to epidural or parenteral routes (Table 40.10).

Table 40.10 Comparison of intrathecal opioids

Opioid	Intrathecal dose	Onset (min)	Duration (hr)	Epidural dose
Morphine (preservative-free)	0.1–0.2mg	15–30	8–24	2–3mg
Pethidine (preservative-free)	10–25mg	<5	1–2	10–50mg
Fentanyl	10–25 micrograms	<10	1–4	50–100 micrograms
Diamorphine	0.25–0.5mg	<10	10–20	2.5–5mg

- The more lipid-soluble the drug, the more rapid the onset and the shorter the duration of action.
- Pethidine has LA, as well as opioid, properties. It can be used as the sole drug for spinal anaesthesia (requires higher doses).
- Delayed or late respiratory depression can occur with the less lipid-soluble drugs (particularly morphine). Increasing patient age, high doses of opioid administered intrathecally, concurrent use of sedatives, and systemic opioids are associated with increased risk of respiratory depression.
- Diamorphine (if available) offers the best combination of duration of analgesia with fewest side effects.

Spinal infection

Extreme vigilance is needed for all patients who have had epidural analgesia because of the risk of spinal infection.[10] Pyrexia and/or backache are the commonest signs and symptoms but are not invariable. Only 13% of patients with an epidural abscess present with the classical triad of fever, backache, and neurological signs and symptoms. **Back pain** is the initial symptom in 75% of cases. **Fever** occurs in 66% of cases. Only two out of three patients have a **leucocytosis**. A raised ESR (>30mm) is a consistent finding. A normal CRP does not exclude spinal infection. Monitoring trends is more important than relying on a single measurement. If there is a suspicion of infection, a full infection screen and blood cultures are mandatory. The epidural catheter should always be removed immediately and sent to the laboratory for microbiological investigation. Ninety per cent of spinal infections are bacterial, mainly *Staphylococcus aureus*. MRI with gadolinium is the investigation of choice. The whole spine should be scanned early, before neurological signs and symptoms occur. Once muscle weakness is present, only 20% of patients regain full function, even after spinal surgery. Poor recovery is predicted by patient age (older patients do worse), extent of cord compression, and duration of neurological symptoms (<36hr has better prognosis). Mortality from an epidural abscess is 10%. Treatment is based on surgical or percutaneous abscess drainage and antibiotics. Steroids are contraindicated.

References

6 Block BM, Liu SS, Rowlinson AJ, *et al.* (2003). Efficacy of postoperative epidural analgesia: a meta-analysis. *JAMA*, **290**, 2455–63.

7 Ballantyne JC, Carr DB, deFerranti S, *et al.* (1998). The comparative effects of postoperative analgesic therapies on pulmonary outcome: cumulative meta-analyses of randomized, controlled trials. *Anesth Analg*, **86**, 598–612.

8 Rigg JRA, Jamrozik K, Myles PS, *et al.* (2002). Epidural anaesthesia and analgesia and outcome of major surgery: a randomised trial. *Lancet*, **359**, 1276–82.

9 Royal College of Anaesthetists (2009). *National audit of major complications of central neuraxial block in the United Kingdom. Report and findings, January 2009.* ℳ http://www.rcoa.ac.uk/nap3.

10 Joshi SM, Hatfield RH, Martin J, *et al.* (2003). Spinal epidural abscess: a diagnostic challenge. *Br J Neurosurg*, **17**, 160–3.

Continuous peripheral nerve blockade

There are many potential benefits of continuous peripheral nerve blockade. The quality of analgesia is better, compared with opioids, and the incidence of post-operative side effects, including nausea and vomiting, is decreased. Compared with epidural analgesia for knee joint arthroplasty, analgesia is of equal quality, but the side effect profile is better with peripheral nerve catheters. A recent development is the use of ultrasound to direct peripheral nerve catheter placement. Successful catheter placement relies on a high degree of skill in a practitioner who is already very familiar with single-shot peripheral nerve blockade.

Table 40.11 suggests typical bolus and infusion rates for peripheral nerve blockade—0.5% or 0.25% ropivacaine or levobupivacaine is commonly used for the initial bolus; 0.1–0.25% levobupivacaine or ropivacaine is used for the continuous infusion. Safe doses must be calculated on a per kg basis for every patient. Do not exceed 0.6mg/kg/hr for either levobupivacaine or ropivacaine.

Table 40.11 Typical bolus and infusion rates for peripheral nerve blockade

Catheter site	Initial bolus (mL)	Basal rate (mL/hr)	Patient-controlled bolus (mL)
Interscalene	25–35	3–5	3–5
Axillary	30	5–10	5
Femoral/fascia iliaca	30	4–6	5–10
Sciatic	15–20	2–4	2–4

Absolute contraindications for this technique include: patient refusal, skin infection at or near the puncture site, systemic infection, pyrexia, bleeding diathesis (including systemic anticoagulation), peripheral neuropathy, and compartment syndrome.

Complications include: bruising, haematoma, LA toxicity, peripheral nerve damage, infection, catheter kinking, and catheter migration.

Stimulation-produced analgesia: transcutaneous electrical nerve stimulation and acupuncture

- Stimulation techniques activate the body's pain modulation systems. The gate control theory of pain by Melzack and Wall in 1965 provided a model to explain this phenomenon.
- Incoming noxious pain signals are reduced by presynaptic and post-synaptic inhibition in laminae 1–5 in the dorsal horn of the spinal cord. Modulatory input arrives via the descending pathways and lateral branches from myelinated afferent A-fibres. A-fibres arise in low-threshold mechanoreceptors activated by TENS, and in high-threshold mechanoreceptors responsive to low-frequency needle manipulation (acupuncture).
- A-fibres are recruited at 50–200Hz and respond to low-intensity stimulation. Pain relief occurs immediately but lasts only as long as stimulation continues. A-fibre stimulation increases levels of the inhibitory neurotransmitters dynorphin A and B in the dorsal horn.
- A-fibres are recruited at 2–4Hz and respond to high-intensity stimulation. Pain relief takes 20–30min but lasts hours or days. A-fibre stimulation also increases inhibitory neurotransmitter met-enkephalin levels in the dorsal horn.

The opioid-dependent patient

The principles of acute pain management in the opioid-dependent patient are similar to those previously described. The aim is to bring acute pain under control. Involvement of a multidisciplinary team will often be necessary to manage behavioural, psychological, psychiatric, and medical problems encountered in this group of patients.

- Tolerance, dependence, addiction, and pseudoaddiction—tolerance is a decrease in sensitivity to opioids, resulting in less effect from the same dose. Physical dependence is a physiological phenomenon characterized by a withdrawal reaction when the drug is withdrawn or an antagonist is administered. Addiction is a pattern of drug abuse characterized by compulsive use to experience a psychological effect and to avoid a withdrawal reaction. Pseudoaddiction is an iatrogenic drug-seeking behaviour normally due to undertreatment of acute pain by the physician.
- Symptoms and signs of withdrawal include yawning, sweating, anxiety, rhinorrhoea, lacrimation, tachycardia, hypertension, diarrhoea, nausea, vomiting, abdominal pain, and cramps. On average, these symptoms peak at 36–72hr after the last dose. Aims of treatment must be the provision of analgesia, prevention of opioid withdrawal, and management of abnormal drug-taking behaviour. Non-opioid analgesics, such as paracetamol and NSAIDs, should be prescribed regularly, if possible.
- Opioid-dependent patients normally fall into one of three groups: opioid addicts, chronic non-cancer pain, and cancer pain. The principles of management are the same for each group.

Opioid requirements will, in general, be much higher than in non-opioid-dependent patients. The initial dose prescribed should take the patient's current opioid requirement into account. It may be difficult to judge current opioid use when illicit drugs have been taken. The GP, local pharmacist, or drug rehabilitation centre may provide helpful information.

- Opioid-tolerant patients report higher pain scores and have lower incidence of opioid-induced nausea and vomiting.
- Opioid-tolerant patients are at risk of opioid withdrawal if non-opioid analgesic regimens or tramadol are used.
- PCA settings may need to include a background infusion to replace the usual opioid dose and a higher bolus dose.
- Total dose should be increased, until acceptable analgesia is achieved or until side effects prohibit any further dose increases. PCA with larger-than-average bolus doses is the preferred means of administrating opioids.[11,12] Opioid rotation may be of use, particularly with an agent of higher intrinsic opioid agonist activity.[13]
- The aim is to eventually discharge the patient on no more opioid than was used before admission. Normally, dose reductions of 20–25% every day towards the pre-admission opioid intake will avoid symptoms of withdrawal.
- Oral or SC **clonidine** (50 micrograms tds) can be used to treat symptoms of opioid withdrawal.

- An objective assessment of function, e.g. the ability to cough, may be a better guide to opioid requirements than pain scores. Patients with an addiction to opioids tend to exaggerate pain, in the hope of receiving increased dosages.[11–13]
- Whenever possible, regional analgesic techniques should be used (e.g. continuous lumbar plexus, brachial plexus, or epidural infusions).
- Liaise with all clinicians involved in the treatment of these patients.

References

11 Macintyre PE, Ready LB (2001). *Acute pain management: a practical guide*, 2nd edn. London: Harcourt Publishers.
12 Mitra S, Sinatra RS (2004). Perioperative management of acute pain in the opioid-dependent patient. *Anesthesiology*, **101**, 212–27.
13 De Leon-Casasola OA, Lema MJ (1994). Epidural bupivacaine/sufentanil therapy for postoperative pain control in patients tolerant to opioid and unresponsive to epidural bupivacaine/morphine. *Anesthesiology*, **80**, 303–9.

The patient with a substance abuse disorder

A substance abuse disorder (SAD) exists when the extent and pattern of substance use interferes with the psychological and sociocultural integrity of the person.[14]

Effective management of acute pain in patients with SAD may be complicated by:

- Psychological and behavioural characteristics.
- Presence of the drug of abuse.
- Presence of tolerance, physical dependence, and the risk of withdrawal.
- Medications used to assist with drug withdrawal or rehabilitation.
- Complications related to drug abuse, including organ impairment.

Ethical dilemmas can arise as a result of the need to balance concerns of undermedication against anxieties about safety and possible abuse or diversion of the drugs.

Management of pain in patients with SAD should focus on:

- Prevention of withdrawal.
- Effective analgesia.
- Symptomatic treatment of affective and behavioural problems.

Patients with SAD may be abusing CNS depressant drugs (alcohol, benzodiazepines, opioids) or CNS stimulant drugs (cocaine, amphetamines, ecstasy, cannabinoids).

Drugs used in the treatment of SAD include:

- Methadone—long-acting pure opioid agonist. In the acute pain setting, methadone should be continued at the same dose. If the patient is unable to take methadone orally, substitution with parenteral methadone or other opioids may be required in the short term.
- Naltrexone—pure opioid antagonist administered orally. Binds to opioid receptors for 24hr following a single dose. May create difficulties in the acute pain setting. It is recommended that naltrexone is stopped 24hr before surgery. Usual maintenance dose is 25–50mg daily.
- Buprenorphine—partial opioid agonist used in the treatment of opioid addiction. Commonly prescribed doses are 8–32mg. Continuation of buprenorphine pre-surgery has been suggested, although it may be difficult to obtain good analgesia with full-agonist opioids. Multimodal analgesic strategies should be used.

Patients in drug-free recovery may be concerned about the risk of relapse into active SAD if given opioids for acute pain management. Use of multimodal analgesic strategies, reassurance that the risk of reversion is small, and information that ineffective analgesia can paradoxically lead to relapses in recovering patients help avoid undertreatment.

Reference

14 American Psychiatric Association (1994). *Diagnostic and statistical manual of mental disorders*, 4th edn. Washington DC: American Psychiatric Association.

Non-opioid-based adjuvant analgesic drugs in perioperative care

The occurrence of persistent pain following surgery is becoming increasingly recognized. Acute post-operative neuropathic pain does not usually occur in isolation; there will also be nociceptive pain as a result of tissue damage/inflammation.

- ~14% of patients presenting to the pain clinic attribute their pain to surgery, with the pain beginning acutely.
- Patients may complain of an unusual type of pain different from the usual post-operative nociceptive pain. Patients often describe the pain as burning or shooting in nature. Pain may extend beyond the territory of a single peripheral nerve.
- The pain is often poorly responsive to opioid analgesia, despite high doses being administered and may be:
  - **Allodynia**—pain following a normal innocuous stimulation
  - **Hyperalgesia**—pain disproportionate to a noxious stimulus
  - **Dysaesthesias**—spontaneous unpleasant abnormal sensations.
- The presence of a neurological deficit, such as brachial plexus avulsion or spinal cord injury, makes the presence of acute neuropathic pain more likely.

Treatment

There is currently no published evidence to guide treatment of acute neuropathic pain.

Mechanisms of neuropathic pain involve CNS changes and increased peripheral nerve excitability. Drug therapy focuses on reducing neuronal hyperexcitability and reducing activity of the *N*-methyl-*D*-aspartate (NMDA) receptor in an attempt to reverse neuronal changes.

- **Ketamine.** NMDA receptor antagonist in the CNS and peripheral nervous system. NMDA receptor activation has a key role in the development of central sensitization, wind-up, and pain memory, resulting in chronic post-surgical pain (CPSP). Ketamine has been used as an adjuvant analgesic in a variety of settings, with a reported reduction of up to 25% in pain intensity and 30–50% in analgesic consumption up to 48hr after surgery.[15] The analgesic effect of ketamine is independent of the type of opioid used, timing of ketamine administration, and dose of ketamine.[16] Major side effects are uncommon. Psychomimetic side effects are commoner in patients undergoing awake procedures, compared to GA.[17] At the present time, there is insufficient evidence to recommend ketamine as a routine perioperative analgesic. More concrete evidence is required to ascertain the role of ketamine in modulating the development of CPSP.
- **Gabapentinoids.** Gabapentin and pregabalin are increasingly used as an adjuvant for perioperative analgesia. They act on presynaptic calcium channels and inhibit neuronal calcium influx. They may prevent central sensitization and subsequent hyperalgesia and allodynia. Gabapentinoids may contribute to better post-operative pain management, enhance opioid analgesia, prevent opioid tolerance, and prevent CPSP, as

well as have useful anxiolytic and sleep modulating properties. They are not likely to be sufficiently effective if used as sole agents for the management of acute post-operative pain.[18] Common side effects are drowsiness, dizziness, and gait disturbance.

- **Lidocaine**. Lidocaine has analgesic, anti-inflammatory, and anti-hyperalgesic properties. IV lidocaine is used for the treatment of neuropathic pain. In acute perioperative pain, IV lidocaine has only been found useful in abdominal surgery where anaesthetic and opioid requirements were significantly reduced in the intra-operative period. There is no clear consensus on the dose, but many studies used a bolus of 100mg or 1.5–2mg/kg at least 30min prior to incision, followed by an infusion of 1.33–3mg/kg/hr intra-operatively and up to 24hr post-operatively. No major complications were reported.[19] IV lidocaine may prevent the development of CPSP by its inhibition of NMDA receptors and polymorphonuclear leucocyte priming.

- **α_2-adrenoceptor agonists**. This group of drugs are a useful adjuvant in perioperative care because of several extra analgesic properties, such as sedation, anxiolysis, analgesia, prevention of post-operative shivering and PONV, mitigation of the stress response, anaesthetic-sparing effect, and to supplement neuraxial and peripheral nerve blocks. Act at supraspinal, spinal, and peripheral sites, causing membrane hyperpolarization and reduced calcium conductance into cells. Clonidine and dexmedetomidine are the two commonly used drugs in this class. Dexmedetomidine is ~8 times more specific at the receptor, but analgesic efficacy seems comparable.[20] A recent review showed that systemic clonidine and dexmedetomidine were associated with a moderate decrease in pain intensity, opioid consumption, and early post-operative nausea. Clonidine was associated with increased intra-operative and post-operative hypotension, and dexmedetomidine with increased incidence of bradycardia. The best dose, timing, and route of administration required to produce maximum benefit and minimum harm are unknown. Currently, there is no evidence to suggest that perioperative use of α_2-agonists has a preventive analgesic effect or reduces the incidence of CPSP.

References

15 Bell RF, Dahl JB, Moore RA, Kalso E (2006). Perioperative ketamine for acute postoperative pain. *Cochrane Database Syst Rev*, **1**, CD004603.

16 Laskowski K, Stirling A, McKay WP, Lim HJ (2011). A systematic review of intravenous ketamine for postoperative analgesia. *Can J Anaesth*, **58**, 911–23.

17 McCartney CJL, Sinha A, Katz J (2004). A qualitative systemic review of the role of N-methyl-D-aspartate receptor antagonists in preventive analgesia. *Anesth Analg*, **98**, 1385–400.

18 Tippana EM, Hamunen K, Kontinen VK, Kalso E (2007). Do surgical patients benefit from perioperative gabapentin/pregabalin? A systemic review of efficacy and safety. *Anesth Analg*, **104**, 1545–56.

19 Vigneault L, Turgeon AF, Cote D, et al. (2011). Perioperative intravenous lidocaine infusion for postoperative pain control: a meta-analysis of randomized controlled trials. *Can J Anaesth*, **58**, 22–37.

20 Blaudszun G, Lysakowski C, Elia N, Tramer MR (2012). Effect of perioperative systemic α-2 agonists on postoperative morphine consumption and pain intensity systemic review and meta-analysis of randomized controlled trials. *Anesthesiology*, **116**, 1312–22.

Post-operative nausea and vomiting

Adrian Dashfield

General principles

Definitions
- Nausea is the subjective sensation of the need to vomit.
- Vomiting is the forced expulsion of GI contents through the mouth.

Incidence
- ~30% overall after GA.
- Up to 80% in high-risk patients.

Associated morbidity
- Decreased patient satisfaction, delayed hospital discharge, unexpected hospital admission.
- Wound dehiscence, bleeding, pulmonary aspiration, oesophageal rupture.
- Fluid and electrolyte disturbances.

Anatomy and physiology
- Activation of $5\text{-}HT_3$ receptors in the gut results in stimulation of vagal efferents. Impulses conducted to the area postrema, in the floor of the 4th ventricle, and the lower pons.
- This area has a poorly developed blood–brain barrier, allowing detection of emetogenic toxins, metabolites, and drugs in blood and CSF.
- Can be considered a 'chemoreceptor trigger zone' (CRTZ).
- Afferents from the CRTZ, vestibular apparatus, vagus nerve, gut, and limbic system project to the nucleus tractus solitarius (NTS).
- Multiple central structures throughout the medulla are involved in vomiting, which is no longer considered a vomiting 'centre', but now designated a 'central pattern generator for vomiting'.
- The CRTZ projects neurons to the NTS, which receives input from vagal afferents and from the vestibular and limbic systems.
- The NTS triggers vomiting by stimulating the rostral nucleus, the nucleus ambiguus, the ventral respiratory group, and the dorsal motor nucleus of the vagus.
- Receptor systems—dopaminergic (D_2), muscarinic, serotonergic ($5\text{-}HT_3$), histaminergic (H_1), and neurokinin (NK_1).

Risk factors contributing to post-operative nausea and vomiting

Key factors
- ♀ (3× risk).
- Previous PONV or motion sickness (2–3× risk).
- Non-smokers (2× risk).
- Use of perioperative opioids.

In adults, the incidence of PONV decreases as patients age; for paediatric patients, age increases the risk, such that children older than 3yr have an increased risk of PONV, compared with children younger than 3yr.

Other factors
- Surgery:
  - Breast, ophthalmic (strabismus repair), ENT, gynaecological, laparoscopic, laparotomy, craniotomy (posterior fossa), genitourinary, orthopaedic (shoulder procedures), thyroid. In general, however, the type of surgery does not provide a reliable, reproducible, and clinically useful means of assessing the risk of PONV in adult patients
  - Disproved risk factors:
    — BMI and menstrual cycle phase have no impact on the incidence of PONV
    — The use of supplemental O_2 (FiO_2) does not reduce the incidence of PONV
    — Gastric tube decompression has no effect on PONV.
- Anaesthetic:
  - Premedication—decreased risk after benzodiazepines and clonidine, increased risk after opioids
  - Type of anaesthesia:
    o Volatile anaesthesia is associated with a 2-fold increase in risk of PONV, with risk increasing in a dose-dependent manner. No significant difference between different volatile agents
    o N_2O increases the relative risk of PONV by 1.4
    o Intra-operative and post-operative opioid use increases the risk of PONV in a dose-dependent manner. Opioids reduce muscle tone and peristaltic activity, thereby delaying gastric emptying, inducing distension, and triggering the vomiting reflex. The use of a short-acting opioid, like remifentanil, does not decrease the incidence of PONV[1]
  - Dehydration increases the risk; also too early resumption of food/fluids.

Risk scores for predicting post-operative nausea and vomiting
- Currently, there are two simplified PONV risk scores for adults, and one simplified PONV risk score for children.
  - Koivuranta's PONV risk score features five risk factors: ♀ gender, non-smoking status, history of PONV, history of motion sickness, and duration of surgery >60 min. If 0, 1, 2, 3, 4, or 5 risk factors are present, the incidence of PONV is 17%, 18%, 43%, 54%, 74%, and 87%, respectively.
  - Apfel et al.[2] developed a simplified risk score that reduced the number of risk factors in the model from five to four. The Apfel simplified score includes: ♀ gender, history of PONV and/or motion sickness, non-smoking status, and post-operative use of opioids. When 0, 1, 2, 3, or 4 factors are present, the risk of PONV is 10%, 20%, 40%, 60%, or 80%, respectively.

- The POVOC score is the simplified risk score for predicting PONV in children. The four independent risk factors are: duration of surgery ≥30min, age ≥3yr, strabismus surgery, and history of PONV in the child or of PONV in his/her relatives. When 0, 1, 2, 3, or 4 risk factors are present, the incidence is 9%, 10%, 30%, 55%, or 70%, respectively.

References

1 Apfel CC, Kortilla K, Abdalla M, *et al.* (2004). A factorial trial of six interventions for the prevention of postoperative nausea and vomiting. *N Eng J Med*, **350**, 2441–51.
2 Apfel CC, Kranke P, Eberhardt LH, Roos A, Roewer N (2002). Comparison of predictive models for postoperative nausea and vomiting. *Br J Anaesth*, **88**, 234–40.

Management of post-operative nausea and vomiting

PONV is multifactorial (multiple pathways and neurotransmitters); therefore, a multimodal approach is most effective (Table 41.1).

Pharmacological methods

- Prophylaxis versus treatment remains controversial.
- Three classes of antiemetic drugs are used 1st-line; serotonin antagonists (ondansetron, palonosetron), corticosteroids (dexamethasone), and dopamine antagonists (droperidol) have a similar efficacy against PONV, with a relative risk reduction of about 25%. Each drug results in similar relative risk reduction, giving an additive, but declining, absolute effect.
- Second-line drugs are metoclopramide (D_2 antagonist), but associated with extrapyramidal and sedative side effects. Cyclizine is an antihistamine and is effective, but associated with a significant rate of side effects such as sedation, dry mouth, visual disturbance, and urinary retention. Transdermal scopolamine is a cholinergic antagonist that reduces the risk of PONV by 40% when applied prior to surgery but carries a 3-fold increased risk of visual disturbance, compared with placebo.

Non-pharmacological methods

- Acupuncture—pericardium (P6) point on the palmar aspect of the wrist. As effective as standard antiemetics, but no side effects (number needed to treat, NNT = 5).[3]
- Others include ginger root extract, hypnosis, suggestion, and homeopathy.

The vomiting patient

- Reassurance.
- Correct vital signs appropriately.
- Ensure adequate analgesia and hydration.
- Look for a surgical cause (e.g. distended abdomen—insert or aspirate via NGT).
- Antiemetics:
  - Check if a prophylactic antiemetic was given. Ondansetron is no more effective than placebo for rescue treatment if the patient received a 5-HT_3 receptor antagonist intra-operatively as prophylaxis.
  - Antiemetics administered as rescue treatment should be of a different class than the drug administered as prophylaxis.[4]

References

3 Lee A, Fan LT (2009). Stimulation of the wrist acupuncture point P6 for preventing postoperative nausea and vomiting. *Cochrane Database Syst Rev*, **2**, CD003281.
4 Gan TJ, Meyer TA, Apfel CC, *et al.* (2007). Society for Ambulatory Anesthesia guidelines for the management of postoperative nausea and vomiting. *Anesth Analg*, **105**, 1615–28.

Table 41.1 Drugs available for the prophylaxis and treatment of PONV

Drug	Action	Dose, route, and frequency	Number needed to treat	Side effects	Other points
Hyoscine hydrobromide	Anticholinergic	0.2–0.4mg SC or IM 6-hourly	3.8	Dry mouth, blurred vision, dizziness, confusion (elderly)	Useful for motion sickness, labyrinth disorders, posterior fossa surgery, opioid-related nausea
Cyclizine	Antihistamine	50mg PO, IM, or IV 8-hourly	10	Sedation, dry mouth, blurred vision. Tachycardia and hypotension when given IV	Useful for motion sickness, labyrinth disorders, opioid-related nausea
Prochlorperazine	D₂ antagonist	12.5mg IM, 3mg buccal 6-hourly		Extrapyramidal, sedation	Useful for opioid-related nausea
Metoclopramide	D₂ antagonist	10mg IM or IV 8-hourly		Extrapyramidal, sedation, abdominal cramping, dizziness	Promotes gastric emptying, ↑ lower oesophageal sphincter barrier pressure. Useful for opioid-related nausea
Droperidol	D₂ antagonist	0.5–1.25mg IV, 2.5–5mg PO 8-hourly	5	Extrapyramidal, sedation, neurolepsis, GI disturbances, abnormal LFTs	Used in technique of neuroleptanalgesia

Ondansetron	5-HT$_3$ antagonist	1–8mg PO, IM, or IV 8-hourly	5	Hypersensitivity reactions, headache, dizziness, transient elevated liver enzymes	Paediatrics—drug of 1st choice due to its reduced side effect profile (0.1mg/kg)
Granisetron	5-HT$_3$ antagonist	1mg IV 12-hourly		Hypersensitivity reactions, transient elevated liver enzymes	
Tropisetron	5-HT$_3$ antagonist	2mg IV 24-hourly	6.7 (nausea), 5 (vomiting)	Hypersensitivity reactions, headache, abdominal pain	
Palonosetron	5-HT$_3$ antagonist	0.075mg single dose		Headache, dizziness, hypersensitivity reactions	Recently licensed in the US for PONV
Dexamethasone	Steroid	2–8mg IV single prophylactic dose	4	Wound infection, adrenal suppression	Better in combination with other drugs

Regional anaesthesia

**Adam Shonfeld and
   William Harrop-Griffiths**

Regional anaesthesia

Regional anaesthesia is ideal for many operations, in particular those on the limbs and lower abdomen. For those who do not wish to be fully awake for surgery, sedation can also be used. For many other operations, regional analgesia can complement GA and provide lasting and effective post-operative pain relief.

Although regional anaesthesia has side effects and complications (see ⊃ p. 1142 and p. 24), it is an excellent option for many patients, especially those with major co-morbidities such as significant heart and lung disease. Spinal and epidural anaesthesia are the techniques of choice for a Caesarean section for the vast majority of women. Current research is investigating whether regional anaesthesia can affect the incidence of chronic post-operative pain and tumour recurrence after cancer surgery.

Regional anaesthesia can be accomplished with basic equipment. The use of a PNS will improve the success of a wide range of blocks (see ⊃ p. 1100). Despite the expense, the use of ultrasound machines is established practice in many countries and improves block quality, decreases LA doses, and reduces complication rates.

A detailed knowledge of the anatomy, good manual dexterity, current resuscitation skills, and the willingness to accept that they will need to be committed to deliver the best results are essential for the practitioner.

Unfortunately, regional anaesthesia can never offer 100% success, and a 'plan B' is essential—this will usually be GA. The knowledge, skills, and facilities necessary to provide safe GA are therefore a prerequisite for the performance of regional anaesthesia.

Desert island blocks

No single anaesthetist can be proficient in all blocks. 'Desert island blocks' are those that ideally all anaesthetists should know how to perform, do not require high-tech equipment, and cover as much of the body as possible. A suggested shortlist would include:

- Interscalene brachial plexus block (for shoulder and elbow surgery)
- Axillary brachial plexus block (for every other part of the arm)
- Labat sciatic nerve block (for almost all the leg)
- Femoral nerve block (for the rest of the leg)
- Spinal anaesthesia (for the abdomen).

Other anaesthetists may choose different blocks, but, if you become competent in these five, there is little that you cannot provide for your patients in the way of regional anaesthesia.

Which blocks to use for which operations?

See Table 42.7 for which blocks to use for which operations.

Fundamentals of safe practice

Patient consent and preparation

In order to provide informed consent, a patient needs to have an understanding of the benefits and risks of the proposed therapy and of alternative treatments available to them. In terms of regional anaesthesia, this will include:

- An explanation of the comparative risks and benefits of regional anaesthesia and GA.
- An explanation of how the block will be performed and a description of the use of sedation or GA in addition to the regional block.

Although most countries (including the UK) do not require specific written consent for anaesthesia, the consent process for regional anaesthesia should be documented in the notes, and mention should be made of the specific risks that have been discussed with the patient. Generic complications relevant to most regional techniques include failure, LA toxicity, and nerve damage, and these should be discussed with patients. Complications specific to particular techniques are described with each block (see also ➲ p. 24).

Equipment

The drugs and equipment necessary for resuscitation and the administration of GA should be immediately available and checked. Equipment necessary for the regional anaesthetic should be prepared, and drugs clearly labelled.

Monitoring

This should include the continuous presence of an anaesthetist and the provision of an ECG, NIBP, and pulse oximetry.[1]

Assistance

Trained assistance is as necessary for the safe and effective conduct of regional anaesthesia as it is for GA.

Environment

Regional anaesthesia should, if possible, be performed in a well-lit, quiet, and calm environment, and in an unhurried manner. Appropriate aseptic precautions should be taken, and ready access to additional assistance should be available.

Documentation

In addition to standard logbook data, the documentation of a regional anaesthetic block should include the following:

- Whether the block performed is on an anaesthetized, sedated, or awake patient.
- Block(s) performed.
- Needle(s) used.
- Location technique used (ultrasound, PNS, loss of resistance, etc.).
- Volume and concentration of LA used, along with adjuncts.

- If using a PNS, the stimulus duration and current threshold, and a comment on whether the start of LA injection was associated with 'positive twitch abolition'.
- A comment on whether the injection(s) was (were) easy and painless.
- A note of any complications that occurred.
- A note on whether the block was successful and whether it needed supplementation.

Training and supervision

The era of regional anaesthesia as a 'have a go' subspecialty is now ended. The acquisition of a detailed knowledge of the anatomy and pharmacology should be followed by a study of the block to be performed. The trainee should then discuss the block with an appropriately experienced teacher and should observe the performance of the block on several occasions. The teacher should closely supervise the trainee in the performance of the block for as many times as is necessary, to be confident that the trainee is both competent and safe in the performance of the block.

Personal audit

Regional anaesthetists should keep an accurate and complete record of the blocks they perform. Difficulties encountered, success rates, and complications should be recorded and should be both compared with available published data and discussed in an appraisal process. Lower success rates or higher complication rates than are currently accepted, or any serious complications, should be discussed with an appropriate colleague.

Local anaesthetics and adjuncts

- The duration of action of an LA is related to the extent of protein binding at the site of action and factors that affect removal of the drug from the site, e.g. blood supply. The speed of onset of an LA depends on the local availability of unionized free base. This can be improved by increasing the concentration of the LA or increasing the pH of the LA by the addition of bicarbonate. The acidic, low-pH environment surrounding infected areas, e.g. abscesses, impairs the action of LAs.
- Table 42.1 gives a comparison of the properties of different LAs.

Table 42.1 Properties of local anaesthetics

Local anaesthetic	pKa	Onset	Protein binding (%)	Duration of action	Maximum dose (mg/kg)
Bupivacaine	8.1	Medium	95	Long	2
Levobupivacaine	8.1	Medium	95	Long	2
Ropivacaine	8.1	Medium	94	Long	3
Prilocaine	7.7	Fast	55	Medium	6 (8 with adrenaline)
Lidocaine	7.7	Fast	65	Medium	3 (7 with adrenaline)
Articaine	7.8	Very fast	70	Medium	7
Tetracaine	8.5	Slow	75	Long	1.5
Procaine	8.9	Slow	6	Short	12
Cocaine	8.6			Short	1.5

Choice of agent

A list of commonly used LAs is given in Table 42.2.

- If rapid-onset peripheral blockade for surgery is needed, use **lidocaine** or **prilocaine** 1–2%. The low pKa of these agents means that more molecules are present in the unionized form, and they are therefore able to cross the cell membrane rapidly. For long-lasting post-operative analgesia, use **bupivacaine** or **levobupivacaine** 0.25–0.5%. **Ropivacaine** has a slightly faster onset and slightly shorter duration than bupivacaine. When using large doses of LAs or injecting into areas of rapid uptake, consider the use of levobupivacaine or ropivacaine, which may be associated with a lesser propensity to produce LA toxicity than racemic bupivacaine. If a continuous infusion is used, a low concentration of LA might be preferred, e.g. levobupivacaine 0.1% or ropivacaine 0.2%. **Articaine** is a relatively recently introduced agent for use in dentistry. It has a rapid onset and high safety profile and appears to diffuse through tissues more readily than other agents.

Table 42.2 Commonly used local anaesthetics

Drug	Characteristics
Lidocaine	Medium-acting amide. Moderate vasodilatation. Cerebral irritation before cardiac depression. Duration: enhanced and peak plasma levels reduced by adrenaline. Available in high concentrations for use in topical airway anaesthesia (4% solution and 10mg/dose spray). A class 1b antiarrhythmic
Prilocaine	Medium-acting amide. No vasodilatation. Rapid metabolism and low toxicity. Metabolized to o-toluidine causing methaemoglobinaemia (care in obstetrics and anaemia), caution with doses >600mg (adult). Used for IV regional anaesthesia due to its rapid metabolism
Bupivacaine	Long-acting amide. Racemic mixture of R- and S-enantiomers. Prolonged cardiotoxicity in higher doses
Levobupivacaine	S-enantiomer of bupivacaine. Slightly reduced intensity and duration of motor block, with less cardiotoxicity, than bupivacaine
Ropivacaine	Long-acting amide, pure S-enantiomer. Less duration of motor block than bupivacaine. Less cardiotoxic than bupivacaine or levobupivacaine
Articaine	Medium-acting amide. Licensed for dental use in the UK. Low toxicity and improved penetration of tissues. Available as 4% solution with adrenaline
Tetracaine	Long-acting ester. Rapid absorption from mucous membranes or transdermal route. Relatively toxic
Benzocaine	Short-acting ester. Low potency. Used as lozenges
Cocaine	Short-acting ester. Slow onset, profound vasoconstriction by preventing noradrenaline reuptake. Limited LA use, toxic (hypertension, convulsions, arrhythmias). Part of Moffett's solution (2mL of 8% cocaine, 2mL of 1% sodium bicarbonate, 1mL of 1:1000 adrenaline)

Mixtures of local anaesthetics

- A mixture of a short-acting LA, e.g. lidocaine or prilocaine, and a long-acting LA, e.g. bupivacaine or levobupivacaine, is often used. However, caution should be exercised—the side effects and toxicity are probably additive, and errors may increase if several drugs are used.
- Table 42.3 provides a list of medications commonly added to LAs to improve their effects.

Topical local anaesthetic preparations

EMLA® (Eutectic Mixture of Local Anaesthetics)

- Contains lidocaine 2.5% plus prilocaine 2.5%, Arlatone (emulsifier), Carbopol (thickener), distilled water, and sodium hydroxide.
- Application 1–5hr before venepuncture.
- Side effects include blanching and vasoconstriction.

Table 42.3 Commonly used adjuncts to regional anaesthesia

Drug	Characteristics
Bicarbonate	Added to increase speed of onset by increasing pH of solution, and therefore fraction of unionized LA. Add 1mL of 8.4% to every 10mL of lidocaine or 20mL of bupivacaine. Discard LA if precipitate forms
Adrenaline (epinephrine)	Decreases vascular uptake, thereby increasing duration of LA effect. Decreases peak plasma levels of lidocaine and mepivacaine. Little benefit if long-acting LAs used. Less effective in epidural than peripheral blocks. Do not exceed total dose of 200 micrograms in adult (halve this during halothane anaesthesia). Do not use for digital or penile blocks. Adding 1mL of 1:10 000 solution (100 micrograms/mL) or 0.1mL of 1:1000 solution (1mg/mL) to 20mL of LA produces a 1:200 000 dilution (5 micrograms/mL)
Clonidine	Prolongs sensory and motor block and duration of post-operative analgesia. Acts on α_2-adrenergic receptors. Effective in epidural, caudal, spinal, and peripheral nerve blocks. Use is limited by hypotension and sedation. Use 1–2 micrograms/kg
Ketamine	An NMDA receptor agonist with weak LA properties; 0.5mg/kg may extend and deepen caudal anaesthesia. S-ketamine has better side effect profile
Opioids	Proven synergism with intrathecal and epidural LA. Beware delayed respiratory depression with intrathecal morphine in particular. All opioids have been used. Of doubtful benefit in peripheral blocks. Intra-articular morphine 2–5mg in knee surgery is used in combination with LA by some surgeons. Evidence is weak for its efficacy. Intrathecal remifentanil is contraindicated due to the presence of glycine
Glucose	Used to increase baricity of LA for intrathecal use. Hyperbaric bupivacaine contains 80mg/mL of dextrose. Allows more consistent spread of block and provides the opportunity to control spread by altering patient position
Hyaluronidase	Used in peribulbar and retrobulbar blocks of the eye to enhance LA spread. Dose 15U/mL

- Avoid on broken skin or mucous membranes and in patients <1yr old.
- Can cause methaemoglobinaemia in at-risk individuals.

Ametop® (topical amethocaine gel)
- Contains amethocaine 4%, xanthan gum, methyl and propyl-*p*-hydroxy-benzoate, water, and saline.
- Application 30min before venepuncture, and 45min before cannulation. Remove the gel after 1hr.
- Side effects are erythema, oedema, and pruritus.
- Not recommended in babies <1 month.
- Lasts for 4–6hr after removal of the cream.

Finding nerves

Anatomical techniques

The safe practice of regional anaesthesia is based on a detailed knowledge of the anatomy and its variations. Even though many techniques, based primarily on surface anatomy and the palpation of deeper structures, have been superseded by the use of ultrasound and nerve stimulation, several purely anatomy-based blocks are still effective and practical. Both ultrasound and nerve stimulation still require surface anatomy as a starting point.

Clicks, pops, and loss of resistance

Some techniques, such as the ilioinguinal, fascia lata, and TAP blocks, when used without ultrasound guidance depend upon the sensation of a blunt or blunted needle passing through a fascial plane to identify the correct anatomical location for injection of the LA. These 'clicks' and 'pops' take experience to appreciate and, even for experienced anaesthetists, do not always guarantee correct placement of the needle tip. Some fascial planes, such as the rectus sheath, will produce a 'scratching' sensation if the needle is moved so as to rub against it—this may also guide correct positioning of the needle. Loss of resistance has been used successfully for many decades to identify the epidural space correctly and can also be used for some other techniques such as the TAP block.

Paraesthesiae

Direct contact between needle and nerve may result in an unpleasant 'electric shock' sensation that is felt in the distribution of the target nerve. This is termed 'paraesthesiae' and, before the introduction of nerve stimulation, was often sought as confirmation of needle proximity to a nerve. A popular adage of the 1960s and 1970s was 'no paraesthesiae, no anaesthesia'. With the availability of nerve stimulators and ultrasound machines, paraesthesiae is now seen as a potential indicator of nerve damage resulting from needle–nerve contact. However, paraesthesiae-based techniques remain safe and effective in experienced hands and, in the absence of nerve stimulators and ultrasound machines, have much to recommend them.

Nerve stimulation

The use of nerve stimulators dominated the art of nerve location in the last 20yr of the last century and is still widely practised. The production of evoked muscle contractions at low current levels (0.2–0.5mA) is thought to confirm the placement of a needle in close proximity to a nerve, while the production of evoked contractions at very low current thresholds (<0.2mA) is thought to indicate possible intraneural needle tip placement. If the target nerve contains sensory fibres, the sensation may be unpleasant. The use of nerve stimulators remains rightly popular, either on their own, if no ultrasound machines are available, or in combination with ultrasound to provide the anaesthetist with reassurance that the structure on the screen being approached by the needle is the target nerve.

Using a peripheral nerve stimulator

- Connect the stimulating needle to the negative lead (black) and ground electrode or the ECG pad to the positive lead (red)—'**negative to needle, positive to patient**'.
- Keep the ECG electrode at least 20cm from the site of injection. Start with a current of 1.0–2.0mA and a frequency of 1–2Hz. In theory, a stimulus duration of 0.1ms will preferentially stimulate motor nerves, rather than sensory nerves, and may be less unpleasant for the patient.
- Insert the insulated needle. At all times, move the needle slowly and gently, watching for signs of nerve stimulation. Aim to move the needle in small, steady steps, no more than 1–2mm at a time.
- When muscle contractions are evoked, try to optimize the position of the needle to obtain a good motor response in the muscles supplied by the target nerve with a stimulating current of 0.2–0.5mA.
- Aspirate to exclude intravascular needle placement, and inject 1mL of LA solution; the motor response should disappear, because the nerve is displaced by fluid. Inject the full volume in small boluses, interspersed by careful aspirations.
- If the motor response does not disappear with the initial 1mL, suspect that the needle may be within the nerve sheath. Reposition the needle before further injection.
- If there is any pain or significant resistance to injection, stop immediately, and reposition the needle—it may be in a nerve.

Ultrasound in regional anaesthesia

Ultrasound[1,2] relies on the piezoelectric effect to produce meaningful images from pulsed sound waves of 1–20MHz. The piezoelectric effect occurs when crystals and certain ceramics are deformed by the passage of an electrical current; they also exhibit the reverse effect—they produce an electrical potential in response to physical compression. This property can be used both to send and receive pressure waves in the form of ultrasound; the ultrasound transducer acts as both transmitter and receiver. The delay between transmitting and receiving a signal corresponds to the tissue depth from which the signal was reflected. The strength of the returning signal indicates the amount of reflected waves, which corresponds to the density of the medium. Bone and air both reflect the ultrasound beam and cause shadowing beyond their position. The frequency of ultrasound used is important; the higher the frequency, the better the resolution of the image. When using higher frequencies, the penetration depth is decreased; thus, the highest frequency that can give acceptable image quality should be used.

In-plane and out-of-plane

When using an in-plane (IP) technique, the ultrasound probe is held parallel to the needle, so that the entire shaft of the needle should be visible (as in Fig. 42.1). This has the advantage that you can keep the tip of the needle visible at all times, and thereby avoid its contact with the nerve or other structures that it would be best not to enter. In the out-of-plane (OOP) technique, the ultrasound beam is perpendicular to the needle, and only a cross-section of the needle is visible as a small white dot. Some blocks and approaches lend themselves to the IP technique, and some to the OOP technique. Inexperienced ultrasound users are probably safer using the IP technique if it is practicable for the block being performed; experienced operators can use either IP or OOP safely.

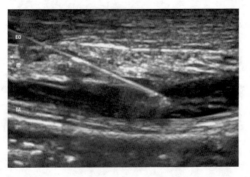

Fig. 42.1 Whole of needle seen with the IP technique for ultrasound (TAP block).
With thanks to Nigel Bedforth.

Practice makes perfect

Manipulating the ultrasound probe and needle, while looking at the displayed image, can be a difficult skill to acquire. While knowledge and experience are important, there are a few tips that will accelerate your passage from novice to expert:

- Get taught properly by experienced ultrasound users.
- Learn from all available media—online videos, ultrasound and cadaver courses, and phantoms, as well as books.
- Do not just scan when performing a block. Use ultrasound machines to scan easily accessible aspects of yourself, colleagues, and consented patients to become familiar with the technology.
- When performing blocks, position yourself, the area being blocked, and the display in a line, so you can easily look from your needle and probe to the display.
- Orientate your probe, so the left and right of the display correspond to the probe.
- The needle needs to be in the beam to be seen; if you cannot see the needle, move the probe, i.e. the beam, to find it; slide it from side to side, and rotate it until the needle is found. You should not advance the needle or inject down it if you cannot see its tip.

Advantages and disadvantages

The use of ultrasound to guide regional anaesthetic techniques has been shown to accelerate block onset, increase block success rate, decrease the dose of LA used, decrease the time taken to perform nerve blocks, and decrease the incidence of certain complications such as vascular puncture. It was hoped, when nerve stimulation techniques became widespread, that there would be evidence of a significant decrease in the incidence of nerve damage when compared to the use of paraesthesiae and landmark methods. While nerve stimulation is now the gold standard, a clear benefit in terms of nerve damage has never conclusively been established. Although it is likely that ultrasound-guided regional anaesthesia will be proven to be associated with a decrease in the incidence of nerve damage, definitive proof is awaited.

References

1 Marhofer P, Harrop-Griffiths W, Willschke H, Kirchmair L (2010). Fifteen years of ultrasound guidance in regional anaesthesia: Part 2—recent developments in block techniques. *Br J Anaesth*, **104**, 673–83.
2 Marhofer P, Harrop-Griffiths W, Kettner SC, Kirchmair L (2010). Fifteen years of ultrasound guidance in regional anaesthesia: Part 1. *Br J Anaesth*, **104**, 538–46.

Needle design

Four types of needle tip design are commonly used for regional anaesthesia, whether PNBs or neuraxial blocks (spinal and epidural blocks). These are:

- **Long-bevelled needles** (usually 10–15°). These are sharp and pass readily through tissues, without giving the operator a clear sensation of passage of the needle through tissue planes and fascial layers. It is argued that, although long-bevelled needles are more likely to enter individual nerves, they are less likely to damage the nerve fascicles if they do so.
- **Short-bevelled needles** (18–45°). These are relatively blunt and give the operator a clearer sensation of the passage of the needle through tissue planes and fascial layers. It is argued that these needles are less likely to enter individual nerves, although they may do more damage to nerve fascicles than long-bevelled needles if they do so.
- **Pencil-point needles**. These are popular for spinal anaesthesia, as they are thought to separate the fibres of the dura mater, rather than cut them as would a bevelled needle. They are associated with a lower incidence of PDPH than the use of the bevelled alternative (often called the Quincke-tip needle). Pencil-point needles used for PNBs are so blunt that they are often difficult to pass through intact skin and provide marked operator feedback—often more than is wanted. It is worth noting that pencil-point needles have an injection orifice proximal to the tip of the needle. This may protect against intraneural injection but may lead to the LA being injected into a different plane to that in which the tip has been placed.
- **Tuohy needle**. This was originally designed to allow epidural catheterization (and remains the most popular epidural needle design in many countries, including the UK), but the tip design has also been adapted for use in placing peripheral nerve catheters.

Other needle tips have been designed, manufactured, and brought into clinical use, but none remains as popular as the four listed above.

Needles designed for use with nerve stimulators are often insulated—coated with a non-conducting material that allows current flow only from a small area at the tip of the needle. Although there is evidence that this increases the current density at the point at which the LA is injected, and thereby may improve the accuracy of nerve location with a PNS, there is also good evidence that uninsulated needles can be successfully used for regional anaesthesia. If available, however, insulated needles should be used.

Continuous regional anaesthesia

Although single-shot PNBs with long-acting LAs can last for many hours, the pain resulting from surgery can outlast them. Continuous regional analgesia (CRA), a technique in which a catheter is placed near a nerve or plexus and LA is injected or infused down the catheter for some hours or even days after surgery, can match the duration of the analgesia to that of the pain. Studies have shown that CRA provides superior analgesia to systemic techniques, while accelerating early mobilization and improving rehabilitation. In addition, the effects of opioid and non-steroidal analgesia are minimized or avoided.

All CRA techniques are based on a single-shot PNB technique. However, the placement of a catheter requires special equipment, scrupulous asepsis, and additional experience. Catheters are placed through a needle, which may be similar in design to a Tuohy needle or may be placed either over a needle or through a cannula that has been positioned close to the nerve. It is possible to confirm the correct placement of a nerve catheter either with the use of ultrasound imaging or by seeking evoked contractions in response to nerve stimulation via a 'stimulating catheter'.

As the catheters are prone to dislodgement, it is wise to insert them through relatively immobile skin and to secure them firmly. Popular sites for catheterization include: interscalene, supraclavicular, and infraclavicular (upper limb); paravertebral (trunk); posterior lumbar plexus, sciatic, femoral, and popliteal sciatic (lower limb).

LA drugs at low concentrations are infused or injected down the catheter to provide analgesia. Bupivacaine 0.1% and ropivacaine 0.2% are popular for this application and seem to be able to provide good analgesia with minimal motor blockade. Pumps that provide a background infusion but have the capacity to provide patient-actuated boluses are increasingly popular. Pumps may be either reusable and electronic or disposable and elastomeric; these latter pumps tend to be lighter and more practicable for post-operative and outpatient use.

Surveillance during CRA is important; the patient needs to be taught how to care for an insensate limb, and both patient and carers need to be taught to identify the signs and symptoms of LA toxicity and catheter sepsis. Nerve catheters can never be 100% successful, and there will need to be a backup plan for analgesia in the event of failure of CRA.

Continuous nerve blocks carry with them all the complications of one-shot blocks, along with additional risks of LA toxicity, catheter misplacement or movement, and bacterial colonization and sepsis. Notwithstanding the fact that the needles used to place catheters are larger than those used in one-shot blocks, there is currently no evidence of an increased incidence of nerve damage associated with CRA.

Nerve blocks: neck

(See Fig. 42.2.)

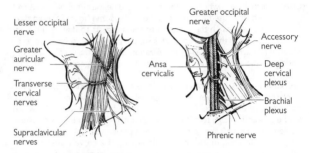

Fig. 42.2 Superficial and deep cervical plexus.

Superficial cervical plexus block

- **Indications**: analgesia or anaesthesia for carotid surgery and other superficial neck procedures.
- **Landmarks**: the superficial cervical plexus comprises four nerves (the lesser occipital, greater auricular, cutaneous cervical, and supraclavicular), which form from the 1° rami of C2–C4 and branch around the posterior border of the sternocleidomastoid muscle (SCM) fanning outwards. The nerves provide sensation to the anterolateral neck. The patient's head should be turned slightly away from the side to be blocked. The point of injection is at the midpoint of the posterior border of the SCM—this is usually at the level of the cricoid cartilage, i.e. the C6 level. After puncturing the 1st fascial layer, LA should be infiltrated 2–3cm cranially and caudally along the posterior border of the SCM, using a total of 10mL.
- **Sono-anatomy**: start by imaging a transverse cross-section of the neck along the posterior border of the SCM. The point of emergence of the nerves around the SCM should be identified. At this point, using an IP posterior approach, LA should be infiltrated just deep under the lateral border of the SCM. The carotid and internal and external jugular should be identified before performing the block to aid avoiding vessel puncture.
- **Side effects of note**: phrenic nerve block, brachial plexus block, vagus nerve block, Horner's syndrome.
- **Complications**: vessel puncture, haematoma formation, intravascular injection.

Deep cervical plexus block

- **Indications**: analgesia or anaesthesia for carotid surgery and other superficial neck surgery.

- **Landmarks**: this will block C2–C4 nerve roots and can be considered a paravertebral block of the cervical region, albeit one accessed from the side of the neck. The patient should be lying supine, with their head turned slightly away from the side of the block. The mastoid process, the transverse process of C6 (Chassaignac's tubercle—at the level of the cricoid, just behind the SCM), and the posterior border of the SCM should be identified. A line should be drawn or marked between the mastoid process and Chassaignac's tubercle. The needle should be inserted at 2, 4, and 6cm distances (this varies with the size of the patient) from the mastoid process along this line to contact the transverse processes of C2, C3, and C4 vertebrae; the transverse processes may be palpable at the appropriate distances. A perpendicular or slight caudad angulation should be used. The needle should not be angulated cephalad, as this will increase the risk of inserting the needle between the vertebrae towards the spinal cord. On contact with the transverse processes, usually within 1–2cm of the skin (rarely >2.5cm), the needle should be withdrawn slightly, and, after careful and repeated aspiration, 3–5mL of LA injected. A single injection at C3 or C4 of 10–15mL may be as effective as multiple injections.
- **Sono-anatomy**: using a transverse plane scan from the base of the neck, moving cranially. After visualizing the C5 root, continue cranially until the C4 root can be seen just posterior to the tip of the shadow of the C4 transverse process, with the shadow of the articular process dorsally. Using an OOP technique with the needle cranial to the probe, advance the needle until it is dorsal to the C4 root, and, after careful aspiration, inject the LA. Scan further cranially, and repeat for C3 and C2.
- **Twitches if using PNS**: C3—scalenus medius, C4—scalenus anterior.
- **LA dose**: 3–5mL per level if multiple injections used or 10–15mL if single injection.
- **Side effects of note**: phrenic nerve block, brachial plexus block, vagus nerve block.
- **Complications**: epidural or intrathecal injection, vertebral artery puncture, injection into the vertebral artery (as going direct to the brain, this may result in immediate seizures).
- **Tips and tweaks**: never perform block on a patient with contralateral phrenic nerve palsy (risk of bilateral phrenic nerve block). The carotid body is innervated by the glossopharyngeal nerve and will require supplemental LA from the surgeon.

Nerve blocks: upper limb

Interscalene brachial plexus block
(See Figs. 42.3 and 42.4.)

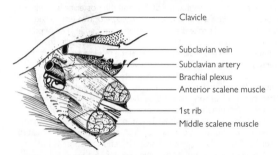

Clavicle
Subclavian vein
Subclavian artery
Brachial plexus
Anterior scalene muscle
1st rib
Middle scalene muscle

Fig. 42.3 Brachial plexus passing over the 1st rib.

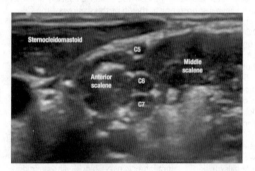

Fig. 42.4 Ultrasound image of the C5, C6, and C7 roots lying in the plane between the two scalene muscles.

With thanks to Nigel Bedforth.

- **Indications**: analgesia or anaesthesia for shoulder, humerus, or elbow surgery.
- **Landmarks**: position the patient with the head slightly turned away from the side of the block. Insertion point is at the level of the cricoid cartilage (C6), lateral to the lateral border of the SCM, in the 'groove' between scalenus anterior and scalenus medius. Winnie describes passing the needle in a 'mesiad, dorsad, and slightly caudad' direction, which can be imitated by directing the needle towards the contralateral elbow. The nerves are very superficial, a depth of no greater than 2.5cm.

- **Sono-anatomy:** the cervical nerve roots can be visualized lateral to the carotid and internal jugular between the scalene muscles, with C5 most superficial and C6, C7, C8, and T1 progressively deeper. A muscle bridge may exist between C7 and C8, which may impair the spread of LA to C8 and T1. Position the probe to give a transverse plane, i.e. a cross-section of the neck. Approach can be IP or OOP. The IP posterior approach requires insertion through scalenus medius and may theoretically risk damage to the dorsal scapular nerve and the long thoracic nerve.
- **Twitches if using PNS:** C5 deltoid, C6 biceps.
- **LA dose:** traditionally ~20mL for analgesia and ~40mL for anaesthesia. If circumferential LA around nerves visualized on ultrasound, these doses may be at least halved.
- **Side effects:** phrenic nerve block (up to 100%), Horner's syndrome, recurrent laryngeal nerve block causing a hoarse voice, subjective dyspnoea.
- **Complications:** vessel puncture, intravascular injection, intrathecal or epidural injection, pneumothorax.
- **Tips and tweaks:**
  - Phrenic nerve stimulation means the needle is too anterior. Levator scapulae stimulation indicates the needle is too posterior (on the dorsal scapular nerve)
  - Triceps or pectoralis major contractions may be acceptable if deltoid or biceps contractions are not found
  - The external jugular may lie over the entry point; note its position, and avoid
  - We recommend that this block only be performed on awake or lightly sedated patients
  - Avoid in patients with severe respiratory disease and contralateral phrenic nerve palsy because of phrenic nerve block.

Supraclavicular block
(See Fig. 42.5.)

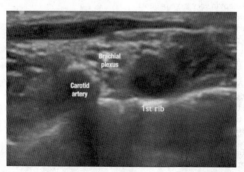

Fig. 42.5 Ultrasound image of the brachial plexus lying adjacent to the subclavian artery as it passes over the 1st rib.

With thanks to Nigel Bedforth.

- **Indications**: analgesia or anaesthesia for elbow, forearm, wrist, or hand surgery. The traditional Kulenkampff technique was abandoned in the 1980s because of the high incidence of pneumothorax. The technique languished until the introduction of ultrasound.
- **Landmarks**: the subclavian artery and brachial plexus are easily visible, as they pass over the 1st rib in the supraclavicular fossa. IP technique with lateral needle entry allows the whole of the needle to be kept in continuous view and to deposit LA accurately around the brachial plexus.
- The subclavian artery is not the only blood vessel in the area, and colour-flow Doppler is advised to identify all vessels close to the plexus.
- Perform injection with an ultrasound image of the artery resting on the 1st rib, not the pleura. This will mean that a needle directed too inferiorly will be more likely to encounter the bone, not the pleura.
- Injection should include the angle between the artery and 1st rib (the 'corner pocket') to increase success rate.
- Pneumothorax still possible, despite the use of ultrasound.
- Rapid onset and good efficacy cause some to call this block 'the arm spinal'.
- **LA dose**: 20–40mL, as necessary, to surround all nerves of the plexus.
- **Side effects of note**: Horner's syndrome, phrenic nerve block.
- **Complications**: pneumothorax, artery puncture, intravascular injection.

Vertical infraclavicular block

- **Indications**: analgesia or anaesthesia for forearm, wrist, or hand surgery.
- **Landmarks**: with the patient lying supine, palpate the sternal notch and the anterior process of the acromion. Mark the midpoint of the clavicle between these two points. The needle should pass just below the clavicle, with the needle placed absolutely vertically—no medial or caudal angulation, as doing so may increase the risk of pneumothorax. The entry point should be moved slightly medially or laterally to achieve appropriate stimulation. Take care with the depth—never go deeper than 5cm, except in very large patients.
- **Sono-anatomy**: position the probe beneath the midpoint of the clavicle to achieve a circular cross-section of the subclavian artery. An IP technique can help to minimize the risk of pneumothorax. It is important to achieve LA deposition posterior and lateral to the artery. This may be achieved with spread from a single injection, or the needle may be repositioned medial, lateral, and posterior to the artery between the artery and each cord to achieve this.
- **Use of ultrasound** allows infraclavicular techniques more distal in the plexus than the vertical infraclavicular.
- **Twitches if using PNS**: lateral cord—elbow flexion (do not accept—too lateral), posterior cord—wrist or finger extension (accept), pectoralis twitch (too superficial).
- **LA dose**: 40mL if single injection, or 10mL per cord, ideally achieve circumferential LA around the cords if they can be visualized with ultrasound.
- **Side effects of note**: Horner's syndrome, phrenic nerve block.
- **Complications**: pneumothorax, artery puncture, intravascular injection.

Coracoid block

- **Indications:** analgesia or anaesthesia for elbow, wrist, or hand surgery.
- **Landmarks:** the arm should be adducted and elbow flexed to 90°, with the forearm placed on the abdomen. The coracoid process of the scapula may be palpated inferior to the lateral 3rd of the clavicle. It must be differentiated from the acromion, which can be palpated as a bony continuation of the distal clavicle. The point of insertion is 1.5cm medial and 1.5cm caudal to the most anterior point of the coracoid. The depth can vary between 3cm and 9cm, depending on body mass.
- **Sono-anatomy:** the use of ultrasound will be technically difficult in patients with a high BMI, as the cords of the brachial plexus will be deep. The ultrasound probe should be positioned in a parasagittal plane just medial to the coracoid process. The subclavian artery and the lateral (musculocutaneous and median nerves), medial (median and ulnar nerves), and posterior (radial nerve) cords should be visualized. Using an IP technique, the needle tip should be advanced until it lies posterior to the artery. Continuous ultrasound monitoring should be used to evaluate the spread of LA while it is injected in 5mL aliquots.
- **Twitches:** pectoralis major—expected at 1–2cm depth (needle too superficial), lateral cord—elbow flexion (do not accept—too lateral), medial cord—wrist flexion (acceptable), posterior cord—wrist or finger extension (optimal).
- **LA dose:** 40mL, less if ultrasound used.
- **Side effects of note:** nil.
- **Complications:** vascular puncture, intravascular injection, pneumothorax.
- **Tips and tweaks:**
  - Never angle the needle medially—increased risk of pneumothorax
  - While proximal spread and anaesthesia around the upper part of the arm may occur, a coracoid block may not block upper arm pain, so, if a tourniquet is used, the block will often need to be combined with a GA.

Axillary block

(See Figs. 42.6 and 42.7.)

- **Indications:** analgesia or anaesthesia for forearm, wrist, or hand surgery.
- **Landmarks:** position the patient with the arm abducted to 90°. Palpate the axillary artery high in the axilla. There are four nerves surrounding the artery that require blocking: the median and musculocutaneous nerves (both above the artery), the radial nerve (usually behind), and the ulnar (usually below). The radial, ulnar, and median nerves are all within the fascial sheath surrounding the artery at ~5–15mm depth. The musculocutaneous nerve has a proximal origin and has usually left the fascial sheath to run in the body of the coracobrachialis muscle at the axillary level at which the block is performed. Membrane compartments may exist and may stop a single-injection technique from blocking all the nerves. A nerve stimulator or ultrasound technique isolating each nerve will have a greater chance of success, but also a greater degree of complexity.

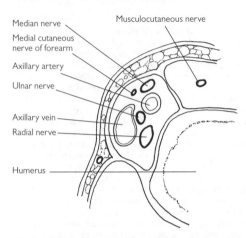

Fig. 42.6 Relationship of the axillary artery and nerves in the axilla.

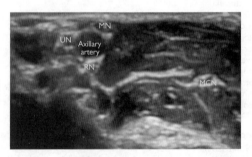

Fig. 42.7 Ultrasound image showing the median nerve (MN), ulnar nerve (UN), and radial nerve (RN) lying around the axillary artery; the musculocutaneous nerve (MCN) lies between the biceps and coracobrachialis muscles.

With thanks to Nigel Bedforth.

- **Sono-anatomy:** the ultrasound probe should be positioned high in the axilla and perpendicular to the humerus. An OOP technique is usually used, but an IP approach can also be used. Following the nerves up from their location at the elbow may help their identification in the axilla. Blocking deeper nerves first will prevent the superficial anatomy from becoming distorted and may prevent air artefacts caused by tiny bubbles in the LA mixture. A distinct 'pop' may be felt on entering the sheath.
- **Twitches:** radial—thumb, wrist, or finger extension; ulnar—adduction of the thumb, little finger flexion; median—finger and wrist flexion

and pronation of the wrist; musculocutaneous—biceps and brachialis contraction (see also ➲ p. 1154).

- **LA dose:** 30–40mL in single or divided doses when using a nerve stimulator—volumes used with ultrasound are much less.
- **Side effects of note:** nil.
- **Complications:** artery puncture (compress for 5min if it occurs), intravascular injection.
- **Tips and tweaks:**
  - Highly variable anatomy exists; the nerve positions may differ, and the musculocutaneous nerve may lie inside or outside the fascial sheath
  - There may be multiple veins within the sheath, and great care should be exercised to avoid IV injection of LA
  - Tourniquet pain is usually caused by axillary nerve and T2 dermatome territory pain, which will not reliably be prevented by axillary nerve blockade
  - Some techniques use intentional arterial transfixion to reach the axillary artery, with 20mL of LA deposited posterior, and 20mL anterior, to the artery. This is now seldom used.

Mid-humeral block

(See Figs. 42.8 and 42.9.)

- **Indications:** analgesia or anaesthesia for forearm, wrist, or hand surgery.
- **Landmarks:** position the patient with their arm abducted to 90°. Palpate the brachial artery one-third of the way along the humerus underneath the biceps. The median, ulnar, and medial cutaneous nerves of the forearm should still be within the fascial sheath with the brachial artery. The median nerve lies above the artery, and the ulnar and median cutaneous nerves lie slightly beneath and superficial to the artery, all within 1–2cm of each other. The musculocutaneous nerve lies above and deep to the artery at 1–3cm. The radial nerve lies on the inferior border of the humerus and is the deepest nerve at 2–5cm.
- **Sono-anatomy:** position the probe to achieve a circular cross-section of the arm one-third of the way from the axilla. An IP technique is appropriate for the more superficial median and ulnar nerves, which are near the artery, and an IP or OOP for the musculocutaneous nerve,

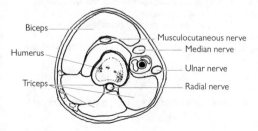

Biceps —
Humerus —
Triceps —
— Musculocutaneous nerve
— Median nerve
— Ulnar nerve
— Radial nerve

Fig. 42.8 Mid-humeral block.

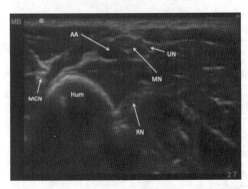

Fig. 42.9 Ultrasound image showing structures at the mid-humeral level: humerus (Hum), axillary artery (AA), median nerve (MN), ulnar nerve (UN), radial nerve (RN), and musculocutaneous nerve (MCN).

With thanks to Nigel Bedforth.

which lies between the biceps and humerus or within the biceps. An IP or OOP technique is appropriate for the deeper radial nerve, which lies between the humerus and the triceps muscle. By rotating the ultrasound probe underneath the arm, the view of the radial nerve may be improved.

- **Twitches if using PNS:** radial—thumb, wrist, or finger extension; ulnar—adduction of the thumb, little finger flexion; median—finger and wrist flexion and pronation of the wrist; musculocutaneous—biceps and brachialis contraction (see also ➲ p. 1154).
- **LA dose:** 5–10mL per nerve, ideally to achieve circumferential LA spread if using ultrasound.
- **Side effects of note:** nil.
- **Complications:** artery puncture (compress for 5min if it occurs), intravascular injection.
- **Tips and tweaks:**
  - Ensure adequate LA infiltration for the needle passing through the muscle for blocking of the musculocutaneous and radial nerves
  - Tourniquet pain will not be prevented
  - Five mL of SC LA over the sheath may help to block the medial cutaneous nerve of the arm
  - Blocking deeper nerves first will prevent image artefacts when using ultrasound.

Elbow block
(See Fig. 42.10.)
- **Indications:** analgesia or anaesthesia for distal forearm, wrist, or hand surgery.
- **Landmarks:**

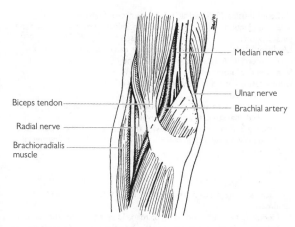

Fig. 42.10 Elbow block (medial, radial, and ulnar) (antecubital fossa, right arm).

- **Median nerve**—position the patient with their arm slightly abducted, elbow slightly flexed, and forearm supinated. Feel the brachial artery at the antecubital fossa crease—the median nerve lies medial and deep to the artery. A pop may be felt on passing through the fascial plane to reach the nerve. It usually lies at 1–2cm depth
- **Radial nerve**—position as for median; nerve lies between the insertion of the biceps and brachioradialis, proximal to the flexor crease in the antecubital fossa. It is slightly deeper than median at 2–4cm depth
- **Ulnar nerve**—the elbow should be slightly flexed, with the arm abducted at the shoulder and externally rotated, so as to expose the ulnar groove at the elbow, or with the hand on the contralateral shoulder and arm across the chest. The ulnar nerve lies in the groove between the medial epicondyle of the humerus and the olecranon process. Pressure neurapraxia may, in theory, develop from blocking at the groove, so the point of injection is often 2–3cm proximal to this, at a depth of 1–3cm.
- **Sono-anatomy**: OOP technique is usually most appropriate; IP may be useful for the median, as the nerve lies near the artery. Following the nerves up from their location at the wrist or axilla may help in their identification.
  - **Median nerve**—seen medial and slightly deeper than the brachial artery.
  - **Radial nerve**—lateral to the biceps tendon lying between the brachialis and brachioradialis.
  - **Ulnar nerve**—trace the nerve from the ulnar groove, 2–3cm proximally. The nerve runs along and then within the triceps.

- **Twitches if using PNS**: radial—thumb, wrist, or finger extension; ulnar—adduction of the thumb, little finger flexion; median—finger and wrist flexion and pronation of the wrist (see also Fig. 42.29).
- **LA dose**: 5–8mL for each nerve. Volumes can be at least halved if circumferential LA achieved with ultrasound.
- **Side effects of note**: nil.
- **Complications**: median nerve—intravascular injection.
- **Tips and tweaks**:
  - A useful block to supplement an axillary brachial plexus block if the required anaesthesia is not achieved
  - Injecting 5–8mL when withdrawing the needle from the median and radial nerves may help in blocking the median and lateral nerves of the forearm.

Wrist block

(See Figs. 42.11 and 42.12.)
- **Indications**: analgesia or anaesthesia for hand surgery.
- **Landmarks**:
  - **Median nerve** passes between palmaris longus (look for the tendon in the middle of the wrist when clenching the fist and flexing the wrist) and flexor carpi radialis. Inject 2–3cm proximal to the wrist creases, at ~1cm depth
  - **Ulnar nerve** runs between the ulnar artery and flexor carpi ulnaris, deep to both. Inject 1–2cm proximal from the wrist creases from the ulnar side of the wrist towards the radius underneath flexor carpi ulnaris, 1cm depth
  - **Radial**—commonly divides above the wrist, purely sensory nerve at this stage. Can be blocked by infiltrating 5–8mL of LA, ~1cm

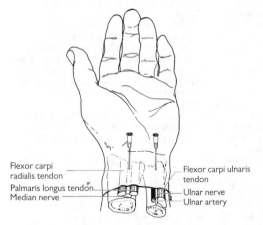

Flexor carpi radialis tendon
Palmaris longus tendon
Median nerve

Flexor carpi ulnaris tendon
Ulnar nerve
Ulnar artery

Fig. 42.11 Wrist block (median and ulnar nerves).

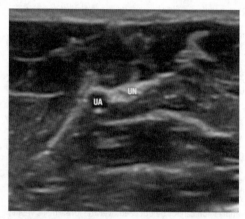

Fig. 42.12 Ultrasound image showing the ulnar nerve (UN) lying adjacent to the ulnar artery (UA) in the forearm.

With thanks to Nigel Bedforth.

proximal to the anatomical snuffbox at the base of the thumb over the dorsum of the radius.
- **Sono-anatomy:**
  - **Median**—follow the median nerve a small distance from the wrist proximally. The nerve may appear to fade at some points. Identify the most superficial and visible point along its path, and, using an OOP technique, inject underneath the nerve, readjusting, if necessary, to achieve circumferential spread
  - **Ulnar**—with the probe just proximal and parallel to the wrist crease, use an IP technique to identify the ulnar artery and nerve; inject beyond the nerve initially, again readjusting to aim for circumferential spread.
- **Twitches:** ulnar—adduction of the thumb; median—minimal 2nd and 3rd finger flexion.
- **LA dose:** median 3–5mL, ulnar 3–5mL, radial 5–8mL.
- **Side effects of note:** nil.
- **Complications:** ulnar artery puncture.
- **Tips and tweaks:**
  - Avoid median nerve block and wrist block in patients with carpal tunnel syndrome.

Digital block

- **Indications:** distal finger/toe surgery.
- **Technique:**
  - The nerves run on either side of the phalanges, two on the palmar side and two on the dorsal side of each finger

- Insert a 25G needle just distal to the metacarpophalangeal joint from the dorsal side (less painful), past the proximal phalanx on either side of the finger to be blocked
- Inject 2–3mL of 1% lidocaine on either side, while withdrawing the needle.
- **Side effects of note:** nil.
- **Complications:** vascular puncture.
- **Tips:** never use adrenaline or other potent vasoconstrictor.

Intravenous regional anaesthesia—Bier's block

- **Indications:** anaesthesia for superficial arm surgery or fracture reduction; maximum operation length of about 30 min. Can be used for lower limb.
- **Technique:**
  - Measure the patient's BP
  - Insert one IV cannula into the limb requiring surgery, and one into another limb
  - Apply a double- or single-cuff tourniquet to the upper arm. Reliable arterial compression cannot be obtained over the forearm, as vessels will be held open between the radius and ulna
  - The limb should be exsanguinated with a compression bandage, such as an Esmarch bandage, or by elevation if fractured
  - The cuff should then be inflated to 50–100mmHg above the patient's systolic BP; if using a double cuff, inflate the distal, then the proximal, cuff; then deflate the distal cuff
  - A non-adrenaline-containing LA with low systemic toxicity should be used such as prilocaine 0.5%—inject slowly; 40mL for small, 50mL for medium, and 60mL for a large arm. Alternatively, lidocaine 0.5% can be used, maximum dose 250mg. Other LAs are not appropriate
  - The patient should be warned that the arm will begin to feel warm and appear mottled
  - Surgery can start within a few minutes
  - On no account should the tourniquet cuff be deflated before 15min for prilocaine and 20min for lidocaine—potentially devastating systemic effects if large volumes of LA are released before it becomes bound or metabolized
  - If tourniquet pain is experienced during the procedure and a double cuff is used, the distal cuff can be inflated before deflating the proximal cuff. The tissue under the distal cuff should be anaesthetized at this stage.
- Technique is contraindicated if pre-existing circulatory difficulties, e.g. crush injury, homozygous SCD, peripheral vascular disease.
- A reliable tourniquet and resuscitation equipment are essential.

Nerve blocks: trunk

Anatomy of the nerve supply to the thorax and abdomen

- The muscles and skin of the chest and abdomen are supplied by the spinal nerves T2–T12, with a contribution from L1 in the inguinal region. These mixed spinal nerves emerge from the intervertebral foramen into the paravertebral space, dividing into the dorsal and ventral rami.
- The dorsal rami supply the deep muscles and skin over the dorsum of the trunk.
- The ventral rami form the intercostal nerves, which pass into the neurovascular plane between the internal and innermost intercostal muscles.
- A lateral cutaneous branch is given off before the costal angle, piercing the intercostal and overlying muscles in the mid-axillary line.
- The intercostal nerves end as an anterior cutaneous nerve.

Thoracic paravertebral block

(See Fig. 42.13.)
- **Indications:** analgesia or anaesthesia for breast surgery, analgesia for thoracic surgery, open cholecystectomy, renal surgery, or fractured ribs.
- **Landmarks:** the paravertebral space lies lateral to the vertebrae and provides access to the thoracic and lumbar nerves that have a minimal fascial covering and can be very effectively blocked. The block can be performed at multiple levels, or a single larger dose will block up to 3–5 levels. To perform the block, position the patient in a sitting or lateral position (block side uppermost). Palpate the spinous processes.

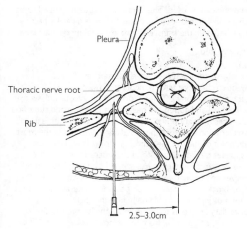

Fig. 42.13 Thoracic paravertebral block.

- The needle insertion point is 2.5cm lateral to the cephalad aspect of the spinous process at the desired block level. The needle should be inserted to contact the transverse process usually at a depth of 2–4cm; note the depth at which this occurs. After contact with bone, withdraw the needle slightly, and change the angle such that the needle will pass cephalad to the transverse process. At this point, a loss of resistance technique can be used, or the needle can be simply inserted 1cm further than the depth at which the transverse process was first encountered. Inject the LA.
- **Ultrasound technique**: the ultrasound probe should be positioned over the spinous processes, with its axis parallel to them. Move the probe 2–3cm laterally to the operative side, so that the transverse processes on either side of the level to be blocked can be seen (hyperechoic edged ovals over large dark shadows). One or more visible lines between the transverse processes indicating the external intercostal muscle or the internal intercostal membrane may be visible. The pleura should be visible between the ribs as a hyperechoic line covering a speckled moving area—the lung tissue. Use an OOP technique, and aim to deposit the LA between the internal intercostal membrane and the pleura. The pleura and lung tissue should be seen to be displaced ventrally as the LA is injected.
- **LA dose**: 5mL per level or 15–20mL at a single level.
- **Side effects of note**: epidural spread, sympathetic block.
- **Complications**: pneumothorax, LA toxicity, intravascular injection.
- **Tips and tweaks**:
  - To reduce the risk of pneumothorax, try to keep the needle tip on the ultrasound image at all times
  - Use small-volume hydrodissection to help gauge when the internal intercostal is passed
  - An IP technique can be used. The ultrasound probe may need to be rotated to a transverse or oblique plane if there is difficulty passing an IP needle between the transverse processes in the sagittal plane.

Intercostal nerve block

(See Fig. 42.14.)

- **Indications**: analgesia for fractured ribs, chest tube insertion, thoracotomy, open cholecystectomy, nephrectomy.
- **Landmarks**: the anterior rami of T1–L1 form the intercostal nerves that supply the intercostal and abdominal muscles and the skin and superficial tissue over the chest and abdomen. The nerves lie underneath each rib in a neurovascular bundle. Before the costal angle, which is at the most posterolateral point of the rib, the nerves give off a lateral cutaneous branch that supplies the lateral trunk and abdomen. There are three intercostal muscle layers—the external, internal, and innermost; the intercostal nerves lie between the internal and the innermost muscles. To perform the block, the patient can be positioned lateral, sitting, or prone. The point of injection should be before the angle of the rib in the posterior axillary line so as to anaesthetize the lateral branch. To identify the rib level, count down from the spinous processes of C7 or

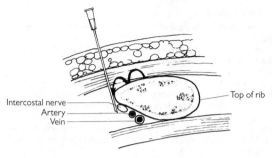

Intercostal nerve
Artery
Vein
Top of rib

Fig. 42.14 Intercostal nerve block.

upwards from the 12th rib or the inferior border of the scapula (T7). After identifying the level to be blocked, the rib should be palpated, and the superior and inferior borders located. The skin should be stretched cephalad slightly, and a 22G needle inserted perpendicularly to touch the tip of the caudad border of the rib. The needle should then be withdrawn 2–3mm, and the cephalad skin stretch released. The needle will now have a caudad angulation and will pass just under the rib. Insert the needle 3–4mm further, feeling for a pop as it pierces the fascia of the internal intercostal muscle. Inject the LA after careful aspiration. In addition, it is normally necessary to block one level above and below the required dermatomes because of crossover innervation.

- **Ultrasound technique**: image the intercostal space with the probe in a sagittal/coronal plane on the posterior axillary line. Identify the two ribs as hyperechoic edged ovals over dark shadows. The pleura should be visible between the ribs as a hyperechoic line covering a speckled moving area—the lung tissue. An IP or OOP technique can be used. If IP, the needle should be caudad to the probe. Insert the needle slowly, keeping the tip visible until it is between the ribs just caudad to the upper rib. LA injection in the correct plane will depress the pleura inwards.
- **LA dose**: 3–5mL per level.
- **Side effects of note**: high LA absorption—risk of toxicity if multiple levels blocked.
- **Complications**: pneumothorax, haematoma formation.
- **Tips and tweaks**:
  - Paravertebral block or thoracic epidural are alternatives if blockade at multiple levels is required
  - Good analgesic option if neuraxial blockade contraindicated due to anticoagulation
  - Avoid if pneumothorax would be catastrophic and chest tube not already in place.

Inguinal field block
- **Indications**: analgesia for inguinal hernia, orchidopexy, or hydrocele surgery.
- **Landmarks**: the ilioinguinal and iliohypogastric nerves are branches of the lumbar plexus, originating from the L1 anterior rami. The nerves run initially in the TAP before piercing first the internal oblique (IO) and then the external oblique (EO) muscles to provide sensory innervation over the lower abdomen and upper thigh. The classical technique relies on performing a plane block between the transversus abdominis (TA) and IO and between the IO and EO to block the ilioinguinal and iliohypogastric, respectively. The point of needle insertion is 2cm medial to the ASIS. Inject after the 1st pop; insert the needle deeper, and inject after the 2nd pop.
- **Ultrasound technique**: ultrasound can be used to identify the correct planes, or it may be possible to locate specific nerves. Place the probe between the ASIS and the umbilicus, and scan caudally. Blood vessels may lie with the nerves and aid in identification. Use an IP technique with the needle medial to the probe. The nerves most commonly lie between the TA and IO, but variations are common.
- **LA dose**: 8mL in each plane.
- **Side effects of note**: femoral nerve block.
- **Complications**: puncture of bowel, intravascular injection.
- **Tips and tweaks**:
  - Fan-wise SC infiltration superficial to the aponeurosis will block the cutaneous supply from the lower intercostals and subcostal nerves
  - SC infiltration at the medial end of incision or fan-wise from the pubic tubercle will block contralateral innervations
  - Five mL injected into the inguinal canal by the surgeon will block the genitofemoral nerve.

Penile block
(See Fig. 42.15.)
- **Indications**: circumcision.
- **Landmarks**: palpate the symphysis pubis above the root of the penis. Insert a 25G needle at the lateral base of the shaft of the penis to just touch the inferior border of the pubis. When contact is made, withdraw slightly; change the needle angle to pass just beneath the pubis—a pop may be felt at 1–2cm when Buck's fascia is pierced. If an assistant pulls down slightly on the end of the penis, the passage through the fascia will become more apparent. Inject 5mL (or 0.1mL/kg of bupivacaine 0.5% in children); repeat on the other side. Performing an additional infiltration SC around the root of the penis onto the scrotum blocks input from the ilioinguinal and genitofemoral nerves but increases the risk of bleeding.
- **Complications**: haematoma.
- **Tips and tweaks**: never use adrenaline-containing solutions. A caudal block may be easier and a more appropriate analgesia for circumcision in infants. If stimulation is noted during the surgery, ask the surgeon to supplement the block (most commonly around the frenulum).

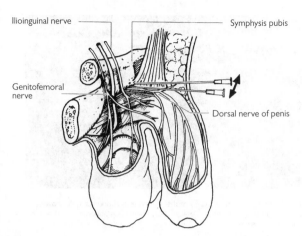

Fig. 42.15 Penile block.

Transversus abdominis plane block

(See Fig. 42.16.)

- **Indications:** analgesia for any surgery on the anterior abdomen.
- **Landmarks:** the anterior abdominal wall is innervated by the anterior rami of T7–L1. The muscle layers from the outside in are the EO, the IO, and the TA. The anterior rami form nerves that pierce the TA and lie in the tissue plane between the IO and the TA. Halfway through their course, the nerves give out lateral cutaneous branches, which travel through the IO and EO to supply the lateral abdominal wall. Therefore, to provide analgesia to the lateral abdominal wall, the nerves must be blocked before this point. After giving off the lateral branch, the nerves finally reach the rectus abdominis, which they perforate to supply the skin of the anterior abdomen. Classically, the block is performed in the triangle of Petit, which is located above the iliac crest, with the muscle of EO forming the anterior border and the latissimus dorsi the posterior border. The EO is still present as fascia in this area, so two pops should be felt as the needle passes perpendicular to the skin, just above the iliac crest before the injection of the LA.
- **Ultrasound technique** (Fig. 42.17): place the ultrasound probe midway between the costal margin and the iliac crest to image in the transverse plane. An IP technique is used, with the probe in the mid-axillary line and the needle anterior to it. The needle should be gradually passed through the skin, SC tissue, the EO, and the IO, until it lies between the IO and TA—this is the TAP. Using hydrodissection and taking care to feel the passage through the EO and IO will aid in achieving an ideal needle position. Inject 30mL here.

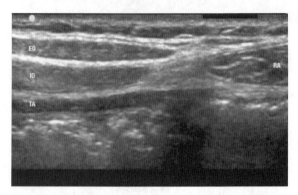

Fig. 42.16 Ultrasound anatomy of the anterolateral abdominal wall, showing the external oblique (EO), internal oblique (IO), transversus abdominis (TA), and rectus abdominis (RA) muscle.

With thanks to Nigel Bedforth.

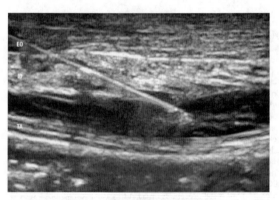

Fig. 42.17 Ultrasound image of TAP block showing the needle and transversus abdominis plane distended by 20mL of local anaesthetic.

EO, external oblique; IO, internal oblique; TA, transversus abdominis. With thanks to Nigel Bedforth.

- **LA dose:** 30mL per side. Care with maximum anaesthetic dose. Volume is more important than concentration, as spread is required to reach multiple nerves.
- **Complications:** puncture of bowel, intrahepatic or intrasplenic injection.
- **Tips and tweaks:** a 2nd injection of 10mL just under the costal margin, using the same technique, may aid in reaching the T7–T10 nerves which are less frequently blocked with a single lower injection.

Rectus sheath block

- **Indications**: analgesia for midline abdominal incisions or anterior laparoscopic port incisions.
- **Landmarks**: the three muscle layers of the lateral abdominal wall combine medially on the anterior abdominal wall and then split to form the anterior and posterior rectus sheaths. The rectus sheath contains the rectus abdominis muscle, which runs craniocaudally from the xiphisternum to the pubic symphysis. The spinal nerves from T7 to L1 lie between the muscle layers of the abdominal wall, before the anterior cutaneous branch enters the rectus sheath and innervates the rectus abdominis, and supplies cutaneous sensation to the skin over the muscle. The aim of the block is to deposit LA anterior to the posterior rectus sheath between it and the rectus abdominis muscle. To perform the block, four points should be marked at 5cm cephalad/5cm lateral and 5cm caudad/5cm lateral on each side of the umbilicus. A short bevelled or blunted 22G needle should be inserted through the skin and SC tissue. The 1st fascial plane is the anterior rectus sheath. A scratch technique of wiggling the needle against the resistance (and feeling a 'scratching' sensation) may make it more apparent before 'popping' through the plane. The needle should then be inserted until a 2nd resistance is felt, but no further, and 10–15mL injected. The technique should be repeated at the other three locations.
- **Ultrasound technique**: perform a scan of the superficial abdomen, using a transverse view across the anterior abdominal wall. Identify the three lateral muscle layers and where they join and divide around the rectus. Roughly at 5cm lateral and 5cm cephalad/caudad from the umbilicus, identify where the anterior and posterior sheath and the rectus muscle are most distinct. Use an IP technique. Insert the needle slowly, until it has passed through the anterior sheath/rectus muscle and lies in the plane in front of the posterior sheath (above the 'tram-lines' of the posterior rectus sheath and peritoneum). Inject 10–15mL of LA here. If the LA tracks along the length of the muscle, a single injection on that side of 20–30mL may be as effective as two separate injections. If inserting a catheter, a 16G Tuohy needle can be used at the cephalad points, and standard epidural catheters passed into the space created with the LA. The catheters may need tunnelling laterally, depending on the surgical site. Alternatively, the surgeon can insert catheters under direct vision following intra-abdominal procedures.
- **LA dose**: 40–60mL in total: 20–30mL per side. Care with maximum LA dose.
- **Complications**: bowel puncture, LA toxicity.

Nerve blocks: lower limb

Lumbar plexus block
(See Figs. 42.18 and 42.19)

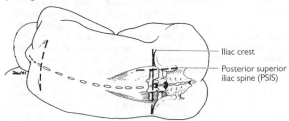

Iliac crest

Posterior superior
iliac spine (PSIS)

Fig. 42.18 Posterior approach to the lumbar plexus (psoas compartment block).

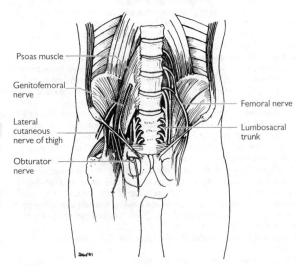

Psoas muscle

Genitofemoral
nerve

Lateral
cutaneous
nerve of thigh

Obturator
nerve

Femoral nerve

Lumbosacral
trunk

Fig. 42.19 Lumbar plexus.

- **Indications**: analgesia or for hip, knee, or femoral shaft surgery.
  Combined with sciatic nerve block, anaesthesia or analgesia for surgery
  to the knee or lower leg.
- **Landmarks**: the lumbar plexus is formed close to the lumbar vertebrae
  and comprises five nerves supplying the lower abdomen and leg: the
  iliohypogastric/ilioinguinal nerve, the genitofemoral nerve, the lateral

cutaneous nerve of the thigh, the femoral nerve, and the obturator nerve. The nerves lie within the body of the psoas muscle. The patient should be in a lateral position, with the limb to be blocked uppermost and the upper hip slightly flexed. Palpate the iliac crests, and mark a line joining them (Tuffier's line—roughly at the L4 level). Mark the spinous processes at this level, and draw a line parallel to them at the level of the posterior superior iliac spine (PSIS). The point of needle insertion is two-thirds of the way between the spinous processes and the PSIS line along Tuffier's line. The needle should be inserted perpendicular to the skin and should contact a transverse process of the vertebrae at about 4–7cm. If this occurs, the needle should be withdrawn slightly and redirected cephalad or caudad, with no change in medial or lateral angulation. The lumbar plexus should be reached at 6–9cm, depending on the body mass, and correct positioning is indicated by quadriceps contraction causing a 'dancing patella' twitch if using a PNS.

- **Sono-anatomy:** a tricky ultrasound block. Due to the depth required, a curved array, low-frequency probe is most suitable. Nerve stimulation should be used alongside ultrasound. Using the position described above, identify the L4 transverse process by scanning cranially from the sacrum. In a transverse plane, deep to the erector spinae and the transversospinal muscles, the psoas major should be visible lateral to the most superficial part of the shadow of the vertebral body. The nerves may be visible within the psoas. If performing the block on an awake patient, use deep infiltration, and use an IP technique with the needle lateral to the probe. Access the posterior part of the psoas muscle, and assess for quadriceps twitch. The depth may be as much as 7–11cm due to the needle angulation.
- **Twitches:** femoral component of the lumbar plexus—quadriceps twitch and patellar dance.
- **LA dose:** 25–35mL.
- **Side effects of note:** epidural spread.
- **Complications:** intrathecal injection, systemic toxicity (nerves located in highly vascular muscle bed), intravascular injection, damage to intra-abdominal organs.
- **Tips and tweaks:**
  - Stimulation currents <0.5mA may indicate the needle tip is within the dural coating of the nerve, and LA injected may track up the nerve sleeve to the epidural or subarachnoid spaces, rather than spreading in the psoas compartment where the rest of the lumbar plexus nerves lie
  - Very difficult in the obese; consider alternatives such as femoral block.

Fascia iliaca block

Fascia iliaca block has become a popular method of providing analgesia, particularly for patients who have suffered from a fractured neck of the femur. While they have a place in providing surgical analgesia, they are also increasingly being used in patients in the emergency department or on the orthopaedic ward before surgery. The block relies on placing a large volume beneath the fascia iliaca plane and allowing spread to give effective analgesia.

- **Indications:** analgesia for patients suffering from a fractured neck of the femur. Combined with spinal or GA, for patients undergoing hip surgery.
- **Landmarks:** at the junction between the middle and lateral thirds of the femoral crease, joining the ASIS and the pubic tubercle. Aim is to be lateral to the femoral nerve. The needle needs to pass through the fascia lata (1st pop) and fascia iliaca (2nd pop).
- **Sono-anatomy:** helpful in ensuring accurate needle tip placement below both layers of fascia. IP-approach needle lateral to the probe, aiming to have a final needle tip position slightly lateral to the femoral nerve. The fascia iliaca runs under the (more lateral) sartorius muscle and on the surface of the iliacus muscle (between sartorius and the femoral artery) and over the femoral nerve. Use small 1–2mL of hydrodissection to ensure the needle tip is below the fascia iliaca before injecting the remaining volume, aspirating between 5mL aliquots.
- **LA dose:** 30–40mL.
- **Side effects of note:** nil.
- **Complications:** nil of note.

Femoral nerve block

- **Indications:** analgesia or for knee or femoral shaft surgery. Combined with sciatic nerve block to produce anaesthesia or analgesia for surgery to the knee or lower leg.
- **Landmarks:** the femoral nerve is best reached after it has passed under the inguinal ligament. The structures here from lateral to medial are: nerve, artery, and vein. The nerve is separated from the vessels by the fascia of the femoral sheath. With the patient lying supine, palpate the pubic tubercle and the ASIS. The inguinal ligament formed from the EO muscle connects to these bones. Palpate the femoral artery beneath the inguinal ligament; ~1–1.5cm lateral to this is the femoral nerve. Insert the needle 1cm distal to the ligament; two 'pops' may be felt as the needle passes the fascia lata, then the fascia iliaca. Depth to nerve of 2–4cm.
- **Sono-anatomy:** IP or OOP can be used. IP needle lateral to probe. Try to deposit the LA deep and medial to the nerve at first. Reposition the needle, if necessary, to try to achieve circumferential spread.
- **Twitches:** femoral nerve—patella dance, if sartorius—needle too medial or superficial; withdraw and redirect laterally, and go slightly deeper.
- **LA dose:** 10–20mL for the femoral nerve (30–40mL for '3-in-1 block', apply pressure 2–3cm distal to the site of injection; the intention is for the LA to spread proximally and block the obturator and lateral cutaneous nerve of the thigh. In reality, the spread of the LA is lateral and does not reliably block the other two nerves.)
- **Side effects of note:** nil.
- **Complications:** arterial puncture, intravascular injection.

Lateral cutaneous nerve of the thigh block

- **Indications:** analgesia for hip or femoral shaft surgery with incision in the lateral thigh.
- **Landmarks:** the nerve runs under the inguinal ligament, just medial to the ASIS and over the sartorius muscle. The nerve can be blocked 2cm

medial and 2cm caudal to the ASIS. Insert the needle perpendicular to the skin to a depth of 1–3cm, until you feel the needle pass through the fascia lata, and inject here.

- **Sono-anatomy:** use an OOP needle distal to the probe or IP with the needle medial. Scan distally, starting just medial to the ASIS, and identify the nerve below the inguinal ligament medial to the sartorius muscle. The nerve is small; hydrodissection may help identify its position between the fascia lata and fascia iliaca.
- **LA dose:** 5–10mL.
- **Side effects of note:** nil.
- **Complications:** femoral nerve block.

Sciatic nerve block

(See Figs. 42.20 and 42.21.)

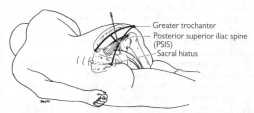

Greater trochanter
Posterior superior iliac spine (PSIS)
Sacral hiatus

Fig. 42.20 Posterior (Labat) approach to the sciatic nerve.

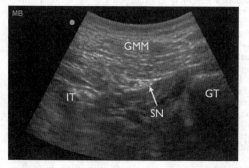

Fig. 42.21 Ultrasound image of the sciatic nerve (SN, arrow) as it passes underneath the gluteus maximus muscle (GMM) and between the greater trochanter (GT) and ischial tuberosity (IT).

With thanks to Nigel Bedforth.

- **Indications**: analgesia for ankle or foot surgery, or for lower limb amputation. Combined with femoral nerve block or lumbar plexus block for total anaesthesia of the leg.
- **Landmarks**: the sciatic nerve is the largest nerve in the body. It is formed from L4 to S3 nerve roots and exits the pelvis via the sciatic foramen before continuing down the leg between the muscles in the posterior thigh.
  - **Labat**—position the patient in the Sims' position/recovery position, with the operative leg uppermost. Identify and mark the PSIS, the greater trochanter (GT) of the femur, and the sacral hiatus (SH). Draw a line between the PSIS and GT, and between the GT and SH. Draw a 3rd line perpendicular from the midpoint between the PSIS and GT to intersect the 2nd line. This is the point of needle insertion perpendicular to the skin to a depth of 5–10cm.
  - **Raj**—with the patient supine, flex the hip and knee to 90°. The point of needle insertion is halfway between the ischial tuberosity (IT) on the inferomedial border and the GT on the inferolateral border of the thigh. With a perpendicular or slightly medial angulation, the nerve should be encountered at a depth of 4–8cm.
- **Ultrasound techniques**:
  - **Labat**—a curved, low-frequency probe is needed due to the depth required. The depth makes the sciatic nerve difficult to visualize. The nerve may be round or flat. Use the landmark technique to position the probe over the traditional needle insertion site. The sciatic nerve lies deep to the gluteus maximus, lateral to the pudendal blood vessels, and runs over the ischial bone. Scan cephalad and caudad from the starting point, and try different angles to optimize the ultrasound image. An IP technique with the needle lateral to the probe or an OOP technique may be used. The depth means that it will be difficult to keep the needle tip under direct vision. Due to the size of the nerve, two needle positions—one medial and one lateral to the nerve—are usually required to achieve circumferential spread.
  - **Subgluteal**—here the sciatic nerve is more superficial, enabling easier ultrasound imaging. Position the patient lateral or semiprone. In the position described in the Raj technique, between the IT and GT, use a curved array probe, and scan across the region, identifying the IT, GT, gluteus maximus muscle (the large superficial muscle under the skin), and quadratus femoris muscle under the gluteus maximus. The sciatic nerve lies in the tissue plane between the gluteus maximus and quadratus femoris. The nerve can be blocked here, or it can be traced to a more superficial position midway down the thigh and blocked passing the needle between the flexor tendons. Nerve stimulation is helpful in confirming nerve location. IP with the needle lateral to the probe or OOP techniques can be used.
- **Twitches**: tibial component—plantar flexion of the foot (optimal); common peroneal component—eversion of the foot (withdraw the needle, and aim more medially); gluteal muscles—direct stimulation; needle too shallow.
- **LA dose**: 15–30mL.

- Side effects of note: nil.
- **Complications**: intravascular injection is not uncommon.
- **Tips and tweaks**:
  - Care with LA maximum doses if performing with femoral or lumbar plexus blocks.

Popliteal sciatic nerve block
(See Fig. 42.22.)

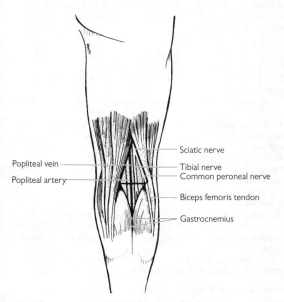

Fig. 42.22 Popliteal fossa block (right leg).

Labels on figure:
- Sciatic nerve
- Popliteal vein
- Tibial nerve
- Common peroneal nerve
- Popliteal artery
- Biceps femoris tendon
- Gastrocnemius

The popliteal fossa is a diamond-shaped area, bounded inferiorly by the medial and lateral heads of the gastrocnemius and superiorly by the long head of the biceps femoris (laterally) and the superimposed heads of the semimembranosus and semitendinosus (medially). The posterior skin crease marks the widest point of the fossa, and, with the knee slightly flexed, the muscular boundaries of the fossa can be identified. This block is indicated for ankle and foot surgery.

Posterior approach
- With the patient prone, flex the knee; identify and mark the muscular borders of the fossa, and then straighten the leg.
- Mark a point 7–10cm proximal to the popliteal skin crease, in the midline between the biceps femoris (laterally) and semitendinosus and semimembranosus (medially).
- Insert a 22G 50mm or 100mm needle (depending on the size of the patient) at this point, directing the needle proximally at an angle of 45°.
- At a depth of 4–8cm, the sciatic nerve or components will be found (tibial—plantar flexion, common peroneal—dorsiflexion).
- Inject 20–30mL of LA.

Lateral approach
- Supine, with the knee slightly flexed, mark the groove between the vastus lateralis (above) and biceps femoris (below).
- Draw a line down from the superior border of the patella where it crosses this groove.
- Insert a 22G 100mm needle, directed posteriorly 25–30° and slightly caudally.
- The needle passes through the biceps femoris into the popliteal fossa—initially encountering the common peroneal nerve, then the tibial nerve.
- Inject 10mL of LA around each nerve.
- **Ultrasound technique**: essentially a lateral approach, but with the knee flexed and the probe placed at the back of the knee; the nerves are readily identified, and an IP technique can be used.
- **Tips and tweaks**:
  - The sciatic nerve is two nerves loosely bound together at this level, commonly dividing into the tibial and peroneal nerves 5–12cm above the popliteal crease. In a small proportion of people, it is separated for its entire course
  - High-volume popliteal techniques—often block both nerves, but individual localization of both nerves may improve success rate.

Saphenous nerve block

Provides analgesia for the medial lower leg and ankle; useful in combination with a sciatic nerve block for foot and ankle procedures.
- **Landmarks**: tibial tuberosity, medial tibial condyle.
- **Technique**: the patient should be supine, with the leg externally rotated. Identify the tibial tuberosity, and inject 10–15mL SC from the tibial tuberosity towards the medial tibial condyle.
- **Ultrasound techniques** allow saphenous nerve block in the thigh.

Ankle block

(See Figs. 42.23 and 42.24.)
- **Indications**: analgesia or anaesthesia for surgery on the foot.
- **Landmarks**: five nerves innervate the foot. The saphenous nerve is the terminal branch of the femoral nerve (innervates the medial aspect of the ankle and foot); the sural (lateral aspect of the foot and the 5th toe), tibial (sole of the foot and many of the intrinsic muscles), and superficial

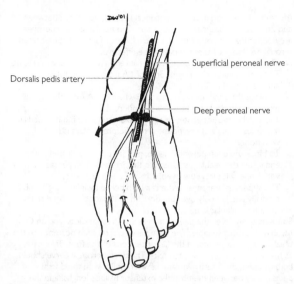

Fig. 42.23 Ankle block I.

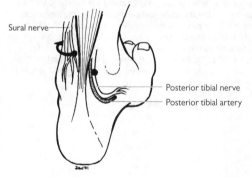

Fig. 42.24 Ankle block II.

(dorsum of the foot) and deep peroneal nerves (web space between 1st and 2nd toe) are branches of the sciatic. The tibial and deep peroneal are deeper than the other nerves, and a layer of fascia must be passed through for block of these nerves to be effective.

- The saphenous nerve usually passes anterior to the medial malleolus. To block it, infiltrate a ring of 5mL of LA from the medial malleolus anteriorly to the tibial ridge.
- To block the sural nerve, raise an SC wheal of LA from the lateral malleolus inferiorly to the Achilles tendon.
- The tibial nerve lies posterior to the tibial artery behind the medial malleolus. Inject just behind the artery before contact is made with bone.
- To block the deep peroneal nerve, palpate the dorsalis pedis artery, and insert the needle just lateral to the artery. When contact is made with bone, withdraw the needle slightly, and inject here.
- The superficial peroneal nerve can be blocked by infiltrating 10mL SC medially and laterally over the dorsum of the foot, 2–3cm distal to the intermalleolar line.

- **Sono-anatomy**: even the deeper nerves are still superficial, and an OOP technique is most suitable. The tibial nerve can be seen posterior to the tibial artery between it and the flexor tendons of the foot. Take care, as many vessels lie in close proximity. The deep peroneal nerve should be blocked at the intermalleolar line where it lies with the dorsalis pedis artery between the tibia, the extensor hallucis longus, and the extensor digitorum longus tendons. If the nerve cannot be visualized, inject 2–3mL on either side of the artery. Again, care should be taken due to the risk of arterial puncture and intravascular injection. While it is possible to visualize the superficial peroneal, sural, and saphenous nerves, they may be very small and have multiple branches. A traditional superficial infiltration, as described above, should be appropriate.
- **LA dose**: 5mL each to the saphenous and sural nerves; 5–10mL to the tibial nerve; 10mL to the superficial peroneal nerve; 3–6mL to the deep peroneal nerve (doses may be reduced if circumferential spread is observed with ultrasound).
- **Side effects of note**: nil.
- **Complications**: arterial puncture, bruising.

Nerve blocks: neuraxial

Spinal and epidural
(See Figs. 42.25 and 42.26.)

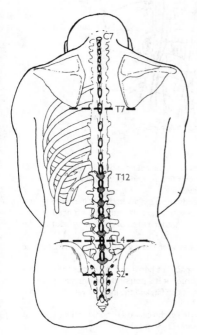

Fig. 42.25 Bony landmarks of the spine.

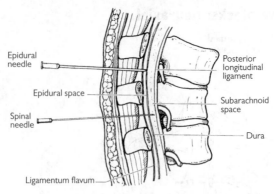

Fig. 42.26 Subarachnoid and epidural spaces.

Spinal and epidural anatomy

- The spinal cord terminates at ~L1 in adults and L3 in infants.
- The line joining the iliac crests (intercristine or Tuffier's line) is approximately at the L4 level.
- The subarachnoid space ends at ~S2 in adults, lower in children (care with paediatric caudal block; use a cannula, rather than a needle).
- The subarachnoid space extends laterally along the nerve roots to the dorsal root ganglia.
- There is a potential space between the dura and arachnoid mater (the subdural space).
- The epidural (extradural) space lies between the walls of the vertebral canal and the spinal dura mater. It is a potential low-pressure space, occupied by areolar tissue, loose fat, and the internal vertebral venous plexus.
- The ligamentum flavum is thin in the cervical region, reaching maximal thickness in the lumbar region (2–5mm).

Spinal block

- Indications for spinal block are:
  - Lower abdominal surgery (Caesarean section, inguinal hernia)
  - Lower limb surgery
  - Perineal surgery
  - More extensive abdominal surgery is possible with experience.
- **Landmarks**: spinous processes of the lumbar vertebrae and the line joining the iliac crests (Tuffier's line).
- **Technique**:
  - The patient should be sitting or lying on their side
  - Mark a line joining the iliac crests
  - Identify the spinous process at the level of this line

- The nearest interspace at this level is L3/4 (there is significant variation)
- Spinal blocks should always be carried out caudal to this space to avoid trauma to the tail end of the spinal cord (the conus).
- After SC infiltration with LA, insert a 24–29G needle of your choice:
  - **Midline**: at the level of the interspace, insert a needle in the midline (coronal plane). With a 15° cephalad angulation, advance until a click or pop is felt, at an approximate depth of 4–6cm.
  - **Paramedian**: 1–2cm lateral to the upper border of the spinous process. Insert a needle perpendicular to the skin to contact the lamina of the vertebra. Withdraw slightly, reinserting the needle 15° medially and 30° cephalad to pass over the lamina through the interlaminar space. Advance until a click or pop is felt (the dura is pierced).
  - After free flow of CSF, connect up the syringe containing the LA. Aspirate before and after injection to confirm correct placement in CSF throughout injection.

Local anaesthetic drugs and doses for spinal anaesthesia

- Dosing of LA in adults depends upon age and pregnancy—the older the patient, the less drug will be needed; pregnant patients need less than their non-pregnant counterparts.
- A volume of 2.5–3.0mL of a hyperbaric solution of LA will reach T6–T10 in most non-pregnant young adults placed in the recumbent position shortly after spinal injection.
- The dose of plain LA needed tends to be a little higher.
- Chloroprocaine 1% is now available in the UK for short-duration spinal anaesthesia. A dose of 40–50mg is recommended for adult use.
- Manufacturers advise against the use of lidocaine due to risks of **cauda equina syndrome** and **transient radicular irritation** and transient neurological symptoms.
- Ropivacaine does not have a product licence for intrathecal use.
- **Bupivacaine** (plain or heavy) can be used (usually 0.5%). 'Heavy' is hyperbaric and contains 8% glucose. 'Plain' is isobaric at body temperature.
- Due to spread in the intrathecal space, hyperbaric solutions can be used to achieve a higher block. Plain solutions will usually produce a lower block height, with consequently less hypotension, under normal conditions.
- See drug additive chart on ➔ p. 811 and p. 1076 (paediatrics).

Clinical tips

- Ideally, the injection should be at the L3/4 interspace; if there is difficulty, go down, not up, as the level of termination of the conus is variable.
- Accurate surface identification of the L3/4 interspace is difficult—70% of clinicians mark it as a higher space.
- A sitting position increases CSF pressure, and hence improves CSF flow with fine needles. It is also easier to find the midline in obese patients in this position.

- Lateral position offers familiarity of practice and possibility of sedation.
- Often problems are due to too short an introducer and a flexible needle. When difficulty is encountered in an elderly and osteophytic patient who would benefit from a spinal, consider a 22G Quincke-tip needle; PDPH is rare in this patient group.
- When repeatedly hitting bone, ask the patient to identify which side you are on. If they state 'middle', you are on a spinous process; if they can identify one side, you are out of the midline.

Contraindications
- Relative contraindications:
  - **Aortic or mitral valve stenosis (hypotension due to sympathetic block)**
  - Hypovolaemia (hypotension)
  - Previous back surgery (technical difficulty)
  - Neurological disease
  - Systemic sepsis (increased incidence of epidural abscess, meningitis).
- Absolute contraindications:
  - **Local sepsis**
  - Patient refusal
  - Anticoagulation (see ➲ p. 1141).

Complications
- Hypotension.
- Bradycardia (if block extends to the mid-thoracic region)—can progress to cardiac arrest.
- High block, compromising breathing, may extend to 'total spinal'.
- Urinary retention.
- Nerve damage (see ➲ p. 24 and p. 1142).
- PDPH (see ➲ p. 732).
- Infection: abscess, meningitis.
- Bleeding: spinal canal haematoma—more likely in patients with disorders of coagulation. Can cause spinal cord compression and permanent paraplegia.
- The serious complications of spinal and epidural anaesthesia have been the subject of a nationwide audit in the UK—the Royal College of Anaesthetists' 3rd National Audit Project (NAP 3). **The incidence of permanent injury due to neuraxial blocks** was 1:25 000–1:50 000, with an incidence of death or paraplegia of 1:50 000–1:140 000. The incidence of complications in children, in obstetric patients, and in those undergoing chronic pain procedures was very low. There was an excess incidence of serious complications in elderly patients with epidurals used during and after surgery, and in patients undergoing CSEs, a finding supported by other large studies. However, the overall incidence of major complications was reassuringly low. There were problems reported with the identification, treatment, and management of the serious complications of neuraxial anaesthesia. See ℘ http://www.rcoa.ac.uk/nap3.

Ultrasound for neuraxial block

The use of ultrasound for spinal or epidural anaesthesia has several benefits. It may reduce the number of failed attempts or traumatic procedures, and also reduces the number of needle reinsertions and redirections.

Ultrasound allows identification of the midline, estimation of the depth to the ligamentum flavum, and the angle of insertion needed to reach the space. While this technique may not be of benefit to all patients, it may be particularly useful in those with an abnormal anatomy or in those whose bony landmarks are not palpable.

Ultrasound can also be used as a teaching aid, as it allows demonstration of the anatomy by the instructor and allows the student to show that they have identified the correct insertion point and maximum depth to insert the needle.

Ultrasound for neuraxial block typically is used to scan the back and identify landmarks before performing the procedure (pre-procedural ultrasound).

Technique for pre-procedural ultrasound

Using a low-frequency, curvilinear probe, there are two acoustic windows that are effective for epidural lumbar spine sonography. Initially, place the probe in the longitudinal paramedian plane by identifying the spinous processes, which can be seen as the most superficial echogenic structure casting an acoustic shadow, typically described as the 'saw sign'. Start by identifying the sacrum, which has a long, flat hyperechogenic structure, then scan upwards, counting the spinous processes. Once the desired level has been reached, the interspinous space can be found, and the depth to the ligamentum flavum/epidural space can be seen. The probe can then be turned to a transverse plane where the most appropriate point and angle of insertion can be found.

Continuous spinal anaesthesia

- Better control over the rate of onset, level, intensity, and duration of block.
- Possibly less hypotension: incremental dosing and reduced total dose.
- The use of small spinal catheters has declined after reports of cauda equina syndrome.
- Low incidence of PDPH in older patients (1–6%).
- This block is indicated for lower abdominal, hip, and knee surgery.
- Technique:
  - Make a dural puncture using your needle of choice, e.g. **18G Tuohy**
  - The level of insertion should be at or below L3/4
  - Insert a catheter 3–5cm into the CSF, and attach a bacterial filter
  - Inject 1–1.5mL of, for example, bupivacaine 0.5% plain. Wait 10min, and test the block
  - Inject a further 0.5–1.0mL as necessary or when the level of block decreases by two segments
  - Dedicated commercial spinal catheter kits are available.

Epidural block

See ➔ p. 724, p. 1074, p. 1141, and p. 1142.

Caudal block

(See ➔ p. 810.)

- Useful in surgery of the perineum in adults.
- Adult dose 20–25mL of bupivacaine plain 0.125–0.5%.
- Use a 21G (green) needle or 20G IV cannula.

Regional anaesthesia and coagulation disorders

(See also ➲ p. 722 and p. 758.)

- Blood vessels are frequently encountered and damaged during the performance of regional anaesthetics. These may be large named vessels, such as the axillary, subclavian, and femoral arteries, or small blood vessels such as epidural veins. Although patients with normal coagulation only very rarely suffer from these vascular encounters, those with abnormalities of coagulation can suffer significantly.
- Haemorrhage can be brisk; haematomas can compress nerves and other anatomical structures, and the presence of even a relatively small haematoma in the non-distensible spinal canal can cause permanent spinal cord and nerve injury.
- Therefore, a coagulopathy is a relative contraindication to the performance of regional anaesthetic techniques. The degree of contraindication will depend upon the extent of the coagulation defect, the block planned, and the likely benefit to the patient of undergoing surgery under regional—rather than general—anaesthesia.
- Full therapeutic anticoagulation in an otherwise fit patient scheduled to undergo minor lower limb surgery would rightly be considered an absolute contraindication to spinal anaesthesia. A mild coagulopathy in a patient with severe lung disease would be only a marginal contraindication to the performance of forearm blocks to allow them to undergo hand surgery without GA. Decisions about the performance of blocks in patients with abnormal coagulation should be taken by experienced clinicians.
- The use of anticoagulant drugs to prevent or treat VTE is increasing rapidly, along with the number and potency of the drugs employed for such purposes.
- Several guidelines for the management of patients with abnormalities of coagulation exist, and the tables reproduced as Tables 42.4, 42.5, and 42.6, are drawn from guidelines recently published by AAGBI. These can be downloaded from http://www.aagbi.org/publications/publications-guidelines/M/R. They are reproduced with permission.

Regional anaesthesia and nerve injury

(See also ➜ p. 24.)

- Estimates of the incidence of nerve damage associated with regional anaesthesia vary.[3,4] From the evidence available, it seems that the incidence of temporary nerve damage (**neurapraxia**) is in the order of 1:100–1:200 and that of **permanent nerve damage** is in the range 1:5000–1:10 000. However, the likelihood of nerve damage depends upon a number of factors, including how the nerve block is performed, which nerve block is performed, the age of the patient, whether they are pregnant, and their co-morbidities.

- Nerve–needle contact can cause nerve damage, and therefore careful technique is very likely to be associated with a low incidence of nerve damage; the needle should always be advanced slowly and gently, and, if the patient complains of paraesthesiae or significant pain, it should be withdrawn, and injection should not be performed. Visualization of the nerves and needle with ultrasound should allow the anaesthetist to achieve a very low incidence of nerve–needle contact, thereby minimizing the chances of nerve damage.

- Although this is intuitively correct, definitive evidence from large-scale studies to support this contention is currently lacking.

- Direct injection of fluid into a nerve—intraneural injection—can be associated with high pressures in the nerve that can lead to ischaemic damage. The hallmarks of intraneural injection are held to include high injection pressures, pain on injection, low current thresholds when using a PNS, failure of the evoked contractions to disappear at the start of LA injection, and swelling of the nerve if visualized with ultrasound. If any of these are encountered, injection should cease immediately.

- Recent studies suggest that intraneural injection is not always painful, not always difficult, and not always dangerous. Indeed, it seems likely that a high proportion of lower limb PNBs using a PNS are, in fact, intraneural injections. Notwithstanding this evidence, intraneural injections should be avoided.

- Nerve damage can also be caused by ischaemia due to hypotension and vascular occlusion, pressure from haematomas, poor patient positioning, stretching or direct trauma during surgery, and the position of the patient's limbs.

- Some blocks seem to be associated with a higher incidence of nerve damage.

- Upper limb blocks seem to attract a higher incidence of reported injury. This may be due to a greater chance of minor neurological deficits being appreciated or may relate to the fact that there is a greater ratio of nerve tissue to connective tissue in upper limb nerves than in lower limb nerves.

- Publications suggest that the interscalene brachial plexus block is the PNB that has the highest capacity to be associated with nerve injury. There has been speculation about whether this is related to the relative tethering of the nerves to the cervical spine, from where they have just emerged at the location of the block. Whatever the reason for this apparent excess incidence of nerve damage, particularly good training

Table 42.4 Recommendations related to drugs used to modify coagulation

Drug	Time to peak effect	Elimination half-life	Acceptable time after drug for block performance	Administration of drug while spinal or epidural catheter in place[1]	Acceptable time after block performance or catheter removal for next drug dose
Rivaroxaban prophylaxis[1] (CrCl > 30 ml.min⁻¹)	3 h	7–9 h	18 h	Not recommended	6 h
Rivaroxaban treatment[1] (CrCl > 30 ml.min⁻¹)	3 h	7–11 h	48 h	Not recommended	6 h
Dabigatran prophylaxis or treatment[2]					
(CrCl > 80 ml.min⁻¹)	0.5–2.0 h	12–17 h	48 h	Not recommended	6 h
(CrCl 50–80 ml.min⁻¹)	0.5–2.0 h	15 h	72 h	Not recommended	6 h
(CrCl 30–50 ml.min⁻¹)	0.5–2.0 h	18 h	96 h	Not recommended	6 h
Apixaban prophylaxis	3–4 h	12 h	24–48 h	Not recommended	6 h
Thrombolytic drugs					
Alteplase, anistreplase, reteplase, streptokinase	< 5 min	4–24 min	10 days	Not recommended	10 days

CrCl, creatinine clearance.

[1] Manufacturer recommends caution with use of neuraxial catheters.

[2] Manufacturer recommends that neuraxial catheters are not used.

Table 42.5 Relative risk related to neuraxial and peripheral nerve blocks in patients with abnormalities of coagulation

	Block category	Examples of blocks in category
Higher risk	Epidural with catheter; Single-shot epidural; Spinal; Paravertebral blocks	Paravertebral block; Lumbar plexus block; Lumbar sympathectomy; Deep cervical plexus block
	Deep blocks	Coeliac plexus block; Stellate ganglion block; Proximal sciatic block (Labat, Raj, sub-gluteal); Obturator block; Infraclavicular brachial plexus block; Vertical infraclavicular block; Supraclavicular brachial plexus block
	Superficial perivascular blocks	Popliteal sciatic block; Femoral nerve block; Intercostal nerve blocks; Interscalene brachial plexus block; Axillary brachial plexus block
	Fascial blocks	Ilio-inguinal block; Ilio-hypogastric block; Transversus abdominis plane block; Fascia lata block
	Superficial blocks	Forearm nerve blocks; Saphenous nerve block at the knee; Nerve blocks at the ankle; Superficial cervical plexus block; Wrist block; Digital nerve block; Bier's block
Normal risk	Local infiltration	

and practice are required to perform this block safely, and great caution should be exercised when placing a needle anywhere near the upper reaches of the brachial plexus.

- Publications suggest that children only very rarely suffer nerve damage from regional anaesthesia and that the incidence of nerve damage in pregnant women undergoing spinal and/or epidural anaesthesia is similarly low. Obese patients seem to be at greater risk than their non-obese counterparts, and there is a substantial excess incidence of adverse sequelae in elderly patients undergoing spinal and epidural anaesthesia and analgesia. It is likely that the elderly, patients with **diabetes**, and those with **pre-existing neurological conditions** are at a higher risk of nerve damage.

- The management of nerve damage involves its early recognition and referral to a neurologist. Nerve conduction studies, MRI, and EMG can all assist in the identification of the severity and location. There

Table 42.6 Relative risks related to neuraxial blocks in obstetric patients with abnormalities of coagulation

Risk factor	Normal risk	Increased risk	High risk	Very high risk
LMWH – prophylactic dose	> 12 h	6–12 h	< 6 h	< 6 h
LMWH – therapeutic dose	> 24 h	12–24 h	6–12 h	
UFH – infusion	Stopped > 4 h and APTTR ≤ 1.4			APTTR above normal range
UFH – prophylactic bolus dose	Last given > 4 h	Last given < 4 h		
NSAID + aspirin	Without LMWH	With LMWH dose 12–24 h	With LMWH dose < 12 h	
Warfarin	INR ≤ 1.4	INR 1.4–1.7	INR 1.7–2.0	INR > 2.0
General anaesthesia	Fasted, not in labour, antacids given		Full stomach or in labour	
Pre-eclampsia	Platelets > 100 × 10⁹·L⁻¹ within 6 h of block	Platelets 75–100 × 10⁹·L⁻¹ (stable) and normal coagulation tests	Platelets 75–100 × 10⁹·L⁻¹ (decreasing) and normal coagulation tests	Platelets < 75 × 10⁹·L⁻¹ or abnormal coagulation tests with indices ≥ 1.5 or HELLP syndrome
Idiopathic thrombocytopenia	Platelets > 75 × 10⁹·L⁻¹ within 24 h of block	Platelets 50–75 × 10⁹·L⁻¹	Platelets 20–50 × 10⁹·L⁻¹	Platelets < 20 × 10⁹·L⁻¹
Intra-uterine fetal death	FBC and coagulation tests normal within 6 h of block	No clinical problems but no investigation results available		With abruption or overt sepsis
Cholestasis	INR ≤ 1.4 within 24 h	No other clinical problems but no investigation results available		

APTTR, activated partial thromboplastin time ratio; FBC, full blood count; INR, international normalized ratio; LMWH, low molecular weight heparin; NSAID, non-steroidal anti-inflammatory drug; UFH, unfractionated heparin.

is little that can be done to hasten the recovery of nerve function or to minimize the extent of the nerve damage once harmed. However, damage resulting from pressure from other structures or spinal abscesses and haematomas can be helped by surgery.

- Recovery of neurological function is mercifully the norm. More than 90% of cases of nerve damage resulting from regional anaesthesia recover within 3 months, and >99% within a year.
- Patients should be told in advance of the incidence of nerve damage; whether to undergo regional anaesthesia or GA is their choice. It is always useful to ask the patient about their jobs and passions. Slight damage to the brachial plexus will have more of a potential impact on the life of a professional or enthusiastic amateur violinist than on a lawyer! The disclosure and consent process should be recorded in the patient's notes.

Awake or asleep?

- The debate about whether nerve blocks should only be placed in awake or lightly sedated patients or whether it is acceptable to perform blocks on anaesthetized patients has raged for some time and shows no signs of abating.
- Supporters of 'awake blocks' argue that nerve–needle contact is associated with pain and paraesthesiae and that the insertion of a needle and the subsequent injection of LA into the nerve is usually painful and often dangerous. Therefore, an awake or lightly sedated patient may warn you of nerve–needle contact. Similarly, awake-block supporters argue that their patients might warn them of the early signs of LA toxicity as a result of inadvertent intravascular injection, thus allowing them to cease injection before plasma LA levels rise to cardiotoxic or convulsive levels. Those anaesthetists happy to perform blocks on the anaesthetized patient argue that the important hallmarks of intraneural injection are sufficiently present to protect the patient, provided the anaesthetist is aware of them and responds appropriately: visualization of intraneural needle placement and LA injection with ultrasound; low-threshold currents if using a PNS; failure of evoked contraction disappearance on injection of the LA; and difficulty of injection. Paediatric anaesthetists argue that, for many of their patients, 'awake' is not an option; they are perhaps fortunate that the incidence of nerve damage associated with PNBs in children is very low indeed.
- Although it is likely that the majority of anaesthetists believe that neuraxial blocks should not be performed on anaesthetized patients, views regarding PNBs are less one-sided. What is beyond doubt is that there is currently no hard evidence definitively to support either the 'awake' or the 'asleep' camps. The American Society of Regional Anesthesia and Pain Medicine (ASRA) recently advised its members not to perform blocks on anaesthetized patients when possible. The guidance also called attention to the suspicion that the performance of a PNB after a marked paraesthesiae has been produced may increase the chances of nerve damage, even though the needle is withdrawn and reinserted. Although not medico-legally binding on anaesthetists outside the US, the opinions expressed and the information presented

in support is worth both reading and heeding. In the authors' opinion, the ASRA advice should be followed.
* The performance of PNBs on the non-anaesthetized patient need not be unpleasant for the patient. Many anaesthetists successfully use sedation with small doses of a benzodiazepine (e.g. midazolam) and/or an opioid (e.g. fentanyl) or infusions of small amounts of propofol or remifentanil. The increasing use of ultrasound for nerve location is known to increase patient comfort if the evoked contractions produced by nerve stimulators are avoided, and it is therefore relatively easy to perform ultrasound-guided blocks on patients who are wide awake.

References

3 Neal JM, Bernards CM, Hadzic A, *et al*. (2008). ASRA Practice Advisory on Neurologic Complications in Regional Anesthesia and Pain Medicine. *Reg Anesth Pain Med*, **33**, 404–15.
4 Szypula K, Ashpole KJ, Bogod D, *et al*. (2010). Litigation related to regional anaesthesia: an analysis of claims against the NHS in England 1995–2007. *Anaesthesia*, **65**, 443–52.

Management of local anaesthetic toxicity

LA systemic toxicity (often referred to as 'LAST') occurs when an excessive amount of LA enters the circulation. Toxicity can be avoided by injecting slowly and in small boluses, interspersed with frequent gentle aspirations to exclude accidental intravascular needle placement, especially when single-site large doses are administered.

Maximum dosages vary, depending on the age and size of the patient, the site to be anaesthetized, vascularity of the tissues, individual tolerance, and the anaesthetic technique, but suggested maximum doses are given on → p. 1097 and 1097 (Table 42.1).

Levobupivacaine and ropivacaine are less toxic than bupivacaine. The higher toxicity of bupivacaine is related to the R-enantiomer, which binds more firmly and is released more slowly from the myocardium.

Toxicity from prilocaine is less likely because of its rapid metabolism, primarily by the liver. Methaemoglobinaemia may occur with high doses (>600mg in an adult) and should be treated with methylthioninium chloride (methylene blue 1–2mg/kg).

Articaine probably has the highest therapeutic ratio and the most rapid metabolism of all commonly used agents.

Allergic reactions to LAs are extremely rare. The ester groups are more prone to exhibit allergic reactions than amides, because they are metabolized to para-aminobenzoic acid (PABA), which acts as a hapten. There is also a cross-sensitivity of ester-type agents with sulphonamides. Allergic reactions range from simple local irritation with rash or urticaria to laryngeal oedema or anaphylaxis.

Presentation

- Light-headedness, dizziness, drowsiness. Tingling around the lips, fingers, or generalized. Metallic taste, tinnitus, blurred vision.
- Confusion, restlessness, incoherent speech, tremors, or twitching, leading to convulsions, with loss of consciousness and coma.
- Bradycardia, hypotension, CVS collapse, and respiratory arrest. ECG changes (prolongation of QRS and PR interval, AV block, and/or changes in T-wave amplitude).

Immediate management

- Discontinue injection.
- ABC … 100% O_2.
- Intubate and ventilate, if required, to prevent hypoxic CVS collapse. Hyperventilation may help by increasing the pH in the presence of metabolic acidosis.
- CPR if pulseless—commence the ALS protocol (see → p. 889).
- Treat convulsions with IV midazolam (3–10mg), diazepam (5–15mg), lorazepam (0.1mg/kg), propofol (20–60mg), or thiopental (50–150mg). Titrate against the patient response.

Lipid emulsion therapy

- Give an IV bolus injection of 20% lipid emulsion, e.g. Intralipid® 20%, 1.5mL/kg over 1 min (100mL for a 70kg patient).

- Start an IV infusion of 20% lipid emulsion at 15mL/kg/hr (1000mL over 1hr for a 70kg patient).
- Repeat the initial bolus twice at 5min intervals if an adequate circulation has not been restored.
- After 5min, double the infusion rate if an adequate circulation has not been restored.
- Continue CPR and infusion, until a stable, adequate circulation has been restored.

Propofol is NOT a suitable alternative to lipid emulsion.

The mechanism of action is thought to be through extraction of lipophilic LAs from aqueous plasma and tissues or by counteracting the LA inhibition of myocardial fatty acid oxidation, although other theories exist.

Anaesthetists should be familiar with guidelines for the treatment of LA toxicity and should practise management drills. AAGBI guidelines are available for download from ℘ http://www.aagbi.org/publications/publications-guidelines/M/R.

Which blocks for which operations?

Table 42.7 Suitable blocks for various regions of the body

Neck	
Carotid surgery	Superficial cervical plexus block, deep cervical plexus block (but some doubt the latter's necessity)
Thyroid surgery	Superficial cervical plexus block (bilateral needed)
Shoulder and upper limb	
Shoulder	Interscalene block
Humerus	Interscalene block
Elbow	Supraclavicular block, infraclavicular block, coracoid block, axillary block
Forearm	Supraclavicular block, infraclavicular block, coracoid block, axillary block, mid-humeral block, elbow blocks (distal forearm), IV regional anaesthesia (IVRA)
Hand surgery	Supraclavicular block, infraclavicular block, coracoid block, axillary block, mid-humeral block, elbow blocks, forearm blocks, wrist blocks, IVRA
Trunk and abdomen	
Thoracotomy	Thoracic epidural, thoracic paravertebral blocks, intercostal blocks
Rib fracture	Intercostal blocks, thoracic paravertebral blocks
Major breast surgery	Thoracic paravertebral blocks (controversial)
Upper abdominal surgery	Thoracic epidural, thoracic paravertebral blocks, intercostal blocks, TAP block
Laparotomy	Epidural, TAP, rectus sheath blocks
Lower abdominal surgery	Spinal, thoracic/lumbar epidural, TAP blocks

(Continued)

Table 42.7 (Contd.)

Inguinal hernia repair	Ilioinguinal/iliohypogastric blocks, spinal, caudal (children)
Circumcision	Penile block, caudal (children)
Haemorrhoid surgery	Spinal/infiltration
Lower limb	
Hip fracture surgery	Spinal, epidural, femoral nerve block, lumbar plexus block, lateral cutaneous nerve of the thigh block
Total hip replacement	Spinal, epidural, femoral nerve block, lumbar plexus block
Above-knee amputation	Spinal, epidural, sciatic nerve block, femoral nerve block, lumbar plexus block
Knee surgery	Spinal, epidural, combined sciatic and femoral nerve blocks
Lower leg surgery	Spinal, epidural, combined sciatic and femoral nerve blocks
Ankle surgery	Spinal, popliteal sciatic, and saphenous
Foot surgery	Ankle blocks/infiltration

Resources

The dermatome map
Figs. 42.27 and 42.28 provide maps of dermatomes and cutaneous innervation in the adult.

Twitches and nerves
See Fig. 42.29.

Further reading
American Society of Regional Anesthesia and Pain Medicine (ASRA). ℰ http://www.asra.com.
e-Learning for Healthcare. *e-learning anaesthesia*. ℰ http://www.e-lfh.org.uk/projects/ela.
European Society of Regional Anaesthesia and Pain Therapy (ESRA). ℰ http://www.esraeurope.org.
New York School of Regional Anesthesia (NYSORA). ℰ http://www.nysora.com.
Regional Anaesthesia—United Kingdom (RA-UK). ℰ http://www.ra-uk.org.
Ultrasound for Regional Anesthesia. ℰ http://www.usra.ca.

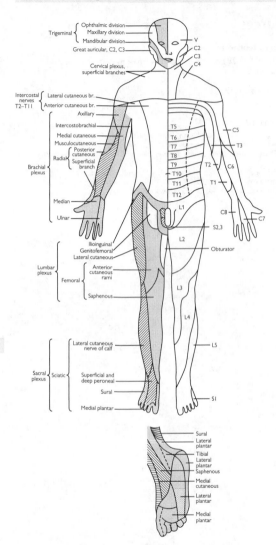

Fig. 42.27 Dermatome map in the adult (front).

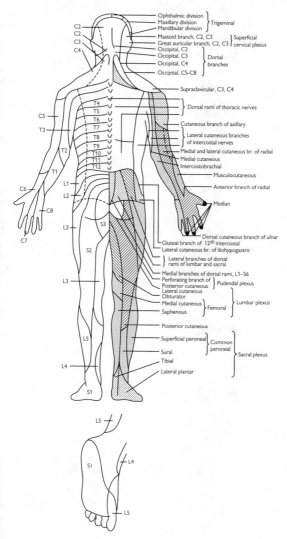

Fig. 42.28 Dermatome map in the adult (rear).

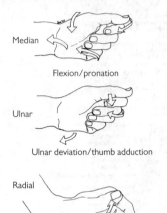

Median

Flexion/pronation

Ulnar

Ulnar deviation/thumb adduction

Radial

Wrist/thumb extension

Fig. 42.29 Typical movements produced by stimulation of nerves in the forearm.

Drug formulary

Joanna Wilson and Ben Ballisat

Introduction

This chapter provides a formulary of selected drugs and doses (Table 43.1) and infusion regimes (Table 43.2). A list of medical gases and cylinders can be found in Table 43.3. The MAC values for inhalational agents are given in Table 43.4, together with graphs showing how MAC changes with age (Fig. 43.1).

Drug formulary

Table 43.1 Drug formulary

Drug	Description and perioperative indications	Cautions and contraindications	Side effects	Dose (paediatric)	Dose (adult)
Abciximab	Synthetic monoclonal antibody. Glycoprotein IIb/IIIa inhibitor (powerful antiplatelet action). Used to prevent ischaemic complications before or during PCI	Intracranial or intraspinal surgery within 2 months, stroke within 2yr, trauma, or neoplasm. Major surgery. Ongoing haemorrhage. Hypertensive retinopathy. Can only be given once	Haemorrhage. Bradycardia, hypotension, nausea and vomiting. Chest and back pain. May provoke hypersensitivity reactions. Increased bleeding in hepatic/renal impairment		250 micrograms/kg bolus over 1min, then infuse at 0.125 micrograms/kg/min (max 10 micrograms/min). Start 10–60min before coronary intervention, and continue for at least 12hr; unstable angina, start 24hr prior to PCI
Acetazolamide	Carbonic anhydrase inhibitor used for acute reduction of intraocular pressure. Weak diuretic	Extravasation causes necrosis. Hypokalaemia/hyponatraemia. Hyperchloraemic acidosis. Avoid in severe hepatic impairment	Thrombocytopenia, nausea, vomiting, flushing, paraesthesiae, rash	1 month–12yr: PO/IV 5mg/kg 2–4 times daily (max 750mg). 12–18yr 250mg 2–4 times daily	IV/PO: 0.25–1g daily in divided doses

(Continued)

IV, intravenous. IM, intramuscular. SC, subcutaneous. PO, per os (oral). SL, sublingual. ET, endotracheal. od, once daily. bd, twice daily. tds, three times daily. qds, four times daily. NR, not recommended. Doses are IV and dilutions in 0.9% NaCl unless otherwise stated.

Table 43.1 (Contd.)

Drug	Description and perioperative indications	Cautions and contraindications	Side effects	Dose (paediatric)	Dose (adult)
Adenosine	Endogenous nucleoside with antiarrhythmic activity. Slows conduction through AV node. Treatment of acute paroxysmal SVT (including WPW) or differentiation of SVT from VT. Duration 10s	2nd- or 3rd-degree heart block. Long QT. Asthma/COPD. Reduce dose in heart transplant or dipyridamole treatment	Flushing, dyspnoea, headache, AV block, angina—transient	1 month–1yr: 0.1mg/kg fast IV bolus, increasing by 0.05–0.1mg/kg every 1–2min to max 0.5mg/kg (max 12mg). >12yr: as adult	6mg fast IV bolus, followed by 12mg at 1–2min, then further 12mg at 1–2min, as necessary. Reduce to quarter of dose if giving with dipyridamole
Adrenaline	Endogenous catecholamine with α and β action: 1. Treatment of anaphylaxis 2. Bronchodilator 3. Positive inotrope 4. Given by nebulizer for croup 5. Prolongation of LA action. 1:1000 contains 1mg/mL, 1:10 000 contains 100 micrograms/mL, 1:200 000 contains 5 micrograms/mL 6. Cardiac arrest	Arrhythmias, especially with halothane. Caution in elderly. Via central catheter whenever possible	Hypertension, tachycardia, anxiety, hyperglycaemia, arrhythmias. Reduces uterine blood flow	1. Refer to paediatric anaphylaxis emergency (see ● p. 937) 2. ETT 0.1mL/kg of 1:1000 (100 micrograms/kg) 3. Infusion 0.05– 1 micrograms/kg/min 4. Neb 0.5mL/kg (up to 5mL) 1:1000 5. Maximum dose for infiltration 2 micrograms/kg 6. 10 micrograms/kg refer to cardiac arrest (see ● p. 926)	1–3. IV/IM/ET 1mL aliquots of 1:10 000 up to 5–10mL (0.5–1mg). Infusion 2–20 micrograms/min (0.04–0.4 micrograms/kg/min) 4. Nebulization 5mL 1:1000 (max 5mg) 5. Maximum dose for infiltration 2 micrograms/kg 6. 1mg (10mL of 1:10 000), every 3–5 min

Alcohol	See ethanol		
Alfentanil	Short-acting, potent, opioid analgesic. Duration 10min Sedation in ICU	Respiratory depression, bradycardia, hypotension. Prolonged half-life in neonates Use IBW	Injection: 5–20 micrograms/kg, then 10 micrograms/kg boluses Infusion: 10–100 micrograms/kg over 10min, then 0.5–1 micrograms/kg/min	250–750 micrograms (5–10 micrograms/kg). Attenuation of CVS response to intubation: 10–20 micrograms/kg Sedation: infusion 2mg/hr
Alimemazine (trimeprazine)	Sedative antihistamine (paediatric premed)		PO: 2mg/kg 1–2hr preop (over 2yr) max 100mg daily	
Ametop®	See tetracaine		
Aminophylline	Methylxanthine bronchodilator used in prevention and treatment of asthma. Converted to theophylline, a phosphodiesterase inhibitor. Serum levels 10–20mg/L (55–110 micromoles/L)	Palpitations, tachycardia, tachypnoea, seizures, nausea, arrhythmias Caution in patients already receiving oral or IV theophyllines. Where serum level known, aminophylline 0.6mg/kg should increase level by 1mg/L	IV 5mg/kg over 20min, then 0.5–1mg/kg/hr infusion according to levels	5mg/kg over 20min, then 0.5mg/kg/hr infusion according to levels

IV, intravenous. IM, intramuscular. SC, subcutaneous. PO, per os (oral). SL, sublingual. ET, endotracheal. od, once daily. bd, twice daily. tds, three times daily. qds, four times daily. NR, not recommended. Doses are IV and dilutions in 0.9% NaCl unless otherwise stated.

(Continued)

Table 43.1 (Contd.)

Drug	Description and perioperative indications	Cautions and contraindications	Side effects	Dose (paediatric)	Dose (adult)
Amiodarone	Mainly class III antiarrhythmic useful in treatment of supraventricular and ventricular arrhythmias	Via central catheter. Sinoatrial heart block, thyroid dysfunction, pregnancy, porphyria, iodine sensitivity. Dilute in dextrose 5% not saline	Commonly causes thyroid dysfunction and reversible corneal deposits	>1yr IV: 5mg/kg over 20–120min. Infusion: 5 micrograms/kg/min, max 1.2g/24hr. 5mg/kg slow IV bolus for defib-resistant VF/VT	5mg/kg over 20–120min, followed by infusion if required, maximum 1.2g in 24hr. 300mg slow IV bolus for defib-resistant VF/VT
Amoxicillin	Broad-spectrum penicillin antibiotic 1. UTI/CAP/infections 2. *Listeria* meningitis or endococcal endocarditis	History of allergy	Nausea, diarrhoea, rash	1. IV/IM: 20–30mg/kg tds (double in severe infections) 2. 50mg/kg max 2g every 4hr	1. PO/IM/IV: 500mg tds, increased to 1g qds in severe infections 2. 2g every 4hr
Atenolol	Cardioselective β-blocker. Long-acting	Asthma, heart failure, AV block, verapamil treatment	Bradycardia, hypotension, and decreased contractility	0.05mg/kg every 5min—max four doses	5–10mg over 10min
Atracurium	Benzylisoquinolinium non-depolarizing muscle relaxant. Undergoes temperature- and pH-dependent Hofmann elimination (to laudanosine), plus non-specific enzymatic ester hydrolysis. Useful in severe renal or hepatic disease. Duration 20–35min	NMB potentiated by aminoglycosides, loop diuretics, magnesium, lithium, ↓ temp, ↓ K⁺, prior use of suxamethonium, volatile agents. Store at 2–8°C	Mild histamine release and rash common with higher doses. Flush with saline before and after	Intubation: 0.3–0.6mg/kg Maintenance: 0.1–0.2mg/kg Infusion: 0.3–0.6mg/kg/hr; monitor NMB	Intubation: 0.3–0.6mg/kg Maintenance: 0.1–0.2mg/kg Infusion: 0.3–0.6mg/kg/hr; monitor neuromuscular blockade Use IBW

Drug	Description	Cautions	Side effects	Dose
Atropine	Muscarinic acetylcholine antagonist. Vagal blockade at AV and sinus node increases heart rate (transient decrease at low doses due to weak agonist effect). Tertiary amine, therefore crosses blood–brain barrier	Obstructive uropathy and CVS disease. Glaucoma, myasthenia gravis	Decreases secretions and lower oesophageal sphincter tone, relaxes bronchial smooth muscle. Confusion in elderly	IV: 10–20 micrograms/kg. Control of muscarinic effects of neostigmine: 20 micrograms/kg. IM/SC: 10–30 micrograms/kg, PO: 40 micrograms/kg	300–600 micrograms. Prevention of muscarinic effects of neostigmine: 600–1200 micrograms
Benzylpenicillin	Broad-spectrum antibiotic	History of allergy	Nausea, diarrhoea, rash	25mg/kg qds. 50mg/kg qds for severe infections (max 2.4g 4-hourly)	600mg–1.2g qds. Higher doses may also be used (max 2.4g 4-hourly)
Bicarbonate (sodium)	Alkaline salt used for correction of acidosis and to enhance onset of action of LAs. 8.4%, 1000mmol/L. Dose (mmol) in acidosis: weight (kg) × base deficit × 0.3	Precipitation with calcium-containing solutions, increased CO_2 production, necrosis on extravasation. Via central catheter if possible	Alkalosis, hypokalaemia, hypernatraemia, hypocalcaemia	Dependent on degree of acidosis. 1mL/kg of 8.4% solution (1mmol/kg)	Dependent on degree of acidosis. Resuscitation: 50mL 8.4%, then recheck blood gases. Bicarbonation of LA: 1mL 8.4% to 20mL bupivacaine. 1mL of 8.4% to 10mL lidocaine/prilocaine
Bupivacaine	Amide-type LA used for infiltration, epidural, and spinal anaesthesia. Slower onset than lidocaine. Duration 3–6hr (slightly prolonged by adrenaline), pKa 8.1	Greater cardiotoxicity than other local agents. Do not use for IVRA. Adrenaline-containing solutions contain preservative and do not prolong action	Toxicity: tongue/circumoral numbness, restlessness, tinnitus, seizures, cardiac arrest	Infiltration/epidural: maximum dose dependent upon injection site—2mg/kg/4hr recommended	0.25–0.75% solution. Infiltration/epidural: maximum dose dependent upon injection site—2mg/kg/4hr (2mg/kg with adrenaline). 0.75% solution contraindicated in pregnancy

IV, intravenous. IM, intramuscular. SC, subcutaneous. PO, per os (oral). SL, sublingual. ET, endotracheal. od, once daily. bd, twice daily. tds, three times daily. qds, four times daily. NR, not recommended. Doses are IV and dilutions in 0.9% NaCl unless otherwise stated.

(Continued)

Table 43.1 (Contd.)

Drug	Description and perioperative indications	Cautions and contraindications	Side effects	Dose (paediatric)	Dose (adult)
Buprenorphine	Opioid with both agonist and antagonist actions. Duration 6hr	May precipitate withdrawal in opioid-dependent patients. Only partially reversed by naloxone	Nausea, respiratory depression, constipation	6 months–12yr: IV 3–6 micrograms/kg tds (max 9 micrograms/kg) 12–18yr: IV 300–600 micrograms tds	Slow IV/IM: 300–600 micrograms qds. SL: 200–400 micrograms qds
Caffeine citrate	Mild stimulant effective in the treatment of post-dural puncture headache. IV preparation available as caffeine sodium benzoate	Monitor levels in neonates	Insomnia, weakly diuretic, excitation, tachycardia	SCBU: loading dose 20mg/kg, then 5mg/kg od	IV/PO: 300–500mg bd. One cup of coffee contains 50–100mg. Soft drinks contain up to 35–50mg
Calcium chloride	Electrolyte replacement, positive inotrope, hypermagnesaemia. Calcium chloride 10% contains Ca^{2+} 680 micromoles/mL	Necrosis on extravasation. Incompatible with bicarbonate	Arrhythmias, hypertension, hypercalcaemia	0.1mL/kg 10% solution, slow IV	2–10mL 10% solution (10mg/kg, 0.07mmol/kg)
Calcium gluconate	As calcium chloride. Calcium gluconate 10% contains Ca^{2+} 225 micromoles/mL	Less phlebitis than calcium chloride	As calcium chloride	0.3–0.5 mL/kg 10% solution (max 20mL)	6–15mL of 10% solution (30mg/kg, 0.07mmol/kg)

Carboprost	Synthetic PGF2α analogue used to treat severe post-partum haemorrhage due to uterine atony (after ergometrine and oxytocin failed)	Asthma, diabetes, epilepsy, jaundice, anaemia, glaucoma. Large doses may cause uterine rupture	Fever, bronchospasm. Nausea, vomiting, flushing. May cause CVS collapse	NEVER GIVE IV. 250 micrograms deep IM or directly into the myometrium. Repeat, if needed, after at least 15min. Max dose 2mg/24hr
Cefotaxime	3rd-generation cephalosporin broad-spectrum antibiotic	10% cross-sensitivity with penicillin allergy		Neonate: 25mg/kg bd. Child: 50mg/kg bd/tds. 50mg/kg qds in severe infections (max 12g daily)	1g bd (up to 12g daily in divided doses in severe infections)
Cefuroxime	2nd-generation cephalosporin broad-spectrum antibiotic	10% cross-sensitivity with penicillin allergy		20–30mg/kg tds (max 1.5g tds)	750mg–1.5g tds
Celecoxib	NSAID with selective inhibition of cyclo-oxygenase 2 (COX-2) enzyme. Reduced gastric, asthma, and platelet side effects	Hypersensitivity to sulphonamides and aspirin, severe renal impairment, peptic ulceration, IHD, inflammatory bowel disease		NR	PO: 100–200mg bd
Cetirizine	Non-sedative antihistamine. Relief of allergy, urticaria	Prostatic hypertrophy, urinary retention, glaucoma, porphyria	Dry mouth	PO: 1–2yr 0.25mg/kg bd. 2–6yr: 2.5mg bd. >6yr: 5mg bd	PO: 10mg od. Half dose if eGFR <50mL/min/m²

IV, intravenous. IM, intramuscular. SC, subcutaneous. PO, per os (oral). SL, sublingual. ET, endotracheal. od, once daily. bd, twice daily. tds, three times daily. qds, four times daily. NR, not recommended. SCBU, special care baby unit. Doses are IV and dilutions in 0.9% NaCl unless otherwise stated.

(Continued)

Table 43.1 (Contd.)

Drug	Description and perioperative indications	Cautions and contraindications	Side effects	Dose (paediatric)	Dose (adult)
Chloral hydrate	Formerly a popular hypnotic in children	Avoid prolonged use. Caution in elderly, gastritis, and porphyria	Gastric irritation, ataxia	PO: 30–50mg/kg as single dose for sedation (up to 1g)	
Chlorphenamine	Sedative antihistamine. Relief of allergy, urticaria, anaphylaxis (see ❐ p. 920 for doses)	Prostatic hypertrophy, urinary retention, glaucoma, porphyria	Drowsiness, dry mouth	PO 0.1mg/kg up to 4mg qds	Slow IV/IM: 10mg qds. PO: 4mg qds
Chlorpromazine	Phenothiazine, antipsychotic. Mild α blocking action. Potent antiemetic and used for chronic hiccups	Hypotension	Extrapyramidal and anticholinergic symptoms, sedation, hypotension	1–6yr: IM/PO 0.5mg/kg tds (max 40mg/d). 6–12yr: IM/PO 0.5mg/kg tds (max 75mg/d). >12yr: adult dose	PO: 10–25mg tds/75mg ON. Deep IM: 25–50mg 6- to 8-hourly
Cisatracurium	Single isomer of atracurium with greater potency, longer duration of action, and less histamine release. Duration 55min	Neuromuscular block potentiated by aminoglycosides, loop diuretics, magnesium, lithium, ↓ temp, ↓ K⁺, ↓ pH, prior use of suxamethonium, volatile agents. Store at 2–8°C	Enhanced effect in myasthenia gravis, effects antagonized by anticholinesterases, e.g. neostigmine. Monitor response with peripheral nerve stimulator	Intubation: (>1 month) 150 micrograms/kg. Maintenance (>2yr) 30 micrograms/kg every 20min. Infusion: (>2yr) 0.06–0.18mg/kg/hr	Intubation: 150 micrograms/kg. Maintenance: 30 micrograms/kg every 20–30min. Infusion: 0.06–0.18mg/kg/hr
Citrate (sodium)	Non-particulate antacid oral premedication. Aspiration prophylaxis				PO: 30mL 0.3M solution

Clonidine	Centrally acting α₂-agonist. Reduces requirement for opioids and volatile anaesthetics. Enhances epidural analgesia	Rebound hypertension on acute withdrawal of chronic therapy	Hypotension, sedation	Over 6 months: 1–3 micrograms/kg slowly. PO premed: 4 micrograms/kg. Caudal: 1 microgram/kg	150–300 micrograms over 5min. Epidural: 75–150 micrograms in 10mL saline
Co-amoxiclav	Mixture of amoxicillin and clavulanic acid. 1.2g contains 1g amoxicillin	See amoxicillin	Cholestatic jaundice, see amoxicillin	30mg/kg (max 1.2g) tds	1.2g tds
Cocaine	Ester-type LA and potent vasoconstrictor. Topical anaesthesia of mucous membranes (nasal passages). Duration 20–30min	Topical use only. Caution with other sympathomimetic agents, halothane, anticholinesterase deficiency. Porphyria, MAOIs	Hypertension, arrhythmias, euphoria	1–3mg/kg topical	4–10% solution. Maximum topical dose 3mg/kg
Co-codamol 8/500	Combination oral analgesic containing codeine 8mg and paracetamol 500mg	See paracetamol	See paracetamol	NR	PO: 1–2 tablets qds (maximum eight tablets per day)
Co-codamol	Combination oral analgesic containing codeine and paracetamol (available as 8/500 or 30/500)	See paracetamol and codeine	See paracetamol and codeine	NR	PO: 1–2 tablets qds (maximum eight tablets per day)

IV, intravenous. IM, intramuscular. SC, subcutaneous. PO, per os (oral). SL, sublingual. ET, endotracheal. od, once daily. bd, twice daily. tds, three times daily. qds. four times daily. NR, not recommended. ON, omni nocte. Doses are IV and dilutions in 0.9% NaCl unless otherwise stated.

(Continued)

Table 43.1 (Contd.)

Drug	Description and perioperative indications	Cautions and contraindications	Side effects	Dose (paediatric)	Dose (adult)
Co-codaprin	Combination oral analgesic containing codeine 8mg and aspirin 400mg	See ibuprofen and codeine		NR	PO: 1–2 tablets qds (maximum eight tablets per day)
Codeine phosphate	Opioid used for mild to moderate pain. Wide variation in capacity to metabolize	<12yr, <18yr with tonsillectomy/ adenoidectomy for OSA	Nausea, vomiting, dysphoria, drowsiness, constipation	>12yr PO/IM/PR: 1mg/ kg 6-hourly (max 240mg/d 4-hourly (maximum for 3 days total) 240mg/d)	PO/IM: 30–60mg
Co-dydramol	Combination oral analgesic containing dihydrocodeine 10mg and paracetamol 500mg	See paracetamol		NR	PO: 1–2 tablets qds (maximum eight tablets per day)
Cyclizine	Antihistamine, antimuscarinic, anti-emetic agent	Caution in severe heart failure	Drowsiness, dry mouth, blurred vision, tachycardia	IV/IM/PO: 1mg/kg up to 50mg tds	IV/IM/PO: 50mg tds
Dabigatran	Direct inhibitor of factor Xa. Uses: 1. Prophylaxis of VTE after major orthopaedic surgery 2. Prophylaxis of stroke in AF	Risk of major bleeding, severe liver disease. Reduce dose in elderly or concomitant use of verapamil or amiodarone. No routine monitoring required	Nausea, haemorrhage	NR	1. PO: 110mg 1–4hr post-operatively, then 220mg daily for 9d 2. PO: 150mg bd

Dalteparin	LMWH used in prevention and treatment of VTE. No routine monitoring required. Complete risk assessment, and follow local policy	Risk of bleeding, renal impairment	HIT rarely	SC prophylaxis: 100U/kg od. >12yr: adult dose	SC prophylaxis: 2500–5000U od. High risk—see local policy
Dantrolene	Direct-acting skeletal muscle relaxant used in treatment of malignant hyperthermia and neuroleptic malignant syndrome. 20mg/vial—reconstitute in 60mL warm water, and give via blood set	Avoid combination with calcium channel blockers (verapamil) as may cause hyperkalaemia and CVS collapse. Crosses placenta	Skeletal muscle weakness (22%), phlebitis (10%)	1mg/kg, repeated every 5min to a maximum of 10mg/kg	1mg/kg, repeated every 5min to a maximum of 10mg/kg. Usually 2.5mg/kg
Desmopressin	Synthetic analogue of vasopressin (ADH) with longer duration of action and reduced pressor effect. Used for neurogenic diabetes insipidus and haemophilia (enhances factor VIII activity)	Caution in hypertension and CVS disease	Hypertension, angina, abdominal pain, flushing, hyponatraemia	Diabetes insipidus: IV/IM/SC 0.5–2 micrograms/d (not per kg). Haemophilia: 0.3 micrograms/kg (in 50mL saline over 30min IV)	Diabetes insipidus: IV/IM/SC 0.5–2 micrograms/d (not per kg). Haemophilia: 0.3 micrograms/kg (in 50mL saline over 30min IV)

(Continued)

IV, intravenous. IM, intramuscular. SC, subcutaneous. PO, per os (oral). SL, sublingual. ET, endotracheal. od, once daily. bd, twice daily. tds, three times daily. qds, four times daily. NR, not recommended. Doses are IV and dilutions in 0.9% NaCl unless otherwise stated.

Table 43.1 (Contd.)

Drug	Description and perioperative indications	Cautions and contraindications	Side effects	Dose (paediatric)	Dose (adult)
Dexamethasone	Prednisolone derivative corticosteroid. Less sodium retention than hydrocortisone. Cerebral oedema, oedema prevention, antiemetic	Interacts with anticholinesterase agents to increase weakness in myasthenia gravis. Dexamethasone 0.75mg, prednisolone 5mg	See prednisolone	IV/IM/SC: 200–400 micrograms/kg bd. Cerebral oedema: see BNFc. Croup: 150 micrograms/kg, ± repeat at 12h. Antiemetic: 150 micrograms/kg (max 8mg)	IV/IM/SC: 4–8mg. Cerebral oedema: 8–16mg initially, then 5mg qds. Antiemesis 2–8mg
Diamorphine	Potent opioid analgesic	Spinal/epidural use associated with risk of respiratory depression, pruritus, nausea	Histamine release, hypotension, bronchospasm, nausea, vomiting, pruritus, dysphoria	IV/SC: 20–100 micrograms/kg, then 15 micrograms/kg/hr. Epidural: 2.5mg in 60mL 0.125% bupivacaine at 0.1–0.4mL/kg/hr. Intranasal: 100 micrograms/kg in 0.2mL saline	IV/IM/SC: 2.5–5mg 4-hourly. Epidural: 2.5mg diluted in 10mL LA/ saline, then 0.1–0.5mg/ hr. Spinal: 0.25–0.5mg
Diazepam	Long-acting benzodiazepine. Sedation or termination of status epilepticus. Alcohol withdrawal	Thrombophlebitis: emulsion (Diazemuls®) less irritant to veins. Reduce in elderly	Sedation, circulatory depression	0.2–0.3mg/kg. Rectal: 0.5mg/kg as Stesolid® or may use IV preparation	IV/IM/PO: 2–10mg, repeat if required (max tds)
Diclofenac sodium	Potent NSAID analgesic for mild to moderate pain	Hypersensitivity to aspirin, asthma, severe renal impairment, peptic ulceration, proctitis	GI upset or bleeding, bronchospasm, tinnitus, fluid retention, platelet inhibition, thrombotic events	>1yr: PO/PR: 1mg/kg tds. Maximum 150mg/d. PR: NR <6 months	PO/PR: 25–50mg tds (or 100mg 18-hourly). Maximum 150mg/d

Digoxin	Cardiac glycoside. Weak inotrope and control of ventricular response in supraventricular arrhythmia. Therapeutic levels 0.8–2 micrograms/L (1.2–2.6nmol/L)	Reduce dose in elderly. Enhanced effect/toxicity in hypokalaemia. Avoid cardioversion in toxicity	Anorexia, nausea, fatigue, arrhythmias, blurred/yellow vision	Rapid IV loading: 250–500 micrograms over 30min. Maximum 1mg/24hr. PO loading: 1–1.5mg in divided doses over 24hr. PO maintenance: 125–250 micrograms/d
Dihydrocodeine tartrate	Opioid used for mild to moderate pain		Nausea, vomiting, dysphoria, drowsiness	PO/IM/PR: +0.5–1mg/kg 4-hourly (max dose 60mg 4-hourly) PO/IM: 30–60mg 4-hourly
Dobutamine	β_1-adrenergic agonist, positive inotrope and chronotrope. Cardiac failure	Arrhythmias and hypertension. Phlebitis, but can be administered peripherally	Tachycardia. Decreased peripheral and pulmonary vascular resistance	Infusion: 2–20 micrograms/kg/min Infusion: 2.5–10 micrograms/kg/min
Domperidone	Antiemetic acting on chemoreceptor trigger zone and peripheral D_2 receptors	Renal impairment, QT interval prolongation. Not recommended for PONV prophylaxis	Raised prolactin. Rarely acute dystonic reactions	PO: 200–400 micrograms/kg 6- to 8-hourly PO: 10–20mg 4- to 6-hourly. PR: 30–60mg 4- to 6-hourly
Dopamine	Naturally occurring catecholamine with α, β_1, and dopaminergic activity. Inotropic agent	Via central catheter. Phaeochromocytoma (due to noradrenaline release)	Tachycardia, dysrhythmias	Infusion: 2–20 micrograms/kg/min Infusion: 2–5 micrograms/kg/min

IV, intravenous. IM, intramuscular. SC, subcutaneous. PO, per os (oral). SL, sublingual. ET, endotracheal. od, once daily. bd, twice daily. tds, three times daily. qds, four times daily. NR, not recommended. Doses are IV and dilutions in 0.9% NaCl unless otherwise stated.

(Continued)

Table 43.1 (Contd.)

Drug	Description and perioperative indications	Cautions and contraindications	Side effects	Dose (paediatric)	Dose (adult)
Dopexamine	Catecholamine with β2 and dopaminergic activity. Inotropic agent.	Via central catheter. Phaeochromocytoma, hypokalaemia	Tachycardia	Infusion: 0.5–6 micrograms/kg/min	Infusion: 0.5–6 micrograms/kg/min
Doxapram	Respiratory stimulant acting through carotid chemoreceptors and medulla. Duration 12min	Epilepsy, airway obstruction, acute asthma, severe CVS disease	Risk of arrhythmia. Hypertension	1mg/kg slowly. Infusion: 0.5–1mg/kg/hr for 1hr. NR <12yr	1–1.5mg/kg over >30s. Infusion: 2–4mg/min
Droperidol	Butyrophenone related to haloperidol. Neuroleptic anaesthesia and potent antiemetic. Duration 4hr	α-adrenergic blocker. Parkinson's disease	Vasodilatation, hypotension. Dystonic reactions	Antiemetic: 25–50 micrograms/kg (max dose 1.25mg qds)	Antiemetic: 0.5–2.5mg
Edrophonium	Anticholinesterase used in diagnostic assessment of myasthenia gravis; 15 times less potent than neostigmine	Short-acting (10min)	Bradycardia, AV block	20 micrograms/kg test dose, then 80 micrograms/kg. >12yr: adult dose	1mg slow IV every 2–4min. Maximum 10mg. Reversal: 0.5mg/kg with anticholinergic
EMLA®	Eutectic mixture of 2.5% lidocaine and 2.5% prilocaine. Topical anaesthesia	Absorption of anaesthetic depends on surface area and duration of application. Avoid use on abrasions or mucous membranes	Methaemoglobinaemia in high doses	NR premature neonates. Apply 1–2g under occlusive dressing 1–5hr before procedure (max two doses/24hr)	Apply under occlusive dressing 1–5hr before procedure (max 60g)

Enoxaparin	LMWH used in prevention of VTE	Once-daily dosing and monitoring not usually required	SC prophylaxis: 500 micrograms/kg bd (max 40mg daily)	SC prophylaxis: 20mg (2000U) od (40mg if high-risk)
Enoximone	Type III phosphodiesterase inhibitor used in cardiac failure with increased filling pressures. Inodilator	Stenotic valvular disease, cardiomyopathy	Arrhythmias, hypotension, nausea	Initial loading dose 500 micrograms/kg, then infusion: 5–20 micrograms/kg/min for 24hr	Infusion: 90 micrograms/kg/min for 10–30min, then 5–20 micrograms/kg/min (max 24mg/kg/d)
Ephedrine	Direct and indirect sympathomimetic (α- and β-adrenergic action). Vasopressor, safe in pregnancy. Duration 10–60min	Caution in elderly, hypertension, and CVS disease. Tachyphylaxis. Avoid with MAOI	Tachycardia, hypertension		3–6mg repeated (dilute 30mg in 10mL saline, 1mL increments). IM: 30mg
Ergometrine	Ergot alkaloid used to control uterine hypotony or bleeding. Syntometrine® = ergometrine 500 micrograms/mL and oxytocin 5U/mL	Severe cardiac disease and hypertension	Vasoconstriction, hypertension, vomiting		IM: 1mL as Syntometrine®. Careful SLOW IV: 250–500 micrograms, with antiemetic cover recommended
Erythromycin	Macrolide antibiotic with spectrum similar to penicillin	Arrhythmias with cisapride, terfenadine, astemizole	Nausea, diarrhoea	12.5mg/kg qds over 20–60min. >8yr: adult dose	250–500mg (6-hourly in divided doses). Max four doses

(Continued)

IV, intravenous. IM, intramuscular. SC, subcutaneous. PO, *per os* (oral). SL, sublingual. ET, endotracheal. od, once daily. bd, twice daily. tds, three times daily. qds, four times daily. NR, not recommended. Doses are IV and dilutions in 0.9% NaCl unless otherwise stated.

Table 43.1 (Contd.)

Drug	Description and perioperative indications	Cautions and contraindications	Side effects	Dose (paediatric)	Dose (adult)
Esmolol	Short-acting cardioselective β-blocker. Metabolized by red cell esterases. Treatment of SVT or intraoperative hypertension. Duration 10min	Asthma, heart failure, AV block, verapamil treatment	Hypotension, bradycardia. May prolong action of suxamethonium	SVT: 0.5mg/kg over 1min, then 50–200 micrograms/kg/min	SVT: 0.5mg/kg over 1min, then 50–200 micrograms/kg/min. Hypertension: 25–100mg, then 50–300 micrograms/kg/min
Ethanol	Useful sedative/hypnotic. Has been tried as an IV induction agent in doses of up to 44g	Administered as dehydrated absolute alcohol BP. Refer to TOXBASE	Diuretic effect		2g (2mL) diluted to 5–10% solution in saline or glucose, repeated as necessary
Etomidate	IV induction agent. Cardiostable in therapeutic doses. Available in lipid emulsion	Pain on injection. Adrenocortical suppression	Nausea and vomiting. Myoclonic movements	0.3mg/kg	0.15–0.3mg/kg
Fentanyl	Synthetic phenylpiperidine derivative opioid analgesic. High lipid solubility and cardiostability. Duration 30–60min	Reduce dose in elderly. Delayed respiratory depression and pruritus if epidural/spinal	Circulatory and ventilatory depression. High doses may produce muscle rigidity	1–5 micrograms/kg, up to 50 micrograms/kg if ventilating post-operatively. Infusion: 2–4 micrograms/kg/hr	1–5 micrograms/kg (up to 50 micrograms/kg). Epidural: 50–100 micrograms (diluted in 10mL saline/LA). Spinal: 5–20 micrograms
Flecainide	Class 1c antiarrhythmic agent used for VT, WPW, and 'chemical cardioversion' of paroxysmal AF	Rise in pacemaker threshold. AV block, heart failure, previous MI	Nausea and vomiting. Pro-arrhythmic effects, AV block	2mg/kg (max dose 150mg) over 15min, with ECG monitoring	'Chemical cardioversion': 2mg/kg up to 150mg (over 15min with ECG monitoring). PO: 200–300mg

Flucloxacillin	Penicillinase-resistant antibiotic active against staphylococci	Hypotension on rapid IV administration	12.5–50mg/kg qds (max dose 2g qds)	500mg–2g qds slow IV. Surgical prophylaxis: 1–2g slow IV
Flumazenil	Benzodiazepine receptor antagonist. Duration 45–90min	Arrhythmia, seizures	10 micrograms/kg (max 200 micrograms), repeat if required (max 50 micrograms/ kg). Infusion: 2–10 micrograms/kg/hr	200 micrograms, then 100 micrograms at 60s intervals (up to max 1mg). Infusion: 100–400 micrograms/hr
Fondaparinux	Synthetic pentasaccharide which inhibits activated factor X. DVT prophylaxis after major lower limb orthopaedic surgery	Active bleeding, severe renal impairment, bacterial endocarditis. Caution with spinal and epidural (see ⊕ p. 1141)	Haemorrhage, thrombocytopenia, oedema, deranged LFTs	NR	Prophylaxis SC: 2.5mg od started 6hr post-operatively for up to 5d. Do not give IM or IV. Monitor platelet count
Fosphenytoin	Prodrug of phenytoin. Can be administered more rapidly. Dosages in phenytoin equivalents (PE): fosphenytoin 1.5mg, phenytoin 1mg	See phenytoin—monitor ECG/BP. Infusion rate: 50–100 mg (PE)/ min (status 100–150mg (PE)/min)	See phenytoin	>5yr: 10–20 mg (PE)/ kg, then 4–5mg (PE)/kg daily in 1–4 divided doses. Infusion rate: 1–2mg (PE)/ kg/min	Infusion: 10–15 mg (PE)/ kg, then 4–5mg (PE)/ kg daily. Status: 20mg (PE)/kg. Can also be administered IM. Infusion rate 50–100mg (PE)/min
Furosemide (frusemide)	Loop diuretic used in treatment of hypertension, CCF, renal failure, fluid overload	Hypotension, tinnitus, ototoxicity, hypokalaemia, hyperglycaemia	0.5–1.5mg/kg bd	10–40mg slowly

IV, intravenous. IM, intramuscular. SC, subcutaneous. PO, per os (oral). SL, sublingual. ET, endotracheal. od, once daily. bd, twice daily. tds, three times daily. qds, four times daily. NR, not recommended. Doses are IV and dilutions in 0.9% NaCl unless otherwise stated.

(Continued)

Table 43.1 (Contd.)

Drug	Description and perioperative indications	Cautions and contraindications	Side effects	Dose (paediatric)	Dose (adult)
Gabapentin	Structural analogue GABA. Indications post-herpetic neuralgia, neuropathic pain, focal seizures	Avoid abrupt withdrawal, elderly, renal impairment	Nausea, vomiting, abdominal pain, malaise	Seizures: day 1 10mg/kg (max 300mg) od, then bd, then tds max 70mg/kg	Pain: day 1 300mg od, day 2 300mg bd, then 300mg tds to max 3.6g/d
Gentamicin	Aminoglycoside antibiotic active against Gram-negative bacteria. Peak level 6–10mg/L. Trough level <1–2mg/L	Impairs neuromuscular transmission—avoid in myasthenia	Ototoxicity, nephrotoxicity	2mg/kg tds or 5mg/kg/d as a single dose (administered over 5min)	3–5mg/kg divided doses or 5–7mg/kg/d as a single dose (administered over 5min)
Glucagon	Polypeptide hormone used in treatment of hypoglycaemia and overdose of β-blocker. Hyperglycaemic action lasts 10–30min. 1U = 1mg	Glucose must be administered as soon as possible. Phaeochromocytoma	Hypertension, hypotension, nausea, vomiting	<25kg: 0.5U (0.5mg). >25kg: 1U (1mg)	SC/IM/IV: 1U (1mg). β-blocker overdose unresponsive to atropine: 2–10mg (max 10mg) in glucose 5%
Glucose	Treatment of hypoglycaemia in unconscious patient	50% solution irritant, therefore flush after administration into large vein. <20% peripherally		0.5mL/kg of 50% solution: use more dilute solutions: bolus 5mL/kg 10%, repeat PRN	25–50g (50–100mL 50% solution). Can use more dilute solutions
Glyceryl trinitrate	Organic nitrate vasodilator. Controlled hypotension, angina, CCF	Remove patches before defibrillation to avoid electrical arcing	Tachycardia, hypotension, headache, nausea, flushing, methaemoglobinaemia	10–30 micrograms/kg/hr, starting dose up to 300 micrograms/kg/hr. Max 600 micrograms/kg/hr	Infusion: 0.5–10mg/hr. SL tabs: 0.3–1mg PRN. SL spray: 400 micrograms PRN. Patch: 5–10mg/24hr

Glycopyrronium bromide (glycopyrrolate)	Quaternary ammonium anticholinergic agent. Bradycardia, blockade of muscarinic effects of anticholinesterases, antisialogogue	Caution in glaucoma, CVS disease. Unlike atropine, does not cross blood–brain barrier	Paradoxical bradycardia in small doses. Reduces lower oesophageal sphincter tone	4–10 micrograms/kg	200–400 micrograms. Control of muscarinic effects of neostigmine: 200 micrograms for each 1mg neostigmine
Granisetron	5-HT$_3$ receptor antagonist. Antiemetic. Long-acting	Pregnancy, breastfeeding, QT interval prolongation	Reduces colonic motility. Headache	NR <12yr	1mg diluted to 5mL with saline. Give over 30s. Max 9mg/d
Haloperidol	Butyrophenone derivative antipsychotic. Useful antiemetic	Neuroleptic malignant syndrome. Half dose in elderly	Extrapyramidal reactions	NR	IM/IV: 2–10mg 4- to 8-hourly (max 18mg/d). Antiemetic: 0.5–2mg IV. PO: 0.5–3mg
Heparin (unfractionated)	Endogenous mucopolysaccharide used for anticoagulation. Half-life 1–3hr. 100U, 1mg	Monitor APTT. Reversed with protamine	Haemorrhage, thrombocytopenia, hyperkalaemia	Low dose: 50–75U/kg IV, then 10–15U/kg/hr. Full dose: 200U/kg IV, then 15–30U/kg/hr, Anticoagulation for bypass 300–400U/kg IV	Low dose SC: 5000U bd. Full dose IV: 5000U, then 18U/kg/hr infusion. Anticoagulation for bypass: 300–400U/kg
Human prothrombin complex (Beriplex®, Octaplex®)	Dried prothrombin complex, prepared from human plasma. Rapid reversal of warfarin anticoagulation.	Risk of thrombotic events	Discuss with haematologist	Discuss with haematologist	

IV, intravenous. IM, intramuscular. SC, subcutaneous. PO, per os (oral). SL, sublingual. ET, endotracheal. od, once daily. bd, twice daily. tds, three times daily. qds, four times daily. NR, not recommended. Doses are IV and dilutions in 0.9% NaCl unless otherwise stated.

(Continued)

Table 43.1 (Contd.)

Drug	Description and perioperative indications	Cautions and contraindications	Side effects	Dose (paediatric)	Dose (adult)
Hyaluronidase	Enzyme used to enhance permeation of injected fluids and LAs. Treatment of extravasation. Hypodermoclysis: 1500U/L	Not for IV administration	Occasional severe allergy	LA: 15U/mL solution	Ophthalmology: 10–15U/mL local. Extravasation: 1500U in 1mL saline infiltrated to affected area
Hydralazine	Direct-acting arteriolar vasodilator used to control arterial pressure. Duration 2–4hr	Higher doses required in rapid acetylators. SLE	Increased HR, cardiac output, stroke volume	0.1–0.5mg/kg 4- to 6-hourly	5mg every 5min to a max of 20mg
Hydrocortisone (cortisol)	Endogenous steroid with anti-inflammatory and potent mineralocorticoid action (steroid of choice in replacement therapy—active form of cortisone). Treatment of allergy	Hydrocortisone 20mg, prednisolone 5mg	Hyperglycaemia, hypertension, psychiatric reactions, muscle weakness, fluid retention	4mg/kg, then 2–4mg/kg qds	IV/IM: 50–200mg qds. Adrenal suppression and surgery: 25mg at induction, then 25mg qds. PO: 10–30mg/d
Hydromorphone hydrochloride	Opioid used for moderate to severe pain in cancer	As morphine	Nausea, vomiting, dysphoria, drowsiness	<12yr: NR. >12yr: adult dose	PO: 1.3mg 4-hourly, increased as necessary. PO slow release: 4mg bd
Hyoscine butylbromide	Antimuscarinic agent used as an antispasmodic (racemic hyoscine)	See atropine	See atropine	2–6yr: IV/IM: 5mg. 6–12yr: IV/IM: 5–10mg. >12yr: adult dose	IV/IM: 20mg slowly, repeated if necessary

Hyoscine hydrobromide	Antimuscarinic sedative, antiemetic agent used as premedication (L-isomer of hyoscine)	See atropine. Avoid in elderly—delirium	See atropine. Sedation	IM/SC: 15 micrograms/kg (max 600 micrograms)	IV/IM/SC: 200–600 micrograms. PO: 300 micrograms tds
Ibuprofen	NSAID analgesic for mild to moderate pain. Best side effect profile of NSAIDs	Hypersensitivity to aspirin, asthma, severe renal impairment, peptic ulceration	GI upset or bleeding, bronchospasm, tinnitus, fluid retention, platelet inhibition	NR <3months/<5kg. PO: 10mg/kg tds or 5mg/kg qds (max 30mg/kg tds)	PO: 400mg qds
Imipenem	Carbapenem broad-spectrum antibiotic. Administered with cilastatin to reduce renal metabolism	Caution in renal failure and pregnancy	Nausea, vomiting, diarrhoea, convulsions, thrombophlebitis	>3 months: 15mg/kg over 30min qds (25mg/kg in severe infections)	Slow IV (1hr): 250–500mg qds. Surgical prophylaxis: 1g at induction, repeated after 3hr
Indometacin	NSAID analgesic for moderate pain. High incidence of side effects. Also used for neonatal ductus arteriosus closure	Hypersensitivity to aspirin, asthma, severe renal impairment, peptic ulceration	GI upset or bleeding, bronchospasm, tinnitus, fluid retention, platelet inhibition	Ductus closure: 200 micrograms/kg, three doses	PO/PR: 25–50mg tds. PR: 100mg bd
Insulin (soluble)	Human soluble pancreatic hormone facilitating intracellular transport of glucose and anabolism. Diabetes mellitus, ketoacidosis, and hyperkalaemia	Monitor blood glucose and serum potassium. Store at 2-8°C	Hypoglycaemia, hypokalaemia	Ketoacidosis: 0.1–0.2U/kg (max 20U), then 0.1U/kg/hr (max 5–10U/hr)	Ketoacidosis: 10–20U, then 5–10U/hr. Sliding scale (see ⬆ p. 148). Hyperkalaemia (see ⬆ p. 176)

IV, intravenous. IM, intramuscular. SC, subcutaneous. PO, per os (oral). SL, sublingual. ET, endotracheal. od, once daily. bd, twice daily. tds, three times daily. qds, four times daily. NR, not recommended. Doses are IV and dilutions in 0.9% NaCl unless otherwise stated.

(Continued)

Table 43.1 (Contd.)

Drug	Description and perioperative indications	Cautions and contraindications	Side effects	Dose (paediatric)	Dose (adult)
Intralipid®	20% emulsion used in the treatment of severe LA toxicity	See ⌖ p. 1148 for LA toxicity guidelines		1.5mL/kg bolus, followed by 15mL/kg/hr	1.5mL/kg bolus, followed by 15mL/kg/hr
Isoprenaline	Synthetic catecholamine with potent β₁-adrenergic agonist activity. Emergency treatment of heart block and bradycardia unresponsive to atropine. β-blocker overdose	IHD, hyperthyroidism, diabetes mellitus. MHRA: NR, unless special requirements	Tachycardia, arrhythmias, sweating, tremor	Bolus: 5 micrograms/kg. Infusion: 0.02–1 micrograms/kg/min	Infusion: 0.5–10 micrograms/min (0.2mg in 500mL 5% glucose at 2–20mL/min or 1mg in 50mL at 1.5–30mL/hr)
Ketamine	Phencyclidine derivative producing dissociative anaesthesia. Induction/maintenance of anaesthesia in high-risk and hypovolaemic patients	Emergence delirium reduced by benzodiazepines. Caution in hypertension. Control excess salivation with antimuscarinic agent	Bronchodilation. Increased ICP, BP, uterine tone, salivation. Respiratory depression if given rapidly	Induction: 0.5–2mg/kg IV, 5–10mg/kg IM. Infusion: 10–45 micrograms/kg/min. Caudal: 0.5mg/kg (preservative-free only)	Induction: 1–2mg/kg IV, 5–10mg/kg IM. Infusion: 1–3mg/kg/hr (analgesia only 0.25mg/kg/hr)
Ketorolac	NSAID analgesic for mild to moderate pain. Not licensed for perioperative use	Hypersensitivity to aspirin, asthma, severe renal impairment, peptic ulceration	GI upset or bleeding, bronchospasm, tinnitus, fluid retention, platelet inhibition	>6 months: slow IV/IM: 0.5mg/kg up to 30mg tds (max 60mg/d)	Slow IV/IM: 10mg, then 10–30mg every 4–6hr (max daily dose 90mg, but 60mg in elderly)

Labetalol	Combined α- (mild) and β-adrenergic receptor antagonist. BP control without reflex tachycardia. Duration 2-4hr	Asthma, heart failure, AV block, verapamil treatment	Hypotension, bradycardia, bronchospasm, liver damage	0.2 mg/kg boluses up to 0.5mg/kg (max 20mg <12yr). Infusion: 0.5-3mg/kg/hr	5mg increments up to 100mg. Infusion: 20-160mg/hr (in glucose)
Lansoprazole	PPI. Reduction of gastric acid secretion	Liver disease, pregnancy	Headache, diarrhoea	PO: 0.5-1mg/kg (max 15-30mg) od	PO: 15-30mg od
Levobupivacaine	Levorotatory (S) enantiomer of bupivacaine with reduced cardiotoxicity	See bupivacaine	See bupivacaine and use IBW	See bupivacaine. 2mg/kg	See bupivacaine. Max dose: 2mg/kg
Lidocaine	Amide-type LA: 1. Treatment of ventricular arrhythmias. 2. Reduction of pressor response to intubation. 3. LA—rapid onset, duration 30-90min (prolonged by adrenaline), pKa 7.7	Adrenaline-containing solutions contain preservative. Max dose dependent upon injection site—3mg/kg/4hr (6mg/kg with adrenaline)	Toxicity: tongue/circumoral numbness, restlessness, tinnitus, seizures, cardiac arrest. Prolongs action of neuromuscular blockers. Use IBW	1. Antiarrhythmic: 0.5-1mg/kg, then 10-50 micrograms/kg/min. 2. Attenuation of pressor response: 1.5mg/kg. 3. LA: 0.5-2% solution	1. Antiarrhythmic: 1mg/kg, then 1-4mg/min. 2. Attenuation of pressor response: 1.5mg/kg. 3. LA: 0.5-2% solution
Loratadine	Non-sedative antihistamine. Relief of allergy, urticaria	Prostatic hypertrophy, urinary retention, glaucoma, porphyria	Dry mouth	<2yr: NR. PO: <30kg: 5mg od. >30kg: 10mg od	PO: 10mg/d

IV, intravenous. IM, intramuscular. SC, subcutaneous. PO, per os (oral). SL, sublingual. ET, endotracheal. od, once daily. bd, twice daily. tds, three times daily. qds, four times daily. NR, not recommended. Doses are IV and dilutions in 0.9% NaCl unless otherwise stated.

(Continued)

Table 43.1 (Contd.)

Drug	Description and perioperative indications	Cautions and contraindications	Side effects	Dose (paediatric)	Dose (adult)
Lorazepam	Benzodiazepine: 1. Sedation or premedication 2. Status epilepticus. Duration 6–10hr	Decreased requirement for anaesthetic agents. Half in elderly	Respiratory depression in combination with opioids. Amnesia	Status 0.1mg/kg: max 4mg	1. PO: 1–4mg 1–2hr preoperatively. IV/IM: 1.5–2.5mg 2. Status: 4mg IV, repeat after 10min if required
Lormetazepam	Benzodiazepine hypnotic sedative premed	Decreased requirement for anaesthetic agents	Respiratory depression in combination with opioid. Amnesia	NR	0.5–1.5mg 1–2hr preoperatively (elderly 0.5mg)
Magnesium sulfate	Essential mineral used to treat: 1. Hypomagnesaemia 2. Arrhythmias 3. Eclamptic seizures 4. Severe asthma. Magnesium sulphate 50%, 500mg/mL, 2mmol Mg²⁺/mL. Normal plasma level Mg²⁺ 0.75–1.05mmol/L. Therapeutic level 2–4mmol/L	Potentiates muscle relaxants. Monitoring of serum level essential during treatment. Myasthenia and muscular dystrophy. Heart block. Magnesium sulphate 1g = Mg²⁺ 4mmol	CNS depression, hypotension, muscle weakness	1. Hypomagnesaemia: 0.2–0.4mmol/kg (max 20mmol/d)—check levels 2. Arrhythmias: 25–50mg/kg over 10min (max dose 2g) once if necessary	1. Hypomagnesaemia: 0.5–1mmol/kg (max 160mmol/5d), check levels. 2. Arrhythmias/asthma: 2g (8mmol) over 10min, repeat once if necessary. 3. Eclampsia: 4g (16mmol) over 10min, then 1g/hr for 24hr (see ➲ p. 760)

Mannitol	Osmotic diuretic used for renal protection and reduction of ICP 20% solution, 20g/100mL	Diuresis, ARF, hypertonicity	Extracellular volume expansion, caution in severe renal and CVS disease	0.25–1.5g/kg	0.25–2g/kg (typically 0.3g/kg of 20% solution)
Metaraminol	Potent direct/indirect acting α-adrenergic sympathomimetic. Treatment of hypotension. Duration 20–60min	Hypertension, reflex bradycardia, arrhythmias, decreased renal and placental perfusion	MAOIs, pregnancy. Caution in elderly and hypertensives. Extravasation can cause necrosis	10 micrograms/kg, then 0.1–1 micrograms/kg/min, >12yr	0.5–2mg. Dilute 10mg in 20mL saline, and give 0.5–1mL increments (increase dilution in elderly)
Methohexital	Short-acting barbiturate induction agent useful for ECT. Duration 5–10min. 1% solution, 10mg/mL	Excitatory phenomenon, hypotension, respiratory depression, hiccups	Porphyria. Premedication reduces excitation at induction	1–2mg/kg	1–1.5mg/kg. Infusion: 50–150 micrograms/kg/min
Methylthioninium chloride (methylene blue)	1. Treatment of methaemoglobinaemia 2. Ureteric identification during surgery (renally excreted) 3. Identification of para-thyroid glands during surgery 4. Identification of sentinel node during cancer surgery	Tachycardia, nausea, stains skin, allergy reported	G6PD deficiency. Blue coloration causes acute changes in pulse oximetry readings	1mg/kg slow IV(max 7mg/kg)	1mg/kg slow IV (max 7mg/kg)

IV, intravenous. IM, intramuscular. SC, subcutaneous. PO, per os (oral). SL, sublingual. ET, endotracheal. od, once daily. bd, twice daily. tds, three times daily. qds, four times daily. NR, not recommended. Doses are IV and dilutions in 0.9% NaCl unless otherwise stated.

(Continued)

Table 43.1 (Contd.)

Drug	Description and perioperative indications	Cautions and contraindications	Side effects	Dose (paediatric)	Dose (adult)
Metoclopramide	Dopaminergic antiemetic which increases gastric emptying and lower oesophageal sphincter tone	Hypertension in phaeochromocytoma. Inhibits plasma cholinesterase. Increases IOP	Extrapyramidal/ dystonic reactions (treat with benztropine or procyclidine)	PO/IM/IV: 0.15mg/kg, up to 5mg tds (>60kg, up to 10mg tds)	PO/IM/IV: 10mg tds
Metoprolol	Cardioselective β-blocker	Asthma, heart failure, AV block, verapamil treatment	Causes bradycardia, hypotension, and decreased cardiac contractility	0.1mg/kg up to 5mg over 10min	1–5mg over 10min, repeat if required (max 15mg)
Metronidazole	Antibiotic with activity against anaerobic bacteria	Disulfiram (Antabuse®)- like effect with alcohol consumption		7.5mg/kg tds (max dose 500mg tds)	500mg tds
Midazolam	Short-acting benzodiazepine. Sedative, anxiolytic, amnesic, anticonvulsant. Duration 20–60min. Oral administration of IV preparation effective, though larger dose required	Reduce dose in elderly (very sensitive)	Hypotension, respiratory depression, apnoea	IV: 0.1–0.2mg/ kg. PO: 0.5mg/kg (use IV preparation in orange squash). Intranasal: 0.2–0.3mg/ kg (use 5mg/mL IV preparation). Infusion: 0.5–20 micrograms/kg/min	Sedation: 0.5–5mg, titrate to effect. PO: 0.5mg/kg (use IV preparation in orange squash). IM: 2.5–10mg (0.1mg/kg)

Milrinone	Selective phosphodiesterase inhibitor used in cardiac failure with increased filling pressures. Inodilator used after cardiac surgery	Stenotic valvular disease, cardiomyopathy	Arrhythmias, hypotension, nausea	50 micrograms/kg over 30–60min, then 0.375–0.75 micrograms/kg/min. Max 1.13mg/kg/d	50 micrograms/kg over 10min, then 0.375–0.75 micrograms/kg/min. Max 1.13mg/kg/d
Mivacurium	Short-acting non-depolarizing muscle relaxant. Metabolized by plasma cholinesterase. Duration 6–16min (often variable). Enhanced duration if low plasma cholinesterase. Antagonized by neostigmine — but avoid giving too early to avoid inhibiting drug metabolism	See cisatracurium. Avoid in asthma	See cisatracurium. Some histamine release	Intubation: 0.15–0.2mg/kg. Maintenance: 0.1mg/kg. Infusion: 8–10 micrograms/kg/min	Intubation: 0.07–0.25mg/kg (doses of 0.07, 0.15, 0.2, and 0.25mg/kg produce block for 13, 16, 20, and 23min, respectively). Maintenance: 0.1mg/kg. Infusion: 0.4–0.6mg/kg/hr
Morphine	Opioid analgesic. Half-life 2–4hr	Prolonged risk of respiratory depression, pruritus, nausea when used via spinal/epidural	Histamine release, hypotension, bronchospasm, nausea, vomiting, pruritus, dysphoria	PO: 0.05–0.3mg/kg 4-hourly. IV boluses: 50–100 micrograms/kg. For PCA, NCA, infusion, see p. 808	IV: 2.5–10mg. IM/SC: 5–10mg 4-hourly. PO: 10–30mg 4-hourly. PCA: 1mg 5min lockout. Infusion: 1–3.5mg/hr. Epidural: 2–5mg preservative-free. Spinal: 0.1–1mg preservative-free

IV, intravenous. IM, intramuscular. SC, subcutaneous. PO, per os (oral). SL, sublingual. ET, endotracheal. od, once daily. bd, twice daily. tds, three times daily. qds, four times daily. NR, not recommended. Doses are IV and dilutions in 0.9% NaCl unless otherwise stated.

(Continued)

Table 43.1 (Contd.)

Drug	Description and perioperative indications	Cautions and contraindications	Side effects	Dose (paediatric)	Dose (adult)
Naloxone	Pure opioid antagonist. Can be used in low doses to reverse pruritus associated with epidural opioids and as depot IM injection in newborn of mothers given opioids	Beware renarcotization if reversing long-acting opioid. Caution in opioid-dependent patients—may precipitate acute withdrawal. Duration of action 30min		5–10 micrograms/kg. Infusion: 5–20 micrograms/kg/hr. IM depot in newborn: 200 micrograms. Pruritus: 0.5 micrograms/kg	200–400 micrograms, titrated to desired effect. Treatment of opioid/epidural pruritus: 100 micrograms bolus plus 300 micrograms added to IV fluids
Naproxen	NSAID analgesic for mild to moderate pain. Juvenile idiopathic arthritis	See ibuprofen	See ibuprofen. Low thrombotic risk profile		PO: 500mg bd. Max 1.25g/d
Neostigmine	Anticholinesterase used for: 1. Reversal of non-depolarizing muscle relaxant 2. Treatment of myasthenia gravis Duration 60min IV (2–4hr PO)	Administer with antimuscarinic agent	Bradycardia, nausea, excessive salivation (muscarinic effects)	50 micrograms/kg with atropine 20 micrograms/kg or glycopyrronium 10 micrograms/kg	1. 50–70 micrograms/kg (max 5mg) with atropine 10–20 micrograms/kg or glycopyrronium 10–15 micrograms/kg 2. PO: 15–30mg at suitable intervals

Drug	Description	Dose (1)	Notes	Dose (2)
Neostigmine and glycopyrronium	Combination of neostigmine metilsulphate (2.5mg) and glycopyrronium (500 micrograms) per 1mL	See neostigmine	See neostigmine	1–2mL over 30s
Nimodipine	Calcium channel blocker used to prevent vascular spasm after subarachnoid haemorrhage (treat for 21 days)	Via central catheter. Cerebral oedema, raised ICP, grapefruit juice. Incompatible with PVC	Hypotension, flushing, headache	PO: 60mg 4-hourly (max 360mg/d). Infusion: 1mg/hr, increasing after 2hr to 2mg/hr
Nitroprusside (sodium—SNP)	Protect solution from light. Metabolism yields cyanide which is then converted to thiocyanate	N_2O generating potent peripheral vasodilator. Controlled hypotension	Methaemoglobinaemia, hypotension, tachycardia. Cyanide causes tachycardia, sweating, acidosis	Infusion: 0.1–0.5 micrograms/kg/min (increased max 2mg/hr)	Infusion: 0.3–1.5 micrograms/kg/min (up to 8 micrograms/kg/min). Max total dose: 1.5mg/kg (acutely)
Noradrenaline	Via central catheter only. Potentiated by MAOI and tricyclic antidepressants	Potent catecholamine α-adrenergic agonist. Vasoconstriction	Reflex bradycardia, arrhythmia, hypertension	Infusion: 0.02–0.5 micrograms/kg/min	Infusion: 0.04–0.4 micrograms/kg/min
Octreotide	Somatostatin analogue used in treatment of carcinoid, acromegaly, and variceal bleeding (unlicensed use)	Pituitary tumour expansion, reduced need for antidiabetic treatments	GI disturbance, gallstones, hyper- and hypoglycaemia	SC: 1–5 micrograms/kg 6- to 8-hourly	SC: 50 micrograms od/bd, increased up to 200 micrograms tds. IV: 50 micrograms diluted in saline (ECG monitoring)

IV, intravenous. IM, intramuscular. SC, subcutaneous. PO, per os (oral). SL, sublingual. ET, endotracheal. od, once daily. bd, twice daily. tds, three times daily. qds, four times daily. NR, not recommended. Doses are IV and dilutions in 0.9% NaCl unless otherwise stated.

(Continued)

Table 43.1 (Contd.)

Drug	Description and perioperative indications	Cautions and contraindications	Side effects	Dose (paediatric)	Dose (adult)
Omeprazole	PPI. Reduction in gastric acid secretion	Liver disease max 20mg od	Headache, diarrhoea, prolonged QT	PO: 0.7–1.4mg/kg up to 40mg od. IV: 0.5mg/kg od	PO/slow IV: 20–40mg od. Premedication PO: 40mg. Bleeding peptic ulcer: 80mg bolus, then 8mg/hr for 3d
Ondansetron	Serotonin (5-HT₃) receptor antagonist antiemetic	QT interval prolongation	Hypotension, headache, flushing	>1/12: slow IV: 100 micrograms/kg (max 4mg) qds	Slow IV/IM/PO: 4mg tds
Oxybuprocaine	LA. Topical anaesthesia to cornea				0.4% solution. 0.5mL eye drops
Oxycodone	Opioid used for moderate pain, often in palliative care. IV preparation available: dose 1–10mg 4-hourly	Porphyria, acute abdomen	Nausea, vomiting, dysphoria, drowsiness	PO: Oxynorm® >1 month: initially 200 micrograms/kg (max 5mg) 4- to 6-hourly. >12yr: adult doses	PO: Oxynorm® 5mg 4- to 6-hourly, increased as required. Oxycontin® 10mg bd, increased as required
Oxytocin	Nonapeptide hormone which stimulates uterine contraction. Induction of labour and prevention of post-partum haemorrhage	Avoid rapid administration. Fetal distress	Vasodilatation, hypotension, flushing, tachycardia		Post-partum slow IV: 5U, followed, if required, by infusion 10U/hr (40U in 40mL 0.9% saline)

Pancuronium	Long-acting aminosteroid non-depolarizing muscle relaxant. Little histamine release. Duration 45–65min	See cisatracurium	See cisatracurium. Increased HR and BP due to vagolysis and sympathetic stimulation	Intubation: 0.1mg/kg. Maintenance: 0.02mg/kg, as required	Intubation: 0.1mg/kg. Maintenance: 0.02mg/kg, as required
Pantoprazole	PPI used to inhibit gastric acid secretion	Liver disease, pregnancy. Renal disease	Headache, pruritus, bronchospasm	NR	PO/slow IV: 40mg od (max 80mg)
Paracetamol	Mild to moderate analgesic and antipyretic	Neonates: PO: 10–15mg/kg 6-hourly (5mg/kg if jaundiced). Max 60mg/kg/d. <10kg: IV: 7.5mg/kg 6-hourly. Max 30mg/kg/d	Liver damage in overdose	Slow IV: 15mg/kg qds (max 60mg/kg/d) (10–50kg max 60mg/kg, >50kg max 4g/d). PO/PR: 20mg/kg qds (max 75mg/kg/d up to 4g/d). PR loading dose. 30–40mg/kg (>44 wk post-conception)	Slow IV: >50kg 1g qds, <50kg 15mg/kg qds. PO: 0.5–1g qds
Paraldehyde	Status epilepticus	Dilute neat solution with equal volume of olive oil before PR administration		Deep IM: 0.2mL/kg. PR: 0.3mL/kg	Deep IM: 5–10mL. PR: 10–20mL
Parecoxib	See celecoxib. Prodrug of valdecoxib. COX-2 inhibitor. Licensed for acute pain	See celecoxib. Reconstitute with 0.9% saline	GI upset, thrombotic events		IV/IM: 40mg, then 20–40mg 6- to 12-hourly (max 80mg/d)

IV, intravenous. IM, intramuscular. SC, subcutaneous. PO, per os (oral). SL, sublingual. ET, endotracheal. od, once daily. bd, twice daily. tds, three times daily. qds, four times daily. NR, not recommended. Doses are IV and dilutions in 0.9% NaCl unless otherwise stated.

(Continued)

Table 43.1 (Contd.)

Drug	Description and perioperative indications	Cautions and contraindications	Side effects	Dose (paediatric)	Dose (adult)
Pethidine	Synthetic opioid: 1. Analgesia 2. Post-operative shivering	Seizures possible in high dosage—max daily dose 1g/d (20mg/kg/d). MAOI	Respiratory depression, hypotension, dysphoria	>12yr: IV/IM/SC: 0.5–1mg/kg (max 100mg). Infusion: 5mg/kg in 50mL5% glucose at 1–3mL/hr (100–300 micrograms/kg/hr)	IM/SC: 25–100mg 3-hourly. IV: 25–50mg. PCA: 10mg/5min lockout. Shivering: 10–25mg
Phentolamine	α_1- and α_2-adrenergic antagonist. Peripheral vasodilatation and controlled hypotension. Treatment of extravasation. Duration 10min	Treat excessive hypotension with noradrenaline or methoxamine (not adrenaline/ephedrine due to β effects)	Hypotension, tachycardia, flushing	0.1mg/kg, then 5–50 micrograms/kg/min	2–5mg (10mg in 10mL saline, 1mL aliquots)
Phenylephrine	Selective direct-acting α-adrenergic agonist. Peripheral vasoconstriction and treatment of hypotension. Duration 20min	Caution in elderly and CVS disease. Hyperthyroidism	Reflex bradycardia, arrhythmias	2–10 micrograms/kg, then 0.1–0.5 micrograms/kg/min	20–100 micrograms increments (10mg in 500mL saline, 1mL aliquots). IM: 2–5mg. Infusion: 30–60 micrograms/min (5mg in 50mL saline at 0–30mL/hr)
Phenytoin	Anticonvulsant and treatment of digoxin toxicity. Serum levels 10–20mg/L (40–80 micromoles/L)	Avoid in AV heart block, pregnancy, and porphyria. Monitor ECG/BP on IV administration	Hypotension, AV conduction defects, ataxia. Enzyme induction	IV loading dose: 20mg/kg over 1hr	20mg/kg (max 2g) over 1hr (dilute to 10mg/mL in saline), then 100mg tds. Arrhythmia: 3.5–5mg/kg (rate <50mg/min)

Pipecuronium	Piperazinium derivative long-acting non-depolarizing muscle relaxant. Duration 45–120min	See cisatracurium	See cisatracurium	Intubation: 0.08mg/kg. Maintenance: 0.01–0.04mg/kg
Piroxicam	NSAID analgesic for inflammatory or degenerative joint pain. High incidence of side effects	Hypersensitivity to aspirin, asthma, severe renal impairment, peptic ulceration. Avoid in porphyria	GI upset or bleeding, bronchospasm, tinnitus, fluid retention, platelet inhibition, skin reactions	NR	PO/PR: 10–20mg od
Potassium chloride	Electrolyte replacement (see ➔ p. 1053 and p. 174)	Dilute solution before administration	Rapid infusion can cause cardiac arrest. High concentration causes phlebitis	0.5mmol/kg over 1hr. Maintenance: 1–2mmol/kg/d	10–20mmol/hr (max concentration 40mmol/L peripherally). With ECG monitoring: up to 20–40mmol/hr via central line (max 200mmol/d)
Pregabalin	Binds to voltage-dependent calcium channels and decreases release neurotransmitters. Adjunct for focal seizures.	Avoid abrupt withdrawal, severe CCF, renal impairment	Dry mouth, constipation, oedema, dizziness		Pain >18yr: 150mg 2–3 divided doses with slow increase. Epilepsy >18yr: 25mg bd increasing

IV, intravenous. IM, intramuscular. SC, subcutaneous. PO, per os (oral). SL, sublingual. ET, endotracheal. od, once daily. bd, twice daily. tds, three times daily. qds, four times daily. NR, not recommended. Doses are IV and dilutions in 0.9% NaCl unless otherwise stated.

(Continued)

Table 43.1 (Contd.)

Drug	Description and perioperative indications	Cautions and contraindications	Side effects	Dose (paediatric)	Dose (adult)
Prednisolone	Orally active corticosteroid. Less mineralocorticoid action than hydrocortisone	Adrenal suppression, severe systemic infections	Dyspepsia and ulceration, osteoporosis, myopathy, psychosis, impaired healing, diabetes mellitus	PO: 1–2mg/kg od. Croup: 4mg/kg, then 1mg/kg tds	PO: initially 20–60mg od, reduced to 2.5–15mg od for maintenance
Prilocaine	Amide-type LA. Less toxic than lidocaine. Used for infiltration and IVRA. Rapid onset. Duration 30–90min (prolonged by adrenaline), pKa 7.9	Adrenaline-containing solutions contain preservative. Significant methaemoglobinaemia if dose >600mg. Use IBW	Toxicity: tongue/circumoral numbness, restlessness, tinnitus, seizures, cardiac arrest	NR <6 months	LA: 0.5–2% solution. Max dose dependent upon injection site—6mg/kg/4hr (9mg/kg with adrenaline)
Prochlorperazine	Phenothiazine antiemetic	Hypotension on rapid IV administration. Neuroleptic malignant syndrome	Tardive dyskinesia and extrapyramidal symptoms	>10kg: PO: 0.25mg/kg tds. IM: 0.1–0.2mg/kg tds	IM: 12.5mg tds. PO: 20mg, then 5–10mg tds
Procyclidine	Antimuscarinic used in acute treatment of drug-induced dystonic reactions (except tardive dyskinesia)	Glaucoma, GI obstruction. Lower dose in elderly	Urinary retention, dry mouth, blurred vision	<2yr: 0.5–2mg. 2–10yr: 2–5mg. >10yr: adult dose	IV/IM: 5–10mg, repeat after 20min if needed
Promethazine	Phenothiazine, antihistamine, anticholinergic, antiemetic sedative. Paediatric sedation		Extrapyramidal reactions	>2yr: sedation/premed. PO: 1–2mg/kg	PO/IM: 10–25mg tds

Propofol	Di-isopropylphenol IV induction agent. Rapid recovery and little nausea. Agent of choice for day surgery, sedation, or laryngeal mask insertion—can be used for ECT	Reduce dose in elderly or haemodynamically unstable. Caution in severe allergy to eggs, peanuts, soya, soybean oil. Caution in epilepsy	Apnoea, hypotension, pain on injection. Myoclonic spasms, rarely convulsions	Induction: 2–4mg/kg. Infusion: 4–15mg/kg/hr. NR induction <1 month. NR maintenance <3yr	Induction: 2–3mg/kg. Infusion: 6–10mg/kg/hr. TCI: initially 4–8 micrograms/mL, then 3–6 micrograms/mL (reduce in elderly)
Propranolol	Non-selective β-adrenergic antagonist. Controlled hypotension, symptomatic treatment of thyrotoxicosis	Asthma, heart failure, AV block, verapamil treatment	Bradycardia, hypotension, AV block, bronchospasm	0.1mg/kg over 5min	1mg increments, up to 5–10mg
Protamine	Basic protein produced from salmon sperm. Heparin antagonist	Weakly anticoagulant and marked histamine release. Risk of allergy	Severe hypotension, pulmonary hypertension, bronchospasm, flushing	Slow IV: 1mg per 1mg heparin (100U) to be reversed	Slow IV: 1mg per 1mg heparin (100U) to be reversed
Proxymetacaine (proparacaine)	LA. Topical anaesthesia to cornea	Less stinging than with other eye drops		Avoid preterms. One drop/eye, then one drop/eye every 10min, max 5–7 doses	0.5% solution. 0.5mL eye drops
Pyridostigmine	Long-acting anticholinesterase used in treatment of myasthenia gravis	See neostigmine	See neostigmine	PO: 1–1.5mg/kg at intervals (4- to 12-hourly)	PO: 30–120mg at intervals through day (maximum 1.2g/d)

(Continued)

IV, intravenous. IM, intramuscular. SC, subcutaneous. PO, *per os* (oral). SL, sublingual. ET, endotracheal. od, once daily. bd, twice daily. tds, three times daily. qds, four times daily. NR, not recommended. Doses are IV and dilutions in 0.9% NaCl unless otherwise stated.

Table 43.1 (Contd.)

Drug	Description and perioperative indications	Cautions and contraindications	Side effects	Dose (paediatric)	Dose (adult)
Ranitidine	Histamine (H$_2$) receptor antagonist. Reduction in gastric acid secretion	Porphyria	Tachycardia	IV: 1mg/kg slowly tds (max 50mg). PO: 2–4mg/kg bd	IV: 50mg (diluted in 20mL saline, given over 2min) qds. IM: 50mg qds. PO: 150mg bd or 300mg od
Remifentanil	Ultrashort-acting opioid used to supplement GA. Metabolized by non-specific esterases (not plasma cholinesterase). Duration 5–10min. Can be used as PCA in labour: 25–75 micrograms bolus, 3min lockout (0.5–1.5mL of 50 micrograms/mL). May be mixed with propofol: 125 micrograms/50mL SV, 250–500 micrograms/50mL IPPV	Muscle rigidity, respiratory depression, hypotension, bradycardia. Use IBW		Slow bolus: up to 1 microgram/kg. Infusion (IPPV): 0.1–0.5 micrograms/kg/min. Start at 0.1 micrograms/kg/min, and adjust dose as necessary	Slow bolus: up to 1 microgram/kg. Infusion (IPPV): 0.1–0.5 micrograms/kg/min. Infusion (SV): 0.025–0.1 micrograms/kg/min. Start at 0.1 micrograms/kg/min, and adjust dose as necessary
Rivaroxaban	Direct inhibitor of factor Xa. Uses: 1. Prophylaxis of VTE after major orthopaedic surgery 2. Prophylaxis of stroke in AF 3. Treatment of VTE and prevention of recurrent VTE	Risk of major bleeding, renal impairment, severe liver disease. No routine monitoring required	Nausea, haemorrhage	NR	1. PO: 10mg od for 14d 2. PO: 20mg od 3. PO: 15mg bd for 21d, then 20mg od

Rocuronium	Rapidly acting aminosteroid non-depolarizing muscle relaxant. RSI (avoiding suxamethonium). Duration 10–40min (variable). Intubating conditions within 1min	See cisatracurium	Mild tachycardia. See cisatracurium	Intubation: 0.6–1mg/kg. Maintenance: 0.1–0.15mg/kg. Infusion: 0.3–0.6mg/kg/hr	Intubation: 0.6–1mg/kg. Maintenance: 0.1–0.15mg/kg/hr. Infusion: 0.3–0.6mg/kg/hr
Ropivacaine	Amide-type LA agent. Possibly less motor block than other agents. Duration similar to bupivacaine, but lower toxicity. pKa 8.1		Toxicity: tongue/circumoral numbness, restlessness, tinnitus, seizures, cardiac arrest	0.2–1% solution. Maximum dose dependent upon injection site—3–4mg/kg/4hr	Infiltration/epidural: max dose dependent upon injection site, 3–4mg/kg/4hr
Salbutamol	β_2 receptor agonist. Treatment of bronchospasm. Larger doses now suggested in paediatrics or IV	Monitor potassium concentration with higher doses	Tremor, vasodilatation, tachycardia, hypokalaemia	Slow IV: 1 month–2 yr 5 micrograms/kg, >2yr 15 micrograms/kg (max 250 micrograms). Infusion: 1–5 micrograms/kg/min. Nebulizer: <5yr 2.5mg, >5yr 2.5–5mg	250 micrograms slow IV, then 5 micrograms/min (up to 20 micrograms/min). Nebulizer: 2.5–5mg PRN
Sufentanil	More potent thiamyl analogue of fentanyl (five times potency). Analgesia. Duration 20–45min	See fentanyl	See fentanyl	Analgesia: 10–30 micrograms (0.2–0.6 micrograms/kg). Anaesthesia 0.6–8 micrograms/kg	Analgesia: 10–30 micrograms (0.2–0.6 micrograms/kg). Anaesthesia 0.6–8 micrograms/kg

IV, intravenous. IM, intramuscular. SC, subcutaneous. PO, per os (oral). SL, sublingual. ET, endotracheal. od, once daily. bd, twice daily. tds, three times daily. qds, four times daily. NR, not recommended. Doses are IV and dilutions in 0.9% NaCl unless otherwise stated.

(Continued)

Table 43.1 (Contd.)

Drug	Description and perioperative indications	Cautions and contraindications	Side effects	Dose (paediatric)	Dose (adult)
Sugammadex	Specific cyclodextrin reversal agent for rocuronium and vecuronium	Wait 24hr after use before using rocuronium/vecuronium in patient; fusidic acid or flucloxacillin may displace relaxant from sugammadex within 6hr	Binds with contraceptive pill	T2 present 2mg/kg. Full reversal NR at present	T2 present 2mg/kg. To reverse full dose of rocuronium or vecuroniumm immediately 16mg/kg
Suxamethonium	Depolarizing muscle relaxant. Rapid short-acting muscle paralysis. Phase II block develops with repeated doses (>8mg/kg). Store at 2–8°C	Prolonged block in plasma cholinesterase deficiency, hypokalaemia, hypocalcaemia. MH, neuromuscular disorders. Increased serum K+ (normally 0.5mmol/L, greater in burns, trauma, upper motor neuron injury)	Increased intraocular pressure. Bradycardia with 2nd dose	IV: 1-2mg/kg. IM: 3-4mg/kg	1–1.5mg/kg. Infusion: 0.5–10mg/min
Tapentadol	Moderate to severe pain managed only by opioids	Reduce in hepatic impairment	Diarrhoea, dyspepsia, weight loss	Consult tertiary consultant	>18yr PO: 50mg 4- to 6-hourly, max 700mg

Teicoplanin	Glycopeptide antibiotic with activity against aerobic and anaerobic Gram-positive bacteria	Renal impairment	Allergic reactions, blood disorders, ototoxicity, nephrotoxicity	>1 month: 10mg/kg for three doses 12-hourly, then 6mg/kg od	IV/IM: 400mg for three doses 12-hourly, then 400mg od
Temazepam	Benzodiazepine. Sedation or premedication. Duration 1–2hr	Decreased requirement for anaesthetic agents	Respiratory depression in combination with opioids. Amnesia	PO: 0.3mg/kg preoperatively. NR <12yr	PO: 10–40mg 1hr preoperatively (elderly 10–20mg)
Tenoxicam	NSAID analgesic for mild to moderate pain	Hypersensitivity to aspirin, asthma, severe renal impairment, peptic ulceration	GI upset or bleeding, bronchospasm, tinnitus, fluid retention, platelet inhibition	NR	PO: 20mg od. IV/IM: 20mg od
Tetracaine (amethocaine)	Ester-type LA. Topical analgesia prior to venepuncture. Ametop® gel contains 4% amethocaine. (Also available as eye drops, but has temporary disruptive effect on corneal epithelium). Duration 4hr	Apply only to intact skin under occlusive dressing. Remove after 45min. Rapid absorption through mucosa		As adult. <1 month NR	Each tube expels 1.5g (sufficient for area 6 × 5cm)

IV, intravenous. IM, intramuscular. SC, subcutaneous. PO, *per os* (oral). SL, sublingual. ET, endotracheal. od, once daily. bd, twice daily. tds, three times daily. qds, four times daily. NR, not recommended. Doses are IV and dilutions in 0.9% NaCl unless otherwise stated.

(Continued)

Table 43.1 (Contd.)

Drug	Description and perioperative indications	Cautions and contraindications	Side effects	Dose (paediatric)	Dose (adult)
Thiopental	Short-acting thiobarbiturate. Induction of anaesthesia, anticonvulsant, cerebral protection. Recovery due to redistribution	Accumulation with repeated doses. Caution in hypovolaemia and elderly. Porphyria	Hypotension. Necrosis if intra-arterial	Induction: neonate 2–4mg/kg, child 5–6mg/kg. Status: 2–4mg/kg, then 8mg/kg/hr	Induction/cerebral protection: 3–5mg/kg. Anticonvulsant: 0.5–2mg/kg PRN
Tramadol	Analgesic thought to have less respiratory depression, constipation, euphoria, and abuse potential than other opioids. Has opioid and non-opioid mechanisms of action	Only 30% antagonized by naloxone. Caution in epilepsy. Previously not recommended for intraoperative use. MAOI	Nausea, dizziness, dry mouth. Increased side effects in conjunction with other opioids	>12yr: adult dose	PO: 50–100mg 4-hourly. Slow IV/IM: 50–100mg 4-hourly (100mg initially, then 50mg increments to max 250mg). Max 600mg/d
Tranexamic acid	Inhibits plasminogen activation, reducing fibrin dissolution by plasmin. Reduced haemorrhage in major trauma, prostatectomy, and dental extraction	Avoid in thromboembolic disease, renal impairment, and pregnancy	Dizziness, nausea	Slow IV: 10–15mg/kg tds. PO: 10–25mg/kg tds	Slow IV: 0.5–1g tds. PO: 15–25mg/kg tds

Triamcinolone acetonide	Relatively insoluble corticosteroid for depot injection. Epidural unlicensed use. Triamcinolone 4mg, prednisolone 5mg	Dose depends upon site of injection. Strict asepsis essential. Dilute 40mg/mL solution prior to use	See prednisolone	Intra-articular or intrasynovial: 2mg/kg, max 40mg	Intra-articular or intrasynovial: 5–40mg. Epidural: 40–60mg diluted with LA
Trimeprazine	See alimemazine				
Vancomycin	Glycopeptide antibiotic with activity against aerobic and anaerobic Gram-positive bacteria. Peak level <30mg/L. Trough level 10–15mg/L	Avoid rapid infusion (hypotension, wheezing, urticaria, 'red man' syndrome). Reduce dose in renal impairment/elderly	Ototoxicity, nephrotoxicity, phlebitis, neutropenia	>1 month: 15mg/kg over 2hr tds (max 2g daily)	1–1.5g over 100min bd (check blood levels after 3rd dose). Reduce 500mg bd elderly
Vasopressin	Synthetic ADH used in treatment of diabetes insipidus, resistant vasodilatory shock, variceal bleeding	Extreme caution in coronary vascular disease	Pallor, coronary vasoconstriction, water intoxication	Diabetes insipidus SC/IM: <12yr 0.1–0.4 micrograms/d. >12yr 1–4 micrograms/d. See BNFc for specific indications	Diabetes insipidus SC/IM: 5–20U 4-hourly. Septic shock infusion: 1–4U/hr. Variceal bleed: 20U over 15min

IV, intravenous. IM, intramuscular. SC, subcutaneous. PO, per os (oral). SL, sublingual. ET, endotracheal. od, once daily. bd, twice daily. tds, three times daily. qds, four times daily. NR, not recommended. Doses are IV and dilutions in 0.9% NaCl unless otherwise stated.

(Continued)

Table 43.1 (Contd.)

Drug	Description and perioperative indications	Cautions and contraindications	Side effects	Dose (paediatric)	Dose (adult)
Vecuronium	Aminosteroid non-depolarizing muscle relaxant. Cardiostable and no histamine release. Duration 30–45min	See cisatracurium	See cisatracurium	Intubation: 80–100 micrograms/kg. Maintenance: 20–30 micrograms/kg. Infusion: 0.8–1.4 micrograms/kg/min	Intubation: 80–100 micrograms/kg. Maintenance: 20–30 micrograms/kg. Infusion: 0.8–1.4 micrograms/kg/min
Warfarin	Coumarin derivative oral anticoagulant. Target INR: 2.5—treatment DVT/PE, AF, mitral valve disease; 3.5—recurrent DVT/PE while on warfarin, mechanical heart valves (lower INR acceptable with low-risk valves)	Previous haemorrhagic stroke, severe renal or liver disease, pregnancy, peptic ulcer disease. Reduce dose in elderly	Haemorrhage	PO: 0.2mg/kg up to 10mg od for 2d, then 0.05–0.2mg/kg od	PO: 10mg od for 2d, then 3–9mg od, dependent on INR

| Zolpidem | Short-acting imidazopyridine hypnotic with little hangover effect | OSA, myasthenia gravis | Nausea, dizziness | NR | PO: 10mg nocte (elderly 5mg) |
| Zopiclone | Short-acting cyclopyrrolone hypnotic with little hangover effect | OSA, myasthenia gravis | Nausea, bitter taste in mouth | NR | PO: 7.5mg nocte (elderly 3.75mg) |

IV, intravenous. IM, intramuscular. SC, subcutaneous. PO, per os (oral). SL, sublingual. ET, endotracheal. od, once daily. bd, twice daily. tds, three times daily. qds, four times daily. NR, not recommended. Doses are IV and dilutions in 0.9% NaCl unless otherwise stated.

Infusion regimes

Table 43.2 Infusion regimes

Drug	Indication	Diluent	Dose	Suggested regime (60kg adult)	Infusion range	Initial rate (adult)	Comments
Adrenaline	Treatment of hypotension	0.9% NaCl, 5% glucose	2–20 micrograms/min (0.04–0.4 micrograms/kg/min)	5mg/50mL (100 micrograms/mL)	1.2–12+ mL/hr	5mL/hr	Via central catheter. Suggest 1mg/50mL for initial intra-operative use (or 1mg/500mL if no central access)
Alfentanil	Analgesia	0.9% NaCl, 5% glucose	0.5–1 micrograms/kg/min	Undiluted (500 micrograms/mL)	0–8mL/hr	4mL/hr	1–2mg can be added to 50mL propofol for infusion
Aminophylline	Bronchodilation	0.9% NaCl, 5% glucose	0.5mg/kg/hr	250mg/50mL (5mg/mL)	0–6mL/hr	6mL/h	After 5mg/kg slow bolus
Amiodarone	Treatment of arrhythmias	5% glucose only	Loading infusion 5mg/kg over 20–120min, then 900mg over 24hr	300mg/50mL (6mg/mL)	25–50mL/hr, then 6mL/hr	25mL/hr	Via central line (peripherally 'in extremis'). Max 1.2g in 24hr. Adjust to therapeutic levels

Atracurium	Muscle relaxant	0.9% NaCl, 5% glucose	0.3–0.6mg/kg/hr	Undiluted (10mg/mL)	1.5–4mL/hr	3mL/hr	Assess rate with nerve stimulator
Cisatracurium	Muscle relaxant	0.9% NaCl, 5% glucose	0.06–0.18mg/kg/hr	Undiluted (2mg/mL)	2–5mL/hr	5mL/hr	Assess rate with nerve stimulator
Digoxin	Rapid control of ventricular rate	0.9% NaCl, 5% glucose	250–500 micrograms over 30–60min; 0.75–1mg over 2hr	250–500 micrograms/50mL	0–100mL/hr	50mL/hr	ECG monitoring suggested
Dobutamine	Cardiac failure/ inotrope	0.9% NaCl, 5% glucose	2.5–10 micrograms/kg/ min	250mg/50mL (5mg/mL)	2–7mL/hr	2mL/hr	
Dopamine	Inotrope	0.9% NaCl, 5% glucose	2–10 micrograms/ kg/min	200mg/50mL (4mg/mL)	2–9mL/hr	2mL/hr	Via central line
Dopexamine	Inotrope	0.9% NaCl, 5% glucose	0.5–6 micrograms/ kg/min	50mg/50mL (1mg/mL)	2–22mL/hr	2mL/hr	May be given via large peripheral vein
Doxapram	Respiratory stimulant	0.9% NaCl, 5% glucose	2–4mg/min	200mg/50mL (4mg/mL)	30–60mL/hr	30mL/hr	Max dose 4mg/kg. NR child
Alternative regimes for any infusion		3mg/kg/50mL, then 1mL/hr = 1 microgram/kg/min; 3mg/50mL, then 1mL/hr = 1 microgram/min. Rate (mL/hr), 60 × rate (micrograms/kg/min) × weight (kg) / concentration (micrograms/mL)					

(Continued)

Table 43.2 (Contd.)

Drug	Indication	Diluent	Dose	Suggested regime (60kg adult)	Infusion range	Initial rate (adult)	Comments
Enoximone	Inodilator	0.9% NaCl only	90 micrograms/kg/min for 10–30min, then 5–20 micrograms/kg/min	100mg/50mL (2mg/mL)	9–36mL/hr	162mL/hr for 10–30min	Max 24mg/kg/d
Esmolol	β-blocker	0.9% NaCl, 5% glucose	50–200 micrograms/kg/min	2.5g/50mL (50mg/mL)	3–15mL/hr	3mL/hr	ECG monitoring
Glyceryl trinitrate	Controlled hypotension	0.9% NaCl, 5% glucose	0.5–12mg/hr	50mg/50mL (1mg/mL)	0.5–12mL/hr	5mL/hr	
Heparin	Anticoagulation	0.9% NaCl, 5% glucose	24 000–48 000U per 24hr	50 000U/50mL (1000U/mL)	1–2mL/hr	2mL/hr	Check APTT after 12hr. See local guidelines
Insulin (soluble)	Diabetes mellitus	0.9% NaCl	Sliding scale	50U/50mL (1U/mL)	Sliding scale	Sliding scale	
Isoprenaline	Treatment of heart block or bradycardia	0.9% NaCl, 5% glucose	1.5–10 micrograms/min	1mg/50mL (20 micrograms/mL)	0.5–30mL/hr	7mL/hr	Special order request required
Ketamine	GA	0.9% NaCl, 5% glucose	1–3mg/kg/hr	500mg/50mL (10mg/mL)	6–18mL/hr	10mL/hr	Induction 0.5–2mg/kg

Ketamine	Analgesia	0.9% NaCl, 5% glucose	0.2mg/kg/hr	200mg/50mL (4mg/mL)	0–6mL/hr	3mL/hr	With midazolam 2–5 mg/hr
Ketamine	'Trauma' mixture	0.9% NaCl	0.5mL/kg/hr	50mL mixture (4mg/mL ketamine)	15–45mL/hr	30mL/hr	200mg ketamine + 10mg midazolam + 10mg vecuronium in 50mL
Lidocaine (lignocaine)	Ventricular arrhythmias	0.9% NaCl	4mg/min for 30min, 2mg/min for 2hr, then 1mg/min for 24hr	500mg/50mL (10mg/mL, 1%)	6–24mL/hr	24mL/hr	After 50–100mg, slow IV bolus. ECG monitoring
Milrinone	Inodilator	0.9% NaCl, 5% glucose	50 micrograms/kg over 10min, then 0.375–0.75 micrograms/kg/min	10mg/50mL (0.2mg/mL)	7–14mL/hr	90mL/hr for 10min	Max 1.13mg/kg/d
Mivacurium	Muscle relaxant	0.9% NaCl, 5% glucose	0.4–0.6mg/kg/hr	Undiluted (2mg/mL)	12–18mL/hr	18mL/hr	Assess rate with nerve stimulator
Morphine	Analgesia	0.9% NaCl	0–3.5mg/hr	50mg/50mL (1mg/mL)	0–3.5mL/hr	2mL/hr	Monitor respiration and sedation hourly. Administer O_2.
Alternative regimes for any infusion	3mg/kg/50mL, then 1mL/hr = 1 microgram/kg/min; 3mg/50mL, then 1mL/hr = 1 microgram/min						
	Rate (mL/hr) = 60 × rate (micrograms/kg/min) × weight (kg) / concentration (micrograms/mL)						

(Continued)

Table 43.2 (Contd.)

Drug	Indication	Diluent	Dose	Suggested regime (60kg adult)	Infusion range	Initial rate (adult)	Comments
Naloxone	Opioid antagonist	0.9% NaCl, 5% glucose	>1 microgram/kg/hr	2mg/500mL (4 micrograms/mL)		100mL/hr	Rate adjusted according to response
Nimodipine	Prevention of vasospasm after SAH	0.9% NaCl, 5% glucose	1mg/hr, increasing to 2mg/hr after 2hr	Undiluted (0.2mg/mL)	5–10mL/hr	5mL/hr	Via central line. Incompatible with polyvinyl chloride
Nitroprusside (sodium)	Controlled hypotension	5% glucose	0.3–1.5 micrograms/kg/min	25mg/50mL (500 micrograms/mL)	2–10mL/hr	5mL/hr	Max dose 1.5mg/kg. Protect from light
Noradrenaline	Treatment of hypotension	5% glucose	2–20 micrograms/min (0.04–0.4 micrograms/kg/min)	4mg/40mL (100 micrograms/mL)	1.2–12+ mL/hr	5mL/hr	Via central line
Octreotide	Somatostatin analogue	0.9% NaCl	25–50 micrograms/hr	500 micrograms/50mL (10 micrograms/mL)	2–5mL/hr	5mL/hr	Use in variceal bleeding unlicensed
Oxytocin	Prevention of uterine atony	0.9% NaCl, 5% glucose	0.02–0.125U/min (10U/hr)	30U in 500mL (0.06U/mL)	30–125mL/hr	125mL/hr	Individual unit protocols vary
Phenylephrine	Treatment of hypotension	0.9% NaCl, 5% glucose	30–60 micrograms/min	5mg in 50mL (100 micrograms/mL)	18–36mL/hr	30mL/hr	Gaining popularity for regional Caesarean

Phenytoin	Anticonvulsant prophylaxis	0.9% NaCl	20mg/kg	900mg/90mL (administer via 0.22–0.5 micron filter)	Up to 50mg/min	180mL/hr	ECG and BP monitoring. Complete within 1hr of preparation
Propofol	Anaesthesia		6–10mg/kg/hr	Undiluted (10mg/mL)		36–60mL/hr	TCI: initially 4–8 micrograms/mL, then 3–6 micrograms/mL
Propofol	Sedation		0–3mg/kg/hr	Undiluted (10mg/mL)		0–20mL/hr	TCI: 0–2.5 micrograms/mL
Remifentanil	Analgesia during GA	0.9% NaCl, 5% glucose	0.1–1.0 micrograms/kg/min	2mg/40mL (50 micrograms/mL)	5–40mL/hr IPPV 2–7mL/hr SV	8mL/hr IPPV 2mL/hr SV	Suggest starting at 0.1 micrograms/kg/min (8mL/hr), then adjust up to 0.25 micrograms/kg/min (20mL/hr) as required
Rocuronium	Muscle relaxant	0.9% NaCl, 5% glucose	0.3–0.6mg/kg/hr	Undiluted (10mg/mL)		1.5–4mL/hr	3mL/hr	Assess rate with nerve stimulator
Alternative regimes for any infusion	3mg/kg/50mL, then 1mL/hr = 1 microgram/kg/min; 3mg/50mL, then 1mL/hr = 1 microgram/min Rate (mL/hr) = 60 × rate (micrograms/kg/min) × weight (kg) / concentration (micrograms/mL)						

(Continued)

Table 43.2 (Contd.)

Drug	Indication	Diluent	Dose	Suggested regime (60kg adult)	Infusion range	Initial rate (adult)	Comments
Salbutamol	Bronchospasm	5% glucose	5–20 micrograms/min	1mg/50mL (20 micrograms/mL)	15–60mL/hr	30mL/hr	After 250 micrograms, slow IV bolus
Sodium bicarbonate	Acidosis		(Weight (kg) × base deficit × 0.3) mmol	Undiluted (8.4% solution)			8.4%, 1000mmol/L. Via central line, if possible
Vancomycin	Antibiotic	0.9% NaCl, 5% glucose	1–1.5g 12-hourly	1g/500mL	500mL/100min	500mL/100min	Elderly 500mg 12-hourly
Vecuronium	Muscle relaxant	0.9% NaCl, 5% glucose	0.05–0.08mg/kg/hr	Undiluted (2mg/mL)	1.5–3mL/hr	2.5mL/hr	Assess rate with nerve stimulator
Alternative regimes for any infusion	3mg/kg/50mL, then 1mL/hr = 1 microgram/kg/min; 3mg/50mL, then 1mL/hr = 1 microgram/min. Rate (mL/hr) = 60 × rate (micrograms/kg/min) × weight (kg) / concentration (micrograms/mL)						

Medical gases

Table 43.3 Medical gases storage and properties

Medical gas	State in cylinder	Body colour	Shoulder colour	Cylinder capacity (L)				Cylinder pressure when full (×100 Pa)	Critical temperature (°C)
				Type C	Type D	Type E	Type F		
Oxygen (O_2)	Gas	White	White	170	340	680	1360	137	−118.4
Nitrous oxide (N_2O)	Liquid	White	Blue	450	900	1800	3600	44*	36.4
O_2:N_2O 50:50 (Entonox®)	Gas	White	Blue and white		500		2000	137	−6†
Medical air	Gas	White	Black and white			640	1280	137	
Carbon dioxide (CO_2)	Liquid	White	Grey	450		1800		50*	30
O_2:CO_2 95:5	Gas	White	Grey and white				1360	137	
Medical helium (He)	Gas	White	Brown		300		1200	137	−268
O_2:He 21:79	Gas	White	Brown and white				1200	137	
Water capacity of cylinder (L)				1.2	2.32	4.68	9.43		

*Where the contents are liquid, the pressure is not a reliable method of judging the contents.

†Entonox® separates into O_2 and N_2O at −6°C—'pseudocritical' temperature.

Pressures quoted for full cylinders are at 15°C.

All medical gas cylinders will change to white body cylinders by 2025. Cylinder colours, pressures, and contents may vary outside the UK.

Minimum alveolar concentration values

Table 43.4 Properties of inhalational agents

	MAC in O₂/air[1] (%)			MAC in 67% N₂O (%)			BP (°C)	SVP (kPa)	Oil:gas part. coeff.	Blood:gas part. coeff	MW	Biotrans. (%)
	1yr	40yr	80yr	1yr	40yr	80yr						
Halothane	0.95	0.75	0.58	0.47	0.27	0.1	50.2	32.5	224	2.3	197.4	25
Enflurane	2.08	1.63	1.27	1.03	0.58	0.22	56.5	22.9	96	1.91	184.5	3
Isoflurane	1.49	1.17	0.91	0.74	0.42	0.17	48.5	31.9	91	1.4	184.5	0.2
Sevoflurane	2.29	1.8	1.4	1.13	0.65	0.25	58.5	21.3	53	0.59	200	2.5
Desflurane	8.3	6.6	5.1	4.2	2.4	0.93	23.5	88.5	18.7	0.42	168	Minimal
Nitrous oxide	133	104	81	NA	NA	NA	−88	5080	1.4	0.47	44	0
Xenon	92	72	57	NA	NA	NA	−107.1	5800	20	0.14	131.3	0

Potency (MAC) correlates with oil:gas partition coefficient (hence lipid solubility).

Speed of onset correlates with blood:gas partition coefficient (lower, faster).

SVP, saturated vapour pressure at 20°C; part. coeff., partition coefficient at 37°C; MW, molecular weight; BP, boiling point; biotrans., biotransformation.

[1] Nickalls RWD, Mapleson WW (2003). Age-related iso-MAC charts for isoflurane, sevoflurane and desflurane in man. *Br J Anaesth* **91**, 170–4.

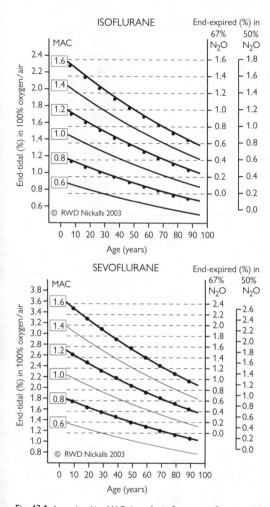

Fig. 43.1 Age-related iso-MAC charts for isoflurane, sevoflurane, and desflurane.

Reasonable ranges of MAC: SV/LMA 1.2–1.6 MAC; IPPV with opioids 1.0–1.3 MAC; IPPV with remifentanil (0.25 micrograms/kg/min) 0.6–0.9 MAC. (Courtesy of Dr RWD Nickalls). Nickalls RWD, Mapleson WW (2003). Age-related iso-MAC charts for isoflurane, sevoflurane and desflurane in man. *British Journal of Anaesthesia*, **91**, 170–174, http://bja.oxfordjournals.org/cgi/reprint/91/2/170.pdf; Lerou JGC (2004). Nomogram to estimate age-related MAC. *British Journal of Anaesthesia*, **93**, 288–291.

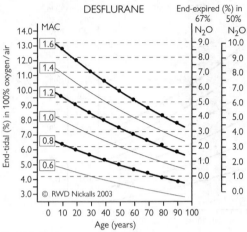

Fig. 43.1 *Contd.*

Antibiotic prophylaxis

Antibiotics are commonly used in elective and emergency surgery to prevent infection resulting from bacterial contamination. The choices of antibiotics are determined by local prevalences and sensitivities.

Surgical antibiotic prophylaxis

Table 43.5 provides a list of surgical procedures and recommended antibiotic prophylaxis.

Timing of prophylactic antibiotics

Antibiotics should be administered before skin incision and not >60 min prior to this event. One exception is with infected patients where it is planned to take surgical samples prior to administering antibiotics.

Penicillin allergy

- How 'allergic'? What happens (e.g. diarrhoea is not an allergy)? Was it anaphylaxis?
- Check old drug charts—may have had a penicillin in the past without problems. This further strengthens the case against a genuine penicillin allergy.
- If penicillin allergy is only a rash, cephalosporins may be used with care (2–5% cross-sensitivity in practice).
- If history of anaphylaxis with penicillin, avoid any β-lactam (i.e. no penicillins, cephalosporins, or carbapenems). Discuss alternatives with a microbiologist. Remember vancomycin and teicoplanin have no Gram-negative cover.

Prophylaxis for perioperative aspiration pneumonia

- General tendency to overtreat 'aspiration pneumonia', much of which is due to chemical pneumonitis. Organisms likely to cause infection are from the oropharynx, mainly anaerobes, but may include Gram-negative aerobes, including *Pseudomonas* species in hospitalized patients.
  If prophylaxis is deemed necessary, choose antibiotics that cover anaerobes:
  - Co-amoxiclav 1.2g IV for three doses 8-hourly
  - Clarithromycin 500mg IV for two doses 12-hourly
  - Where Gram-negative bacteria may be problematic—cefuroxime 1.5g IV tds ± metronidazole 500mg IV tds.

Patients known to be previously colonized with meticillin-resistant *Staphylococcus aureus*

Such patients can never be assumed free, despite negative screens, so flucloxacillin and related cephalosporins or carbapenems will be ineffective. Check the previous organisms' sensitivities, and, if in doubt, give either vancomycin 1g IV or teicoplanin 400mg IV.

Endocarditis prophylaxis

Infective endocarditis (IE) primarily affects heart valves and is caused mainly by bacteria, but occasionally by other infectious agents. It is a life-threatening disease, with significant mortality (around 20%) and morbidity.

Table 43.5 Recommended surgical antibiotic prophylaxis

Procedure	1st choice	2nd choice (mild penicillin allergy)	2nd choice (severe penicillin allergy)	MRSA positive
General surgery				
Appendicectomy, gastro-oesophageal, open biliary tract, pancreato-biliary colorectal, complex laparoscopic cholecystectomy	Cefuroxime 1.5g IV	Cefuroxime 1.5g IV and metronidazole 500mg IV	Gentamicin 3mg/kg IV and teicoplanin 400mg IV	Add teicoplanin 400mg IV (unless already given)
Laparoscopic cholecystectomy (uncomplicated), thyroid surgery	Prophylaxis not routinely recommended			
Inguinal hernia repair (laparoscopic or open)	Prophylaxis not routinely recommended (with or without mesh)			
Splenectomy	Prophylaxis not routinely recommended; however, will require lifelong oral antibiotics and immunization			
Breast surgery				
Breast surgery	Prophylaxis not routinely recommended; however, consider for the following—wire-guided excision, re-operation, and reconstructive surgery. Surgery with implant (consider also adding teicoplanin 400mg IV with implants)			
	Co-amoxiclav 1.2g IV	Cefuroxime 1.5g IV	Gentamicin 3mg/kg IV and teicoplanin 400mg IV	Add teicoplanin 400mg IV (unless already given)

Vascular surgery		
Vascular surgery (abdominal and lower limb) and lower limb amputation	Co-amoxiclav 1.2g IV and two post-operative doses 8-hourly	Gentamicin 3mg/kg IV and teicoplanin 400mg IV and one post-operative dose of teicoplanin at 8hr	Add teicoplanin 400mg IV and one post-operative dose at 8hr (unless already given)
ENT and maxillofacial surgery		
Tonsillectomy, adenoidectomy, grommet insertion, routine nasal and sinus surgery, head and neck (clean), facial (clean), ear (clean), and dentoalveolar	Prophylaxis not routinely recommended	
Major head and neck, facial or bony surgery (contaminated/ clean-contaminated)	Co-amoxiclav 1.2g IV	Gentamicin 3mg/kg IV and metronidazole 500mg IV	Add teicoplanin 400mg IV
Urological surgery		
Transurethral resection of the prostate (TURP)	Send preoperative MSU, and check sensitivities	Add teicoplanin 400mg IV
	Gentamicin 3mg/kg IV (unless resistant organism)	
Transrectal prostate biopsy	Ciprofloxacin 500mg bd PO (1st dose 1hr before operation, continue for 48hr)	

(Continued)

Table 43.5 (Contd.)

Procedure	1st choice	2nd choice (mild penicillin allergy)	2nd choice (severe penicillin allergy)	MRSA positive
Transurethral resection of bladder tumours (TURBT) and other transurethral procedures (bladder neck incision, cystoscopy), shockwave lithotripsy	Prophylaxis not routinely recommended. If positive MSU, then treat according to sensitivities			
Open or laparoscopic procedures, open cystectomy, nephrectomy and radical prostatectomy	Cefuroxime 1.5g IV and metronidazole 500mg IV		Gentamicin 3mg/kg IV and metronidazole 500mg IV	Add teicoplanin 400mg IV
Ophthalmic surgery				
Intraocular and cataract surgery	Systemic prophylaxis not routinely recommended. Intracameral cefuroxime at the discretion of the surgeon			
Plastic surgery				
Non-infected lesions and minor excisions, hand surgery (without implants)	Prophylaxis not routinely recommended			
Procedures on the breast, groin/axilla/neck dissections, hand implants and other procedures requiring implants	Co-amoxiclav 1.2g IV	Cefuroxime 1.5g IV	Gentamicin 3mg/kg IV and teicoplanin 400mg IV	Add teicoplanin 400mg IV (unless already given)
Thoracic surgery				
Lung resection and VATS	Cefuroxime 1.5g IV		Gentamicin 3mg/kg IV and teicoplanin 400mg IV	Add teicoplanin 400mg IV

Orthopaedic surgery			
Orthopaedic surgery	Ciprofloxacin 500mg bd PO (1st dose 1hr before operation, continue for 48hr)		
Surgery without prosthetic device	Prophylaxis not routinely recommended. If positive MSU, then treat according to sensitivities		
Minor metal work	Cefuroxime 1.5g IV Consider further dose at 8hr if high risk (revision, obesity, diabetes)	Gentamicin 3mg/kg IV and metronidazole 500mg IV	Add teicoplanin 400mg IV
Prosthetic joint surgery and spinal surgery	Gentamicin 3mg/kg IV and teicoplanin 400mg IV (consider further dose at 8hr if high risk)		
Obstetrics			
Caesarean section	Co-amoxiclav 1.2g IV	Cefuroxime 1.5g IV	Gentamicin 3mg/kg IV and clindamycin 600mg IV	Add teicoplanin 400mg IV
Manual removal of placenta and perineal tears involving anus/rectum	Co-amoxiclav 1.2g IV	Cefuroxime 1.5g IV and metronidazole 500mg IV	Gentamicin 3mg/kg IV and metronidazole 500mg IV	Add teicoplanin 400mg IV
Gynaecological surgery			
Diagnostic/operative laparoscopy, laparoscopic/hysteroscopic sterilization, hysteroscopy, endometrial biopsy or ablation	Prophylaxis not routinely recommended		

(Continued)

Table 43.5 (Contd.)

Procedure	1st choice	2nd choice (mild penicillin allergy)	2nd choice (severe penicillin allergy)	MRSA positive
Hysterectomy (vaginal, laparoscopic, and abdominal), laparotomy and vaginal repair	Co-amoxiclav 1.2g IV	Cefuroxime 1.5g IV and metronidazole 500mg IV	Gentamicin 3mg/kg IV and metronidazole 500mg IV	Add teicoplanin 400mg IV
Surgical termination, evacuation of retained products of conception (ERPC), hysterosalpingogram, laparoscopy with dye hydrotubation	Metronidazole 400mg PO or 1g PR and azithromycin 1g PO (to cover *Chlamydia*) 1hr preoperatively			

Adapted from the Royal Devon and Exeter NHS Foundation Trust 'Adult Surgical Antibiotic Prophylaxis' guideline.

IE usually arises through haematogenous spread of bacteria. Invasive procedures often result in a transient bacteraemia; however, there is no clear evidence to suggest this event increases the risk of developing IE. Studies suggest that transient bacteraemias are a common occurrence, e.g. as a consequence of regular tooth brushing. As a result, guidelines published in recent years have discouraged the routine use of antibiotic prophylaxis.

National Institute for Health and Care Excellence 2008 guideline on endocarditis prophylaxis

In England, in 2008, NICE issued guidelines[1] on the prevention of IE which concluded:

- Patients with certain cardiac conditions are at a higher risk of developing IE (Box 43.1).
- The clinical effectiveness of antibiotic prophylaxis is not proven and may overall lead to harm (due to risk of anaphylaxis).
- Antibiotic prophylaxis against IE is no longer recommended for any patients undergoing dental, GI, genitourinary, or upper and lower respiratory tract procedures.
- If a person at risk of IE is receiving antimicrobial therapy because they are undergoing a procedure at a site where there is a suspected infection, then the person should receive an antibiotic that covers organisms causing IE.
- Maintaining good oral hygiene is important and effective at reducing the risk of IE.

Box 43.1 Cardiac conditions at highest risk of infective endocarditis

- Prosthetic cardiac valve or prosthetic material used for cardiac valve repair.
- Previous IE.
- Unrepaired cyanotic CHD, including palliative shunts and conduits.
- Completely repaired congenital heart defect with prosthetic material or device, whether placed by surgery or by catheter intervention, during the first 6 months after the procedure.
- Repaired cyanotic CHD with residual defects at the site or adjacent to the site of a prosthetic patch or prosthetic device (which inhibit endothelialization).
  Note: Endothelialization of prosthetic material occurs within 6 months of the procedure.

European Society of Cardiology 2009 guideline

Published after the NICE guideline and similar to the advice of the American Heart Association, it suggests:[2]

- Avoidance of extensive use of antibiotic prophylaxis.
- Prophylaxis should be considered for high-risk patients (Table 43.5) who are undergoing dental procedures that require manipulation of the gingival or periapical region of the teeth or perforation of the oral mucosa.

General recommendations

- Antibiotics indicated for surgical procedures should be given as normal.
- For 'infected surgery' in patients at risk of IE, appropriate antibiotic prophylaxis should be administered.
- In patients at high risk of IE, the decision to provide prophylactic antibiotics for dental treatment should be made by treating clinicians after discussion with the patient.
- Administration of antibiotics is not risk-free, and local protocols should be followed.

References

1 National Institute for Health and Care Excellence (2008). *Prophylaxis against infective endocarditis: antimicrobial prophylaxis against infective endocarditis in adults and children undergoing interventional procedures. NICE CG64.* ℘https://www.nice.org.uk/guidance/cg64.
2 Habib G, Hoen B, Tornos P, *et al.*; ESC Committee for Practice Guidelines (2009). Guidelines on the prevention, diagnosis, and treatment of infective endocarditis (new version 2009): the Task Force on the Prevention, Diagnosis, and Treatment of Infective Endocarditis of the European Society of Cardiology (ESC). Endorsed by the European Society of Clinical Microbiology and Infectious Diseases (ESCMID) and the International Society of Chemotherapy (ISC) for Infection and Cancer. *Eur Heart J*, **30**, 2369–413.

Further reading

Glenny AM, Oliver R, Roberts GJ, Hooper L, Worthington HV (2013). Antibiotics for the prophylaxis of bacterial endocarditis in dentistry. *Cochrane Database Syst Rev*, **10**, CD003813.
Richey R, Wray D, Stokes T (2008). Prophylaxis against infective endocarditis: summary of NICE guidance. *BMJ*, **336**, 770–1.

Anaesthesia data

Charles Gibson and Fred Roberts

ASA/CEPOD classifications

ASA classifications of physical status are given in Table 44.1. CEPOD classifications of surgical urgency are given in Table 44.2.

Table 44.1 ASA physical status classification system for assessing fitness for surgery

Grade	Description
1	A healthy patient with no systemic disease
2	Mild to moderate systemic disease
3	Severe systemic disease imposing functional limitation on patient
4	Severe systemic disease which is a constant threat to life
5	Moribund patient who is not expected to survive with or without the operation
6	A brainstem-dead patient whose organs are being removed for donor purposes

For emergency cases, the suffix 'E' is used,

ASA, American Society of Anesthesiologists

Table 44.2 CEPOD classification of the urgency for surgery

Description of surgery	
Elective	Intervention planned or booked in advance of routine admission to hospital. Timing to suit patient, hospital, and staff
Expedited	Patient requiring early treatment where the condition is not an immediate threat to life, limb, or organ survival. Normally within days of decision to operate
Urgent	Intervention for acute onset or clinical deterioration of potentially life-threatening conditions, for those conditions that may threaten the survival of limb or organ, for fixation of many fractures, and for the relief of pain or other distressing symptoms. Normally within hours of decision to operate
Immediate	Immediate life-, limb-, or organ-saving intervention—resuscitation simultaneous with intervention. Normally within minutes of decision to operate: a. Lifesaving b. Other, e.g. limb- or organ-saving

CEPOD, (National) Confidential Enquiry into Patient Outcome and Death.

Breathing systems

Anaesthetic breathing systems can be classified into **open** (e.g. air), **semi-open** (e.g. Hudson mask), **semi-closed** (Mapleson classification; Fig. 44.1), and **closed** (circle; Fig. 44.2). The FGFs required to prevent rebreathing in a Mapleson system are given in Table 44.3, and the FGFs required in a circle system are given in Table 44.4.

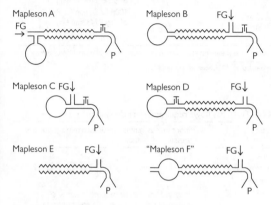

Fig. 44.1 Mapleson classification of breathing systems.
FG, fresh gas; P, patient.

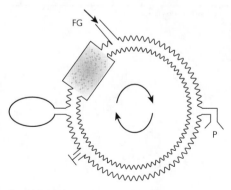

Fig. 44.2 The circle system.

Table 44.3 Fresh gas flows required in Mapleson breathing systems

Breathing system	Spontaneous ventilation	Intermittent positive pressure ventilation
A (Lack or Magill)	Equal to V_A 70mL/kg/min	2.5 × MV 250mL/kg/min
D (Bain) E (Ayre's T-piece) F (Jackson Rees modification)	2 × MV 200mL/kg/min[1]	70mL/kg/min for $PaCO_2$ of 5.3kPa (40mmHg) or 100mL/kg/min for $PaCO_2$ of 4.3kPa (32mmHg) Minimum of 3L/min

[1] In young children, the greater MV/kg may require a fresh gas flow of up to 300mL/kg/min

MV, minute ventilation; V_A, alveolar minute ventilation.

Table 44.4 Fresh gas flows required in a circle system

Stage of case	Spontaneous ventilation or intermittent positive pressure ventilation
Initial uptake Rapid change in depth Washout (emergence)	Equal to MV 100mL/kg/min
Maintenance	Fresh gas flow can be reduced, but the percentage of O_2 and volatile agent must be increased to produce same concentrations in the final inspired gas (due to patient uptake).[1] A total flow of at least 1L/min is generally used

[1] O_2 and agent monitoring are essential at low flows.

MV, minute ventilation.

Pulmonary function tests

This section provides data on normal PFT results (Table 44.5), normal arterial and mixed venous blood gas results (Table 44.6), units of pressure (Table 44.7), lung volumes (Table 44.8 and Fig. 44.3), and the gas laws (Table 44.9).

Table 44.5 Pulmonary function tests

Age (yr)	FEV$_1$ (L)		FVC (L)		FEV$_1$/FVC (%)		PEFR (L/min)	
	M	F	M	F	M	F	M	F
20	4.15	3.09	4.95	3.83	82.5	81.0	625	433
30	4.00	2.94	4.84	3.68	80.6	79.9	612	422
40	3.69	2.64	4.62	3.38	76.9	77.7	586	401
50	3.38	2.34	4.40	3.08	73.1	75.5	560	380
60	3.06	2.04	4.18	2.78	69.4	73.2	533	359
70	2.75	1.74	3.96	2.48	65.7	71.0	507	338

M, ♂ assuming height of 175cm; F, ♀ assuming height of 160cm.

Table 44.6 Arterial/mixed venous blood gases

	Mixed venous	Arterial
pH	7.32–7.42	7.36–7.44
PO$_2$	4.9–5.6kPa (37–42mmHg)	12.0–14.7kPa (90–110mmHg)
PCO$_2$	5.3–6.9kPa (40–52mmHg)	4.5–6.1kPa (34–46mmHg)
SaO$_2$	>75%	>97%
HCO$_3^-$		24–30mmoL/L
Lactate		<2mmoL/L
Base excess		± 2mmoL/L
Anion gap	8–12mmoL/L (calculated from $(Na^+ + K^+) - (HCO_3^- + Cl^-)$)	

Table 44.7 Pressure conversion chart

100kPa is equal to:
1 bar
750mmHg (torr)
1020cmH$_2$O
0.987atm
14.5psi

atm, atmosphere; psi, pounds per square inch.

Respiratory physiology data

Table 44.8 Lung volumes

	Fit young ♂	For 70kg (approx)
Dead space (V_D)	2mL/kg	150mL
Tidal volume (V_T)	7mL/kg	500mL
Alveolar minute ventilation (V_A)	70mL/kg/min	5000mL/min
Minute ventilation (MV)	100mL/kg/min	7000mL/min
Vital capacity (VC)	70mL/kg	5000mL
Respiratory rate (RR)	14/min	14/min
Total lung capacity (TLC)	80mL/kg	6000mL
Inspiratory reserve volume (IRV)	40mL/kg	3000mL
Expiratory reserve volume (ERV)	20mL/kg	1500mL
Functional residual capacity (FRC)	35mL/kg	2500mL
Residual volume (RV)	15mL/kg	1000mL

Table 44.9 Gas laws

Boyle's law	Pressure is inversely proportional to volume (at a constant temperature)	$P \propto 1/V$
Charles' law	Volume is proportional to temperature (at a constant pressure)	$V \propto T$
Gay–Lussac's law	Pressure is proportional to temperature (at a constant volume)	$P \propto T$
Dalton's law of partial pressure	If a container holds a mixture of gases, the pressure exerted by each gas (i.e. the partial pressure) is the same as if it alone occupied the container	
Avogadro's law	One mole of an ideal gas occupies 22.4L at standard temperature and pressure	

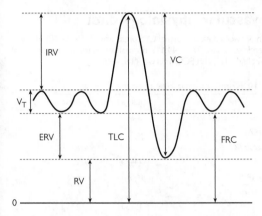

Fig. 44.3 Lung volumes on a spirometer trace.

ERV, expiratory reserve volume; FRC, functional residual capacity; IRV, inspiratory reserve volume; RV, residual volume; TLC, total lung capacity; VC, vital capacity; V$_T$, tidal volume.

Cardiovascular physiology data

This section provides data on normal CVS pressures (Table 44.10), derived haemodynamic variables (Table 44.11), normal values for the oesophageal Doppler (Table 44.12), and ECG intervals (Table 44.13).

Table 44.10 Normal cardiovascular pressures

	Range (mmHg)	Mean (mmHg)
Central venous pressure (CVP)	0–8	4
Right atrial (RA)	0–8	4
Right ventricular (RV):		
Systolic	14–30	25
End-diastolic (RVEDP)	0–8	4
Pulmonary arterial (PA):		
Systolic	15–30	23
Diastolic	5–15	10
Mean (PAP)	10–20	15
Mean pulmonary artery occlusion pressure (PAOP)	5–15	10
Left atrial (LA)	4–12	7
Left ventricular (LV): Systolic	90–140	120
End-diastolic (LVEDP)	4–12	7

Table 44.11 Derived haemodynamic variables

Variable	Formula	Normal values
Cardiac output (CO)	SV × HR	4.5–8L/min
Cardiac index (CI)	CO/BSA	2.7–4L/min/m^2
Stroke volume (SV)	(CO/HR) × 1000	60–130mL/beat
Systemic vascular resistance (SVR)	80 × (MAP − CVP)/CO	770–1500dyn.s/cm^5
Pulmonary vascular resistance (PVR)	80 × (PAP − PAOP)/CO	100–250dyn.s/cm^5
Ejection fraction (EF)	(EDV − ESV)/EDV	>0.6
Mean arterial pressure (MAP)	MAP = CO × SVR	80–90mmHg
Estimated MAP (MAP$_{est}$)	MAP$_{est}$ = diastolic BP + 1/3 pulse pressure	
Cerebral perfusion pressure (CPP)	CPP = MAP − ICP	70–75mmHg

BSA, body surface area; CVP, central venous pressure; EDV, end-diastolic volume; ESV, end-systolic volume; HR, heart rate; MAP, mean arterial pressure; PAP, mean pulmonary arterial pressure; PAOP, pulmonary artery occlusion pressure.

Table 44.12 Normal values for the oesophageal Doppler

Index	Value
Cardiac output	5L/min
Stroke volume	70mL
Flow time corrected (FTc)	330–360ms
Peak velocity:	
20yr	90–120cm/s
50yr	70–100cm/s
70yr	50–80cm/s

Table 44.13 Normal ECG data

Normal height is 1mV = 1cm
Normal speed is 25mm/s

Mean frontal axis	−30 to +90
PR interval	0.12–0.20s
QRS duration	0.04–0.12s
QT corrected	0.38–0.42s

Correction = QT/√RR interval

Useful equations and definitions

Alveolar gas equation

$$P_AO_2 = PiO_2 - P_ACO_2/RQ$$

where P_AO_2 = alveolar O_2 partial pressure (pp), PiO_2 = inspired O_2 pp, P_ACO_2 = alveolar CO_2 pp, RQ = respiratory quotient.

Dead space is the part of the tidal volume that does not take part in gas exchange; physiological (total) dead space consists of anatomical dead space (upper airways) and alveolar dead space (unperfused alveoli).

Alveolar volume is the part of the tidal volume reaching the lower airways = tidal volume (V_T) − anatomical dead space (V_D).

Alveolar minute ventilation (V_A) is the volume of gas reaching the lower airways per min = $(V_T - V_D)$ × respiratory rate.

Oxygen content of blood per 100mL = (O_2 bound to Hb) + (O_2 dissolved).

Arterial O_2 content CaO_2 = (SaO_2 × 1.34 × Hb) + (0.023 × PO_2 (kPa))

Oxygen flux (O_2 delivery) = cardiac output × arterial O_2 content.

Shunt is the pulmonary blood flow that bypasses ventilated alveoli.

Shunt (fraction) equation

$$Qs/Qt = (CcO_2 - CaO_2)/(CcO_2 - CvO_2)$$

where Qs = shunt flow, Qt = total flow, CcO_2 = pulmonary end-capillary O_2 content, CaO_2 = arterial O_2 content, CvO_2 = mixed venous O_2 content.

Compliance is the volume change per unit pressure change.

Laplace's law for a sphere Pressure across the wall = 2 × tension/radius.

Reynold's number predicts whether gas flow is likely to be laminar or turbulent:

$$Re = (Diameter × velocity × density)/viscosity$$

<1000 = laminar flow

>2000 = turbulent flow.

Hagen–Poiseuille law describes laminar flow in tubes:

$$Flow\ rate = (Pressure\ difference × \pi × radius^4)/(8 × length × viscosity)$$

Henderson–Hasselbalch equation describes how the pH is derived from pKa and the ratio of dissociated and undissociated acid/base. For H_2CO_3/CO_2:

$$pH = pKa + log_{10} (HCO_3^-/H_2CO_3)$$

Normal values

This section provides tables of normal haematological blood results (Table 44.14) and biochemical blood results (Table 44.15).

Table 44.14 Normal blood results (haematology)

Measurement	Reference range
White cell count	4.0–11.0 × 10^9/L
Red cell count	♂ 4.5–6.5 × 10^{12}/L, ♀ 3.9–5.6 × 10^{12}/L
Haemoglobin	♂ 135–180g/L, ♀ 115–160g/L
Packed red cell volume (haematocrit)	♂ 0.4–0.54L/L, ♀ 0.37–0.47L/L
Mean cell volume	76–96fL
Mean cell haemoglobin	27–32pg
Neutrophils	2.0–7.5 × 10^9/L (40–75% of WCC)
Lymphocytes	1.3–3.5 × 10^9/L (20–45% of WCC)
Eosinophils	0.04–0.44 × 10^9/L (1–6% of WCC)
Basophils	0.0–0.10 × 10^9/L (0.1% of WCC)
Monocytes	0.2–0.8 × 10^9/L (2–10% of WCC)
Platelet count	150–400 × 10^9/L
Prothrombin time (factors I, II, VII, X)	10–14s
Activated partial thromboplastin time (VIII, IX, XI, XII)	35–45s
INR:	
Normal	1
Anticoagulation targets:	
AF	2.5 (± 0.5)
Treatment DVT/PE	2.5 (± 0.5)
Prosthetic valve	3.5 (± 0.5)

Table 44.15 Normal blood results (biochemistry)

	Specimen	Reference interval
Adrenocorticotrophic hormone	P	<80ng/L
Alanine aminotransferase (ALT)	P	5–35IU/L
Albumin	P	35–50g/L
Aldosterone	P	100–500pmol/L
Alkaline phosphatase	P	30–300IU/L (adults)
Amylase	P	0–180 Somogyi units/dL
Antidiuretic hormone (ADH)	P	0.9–4.6pmol/L
Aspartate transaminase (AST)	P	5–35IU/L
Bicarbonate	P	24–30mmol/L
Bilirubin	P	3–17 micromoles/L
Calcitonin	P	<0.1 micrograms/L
Calcium (ionized)	P	1.0–1.25mmol/L
Calcium (total)	P	2.12–2.65mmol/L
Chloride	P	95–105mmol/L
Cholesterol	P	3.9–7.8mmol/L
Very-low-density lipoprotein (VLDL)	P	0.128–0.645mmol/L
Low-density lipoprotein (LDL)	P	1.55–4.4mmol/L
High-density lipoprotein (HDL)	P	0.9–1.93mmol/L
Cholinesterase	P	♂ 5900–12220U/L
		♀ 4650–10440U/L
Cortisol	P	a.m. 450–700nmol/L
		Midnight 80–280nmol/L
Creatine kinase (CK)	P	25–195IU/L
Creatinine (related to lean body mass)	P	♂ 70–110 micromoles/L
		♀ 60–100 micromoles/L
CRP	P	0–12mg/L
Ferritin	P	12–200 micrograms/L
Folate	S	2.1 micrograms/L
Gamma-glutamyl transpeptidase	P	11–51IU/L
Glucose (fasting)	P	3.5–5.5mmol/L
Growth hormone	P	<20mu/L
HbA1c (= glycosylated Hb)	B	2.3–6.5%
Iron	S	♂ 14–31 micromoles/L
		♀ 11–30 micromoles/L

	Specimen	Reference interval
Magnesium	P	0.7–1mmol/L
Osmolality	P	278–305mOsmol/kg
Parathyroid hormone (PTH)	P	<0.8–8.5pmol/L
Phosphate (inorganic)	P	0.8–1.45mmol/L
Potassium	P	3.5–5.0mmol/L
Protein (total)	P	60–80g/L
Red cell folate	B	0.36–1.44 micromoles/L (160–640 micrograms/L)
Renin (erect/recumbent)	P	2.8–4.5/1.1–2.7pmol/mL/hr
Sodium	P	135–145mmol/L
Thyroid-binding globulin (TBG)	P	7–17mg/L
Thyroid-stimulating hormone (TSH)	P	0.5–5.7mu/L
Normal range widens with age		
Thyroxine (T_4)	P	70–140mmol/L
Thyroxine (free)	P	9–22pmol/L
Total iron binding capacity	S	54–75 micromoles/L
Triglyceride	P	0.55–1.90mmol/L
Tri-iodothyronine (T_3)	P	1.2–3.0nmol/L
Troponin T (taken at least 12hr after onset of chest pain)	P	0–0.01 micrograms/L normal 0.01–0.1 micrograms/L suspicious >0.1 micrograms/L diagnostic of MI
Urate	P	♂ 210–480 micromoles/L ♀ 150–390 micromoles/L
Urea	P	2.5–6.7mmol/L
Vitamin B12	S	0.13–0.68nmol/L (>150ng/L)

Renal

	Reference interval
Glomerular filtration rate	4>120mL/min
Renal blood flow	1200mL/min
Urine output	0.5–1.0mL/kg/hr
Urine osmolality	350–1000mOsmol/kg

B, whole blood (edetic acid EDTA bottle); P, plasma (e.g. heparin bottle); S, serum (clotted; no anticoagulant).

Note: there is minor variation in the normal ranges quoted by different laboratories.

Useful websites

Table 44.16 is a list of websites which contain useful information about the practice of anaesthesia. Oxford University Press is not responsible for the content of these websites.

Table 44.16 Useful websites

http://www.rcoa.ac.uk	The Royal College of Anaesthetists
http://www.aagbi.org	The Association of Anaesthetists of Great Britain and Ireland
http://www.anaesthesiologists.org	World Federation of Societies of Anaesthesiologists
http://www.asahq.org	American Society of Anesthesiologists
http://www.anzca.edu.au	Australian and New Zealand College of Anaesthetists
http://www.esahq.org	European Society of Anaesthesiology
http://www.apagbi.org.uk	Association of Paediatric Anaesthetists of Great Britain and Ireland
http://www.vasgbi.com	The Vascular Anaesthesia Society of Great Britain and Ireland
http://www.acta.org.uk	Association of Cardiothoracic Anaesthetists
http://www.oaa-anaes.ac.uk	Obstetric Anaesthetists' Association
http://www.boas.org	British Ophthalmic Anaesthesia Society
http://www.nasgbi.org.uk	The Neuroanaesthesia Society of Great Britain and Ireland
http://www.snacc.org	Society for Neuroscience in Anesthesiology and Critical Care
http://www.esraeurope.org	The European Society of Regional Anaesthesia and Pain Therapy
http://www.asra.com	American Society of Regional Anesthesia and Pain Medicine
http://www.britishpainsociety.org	The British Pain Society
http://www.siva.ac.uk	The Society for Intravenous Anaesthesia
http://www.das.uk.com	Difficult Airway Society
http://www.resus.org.uk	Resuscitation Council (UK)
http://www.bja.oxfordjournals.org	*British Journal of Anaesthesia*
http://www.anesthesia-analgesia.org	*Anesthesia & Analgesia*
http://anesthesiology.pubs.asahq.org/	*Anesthesiology*

✍ http://www.cochrane.org	The Cochrane Collaboration
✍ http://www.nice.org.uk	National Institute for Health and Care Excellence
✍ http://www.virtual-anesthesia-textbook.com	*Virtual Anaesthesia Textbook*
✍ http://www.frca.co.uk	Anaesthesia UK
✍ http://www.gmc-uk.org	General Medical Council
✍ http://www.bma.org.uk	British Medical Association
✍ http://www.histansoc.org.uk	History of Anaesthesia Society

Checklist for anaesthetic equipment

Because of the specific and complex nature of modern anaesthetic equipment, preoperative checks should include both the manufacturer's testing sequence and a generic check of the range of normal functions. A written record of the check should be made both in the patient record and machine log.

The following summarizes the items in the equipment checklist of AAGBI:[1]

- Self-inflating bag available
- Manufacturer's (automatic) machine check
- Power supply:
  - Plugged in/switched on/backup battery charged
- Gas supplies and suction:
  - Pipelines/cylinders/suction
  - Flow meters with hypoxic guard
  - Vaporizer
  - O_2 flush
- Breathing system:
  - Securely connected, patent, and leak-free
  - 'Two-bag' test*
  - Soda lime
  - Correct gas outlet selected
- Ventilator
- Scavenging
- Monitors (including alarms)
- Airway equipment.

In addition, the anaesthetist should:
- Prepare and check equipment relating to any special techniques planned (TIVA, regional blocks, invasive monitoring)
- Be aware of how to access emergency equipment (difficult airway devices, defibrillator).

Reference

1 Association of Anaesthetists of Great Britain and Ireland (2012). *Checklist for anaesthetist equipment 2012. AAGBI safety guideline.* ℛ http://www.aagbi.org/sites/default/files/checklist_for_anaesthetic_equipment_2012.pdf.

* The 'two-bag' test uses one bag as a test lung to check for leaks, patency, and unidirectional flow in the breathing system.

Index